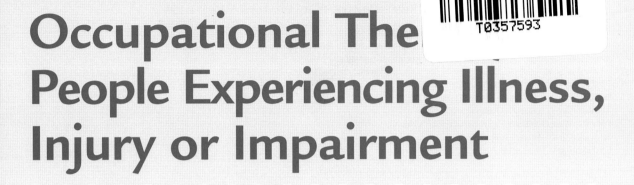

Occupational Therapy for People Experiencing Illness, Injury or Impairment

PROMOTING OCCUPATIONAL PARTICIPATION

Eighth Edition

Edited by

MICHAEL CURTIN EdD, MPhil, BOccThy
Head of School and Associate Professor, School of Allied Health, Exercise and Sports Sciences, Charles Sturt University, Albury, NSW, Australia

MARY EGAN PhD, OT Reg. (Ont.), FCAOT
Professor, School of Rehabilitation Sciences, University of Ottawa, Ottawa, Ontario, Canada

YELIZ PRIOR PhD, BSc, FHEA, HCPC, MRCOT
Professor of Clinical Rehabilitation, School of Health and Society, The University of Salford, Salford, Greater Manchester, United Kingdom

TRACEY PARNELL, PhD, MOT, BaAppSc(OT), GCLTHE, SFHEA
Associate Head of School and Senior Lecturer in Occupational Therapy, School of Allied Health, Exercise and Sports Sciences, Charles Sturt University, Albury, NSW, Australia

ROSHAN GALVAAN, PhD, MSc(OT), BSc(OT)
Professor of Occupational Therapy, Department of Health and Rehabilitation Sciences, University of Cape Town, Cape Town, South Africa

KATRINE SAUVÉ-SCHENK PhD, OT Reg. (Ont.)
Assistant Professor, School of Rehabilitation Sciences, University of Ottawa, Ottawa, Ontario, Canada

DANIEL CEZAR DA CRUZ, PhD, MSc, BSc, FHEA, MRCOT
Senior Lecturer in Occupational Therapy Programme, School of Health, Leeds Beckett University, Leeds, West Yorkshire, United Kingdom

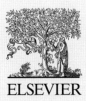

ELSEVIER

First edition © Longman Group Limited 1981
Second edition © Longman Group Limited 1987
Third edition © Longman Group Limited 1992
Fourth edition © Pearson Professional Group 1996
Fifth edition © Elsevier Limited 1999
Sixth edition © Elsevier Limited 2010

Notice

Practitioners and researchers must always rely on their own experience and knowledge in evaluating and using any information, methods, compounds or experiments described herein. Because of rapid advances in the medical sciences, in particular, independent verification of diagnoses and drug dosages should be made. To the fullest extent of the law, no responsibility is assumed by Elsevier, authors, editors or contributors for any injury and/or damage to persons or property as a matter of products liability, negligence or otherwise, or from any use or operation of any methods, products, instructions, or ideas contained in the material herein.

ISBN: 978-0-323-88292-7

Content Strategist: Trinity Hutton
Content Project Manager: Tapajyoti Chaudhuri
Design: Christian Bilbow
Marketing Manager: Deborah J. Watkins

Printed in India
Last digit is the print number: 9 8 7 6 5 4 3 2 1

Working together to grow libraries in developing countries

www.elsevier.com • www.bookaid.org

CONTENTS

SECTION 3

SKILLS AND STRATEGIES TO PROMOTE
OCCUPATIONAL PARTICIPATION

SECTION 4

SKILLS AND STRATEGIES TO SUPPORT
THE PROMOTION OF OCCUPATIONAL
PARTICIPATION

Occupational Therapy for People Experiencing Illness, Injury or Impairment

SECTION 5

PRACTICE STORIES – PROMOTING OCCUPATIONAL PARTICIPATION

FOREWORD

In the journey of studying occupational therapy, there are moments when one feels both excited and overwhelmed by the vast knowledge and practice that lies ahead. This book stands out as a beacon of clarity and inspiration in this complex field. *I wish it had been a prescribed textbook in my first year*. It's a valuable resource that brings together the theory I've learned in a more understandable way while offering new insights that have deepened my understanding of various concepts.

What I appreciate most about this book is its ability to engage readers in the conversation. I recall struggling in class with complex topics and feeling hesitant to ask questions, which often left me feeling excluded from discussions. This book addresses such challenges effectively, breaking down intricate concepts into clear, relatable examples that make it easier to follow and critically reflect on.

Beyond providing a comprehensive overview of important concepts, the book has validated my evolving thoughts and questions. From the first section, I felt understood because some of the conflicts I believe most of us face as students were addressed. It serves not only as an educational tool but also as a guide for those at the beginning of their careers, those seeking direction, and like me, those needing a reminder that occupational therapy is evolving and there is room to challenge Western perspectives that do not align with your reality.

With contributions from a diverse range of writers worldwide, each drawing on their own perspectives, the book allows readers to find relatable experiences, and learn from experiences that differ from their own.

I wholeheartedly recommend this book to anyone seeking to understand and navigate the intricate world of occupational therapy. It is a testament to the evolving nature of our field and a reminder that our core values remain at the heart of what we do.

Keoratile Segoe,
University of Cape Town, South Africa

The 8th edition of *Occupational Therapy for People Experiencing Illness, Injury or Impairment: Promoting Occupational Participation* continues to highlight the ever-changing landscape of occupational therapy on an international scale. It aptly opens with a series of chapters detailing contemporary areas of occupational therapy theory and practice. It calls for an increased focus on decolonising our work, prioritising a collaborative relationship-focused approach to practice and continuing to challenge political, social, institutional and environmental factors. All of these amplify the need for occupational therapy students, educators and clinicians to promote and enable occupational participation as a key pillar of our role. Considering these contemporary concerns, a new and updated model, framework and practice process are introduced, with the remaining chapters detailing how these are applied to practice through theoretical discussion and insightful practice stories.

Occupational therapy practice needs to hold collaborative relationship-focused practice as the central component, tying together and sustaining therapeutic relationships across our broad scope of practice. This centralises the goals of the individuals and collectives we work with and supports occupational therapists in decolonising power imbalances.

Students, educators and clinicians are not the gatekeepers of improved health, well-being, and occupational participation; rather they act as collaborative facilitators and supporters. The focus on building therapeutic self-direction further advocates for the empowerment of people with injury, illness or impairment to have control over their own fulfilling occupational participation.

As a recent graduate, it has been refreshing to read the eighth edition and see how occupational therapists are continuing to challenge, re-evaluate and call attention to the important issues confronting our work. It has been an honour to be included in this new edition – one voice joining a myriad of others in the important and ongoing dialogue surrounding our profession. May you enjoy reading the eighth edition as much as I have!

Sarah Sheely,
Charles Sturt University, Australia

It is a privilege to contribute to the Foreword of the 8th edition of *Occupational Therapy for People Experiencing Illness, Injury or Impairment: Promoting Occupational Participation*, having found the previous editions to be an invaluable reference point and source of knowledge throughout my studies. This book encourages the audience to reflect on and deeply consider their approach to practice and the numerous influential factors that impact practice. It is structured to first provide core occupational therapy knowledge, history and theory. Readers are then guided through complex processes and approaches in a simple and easier-to-digest way that can be replicated, practiced and built upon by students and new graduates. The sections that follow dive deeper into specific skills and areas where occupational therapists can support individuals, providing guidance and practice stories to assist with practical application.

As a new graduate who is emigrating to another country, I particularly appreciate the book's international focus, open approach and the influence and knowledge from contributors across the globe. I have found the chapters on skills and strategies to support the promotion of occupational participation especially interesting. Throughout this book, the wide-ranging scope of occupational therapy is highlighted, and the reader is reminded to keep exploring boundaries and ways to work with individuals and collectives to achieve their occupational participation goals.

As a new graduate, the transition from a student to a new practitioner can be daunting. It can be difficult to remember the essential knowledge that underpins practice and apply it in real-world scenarios. This book will be an extremely useful practical resource to support students and new practitioners on this journey.

Laura Sexton,
Leeds Beckett University, England

It is an incredible honour to contribute to the foreword for the 8th edition of *Occupational Therapy for People Experiencing Illness, Injury or Impairment: Promoting Occupational Participation*. As a recent graduate of the occupational therapy program at the University of Ottawa, I am cognizant of the imposter syndrome that comes with limited experience in the occupational therapy field. Therefore, finding resources that enable continuing education, whether as a student or an early career occupational therapist, on contemporary topics in occupational therapy are greatly valued to further knowledge and confidence in practice.

The content of the 8th edition embraces the change in occupational therapy philosophy by focusing on the importance of occupational participation, as well as incorporating different occupational therapy practices and views that new and future occupational therapists may encounter in practice. The content includes practice stories, reflexive and reflection questions, people-focused occupational therapy practice theories, assessments and interventions and allows readers to develop their professional reasoning.

Many chapters stood out to me as they allow readers to develop their knowledge regarding the impact of psychosocial and socio-political factors on occupation, develop their ability to critically analyse how their internal or external biases may impact a therapeutic relationship and develop their advocacy and cultural humility skills, all of which are of utmost importance for prioritising a collaborative relationship-focused approach to practice.

This book is a wonderful way to learn about a variety of contemporary topics that both early career and future occupational therapists will benefit from to promote person-focused occupational participation and enhance professional reasoning.

Kaitlyn Duquette,
University of Ottawa, Canada

PREFACE

The editors of this book aspire towards a critical praxis, acknowledging the value of decolonial perspectives in the widespread context of settler colonialism. We gratefully thank and honour the deep social relations, knowledges, and languages that arise from the First Nations peoples' lands on which we live, travel, and learn.

THE RIGHT ATTITUDE (REVISITED) AND CRITICAL THINKING

The Preface for the previous edition of this book started with the story of Matthew deciding, when he was 18 years old, to move out of his family home to live by himself. Matthew had not decided to move out because he was unhappy at home but because he just 'thought it was about time'. However, it took another 3 years, until he was 21 years old, to make the move into a place of his own. Matthew was diagnosed with cerebral palsy. Matthew used a powered wheelchair to move around, a communication device to talk with people and physical assistance to accomplish many of his personal care and daily activities. Matthew felt that in making the decision to live on his own he became more confident in making his own arrangements and doing the things he wanted to do the way he liked to do them. He had control of *how* and *when* he participated in occupations.

Based on his experiences, Matthew offered the following advice: 'You just do not know the possibilities, until you try it. Whatever your disability is, whatever your fear is, whatever your abilities are […] anything is possible'. Cathy, Matthew's mother and advocate, adds a caveat to Matthew's statement, explaining, 'It took a lot more than Matthew's great attitude and determination to achieve his goals. It required the support of others, both family and professionals and a context in which supports were available to facilitate his participation. He required people who shared this can-do attitude, shared his vision, believed in him and were willing to work with him to make his dream a reality. Anything is possible, when people have the *right attitude!*'

Matthew's story of moving out on his own, and his and Cathy's belief that anything is possible, when people have the right attitude, provides an *essential lesson* for the readers of this book. Although this book has garnered the wisdom of a range of skilled and experienced occupational therapists and other professionals from around the world, and offers readers numerous approaches and strategies that can be used when working with people who have an illness, injury or impairment, all of the content rests on the reader establishing genuine collaborative relationships with the people they work with, and being open to exploring and enacting an openness to expanding their professional horizons and contribute to critical orientations of occupational therapy practice.

Occupational therapists with an openness to critical occupational therapy have a commitment to expanding an individual, group, community and population's 'opportunities to engage in meaningful occupations that contribute positively to their own wellbeing and the wellbeing of their communities' (Whalley Hammell, 2021, p. 7). These occupational therapists have developed critical thinking, which is essential 'to resist conformity, question the assumptions and ideologies that are presented as "truth", and discern the systems of oppression that shape [people's] occupational lives' (Whalley Hammell, 2021, p. 8). Moreover, to facilitate well-being, social inclusion and participatory citizenship, occupational therapists must be critically reflexive and consider whether what they think, say, and do is consistent with what we believe (Whiteford et al., 2021). Critical thinking is key to recognising and understanding how power structures and systems 'of oppression and domination can negatively affect [the health and wellbeing of people] through restriction of their occupational participation. Such understanding will illuminate the structural determinants of health, thereby opening new pathways for intervention' (Bailliard, 2016, p. 13).

As editors of this book, we trust that readers will approach it as critical thinkers and have the capacity to go beyond existing attitudes, assumptions, practices, and services to meet the needs, desires, hopes and dreams of the individuals, groups, communities, and populations with whom they work. In this way, we invite readers to practice in a way that genuinely promotes occupational participation.

KEY FEATURES OF THE EIGHTH EDITION

Occupational Therapy for People Experiencing Illness, Injury or Impairment has played a key part in pre-registration occupational therapy education since 1981. For the first six editions, it was called *Occupational Therapy for Physical Dysfunction*, with editions one to five edited by Annie Turner, Marg Foster and Sybil Johnson and edition six edited by Michael Curtin, Matthew Molineux and Jo Supyk.

When Elsevier Publisher commissioned a 7th edition of the book the three editors, Michael Curtin (Charles Sturt University, Australia), Mary Egan (University of Ottawa, Canada) and Jo Adams (University of Southampton, England), instigated changes to the book to have a broader international focus. To acknowledge that the book was taken in a new direction, and to ensure a contemporary focus, the book was given a new title, *Occupational Therapy for People Experiencing Illness, Injury or Impairment: Promoting Occupation and Participation*. This edition was published in 2017.

Elsevier Publishers have commissioned this 8th edition of the book and have supported the move to widen the international relevance and appeal of the book.

This has involved increasing the number of editors from three to seven. Joining Michael Curtin (Charles Sturt University, Australia) and Mary Egan (University of Ottawa, Canada), the additional editors for the 8th edition (listed in alphabetical order) are Daniel Cezar da Cruz (Leeds Beckett University, United Kingdom), Roshan Galvaan (University of Cape Town, South Africa), Tracey Parnell (Charles Sturt University, Australia), Yeliz Prior (The University of Salford, United Kingdom) and Katrine Sauvé-Schenk (University of Ottawa, Canada).

This new edition reflects significant international developments within the occupational therapy profession and the contexts of the delivery of health and social care. It has been built around the professional concepts and processes presented in Egan and Restall's *Promoting Occupational Participation: Collaborative Relationship-focused Occupational Therapy* (2022), a publication by the Canadian Association of Occupational Therapists. We believe that the approach, framework and model presented in this book support occupational therapists to practice in a critically reflexive way.

This edition continues the goal of contributing to preparing the next generation of occupational therapists for the ever-evolving world of practice. This edition:

- Has retained the title *Occupational Therapy for People Experiencing Illness, Injury or Impairment,* and changed the subtitle to *Promoting Occupational Participation.* The title and sub-title acknowledge that:
  - Occupational therapists work with people and not medical conditions and diagnoses – the term *people* here is inclusive of individuals, groups, communities and populations;
  - Occupational therapists are interested in the lived experiences of people;
  - Illness, injury and impairment are not the same as, and are not the primary cause, of disability (or dysfunction) and do not define the person; and
  - The goal of occupational therapy is to promote occupational participation.
- Has been written with particular relevance for occupational therapy students and early career occupational therapists.

- Acknowledges that occupational therapists work in collaboration with individuals, families, groups, communities and populations. The term 'collective' is used throughout this edition to refer to groups, communities and populations.
- Embraces and incorporates a diverse range of occupational therapy views and practices, taking into consideration different cultures, knowledges, values and beliefs. There are over 100 contributors to this edition from many countries around the world.
- Explores the core work of occupational therapists to '[promote] access to, initiation of, and sustained participation in valued occupations within meaningful relationships and contexts' (Egan & Restall, 2022, p. 1).
- Is underpinned by 'a capabilities approach [that] shifts the focus away from a preoccupation with identifying, categorizing and classifying impairments […] and encourages occupational therapists to work towards equalizing people's possibilities and choices' (Whalley Hammell, 2020, p. 13). This approach is explained further in Chapter 10.
- Seeks to provide practical application of the processes and concepts presented in the Canadian Association of Occupational Therapist's 2022 publication *Promoting Occupational Participation: Collaborative Relationship-Focused Occupational Therapy* edited by Mary Egan and Gayle Restall.
- Includes chapters on promoting occupational participation in practice to illustrate key concepts and processes with different individuals and collectives. Chapters that present practice stories on promoting occupational participation are in Section 5.
- Reflects contemporary research evidence that underpins occupational therapy practice.
- Uses inclusive and strengths-based language. Examples include the following:
  - The term *disabled person* or *person with disability* has been used depending on the preference of the contributor. This reflects the preferred terminology of disability advocates in each contributor's country. For example, *disabled person* is the preferred term of disability advocates in the United Kingdom, as a means

of politicising that disability is caused by attitudinal and environmental barriers rather than a person's impairment; in Australia, disability advocates prefer to use the term *people with disability* to promote people-first language; and in Canada, both terms may be used. The decision to use both terms in this book depending on a contributor's preference is to reflect the global dialogue on disability. Readers will note that in many cases neither term is used as the preference was to use the phrase *a person (or people) with an illness, injury or impairment*.
  - The term *person* or *individual* has been utilised to refer to an individual engaged in a collaborative relationship with, and using the services of, an occupational therapist.
- The term *practice setting* is used to recognise that occupational therapists provide services in a variety of workplaces.
- *Professional reasoning*, which encompasses *occupational reasoning*, is used rather than *clinical reasoning*, as the term *clinical* has medical connotations and the reasoning of occupational therapists embraces more than just the medical implications of an illness, injury or impairment on a person or collective.

STRUCTURE OF THE EIGHTH EDITION

The fifty chapters in this edition are laid out in five sections.

Section 1: Contemporary Reflections on Occupational Therapy

The chapters in this section present a number of key contemporary issues that occupational therapists must consider as they promote occupational participation and become critical thinkers, understanding the historical, political and social influences *on* the profession and practice, and the historical, political and social impact *of* the profession and practice.

- *Chapter 1* addresses decolonising occupational therapy practice, 'inviting current and future occupational therapy practitioners, researchers and educators, to understand and apply essential aspects of decoloniality including understanding social positioning, examining beliefs, supporting first nations' colleagues and building antiracist collectives'.

- *Chapter 2* applies critical theory to question and (re)formulate professional practice 'to envision possibilities for practices that build on individual and collective strengths and allow for fostering collaborative relationships that are socioeconomically, culturally and historically informed'.
- *Chapter 3* challenges occupational therapists to address and reduce moral and political inequalities by aligning with the political project of the profession.
- *Chapter 4* defines and presents the development and application of social occupational therapy.
- *Chapter 5* provides an analysis of the practice context and proposes an approach for occupational therapists to analyse the context in which their practice is situated, and its influence on their practice.
- *Chapter 6* focuses on the conceptualisation and assumptions related to the concept of occupation that guide occupational therapy practice and occupational science research.
- *Chapter 7* provides a reflection on the concept and complexity of the physical, virtual, social, cultural, economic and political dimensions of the environment.
- *Chapter 8* provides a history of occupational therapy to illustrate the continual evolution of the profession, and the contemporary issues and critiques that challenge the sustainability and relevance of the profession.

Section 2: Understanding and Exploring Occupational Participation

The chapters in this section provide an overview of the foundations for occupational therapy practice.

- *Chapter* 9 explains professional reasoning, 'a key skill for occupational therapists to use throughout the occupational therapy process'.

- *Chapter 10* articulates the Occupation, Capability and Wellbeing Framework, a Framework that is underpinned by a rights- and strengths-based approach to practice.
- *Chapters 11 and 12* provide an overview of the Canadian Model of Occupational Participation (CanMOP), collaborative relationship-focused practice, and the Canadian Occupational Therapy Inter-relational Practice Process Framework (COTIPP).
- *Chapter 13* provides an overview of exploring occupational participation stressing that the purpose is 'to identify and document well being aspirations, skills, strengths, meanings, relationships, assets, resources and abilities of individuals and collectives'.
- *Chapters 14 to 18* present different approaches to, and considerations of, exploring occupational participation.
- *Chapter 19* focuses on the importance of co-designing plans for occupational participation.
- *Chapter 20* explores the concepts of safety and risk, encouraging occupational therapists to balance 'the benefits and the potential harm in everyday occupations' when co-designing 'plans that assist people to realise their goals'.

Section 3: Skills and Strategies to Promote Occupational Participation

The chapters in this section present key occupational skills and strategies used to promote occupational participation. The topics covered in this section include:

- Advocacy (*Chapter 21*),
- Education (*Chapter 22*),
- Health promotion (*Chapter 23*),
- Lifestyle and self-management (*Chapter 24*),
- Sexuality (*Chapter 25*),
- Work participation (*Chapter 26*),
- Occupational performance coaching (*Chapter 27*),
- Cognitive orientation to daily occupational performance (CO-OP) (*Chapter 28*),
- Home modifications (*Chapter 29*) and
- Community development (*Chapter 30*).

Section 4: Skills and Strategies to Support the Promotion of Occupational Participation

The chapters in this section present a range of skills and strategies that occupational therapists may use to assist with their goal of promoting occupational participation. The skills and strategies included are not exhaustive, and are not specifically occupation-focused. *It is important for readers to understand that these skills and strategies should only be used with occupation-based approaches to achieve co-designed occupational participation goals.* The skills and strategies included in this section are:

- Assistive technology (*Chapter 31*),
- Mobility (*Chapters 32, 33 and 34*),
- Moving and positioning (*Chapter 35*),
- Biomechanics (*Chapter 36*),
- Managing fatigue and pain (*Chapters 37 and 38*),
- Optimising motor performance (*Chapter 39*),
- Hand therapy and orthotics (*Chapter 40*) and
- Vision, cognition and perception (*Chapters 41 and 42*).

Section 5: Practice Stories – Promoting Occupational Participation

Eight detailed practice stories are included in this section to provide examples of the application of the concepts presented in this book when working as an occupational therapist in collaboration with individuals and collectives.

REFERENCES

Bailliard, A. (2016). Justice, difference, and the capability to function. *Journal of Occupational Science, 23*(1), 3–16. https://doi.org/10.1080/14427591.2014.957886.

Egan, M., & Restall, G. (Eds.). (2022). *Promoting occupational participation: Collaborative relationship-focused occupational therapy.* Rockland: Canadian Association of Occupational Therapists.

Egan, M., & Restall, G. (2022). Introduction. In M. Egan, & G Restall (Eds.), *Promoting occupational participation: Collaborative relationship-focused occupational therapy* (p. 1). Rockland: Canadian Association of Occupational Therapists.

Whalley Hammell, K. (2020). *Engagement in living: Critical perspectives on occupation, rights and wellbeing* (p. 213). Rockland: Canadian Association of Occupational Therapists.

Whalley Hammell, K. (2021). Building back better: Imagining an occupational therapy for a post-COVID-19 world. *Australian Occupational Therapy Journal*, 1–10. https://doi.org/10.1111/1440-1630.12760.

Whiteford, G., Parnell, T., Ramsden, L., Nott, M., & Vine-Daher, S. (2021). Understanding and advancing occupational justice and social inclusion. In P. Liamputtong (Ed.), *Handbook of social inclusion.* Cham: Springer https://doi.org/10.1007/978-3-030-48277-0_10-1.

ACKNOWLEDGEMENTS

We are incredibly grateful to the many contributors from around the world who have kindly and enthusiastically given their time to share their expertise in writing the chapters for this book. We acknowledge the individuality of each contributor, which is why there is some variance in the style of each chapter.

We are also appreciative of the four students/recent graduates who reviewed this book and wrote the Foreword. Thank you, Kaitlyn Duquette (University of Ottawa), Keoratile Segoe (University of Cape Town), Laura Sexton (Leeds Beckett University), and Sarah Sheely (Charles Sturt University).

Thank you to the staff at Elsevier who have supported the planning, development and creation of this book. Your support and guidance have been key to achieving the goal of the publication of this book.

Our aim for this book is for it to serve as a valuable reference for occupational therapy students and new practitioners. We trust that it stimulates reflection on the knowledge, skills and attitudes that inform their practice and on their capabilities to collaborate with individuals and collectives to promote occupational participation.

It is an honour to be editors of this eighth edition.

Michael Curtin
Mary Egan
Yeliz Prior
Tracey Parnell
Roshan Galvaan
Katrine Sauvé-Schenk
Daniel Cezar da Cruz

CONTRIBUTORS

KASHIFA ABRAHAMS, BSc(OT), MSc(OT)
Content Advisor, Women, Youth & Persons with Disabilities, Committee Section of Parliament RSA, Parliament of Republic of South Africa, Cape Town, South Africa

REBECCA M. ALDRICH, PhD, OTR/L
Professor of Clinical Occupational Therapy, Mrs. T. H. Chan Division of Occupational Science and Occupational Therapy, University of Southern California, Los Angeles, California, United States

DIEGO EUGÊNIO ROQUETE GODOY DE ALMEIDA, PhD, MSc(EDUCATION AND HEALTH), BSc(OT)
Professor, Federal University of Espírito Santo, Occupational Therapy, Federal University of Espírito Santo, Vitória, Espírito Santo, Brazil

LILIANA ALVAREZ, PhD, MSc, OT REG.(ONT.)
Associate Professor, School of Occupational Therapy, Western University, London, Ontario, Canada

SARAH ASH, BSc(OT), BSc(SOCIAL POLICY)
Team Lead Occupational Therapist, West Berkshire Council, Adult Social care, Berkshire, United Kingdom

GIOVANNA BARDI, PhD(SOCIAL POLICY), MSc(OT), BSc(OT)
Professor, Occupational Therapy Department, Federal University of Espírito Santo (UFES), Vitória, Espírito Santo, Brazil

CHARMAINE BERNIE, PhD
Senior Research Fellow, Faculty of Education, Southern Cross University, Gold Coast, Queensland, Australia

JENNIFER BERTONI, DSC RHL(CANDIDATE), MPH, OT REG.(ONT.)
School of Rehabilitation Therapy, Queen's University, Kingston, Ontario, Canada

PATRÍCIA LEME DE OLIVEIRA BORBA, PhD MASTER'S DEGREE IN EDUCATION, GRADUATE AND POS-PhD IN OCCUPATIONAL THERAPY
Professor, Health, Education and Society, Federal University of São Paulo, Santos, São Paulo, Brazil

JAIMIE BORISOFF, PhD
Director, MAKE+, Applied Research, British Columbia Institute of Technology, Burnaby, British Columbia, Canada

CATHERINE ELIZABETH BRIDGE, BAppSc(OT), MCogSc, PhD(ARCH)
Emeritus Professor, School of the Built Environment, University of New South Wales, Australia, Kensington, New South Wales, Australia

ROB BROOKS, PhD, PGDIP, BSc(HONS)
Associate Professor, Occupational Therapy, University of Bradford, Bradford, West Yorkshire, United Kingdom

CHLOE BRYANT, PhD, BOccThy(HONS)
Lecturer in Occupational Therapy, School of Health and Rehabilitation Sciences, Faculty of Health and Behavioural Sciences, The University of Queensland, St Lucia, Queensland, Australia

LUCIANA BUIN, PhD
Occupational Therapy Postgraduate Programme, Federal University of Sao Carlos, Sao Carlos, Brazil

GUNILLA CARLSSON, PhD, REG OT
Associate Professor, Department of Health Sciences, Lund University, Lund, Sweden

PHILLIPPA CARNEMOLLA, BDES, MDES, PhD
Associate Professor, Faculty of Design Architecture and Building, University of Technology Sydney, Sydney, New South Wales, Australia

CHRISTINE J CHAPPARO, PhD, MA, DipOT(NSW), FAOTA
Associate Professor (Honorary), Discipline of Occupational Therapy, Faculty of Medicine and Health, The University of Sydney, Sydney, New South Wales, Australia

CHI-WEN CHIEN, PhD
Associate Professor, Department of Rehabilitation Sciences, The Hong Kong Polytechnic University, Kowloon, Hong Kong

PEÑAFRANCIA E. CHING, MCOMM DEV, OTRP
Assistant Professor, Department of Occupational Therapy, College of Allied Medical Professions, University of the Philippines Manila, Manila, Philippines

LAUREN J. CHRISTIE, PhD, BAppSc(OT)
Senior Implementation Science Research Fellow, Allied Health Research Unit, St Vincent's Health Network Sydney, Darlinghurst, New South Wales, Australia
Clinical Fellow, Faculty of Health Sciences, Australian Catholic University, North Sydney, Australia
Occupational Therapist, The StrokeEd Collaboration, Sydney, New South Wales, Australia

LINDY MAXTED CLEMSON, PhD, MAppSc(RESEARCH), BAppSc(OT), Dip(OT), FOTARA
Professor Emeritus, Faculty of Medicine and Health, The University of Sydney, Sydney, New South Wales, Australia

HEATHER COLQUHOUN, BSc OT, PhD
Associate Professor, Occupational Science and Occupational Therapy, University of Toronto, Toronto, Ontario, Canada

GILL CREIGHTON, BSc(HONS) OCCUPATIONAL THERAPY
Occupational Therapist and Moving and Handling Advisor, Moving and handling, GillCreighton Ltd, Winchester, United Kingdom
Occupational Therapy Expert Witness, MaggireSargeant & Associates, United Kingdom

MICHAEL CURTIN, EdD, MPHIL, BOccThy
Head of School and Associate Professor, School of Allied Health, Exercise and Sports Sciences, Charles Sturt University, Albury, NSW, Australia

MONIA D'AMOURS, MSc
Research Associate, Research Centre on Aging, CIUSSS de l'Estrie-CHUS, Sherbrooke, Québec, Canada

KATE D'CRUZ, PhD, M(OT), B(OT)
Senior Research Fellow, Research, Summer Foundation, Box Hill, Victoria, Australia
Adjunct, Occupational Therapy, La Trobe University, Melbourne, Victoria, Australia

DANIEL CEZAR DA CRUZ, PhD, MSc, BSc
Senior Lecturer in Occupational Therapy Programme, School of Health, Leeds Beckett University, Leeds, West Yorkshire, United Kingdom

SIMONE DORSCH, BAppSci(PHYSIO), MHlthSci, PhD
Associate Professor, School of Allied Health, Australian Catholic University, Sydney, New South Wales, Australia
Director, StrokeEd, Sydney, New South Wales, Australia

VAGNER DOS SANTOS, PhD, MSc, BSc
Senior Lecturer in Occupational Therapy, Head of Discipline, School of Allied Health, Exercise & Sports Sciences, Charles Sturt University, Port Macquarie, New South Wales, Australia

R LYLE DUQUE, MSOT, OTRP, FPAOT
Executive Director, Therapy and Education Services, Life Skills Therapy Center, Tarlac City, Philippines

Professional Regulatory Board Member, Professional Regulatory Board of Occupational Therapy, Professional Regulation Commission, Manila, Philippines

MARY EGAN, PHD, OT REG.(ONT.)
Professor, Rehabilitation Sciences, University of Ottawa, Ottawa, Ontario, Canada

ISLA EMERY-WHITTINGTON, BHSC, MHSC, PHD
Consultant, Consultant Occupational Therapist, Emery-Whittington Consultants Ltd, Auckland, New Zealand

ERIN E. EPLEY, OTD, OTR/L
Assistant Professor, Master of Occupational Therapy, Elmhurst University, Elmhurst, Illinois, United States

LISETTE FARIAS, PHD, MSC, OT REG.
Assistant Professor, Department of Neurobiology, Care Sciences and Society (NVS), Karolinska Institutet, Stockholm, Sweden

ANDREW R. FREEMAN, BSC(OT) (HONS), MSC(OT), PHD(REHABILITATION SCIENCES)
Associate Professor, École des sciences en réadaptation (Faculté de médecine), Université Laval, Quebec City, Quebec, Canada

ROSHAN GALVAAN, PHD, MSC(OT), BSC(OT)
Professor of Occupational Therapy, Department of Health and Rehabilitation Sciences, University of Cape Town, Cape Town, South Africa

FADIA GAMIELDIEN, BSC(OT), MSC(OT)
Senior Clinical Educator, Division of Occupational Therapy, Inclusive Practices Africa Research Unit, Department of Health and Rehabilitation Sciences, Faculty of Health Sciences, University of Cape Town, Cape Town, Western Cape Province, South Africa

EMMA ELIZABETH GEE, BSC(OT)
Lived Experience Consultant and Author, Kew, Australia
Lived Experience Advisor and Information Service, Co-design Team, Summer Foundation, Australia

MONICA VILLAÇA GONÇALVES, PHD(OT), MSC(PUBLIC HEALTH), BSC(OT)
Professor, Occupational Therapy Department, Federal University of Espírito Santo (UFES), Vitória, Espírito Santo, Brazil

FI GRAHAM, PGDIP HE, PHD, BOCCTHY
Associate Professor, Rehabilitation Teaching and Research Unit, Department of Medicine, University of Otago, Wellington, New Zealand

MARIE GRANDISSON, ERG., PHD
Professor, School of Rehabilitation Sciences, Université Laval, Quebec City, Quebec, Canada

ELE GRIMWOOD, BHSC(HONS) OT
Occupational therapy team manager, Department of Adult Social Care, City of Bradford Metropolitan District Council, Bradford, United Kingdom

CHRISTINE GUPTILL, PHD, OT REG.(ONT.)
Associate Professor, Rehabilitation Sciences, University of Ottawa, Ottawa, Ontario, Canada

SUZANNE HENSHALL, BHSC(HONS) SOCIAL SCIENCE, BHSC(HONS) OCCUPATIONAL THERAPY
Senior Occupational Therapist, Community Neuro Rehab Service, Leeds Community Healthcare, Leeds, United Kingdom
Primary Care Educator, Faculty of Primary Care Wider Workforce, Health Education England/NHS England, Leeds, United Kingdom

CLARE HOCKING, PHD, MHSC
Professor, Occupational Science and Therapy, Auckland University of Technology, Auckland, New Zealand

ANNE W. HUNT, PHD
Assistant Professor Teaching Stream, Occupational Science & Occupational Therapy, University of Toronto, Toronto, Ontario, Canada

DOROTHY KESSLER, PHD
Associate Professor, School of Rehabilitation Therapy, Queen's University, Kingston, Ontario, Canada

DEBBIE LALIBERTE RUDMAN, PHD, MSC, BSC(OT)
Distinguished University Professor, School of Occupational Therapy, University of Western Ontario, London, Ontario, Canada

NATASHA A. LANNIN, PHD, BSC(OT)
Professor, Department of Neuroscience, Monash University, Melbourne, Victoria, Australia
Professor, Occupational Therapy Department, Alfred Health, Melbourne, Victoria, Australia

NATASHA A. LAYTON, PHD
Senior Research Fellow, RAIL Research Centre, Monash University, Clayton, Victoria, Australia

JENICA LEE, OTD, OTR/L
Clinical Associate Professor, Occupational Therapy, University of Illinois Chicago, Chicago, Illinois, United States

JAIME DANIEL LEITE JUNIOR, PHD, BSC(OT)
Lecturer in Occupational Therapy, Department of Occupational Therapy, Federal University of São Carlos, São Carlos, São Paulo, Brazil

ROSELI ESQUERDO LOPES, PHD, MSC, BSC(OT)
Full Professor, Department of Occupational Therapy, Federal University of São Carlos, São Carlos, São Paulo, Brazil

DANIEL LOWRIE, PHD, MSC, BHSC(OT)
Senior Lecturer, Occupational Therapy, James Cook University, Townsville, Queensland, Australia

CLAIRE LYNCH, DOCTOR OF CLINICAL SCIENCE
Senior Lecturer in Occupational Therapy, Allied Health, Australian Catholic University, Melbourne, Victoria, Australia

HEATHER MACLEOD, OT REG. (ONT.), MSC, DSC(C)
Manager, Programs and Partnerships, Provincial Geriatrics Leadership Ontario, Toronto, Ontario, Canada
Doctoral Student, Rehabilitation Therapy, Queens University, Kingston, Ontario, Canada

ANA PAULA SERRATA MALFITANO, PHD
Associate Professor, Occupational Therapy, Federal University of Sao Carlos, Sao Carlos, Sao Paulo, Brazil

AGNETA MALMGREN FÄNGE, PHD, REG.(OT)
Associate Professor, Department of Health Sciences, Lund University, Lund, Sweden

ROSE MARTINI, PHD, OT REG.(ONT.)
Professor and Program Director, Occupational Therapy, University of Ottawa, Ottawa, Ontario, Canada

ALAN MATHEW, BSC(OT), MSC, HCPC, FHEA, PGCERT, MRCOT
Lecturer in Occupational Therapy, Department of Occupational Therapy, Directorate of Allied Health, University of Salford, Salford, United Kingdom

AMY MATHEWS, BSC(OT)
Occupational Therapist, Vision Australia, Victoria, Australia

ANNIE MCCLUSKEY, PHD, MA, DIPCOT
School of Health Sciences, Faculty of Medicine and Health, The University of Sydney, Sydney, New South Wales, Australia

VALERIE METCALFE, BSC(OT), MHSC(OT)
Part-time Professor, Facutly of Health Sciences, Department of Occupational Therapy, University of Ottawa, Ottawa, Ontario, Canada

FRANCINE MILLER, BSCOT
Seating and Mobility Program, Access Community
    Therapists Ltd, Vancouver, British Columbia,
    Canada

WILLIAM C. MILLER, BSCOT, MSCOT, PHD
Professor, Occupational Science and Occupational
    Therapy, University of British Columbia,
    Vancouver, British Columbia, Canada
Principle Investigator, Rehabilitation Research
    Program, GF Strong Rehabilitation Centre,
    Vancouver, British Columbia, Canada
Principle Investigator, Centre for Aging SMART,
    University of British Columbia, Vancouver, British
    Columbia, Canada
Principle Investigator, Vancouver Coast Research
    Institute, University of British Columbia,
    Vancouver, British Columbia, Canada

**W. BEN MORTENSON, BSCOT, MSC, PHD,
FCAOT, OT**
Professor and Department Head, Occupational
    Science and Occupational Therapy, University of
    British Columbia, Vancouver, Canada

JANET M. MURCHISON, BSCOT, BFA
Occupational Therapist, Ambulatory Mental Health,
    Baycrest, Toronto, Ontario, Canada
Lecturer, Occupational Science and Occupational
    Therapy, University of Toronto, Toronto, Ontario,
    Canada

ANGELA M. MURPHY, BSC(OT), MSC, EDD
Senior Lecturer in Occupational Science and
    Occupational Therapy, School of Health, Leeds
    Beckett University, Leeds, United Kingdom

**SITHEMBELENKOSINI BEAUTY NGCOBO,
BSC(OT)**
Lecturer, Department of Health and Rehabilitation
    Sciences, University of Cape Town, Cape Town,
    South Africa

MELISSA THERESE NOTT, PHD, BAPPSC(OT)
Principal Research Fellow, Three Rivers Department
    of Rural Health, Charles Sturt University, Albury,
    New South Wales, Australia

**KATIE O'DONNELL, BSC(HONS) OCCUPATIONAL
THERAPY, PGDIP, ACCREDITED HAND
THERAPIST**
Advanced Clinical Specialist Occupational Therapist,
    Outpatient Therapy Department, University Hospital
    of Southampton, Southampton, United Kingdom

ROSANA TERESA ONOCKO-CAMPOS, PHD
Associate Professor, Public Health Department,
    Faculty of Medical Sciences, Unicamp, Campinas,
    Sao Paulo, Brazil

**TRACEY PARNELL, PHD, MOT, BAAPPSC(OT),
GCLTHE, SFHEA**
Associate Head of School/Senior Lecturer-Occupational
    Therapy, School of Allied Health, Exercise & Sports
    Sciences, Faculty of Science & Health, Charles Sturt
    University, Albury, New South Wales, Australia

CYNTHIA PERLMAN, BSC(OT), MED
Assistant Professor (Professional), School of Physical
    and Occupational Therapy
Director, Office of Interprofessional Education,
    Faculty of Medicine & Health Sciences, McGill
    University, Montreal, Quebec, Canada

**MARIA DENISE PESSOA SILVA, BSC, PGDIP,
MSC, MRCOT**
Associate Lead for Therapies and Professional Lead
    for Occupational Therapy, Occupational Therapy,
    The Royal Marsden NHS Foundation Trust,
    London, United Kingdom

LIESL PETERS, BSC(OT), M(OT)
Senior Lecturer, Health and Rehabilitation Sciences,
    University of Cape Town, Cape Town, Western
    Cape, South Africa

**ANGELA PHENIX, MASTERS OF OCCUPATIONAL
THERAPY, MASTERS OF INDIGENOUS EDUCATION**
Occupational Therapist, Phenix OT Consulting,
    Regina, Canada

ALISON CATHERINE PIGHILLS, MSC, PHD
Mackay Hospital and Health Service, Mackay Institute
    of Research and Innovation, Mackay Hospital and
    Health Service, Mackay, Queensland, Australia

James Cook University, School of Occupational Therapy, James Cook University, Townsville, Queensland, Australia

HELENE J. POLATAJKO, BOT, MEd, PhD, OT(C), FCAOT, FCAHS, LLD(h.c.), OC
Professor Emeritus, Occupational Science and Occupational Therapy, Rehabilitation Sciences Institute, University of Toronto, Toronto, Ontario, Canada

MIKE PRESCOTT, PhD, MA, MBA, BSc
Post-doctoral Fellow, Occupational Sciences and Occupational Therapy, University of British Columbia, Vancouver, Canada

YELIZ PRIOR, PhD, BSc, FHEA, HCPC, MRCOT
Professor of Clinical Rehabilitation, School of Health and Society, The University of Salford, Salford, Greater Manchester, United Kingdom

VÉRONIQUE PROVENCHER, PhD
Professor, School of Rehabilitation, Université de Sherbrooke, Sherbrooke, Quebec, Canada

DANIELLE RAE, BEd, MOT
Occupational Therapist and Clinical Faculty, Occupational Therapy, University of British Columbia, Vancouver, Canada

JUDY L. RANKA, BSc(OT), MA(EDUC&WORK), HLTHSCD
Director and Principal Occupational Therapist, Occupational Therapy, Occupational Performance Network, Sydney, New South Wales, Australia
Honorary Academic Affiliate, School of Occupational Therapy, University of Sydney, Camperdown, New South Wales, Australia

GAYLE RESTALL, BMR(OT), MSc, PhD, OT REG(MB)
Professor Emerita, Occupational Therapy, University of Manitoba, Winnipeg, Canada

CARLIA RIX, BACHELOR OF OCCUPATIONAL SCIENCE AND THERAPY
Senior Practitioner Occupational Therapist, Client Services, Vision Australia, Bendigo, Victoria, Australia

KATIE ROBINSON, PhD, MSc(DISABILITY MANAGEMENT), BSc(OT)
Professor, Ageing Research Centre, Health Research Institute, School of Allied Health, University of Limerick, Limerick, Ireland

KRISTY MAREE ROBSON, PhD, MHSc(ED), DIP HSc(POD)
Dr, Three Rivers Department of Rural Health, Charles Sturt University, Albury, New South Wales, Australia

RUHEENA SANGRAR, PhD OT REG.(ONT.)
Assistant Professor, Teaching Stream, Department of Occupational Science and Occupational Therapy, University of Toronto, Toronto, Ontario, Canada

KATRINE SAUVÉ-SCHENK, OT REG.(ONT.), PhD
Assistant Professor, School of Rehabilitation Sciences, University of Ottawa, Ottawa, Ontario, Canada

BONITA SAWATZKY, PhD
Associate Professor, Orthopaedics, University of British Columbia, Vancouver, British Columbia, Canada

KARL SCHURR, MAppSc, BAppSc
Karl Schurr, Physiotherapist, StrokeEd Collaboration, Sydney, New South Wales, Australia

SALVADOR SIMÓ ALGADO, PhD(INCLUSIVE EDUCATION
Deputy Director of Mental Health, ISAMBES, UVic-UCC, Vic, Barcelona, Spain

SUSAN STARK, PhD, OTR/L
Professor, Occupational Therapy and Neurology, Washington University, St. Louis, United States

JENNY STRONG, PhD, MOccThy, BOccThy, FOTARA
Emeritus Professor, School of Health & Rehabilitation Sciences, The University of Queensland, Brisbane, Queensland, Australia

MIRANDA MICHELLE M. THEW, MSc, BHSc(HONS), DipCOT, CMS
Senior Lecturer Occupational Therapy, School of Science, Technology and Health, York St John University, York, United Kingdom

KAARINA VALAVAARA, MScOT, BA(HONS)
Instructor, School of Occupational Therapy, Dalhousie, Halifax, Canada

CATHERINE VALLÉE, PhD
Professor, School of Rehabilitation Sciences, Université Laval, Quebec City, Quebec, Canada

APRIL VANDER VEEN, PhD(CANDIDATE), MSc(OT), BA
Health and Rehabilitation Sciences, Western University, London, Ontario, Canada

MICHELLE VILLENEUVE, PhD
Associate Professor, Centre for Disability Research and Policy, University of Sydney, Sydney, New South Wales, Australia

KAREN WHALLEY HAMMELL, PhD, MSc, DipCOT
Honorary Professor, Occupational Science & Occupational Therapy, University of British Columbia, Vancouver, British Columbia, Canada

ARISTELA ZANONA, DOCTOR IN NEUROSCIENCES, MASTER IN PHYSICAL EDUCATION, BACHELOR IN OCCUPATIONAL THERAPY
Professor, Occupational Therapy, Universidade Federal de Sergipe, Aracaju, Brazil

Section 1

CONTEMPORARY REFLECTIONS ON OCCUPATIONAL THERAPY

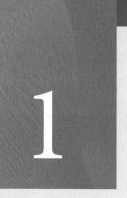

1

DECOLONIALITY IN OCCUPATIONAL THERAPY PRACTICE: PREPARATION AND READINESS

ISLA EMERY-WHITTINGTON

CHAPTER OUTLINE

Overview

Calls for decoloniality across occupational therapy and occupational science practice, education and research are increasing in frequency. Yet white supremacy and coloniality continue to delay and impede growth and opportunities to centre justice and equity within and beyond the profession. Importantly, decoloniality is a process that relies on honesty; the searing kind, that discomforts and inconveniences because both unlearning and learning are required. Decoloniality finds oxygen within conversations and relationships forged and strengthened to centre equity and end coloniality.

Hence, this chapter responds to calls for decoloniality by inviting current and future occupational therapy practitioners, researchers and educators, to a readiness conversation. Preparation and readiness tasks outlined here include building knowledge of key elements of coloniality, such as racism and privilege. In addition, essential aspects of decoloniality, including understanding social positioning, examining beliefs, supporting BIPOC colleagues and building antiracist collectives, facilitate both intimate and collaborative preparation for engagement in decolonial praxis.

KEY POINTS

- Decoloniality requires learning about colonisation, coloniality, racism and privilege.
- Preparation for decolonial praxis can be discomforting as recognition of benefits and harms from coloniality increases.
- Occupational therapists and occupational scientists are exploring many aspects of coloniality as expressed within the profession.
- Unlearning colonial ways of being means finding new ways to learn, educate, research and practice.
- Decolonial tasks differ depending on knowledge, privilege and willingness to share power.

- BIPOC collectives and critical allies are supporting the occupational therapy profession's growth using a number of strategies and platforms.
- Antiracist collectives organised and networked across the occupational therapy profession can move decolonial work from preparation to action.

Positioning

I acknowledge the lands and waters where you are and the people who have looked after those spaces for millennia. I acknowledge the generosity of colleagues, mentors and guides, yours and mine. I acknowledge the energy you bring to this conversation.

I am a Māori cis woman from Ngāti Kauwhata, Ngāti Maniapoto, Ngāti Kahungunu ki Wairarapa peoples from the North Island Te Ika-a-Māui, Aotearoa New Zealand. I trained as an occupational therapist 30 years ago. I live with my three children and husband in Auckland city and am able bodied. I teach about colonisation, antiracism, Te Tiriti o Waitangi (New Zealand's treaty), mental health and addictions, and Indigenous theory and practice of occupational therapy. Like many, I write to both understand the coloniality that is being reproduced by way of everyday occupations and share strategies used to end racialised harming. I believe in the distinctive healing contributions that decolonial praxis in concert with BIPOC[1] and critical ally collegiality can make.

I acknowledge contributions by academics, researchers and practitioners from every continent who disrupt racism, patriarchy, ableism and other manifestations of colonialism. I acknowledge especially peer networks and collaborations who strategise and organise to respond with dignity, humility and strength to coloniality. The text *Promoting Occupational Participation: Collaborative Relationship-Focused Occupational Therapy* (Egan & Restall, 2022) is a solid example of collegiality, strategy and organisation. This chapter builds on and adds to the profession's network of collegiality, trust and work to undo oppression. As such, similar publications citing BIPOC colleagues and critical allies are engaged and highlighted.

---

[1]BIPOC is an acronym for Black, Indigenous, People of Colour. It is imperfect and not meant to imply similarity in experiences of coloniality or decoloniality.

INTRODUCTION

Welcome to this 'decolonial readiness' text. This text is purposefully written to support serious consideration for change – decolonial change – and therefore it can be considered a readiness conversation of a sort. However, decoloniality work is no small undertaking as centuries of doing, being, belonging to and becoming agents of coloniality need to be reckoned with. Some careful preparation is called for which requires new skills, experiences, alliances and ways of learning and sharing, researching and practicing occupational therapy. Occupational therapy has unique and much-needed perspectives of coloniality and decoloniality in relation to everyday occupation, but first there is some internal work to do.

Readiness conversations require assessment of the 'current situation', acquisition and practice of new skills and knowledge, while possibly decentring other skills and unlearning. The reader is encouraged to foreground their own cultural lens and social positioning especially if it is a 'yet to be heard' perspective. Therefore take care and take note of what feels discomforting and schedule rest breaks to centre moments of peace before returning to tricky parts. The reader is encouraged to dialogue about what they notice or have come to think further on especially with a trusted person or group. Please refrain from finding comfort or attempting to domesticate decoloniality by making it palatable or bite sized. In truth, decoloniality is not a chapter, research approach or public statement, but for some, it is the difference between life, opportunities for recovery and death. There are some important assumptions that have shaped this chapter:

1. Occupational therapy and occupational science are raced and classed and have developed in spaces that have favoured white supremacy and coloniality while denying and silencing global knowledges (Emery-Whittington, 2021). There are many knowledges and many ways to know, hold and share knowledge.
2. Not all knowledges are commensurate with what knowledge individuals already hold, and therefore it is not always possible or fruitful to define and compare knowledges. Some knowledges just *are*.

3. The path to knowledge acquisition may be uncomfortable and only attainable through unlearning, grit and humility.
4. Occupational therapy is not necessarily healing, but land back and reparations are.
5. It is assumed that to a greater or lesser extent, most people carry racist beliefs due to the raced social, economic and political foundation of modern societies.

This chapter sits with the conundrum that is decoloniality while working for, studying within and/or practicing within institutions that uphold coloniality. Despite all, this chapter aims to support the occupational therapists to prepare to make the next personal-political step a decolonial one.

In the next section, the reader is encouraged to examine their lens by exploring their social positioning and then building knowledge by exploring definitions and language of decoloniality. Language and definitions regarding coloniality and racism can help hone a focus on both what coloniality and racism are as well as what they do (Azarmandi, 2022). The conversation continues with an explication of colonial expansion history including the doctrine of discovery, privilege and decoloniality. Then, decoloniality tasks for study are explored along with tools to support anti-racist practice. The chapter concludes with two sections, the first section is written to BIPOC Colleagues, as our social positioning means our decolonial tasks and processes differ from critical allies. The second specific section is written for educators and practitioners and addresses the tension of decolonial work in colonial institutions.

WHAT IS THE SHAPE AND NATURE OF YOUR LENS?

Prior to beginning a process of examining and growing a critical lens, it is useful to think about who we are in relation to each other and the world around us. Western notions of occupation and health have been constructed from individual or particulate views of the self (Iwama, 2006). However, decolonial work relies on the notion of connectedness and relationship to all other things is the opposite of colonialism where categorisations, splits, silos, reductions and

---

BOX 1.1

THREE QUESTIONS USED BY THE AUTHOR TO SUPPORT A FOCUS ON CONNECTEDNESS USED IN A CLASSROOM TEACHING SCENARIO

Question 1: 'Before setting out from home, who checked the traffic situation, perhaps on an app or listened for traffic report updates on the radio?' A few hands rise.

I say to the students, 'This makes sense because we don't want to be stuck in traffic'. I suggest to them that 'Perhaps there is another way to think about traffic; a social way. For instance, when we are stuck or sitting in traffic, we are not in traffic, we **are** the traffic, one part of the whole that is "the traffic jam"'.

Question 2: My second question is 'Where is outer space?' Usually, a few fingers point upwards. I pose that '"Outer Space" is a relative and imprecise term and from a non-Earth perspective we are presently **in** outer space'.

Question 3: 'Where is Nature?'

By this stage, some students have comprehended the point of the questions, although some fingers point outside towards trees, hills or even the sea outside the window. I suggest that 'Nature is right here, all around us', gesturing to myself and everyone in the room. 'We **are** nature. Even if we follow the colonial convention that we are "conquerors" of nature or '**the** apex predator', we are still very much Nature'.

---

simplifications are created and nurtured (Emery-Whittington, 2021). Socially constructed separations can create division, fear, otherness, uncertainty, and so decolonial work takes and makes opportunities to think about connectedness to each other within our shared spaces. Decolonial practices can be small, everyday, habitual as well as impactful, disrupting and collaborative. For myself, a decolonial practice before I write is to take a moment to connect to my purpose, and I might bring to mind a proverb, ancestral teachings or prayers that bring a sense of peace and clarity. Decoloniality is about *how* daily deeds are done as much as *what* is done, and so you are encouraged to think about ways that study and collegiality can reflect this. To this point, this reading will be greatly enhanced through conversation – exploration of ideas, following sparks, sitting with new ideas and seeking clarifications. The story presented in Box 1.1 captures a classroom teaching scenario using three questions used to support focus on connectedness.

The lens through which the world is experienced is very much shaped by the relationships and connections we are surrounded with and those we choose to foster. Through intentional consideration of connections, people can momentarily deeply consider their relationship with each other, their shared home spaces and their planet. In so doing, they can reverently reconnect to something greater than their learned individualism – their spirit, purpose and contribution (Emery-Whittington, 2021). The next section builds on considerations of connections by focusing on critical self-awareness via social positionality and land acknowledgement.

Developing a Statement of Social Positionality and Land Acknowledgements

What we say comes from somewhere, and how we view something also comes from somewhere (Hammell, 2020). Social positioning statements allow others to have a sense of who the person is in relation to what is being spoken about. A statement of positionality signals knowledge, capability and/or experience with respect to a topic which can reduce the risk of assumptions about who the person is and what and how much the person knows. Where conversation requires building trust or taking more care, statements of social positioning can be useful. Demonstrating care by explaining one's view on the terms used assists with building trust and creating spaces for dialogue. This is an area that occupational therapy practitioners often assume is unnecessary to explain.

It is a good idea to listen carefully to a range of people introduce themselves and/or state their positionality, for example, keynote speakers, faculty leaders, and even musicians and artists (e.g. Beagan et al., 2023; Hammell, 2021). Drafting sentences, practicing with trusted peers and educators and curating statements to different situations are important steps to building a connection to space and situation. Social positioning statements must feel emotionally honest, be humble in delivery and be matter of fact. Fostering a strong sense of who you are supports the explication of social positioning that feels like a good fit. Questions that may help prompt positionality reflections are presented in Box 1.2.

From an Indigenous vantage, land and waters are vital to existence. Therefore, when entering into new

---

BOX 1.2
QUESTIONS PROMPT POSITIONALITY

What was your pathway to training?
What attracted you?
What made you think that this profession was a good fit for you?
When you told family, friends and trusted people about wanting to be an occupational therapist or scientist what did they say?
How do you sustain this goal – especially when things feel overwhelming – and who sustains it with you?

---

territories and waters, acknowledgement of the people who have cared for and lived in good relation with the space is vital and is considered good manners. Land acknowledgements are becoming part of welcome and connection rituals and ceremonies for many universities in settler-colonial states. Land acknowledgements are highly geographical, context-specific rituals, so there are no universal processes to follow. Decolonial praxis includes learning about the expectations and processes of the locality where one studies and practices in, as this is central to being in relation and connected to the space. Stewart-Ambo and Yang (2021) implore deeper reflection and conversation about institutional use of land acknowledgement and agree that thoughtful land acknowledgements in settler-colonial institutions can centre a fuller awareness of Indigenous peoples – their names, desires and futurity. Conversely, land acknowledgements can ring hollow if recited by rote, treated as a performance, or misinterpreted as *the only* decolonial task of the meeting, lecture or gathering (Beagan et al., 2023; Stewart-Ambo & Yang, 2021). Key to the authenticity of land acknowledgements is collaborative living relationships where strategy and organisation of multiple decolonial actions, including landback, are routine.

DEFINITIONS: GROWING A SHARED LANGUAGE OF DECOLONIALITY

Race and Racism

The American Anthropological Association's (AAA's) 1998 Statement on Race clarified that the concept of race as a biological concept is disproven (AAA, 1998) and that 'Racial myths bear no relationship to the reality of human capabilities or behaviour. Scientists today find that reliance on such folk beliefs about human differences in research has led to countless errors'. Physical features do not predetermine human behaviour. Kendi (2019) described race as a 'power construct of collected or merged difference that lives socially' (p. 35). Whereas racism is a social system that interacts with other social systems and is 'based on an ideology of inferiority and superiority, that drives that categorisation of people by race/ethnicity and structures opportunity according to those categorisations, resulting in the inequitable distribution of power, goods and resources in society' (Harris et al., 2012, pp. 408–409). Further, racism is a way to deny connection to other humans and Nature, thus denying relationship and responsibility to each other.

It is already well established that racism is a social determinant of health (Commission on Social Determinants of Health, 2007; Williams & Mohammed, 2013). Racism can be measured for physiological impacts and psychological distress (e.g. Marsh et al., 2010), social opportunities cost and direct violence, which have causal relationships to poor health and wellbeing (Priest et al., 2013; Williams et al., 2019). Moreover, harm, damage and violence from racism are entirely avoidable (Borell et al., 2009). Researchers have studied racism using a variety of theoretical frameworks to explain ways that racism impacts people's lives. Depending on the depth of analysis required, some researchers use three levels of analysis of racism, and some use four. The four levels of analysis are structural racism, institutional racism, interpersonal/personally mediated racism and internalised racism.

James Nazroo and colleagues (2020) defined 'structural racism' as a societal circulation of 'ideas and representations that produce race and ethnic groups as different, but also as threatening and inferior', which are then used to rationalise and justify inequitable resource distribution (Nazroo et al., 2020, p. 265). Kevin Nadal and colleagues (2021) elaborated to include actions and inactions that can be habitual, direct or vicarious, sometimes malicious and violent, cumulative and intersecting. Camara Jones (2000) defined three levels of racism: institutional racism, personally mediated racism/interpersonal racism and internalised racism. Jones used the allegory of a garden, where some flowers are watered and others are not, and that over time such attention becomes expected, proceduralised and

institutionalised; 'normative, sometimes legalised, and often manifests as inherited disadvantage' (2000, p. 1212).

Personally mediated/interpersonal racism is the level that many automatically think about when discussing racism because it is perhaps at first glance the most obvious form. Personally mediated/interpersonal racism refers to differential assumptions and actions (intentional and unintentional, verbal and nonverbal) based on (presumed) race. As well, such differential assumptions and actions can be expressed and/or withheld, for example, 'everyday avoidance' such as street crossing or purse clutching, poor or no service and police brutality (Jones, 2000, pp. 1212–1213). Because this level of racism is overt, antiracism efforts can often be overly focused on addressing only this level of racism, yet scholars argue that structural and institutional racism has a greater impact on population health (Came, 2014).

Internalised racism is the most devasting kind of racism because it is the least discussed (Pyke, 2010). Yin Paradies (2006) used the concept of two intertwined parts – internalised oppression (self-subordination) and its opposite, internalised dominance (privilege) – to explicate internalised racism. Both manifestations require the 'incorporation of racist attitudes, beliefs or ideologies within an actor's worldview' (Paradies, 2006, p. 151). It is worth noting that what Paradies refers to as 'internalised oppression', other authors refer to as 'internalised racism'. Internalised racism is 'acceptance […] of negative messages about […] own abilities and intrinsic worth' that can manifest as muted self-expression, changing appearance to appear whiter, fratricide, among other expressions (Jones, 2000, p. 1213), self-doubt and feelings of inferiority (Fanon, 1961). Racial distress can be transmitted further amongst a person's own communities due to racial targeting (Memmi, 1965) with varying levels of awareness of self-hate (David et al., 2019). Hence, internalised oppression can be both a source and consequence of structural, institutional and interpersonal racism (James, 2022).

Occupational therapists and occupational scientists have under-theorised oppression including racism (Johnson & Lavalley, 2021; Pooley & Beagan, 2021). Yet, it is clear that there is an important element to the expression and transmission of oppression including racism, that is, occupation itself (Emery-Whittington & Davis, 2023). That is, racism is transmitted and role modelled via everyday occupations, firstly amongst families, then networks and communities (Emery-Whittington, 2024). A proposed occupational perspective of racism is the *habituated expression of white supremacist ideology transmitted via everyday deeds and activities.*

A summary of each level of racism analysis is presented in Box 1.3

Understanding Coloniality and Decoloniality

To understand the very vital role of racism as occupationally expressed in this day and age, it is important to understand colonisation. Colonisation is the business of dispossessing Indigenous nation states of their territories and assuming a right to control their lives (Jackson, 2018). The European style of colonisation peaked in the final few centuries of the last millennium, but it does not follow that it suddenly ended. Contributing to

the unprecedented and diabolical success of theft and genocide with impunity globally, were several crucial factors including the monarchy, church and capitalists (Pitman, personal communication, June 13, 2022). Fifteenth-century monarchs gave explorers civil orders and provided means to colonise, while the church gave moral justification (Pitman, personal communication, June 13, 2022) through the issuing of papal orders, which have come to be known as the Doctrine of Discovery. Trade, profit and extraction at all costs, backed up by science, religion, philosophy and race-based policies, set in motion the very situation that has led to the present day: climate change, poverty and conversely, concentrated wealth held by just a few and supported by governments (Paradies, 2020; Smith, 2012).

Colonisation is sometimes thought of as a past event, a structure or a phase in history. Instead, colonisation establishes white supremacy, white privilege and racism (Te Kāhui Tika Tangata Human Rights Commission, 2022) so that it endures through time shapeshifting as needed. Hence, coloniality is a term that captures the ongoing, fluid yet hidden character of colonisation (Cooper, 2012). Occupational therapy descends from this thought heritage and praxis, and unless theories, frameworks or practice models are explicitly decolonial, it can be assumed that colonialism is built in. Kronenberg (2021) highlighted the occupational therapy profession's perplexing habit of calling for antiracism while actively maintaining racist status quo structures and processes, thus revealing a core element of colonialism: privilege (Box 1.4).

Decoloniality is based on contextual understandings of colonisation, coloniality and their impacts and power (Ramugondo, 2018) and is therefore beyond awareness and sensitivity about 'other' cultures. Decoloniality is about eschewing the status quo that is societal amnesia about colonialism and the many kinds of oppressions it fuels, because it demands critical thinking and attention on privilege and antiracism. The racism that stops equipment being prescribed, visits being offered or delayed, referrals being made and accepted, clinical assessment reports being completed in a timely fashion, support letters being written, and welcoming smiles being offered is the same racism that withholds sharing of lecture notes, study group availability and attention in tutorials. It is the same racism that leverages privilege so that statements like 'there is no budget

BOX 1.4
PRIVILEGE – 'LIKE RUNNING WITH SCISSORS'

Privilege 'refers to systematic and interpersonal advantage that works in concert with systemic discrimination and marginalization to produce population group differentials in access to, among other things, societal goods and services, and exposure to stressors' (Borell et al., 2009, p. 31). Using the allegory of an invisible backpack, McIntosh described privilege from initial research observations regarding gender privilege. McIntosh observed that as much as subjects who identified as men could acknowledge that women generally experience disadvantage, they did not think that they were comparatively advantaged (McIntosh, 1990). It was as if the 'backpack of privilege' was invisible to them. McIntosh's focus then extended to consider ethnicity and began to record and list the everyday ways that their skin colour afforded advantage and ease, that is, if McIntosh asked to see 'the manager' they could be sure to meet someone of their ethnicity and who also spoke the same language.

Privilege ensures that 'inter-generational political, economic, social and cultural benefits and advantages [...] accumulate through the appropriation of Indigenous lands, natural resources and wealth' (HRC, 2022, p. 22). Privilege is the part of oppression that gets to slink into the background and over time comes to be so universally accepted that it becomes invisible. In their work to theorise privilege, Moewaka Barnes and colleagues refer to privilege not as 'the elephant in the room' but as 'the elephant on the sofa' (2014, p. 6). It has been noted that people with privilege can find it difficult to recognise their privilege until they meet people without it (Gerlach, 2015; Nelson, 2007). Certainly, it is much easier for people to recognise those who have more power than themself, and harder to recognise those who have less. Unrecognised privilege is 'like running with scissors' (Hantke, personal communication, March 21, 2022), that is, power in the hands of someone oblivious to its potential for harm is dangerous. In occupational therapy training spaces, privilege shows up in multiple spaces but especially in the setting of curricula – which is essentially a selection of knowledge – and manifests in which knowledge is included and which is excluded, how knowledge is treated, cared for and tested.

Returning to Paradies' (2006) definition of racism, some authors ensure that discussion about various levels of oppression (e.g. racism, sexism, ableism and more) occurs alongside analysis of privilege. However, privilege is much more than the flipside of oppression and marginalisation (Moewaka Barnes et al., 2014); it is fresh fuel for coloniality. That is, for every square mile of land confiscated or taken from Indigenous Māori in New Zealand, a settler or a settler's family, descendants or settler government was – and continues to be – privileged economically, politically and socially. Privilege is a direct challenge to the myth of meritocracy or the idea that success occurs through an individual's effort (Borell et al., 2009) and phrases like 'there would be more women around the board table if they put themselves forward, but they don't' would be seen for the half-truth that they are. The following questions might support reflection on structural, institutional, interpersonal and internalised privilege and are from Moewaka Barnes and colleagues 2014 analysis of privilege.

Reflection questions (Moewaka Barnes et al., 2014, pp. 7–9):

How is your culture treated in stories of national life?
How well does your education system meet the needs of all ethnic groups?
How welcome and 'normal' do you feel in everyday public settings?
How often do you question your sense of identity and self-worth?

---

for that project', 'no policy for that kind of issue' and 'yes there's a policy, but it is out of date and the guidelines we follow are' occur with impunity.

Therefore decoloniality necessitates wholesale structural change, organisation and strategy, which means that any solutions to our current realities devoid of decoloniality, are flawed (Wilkerson, 2020). Decoloniality requires collective, collaborative relationships because actions are aimed at every level of oppression and every occupation (Ramugondo, 2018). Decolonial praxis requires living in ways that uphold and generate humanising occupations. All aspects and expressions of life are included; thus decolonising curriculum for instance is merely an extension or natural next step to decolonising educational institutions which is a natural part of decolonising pedagogies, research and practice.

Being both health practitioners and people who access health services affords a useful perspective that informs practice. The exercises in Boxes 1.5 and 1.6 invite the reader to consider this position in relation to power and cultural safety. Box 1.6 specifically addresses clinical note taking as a potentially everyday sites of antiracism.

Antiracism

Antiracism *requires 'naming, reducing, disrupting, preventing, dismantling and eliminating racism. It [...] centres around solidarity with those targeted by racism, an analysis of power and a commitment to reflective, transformative practice'* (Stop Institutional Racism [STIR] & New Zealand Public Health Association [NZPHA], 2021, p. 9).

Antiracism includes a range of theories, strategies, practices, actions and methods that contribute to eliminating antiracism, which by and large are educational processes leading to action (Came & Griffith,

2018). Instead, antiracism praxis desires the end to all forms of oppression acknowledging that oppression is not a list of 'states' but a multiaxial, simultaneous, compounding and overlapping expression of dehumanisation. Certainly, dehumanisation of any kind is unlikely to respect discrete confines and definitions of singular expressions of oppression. In this way, antiracism is intersectional and needs to be understood, analysed and pitched at multiple levels but crucially must include both personal and institutional levels (Came & Griffith, 2018; Hantke et al., 2022). Antiracism can include bespoke design, such as antiracism marking rubrics or embedded in national policy, such as registration competencies. Good policy guides sound decision making, protects against unfair, unjust, violent harms and provides scaffolding for the times when we are not at our best. From waiting list guidelines to hospital welcome procedures, antiracism policy can guide the usual, typical and expected way of working and learning.

Also, antiracism – and humanity – can be expressed many moments a day, for example, ensuring the person who arrived first in the queue is served first, a person using their privilege to ask a question to power rather than waiting for people from historically excluded communities to do so; not engaging in gossip or stereotyping; not laughing at racist/oppressive jokes; not streaming content where someone is dehumanised. Antiracism can start early in life (Page-Gould, 2010). Adults may think about a time when they explained, or role modelled to children how to respond to a new situation, for example, when a child notices a person using a knee scooter or someone with a bright hairstyle. Typically the adult can convey calmness, openness and a desire to hear and understand. Strengths-based conversation conveys safety, for example, 'Wow, you're so lucky to have seen this today' or 'These are so helpful for moving around the supermarket'. When a child seems frightened or unsure of the 'new' situation, the adult might offer assurance through humanising the situation, that is, wondering about the person's favourite fruit. Conversely, judgemental or closed responses, such as 'They're not like us', 'Don't stare' or 'I would not employ them', can fix or cause a state of unnecessary fear that over time can lead to chronic ill-health (Page-Gould, 2010). In this way, stigma and discrimination diminish opportunities to experience difference as positive, connection enabling and interesting, with an overall reduction in capability and human potential for both the target and perpetrator.

In contrast, when practitioners of antiracism talk about their work, there are several observable characteristics to the conversation. For instance, they share the speaking time and space purposefully with historically excluded communities, the phrase 'we' is heard more than 'I' and there is a drive to precisely describe colonial phenomena. As well misfires, underestimations, and failures are openly reflected on as ways to support each other's learning. There is also genuine pleasure in sharing time along with a palpable sense of commitment, community and cohesion. Antiracism agents know where power lies and understand their sphere of influence, having figured out the specific

levers they can pull (Came-Friar, personal communication, September 29, 2022). In essence, they sense the shape of their particular contribution and how it fits within a bigger plan of curating culturally safe spaces. Clever design and strategy are celebrated, emotional maturity stands out, and some practitioners of antiracism seem to radiate an unshakeable belief that things can improve.

An example of antiracist praxis is described in Box 1.6 in relation to ensuring cultural safety.

Encouragingly, occupational therapists are not shying away from grappling with coloniality. For example, resisting theoretical imperialism (Hammell, 2011), developing occupational consciousness (Ramugondo, 2015), advocacy (Ryan et al., 2020), leadership (Gibson, 2020), occupational justice as coloniality (Emery-Whittington, 2021; Guajardo Córdoba, 2020), white supremacy in occupational therapy education (Davis & Came, 2022; Grenier, 2020; Pride et al., 2022), disobedience (Turcotte & Holmes, 2021), resisting 'laying low' (Bailliard et al., 2021), epistemological antiracism (Wijekoon & Peter, 2022), trauma-informed care and racism (Abou-Arab & Mendonca, 2021), and internalised oppression (Emery-Whittington et al., 2023). In addition, Zafran (2021) suggested that practitioners pay attention to developing a language of decoloniality and regularly check and update vocabulary and language. For instance, is the term 'culture' used to mean 'race', is the term 'cultural safety' used to mean 'culture'? When the phrase 'Global North' is used to describe a 'developed' country's power and access to resources, is it assumed that everyone from that country has the same power and access to resources? (Smith & Smith, 2018).

DECOLONIAL APPROACHES: IMAGINATION, BELIEFS AND VALUES

Decolonial approaches to learning include developing decolonial imagination, allowing for uncertainty (Galvaan et al., 2022), failure and mistakes, refusing the hegemony of a 'neutral position' (Hantke et al., 2022), taking opportunities to think and act as collectives and in varied contexts, standing with the least powerful and most harmed, and thinking deeply about how knowledge is treated and encountered. Decolonial

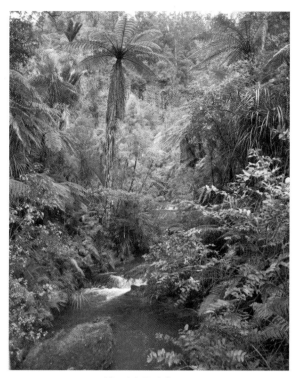

Fig. 1.1 ■ A forest.

learning can be supported by art and imagery because they can provoke deeper awareness of how new experiences and pieces of knowledge are encountered. For instance, the image in Fig. 1.1 taken in Waitākere Ranges, North Island, Aotearoa (New Zealand), brings to mind the moment a person encounters a stream or enters a forest. Upon entering a forest, senses are often heightened, and a person might begin to take notice of smells, humidity, sounds, flora and fauna, proximity and relative distance. For myself, I often do not wish to speak for a time and instead want to allow time for my mind to quieten and my body to acclimatise. Entering a forest space with reverence, humility and preparation is a useful metaphor for encountering knowledge in a decolonial manner, especially knowledge that is ancient but new.

To support the development of decolonial imagination and exploration, techniques like thought experiments, such as 'What if...?' questions can be useful. For example, 'What if equitable representation of your nation's population was represented across your cohort?' and 'What if all assignments were group based?' Expanding on the possibilities this last question raises, if all assignments were group based it is possible that occupational therapy training would provoke a strong social cohesion focus where every learner's needs are everyone's responsibility. As well, an open approach to learning would be necessary as opposed to a super competitive approach. Difficulties and conflicts would have to be managed, negotiated, mediated and led out of. Alternatively, the cohort might increase pressure on those who struggle, and move to quickly exclude or expel learners that could 'let the team down'. By and large, it could be argued that colonially structured institutions already embrace the second approach by allowing overrepresentation of individualistic learning approaches for certain demographics, socially excluding and minimising the needs of particular communities (Beagan et al., 2022; Davis & Came, 2022).

A technique from occupational therapy practice that supports decolonial exploration is the three questions technique utilised in the co-existing mental health and substance use field by Graham and colleagues (2004) (Box 1.7). The technique facilitates the exploration of beliefs held.

The three-questions technique is a way to invite a rethink of what is believed and what a person states is true. In addition, a gentle reflection of a given reply or sentiment as a question can be a safe nonjudgemental method that honours connection while allowing the possibility of exploring the response further. It is possible to apply this technique to beliefs around colonial history and oppression. As people become cognisant of their beliefs and values it can be a bridge to noticing and recognising how societally held beliefs and notions have been incorporated, which in turn provides a choice to continue or update those beliefs and values. Spending time learning about personal values

---

BOX 1.7
THREE QUESTIONS TECHNIQUE (GRAHAM ET AL., 2004)

1. What is the evidence for that (belief)?
2. Is it true all of the time?
3. Are there times when it is not true and what does that mean?

BOX 1.8
TWO SUGGESTIONS FOR REFLECTING ON PERSONAL VALUES AND BELIEFS

1. Values card sort activities can be fun, effective and encourage cohesion and deep listening with peers. Values activities are a useful foundation for imagining, theorising and planning decolonial actions and goals both as individuals and collectives.
2. Keep a simple log or table of antiracism and decolonial actions to support imagination, strategy and organisation. An example of this is provided from the perspective of an individual in Table 1.1. The same table can be used as a group.
   - Start with the 'Where I am/where we are' column;
   - Continue onto the 'Where I/we want to be' column; and
   - Complete the 'Next step/s' column.
   Setting dates to review the log or table with a supervisor, mentor or peer group and recording reflections can contribute to a broader and deeper comprehension of power structures, antiracism and decolonial actions.

---

and beliefs is important for clarifying focus and managing when things do not go as planned. Two suggestions for reflecting on personal values and beliefs are presented in Box 1.8.

Collaboration and network building are also vital decolonial processes that can be intentionally developed and nourished while studying and strengthened throughout practice. For instance, developing a habit of acknowledgement of people who inspire, challenge and support can build networks and create support structures across the globe. Sustaining relationships over time is central to decolonial praxis as is citing purposefully as a way to foreground and elevate thinkers, authors, and art with an aligned worldview. Critical activist scholars and practitioners often include their positioning in their writings, see themselves as part of a community and therefore welcome, and cite and build upon each other's thinking and work.

Tasks and roles in decoloniality differ depending on a person's position. Yet, being indignant to injustice is vital to all roles. People in powerful roles may be unlikely to support decoloniality unless there is a track record of being indignant about inequities, strategising against the status quo, and rallying collective action. In addition, it is important to not expect success in every endeavour and to regroup if allies express fear and revert to silence when racist colleagues are promoted and kinfolk work against their own interests. Certainly, doing nothing in the face of oppression guarantees more oppression, but where collectives united in social justice rally, power can build.

Critical reflexivity is another tool often discussed in occupational therapy literature. Critical reflexivity is important but only insofar as it is part of a continuous cycle of action-reflection-action. Critical reflexivity is a dynamic never-ending moment that can move a person from feeling indignant and into action. For example, critical questions can be posed about assessment tools and frameworks (e.g. MacLachlan et al., 2019; Richards & Galvaan, 2018). Lastly, guarding against

---

TABLE 1.1
A Table to Keep a Plan of Antiracism and Decolonial Actions

Date:

Name/s:

	Where I am /where we are	Next step/s	Where I/we want to be
Equity	Not certain that there is equity in work placement opportunities.	Find numbers and monitor.	Know for sure that everyone has equitable access.
Justice	Aware that reporting of racialised targeting is unsafe.	Offer support to peers and listen deeply. Strategise with peers.	Contribute to policy for safe reporting processes.
Antiracism	Feel unprepared for racist targeting of peers.	Learn phrases that deescalate situations. Do not excuse or laugh at racist jokes.	Feel skilled and practiced at responding to racism in real time.

Review Date:

the domestication of decoloniality includes regular assessment of comfort and convenience because decoloniality done well is discomforting (Tuck & Yang, 2012).

A MESSAGE TO BIPOC COLLEAGUES

If readings on colonialism are new, welcome colleague. It is your right to grow literacy around the causes of injustices and oppressions, as well as what reproduces them every day, but do take care. If instead you have been thinking critically and developing antiracist practices already, I deeply appreciate and thank you for your work and vision. For myself, decoloniality is a two-pronged approach. This chapter is an example of the first prong, that is, supporting mostly non-Indigenous people to grow critical consciousness and provide opportunities and tools for practice. However, this current section is an example of the second prong to create and support opportunities to centre our particular pieces of knowledge and practices so that we can grow, share and heal together. The latter is best done away from the colonial gaze and the former requires cultural capital and critical allies to keep the work safe. Decolonial approaches for BIPOC colleagues require both decentring colonial thinking as well as a profound belief and enduring hope in our own pieces of knowledge and healing.

Another example of the second prong is a support network created by and for Māori practitioners. We meet regularly to support each other and centre Māori pieces of knowledge of occupation and spend time with ancestor stories and guidance untouched by a colonial gaze. Our rituals honour the toil and resistance of previous generations and centre our language, our hopes and futurity. Forming and nurturing a group of like-minded supportive peers has been key to surviving and thriving in a profession that reproduces coloniality. The opportunities to be career and lifelong supporters, cheerleaders, mentors, supervisors and friends, centre our sovereignty and allow fuller expression of our epistemic range. The ability to hold multiple perspectives/cultures/languages is a unique treasure to nurture and guard.

Too often, BIPOC learners are expected to be 'cultural experts'. Informal requests for cultural advice place us in impossible situations because a 'no' can risk grades, reputation and being seen as 'difficult' and a 'yes' can risk becoming a 'functional object of coloniality' (Seet, 2021). In such cases, it is important to remember that adjacency to colonial power is adjacency to white supremacy. It is not a step towards freedom. Compliments, special treatment or 'opportunities' can be short-term, shallow performances of consultation with BIPOC people. Be wary too of calls for help that are 'time critical', especially if your relationships with your own communities are being leveraged for someone else's project. Instead, find strong advocates and join or start safe spaces to help navigate such unnecessary ethical dilemmas. Experienced BIPOC practitioners have been where you are, and there are professional groups that can take the heavy lifting so that you can concentrate on learning.

As a learner, I was racially targeted in the classroom, and as an activist scholar 30 years later, I am racially targeted in the board room. Hence, I am sure that racism is occurring in classrooms, lecture halls and fieldwork placements today, and I acknowledge the dehumanisations you have observed and experienced. Please support the targeted, and if you have experienced dehumanisation in your training, you are seen. You, like me, like many, do not deserve it. There is support, so I implore you to keep reaching out until you find supportive spaces and colleagues. Your community will benefit greatly from your work, and the profession is already better with you in it.

DECOLONIALITY IS A TEAM SPORT: A MESSAGE FOR OCCUPATIONAL THERAPY EDUCATORS AND PRACTITIONERS

Being an educator for decoloniality within Western structures that affirm and uphold coloniality is both challenging and contradictory (Smith & Smith, 2018). Educational institutions are seen as spaces that both perpetuate problematic discourses of diversity and hold the potential for dismantling such discourses (Grenier et al., 2020). Joseph-Salisbury and Connelly (2021) argue that such contradictions and tensions can be exploited for good and that educational institutions are becoming sites of scholar activism. Activist-scholars attest to the importance of navigating institutional racism and backlash alongside trusted peer groups and strong community (Came & Griffith, 2018; Joseph-Salisbury & Connelly, 2021). Also, creating cohesion, joining and serving alongside the community is deeply understood and reflected in the rise of affinity groups within the profession, such as the Māori OT Network, Indigenous International OT Consortium, DisruptOT, BAMEOTUK, ABLEOTUK, Decolonising OT Curriculum group and many others.

There are three tasks that I believe are quite urgent with regards to preparing for antiracism praxis and decoloniality, and they require the collective efforts of occupational therapy educators, researchers, practitioners and leaders alike. First, to address the demographic mismatch between who we train and the global population; second, to grow and nurture antiracism communities of practice; and third, teaching as critical conversations. With regards to the first task, it is an interesting thought experiment to imagine programmes that meet contextual needs as opposed to programmes that mimic the global minority. There is an urgent need in certain programmes to increase the epistemological range so that the needs of the local and global population can be met. Yet plans to encourage, actively recruit and support BIPOC colleagues as educators appear to only extend to BIPOC students or new graduates. Reliance on BIPOC learners to bring epistemological range and knowledge can only be a stop-gap measure at best because there are power differentials that are unjust, making such systemic reliance unethical. Instead, centring and addressing the needs of the most vulnerable communities can help to manage the tension rather than feeding the insatiable demands of the neoliberal academy. In occupational therapy practice settings, BIPOC colleagues need to be recruited into culturally safe spaces ready for their epistemological range and given fair and timely compensation.

The second task is to 'grow and nurture antiracism communities of practice'. As there are currently no global plans or strategies to end racism across occupational therapy and occupational science settings, the work of planning to end racism is left to smaller collectives. However, antiracism communities of practice can be interdependent and local and operate in equal parts support and accountability while crossing institutions. Despite the education and health sector heritage of being colonial silos that rarely coordinate or share decolonial efforts beyond conference presentations or publications, antiracist communities of practice can provide mentorship, role models for power sharing, support when facing racism in real time, and safe places to grow. Examples of team reflexivity as part of research, education and practice include Johnson and Lavalley (2021), Galvaan and colleagues (2022) and Park and Zafran (2018). Conversations inside antiracism communities of practice may be the most 'real' conversations you experience outside of family and close friends.

Delays and derailments to antiracism are frustratingly usual and can be attributed in part to undereducation of beneficiaries of colonialism about coloniality and social determinants of health *prior* to attending professional training. Educators are left with the job of teaching elementals of citizenship (with some learning local history for the first time) while developing concern and compassion for the global community. As well, content focused on culture, cultural occupations, settler-colonial history (where appropriate), diversity and justice have yet to prove liberation and instead appear to maintain the status quo. This leads us to the third task. bell hooks (2010) reminded educators that in their grasp is the ability to curate just learning spaces through critical praxis of conversation. Moreover, the classroom is a powerful place to role model equity and positive social relationships, managing tough conversations and tension in real time (Blaise, 2010). Teaching as critical conversations is exemplified by Galvaan and colleagues (2022) who intentionally stand alongside learners to ensure the *process* of teaching and learning was valued equally if not more than the curriculum content. Turcotte and Holmes (2021) suggest that by 'using disobedient thought instead of perpetuating the rules of an unhealthy capitalist society, occupational therapists have the obligation to express dissent […] and mount a theoretical and critical revolt' (p. 16) whether in the classroom, workplace, conference presentation or home.

CONCLUSION

Preparing to '[promote] access to, initiation of, and sustained participation in valued occupations within meaningful relationships and contexts' (Egan & Restall, 2022, p. 1) includes knowing our histories and ourselves. Leaning into uncertainty, unlearning colonial praxis, seeking and responding to critique, failing and standing again with the community are part and parcel of the discomfort and joy of decolonial work (Galvaan et al., 2022; Gibson, 2020). Indeed, colonial systems that require complicity with hegemony must not be our continued professional legacy.

This chapter aims to support students, educators and practitioners' preparedness for working well with any person or collective who seeks assistance to participate fully in their contexts. While there is much to do to make the occupational therapy profession antiracist and culturally safe (Beagan et al., 2022; Davis & Came, 2022; Pride et al., 2022), a number of tools have been developed and shared to support readiness for decoloniality. Understanding social positioning and privilege, and examining beliefs and knowledge of coloniality are important preparation tasks for the budding decolonial practitioner. In addition, developing foundational knowledge and language of racism and health impacts, making antiracism praxis routine and nurturing global pieces of knowledge are all examples of decolonial praxis that can start today.

Importantly, opportunities for decoloniality are grown within long-term trusting relationships, working alongside and with colleagues addressing local needs while keeping abreast of global big picture concerns. Interdependent collectives in antiracism praxis and research anticipate derailments and barriers to justice and share experience in how to analyse power and dismantle oppressive structures (Came & Griffith, 2018). For colleagues actively working to bring justice and equity, it is hoped this text both sparks further ideas for conversations and provides encouragement for your vital work. Indeed, decoloniality in practice is tied to the decoloniality of the profession itself and its accountability to all communities who share this planet.

REFERENCES

Abou-Arab, A., & Mendonca, R. (2021). Exploring implicit and explicit racial bias in OT professionals. *The American Journal of Occupational Therapy, 74*(Supplement 1). https://doi.org/10.5014/ajot.2020.74S1-PO2314.

American Anthropological Association. (1998). *Statement on race*. American Anthropological Association. https://tinyurl.com/53kadh3v.

Azarmandi, M. (2022). The limits of Pākehā treaty work: Why race matters to anti-racism. In A. Tecun, L. Lopesi, & A. Sankar (Eds.), *Towards a grammar of race in Aotearoa New Zealand* (pp. 138–150). Bridget Williams Books.

Bailliard, A., Carroll, A., & Peak, K. (2021). Laying low: Unmasking the contributions of science and education to racism. *Journal of Occupational Science, 28*(3), 441–448. https://doi.org/10.1080/14427591.2021.1893109.

Beagan, B. L., Bizzeth, S. R., Pride, T. M., & Sibbald, K. R. (2023). Racism in occupational therapy: 'It's part of who we are …'. *British Journal of Occupational Therapy, 86*(3), 171–175. https://doi.org/10.1177/03080226231153345.

Beagan, B. L., Sibbald, K. R., Bizzeth, S. R., & Pride, T. M. (2022). Systemic racism in Canadian occupational therapy: A qualitative study with therapists. *Canadian Journal of Occupational Therapy, 89*(1), 51–61. https://doi.org/10.1177/00084174211066676.

Blaise, D. (2010). The perils of colour blindness. In J. Marsh, R. Mendoza-Denton, & J. A. Smith (Eds.), *Are we born racist? New insights from neuroscience and positive psychology* (pp. 71–74). Beacon Press.

Borell, B. A. E., Gregory, A. S., McCreanor, T. N., Jensen, V. G. L., & Moewaka Barnes, H. (2009). It's hard at the top but it's a whole lot easier than being at the bottom: The role of privilege in understanding disparities in Aotearoa/New Zealand. *Race/Ethnicity: Multidisciplinary Global Contexts, 3*(1), 29–50. https://www.jstor.org/stable/25595023.

Came, H. (2014). Sites of institutional racism in public health policy making in New Zealand. *Social Science and Medicine, 106*, 214–220. https://doi.org/10.1016/j.socscimed.2014.01.055.

Came, H., & Griffith, D. (2018). Tackling racism as a 'wicked' public health problem: Enabling allies in anti-racism praxis. *Social Science and Medicine, 199*, 181–188. https://doi.org/10.1016/j.socscimed.2017.03.028.0.

Commission on Social Determinants of Health. (2007). Achieving health equity: From root causes to fair outcomes. *The Lancet, 370*(9593), 1153–1163. https://doi.org/10.1016/S0140-6736(07)61385-3.

Cooper, G. (2012). Kaupapa Māori research: Epistemic wilderness as freedom? *New Zealand Journal of Educational Studies, 47*(2), 64–73.

David, E. J. R., Schroeder, T. M., & Fernandez, J. (2019). Internalized racism: A systematic review of the psychological literature on racism's most insidious consequence. *Journal of Social Issues, 75*(4), 1057–1086. https://doi.org/10.1111/josi.12350.

Davis, G., & Came, H. (2022). A pūrākau analysis of institutional barriers facing Māori occupational therapy students. *Australian Occupational Therapy Journal, 69*(4), 414–423. https://doi.org/10.1111/1440-1630.12800.

Egan, M., & Restall, G. (2022). *Promoting occupational participation: Collaborative, relationship-focused occupational therapy*. Ottawa: Canadian Association of Occupational Therapists.

Emery-Whittington, I. G. (2021). Occupational justice – Colonial business as usual? Indigenous observations from Aotearoa New Zealand. *Canadian Journal of Occupational Therapy, 88*(2), 153–162. https://doi.org/10.1177/2F00084174211005891.

Emery-Whittington, I., & Davis, G. (2023). Rapua te kurahuna: An occupational perspective of internalised oppression. *AlterNative: An International Journal of Indigenous Peoples, 19*(4), 762–770. https://doi.org/10.1177/11771801231206209.

Emery-Whittington, I., Leite, J. Jr., & Ivlev, S. (2023). Antiracism as means and ends. In M. Ahmed-Landeryou (Ed.), *Antiracism in occupational therapy*. (pp. 119–136). Jessica Kingsley Publishers.

Emery-Whittington, I., (2024). *Decoloniality in action: A Kaupapa Māori occupational analysis of colonization*. In S. Baptiste & S. Shann (Eds.). Routledge International handbook of Occupational Therapy. London: Taylor and Francis.

Fanon, F. (1961). *The wretched of the earth*. Grove Press.

Galvaan, R., Peters, L., Richards, L. A., Francke, M., & Krenzer, M. (2022). Pedagogies within occupational therapy curriculum: Centering a decolonial praxis in community development practice. *Cadernos Brasileiros de Terapia Ocupacional, 30*. https://doi.org/10.1590/2526-8910.ctoAO24023133.

Gerlach, A. J. (2015). Sharpening our critical edge: Occupational therapy in the context of marginalized populations. *Canadian Journal of Occupational Therapy, 82*(4), 245–253. doi: 10.1177/0008417415571730.

Gibson, C. (2020). When the river runs dry: Leadership, decolonisation and healing in occupational therapy. *New Zealand Journal of Occupational Therapy, 67*(1), 11–20. https://doi.org/10.3316/informit.162982618221927.

Graham, H., Copello, A., Birchwood, M. J., Mueser, K. T., Orford, J., McGovern, D., Atkinson, E., Maslin, J., Preece, M., Tobin, D., & Georgiou, G. (2004). *Cognitive-behavioural integrated treatment (C-BIT): A treatment manual for substance misuse in people with severe mental health problems*. Wiley.

Grenier, M.-L. (2020). Cultural competency and the reproduction of white supremacy in occupational therapy education. *Health Education Journal, 79*(6), 633–644. https://doi.org/10.1177/0017896920902515.

Grenier, M.-L., Zafran, H., & Roy, L. (2020). Current landscape of teaching diversity in occupational therapy education: A scoping review. *American Journal of Occupational Therapy, 74*(6), 1–15. https://doi.org/10.5014/ajot.2020.044214.

Guajardo Córdoba, A. (2020). About new forms of colonization in occupational therapy. Reflections on the idea of occupational justice from a critical-political philosophy perspective. *Cadernos Brasileiros de Terapia Ocupacional, 28*, 1365–1381. https://doi.org/10.4322/2526-8910.ctoARF2175.

Hammell, K. W. (2011). Resisting theoretical imperialism in the disciplines of occupational science and occupational therapy. *British Journal of Occupational Therapy, 74*(1), 27–33. https://doi.org/10.4276/030802211X12947686093602.

Hammell, K. W. (2020). *Engagement in living: Critical perspectives on occupation, rights, and wellbeing*. Canadian Association of Occupational Therapists.

Hammell, K. W. (2021). Building back better: Imagining an occupational therapy for a post-COVID-19 world. *Australian Occupational Therapy Journal, 68*(5), 444–453. https://doi.org/10.1111/1440-1630.12760.

Hantke, S., St. Denis, V., & Graham, H (2022). Racism and anti-racism in nursing education: Confronting the problem of whiteness. *BMC Nursing, 21*(1), 146. https://doi.org/10.1186/s12912-022-00929-8.

Harris, R., Cormack, D., Tobias, M., Yeh, L.-C., Talamaivao, N., Minster, J., & Timutimu, R. (2012). The pervasive effects of racism: Experiences of racial discrimination in New Zealand over time and associations with multiple health domains. *Social Science & Medicine, 74*(3), 408–415. https://doi.org/10.1016/j.socscimed.2011.11.004.

Hooks, B. (2010). *Teaching critical thinking: Practical wisdom*. Routledge.

Iwama, M. K. (2006). *The Kawa model: Culturally relevant occupational therapy*. Elsevier.

Jackson, M (2018). In the end "The Hope of Decolonisation". In E. A. McKinley & L. T. Smith (Eds.), *Handbook of indigenous education* (pp. 1–11). Springer https://doi.org/10.1007/978-981-10-1839-8_59-1.

James, D. (2022). An initial framework for the study of internalized racism and health: Internalized racism as a racism-induced identity threat response. *Social and Personality Psychology Compass, 16*(11), e12712. https://doi.org/10.1111/spc3.12712.

Johnson, K. R., & Lavalley, R. (2021). From racialized think-pieces toward anti-racist praxis in our science, education, and practice. *Journal of Occupational Science, 28*(3), 404–409. https://doi.org/10.1080/14427591.2020.1847598.

Jones, C. P. (2000). Levels of racism: A theoretic framework and a gardener's tale. *American Journal of Public Health, 90*(8), 1212–1215. https://doi.org/10.2105/ajph.90.8.1212.

Joseph-Salisbury, R., & Connelly, L. (2021). *Anti-racist scholar-activism*. Manchester University Press.

Jungersen, K. (2002). Cultural safety: Kawa Whakaruruhau–an occupational therapy perspective. *New Zealand Journal of Occupational Therapy, 49*(1), 4–9.

Kendi, I. X. (2019). *How to be an antiracist*. One World.

Kronenberg, F. (2021). Commentary on JOS editorial board's anti-racism pledge. *Journal of Occupational Science, 28*(3), 398–403. https://doi.org/10.1080/14427591.2020.1827483.

MacLachlan, J., & Grenier, M.-L. (2022). Accounting for our words: Anti-oppressive documentation in occupational therapy practice. *Occupational Therapy Now, 25*, 27–30.

MacLachlan, J., Phenix, A., & Valavaara, K. (2019). *Can occupational therapy assessments be culturally safe? A critical exploration [Paper presentation]*. Canadian Association of Occupational Therapists Conference, Niagara Falls.

Marsh, J., Mendoza-Denton, R., & Smith, J. A. (Eds.). (2010). *Are we born racist? New insights from neuroscience and positive psychology*. Beacon Press.

McIntosh, P. (1990). White privilege: Unpacking the invisible backpack. *Independent School, 49*(2), 31–36. www.insightpv.org/storage/.

Memmi, A. (1965). *The colonizer and the colonized*. Beacon Press.

Moewaka Barnes, H., Borell, B., & McCreanor, T. (2014). Theorising the structural dynamics of ethnic privilege in Aotearoa: Unpacking "this breeze at my back" (Kimmell and Ferber 2003). *International Journal of Critical Indigenous Studies, 7*(1), 1–14. https://doi.org/10.5204/ijcis.v7i1.120.

Nadal, K. L., King, R., Sissoko, D. R. G., Floyd, N., & Hines, D. (2021). The legacies of systemic and internalized oppression: Experiences of microaggressions, imposter phenomenon, and stereotype threat on historically marginalized groups. *New Ideas in Psychology, 63*, 100895. https://doi.org/10.1016/j.newideapsych.2021.100895.

Nazroo, J. Y., Bhui, K. S., & Rhodes, J. (2020). Where next for understanding race/ethnic inequalities in severe mental illness? Structural, interpersonal and institutional racism. *Sociology of Health & Illness, 42*(2), 262–276. https://doi.org/10.1111/1467-9566.13001.

Nelson, A. (2007). Seeing white: a critical exploration of occupational therapy with Indigenous Australian people. *Occupational Therapy International, 14*(4), 237-255. doi: 10.1002/oti.236.

Page-Gould, E. (2010). The unhealthy racist. In J. Marsh, R. Mendoza-Denton & J. A. Smith (Eds.), *Are we born racist? New insights from neuroscience and positive psychology* (pp. 41–44). Beacon Press.

Paradies, Y. C. (2006). Defining, conceptualizing and characterizing racism in health research. *Critical Public Health, 16*(2), 143–157. https://doi.org/10.1080/09581590600828881.

Paradies, Y. C. (2020). Unsettling truths: Modernity, (de-)coloniality and Indigenous futures. *Postcolonial Studies, 23*(4), 438–456. https://doi.org/10.1080/13688790.2020.1809069.

Park, M., & Zafran, H. (2018). View from the penthouse: Epistemological bumps and emergent metaphors as method for team reflexivity. *Qualitative Health Research, 28*(3), 408–417. https://doi.org/10.1177/1049732317746379.

Pooley, E. A., & Beagan, B. L. (2021). The concept of oppression and occupational therapy: A critical interpretive synthesis. *Canadian Journal of Occupational Therapy, 88*(4), 407–417. https://doi.org/10.1177/00084174211051168.

Pride, T., Beagan, B. L., MacLeod, A., & Sibbald, K. (2022). Educational experiences of health professionals from marginalized groups: "It definitely takes more work". *Diaspora, Indigenous, and Minority Education, 18*(1), 51–67. https://doi.org/10.1080/15595692.2022.2149485.

Priest, N., Paradies, Y., Trenerry, B., Truong, M., Karlsen, S., & Kelly, Y. (2013). A systematic review of studies examining the relationship between reported racism and health and wellbeing for children and young people. *Social Science & Medicine, 95*, 115–127. https://doi.org/10.1016/j.socscimed.2012.11.031.

Pyke, K. D. (2010). What is internalized racial oppression and why don't we study it? Acknowledging racism's hidden injuries. *Sociological Perspectives, 53*(4), 551–572. https://doi.org/10.1525/sop.2010.53.4.551.

Ramugondo, E. L. (2015). Occupational consciousness. *Journal of Occupational Science, 22*(4), 488–501. https://doi.org/10.1080/14427591.2015.1042516.

Ramugondo, E. L. (2018). Healing work: Intersections for decoloniality. *World Federation of Occupational Therapists Bulletin, 74*(2), 83–91. https://doi.org/10.1080/14473828.2018.1523981.

Richards, L.-A., & Galvaan, R. (2018). Developing a socially transformative focus in occupational therapy: Insights from South African practice. *South African Journal of Occupational Therapy, 48*(1), 3–8. https://doi.org/10.17159/2310-3833/2017/vol48n1a2.

Ryan, A., Gilroy, J., & Gibson, C. (2020). Changethedate: Advocacy as an on-line and decolonising occupation. *Journal of Occupational Science, 27*(3), 405–416. https://doi.org/10.1080/14427591.2020.1759448.

Seet, A. Z. (2021). Serving the white nation: Bringing internalised racism within a sociological understanding. *Journal of Sociology, 57*(2), 213–230. https://doi.org/10.1177/1440783319882087.

Smith, G. H., & Smith, L. T. (2018). Doing indigenous work: Decolonizing and transforming the academy. In McKinley, E. A., & Smith, L. T. (Eds.), *Handbook of indigenous education* (pp. 1074–1101). Springer.

Smith, L. T. (2012). *Decolonizing methodologies: Research and indigenous peoples* (2nd ed.). Zed Books.

Stewart-Ambo, T., & Yang, K. W. (2021). Beyond land acknowledgment in settler institutions. *Social Text 146, 39*(1), 21–46. https://doi.org/10.1215/01642472-8750076.

Stop Institutional Racism & NZ Public Health Association. (2021). *Briefing paper on the forthcoming national action plan against racism.* STIR & NZ PHA and Auckland University of Technology.

Te Kāhui Tika Tangata Human Rights Commission. (2022). *Maranga Mai! The dynamics and impacts of white supremacy, racism, and colonisation upon tangata whenua in Aotearoa New Zealand.* Te Kāhui Tika Tangata Human Rights Commission. https://tikatangata.org.nz/our-work/maranga-mai.

Tuck, E., & Yang, K. W. (2012). Decolonization is not a metaphor. *Decolonization: Indigeneity, Education & Society, 1*(1), 1–40. https://tinyurl.com/4r4mftf6.

Turcotte, P. L., & Holmes, D. (2021). The (dis)obedient occupational therapist: A reflection on dissent against disciplinary propaganda. *Cadernos Brasileiros de Terapia Ocupacional, 29*, e2924. https://doi.org/10.1590/2526-8910.ctoARF2211.

Wijekoon, S., & Peter, N. (2022). Examining racial, ethnic, and cultural diversity in occupational science research: Perspectives of persons of color. *Journal of Occupational Science, 30*(3), 322–341. https://doi.org/10.1080/14427591.2022.2119269.

Wilkerson, I. (2020). *Caste: The lies that divide us.* Random House.

Williams, D. R., Lawrence, J. A., & Davis, B. A. (2019). Racism and health: Evidence and needed research. *Annual Review of Public Health, 40*(1), 105–125. https://doi.org/10.1146/annurev-publhealth-040218-043750.

Williams, D. R., & Mohammed, S. A. (2013). Racism and health 1: Pathways and scientific evidence. *American Behavioral Scientist, 57*(8), 1200–1226. https://doi.org/10.1177/0002764213487340.

Zafran, H. (2021). Lost in translation. *Occupational Therapy Now, 23*(6), 23–25.

REFLECTION

Developing a sense of your standpoint

Central to decolonial praxis is understanding your history, social positioning, how you benefit from or are impacted by coloniality, connections (social, geographical, spiritual) and purpose.

You are invited to explore, signal, question and present your understanding so far.

2

CRITICAL PERSPECTIVES IN OCCUPATIONAL THERAPY: PROBLEMATISING PRACTICE TO ADDRESS THE SOCIO-POLITICAL SHAPING OF OCCUPATION

LISETTE FARIAS

■ ■ ■ ■ ■ ■ ■ ■ ■ ■ ■ ■ ■ ■ ■ ■ ■

CHAPTER OUTLINE

Overview

When reading this chapter readers are encouraged to incorporate the perspectives and values underlying critical theory to question and (re)formulate professional practice. The occupational therapy profession is based on values and assumptions that shape practice, understandings of occupation, and individuals' and collectives' situated possibilities and choices. Without questioning these values and assumptions, occupational therapists risk perpetuating deficit approaches and an individualistic view that focuses on identifying and classifying impairments as personal responsibility. By adopting critical theories into practice, it is possible to envision possibilities for practices that build on individual and collective strengths and allow for fostering collaborative relationships that are socioeconomically, culturally and historically informed. The chapter starts with an introduction to critical theory

as a theoretical umbrella with common values and distinguished points of departure for practice. Then, reflections and examples of theoretical application to practice are provided to illustrate ways of altering the boundaries of student–supervisor relations, practice and institutional culture.

KEY POINTS

Critical theory can allow occupational therapists to

■ Question assumptions, values and systems that shape practice, providing a specific lens to examine the intersections between ability, age, gender, race and class.

■ Understand how sociopolitical processes can exclude or prohibit forms of occupational participation beyond individual control.

■ Develop more socially transformative and responsive practices

■ Support people's efforts of resistance and reclaiming of Indigenous, traditional and rural occupations.

■ Disrupt the expert position and traditional practitioner-client power relations.

INTRODUCTION

Increasingly in the occupational therapy and occupational science literature, authors have examined the potential of critical theory to enhance understanding of occupation, explore the ways in which knowledge is produced, and how this knowledge shapes practice (Farias & Laliberte Rudman, 2016, 2019; Gerlach et al., 2018; Laliberte Rudman, 2013; Njelesani et al., 2013). The structure of this chapter is guided by the following questions: What are the origins of critical theory? What is critical theory? What would occupational therapy practice underpinned by critical theory look like? What are the implications of using critical theory in occupational therapy practice? These questions are used to argue for the incorporation of critical theory into practice to make a difference in the way occupational therapy practice is enacted and occupation is understood. This is not to say that critical theory is sufficient as a singular base for the discipline of occupational science and the profession of occupational therapy, or that it, replaces specialised modes of practice, such as participatory and collaborative approaches. Instead, critical theory forwards situated and socially relevant understandings of occupation. Thus, critical theory is presented here to expand current ways of thinking within the occupational therapy profession to address relevant social issues.

WHAT ARE THE ORIGINS OF CRITICAL THEORY?

To present the specific features that critical theories have in common, a brief historical introduction to the emergence of this theoretical framework is necessary. The term 'critical theory' originates from a group of theorists that established the Frankfurt School (also called the Institute for Social Research) in Germany in 1923. The Frankfurt school was not a political party, but a structured programme focused on social research. The first group of exponents of the Frankfurt School included Immanuel Kant, Georg Hegel, Karl Marx,

Marx Horkheimer, Theodor Adorno, Herbert Marcuse, Friedrich Pollock, Leo Lowenthal and Walter Benjamin (Agger, 1991). Then, Habermas, and other theorists, such as Nikolas Kimpridis, Raymond Guess and Axel Honneth joined as part of the second and third generations of critical theorists. Together they argued for the problematisation of social problems as necessary to reformulate inflexible systems of social organisation, such as capitalism, and support the development of inclusive and equal societies (Crotty, 2010). Although this problematisation was in the beginning, mostly theoretical, it was framed as emerging from human needs and interests and connected to practice, avoiding the construction of 'knowledge for the sake of knowledge' (Habermas, 1968, p. 203).

The group of academics who founded the Frankfurt School often expressed their discontent with the contemporary socio-economic system of that period. The 1930s were characterised by the end of the First World War and the beginning of the Second World War. This interwar period (1918–1939) faced many significant social political, and economic changes in the world, such as the rise of communism in Russia, the great economic depression in the United States in 1929, and the rise of fascism and extreme nationalism, particularly in Italy and Germany (Wyn Jones, 2001). Fascism was supported by right-wing groups including extreme nationalists and militarists that incited threats, human rights violations, and aggression toward ethnic groups and neighbouring countries, spreading values based on male superiority, race superiority and natural hierarchy (Wyn Jones, 2001). Fascism also led to the rise of dictators, such as Benito Mussolini (1922–1943) in Italy and Adolf Hitler (1933–1945) in Germany.

During this period, the great depression greatly affected many of the world's largest economies in Europe and Latin America and lasted until the beginning of the Second World War. This economic crisis resulted in distrust in democracy, leading to its collapse and the rise of antidemocratic regimes in Europe and several countries in Latin America.

The societal changes of the interwar period (1918–1939) shaped the development of the critical theory of the Frankfurt School, probably in part as a reaction to the social and political regimes that increased violence and polarisation within Europe and other regions. Critical theory used theory as 'an act of imagining and it is through theory that we hope, see, think, and know' (Wilson-Thomas, 1995, p. 574). As such, critical theory provides a forum in which academics from the Frankfurt school could develop social critique, visualise a better world, and try to find alternative ways of thinking and acting that would support societies in reconnecting with humanity, peace and equity.

WHAT IS CRITICAL THEORY?

Critical theory is a theoretical umbrella that comprises numerous theoretical critical perspectives that share common features (e.g. Marxism, work from the Frankfurt School, decolonialism, radical feminism, queer theory and others). Some of these features are that critical theory:

1. Aims to generate knowledge that is far from being neutral and objective.
2. This means that knowledge is seen as partial and situated within specific socio-political and historical conditions.
3. Acknowledges power relationships as embedded in societal structures and shaping society.
4. This implies that critical theorists recognise the existence of power imbalances that create and perpetuate domination and oppression as being outside the individual's control. For example, poverty is often attributed to those affected by poverty as supposing that they lack the willingness to work or that they make bad decisions, instead of looking at the social structures that create systemic disadvantages, such as inequitable access to education, unemployment and housing.
5. Seeks to liberate/emancipate individuals and groups from unconscious and conscious constraints that hinder their social participation.
6. This is based on an understanding that power imbalances lead to domination and oppression and that this relationship becomes normalised and accepted as 'the way things are' (Agger, 1991). For a person to reveal their understanding of power imbalances, unquestioned and accepted assumptions need to be examined, such as who constructs and maintains barriers to social participation, and whose interests are

served by the social structures (Wilson-Thomas, 1995). For instance, becoming aware of how society constrains a disabled person's possibilities to engage in occupations as a 'person in need of support' can be liberating as it allows the person to realise that the source of the problem lies in how society perpetuates the idea that disability/disabled is intrinsic to the person, instead of being created by social arrangements that can be transformed (Farias, 2020).

REFLEXIVE QUESTION

Have you reflected on your assumptions about dependence/independence?

From a critical perspective, occupational therapy can be seen as a profession that maintains power imbalances since it is based on societal assumptions about *disability, autonomy, and independence*, which tend to categorise people as 'dependent versus independent', thereby serving the categorisation of people in disempowering groups. This categorisation can create unconscious constraints for those categorised as 'dependent' since it will be assumed that they need to receive support to participate in society instead of changing society to fit the needs of all people.

7. Assumes that a critique of power imbalances and taken-for-granted assumptions can reformulate dominant perspectives and practices that perpetuate privilege and disadvantages.

A commitment to questioning power imbalances and what seems to be 'the way things are', is a key element shared among the theories included in the critical theory umbrella (Cannella & Lincoln, 2009). Hence, critical theory aims to expose, address and transform practices that perpetuate social inequality by challenging the assumptions and values supporting these practices (Farias et al., 2016). As an example, Hammell (2009) has criticised what she calls occupational therapy's 'sacred texts', that is, underpinning assumptions about occupation that have become taken for granted as universal. One of these assumptions is the categorisation of occupation into self-care, productivity and leisure which overlooks occupations that do not fit these (Western) culturally specific and class-bound categories (e.g. praying or meditation, artistic expressions of resistance, such as protests, and rites of passage). Moreover, these assumptions have been developed in urban areas of English-speaking countries located in the Western countries that constitute only 17% of the population, that is, the minority of the world (Hammell, 2009).

REFLEXIVE QUESTIONS

Have you reflected on your assumptions about the term disability?

What do you think about the term disability?

How is your view informed by what is portrayed in commercials, propaganda, TV shows, and other social media in your local context?

How do you think that your view on the term disability is shaped by your context?

Can you come up with occupations that may be performed in your local context that are not possible to categorise into self-care, productivity and leisure?

Although the above-mentioned points are shared assumptions across the theories included in the critical theory umbrella, it is important to highlight the diversity and growing development of this group of theories that adds to its richness and pluralistic nature. This diversity may entail some difficulties when a person is trying to orient themselves for the first time. A suggestion would be for the person to ask themselves which aspects of power imbalances or dominant-oppression relationships they are interested in examining or seeing as important to consider in their practice. A few examples of critical theories that illustrate their diverse focus and scope are included in Table 2.1. An example of using a feminist perspective to consider occupational balance is provided in Box 2.1.

WHAT WOULD OCCUPATIONAL THERAPY PRACTICE UNDERPINNED BY CRITICAL THEORY LOOK LIKE?

Engaging with critical theory allows occupational therapists to critically examine the assumptions and values that underpin their practices, the systems via which their practices occur, and the broader socio-historical, economic and cultural conditions that shape people's opportunities for occupational participation (Farias & Aldrich, 2021). Critical theory also offers theoretical lenses (Table 2.1) that expand the notion of context beyond the local situation and immediate physical environment by including the socio-historical and cultural conditions that shape practice (Ramugondo, 2018). Consistent with this focus, critical theory can expose the intersections of ability/disability with race, gender, age and other identities that place occupational therapy practice, if holistic, into the realm of the social. But if practice is considered as embedded within socio-economic and historical events, what would practice look like? The following examples illustrate that the application of critical theories in diverse aspects of practice is not only beneficial to question practice but also to reveal issues of importance that can guide changes and actions to address these issues in practice.

Example 1: Revealing Occupational Therapy Supervisors' Hidden Expectations

Based on ongoing discussions about decolonisation of practice through infusing non-Western ideas into occupational therapy education (e.g. Mahoney & Kiraly-Alvarez, 2019), Farias and colleagues (2023) present their reflections on decolonising of fieldwork based on qualitative interviews with supervisors receiving international occupational therapy students in Sweden. Using decolonial theory (DiAngelo, 2018; Mignolo, 2011, 2017; Quijano, 2007), they examine tensions that emerged in fieldwork among supervisors' expectations, students' values, and sociocultural situations. For instance, they highlight that Western supervisors tend to use a deficit model to understand international students learning and behaviours, comparing them to domestic students that share the same cultural values and understanding of power as their supervisors (i.e. egalitarian in the Swedish context).

[Some students expect from me] that I will be sharp, decide, it is me who decides. For some, they think I will judge them [...] But if the student has a 10-year habit of the teacher deciding, the student will not question anything more. So, they come here, and I ask, 'What do you think'? It will be different. What

TABLE 2.1
Examples of Critical Theories

Critical Theory	Feminist Theory	Critical Race Theory	Decolonial(ism) Theory
Shared goal	Examine power relations sustained by social structures to support the liberation/emancipation of the oppressed, reformulation of practices and social transformation		
Focus on	■ Understands knowledge as situated, that is, as embedded in time, context, and the social positioning of individuals ■ Challenges the universal nature of women's experiences and how these are socially created as different from men's experiences (roles, opportunities, social expectations) (Young, 1990) ■ Argues for gender equality between men and women and among women by including an examination of race and class (Hooks, 1984)	■ Understands race as socially and historically constructed ■ Challenges the positioning of whiteness as the norm and the categorisation of others in relation to this norm (Moreton-Robinson, 2000) ■ Whiteness is defined as the dominant way of seeing the world in Western culture (Moreton-Robinson, 2000) ■ Seeks to deconstruct the (un)conscious oppressive ways of thinking that limit opportunities for Black and Indigenous people (Ladson-Billings, 1999) ■ Challenges the advantaged position of the white person to empower those classified as others (Ladson-Billings, 1999)	■ Argues that because of coloniality and European domination from the 16th century, the world was divided into two groups: superior-inferior, primitive-modernised/civilised, and traditional-modern/enlightened ■ Such classifications have organised social relations through a hierarchy of groups, keeping domination as the norm (Mignolo, 2017; Quijano, 1999) ■ Seeks to resist the patterns of power that shape power relations and disrupt them to reclaim pluriverse knowledge
Examples from occupational therapy literature	Gilligan, 1976; Hamlin, 1992; Hammell, 2006; Hammell, 2011; Kelly, 1996; Miller, 1992; Morrison, 2016; Pierce & Frank, 1992; Pollard & Walsh, 2000; Primeau, 1992; Taylor, 1995	Beagan et al., 2022; Grenier, 2020; Kitchens et al., 2022; Lerner & Kim, 2022; Nelson, 2007; Owens, 2017; Ramugondo, 2000; Sterman & Njelesani, 2021; Sterman et al., 2022	Córdoba, 2020; Emery-Whittington, 2021; Galvaan et al., 2022; Hendricks et al., 2023; Ramugondo, 2018; Ramugondo & Emery-Whittington, 2022; Ramugondo, 2015; Silva et al., 2022
Reflexive questions	What are the roles and activities that are promoted as ideal for women and men in occupational therapy? Are they equal/unequal to some degree?	What are the dominant ways of doing and being that are promoted in your occupational therapy education and fieldwork? Are there ways of being and doing that are excluded?	What do you know about the process of colonisation and decolonisation? How diverse are the texts and cases that are promoted in your education?

kind of culture do they have behind them? Some students will have to turn around the fact that they have never been allowed to question [someone/something].

(Farias et al., 2023, p. 274)

Neglecting the existence of power imbalances between students and supervisors risks obscuring the fact that some students may need to feel safe by trusting the supervisors' higher expertise as a safety net that can 'catch' their potential mistakes in practice. It is also relevant that supervisors consider students' needs concerning power dynamics and reflect on the power that is attributed to them and use it in ways that acknowledge students' beliefs and values. For instance, there was an occasion in which a supervisor expressed an implicit desire to teach international students about the LGBTQ community in the Swedish context without taking into consideration students' previous experiences or beliefs.

BOX 2.1
AN EXAMPLE OF INTERPRETING OCCUPATIONAL BALANCE FROM A FEMINIST PERSPECTIVE

The representation of a 'good' mother and a father prevalent in social media, policy and social norms, shapes parents' choices and involvement in gendered occupations in ways that differently impact their well-being and balance (Berger et al., 2020). For example, Uthede and colleagues (2023) analysed the answers of working parents in Sweden with at least one child under seven years of age by using the Occupational Balance Questionnaire (OBQ11). The authors chose to focus on parents of young children (≤8 years old) since this group has a higher risk of sick leave and poor perceived health compared with parents of older children and adults without children in Sweden (Borgh et al., 2018). The results of this study show that caring for preschool children can negatively impact both parents' occupational balance, yet significant differences indicate that mothers experience a lower occupational balance than fathers. These differences were interpreted as mothers having conflicts between their expected roles and gender ideologies[1] that includes both caring for children and pursuing a career, regardless of their personal or household gender ideology. As such, working mothers may be confronted with highly diverse (i.e. personal, partner's and societal), and controversial expectations and attitudes concerning their doing and being as a mother, which can lead to low occupational balance.

Using a feminist perspective (i.e. including an understanding of the impact of gender ideologies on how people engage in occupations) and the findings from the OBQ11, occupational therapy interventions could be used to raise awareness about the importance of occupational balance for mothers, including reflections on their personal and societal values to examine if their doing is (in)congruent with what they would like to do, are expected to do or feel that they must do based on individual, institutional and interactional gender ideologies. According to Uthede and colleagues (2023), gender ideologies shape parental attitudes related to domestic, paid occupations, role expectations, and therefore parents' engagement and the degree of their participation in certain occupations.

---

[1]Gender ideology shape occupations at three levels: individual, institutional, and interactional. At the individual level, understanding and internalising gender ideology through socialisation, people develop their identity as a woman or a man. At the institutional level, gender ideology shared in a social and cultural context constructs gender norms and informs social resources that assist people in living in a manner that accommodates to those norms. Interactions between individuals and expectations from others also construct and structure gender (Wada et al., 2010)

This was a student with a completely different background, who had never been abroad before and probably never seen a naked woman before [...] or being in contact with LGBTQ clients. He [the student] was shocked. It was like telling him it is ok to be a paedophile almost.

(Farias et al., 2023, p. 273)

This desire for 'teaching' the international students about the Swedish context as 'superior', may position supervisors as 'saviours' by using their power to 'rescue' students, in this case, from homophobic or traditional social values. The underlying beliefs connected to the saviour or hero complex are expressed in supervisors' comments that value Swedish social norms as potentially more developed than that of students' countries of origin. In this case, even when unconsciously or well-intended, supervisors can benefit from

applying a decolonising lens to fieldwork to open up a dialogue with students about learning expectations and reflect together on how these expectations mirror their socio-historical context. Disrupting supervisors' expectations and desires for students' learning is key to critically reflect on education and deliberatively resisting the hierarchical order upheld through supervisor-student relationships.

Example 2: Raising Awareness of Assumptions Limiting Occupational Therapy Practice

Farias and colleagues (2016, 2019) draw upon critical theory to question the type of knowledge and values underpinning occupational therapy practice to engage with approaches that can support an understanding of the socio-political shaping of occupational injustices. Specifically, they use Freire's dialogical action theory

(1970) based on the concepts of conscientisation[1] and dialogue to engage in the problematisation of practice that intends to work towards social transformation. Freire was a Brazilian critical theorist and adult educator who launched literacy programmes among peasant people in the 1960s. He viewed dialogue as a means to engage with processes that seek to (re)invent knowledge, rather than only as a way to exchange ideas (Farias & Aldrich, 2021).

> *Dialogue is a moment where humans meet to reflect on their reality as they make and remake it. To the extent that we are communicative beings who communicate to each other as we become more able to transform our reality, we are able to know that we know, which is something more than just knowing. [...] Through dialogue, reflecting together on what we know and don't know, we can then act critically to transform reality.*
>
> *(Shor & Freire, 1987, p. 13)*

Based on this understanding of dialogue, Farias and Laliberte Rudman invited five occupational therapists to reflect on their practice through 'dialogue which in turn can give rise to (new) knowledge about power relations and socio-political conditions specific to the problems people are facing, including actions for improving their situation' (Farias et al., 2019, p. 235). This process entailed having in-depth rounds of dialogical sessions with each of the practitioners, followed by sharing the transcripts of those sessions attached to the critical reflections of the person with whom they had the dialogue. This was done to ensure transparency and democratisation of the process and avoid a unidirectional dialogue. From this perspective, the dialogue was taken up in ways that would enable raising awareness (also known as conscientisation[2]) regarding the frames for action used in these practices. Resulting from this dialogue was an awareness of the power of individualisation in practices aimed to embrace more

collective understandings of occupation. As described by one practitioner:

> *Many people said social change—well, in many cases it's remained very individualistic. It can start from an individual person, of course, that's no problem, but [what we do as occupational therapists] has remained so near what we have [done so far].*
>
> *(Farias & Laliberte Rudman, 2019, p. 247)*

Drawing on critical theory to question practice, occupational therapists described how this individualistic tendency neglects ways in which people's social and physical environments support harmful occupations. Another practitioner described this happening in a project trying to promote social transformation:

> *This was about women who drink a lot—they described very well how that comes, from history and structures, and then what they do is, well, we teach people not to drink and to do occupations. But that is still not focusing also on the structures. So then they are still in this environment [that] is forcing them more or less to drink.*
>
> *(Farias & Laliberte Rudman, 2019, p. 247)*

By challenging the values underpinning practices that aim to support people's efforts for resistance or social change, occupational therapists can realise how their practices, although well-intentioned, risk perpetuating an individualistic focus. In doing so, practices will link social problems to personal responsibility (i.e. people's behaviours and lifestyle as personal choices) instead of looking at the socio-political shaping of occupations. Problematising these tendencies is essential for promoting practices that enact action addressing the socio-political, historical and cultural situatedness of occupations. In this case, critical theories were used to problematise and reveal the challenges that occupational therapists face when resisting to frame social problems, such as alcoholism or unemployment, as individual problems.

Example 3: Shifting Power Dynamics at a Nursing Home

Mondaca and colleagues (2018, 2019) explored the possibilities for older adults to influence and engage in

---

[1]Freire believed that marginalisation of a certain group in society is made through establishing a *culture of silence* by those in power with the aim of oppression and is perpetuated by the absence of reflective participation by those who are disempowered (Freire, 1970). Thus, to break this culture, he argued that people need to be empowered through *conscientisation*, that is, encouraging individuals to transform their reality through dialogue, reflection, and action.

available occupations in a nursing home. The limited possibilities to influence occupations were associated with stereotyped views of older adults' interests and preferences. By drawing on critical theory, Mondaca and colleagues' work shifted the view of adults as passive recipients to resourceful, challenging individualistic views of engagement and proposing doing as a collective and democratic process. The nursing home in which this project was based, had a weekly group activity scheduled in which the residents would gather together for two hours to participate in singing and playing bingo or memory games. Other activities were gymnastics, reading newspapers, or watching TV, but these were lacking the active influence of older adults living in this residence. Besides these group activities, the setting was generally lacking opportunities for the older adults to decide on what type of activities and how they would like to be involved. To shift the power dynamics and ways that older people were viewed in the nursing home, Mondaca and colleagues, draw on critical theorist Bhabha's concept of third space (1994) which originally emerged in postcolonial research to enact collaboration, contestation and negotiation. Bhabba is an Indian-British scholar and critical theorist who proposes the third space as an in-between space that allows for rethinking culture as (re)negotiated through doing and interactions, deconstructing hierarchy, and allowing for ambiguity and uncertainty. He places the third space as an in-between space beyond the past and the present and as an innovative act of conversation and negotiation:

> *Such act does not merely recall the past as social cause or aesthetic precedent; it renews the past, refiguring it as a contingent 'in-between' space, that innovates and interrupts the performance of the present. The past-present becomes part of necessity, not the nostalgia, of living.*
>
> **(Bhabba, 1994, p. 7)**

The third space in Mondaca and colleagues' work (2018, 2019) is defined as a co-created practice outside the regular culture of the nursing home. Using this concept to create a (new) practice, a book club was formed to grant access to situations where the residents could have an active space within the institutional culture for having their voices, interests, and preferences heard. The book club meetings were held in the residents' rooms so that they could communicate without interference from staff. This was key for the group to prompt resistance and an opening for new ways of doing that were not established in the institutional culture, as stated by one older adult:

> *'But are you sure we can invite people to our flats?' Yes, I am sure, replied the first author. 'Well I think you need to check with the staff if it is possible anyway, I am not sure we can!' was her reaction. Another resident participating in this conversation added: 'It will be better if you ask if it is possible', agreeing with this hesitation.*
>
> **(Mondaca et al., 2019, p. 444)**

The idea of co-creating an occupation such as the book club that resisted following and perpetuating institutional culture was not only new for the residents but also challenging since their power and position within the institution were being shifted. Mondaca and colleagues (2018, 2019) also describe how the book club provided a (new) sense of familiarity, fellowship and connectedness to the residents that were interpreted as altering the boundaries of the institutional routines and occupations available to them. In contrast to occupations that were available at the nursing home, the book club was specifically formed to fulfil the needs and interests of the residents of a nursing home, providing an occupation in which older adults could participate, co-create and feel connected with others based on their capacities.

WHAT ARE THE IMPLICATIONS OF USING CRITICAL THEORY IN OCCUPATIONAL THERAPY PRACTICE?

Critical theory is a group of theories that aim to mobilise work towards equity and social transformation. Integrating critical theory into practice can help occupational therapists to ensure that research, education and practices are developed in line with understandings of occupation that do not seek to unify or impose a definition of occupation. Yet, critical theory can support openness to diverse worldviews and resisting dominant views that present occupation as representing the interest of only a few groups. By challenging dominant views of occupation, practitioners can avoid enacting colonial agendas that maintain the dominant social order.

Occupational therapy practices that are based on the values and assumptions underlying critical theory can foster (new) conceptualisations of occupation that emerge in practice in diverse contexts. This type of practice understands occupation as shaped by sociopolitical and economic conditions and not as a product of individual choice. This practice is also open to supporting occupations of resistance, that aim to alter or disturb social norms and challenge the categorisation of occupations that neglect ways of living that exist within contexts outside the Western, Anglophone dominant regions. Ultimately, critical theory can support the development and enactment of relevant and socially responsive actions, practices and encounters among occupational therapists and people in diverse settings.

REFERENCES

Agger, B. (1991). Critical theory, poststructuralism, postmodernism: Their sociological relevance. *Annual Review of Sociology, 17*, 105–131. http://www.jstor.org/stable/2083337.

Beagan, B. L., Sibbald, K. R., Bizzeth, S. R., & Pride, T. M. (2022). Systemic racism in Canadian occupational therapy: A qualitative study with therapists. *Canadian Journal of Occupational Therapy, 89*(1), 51–61. https://doi.org/10.1177/00084174211066676.

Berger, M., Asaba, E., Fallahpour, M., & Farias, L. (2020). The sociocultural shaping of mothers' doing, being, becoming and belonging after returning to work. *Journal of Occupational Science, 29*(1), 7–20. https://doi.org/10.1080/14427591.2020.1845226.

Bhabha, H. (1994). *The location of culture*. Routledge.

Borgh, M., Eek, F., Wagman, P., & Håkansson, C. (2018). Organisational factors and occupational balance in working parents in Sweden. *Scandinavian Journal of Public Health, 46*(3), 409–416. https://doi.org/10.1177/1403494817713650.

Cannella, G. S., & Lincoln, Y. S. (2009). Qualitative inquiry and social justice: Toward a politics of hope. In N. K. Denzin, & M. D. Giardina (Eds.), *Deploying qualitative methods for critical social purposes* (pp. 53–72). Left Coast Press, Inc.

Córdoba, A. G. (2020). About new forms of colonization in occupational therapy. Reflections on the Idea of Occupational Justice from a critical-political philosophy perspective. *Cadernos Brasileiros de Terapia Ocupacional, 28*(2869), 1365–1381. https://doi.org/10.4322/2526-8910.ctoarf2175.

Crotty, M. (2010). *The foundations of social research. Meaning and perspective in the research process*. Allen & Unwin.

DiAngelo, R. J. (2018). *White fragility: Why it's so hard for white people to talk about racism*. Beacon Press.

Emery-Whittington, I. G. (2021). Occupational justice – Colonial business as usual? Indigenous observations from Aotearoa New Zealand. *Canadian Journal of Occupational Therapy, 88*(2), 153–162. https://doi.org/10.1177/00084174211005891.

Farias, L. (2020). The (mis)shaping of health: Problematizing neoliberal discourses of individualism and responsibility. In H. Hosseini, J. Goodman, S. C. Motta, & B. K. Gills (Eds.), *The Routledge handbook of transformative global studies* (pp. 268–281). Routledge.

Farias, L., & Aldrich, R. (2021). Critical theory: Resources for questioning and transforming everyday life. In S. Taff (Ed.), *Philosophy and occupational therapy: Informing education, research, and practice* (pp. 155–162). Slack.

Farias, L., Brodin, H., & Bergström, A. (2023). Supervisors of international occupational therapy students on clinical placement: Perceived tensions and hidden expectations. *Scandinavian Journal of Educational Research, 67*(2), 268–280. https://doi.org/10.1080/00313831.2021.2006304.

Farias, L., & Laliberte Rudman, D. (2016). A critical interpretive synthesis of the uptake of critical perspectives in occupational science. *Journal of Occupational Science, 23*(1), 33–50. https://doi.org/10.1080/14427591.2014.989893.

Farias, L., & Laliberte Rudman, D. (2019). Practice analysis: Critical reflexivity on discourses constraining socially transformative occupational therapy practices. *British Journal of Occupational Therapy, 82*(11), 693–697. https://doi.org/10.1177/0308022619862111.

Farias, L., Laliberte Rudman, D., & Magalhães, L. (2016). Illustrating the importance of critical epistemology to realize the promise of occupational justice. *OTJR: Occupation, Participation and Health, 36*(4), 234–243. https://doi.org/10.1177/1539449216665561.

Freire, P. (1970). *Pedagogy of the oppressed*. Seabury Press.

Galvaan, R., Peters, L., Richards, L. A., Francke, M., & Krenzer, M. (2022). Pedagogies within occupational therapy curriculum: Centering a decolonial praxis in community development practice. *Cadernos Brasileiros de Terapia Ocupacional, 30*. https://doi.org/10.1590/2526-8910.ctoAO24023133.

Gerlach, A., Teachman, G., Laliberte-Rudman, D., Aldrich, R. M., & Huot, S. (2018). Expanding beyond individualism: Engaging critical perspectives on occupation. *Scandinavian Journal of Occupational Therapy, 25*(1), 35–43. https://doi.org/10.1080/11038128.2017.1327616.

Gilligan, M. B. (1976). Developmental stages of occupational therapy and the feminist movement. *American Journal of Occupational Therapy, 30*, 560–567.

Grenier, M.-L. (2020). Cultural competency and the reproduction of white supremacy in occupational therapy education. *Health Education Journal, 79*(6), 633–644. https://doi.org/10.1177/0017896920902515.

Habermas, J. (1968). *Knowledge and human interests (J. J. Shapiro, Trans.)*. Beacon Press.

Hamlin, R. B. (1992). Embracing our past, informing our future: A feminist re-vision of health care. *The American Journal of Occupational Therapy, 46*(11), 1028–1035. https://doi.org/10.5014/ajot.46.11.1028.

Hammell, K. W. (2006). *Perspectives on disability and rehabilitation. Contesting assumptions; Challenging practice*. Churchill Livingstone Elsevier.

Hammell, K. W. (2009). Sacred texts: A sceptical exploration of the assumptions underpinning theories of occupation. *Canadian Journal of Occupational Therapy, 76*(1), 6–22. https://doi.org/10.1177/000841740907600105.

Hammell, K. W. (2011). Resisting theoretical imperialism in the disciplines of occupational science and occupational therapy. *British Journal of Occupational Therapy, 74*(1), 27–33. https://doi.org/10.4276/030802211X12947686093602.

Hendricks, F., Singleton, M., Clark, A., Mishin, M., & Epps, M. (2023). A narrative review of student evaluations of teaching in decolonial praxis: Implications for occupational therapy higher education. *The Open Journal of Occupational Therapy, 11*(1), 1–16. https://doi.org/10.15453/2168-6408.1969.

Hooks, B. (1984). *Feminist theory: From margin to center.* (First) Boston, MA: South End Press.

Kelly, G. (1996). Feminist or feminine? The feminine principle in occupational therapy. *British Journal of Occupational Therapy, 59*(1), 2–6. https://doi.org/10.1177/030802269605900102.

Kitchens, R. F., Armstead, A. B., Mani, K., Ghulmi, L., & Collins, D. M. (2022). Exploring the experiences of Black/African American students in entry level occupational therapy and occupational therapy assistant programs: A survey study. *Journal of Occupational Therapy Education, 6*(11236), 2–16. https://doi.org/10.26681/jote.2022.060202.

Ladson-Billings, G. (1999). Just what is critical race theory, and what's it doing in a nice field like education? In L. Parker, D. Deyhle, & S. Villenas (Eds.), *Race is—Race isn't: Critical race theory and qualitative studies in education* (pp. 7–30). Westview Press.

Laliberte Rudman, D. (2013). Enacting the critical potential of occupational science: Problematizing the 'individualizing of occupation. *Journal of Occupational Science, 20*(4), 298–313. https://doi.org/10.1080/14427591.2013.803434.

Lerner, J. E., & Kim, A. (2022). Developing an anti-racist practice in occupational therapy: Guidance for the occupational therapist. *The Open Journal of Occupational Therapy, 10*(4), 1–13. https://doi.org/10.15453/2168-6408.1934.

Mahoney, W. J., & Kiraly-Alvarez, A. F. (2019). Challenging the status quo: Infusing non-western ideas into occupational therapy education and practice. *The Open Journal of Occupational Therapy, 7*(3), 1–10. https://doi.org/10.15453/2168-6408.1592.

Mignolo, W. D. (2011). *The darker side of Western modernity: Global futures, decolonial options.* Duke University Press. https://doi.org/10.2307/j.ctv125jqbw.

Mignolo, W. D. (2017). Coloniality is far from over, and so must be decoloniality. *Afterall: A Journal of Art, Context, and Enquiry, 43,* 38–45. https://doi.org/10.1086/692552.

Miller, R. J. (1992). Interwoven threads: Occupational therapy, feminism, and holistic health. *The American Journal of Occupational Therapy, 46*(11), 1013–1019. https://doi.org/10.5014/ajot.46.11.1013.

Mondaca, M., Josephsson, S., Borell, L., Katz, A., & Rosenberg, L. (2019). Altering the boundaries of everyday life in a nursing home context. *Scandinavian Journal of Occupational Therapy, 26*(6), 441–451. https://doi.org/10.1080/11038128.2018.1483426.

Mondaca, M., Josephsson, S., Katz, A., & Rosenberg, L. (2018). Influencing everyday activities in a nursing home setting: A call for ethical and responsive engagement. *Nursing Inquiry, 25*(2), e12217. https://doi.org/10.1111/nin.12217.

Moreton-Robinson, A. (2000). *Talkin' up to the white woman. Aboriginal women and feminism.* University of Queensland Press.

Morrison, R. (2016). Pragmatist epistemology and Jane Addams: Fundamental concepts for the social paradigm of occupational therapy. *Occupational Therapy International, 23*(4), 295–304. https://doi.org/10.1002/oti.1430.

Nelson, A. (2007). Seeing white: A critical exploration of occupational therapy with Indigenous Australian people. *Occupational Therapy International, 14*(4), 237–255. https://doi.org/10.1002/oti.236.

Njelesani, J., Gibson, B. E., Nixon, S., Cameron, D., & Polatajko, H. J. (2013). Towards a critical occupational approach to research. *International Journal of Qualitative Methods, 12*(1), 207–220. https://doi.org/10.1177/160940691301200109.

Owens, L. (2017). Our professional existence is political: Critical reflections on 'seeing white' in occupational therapy. In D. Sakellariou & N. Pollard (Eds.), *Occupational therapies without borders: Integrating justice with practice* (2nd ed.). Elsevier.

Pierce, D., & Frank, G. (1992). A mother's work: Two levels of feminist analysis of family-centered care. *The American Journal of Occupational Therapy, 46*(11), 972–980. https://doi.org/10.5014/ajot.46.11.972.

Pollard, N., & Walsh, S. (2000). Occupational therapy, gender and mental health: An inclusive perspective? *The British Journal of Occupational Therapy, 63*(9), 425–431. https://doi.org/10.1177/030802260006300904.

Primeau, L. A. (1992). A woman's place: Unpaid work in the home. *The American Journal of Occupational Therapy, 46*(11), 981–988. https://doi.org/10.5014/ajot.46.11.981.

Quijano, A. (1999). Colonialidad del poder, cultura y conocimiento en America Latina. *Dispositio, 24*(51), 137–148. http://www.jstor.org/stable/41491587.

Quijano, A. (2007). Coloniality and modernity/rationality. *Cultural Studies, 21*(2–3), 168–178. https://doi.org/10.1080/09502380601164353.

Ramugondo, E. (2000). *The experience of being an occupational therapy student with an underrepresented ethnic and cultural background* [University of Cape Town]. OpenUCT. http://hdl.handle.net/11427/3455.

Ramugondo, E. (2018). Healing work: Intersections for decoloniality. *World Federation of Occupational Therapists Bulletin, 74*(2), 83–91. https://doi.org/10.1080/14473828.2018.1523981.

Ramugondo, E. L. (2015). Occupational consciousness. *Journal of Occupational Science, 22*(4), 488–501. https://doi.org/10.1080/14427591.2015.1042516.

Ramugondo, E., & Emery-Whittington, I. (2022). A decolonising approach to health promotion. In S. Kessi (Ed.), *Decolonial enactments in community psychology* (pp. 191–211). Springer Nature https://doi.org/10.1007/978-3-030-75201-9_10.

Shor, I., & Freire, P. (1987). What is the 'dialogical method' of teaching? *Journal of Education, 169*(3), 11–31. https://doi.org/10.1177/002205748716900303.

Silva, R. S., Elesbão, K. F., Chagas, M.d., & Almeida, D. E. (2022). Feminismo decolonial e terapia ocupacional: Relato de experiência de um estágio curricular no contexto da pandemia. *Cadernos*

Brasileiros de Terapia Ocupacional, 30(530), 1–11. https://doi.org/10.1590/2526-8910.ctore250532781.

Sterman, J., & Njelesani, J. (2021). Becoming anti-racist occupational therapy practitioners: A scoping study. *OTJR: Occupational Therapy Journal of Research, 41*(4), 232–242. https://doi.org/10.1177/15394492211019931.

Sterman, J., Njelesani, J., & Carr, S. (2022). Anti-racism and occupational therapy education: Beyond diversity and inclusion. *Journal of Occupational Therapy Education, 6*(11236), 2–22. https://doi.org/10.26681/jote.2022.060103.

Taylor, J. (1995). A different voice in occupational therapy. *British Journal of Occupational Therapy, 58*(4), 170–174. https://doi.org/10.1177/030802269505800409.

Uthede, S., Nilsson, I., Wagman, P., Håkansson, C., & Farias, L. (2023). Occupational balance in parents of pre-school children: Potential differences between mothers and fathers. *Scandinavian Journal of Occupational Therapy, 30*(8), 1119–1208. https://doi.org/10.1080/11038128.2022.2046154.

Wada, M., Backman, C. L., & Forwell, S. J. (2010). Theoretical perspectives of balance and the influence of gender ideologies. *Journal of Occupational Science, 17*(2), 92–103. https://doi.org/10.1080/14427591.2010.9686680.

Wilson-Thomas, L. (1995). Applying critical social theory in nursing education to bridge the gap between theory, research and practice. *Journal of Advance Nursing, 21*(3), 568–575. https://doi.org/10.1111/j.1365-2648.1995.tb02742.x.

Wyn Jones, R. (2001). *Critical theory and world politics.* Lynne Rienner.

Young, I. M. (1990). *Justice and the politics of difference.* University Press.

3

A POLITICAL PROJECT FOR OCCUPATIONAL THERAPISTS

VAGNER DOS SANTOS

Overview

The chapter defines the central issue related to the exclusion and exploitation of human life – namely, moral and political inequalities. The prominence of moral and political inequalities becomes evident in understanding that not all lives are treated equitably. These inequalities are intricately tied to the ethics of life and the attributed meaning of life. Historical and current examples of moral and political inequalities and their connection with the profession are presented to support occupational therapists in generating social and cognitive critiques of society. Occupational therapists are encouraged to reconsider their own perspectives on politics and, consequently, life and generate critiques of society. Addressing and reducing moral and political inequalities is at the forefront of the occupational therapy political project.

KEY POINTS

- Political projects regulate and assign meaning and value to human life.

- The meaning and value of human life underpin governance frameworks and the implementation of political ideas in interventions.

- The prominence of moral and political inequalities means that not all lives are treated equitably.

- Understanding and reducing moral and political inequalities are fundamental to and should take a central role in the occupational therapy political project.

- Occupational therapists should assess what needs to change in society and critically reflect on what they need to modify in their own perspectives and understanding of life.

INTRODUCTION

The idea of a 'political project', mentioned in the chapter title, does not refer to a clear set of actions required to become a politically engaged occupational therapist or a prescription of what to do. This chapter does not aim to educate, inform, or provide guidance on how to vote, what democracy is or its diverse arrangements in Western society, how political parties operate, or how legislative measures are implemented. It is a more ambiguous and ambitious resource to support occupational therapists in producing critiques, an invitation to engage with social and cognitive critiques of society. The former refers to our commitment to changing the world, and the latter refers to the task of changing the way we understand the world.

> *Rather than a metaphysics of alterity, what is at stake is a physics of inequality – as is attested by the fact that the biological and biographical dimensions are tightly bound in forms of life, and that ethics of life cannot be thought independently of politics of life.*
>
> *(Didier Fassin, 2018)*

As indicated in the quote, politics is integral to human existence and experiences (Fassin, 2010, 2018). Similarly, a profession, such as occupational therapy, invokes a political project that encompasses a clear understanding of governance frameworks, power interventions, as well as the assignment of meaning and values to human life. This political project influences professional theories, education and practices.

Politics refers to the characteristics of governance and their associated bureaucracies, regulating and attributing meaning and value to human life (Unger, 1987). Politics are articulated into ideas, ideologies, policies and practices (Unger, 1997). Over time, enacting political decisions and actions inevitably produces certain forms of inequalities (Fassin, 2010, 2018). Within politically shaped structures, diverse forms of disparities are intricately tied to how power is allocated through governance to various groups, as well as the subsequent utilisation of that power. This is further intertwined with the meaning and values of human life that underpin those frameworks of governance of populations and the implementation of political ideas into political interventions. These politically associated inequalities should be at the core of what occupational therapists need to understand and change. Inequalities ultimately result from a process of producing exclusion and exploitation of human lives. This is not new or related to only one society – examples can be found throughout history and across regions. Within this chapter, examples to understand the precarious circumstances in which lives existed both centuries ago and today will be used.

The Value of Life Framing Politics

Understanding and reducing inequalities are core elements of producing social and cognitive critiques of society. A person might not declare or be aware of it, but their life actions, including professional decisions, are politically influenced; this political influence aims to regulate and attribute meaning and value to human life – beyond codes of conduct. This political influence refers to an ethics of life which corresponds with the meaning attributed to life. The ethics of life, then, is brought to the heart of the political discussion. The ethics of life is a necessary element to consider when critiquing the nature of inequalities in postcolonial and Western societies where occupational therapy education and services are mostly present. Thus, this chapter invites occupational therapists to examine what they need to change in society as much as what they need to change in their own views and understanding of life.

The political dimension of life compels occupational therapists to transcend taken-for-granted assumptions and dynamics. It requires occupational therapists to unveil the intricate political nuances permeating human biological existence and biographical experiences. Biological existence refers to the physical body and its anatomical structures and physiological cycles, while the biographical experience refers to the events that shape each person's life history. Biological existence and the biographical experience are intertwined and connected, and the inequalities of life will influence both biological existence and biographical experience. While this argument may appear simplistic, it holds a degree of complexity in its relevance to occupational therapy theory, education and practice, as illustrated in the following two examples. The examples highlight the governance of populations and how value is attributed to life. Governance and personal dimensions relate to understanding how inequalities shape the way that human life is conceptualised, regulated, and, consequently, experienced.

Example 1: Sweden's reduction of mortality rates during the early 19th century was propelled by a political governance framework known as 'peace, vaccine and potatoes'. This Swedish framework aimed to protect human life in the Swedish territory by adopting an approach that prioritised access to food, embraced scientific discoveries to improve the population health, and minimised state conflicts to mitigate soldier deaths, the spread of diseases, and the depletion of essential resources for collective civil welfare (Sundin & Willner, 2007).

Example 2: Political interventions within the European context in the same historical period showed that governance can be based on different ethics and, consequently, politics of life. For example, many European nations (e.g., Portugal and Spain) pursued colonial political projects to sustain or expand their empires over the same period. Colonial politics were predominantly characterised by attempts at international governance systems that resulted in the dehumanisation, enslavement, and genocide of First Nations peoples and Africans, epistemicide, and accumulation of material goods, wealth, and military resources (de Susa Santos, 2002b).

These examples demonstrate that politics can change social realities based on the way that the world and human life are understood. The governance in both examples directly exemplify the strategies regulating people's lives, respectively aiming to reduce and create inequalities. While both governance interventions started with Christian notions and values of human life, they have different implications for people's existences and experiences outside the European context. The latter example illustrates the birth of most racial, economic and social inequalities prevalent in postcolonial societies nowadays (Grosfoguel & Rodriguez, 2018; de Susa Santos, 2002a). These inequalities are rooted in a historical and ongoing colonial and imperialistic understanding of life and political-economic interventions. The inequalities reflect societal and political dynamics that intricately intersect with contemporary society's fabric. The point is that history demonstrates that inequalities are present and shaped by the politics of life over time, encompassing governance and the meaning attributed to life (Fassin, 2010, 2018). Inequalities are central to understanding that not all lives are treated equally. This notion guides the central relevance of this assertion to occupational therapists who rhetorically claim themselves as inclusive and compassionate but lack understanding and commitment to address the exclusion and exploitation of individuals and collectives in contemporary society (Dos Santos, 2022; Farias & Lopes, 2022; Hammell, 2023a). Yet, some occupational therapists will resist giving up the benevolently repressive nature of their ideas and practices.

In the following sections a philosophical definition of inequalities is provided, the understanding of which is central to guiding the occupational therapy political project as proposed in this chapter. This is followed by examples showing the occupational therapy profession's limited scope that has traditionally demonstrated little interest in those exposed to the most precarious social conditions. Finally, the chapter focuses on a political project to change occupational therapists' views of the world and to reduce inequalities, drawing attention to the following questions: What needs to be changed in the world? And, what needs to be understood to inform an ethical political project?

UNDERSTANDING INEQUALITY AND ITS SIGNIFICANCE IN THE POLITICAL PROJECT FOR OCCUPATIONAL THERAPY

Inequality encompasses variations in individuals' and collectives' access to various concrete and symbolic goods and life experiences (Almeida-Filho et al., 2004; Marmot, 2003). This chapter adopts a philosophical stance, similar to the approach taken by physician, anthropologist, and sociologist Didier Fassin's 'politics of life' to interpret, analyse and define inequality (Fassin, 2010, 2018). Adopting a philosophical approach based on Jean-Jacques Rousseau's 18th-century ideas (2009), as outlined in 'Discourse on the Origin and Basis of Inequality Among Men', inequality can be understood by two interconnected forms (Fassin, 2018):

- Natural and physical inequalities encompass variations in age, illness, abilities, physical strength and character qualities.
- Moral and political inequalities stem from societal norms, granting privileges that harm some, and creating hierarchies valuing certain individuals over others.

This philosophical insight guides how occupational therapists can understand and then prioritise the reduction of these inequalities in the profession's political project. The distinction is useful for the profession, as many professionals prefer to refer to and start from the realm of the first category of inequality, natural and physical inequalities, to explain occupational therapy's relevance. This is rooted in the ongoing existence of 'natural and physical' variations, such as illness, injury and impairment, which largely justify the scope of the profession's practice. This standpoint supports the clinical relevance of occupational therapy, aligning with individualistic biomedical education and practice. From this perspective, life is perceived as a biological phenomenon, and the biological, that is, 'natural and physical', variations highlight human strengths and vulnerabilities. The emphasis on these variations bestows upon occupational therapy the characteristics of a profession grounded in objectivity, conveyed through deductive reasoning and a neutral political identity (Farias & Lopes, 2023).

The commitment and discussion surrounding the second form of inequality, moral and political inequalities, has traditionally had little attention within the profession. A clear example is presented in the professional content on ageing, in which biological ageing is presented as primarily responsible for levels of functionality and related illness, injury and impairments. This contradicts the wide quantitative evidence that social-demographic variables are associated with early mortality and functional outcomes in late life (Ferraro & Shippee, 2009). A more in-depth exploration of this idea, using a different example, will be presented in the subsequent section, illustrating how the profession's engagement with political projects to mitigate both forms of inequality has not been consistently committed to the ethics of life.

The argument here is that the occupational therapy profession, unfortunately, tends to overlook the most pressing political issues, as well as neglect the embodiment of those experiences (Dos Santos, 2016; Dos Santos et al., 2022; Lopes & Malfitano, 2020). This implies, ultimately, that the professional political perspectives are predominantly shaped to maintain the *status quo*, that is, culturally specific, ableist, White, Anglophone, Judeo-Christian, Western, middle-class norms and values (Hammell, 2023b). The evolution of occupational therapy in the United States is used as an example to showcase some of the issues raised in relation to occupational therapy's alignment with the *status quo*.

The Birth of Occupational Therapy in The American Progressive Era and The Moral-Political Inequalities of Jim Crow

Not everything that is faced can be changed, but nothing can be changed until it is faced.
(James Baldwin, 1962)

African Americans living in the United States during the early decades of the development of the occupational therapy profession had their lives entangled in political and economic systems put in place to segregate them from political and social experiences, such as voting, working rights, reproductive rights, access to care, housing and education, to name a few. The Jim Crow laws were introduced in the late 19th and early 20th centuries to enforce racial segregation. These laws epitomise a governance system designed to subjugate and devalue African Americans' lives by regulating access to resources and assigning value through a dehumanising process (West, 2019). However, only in recent times has the profession started to examine the profound implications of racial segregation, including the Jim Crow laws, on the social structure and subjective experiences of African Americans (Lavalley & Johnson, 2022). At the inception, and for many decades, of the expansion of occupational therapy in the United States, African Americans faced profound moral and political inequalities, often disregarded in the profession's political narrative. It can be argued that the early pragmatic tradition that influenced occupational therapy failed to adequately address the critical concerns of marginalised groups, overlooking matters of race, economics and social dynamics, which inherently shape the meaning and value attributed to human life (Dieleman et al., 2017; Dos Santos & Frank, Forthcoming). Regrettably, minimal consideration has been granted to the profession's historical relation with those exposed to such inequalities.

The foundations of occupational therapy are often considered to be closely aligned with democratic ideals, notably during the Progressive Era (1890–1920) in the United States. The origins of the profession were intricately woven with political activism, as exemplified by the Hull House movement in Chicago, in the north of the United States. Figures like Julia Lathrop, Adolf Meyer and Eleanor Clarke Slagle initially directed their efforts towards reforming the treatment of people who were identified as being mentally ill. A historical exploration of occupational therapy unveils a strong connection between pragmatist philosophy and democratic political reforms, characteristic of the profession's alignment with the Progressive Era. The birth of occupational therapy in Chicago often stands as a compelling case study of political initiatives embedded within a profession's trajectory.

Numerous narratives of the professional history in the United States incorporate political dimensions regarding the backdrop in which occupational therapy education and practice came into being. These accounts contend that the political milieu was characterised by a growing commitment to social justice and reforms. However, these analyses often overlook the necessity for a critical examination of the inequalities that represented the pressing exclusion and exploitation of human lives during that period. They neglect to examine the value attributed to human life as well as the understanding of social views that legitimise political decisions used to justify the exclusion and exploitation of human lives, such as the Jim Crow laws.

To link the creation of occupational therapy to the democratic project in the United States, often a connection is made to the work of pragmatists such as John Dewey. Indeed, these ideas have demonstrated the potential to inspire and inform new theoretical and practical professional projects to address the inequalities of life within the profession (Dos Santos & Frank, 2024; Dos Santos et al., 2020; Frank, 2022; Østergaard Madsen et al., 2024). However, since the Progressive Era occurred almost entirely within the Jim Crow Era that legislated segregation of African Americans, it means that what is considered progressive largely, if not solely, refers to the white American working class. This contributes to making it impossible to identify particular racial attitudes in the South as 'Progressive' or simply as inherited features of long-held Southern racial ideas.

In exploring the history of occupational therapy in the United States, it's essential to consider its evolution within the overlying but distinct Jim Crow Era and Progressive Era to understand the profession's early – and arguably remaining – commitment to inequalities. The chronological approach to understanding occupational therapy history requires a critical approach of incorporating racial, economic, geographical and biographical dimensions to consider how governance and, consequently, the embodiment of those experiences

were shaped in different regions and by individuals of minority social groups in the United States.

To further illustrate this argument, a historical study on the Mississippi School of Occupational Therapy and Department is presented. Reed (2023) indicates that the institution operated from 1921. Notably, the Mississippi School of Occupational Therapy and Department was situated in a southern state of the United States, where the impact of the Jim Crow Era was deeply felt by the early 20th century. According to Reed's (2023) interpretation, racial segregation imposed by the Jim Crow Laws was solely the 'social norm' of those times. This definition is troublesome, as racial segregation goes beyond a social norm; it reflects a political project in which lives were regulated, and not all lives held a similar value in society.

The history of occupational therapy in the United States highlights the profession's insufficient commitment to addressing critical issues of inequalities. This serves as an analysis to illustrate that, while the profession may celebrate political engagement, it often fell short in addressing the extent to which governance and power, through its interventions, perpetuated moral and political inequalities. In this case, the alignment to the *status quo* leads to moral and political inequalities and, as Baldwin (1989) argues, results in inequalities not being faced and, consequently, not being changed.

To complete this argument, it is worth mentioning that Jim Crow laws (1877–1954) existed in the United States at the same time as the birth and expansion of occupational therapy; however, this is not the only example. Similarly, the arrival of occupational therapy and its expansion in South Africa was during the Apartheid Era (1948–1994). Drawing parallels between the development of occupational therapy and the existence of discriminatory laws like Jim Crow and Apartheid provides serious questions into the profession's expansion and its underdeveloped political project in addressing moral-political inequalities.

Neoliberal Orthodoxy and the Economic Face of Moral and Political Inequalities

Caregiving is one of the foundational moral meanings and practices in human experience everywhere: it defines human value and resists crude reduction to counting and costing.

(Arthur Kleinman, 2009)

The case of the birth of occupational therapy in the United States relates to racial segregation and how the profession neglected to properly engage with the most pressing moral and political issue that held specific meaning and value attributed to human life through the dehumanising treatment of Black people for many decades. Racial, ethnic, religious and gender segregation are no longer a part of Western politics that produce moral and political inequalities. Such segregation is no longer acceptable in society and, consequently, in the professional training, discourse and practice. Yet, moral and political inequalities still exist today.

The subtle yet pervasive political-economic ideology of our times does not have those segregation labels, but it similarly aims to regulate governance and attribute value and meaning to human life, contributing to the production of moral and political inequalities. Segregation labels of the 19th and 20th centuries aiming to regulate and attribute meaning and value to lives have changed towards a more subtle yet effective mechanism of control – neoliberalism.

While exploring historical perspectives to better understand the profession and its political projects, it is important to highlight that the political dimensions of life are ubiquitous to all, including occupational therapists and the individuals and collectives whom they work with and for. For example, many, if not most, occupational therapists in the Anglo-Saxon tradition today refer to the people they work with and/or for as clients (Hammell, 2013). The use of market-related vocabulary is a deliberate intervention of power expressed through language and practices. Indeed, this example demonstrates that language can be used as a way of communicating ideas and asserting or maintaining power, including the logic of thinking, over others.

This language (or ideology) of service provision with market-related language is at the centre of specific political-economic contexts of education and practice that are linked to consumerism in healthcare (Winkler, 1987). According to Farias et al. (forthcoming), consumerism in healthcare indicates that individual health issues and access to services are based on their merits, emphasising economic assets. Thus the free market or marketplace language refers to a specific economic-political context of education, practice

and life itself that regulates values and gives meaning to what is done.

It is argued that neoliberal politics and ideology influence the way of thinking and practising occupational therapy (Dos Santos, 2022; Farias et al., Forthcoming), which in turn reinforces the *status quo*. The concern about reinforcing the *status quo* is that many of its beliefs and rituals become accepted and are not questioned, consequently becoming dogmas (Unger, 2000). Aihwa Ong (2007) discusses the plural forms of neo-liberalisms globally and the pervasive effect of this. According to Ong, neo-liberalism is conceived as 'a logic of governing that migrates and is selectively taken up in diverse political contexts' (Ong, 2007, p. 3). As such, neoliberalism is not a cohesive set of ideas that are uniformly imposed worldwide; instead, it takes on various manifestations but will mainly relate to (1) tax cuts, (2) deregulation of corporations, (3) privatisation of nature and utilities, and (4) limited public spending on goods and services (Ong, 2007; Unger, 2000). Neoliberal policies can influence social, educational, housing and healthcare systems by promoting privatisation and market competition. While this approach may increase efficiency and innovation for those with higher incomes and greater access, it exacerbates inequalities and hinders efforts to achieve equity.

Neoliberalism's focus on individual responsibility overlooks the impact of social determinants of health, historical colonialism, racism, discrimination and violence, to name but a few social issues, thus neglecting the intertwined forms of inequality. It emphasises personal choices and behaviours as the primary factors influencing social, educational, economic and health outcomes while neglecting the influence of moral and political inequalities that shape people's experiences in life. Consequently, it celebrates people with privilege and neglects those facing precarious conditions of life. Critical scholars have challenged taken-for-granted occupational therapy assumptions and positions to facilitate change in the profession's values and practices (Correia et al., 2021; Farias & Lopes, 2023; Galvaan, 2015; Grenier, 2021; Hammell, 2020; Lopes & Malfitano, 2020; McGrath, 2019). These changes are aimed to overcome, among other issues, the allegedly political neutrality of the occupational therapy profession.

Individual responsibility and market models currently permeate professional theory, education, research and practice. The economic rationale has become an imperative to reduce costs and increase efficiencies, often translated into the wording of cost-effectiveness as a measure of professional commitment (O'Shea & McGrath, 2019). While appealing in corporate healthcare systems and largely applied, it has limited value as it neglects to consider the emotional, spiritual and aesthetic expressions of the life of occupational therapists and the people they work with. This is not to say that occupational therapy has created this complex economic and social problem leading to moral and political inequalities. Indeed, neoliberal politics create systems that neglect the voices of professionals, such as occupational therapists. Yet, if Kleinman's (2009, p. 1550) argument that 'caregiving is one of the foundational moral meanings and practices in human experience everywhere', is accepted, then the question of which moral compass is used to allow and justify the reproduction of political inequalities in contemporary society within a person's own professional practice has to be addressed. Caring qualities use a language of love and move beyond economic reasoning. To care and be cared for are rights, not products, as Kleinman (p. 1550) argues, 'everyone who has been in love or built a family knows that there are things, essential things, that money can't buy [...] because those things that really matter to us are threatened and must be defended'.

AN ETHICAL COMMITMENT TO ADDRESS MORAL AND POLITICAL INEQUALITIES

Becoming an occupational therapist can be understood as a process of translating caring qualities into professional competencies. These caring qualities relate to human attributes and necessitate consideration of a specific ethical approach towards human life. This implies that one of the primary reasons why occupational therapists exist, which is to care, cannot be overlooked. To care is demanding, often mundane, and emotionally intense, yet profoundly meaningful. Providing care, being emotionally available, and expressing kindness constitute emotional and ethical engagements aligning with our fundamental values (Dos Santos et al., 2022). Caregiving provides

enlightenment about life's essence and unveils the true nature of humanity (Kleinman, 2020). Thus the caring role can be interpreted as that of an actor contributing to reducing inequalities in their physical and political forms.

Over recent decades the profession's political project has started to shift away from its alignment with the *status quo* and progressed to identifying and addressing pressing moral and political inequalities. These changes have been influenced by social, political and scientific shifts in the conception of governance, health and well-being. This includes the emergence of democratic countries (Huntington, 2012), epidemiological studies (Haddon, 1980), and the Alma-Ata Declaration (Organization, 1978) (and its related actions, e.g., Ottawa Charter [Organization, 1986], Caracas Declaration [Bolis, 2002]) that uphold democratic and human rights in its notion of health for all, equity and participation.

Similarly, and more recently, Global South perspectives of occupational therapy have emerged with changes in the profession's epistemological foundations, coinciding with significant political transformations, including the (re)democratisation of South American countries. Occupational therapy arrived in Latin American countries during a period of military dictatorship; however, a large number of professionals were committed to political, health, economic and social reforms and used the political dimension of the profession to advocate for democracy and guarantee citizen rights (Dos Santos & Gallassi, 2014; Dos Santos, 2016; Dos Santos et al., 2022). For instance, many Brazilian occupational therapists contested the military dictatorship regime, challenging long-held assumptions and the profession's scope (knowledge) and jurisdiction (regulatory boundaries of knowledge application). This commitment led to an ethical political project and the development and implementation of an innovative approach known as social occupational therapy (refer to Chapter 4) that ultimately seeks to understand and address moral and political inequalities (Lopes & Malfitano, 2020). An opportunity arose to envision an occupational therapy theory, education, research and practice through an imaginative process that was ethically grounded in understanding and reducing inequalities of human life; a commitment to identify pressing social issues and expand the scope and jurisdiction of occupational therapy professional practice.

A POLITICAL PROJECT FOR OCCUPATIONAL THERAPY

Occupational therapy scholars and practitioners have become increasingly involved in political activism, political economy and biopolitical analysis. Concurrently, they explore the philosophical foundations of governance and the interpretation of meaning and values attributed to life. This emerging movement's growth relies on the comprehension of the profession's scope and jurisdiction. Similarly, it relies on the political landscape shaping the lives of individuals and social groups, including occupational therapists, which regulates through governance and the attribution of meaning and value to life. This chapter has placed emphasis on the significance of governance and power at the structural level, integrated with a person's biological existences and biographical experiences; in other words, what politics does to human life (Box 3.1), and how reflection can lead to actions.

Fassin (2010, 2018) proposed the notion of the 'Politics of Life' – an ethical space for reflection and action bridging biological and biographical, physical and political aspects. These aspects are at – the core of occupational therapy's interest in the human experience of being and doing, and the causes and consequences of inequalities of life, which will be ultimately related to the meaning and values attributed to life itself. Consequently, an understanding of how to approach politics is required, and for Fassin (2009, p. 44) this implies four shifts:

1. Politics is not only about the rules of the game of governing but also about its stakes.
2. More than the power over life, contemporary societies are characterised by the legitimacy they attach to life.
3. Rather than a normalising process, the intervention in lives is a production of inequalities.
4. The politics of life, then, is not only a question of governmentality and technologies but also of meaning and values.

Similar to Fassin's work (2009, 2010, 2018) and a large body of evidence from diverse disciplines, there is an interconnected nature between the two forms of inequality – natural/physical and moral/political. Readers are invited to reflect and discuss the meaning

---

BOX 3.1

A REFLECTION ON THE VALUE ATTRIBUTED TO HUMAN LIFE.

WHAT POLITICS DOES DO TO HUMAN LIVES?

On December 5, 2012, the Brazilian architect Oscar Niemeyer passed away at the age of 104. His social, political and artistic influence is evident in more than 600 buildings across numerous regions and continents, and his death made headlines in Brazil and around the world. In the same week that he passed away, two young people also lost their lives on the outskirts of Brasilia, a city close to the one adorned with Niemeyer's buildings.

I am working on the decentralised campus of the University of Brasilia in Ceilândia, and as I arrive at work, I notice that the flags are being flown at half-mast near a couple of university security guards, signifying mourning. I inquire as to whom they are mourning, and they look surprised and ask me if I haven't heard that Oscar Niemeyer has passed away. I confirm my knowledge, and with some disappointment, I reflect on how Niemeyer lived a full life while lamenting that two more lives have been lost.

I contemplate these events to draw attention to a central theme of occupational therapy: the quotidian – the essence of ordinary life, including the tragedy of death. The deaths of underprivileged people in Brazil and elsewhere often do not make the headlines as it has become an ordinary part of the social life. These early deaths, and their former precarious lives, reflect an inequality that is grounded on a history of colonialism and current economic disparity that legitimatise less value to certain individuals and groups. These highlight a dehumanised treatment that is not only based on repression but also fear and avoidance by many sectors of society, including occupational therapists, of those severely exposed to moral and political inequalities.

---

and value attached to each form of inequality in ordinary life.

In this chapter, attention was drawn to the troubling treatment of individuals and collectives. Thus, an occupational therapy political project encompasses engagement with those who are often forgotten, whose lives do not seem to hold the same value within and outside the systems of governmentality or economics. Given that inequalities are pervasive within our existence and experience, they inherently warrant the consideration of societal and political agents to address them. This encompasses professionals, like occupational therapists, who are arguably committed to enhancing people's everyday life existence and experience.

CONCLUSION

The political project of occupational therapy is growing in its focus and scope. The profession demonstrates an interest in addressing moral and political inequalities and their consequences on individual's and collectives' lives, encompassing their existences and experiences. These interests are sustained with a critical perspective and a large body of evidence. This evidence comes from public health, political economy and education, all showing that inequality has a negative impact on individual's and collectives' social, educational, economic and health experiences. The occupational therapy profession is beginning to develop its future political project based on an understanding that inequality is not merely a product of governance, but that specific meanings and values can engender oppression, marginalisation, and forgetting of individuals and collectives and their biographical lives, that is, the everyday lives that are not accounted for, acknowledged, and cared for.

REFERENCES

Almeida-Filho, N., Lessa, I., Magalhães, L., Araújo, M. J., Aquino, E., James, S. A., & Kawachi, I. (2004). Social inequality and depressive disorders in Bahia, Brazil: Interactions of gender, ethnicity, and social class. *Social Science & Medicine, 59*(7), 1339–1353.

Baldwin, J. (1962). A letter to my nephew. *The Progressive, 1*, 160–164.

Bolis, M. (2002). *The impact of the Caracas Declaration on the modernization of mental health legislation in Latin America and the English-speaking Caribbean.* Citeseer.

Correia, R. L., Wertheime, L. G., Morrison, R., & Silva, C. R. (2021). Contemporary perspectives of occupational therapy in Latin America: Contributions to the glocal dialogue. *South African Journal of Occupational Therapy, 51*(4), 41–50.

de Sousa Santos, B. (2002a). Between Prospero and Caliban: Colonialism, postcolonialism, and inter-identity. *Luso-Brazilian Review, 39*(2), 9–43.

de Sousa Santos, B. (2002b). Para uma sociologia das ausências e uma sociologia das emergências. *Revista Crítica de Ciências Sociais, 63*, 237–280.

Dieleman, S., Rondel, D., & Voparil, C. (2017). *Pragmatism and justice.* Oxford University Press.

Dos Santos, V. (2016). *Occupational therapy across South America: An overview of its backgrounds, current situation and some contemporary issues.* In *Occupational Therapies Without Borders: Integrating Justice With Practice, 2*(1), 203–210. Elsevier.

Dos Santos, V. (2022). Social transformation on the neoliberal university: Reconstructing an academic commitment. *Journal of Occupational Science, 29*(4), 482–486. https://doi.org/10.1080/14427591.2022.2110660.

Dos Santos, V., Bezerra, W. C., Godoy, A., & Terra, E. (2022). A terapia ocupacional de um Brasil democrático e livre. In V. Dos Santos, I. Muñoz, & M. Farias (Eds.), *Questões e práticas contemporâneas da terapia ocupacional na América do Sul* (2nd ed., pp. 41–52). CRV.

Dos Santos, V., & Frank, G. (2024). *Creativity, hope and collective emancipatory-experimentation: Tools for social transformation through occupational therapy.* Taylor and Francis.

Dos Santos, V., & Frank, G. (2024). Creativity, hope and collective emancipatory experimentation: Tools for social transformation through occupational therapy. In T. Brown, S. Isbel, L. Gustafsson, S. Gutman, D. Powers Dirette, B. Collins, & T. Barlott (Eds.), *Human occupation: Contemporary concepts and lifespan perspectives* (1st ed., pp. 249–266). Routledge.

Dos Santos, V., Frank, G., & Mizue, A (2020). Candangos: Teoria da reconstrução ocupacional como uma ferramenta para a compreensão de problemas sociais e ações transformativas na utópica cidade de Brasília. *Cadernos Brasileiros de Terapia Ocupacional, 28*, 765–783.

Dos Santos, V., & Gallassi, A. (2014). *Questoes contemporáneas da terapia ocupacional na América do sul.* CRV Editora.

Dos Santos, V., Muñoz, I., & Farias, M. (2022). *Questões e práticas contemporâneas da terapia ocupacional na América do Sul.* CRV Editora.

Farias, L., Lapierre, M., & Dos Santos, V. (Forthcoming). The neoliberal framing of occupational therapy practices and the rising of the health consumer. In P. Talero, N. Pollard, & V. Dos Santos (Eds.), *Revealing practice: Learning from occupational therapy across Latin America* (1st ed.). Jessica Kingsley Publishers.

Farias, M. N., & Lopes, R. E. (2022). Terapia ocupacional social, antiopressão e liberdade: Considerações sobre a revolução da/na vida cotidiana. *Cadernos Brasileiros de Terapia Ocupacional, 30*, e3100.

Farias, M. N., & Lopes, R. E. (2023). Terapia ocupacional e a armadilha neoliberal progressista: Desafios para uma práxis antiopressiva. *Revista de Terapia Ocupacional Da Universidade de São Paulo, 33*(1), e209610.

Fassin, D. (2009). Another politics of life is possible. *Theory, Culture & Society, 26*(5), 44–60.

Fassin, D. (2010). Ethics of survival: A democratic approach to the politics of life. *Humanity: An International Journal of Human Rights, Humanitarianism, and Development, 1*(1), 81–95. https://doi.org/10.1353/hum.2010.0000.

Fassin, D. (2018). *Life: A critical user's manual* (1st ed.). Polity.

Ferraro, K. F., & Shippee, T. P. (2009). Aging and cumulative inequality: How does inequality get under the skin? *The Gerontologist, 49*(3), 333–343.

Frank, G. (2022). Occupational science's stalled revolution and a manifesto for reconstruction. *Journal of Occupational Science, 29*(4), 455–477.

Galvaan, R. (2015). The contextually situated nature of occupational choice: Marginalised young adolescents' experiences in South Africa. *Journal of Occupational Science, 22*(1), 39–53.

Grenier, M.-L. (2021). Patient case formulations and oppressive disability discourses in occupational therapy education. *Canadian Journal of Occupational Therapy, 88*(3), 266–272. https://doi.org/10.1177/00084174211005882.

Grosfoguel, R., & Rodriguez, J. (2018). What is Racism? Zone of being and zone of non-being in the work of Frantz Fanon and Boaventura de Sousa Santos. In J. Cupples & R. Grosfoguel (Ed.), *Unsettling Eurocentrism in the westernized university* (pp. 264–273). Routledge.

Haddon, W. (1980). Advances in the epidemiology of injuries as a basis for public policy. *Public Health Reports, 95*(5), 411.

Hammell, K. (2020). Ações nos determinantes sociais de saúde: Avançando na equidade ocupacional e nos direitos ocupacionais. *Cadernos Brasileiros de Terapia Ocupacional, 28*(1), 387–400. https://doi.org/10.4322/2526-8910.ctoARF2052.

Hammell, K. W. (2023a). A call to resist occupational therapy's promotion of ableism. *Scandinavian Journal of Occupational Therapy, 30*(6), 745–757.

Hammell, K. W. (2023b). Focusing on 'what matters': The occupation, capability and wellbeing framework for occupational therapy. *Cadernos Brasileiros de Terapia Ocupacional, 31*, e3509.

Hammell, K. R. W. (2013). Client-centred practice in occupational therapy: Critical reflections. *Scandinavian Journal of Occupational Therapy, 20*(3), 174–181. https://doi.org/10.3109/11038128.2012.752032.

Huntington, S. P. (2012). *The third wave: Democratization in the late 20th century (Vol. 4).* University of Oklahoma Press.

Kleinman, A. (2009). Caregiving: The odyssey of becoming more human. *The Lancet, 373*(9660), 292–293.

Kleinman, A. (2020). *The soul of care: The moral education of a husband and a doctor.* Penguin.

Lavalley, R., & Johnson, K. R. (2022). Occupation, injustice, and anti-black racism in the United States of America. *Journal of Occupational Science, 29*(4), 487–499.

Lopes, R. E., & Malfitano, A. P. S. (2020). *Social occupational therapy: Theoretical and practical designs.* Elsevier Health Sciences.

Marmot, M. G. (2003). Understanding social inequalities in health. *Perspectives in Biology and Medicine, 46*(3), S9–S23.

Ong, A. (2007). Neoliberalism as a mobile technology. *Transactions of the Institute of British Geographers, 32*(1), 3–8. https://doi.org/10.1111/j.1475-5661.2007.00234.x.

O'Shea, J., & McGrath, S. (2019). Contemporary factors shaping the professional identity of occupational therapy lecturers. *British Journal of Occupational Therapy, 82*(3), 186–194.

Østergaard Madsen, J., Morrison, R., Dos Santos, V., & Barlott, T. (2024). Pragmatism: Current and future influence on occupational therapy and occupational science. In T. Brown, S. Isbel, L. Gustafsson, S. Gutman, D. Powers Dirette, B. Collins, & T. Barlott (Eds.), *Human occupation: Contemporary concepts and lifespan perspectives* (1st ed., pp. 283–298). Routledge.

Rousseau, J. J. (2009). *Discourse on inequality: On the origin and basis of inequality among men* (p. 115). The Floating Press.

Sakellariou, D., & Pollard, N. (2016). *Occupational therapies without borders e-book: Integrating justice with practice.* Elsevier Health Sciences.

Sundin, J., & Willner, S. (2007). *Social change and health in Sweden: 250 years of politics and practice.* Swedish National Institute of Public Health.

Unger, R. M. (1987). *False necessity: Anti-necessitarian social theory in the service of radical democracy.* Cambridge University Press.

Unger, R. M. (1997). *Politics: The central texts.* Verso.

Unger, R. M. (2000). *Democracy realized: The progressive alternative.* Verso.

West, C. (2019). Race Matters. In J. Arthur & A. Shapiro (Eds.). Color-Class-Identity: The New Politics of Race. (pp. 169-178). Routledge.

Winkler, F. (1987). Consumerism in health care: Beyond the supermarket model. *Policy & Politics, 15*(1), 1–8. https://doi.org/10.1332/030557387782514609.

World Health Organization. (1978). *Declaration of alma-ata.* World Health Organization.

World Health Organization. (1986). *Ottawa charter for health promotion, 1986.* World Health Organization.

REFLECTION

1. Discriminatory laws have been implemented in many countries, and these practices remain today.
    a. Consider whether you are aware of any governance strategy in your country that discriminates against its people.
    b. Describe the nature of this moral-political inequality in terms of the meaning attributed to life and the associated practices.
    c. Reflect on whether occupational therapy has had any political, theoretical, or practical engagement in addressing these ideas and practices.

2. The following questions invite you to reflect on the use and impact of the language of service provision:
    a. In your region, how is access to safe housing, inclusive and participatory education, and adequate healthcare secured? Are these aspects of social life considered 'services' (i.e. products in the marketplace) or 'rights' (i.e. based on policies designed to share them among citizens)?
    b. What are the implications of viewing these as services, that is, within Neoliberal vocabulary or within a lens of commitment to their relation

to the ethics and politics of life, in which opportunities are citizens' rights to be shared?

3. Use the following questions to reflect on and explore existing occupational therapy political practice projects.
   a. What are the political projects that accommodate those often-professed professional goals of occupational therapists, that is, social participation and engagement, inclusion, combatting exclusion and exploration of human life, to name a few?
   b. Is political neutrality possible for a profession with such goals?

4

SOCIAL OCCUPATIONAL THERAPY: PRINCIPLES FOR ACTION TOWARDS PARTICIPATION

ROSELI ESQUERDO LOPES ■ ANA PAULA SERRATA MALFITANO ■ PATRÍCIA LEME DE OLIVEIRA BORBA

CHAPTER OUTLINE

Overview

In this chapter the development of social occupational therapy from the 1970s in Brazil until nowadays is presented. Two foci of social occupational therapy are described. The first focus advocates the need for all actions in occupational therapy to highlight the social contexts. The second focus emphasises the actions in the social field, exemplifying target populations, contexts, services, resources and social technologies. Then the four social technologies of social occupational therapy are explained: (1) workshops of dynamics, activities and projects, (2) individual and territorial follow-up, (3) articulation of resources in the social field, (4) dynamisation of the social care network. They are understood as products, techniques and replicable methodologies co-created with communities, representing alternatives for social transformation towards a more just and equal society. It is necessary to continuously and critically reflect on the work process, assuming the technical, ethical and political dimensions that comprise the professional qualification of social occupational therapists.

KEY POINTS

- Social occupational therapy approaches two main points: all actions in occupational therapy focusing on social contexts, and a specificity of actions in the social field.
- Social technologies can be applied to develop alternatives for social transformation through methodologies co-create with communities.
- Occupational therapists need to have a critical reflection about their role assuming their technical, ethical and political actions.

INTRODUCTION

Occupational therapy in Brazil began with the creation of the first professional education programs in the mid-1950s, as part of a movement by international organisations (such as the United Nations, the World Health Organization and the International Labor Organization) to expand rehabilitation efforts around the world. This process was influenced by economic, political and cultural interests that marked the relations between core capitalist countries and the so-called peripheral ones in the scenario that followed World War II, between the 1940s and 1960s, the polio epidemic in Latin America, and the advancement of industrialisation in Brazil (Bezerra et al., 2023; Soares, 1991). These initial education programs were guided by the technical-political orientation of occupational therapists who had studied in the United States of America – Americans serving the aforementioned international organisations (Drummond & Cruz, 2018; Reis & Lopes, 2018; Soares, 1991).

Like many Latin American countries, Brazil experienced a civil-military dictatorship between 1964 and 1985, directly affecting the possibility for its population to experience rights and citizenship. In that context, on one hand, the professional practice that was established operated around a discourse that took supposed scientific neutrality as a parameter, marking actions of a predominantly biomedical approach. On the other hand, during the same period, there was the combined action in the country of social movements in defense of a democratic state and rights related to citizenship – whether civil, political or social. These movements included the participation of occupational therapists. Occupational therapists began to critically debate the established prevailing order and the role of their technical-professional actions (Bezerra et al., 2023), positioning the profession in the fight to end the dictatorship and establish social rights.

In a space of curtailment of freedom and exacerbation of social inequalities, the first publications on social occupational therapy began in the late 1970s (Barros et al., 2011). Discussion on social occupational therapy ensued, highlighting the social dimension as a focus of occupational therapy practice, based mainly on two complementary theoretical perspectives.

The first theoretical perspective refers to the necessary analysis of social processes that affect the work of occupational therapists, recognising that the social context is an inherent part of professional action. In this case, social occupational therapy is advocated as a critical reading key applicable to any professional practice in occupational therapy (Barros et al., 1999).

The second theoretical perspective arises from questioning medical-psychological knowledge and simplifying social problems to the health-disease binominal (Barros et al., 1999). From this standpoint, the need for occupational therapists to work beyond the health sector is promoted as they engage in the everyday lives of individuals through their insertion/inclusion and participation in the social field. It is acknowledged that occupational therapy could be provided to collectives utilising social care/welfare, education, social security, justice, culture services and other public policy sectors, especially social policies. From this perspective, social occupational therapy refers to politically and ethically framed practices that target individuals, collectives and/or systems to enable justice and social rights. This second theoretical perspective specifically focuses on people experiencing disadvantageous social conditions (Barros et al., 2005).

The Metuia Network – Social Occupational Therapy

Brazilian social occupational therapy has developed theoretical knowledge and professional practices in various fields of activity, to underpin practice that is ethically and politically committed to the context in which it is carried out (Lopes & Malfitano, 2021). In this context, in 1998, the Metuia Project[1] was created, resulting from an interinstitutional initiative of occupational therapy academics from three universities in the state of São Paulo, Brazil. The aim of this collaboration was to develop studies, education and actions to foster the citizenship of socially vulnerable individuals undergoing processes of disruption of their social support networks (Barros et al., 2005). The experiences and elaborations of the Metuia Project constructed the theoretical-methodological framework of social occupational therapy, combined with research and actions in different social policies; 'learning from practice' (Barros et al., 2005; Lopes & Malfitano, 2021).

Currently, the Metuia Project is named Metuia Network – Social Occupational Therapy. It is composed of ten active centres: eight located in different regions of Brazil and two in other countries – Mozambique and France. Each of the Metuia Network centres has unique characteristics, reflecting the local needs and demands combined with the academic/professional interests of the people and institutions involved. In a

---

[1] *Metuia* is a word from the native Brazilian indigenous language of the Bororo community that means friend, companion.

decentralised way, other researchers and professionals also participate in this network. Every 2 years, there is a meeting organised by its members – the Social Occupational Therapy International Symposium. To date five symposiums have been held: the first in 2007 and the most recent in 2022.[2]

The Metuia Network and the symposiums, along with academic and professional debates and discussions with occupational therapists around the world, and recognition of the critical importance and influence of the social dimension on practice, have all contributed to social occupational therapy expanding beyond Brazil.

Focus of the Chapter

Social occupational therapy has become a critical reference perspective for the profession, considering the growing and necessary debate about the social life dimension for occupational therapy practice (Costa et al., 2023). This chapter focuses on two central dimensions of social occupational therapy: the need for all actions in occupational therapy to focus on social contexts; and occupational therapy actions in the social field, exemplifying target populations, contexts, services, resources and social technologies with which this practice has been constituted. Social occupational therapy is presented as a reference for a critical practice committed to the challenges of contemporary times.

THE SOCIAL CONTEXT

Occupational therapy researchers and professionals have increasingly debated the need for a critical perspective (Farias & Aldrich, 2021; Laliberte-Rudman, 2013; Taff & Putnam, 2022), that more authentically focuses on the contexts of people's lives, seeking more responsive action to the real needs of individuals. The centrality of contexts and environments has been discussed in occupational therapy for several decades (Law, 1991) and has been present in different models guiding professional practice (e.g. American Occupational Therapy Association, 2002; Kielhofner, 2009; Teoh & Iwama, 2015; Townsend & Polatajko, 2007), including

the recent Canadian Model of Occupational Participation (Egan & Restall, 2022) (refer to Chapter 11).

However, a discussion is needed about which theoretical framework informs professionals regarding the analysis and action on contexts. It is common for the context to be seen as a 'backdrop' to interventions, that is, just an element present in the everyday life of individuals but not part of the occupational-therapeutic practice (Malfitano & Lopes, 2018). Moreover, there is also a functionalist approach to contexts, understanding them as one of the checklist components of assessments, interventions and/or evaluations. In contrast to both propositions, which do not deepen the theoretical understanding of what context is and its connection with some practice, a socio-historical view that reflects and is always present in the everyday life of all individuals is proposed.

Starting from a historical-dialectical materialist perspective (Marxists Internet Archive Encyclopedia, 2023),[3] it is understood that social relations are determinants of our time, and human beings socially construct this historical time. From this theory, there are three elements to consider:

1. *Materialist*: economic production relations are central in a society organised by capitalism; they are its infrastructure, that is, the material conditions direct the possibilities of life;
2. *Historical*: society is formed by the concrete social action of human beings in their time, in a specific place, and under specific conditions; and
3. *Dialectical*: social processes are transformed by the contradictions that material and existence conditions offer, in the light of human social action in its time.

A historical-dialectical materialist view of the contexts in which people live addresses the economic, political, cultural and social aspects; the relationship between the singular and the totality (Gramsci, 1994).

Based on this assumption, the context cannot be just a 'background', in that it is an essential part of each individual's life, as everyone is inserted into society, with central characteristics of the material

---

[2]The lectures that were part of the program of the 5th International Symposium on Social Occupational Therapy are available on the website: https://www.youtube.com/@metuiaufscar/featured.

[3]Theory that posits an understanding of society, originally formulated by Karl Marx (1818–1883) and Friederich Engels (1920–1895).

reproduction of life, in a historical period when conflict is an inherent condition. Nor can it be only an element of the checklist, since, regardless of the condition and/or need of the individual, life will always be shaped by the context in which a person lives. The centrality of context is recognised as an essential aspect of all occupational therapy practice, regardless of the practice area or people receiving occupational therapy services. A reflective approach is always needed to grasp the context as a starting point for any occupational therapy action, as well as the need for action that primarily combines individuals and/or collectives and their contexts.

Social occupational therapy can be characterised as a critical approach, which has the combination of the macro and micro-social dimensions as one of its principles (Lopes & Malfitano, 2021). Based on this assumption, Malfitano (2021, p. 28) explains

Professional intervention will occur for the expansion of social support networks, individual and social, as described by Castel (2003). In the individual sphere, strategies will be developed to assist people with finding support for their social inclusion and participation, respecting their choices and autonomy. As for the collective sphere, practice is connected to social policies and action in public spaces aimed at the maintenance and/or extension of the recognition of certain needs, intervening in the expansion of services and other spaces that allow access to the rights of this group. It thus comprises the arduous task of articulating individual and collective actions – of a personalized and individualized work that is, at the same time – integrated with political actions.

(Malfitano, 2021, p. 48)

It is a socio-historical perspective that recognises, on the one hand, how the macro-social structure affects the everyday life of individuals and, on the other hand, how the possibility of tensioning the macrostructure resides in this everyday life – the microsocial universe. The challenge is to reveal social life in the fabric of the 'apparent' everyday life, using that same routine as a path to self-knowledge and understanding of the world, understanding social needs (Pais, 1993). Social needs are present in everyday life,

related to the conditions they occur and how individuals are affected by them. Issues, such as inequalities, illnesses and suffering situations, marked by desires and possibilities, need to be understood as social needs.

To deal with both the historical-dialectical materialist and socio-historical theoretical perspectives in social occupational therapy, approaching different social needs, it is necessary to create action methodologies that mediate processes for greater social participation. It will then be possible to understand the processes of oppression experienced by these individuals (Farias & Lopes, 2022) and outline joint propositions that consider the context, along with attention to people's demands, taken both individually and collectively. For example:

- Rehabilitation actions in occupational therapy are not possible unless they analyse where an individual lives, their access to urban mobility, their socioeconomic possibilities, along with the interventions needed for their functional recovery.
- Action in mental health in occupational therapy will only materialise in the direction of the everyday lives of individuals if it addresses social stigma, the possibilities and impossibilities of social belonging, and the specific intervention approaches and the impact of the condition on each person.
- A clinical proposal for children with autism should prioritise their access, or lack thereof, to school, to spaces for socialising and leisure with other children, as well as their cognitive, affective and behavioural needs, regardless of the preestablished diagnosis.

Social occupational therapy is characterised by an understanding of reality applicable to all areas of professional action, with different populations, aiming to emphasise the inseparability between the macro- and micro-social levels of life. It aims to develop theoretical and methodological frameworks that enable actions that always centrally consider individuals in their social contexts, alongside interventions that address the demands of these individuals and that are targeted at their social context, in their political, cultural and social dimensions.

WORKING IN THE SOCIAL FIELD

Occupational therapists have as their locus of action the activities, everyday lives, occupations, and ways of life of people, to promote occupational and social participation, social insertion/inclusion, emancipation and autonomy (Malfitano et al., 2023; Malfitano, 2022). It is not possible to restrict the action of occupational therapists to the health field; so occupational therapists can and should expand their scope of action to other sectors, services and policies, such as those aimed at populations using and/or impacted by social care/welfare, education, social security, justice, city planning and culture services and policies (Lopes & Malfitano, 2021).

Many people live in a capitalist society in which inequalities are social determinations that shape life and its possibilities. The word 'determinations', instead of 'determinants', has been deliberately used because determinations are multiple, such as social class, race/ethnicity, gender and sexuality, generation and place of residence, but with differences in their dynamics of intersection, consubstantiality and incidence, depending on the established political and cultural contexts. Social determination recognises that the forces of social inequities are in social life, beyond randomly added determining factors (in a perspective similar to the critique by Harvey et al. (2022) and Spiegel et al. (2015), regarding the social determinants of health). The processes of the social determination of life and directing professional knowledge towards action that properly focuses on them, is a result of understanding the ethical-political commitment and responsibilities of occupational therapists.

The ethical dimension refers to the impossibility of being indifferent in such an unequal world. It is an ethical responsibility to apply knowledge developed for action related to the activities, everyday lives, occupations, and ways of life of individuals to confront social inequities. One of the ways to approaching it professionally is to work together with groups and populations to mediate the process of accessing rights and of participating in a citizenship perspective. Based on Gramsci (1971), specifically in his discussions about organic intellectuals, occupational therapists' ethical commitment means that they should be seeking to transform the living conditions of individuals (always

considering the structural limits of capitalism). This necessarily aligns with a political perspective, insofar as politics is the collective pact that outlines the conditions for the social determination of life and the possibilities of access to more or less unequal means for its realisation. Therefore emphasising an ethical-political commitment with historical time refers to the responsibility for how occupational therapists expect 'to do occupational therapy' (Pollard et al., 2008).

Brazilian social occupational therapy has led to the development of theoretical and methodological contributions that have facilitated concrete actions in the social field so that occupational therapists can employ their knowledge with various population groups. It emphasises the inseparability between the macro- and micro-social dimensions and a collective perspective of apprehending reality, and in this way, of not individualising social problems, in an approach contrary to social medicalisation (Malfitano, 2021).

The populations, contexts and resources that have been developed by different occupational therapists, academics, researchers and professionals promoting social occupational therapy are presented in the following section. This is done to offer a set of words/images that convey and evoke the numerous possibilities that this field has been creating.

CONNECTING TARGET POPULATIONS AND CONTEXTS IN/OF SOCIAL OCCUPATIONAL THERAPY

At the end of the 1990s, Brazilian academics began to construct a theoretical-methodological framework dedicated to combining the area of occupational therapy with the social question in a structurally unequal society. Named 'Social Occupational Therapy', it focused on informing professional actions aimed at dealing with the impediments experienced by individuals and collectives to their participation in social life (Barros et al., 1999, 2005; Lopes & Malfitano, 2023). As previously mentioned, the Metuia Network – Social Occupational Therapy has played a central role in this construction, and from local demands, social occupational therapeutic propositions targeting different populations in various services have been developed. Regarding the target population, social occupational therapy has been used with poor youth and children in public schools (refer to Chapter 21), young offenders, community actions (refer to Chapter 21), work in social assistance services, street dwellers, illicit drug users, migrants, gender and sex dissent populations (refer to Chapter 49), traditional communities, *quilombola* and Indigenous communities, among others (Lopes & Malfitano, 2021; Lopes & Borba, 2022).

Three unique central elements of the Brazilian experience also enabled the creation and strengthening of social occupational therapy actions – diversifying the target populations and contexts of proper action.

1. *'University extension' projects, a type of 'service assistance'.* It is a service provided by universities in partnership with the local communities, with the purposes of teaching, research, and joint action with community partners, both government and nongovernment. In many universities located in some Latin American countries – influenced by the Paulo Freire postulates – university extension expands and surpasses the understanding of 'service provision'. Even though it is a service, it advocates joint action, constant exchange of knowledge, and the necessary dialogue between academic and popular knowledge, in which both benefit from the meeting space. This is enabled by actions taken in 'university extension' projects (Freire, 1979). These actions are characterised by dialogue with society and seek not only to strengthen the exchange of knowledge with the working classes but also the permanent emancipation of people. In general, strategies to be shared seek access to rights and a more comprehensive understanding of their given realities, in addition to invigorating democracy, elucidating the role of political subjects, and making the construction of the exercise of citizenship tangible. University extension projects call for the university to fulfil its role of commitment to social transformation towards expanding justice and social equity (Gadotti, 2017).

   Many projects carried out by the social occupational therapists of the Metuia Network are university extension projects. Most of the Network's centres were created in public universities that, in partnership with social movements and

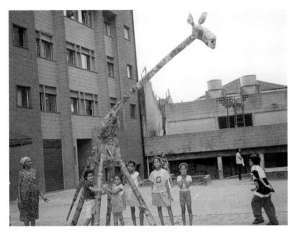

Fig. 4.1 ■ *'Projeto Casarão – Centro de Cultura e Convivência da Celso Garcia'* (Big House Project – Celso Garcia Center for Culture and Coexistence). Communitarian project directed by occupational therapists academics from the Universidade Federal de São Carlos (UFSCar) and Universidade de São Paulo (USP) (Brazil). (From UFSCar-USP Center Metuia Network Archive.)

public services, built actions in favour of individuals and collectives. The first project of the Metuia Network was created in 1998 and titled *'Projeto Casarão – Centro de Cultura e Convivência da Celso Garcia'* (Big House Project – Celso Garcia Center for Culture and Coexistence). This project was characterised by a partnership between the university and the social movement for urban housing rights in São Paulo city (Brazil). The project focused on working with children, young people, and their families, who resided in a public housing complex, and whose *'Casarão'* (Big House), was a fundamental part of their struggle for dignified housing (Barros et al., 2008, 2023) (Fig. 4.1).

It has been 25 years of many achievements, a significant part of which is described in the book *'Social Occupational Therapy: Theoretical Designs and Practical Contours'* (Lopes & Malfitano, 2016), now in its 2nd revised and expanded edition in Portuguese (Lopes & Malfitano, 2023), with an English version published in 2021 by Elsevier (Lopes & Malfitano, 2021). The work of Pan (2019) that chronicled the projects carried out by the Federal University of São Carlos Centre of the Metuia Network was also highlighted.

This work primarily focused on young people and their relationship with public schools and their territories and communities. Additionally, in the book *'Occupational Therapy, Youth, and Education: Understanding Practices and Recognizing Knowledge'* (Lopes & Borba, 2022), published in Portuguese, a series of social occupational therapy experiences in the education sector, particularly in high school and higher education, are described. Aspects of these projects can be accessed in articles and other publications (Borba et al., 2021; Pan & Lopes, 2022).

In addition to creating and implementing resources and technologies for this set of projects, it is through encounters with communities and individuals in their everyday lives and contexts, as well as through the practice of university extension, that occupational therapists are educated. It is also during these encounters that the 'research questions' arise, and thus, university teaching, research and extension activities are combined, not necessarily in this order, but with this triple intent.

2. *The recognition of occupational therapy as one of the professions involved in the teams and management of social assistance services/welfare at all levels of social protection.* In Brazil, the legislation on this protection stems from the political articulation that resulted in the Unified Social Assistance System (SUAS), characterised as a noncontributory national policy of rights to all citizens who need it (Almeida et al., 2012; Almeida & Soares, 2021). This legal recognition was only possible through the theoretical and practical trajectory of social occupational therapy, which preceded the existence of this legislation, and professionals who worked with the regulatory bodies of the profession in Brazil so that this specific area of action could be recognised and incorporated, occurring in a way very distinct from that of the health and rehabilitation sectors.[4] The national social assistance

policy provides a series of services and programs organised at levels of complexity, namely, Basic Social Protection (PSB) and Special Social Protection (PSS). PSB aims to help prevent situations of social risk and violation of rights, while PSS – divided into medium and high complexity – aims to assist families and individuals who have had their rights violated. What differentiates medium and high complexities is the existence, or lack of, family and/or community ties, with these being broken in the latter situation (Brazil, 2004). The following are among the set of services that compose these protections: Social Assistance Reference Centres, Specialised Social Assistance Reference Centres (which include the application of open-environment socio-educational measures for young offenders), Pop Centres (community centres for homelessness), Institutional Sheltering Units (known as shelters – long-term institutions), Community Centres, Day Centres (targeting people with disabilities) and Foster Families (Brazil, 2004).

The presence of occupational therapists in the teams and management of all these services, which cover a diversity of populations and demands, is provided for by law. This has greatly expanded the inclusion of occupational therapy within the social field (Oliveira & Malfitano, 2021).

Another aspect that needs to be pointed out is that occupational therapists, once included in the social assistance policy, seek to align their practice with the theoretical-methodological framework of social occupational therapy. This has stimulated growth in the area and the search for research and courses that assist in this process.

3. *The knowledge production engendered by the Graduate Studies Program in Occupational Therapy at UFSCar, more specifically, by the Networks and Vulnerabilities research line has contributed to the consolidation of social occupational therapy.* This Program started in 2010 at the master's level and began to offer the doctoral course in 2015. Since then, it has accumulated a series of research projects that foster a greater understanding and critique of contemporary reality, as well as the

---

[4]In 2011, the Federal Council of Physical Therapy and Occupational Therapy (COFFITO) published Resolution No. 406 that recognises the professional specialty of occupational therapy in social contexts, establishing large areas of competence for action in the social field.

description and analysis of different resources and technologies of social occupational therapy that, beyond practical interventions, are tested and have been employed within the methodological procedures of research (Pan et al., 2022; Pereira & Malfitano, 2014; Silva & Malfitano, 2021).

Thus, in this journey, the development of social resources and technologies that can be used by occupational therapists in their professional daily practice has become, and remains, necessary. In the following section, some of these developments created throughout this journey are presented.

SOCIAL RESOURCES AND TECHNOLOGIES OF/FOR SOCIAL OCCUPATIONAL THERAPY

The term 'social technologies' was adopted in 2011, initially published in an abstract by some authors of the group in an Occupational Therapy Brazilian Congress (Lopes et al., 2011), and published in articles in 2014 (Lopes et al., 2014). This discussion was later translated into Spanish (Lopes et al., 2016) and English (Lopes et al., 2021). The commitment to 'social technology' terminology is primarily due to three reasons. Social technologies:

1. Refer to a set of techniques and methodologies focused on social transformation and inclusion;
2. Are co-created, implemented and evaluated in partnership with local communities; and
3. Can be reproduced in different contexts and by other actors (Dagnino, 2009).

The choice of the term 'social technologies' can initially be somewhat startling, especially since the tradition in occupational therapy, which stems from the health area, is more familiar with treatment protocols and assessments. However, this proposition is deemed significant as it challenges the vocabulary used by professionals, incorporating words and concepts suited for the social field. Lopes et al. (2021), propose four social technologies:

1. *Workshops of activities, dynamics and projects*: This refers to social technology for collective interventions that originate from the proposition and use of activities. These are inserted into a process that involves various individuals, both on individual and collective levels. Within this context, unique dynamics emerge, and projects can be built collaboratively. They may even extend beyond the workshop setting to be fully achieved. The formative and transformative potential of activity is tapped into since the sociopolitical and cultural dimensions of different tasks permeate everyday life. This promotes the self-worth of individuals and enables the production of a meaningful life, aiming at personal and social emancipation (Fig. 4.2).

2. *Individual territorial follow-ups*: Starting from attentive listening to the needs of individuals and collectives, this social technology seeks to address essential issues in their lives, often determined by social inequality and lack of access to social services and goods. It is worth noting that for individual territorial follow-ups to be implemented there is a requirement to move beyond the collective space of the workshops of activities, dynamics and projects. This demands various relocations and time to jointly search for alternative solutions, strategies and paths (Lopes et al., 2014, 2016, 2021) (Fig. 4.3).

3. *Articulation of resources in the social field*: This refers to social technology that underpins the intervention strategy that is woven through actions focused on specific individuals and collectives, up to those focused on the level of civil society, political action and management. This social technology involves managing the practices at different levels of assistance involving common goals and using possible resources, understood as the financial, material, relational and affective devices, either macro- or microsocial, to compose the interventions.

4. *Dynamisation of support networks:* This social technology refers to an intervention strategy aimed to interact and integrate policies, programs, projects and services oriented towards the targeted population groups, that is, it involves the direct organisation of meetings, conferences and/or movements arising from an issue or theme demanded by the group of individuals or

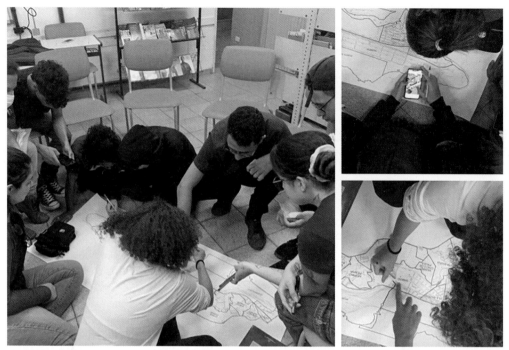

Fig. 4.2 ■ The team working on the 'Active and Democratic Care: Theoretical-Practical Subsidies for the Implementation of Policies to Support the Return and Permanence of Young People to School in the Post-Pandemic Context' project organised their work on the active searches of young people who have dropped out of school using a city map. (From Project file from Núcleo UNIFESP Core/Metuia Network.)

collective assisted by occupational therapists. A good example of this strategy was, for some years, the collaboration that the METUIA/UFSCar Laboratory had in organising the Playful Conferences and the Municipal Conferences on the Rights of Children and Adolescents that were held in the city of São Carlos, Brazil. The objective was the integration of different actors and services, such as professionals, managers, and children and adolescents, involved in developing social policies. This integration would intend to debate solutions created together for children and adolescents care, through a participatory process.

In addition to social technologies, Pan et al. (2022) described four dimensions that intersect and inform the actions of social occupational therapy. To provide an illustration of each of these dimensions, the example of their use when applied to schools and their communities is used. The schools are used here as an important example of a social setting of occupational

therapy practice focusing on the institutional social dimension. The four dimensions are:

■ *Dealing with conflicts:* Conflict is inherent in the construction of democratic and participatory spaces. Therefore knowing how to mediate and find solutions to address such situations is part of the work of occupational therapists, requiring active listening and dialogue-silence as essential resources to operate within this context. Based on Freire's principles, occupational therapists are guided by the principle of speaking with people rather than at them, consciously placing themselves on a horizontal relationship level, aiming to dismantle the historical authoritarianism that characterises vertical relationships. Another significant aspect of dealing with conflicts is the careful use of silence. Through this, occupational therapists can truly listen to the parties involved in the conflict, seeking to understand each person's perspective, as well as the origins and reasons behind the conflicts.

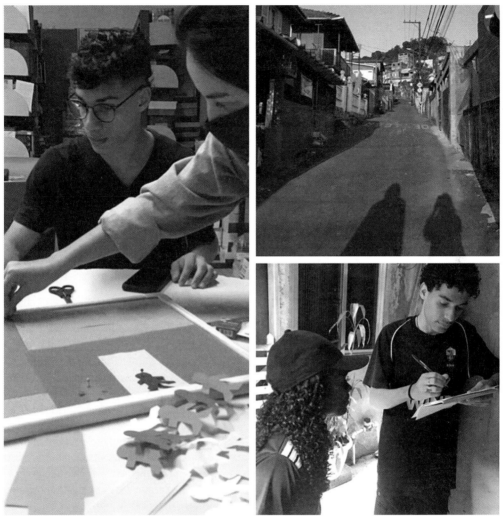

Fig. 4.3 ■ The project team for the 'Active and Democratic Care: Theoretical-Practical Subsidies for the Implementation of Policies to Support the Return and Permanence of Young People to School in the Post-Pandemic Context' project engaged in individual territorial follow-ups related activities. (From Project file from UNIFESP Core/Metuia Network.)

Therefore these principles should strive for a careful clarification of different understandings, negotiate solutions, and pursue a course of action that promotes conflict resolution.

■ *Sensitisation for working with adolescents and youth:* This is based on the dialogical principles of Freire (1979). The role of dialogue within the relationship between occupational therapists and teachers/educators and between occupational therapists and school principal is emphasised.

This is because the adolescent and youth generational phase is commonly perceived as a challenging period to navigate. Additionally, there is limited space for discussion and study about this generation in the curriculum of teacher education programs, which predominantly form the school staff. As a result, perceptions and stereotypes about young people are brought into the work with this population, leading to strained relationships and conflicts.

- *Project management*: This refers to the creation, consultation and management of projects – whether or not they involve execution, monitoring and evaluation. It aims at addressing specific needs selected through dialogue, involving many partners, including young people, school professionals, professionals from other services, and managers from different levels and sectors.
- *Production of care*: Care is understood as an intense support for the maintenance of collective life with the purpose of making society more democratic (Tronto, 2007). To develop care actions, it is considered essential that individuals are actively engaged in this process, and it involves various actors and professionals.

Using the four social technologies and the four dimensions present in their actions, both 'workshops of activities, dynamics, and projects' and 'individual territorial follow-ups' have been widely used as methodological resources in different professional practices. In addition, they have been used also for participatory research, demonstrating richness in the materials accessed and gathered by these technologies (Pan et al., 2022; Pereira & Malfitano, 2014; Silva & Malfitano, 2021).

CONCLUSION

Reflecting on what has been achieved so far and where social occupational therapy stands as a field of professional practice and knowledge production, the following lessons have been learnt:

1. Everything is achieved through reflection and action, dialectically, as Paulo Freire suggested many years ago. Social occupational therapy is the culmination of a history marked by numerous political strategies and collective efforts. It has been developing in Brazil since the mid-1970s, with its principles reformulated at the end of the 1990s, and which gained academic and professional legitimacy throughout the 21st century. In some forums, foreign colleagues have indicated that, in their countries, social occupational therapy cannot exist due to 'local legislation' that prohibits this type of practice. It is crucial to remember that the creation of legislation is a product of historical struggles, and laws can be modified based on the prevailing forces that shape their evolution. The pressing questions then become:

   Can occupational therapy be envisioned to delve into policies and programs beyond the healthcare system?

   Can the potential contributions and, hence, the need for occupational therapy initiatives be backed by policies and programs from other sectors, such as social assistance/welfare, socio-juridical services, or the cultural sector?

   What collective efforts are required from occupational therapists to reshape laws and policies?

   And, importantly, do occupational therapists understand this as integral to their professional responsibilities?

2. The concept of the collective is pivotal in social occupational therapy. As programs/services have a myriad of demands, it is only natural that glimpses into these practices unfold within the context of collectives. This often gives rise to misunderstandings. While there is a prominent focus on collective endeavours, individual follow-ups play a significant role, closely intertwined with collectives in their unique territories. Yet, beyond the performative imagery of interventions, social occupational therapy seldom operates on an individual basis. The act of collectivising authorships, deeds and knowledge also counters the prevailing winds of academic individualisation and a historical era that prioritises the individual.

3. Nothing is truly complete, fully understood, or stagnant. Recognising this incompleteness is crucial because it drives occupational therapists towards seeking solutions. Gaps remain to be filled, despite the many significant advances in the social occupational therapy field and the vast accumulated work. For instance, there is a noticeable lack of studies and initiatives focusing on older people and people with disabilities, especially when these populations are intersected with matters of class, race, gender and religiosity.

Our journey continues to unfold, encompassing the paths we have traversed and those we have yet to explore in the future we envision.

REFERENCES

Almeida, M. C., & Soares, C. R. S. (2021). Occupational therapy and social assistance: Building a critical thinking about the field. In Lopes, R. E., & Malfitano, A. P. S. (Eds.), *Social occupational therapy: Theoretical and practical designs* (pp. 69–79). Elsevier.

Almeida, M. C., Soares, C. R. S., Barros, D. D., & Galvani, D. (2012). Processos e práticas de formalização da terapia ocupacional na assistência social: Alguns marcos e desafios [Formalization processes and practices of occupational therapy in social assistance: Landmarks and challenges]. *Brazilian Journal of Occupational Therapy, 20*(1), 33–41.

American Occupational Therapy Association (AOTA). (2002). Occupational therapy practice framework: Domain and process. *American Journal of Occupational Therapy, 56*, 609–639.

Barros, D. D., Ghirardi, M. I. G., & Lopes, R. E. (1999). Terapia ocupacional e sociedade [Occupational therapy and society]. *Revista de Terapia Ocupacional da Universidade de São Paulo, 10*(2–3), 71–76.

Barros, D. D., Ghirardi, M. I. G., & Lopes, R. E. (2005). Social occupational therapy: A socio-historical perspective. In F. Kronenberg, S. S. Algado, & N. Pollard (Eds.), *Occupational therapy without borders: Learning from the spirit of survivors* (1st ed., pp. 140–151). Elsevier Science/Churchill Livingstone.

Barros, D. D., Ghirardi, M. I. G, Lopes, R. E., & Galheigo, S. M. (2011). Brazilian experiences in social occupational therapy. In F. Kronenberg, N. Pollard, & D. Sakellariou (Eds.), *Occupational therapy without borders* (Vol 2): *Towards an ecology of occupation-based practices* (1st ed., pp. 209–215). Elsevier.

Barros, D. D., Lopes, R. E., Galheigo, S. M., & Galvani, D. (2005). The metuia project in Brazil: Ideas and actions that bind us together. In F. Kronenberg, S. S. Algado, & N. Pollard (Eds.), *Occupational therapy without borders: Learning from the spirit of survivors* (1st ed., pp. 402–413). Elsevier Science/Churchill Livingstone.

Barros, D. D., Lopes, R. E., Galheigo, S. M., & Galvani, D. (2008). Territoires de l'enfance au Brésil [Territories of childhood in Brazil]. *Ergothérapies (Montaigu), 31*, 47–56.

Barros, D. D., Lopes, R. E., Galheigo, S. M., & Galvani, D. (2023). Projeto casarão: Marco histórico, conceitual e do fazer em terapia ocupacional social [Big house project: Historical, conceptual and doing framework in social occupational therapy]. In A. Cavalcanti, & C. Galvão (Eds.), *Terapia ocupacional: Fundamentos e práticas [Occupational therapy: Fundamentals and practice]* (2nd ed., pp. 351–357). Guanabara Koogan.

Bezerra, W. C., Reis, S. C. C. A. G., & Lopes, R. E. (2023). Dos caminhos postos aos caminhos feitos: a trajetória sócio-histórica da terapia ocupacional no Brasil [From laid paths to made paths: The socio-historical trajectory of occupational therapy in Brazil]. In A. C. Guajardo, A. P. S. Malfitano, P. L. O. Borba, & R. E. Lopes (Eds.), *Historiografias en terapia ocupacional desde América del Sur [Historiographies in occupational therapy from South America].* In press.

Borba, P. L. O., Pereira, P. B., & Lopes, R. E. (2021). Offenses, school and professionals roles: complex Complex plots in fragile relations. *Pró-Posições, 32*, e20180099.

Brazil. (2004). Política Nacional de Assistência Social [*National Policy of Social Assistance/Welfare*]. Brasília: MDS.

Castel, R. (2003). *From manual workers to wage laborers: transformation of the social question* (Richard R. Boyd, Ed ed., & Translation). Routledge.

Costa, L. A., Pollard, N., dos Santos, E. F., Campos, M. C. R., & Silva, H. R. (2023). Mapping intervention practices in social occupational therapy in Brazil. *Scandinavian Journal of Occupational Therapy, 30*(7), 970–991. https://doi.org/10.1080/11038128.2023.2198332.

Dagnino, R. (2009). *Tecnologia social: Ferramenta para construir outra sociedade [Social tecnology: Tool to build another society]* (pp. 95). Unicamp.

Drummond, A. F., & Cruz, D. M. C. (2018). History of occupational therapy in Brazil: Inequalities, advances, and challenges. *Annals of International Occupational Therapy, 1*(2), 103–112.

Egan, M., & Restall, G. (2022). *The Canadian model of occupational participation.* In M. Egan and G. Restall (eds). *Promoting occupational participation: Collaborative relationship-focused occupational therapy* (pp. 73–95). Ottawa: Canadian Association of Occupational Therapists.

Farias, L., & Aldrich, R. (2021). Critical theory: Resources for questioning and transforming everyday life. In S. Taff (Ed.), *Philosophy and occupational therapy: Informing education, research, and practice* (pp. 155–162). Slack.

Farias, M. N., & Lopes, R. E. (2022). Social occupational therapy, anti-oppression and freedom: Considerations about the revolution of/in everyday life. *Brazilian Journal of Occupational Therapy, 30*(spe), e3100.

Freire, P. (1979). *Extensão ou comunicação? [Service assistance or comunication].* Paz e Terra.

Gadotti, M. (2017). *Extensão universitária: Para quê? [Service assistance: for what?].* Instituto Paulo Freire.

Gramsci, A. (1971). *Selections from the prison notebooks.* International Publishers.

Gramsci, A. (1994). *Concepção dialética da História [Dialectical conception of History]* (2ª. Edição). Civilização Brasileira.

Harvey, M., Piñones-Rivera, C., & Holmes, S. M. (2022). Thinking with and against the social determinants of health: The Latin American social medicine (collective health) critique from Jaime Breilh. *International Journal of Health Services, 52*(4), 433–441.

Kielhofner, G. (2009). The early development of occupational therapy practice: The preparadigm and occupation paradigm period. In G. Kielhofner (Ed.), *Conceptual foundations of occupational therapy practice* (pp. 15–29). F.A. Davis Co.

Laliberte-Rudman, D. (2013). Enacting the critical potential of occupational science: Problematizing the 'Individualizing of Occupation'. *Journal of Occupational Science, 20*(4), 298–313.

Law, M. (1991). The environment: A focus for occupational therapist. *Canadian Journal of Occupational Therapy, 58*(4), 171–180.

Lopes, R. E., Malfitano, A. P. S., Silva, C. R., & Borba, P. L. O. (2011). Redes Sociais, Espaços Públicos e Cidadania: Políticas e Ações com a Juventude [Social Networks, Public Spaces and Citizenship: Policies and Actions with Youth]. In: IX Congresso Latino-Americano de Terapia Ocupacional e XII Congresso Brasileiro de Terapia Ocupacional, 2011, São Paulo. Brazilian Journal of Occupational Therapy – Congress proceedings – 19(1–10).

Lopes, R. E., Malfitano, A. P. S., Silva, C. R., & Borba, P. L. O. (2014). Recursos e tecnologias em terapia ocupacional social: ações com jovens pobres na cidade [Resources and technologies in Social Occupational Therapy: actions with the poor youth in town]. *Cadernos de Terapia Ocupacional da UFSCar [Brazilian Journal of Occupational Therapy], 22*(3), 591–602.

Lopes, R. E., & Borba, P. L. O. (2022). *Terapia ocupacional, educação e juventudes: Conhecendo práticas e reconhecendo saberes [Occupational therapy, education and youth: Knowing practices and recognizing knowledge].* EdUFSCar.

Lopes, R. E., & Malfitano, A. P. S. (2021). *Social occupational therapy: Theoretical and practical designs*. Elsevier.

Lopes, R. E., Cardoso Duarte, M. L. M., Pereira, B. P., Oliver, F. C., & Malfitano, A. P. S. (2016). A divulgação do conhecimento em terapia ocupacional no Brasil: Um retrato nos seus periódicos [Knowledge dissemination in occupational therapy in Brazil: A portrait in its journals]. *Brazilian Journal of Occupational Therapy, 24*(4), 777–789.

Lopes, R. E., Malfitano, A. P. S., Silva, C. R., & Borba, P. L. O. (2021). Resources and technologies in social occupational therapy: Actions with poor youth. In R. E. Lopes, & A. P. S. Malfitano (Eds.), *Social occupational therapy: Theoretical and practical designs* (pp. 164–176). Elsevier.

Lopes, R. E. & Malfitano, A. P. S. (2016). Terapia ocupacional social: desenhos teóricos e contornos práticos [*Social Occupational Therapy: Theoretical Designs and Practical Contours*]. EdUFSCar, Brazil.

Lopes, R. E. & Malfitano, A. P. S. (2023). Terapia ocupacional social: desenhos teóricos e contornos práticos [*Social Occupational Therapy: Theoretical Designs and Practical Contours*]. 2nd ed. EdUFSCar, Brazil.

Malfitano, A. P. S. (2021). Social context and social actions: Generalizations and specificities in occupational therapy. In R. E. Lopes, & A. P. S. Malfitano (Eds.), *Social occupational therapy: Theoretical and practical designs* (pp. 48–56). Elsevier.

Malfitano, A. P. S. (2022). An anthropophagic proposition in occupational therapy knowledge: Driving our actions towards social life. *World Federation of Occupational Therapists Bulletin, 78*(2), 70–82.

Malfitano, A. P. S., Borba, P. L. O., & Lopes, R. E. (2023). Palavras, conceitos e contextos históricos e culturais: A pluralidade na terapia ocupacional [Words, concepts, and cultural and historical contexts: Plurality in occupational therapy]. *Revista Ocupación Humana, 23*(2), 104–119.

Malfitano, A., & Lopes, R. (2018). Social occupational therapy: Committing to social change. *New Zealand Journal of Occupational Therapy, 65*(1), 20–26.

Marxists Internet Archive Encyclopedia. (2023). *Encyclopedia of Marxism*. Retrieved May 29, 2022, from https://www.marxists.org/glossary/index.htm.

Oliveira, M. L., & Malfitano, A. P. S. (2021). O Sistema Único de Assistência Social e os trabalhadores na Política Nacional Assistência social: Um enfoque às terapeutas ocupacionais [The unified social assistance system and workers in the national social assistance policy: An approach to occupational therapists]. *Serviço Social em Revista, 24*, 148–169.

Pais, J. M. (1993). *Nas rotas do quotidiano [On everyday life routes]* Revista Crítica de Ciências Sociais, Portugal.

Pan, L. C. (2019). *Entrelaçando pontos—de De fora para dentro, de dentro para fora: Ação e formação da terapia ocupacional social na escola pública [Interweaving points—From the outside in, from the inside out: Action and education in social occupational therapy in public schools]*. Doctoral Thesis. Post-graduate Program in Occupational Therapy. Federal University of São Cralos. Available on: https://repositorio.ufscar.br/handle/ufscar/11980.

Pan, L. C., & Lopes, R. E. (2022). Action and formation of social occupational therapy with young people in public schools. *Brazilian Journal of Occupational Therapy, 30*, e2810. https://doi.org/10.1590/2526-8910.ctoAO21252810.

Pan, L. C., Borba, P. L. O., & Lopes, R. E. (2022). Recursos e metodologias para o trabalho de terapeutas ocupacionais na e em relação com a escola pública [Resources and methodologies for the work of occupational therapists in and in relation to public schools]. In R. E. Lopes, & P. L. O. Borba (Eds.), *Terapia ocupacional, educação e juventudes: Conhecendo práticas e reconhecendo saberes [Occupational therapy, education and youth: knowing practices and recognizing knowledge]* (pp. 97–126). EdUFSCar.

Pereira, P. E., & Malfitano, A. P. S. (2014). Olhos de ver, ouvidos de ouvir, mãos de fazer: Oficinas de atividades em Terapia Ocupacional como método de coleta de dados. [Eyes to see, ears to hear, hands to do: Activity workshops on Therapy Occupacional as a data-gathering method]. *Interface Botucatu Online, 18*(49), 415–422.

Pollard, N., Sakellariou, D., & Kronenberg, F. (2008). *A political practice of occupational therapy*. Elsevier /Churchill Livingston.

Reis, S. C. C. A. G., & Lopes, R. E. (2018). The beginning of the trajectory of occupational therapy academic institutionalization in Brazil: What pioneer professors tell about the creation of the first courses. *Brazilian Journal of Occupational Therapy, 26*(2), 255–270.

Silva, M. J., & Malfitano, A. P. S. (2021). Oficinas de atividades, dinâmicas e projetos em terapia ocupacional social como estratégia para a promoção de espaços públicos [Activities workshops, dynamics and projects in social occupational therapy as a strategy for the promotion of public spaces]. *Interface Botucatu Online, 25*, e200055.

Soares, L. B. T. (1991). *Terapia Ocupacional: Lógica do capital ou do trabalho? [Occupational therapy: Logic of capital or work?]*. Editora Hucitec.

Spiegel, J. M., Breilh, J., & Yassi, A. (2015). Why language matters: Insights and challenges in applying a social determination of health approach in a North-South collaborative research program. *Globalization and Health, 11* Article 9.

Taff, S. D., & Putnam, L. (2022). Northern philosophies and professional neocolonialism in occupational therapy: A historical review and critique. *Brazilian Journal of Occupational Therapy, 30*, e2986.

Teoh, J. Y., & Iwama, M. K. (2015). *The Kawa model made easy: A guide to applying the Kawa Model in occupational therapy practice* (2nd ed.). www.kawamodel.com.

Townsend, E. A., & Polatajko, H. J. (2007). *Enabling occupation II: Advancing an occupational therapy vision for health, well-being, & justice through occupation*. CAOT Publications ACE.

Tronto, J. (2007). Assistência democrática e democracias assistenciais [Democratic assistance and welfare democracies]. *Sociedade e Estado, 22*(2), 285–308.

REFLECTION

1. Why is 'social context' important to occupational therapy practice?

2. How would you define social occupational therapy?

3. What is the relevance of critical perspectives in occupational therapy practices?

5

ANALYSING THE PRACTICE CONTEXT: A CRITICAL STEP IN MEETING PROFESSIONAL OBLIGATIONS

ANDREW R. FREEMAN

Overview

Although occupational therapists, like other health professionals, must satisfy several obligations (e.g. legal, ethical, research-informed), meeting these obligations is not necessarily straightforward. Significant challenges can exist for occupational therapists related to the context in which their practice is carried out. The objective of this chapter is to describe contextual trends that can contribute to these challenges, and to propose how the practice context can be analysed. Understanding contextual trends includes recognising the influence of three competing overarching logics – professionalism, managerialism and consumerism – and the tensions between them. A four-step analysis process of the context in which occupational therapists' practice is situated is described, which incorporates three theoretical perspectives – accountability, ethical and professional-as-worker. The ability of occupational therapists to analyse the context in which their practice is situated, and its influence on their practice, is an essential step towards meeting their professional obligations.

KEY POINTS

- Significant challenges exist for occupational therapists to meet their professional obligations related to the context in which their practice is carried out.

- Occupational therapists' ability to analyse their practice context is an essential step towards meeting their obligations.

- It is important to understand the potential influence on the practice of three competing overarching *logics* – professionalism, managerialism and consumerism – and the tensions between them.

■ Occupational therapists' practice can be analysed using a four-step process, which incorporates three theoretical perspectives – accountability, ethical and professional-as-worker.

■ Part of occupational therapists' analysis of the indirect influence of the context on their practice should include *critical reflexivity*, that is, the identification of their own values and assumptions, and their potential influence on their practice.

INTRODUCTION

Occupational therapists, like other health professionals, must satisfy multiple obligations; for example, providing collaborative relationship-focused and research-informed practice, and meeting ethical and legal responsibilities. For various reasons, meeting these obligations is not necessarily straightforward (Freeman et al., 2009). Although new graduates have reported experiencing challenges meeting their obligations in their transition to practice (Gray et al., 2012; Jones et al., 2022; Moir et al., 2021), significant challenges can exist for all occupational therapists related to the context in which their practice is carried out (Carrier et al., 2015; Freeman et al., 2009; Murray et al., 2015). The focus of this chapter is to describe contextual trends that contribute to the challenges of meeting professional obligations and propose how the practice context can be analysed. In this chapter, the term *practice context* is used to refer both to the immediate context in which services are provided (e.g. organisation level) and the broader policy, funding and societal contexts within which services are situated.

It has long been understood that considering the various components of the environment of individuals and collectives is an intrinsic part of occupational therapists' practice to support these individuals and collectives' attainment of their occupational goals (Law, 1991). This notion is integrated into various occupational therapy models, such as the Canadian Model of Occupational Participation (Egan & Restall, 2022) (refer to Chapter 11). This understanding of the role of the environment has evolved to include recognition of its influence on occupational therapists' practice including, in recent years, the influence of certain overarching philosophies within the societal context, for example, neoliberalism and colonialism (Trentham et al., 2022). This chapter's

orientation regarding the interface between occupational therapists' practice and the context in which it is carried out can be summarised as follows: professional practice is carried out in, and inevitably influenced (positively and negatively) by, a context, which is socially and historically constructed.

Some authors' focus on the practice context has been more proximal, for example, practice within acute care hospitals (Britton et al., 2015) or the influence of organisational social processes (Krusen, 2011), and other authors have used a more distal, macro-level orientation, for example, the influence on occupational therapy practice of global reimbursement approaches (Jongbloed & Wendland, 2002), legislation (Fisher & Friesema, 2013) or policy (Lencucha & Shikako-Thomas, 2019). The focus of this chapter is not on a specific practice sector nor environmental element. Rather, its perspective is that occupational therapists' ability to analyse the context in which their practice is situated, and its influence on their practice, is an essential step towards meeting professional obligations.

CONTEXTUAL TRENDS THAT CAN INFLUENCE OCCUPATIONAL THERAPY PRACTICE

The health care context in many countries is characterised by resource pressures. For example, in 2019, Organisation for Economic Co-operation and Development (OECD) countries used, on average, around 8.8% of their gross domestic product on health care (Organisation for Economic Co-operation and Development, 2021). In one specific country example, Canada, health care expenditure comprised between 30% and 40% of provincial and territorial budgets (Canadian Medical Association, 2022). There are ongoing upward pressures on health resources associated with technology (Callahan, 2009), potential contributions to resource demands associated with an ageing population (World Health Organization, 2015), and an increased prevalence of noncommunicable diseases (World Health Organization, 2005, 2013). Although some of these pressures reflect elements that are possibly universal (e.g. technology), they can also reflect the prioritisation of approaches, for example, hospital and other biomedically oriented services. Health care systems are subject to considerable ongoing resource pressures. It is relevant to note that some jurisdictions have insufficient human resources (World Health Organization, 2016); ironically, therefore, although there might be adequate funding, sufficient personnel are not necessarily available to provide the services.

One consequence of resource pressures includes increased external administrative controls on professional practice that are exercised by health service funders and managers (Flood, 2018; Nancarrow & Borthwick, 2021). These controls can be explicit, for example, a specific restriction on the nature of the services that can be offered. They also can be implicit, for example, despite no explicit restriction on the services to be offered, a very high caseload can oblige an occupational therapist to restrict services.

In addition to resource pressures, several factors have contributed to the tendency towards increased external controls on health professionals' practice, and in some instances, also on professions. These factors include concerns about safety (Baker, 2012), and insufficiently justified variability in professional practice (Wennberg & Thomson, 2011). At the broader profession level, concerns have arisen in some jurisdictions about ethical lapses by some professionals and, in turn, about the effectiveness of professional licensing bodies in ensuring the quality of their members' practice (Baker, 2004; The Canadian Press, 2017). As one example of a response to this type of concern, in 2017 the provincial Quebec (Canada) government adopted the *Loi modifiant diverses lois concernant principalement l'admission aux professions et la gouvernance du système professionnel* [Act to amend various statutes mainly concerning admission to the professions and the governance of the professional system]. This law made education in ethics and professional conduct mandatory both for candidates to the professions and individuals in leadership positions of the professional licensing bodies (e.g. Board of directors), as well as requiring certain adjustments in how these organisations function.

There is frequently an interplay among the contextual trends, for example, human resource-related pressures and concerns about safety, and the subsequent responses. As well, given the considerable variability across the world in the development and organisation of the occupational therapy profession and its services (Freeman et al., 2022), the presence and degree of influence of the various contextual trends, and responses to these trends, most likely vary.

THE GLOBAL CONTEXT FOR PROFESSIONAL PRACTICE: THREE COMPETING LOGICS

As the sociologist Eliot Freidson (2001) explained, the societal context in which health professionals practise is situated includes three competing overarching logics: *professionalism*, *managerialism* and *consumerism*. Logics can be thought of as global orientations. Freidson discussed the importance of recognising the influence of, and tensions among, these logics.

Professionalism is situated within the contract between the professions and society. That is, in return for professions' right to regulate themselves and maintain exclusivity (e.g. only those with an appropriate occupational therapy qualification are eligible for occupational therapy positions), they must ensure that their members maintain certain service standards. Consistent with this premise, professionals use various types of information (e.g. research, professional reasoning, experience) to recommend the best course of action for individuals and collectives. In exchange for this autonomy, they must be able to account for their actions (e.g. to the professional licensing body).

Klikauer (2015, p. 1105) provided the following definition of *managerialism*:

> *Managerialism combines management's generic tools and knowledge with ideology to establish itself systemically in organizations, public institutions and society while depriving business owners (property), workers (organizational-economic) and civil society (social-political) of all decision-making powers. Managerialism justifies the application of its one-dimensional managerial techniques to all areas of work, society, and capitalism on the grounds of superior ideology, expert training and the exclusiveness of managerial knowledge necessary to run public institutions and society as corporations.*

According to this logic, hierarchical authority is privileged to identify, distribute, supervise and control the execution of specialised tasks in organisations (Freidson, 2001). Consistent with this premise, the virtue, for example, of efficiency through standardisation is favoured. Many manifestations of managerialism exist within the healthcare system, including the use of management tools and performance indicators to document professionals' productivity. The widespread use of the *Lean* management approach, which is aimed at developing systems that consume fewer resources while delivering superior results (Parkhi, 2019), is an example of the managerialist logic.

Consumerism refers to the privileging of consumer interests: 'In consumer societies, consumers gain power and authority at the expense of producers, whether these are producers of goods or professionals offering a service' (Abercrombie et al., 2000, p. 71). One might use the following well-known expression to sum up this logic: 'the customer is always right'. Consistent with this perspective, an individual might, for example, insist that the occupational therapist provide a specific adaptive device, indicating that the request should be supported because 'the occupational therapist works for the consumer'. It is important to note the distinction between consumerism and collaborative relationship-focused practice (refer to Chapter 12); this latter orientation includes the use of the expertise of both individuals and collectives about their own lives and therapists' expertise based on, for example, research, professional reasoning and experience (Restall & Egan, 2022).

From professionals' perspectives, both managerial and consumerist logics are antithetical. Regarding managerialism, a standardised approach, for example, is contrary to one of the essential characteristics of professional practice, the use of discretionary judgement to ensure that the needs of the individual and collective are responded to. Regarding consumerism, this logic minimises the importance of professionals' expertise. The recognition of this latter risk is reflected, for example, in the restriction in some jurisdictions on direct advertising of prescription drugs, which can be associated with undue pressure on physicians (Mintzes, 2009).

Despite these reservations, it is highly likely that all three logics will continue to influence the landscape in which professional practice is carried out. To a certain extent, this situation is probably justified. As noted earlier, professionals and professions have not always fully respected their contract with society. Furthermore, as Morreim (2001) has argued, that given the various important upward pressures on costs associated with contemporary professional practice, for example, the use of technology (e.g. adaptive equipment, home modifications), it is not reasonable to presume that professionals should be the sole arbiters of how society's resources are used.

These considerations highlight the need to arrive at definitions, agreed upon across stakeholders (e.g. professionals, managers, funders, professional licensing bodies), regarding the nature and amount of services that can be provided, and the necessary level of professional autonomy required to meet this standard (Côté & Freeman, 2023). Although some limits on professional practice are probably inevitable, some of these are reasonable. For example, while continuing to recognise the need for discretionary judgement, the standardisation of best practices can be very helpful both for enhancing practice quality and maximising efficiency (Swan et al., 2010). Nevertheless, care must be taken not to 'throw the baby out with the bathwater' regarding the importance both of professionals' discretionary judgement and their relationships with individuals (Morreim, 2001). To find the right balance professionals must respect certain principles: resources should be used as efficiently as possible, each profession's scope of practice should be optimised within inter-professional teams (Nelson et al., 2014), the benefits of technology must be fully exploited (Liu, 2018), legal and ethical standards must be adhered to, and, finally, citizens have a pivotal role to play in decisions about their care (Britnell, 2015).

There is considerable debate regarding how the health professional role should be defined in contemporary societies (Saks, 2021). For example, greater clarity regarding professionals' and professions' social responsibility, and the associated roles, is being promoted (Boelen, 2016); this orientation is consistent with the evolution taking place in occupational therapy (Egan & Restall, 2022). Some commentators have proposed that a modified form of professionalism is evolving that incorporates organisational and managerial logics (Noordegraaf, 2015). At the more extreme end of the continuum of ideas, some commentators have suggested that the professions and professional practice as they are currently known will evolve into something quite different given, among other factors, advances in technology (e.g. artificial intelligence) and citizens' access to knowledge via the Internet (Susskind & Susskind, 2015).

TABLE 5.1	
Describing Your Practice	
Component	**Example**
Describe access to your services (e.g. eligibility criteria, waiting times)	■ Eligibility criteria for services include imminent safety risks and compromised autonomy in self-care and mobility. ■ The average waiting time to receive services is two months, although individuals experiencing imminent safety risks receive services more quickly.
Describe the precise scope of services offered	■ To primarily address challenges related to safety risks and autonomy in self-care and mobility.
Time – duration of each appointment and total number of appointments	■ There are no explicit restrictions. ■ However, occupational therapists are expected to work as quickly as possible given the waiting list. ■ Occupational therapists must complete statistics regarding the services provided.
The approach used for providing services *Direct* services: include evaluation followed by direct intervention. *Consultative* services: evaluation is followed only by recommendations to be implemented by third parties (e.g. family member, teacher).	■ Consultative services: assessment, recommendations, and follow-up as necessary to ensure that recommendations (e.g. modifications, technical aids) are implemented.

In summary, within the global societal context, professional practice is subject to several pressures, overarching logics and the tensions between them. It is important for occupational therapists, in their efforts to maximise the quality of their services, to recognise and respond to these elements. The underlying premise of this exercise is that the context in which their professional practice is carried out is historically and socially constructed. Consistent with this premise, it is pertinent for occupational therapists to ask why contextual elements exist as they do.

ANALYSING THE PRACTICE CONTEXT: FOUR STEPS

Having considered these macro-level contextual influences on professional practice, the focus now moves to a four-step micro-level analysis of the interface between practice and the context in which it is situated. Further details of this analysis process can be found in Freeman and Jauvin (2019) and Freeman and colleagues (2023).

Step 1: Describing Your Practice

As summarised in Table 5.1, the first step is to describe the access to, nature of, and approach used to provide services.

Step 2: Describing How the Context Directly Influences Practice

The second step is to describe the specific mechanisms in place that influence the access to, the nature of, and the approach used in the services provided. Mechanisms refer to the processes by which the influence takes place, for example, a referral form. It also is helpful to identify at which of the following levels each mechanism is situated (Carrier et al., 2013):

1. Legislative level: legislation and case law.
2. Regulatory level: regulations associated with the laws.
3. Administrative level: policies and directives.
4. Organisational level: the organisation of work (e.g. waiting list policy).

Table 5.2 provides examples of mechanisms and associated levels.

Step 3: Reasons for the Mechanisms that Are in Place

The third step is to identify why the identified mechanisms are in place. Various explanations are possible, for example:

■ Limiting resource allocation.
■ Maximising the efficiency of resource use.
■ Underlying paradigm (e.g. biomedical) guiding the services.

TABLE 5.2		
Examples of Mechanisms that Influence Practice and Associated Levels		
Mechanism	**Purpose**	**Level**
Canada Health Act, L.R.C. (1985), ch. C-6	In comparison to medically necessary services, there is a highly limited inclusion of rehabilitation services in this federal law that underpins the public health insurance system (Medicare) in Canada.	Legislative
Règlement sur les appareils suppléant à une déficience physique et assurés, R.R.Q., ch. A-29, r. 4 (Regulation respecting devices for physical impairment and insured persons), Quebec (Canada)	This regulation, which is associated with the *Loi sur l'assurance-maladie L.R.Q., ch. A-29* (Heath Insurance Act), specifies the nature of assistive devices that can be funded by public health insurance for individuals.	Regulatory
Ministry of Health productivity guidelines	Requires therapists to provide data regarding how many individuals receive direct services/month, and how much time is spent with each individual. Does not include data regarding the supervision of occupational therapy students.	Administrative
Referral form for occupational therapy services	Criteria for referral include an individual's safety or autonomy in personal care and mobility.	Organisational

It is not always possible to be certain about the reasons. However, it is important to gain as much clarity as possible because this understanding will maximise occupational therapists' ability to respond strategically. For example, occupational therapists in an organisation might believe that the productivity requirements that they are required to satisfy are problematic insofar as they only capture a limited range of possible services that the therapists could provide. However, if these requirements, despite being applied at the organisational level, are in fact based on Ministry-level policies, occupational therapists' advocacy efforts to modify the requirements would need to take this into account.

Step 4: Thinking About the Direct and Indirect Influence on Professional Practice Using Three Theoretical Perspectives

As noted earlier, external controls on professional practice can be explicit or implicit. Furthermore, the influence may be direct, for example, a reduced scope of service (Carrier et al., 2015), or indirect due to the negative effects on professionals (e.g. burnout) (Braithwaite et al., 2017).

The following three theoretical lenses are useful for analysing the impact of the practice context on occupational therapy practice: *accountability*, *ethical* and *professional-as-worker*. For a detailed explanation of these perspectives, see Freeman and Jauvin (2019).

Briefly, the *accountability* perspective is consistent with the premise that occupational therapists must account for their autonomy in the use of expert knowledge in the service of others (Saks, 2021). Meeting this obligation is not simple (Cronqvist et al., 2001; Freeman et al., 2009), particularly as occupational therapists may have to respond to different expectations from multiple stakeholders (e.g. employer, professional licensing body). This could lead to undesirable consequences, such as being held responsible for outcomes over which they have limited control (e.g. incongruent documentation obligations) (Adams, 2002).

Professional practice is an *ethical* undertaking (Drolet, 2018). An ethical dilemma confronting many occupational therapists concerns the determination of the resources to which each individual is entitled versus the rights to services of the broader population (Shortell et al., 1998), and which services are privileged in the attribution of resources (Hughes & Light, 2002). Occupational therapists and other health professionals have reported ethical tensions, and the accompanying ethical distress (Austin, 2016), associated with the quality of services they can provide to individuals (Durocher et al., 2016; Penny et al., 2019).

The third theoretical perspective, *professional-as-worker*, permits professionals to analyse the practice context with respect to organisational imperatives and workers' access to conditions that allow them to

	TABLE 5.3	
	Analysis Questions Using Three Theoretical Perspectives	
Accountability Lens	**Ethical Lens**	**Professional-as-Worker Lens**
<ul><li>To which stakeholders are occupational therapists accountable and what are their obligations?</li><li>What difficulties are occupational therapists experiencing in satisfying their accountability obligations to different stakeholders?</li></ul>	<ul><li>What is the nature of the occupational therapy services available to individuals and collectives and the access to these services?</li><li>What difficulties are occupational therapists experiencing in providing the quality of services that they believe individuals and collectives should receive?</li></ul>	<ul><li>What are the organisational conditions (e.g. workload relative to resources available) in place that permit occupational therapists to carry out their mandate while maintaining their well-being?</li><li>What difficulties are occupational therapists experiencing in maintaining their well-being in the process of carrying out their job?</li></ul>

maintain their well-being while meeting their obligations. This analysis lens enables a reflection of work conditions in relation to the transformation in management practices that have occurred over recent decades and how these new norms (e.g. 'do more with less') (De Gaulejac, 2009) affect the subjective experience of work.

As illustrated in Table 5.3, a structured approach can be used to consider these perspectives in the analysis of the practice context (Freeman & Jauvin, 2019).

Applying these three lenses allows occupational therapists to focus on particular dimensions of their practice context. Although each of these lenses offers a useful perspective, the use of all three permits professionals to conduct a comprehensive analysis.

Examples of potential responses to occupational therapists' questions of their analysis are provided in Table 5.4 (Freeman et al., 2023). It is important to recognise that the influence of the context on practice can both be positive and negative. In other words, responding strategically following the analysis of this influence may well include both elements that require change but also existing strengths that can be reinforced.

CRITICAL REFLEXIVITY

Early in the chapter, reference was made to the influence of certain overarching notions within the societal context, for example, neoliberalism and colonialism. Subsequently, the influence of three logics (professionalism, managerialism and consumerism) and three theoretical perspectives (accountability lens, ethical lens, and professional-as-worker lens) useful for reflecting on the impact on professional practice of the context in which it is situated, were presented. A final element to mention

concerns the influence on professional practice of occupational therapists' own values and assumptions. These elements are part of the practice context as occupational therapists, as members of the respective societies in which they have grown up and live, are inevitably influenced by their values and assumptions (e.g. colonialism, neoliberalism) (Restall & Egan, 2022). In turn, consistent with the point made earlier about the importance of recognising both the positive and negative influences of the context on practice, occupational therapists' values and assumptions can exert both a positive and negative influence. Therefore part of occupational therapists' analysis of the indirect influence of the context on their practice, including their ability to satisfy their professional obligations, should include the identification of their own values and assumptions, and the potential influence these have on their practice. This process is known as *critical reflexivity*: 'A process of recognizing one's own position in the world in order both to better understand the limitations of one's knowing and to better appreciate the social realities of others' (Ng et al., 2019, p. 1123). Various processes have been proposed to assist health professionals in this reflection process, for example, Nixon and colleagues' (2017) *Seven-Step Framework for Critical Analysis*. Readers are invited to avail themselves of this and similar excellent resources.

RESPONDING FOLLOWING ANALYSIS

Occupational therapists' motivation for analysing the context in which their practice is situated is to satisfy their professional obligations. Based on their analysis, various possibilities exist for how they might respond. A detailed explanation of these possibilities and how

TABLE 5.4		
Analysis of Positive and Negative Impacts (Freeman et al., 2023)		
Question	**Explanation**	**Example**
What are the DIRECT impacts on the quality of your services?	The impacts, both positive and negative, of the practice context on the quality of services are explored (e.g. access to services, service offer, time available, approach used to provide services).	**Positive impacts** ■ An increased clarity regarding the use of the appropriate services according to the needs of individuals and collectives. ■ There is an attempt to balance the demand associated with providing sufficient services to individuals versus providing reasonable access for the collective population. ■ Minimising the need for individuals to be hospitalised. **Negative impacts** ■ The possibility is ignored that providing truly collaborative relationship-based services could be more effective and efficient in the long term. ■ The occupational therapy role is reduced, thus both limiting opportunities for individuals and collectives and underutilising professional competencies.
What are the INDIRECT impacts on the quality of your services?	What difficulties are you experiencing in meeting your obligations (e.g. ethical, legal) to relevant stakeholders (e.g. professional licensing body, employers)?	Many occupational therapists are concerned about the quality of the services they can provide to individuals and collectives. It may feel like a limited version of occupational therapy and that they will not necessarily be able to address the expressed needs of individuals and collectives. Difficulties in providing collaborative relationship-based practice can make it challenging for occupational therapists to meet their ethical obligations.
	What difficulties are you experiencing in maintaining your well-being in the performance of your professional role?	Although the therapists understand funding pressures and the associated challenges in responding to the range of occupational goals of individuals and collectives, they feel frustrated and disheartened about these changes, believing they cannot do authentic occupational therapy.
	What are the organisational conditions (e.g. workload in relation to available resources) in place that allow you to perform your duties while maintaining your well-being?	Although the service priorities might streamline the occupational therapists' practice with each individual and collective, there may be concerns that these limits will dilute their sense of accomplishment in their job. They are worried about having considerably less autonomy in being able to use their professional judgment in determining how best to address the needs of individuals and collectives, including their expressed needs. The occupational therapists may also be worried about the daily pressures associated with productivity requirements.

TABLE 5.5
Potential Actions Emerging from an Analysis

What actions could you take in the face of any difficulties identified related to:

■ Meeting your professional obligations?	■ Clarify with your professional licensing body and your organisation the barriers to meeting your professional obligations (e.g. documentation standards).
■ The quality of your services?	■ Provide a summary of the evidence (including economic evidence if available) regarding the occupational therapy role to the manager.
	■ Ensure that the distinct contribution of occupational therapy is identified.
	■ Propose adjustments to the referral form to better capture the distinct occupational therapy contribution.
■ Your well-being	■ Contact other occupational therapists working in a similar role to share ideas.
	■ To the extent possible, work in collaboration with other occupational therapists and other health professionals, do not act alone.

to maximise the impact of any actions undertaken. is beyond the scope of this chapter. However, an illustration of some possible orientations that might emerge from an occupational therapist's analysis is provided in Table 5.5 (Freeman et al., 2023).

CONCLUSION

The complexity of the contexts in which many occupational therapists' practice is situated is well documented (Fortune et al., 2013). As explained in this chapter, these contexts are subject to many influences. In occupational therapists' ongoing efforts to meet their obligations and to provide the best possible quality of service, a critical first step is that of carefully analysing the influence of the context on their practice. Although such an analysis does not guarantee occupational therapists will subsequently be able to change elements they believe are problematic, a thorough and considered analysis increases the likelihood of maximising the strategic nature of their approach.

REFERENCES

Abercrombie, N., Hill, S., & Turner, B. S. (2000). *The penguin dictionary of sociology* (4th ed.). Penguin Books.

Adams, B. (2002). Accountable but powerless. *Health Affairs, 21*(1), 218–223.

Austin, W. (2016). Contemporary healthcare practice and the risk of moral distress. *Healthcare Management Forum, 29*(3), 131–133. https://doi.org/10.1177/0840470416637835.

Baker, G. R. (2012). The challenges of making care safer: Leadership and system transformation. *Healthcare Quarterly, 15*(Special Issue), 8–11. https://doi.org/10.12927/hcq.2012.22848.

Baker, R. (2004). Implications of Harold Shipman for general practice. *Postgraduate Medical Journal, 80*(944), 303–306. https://doi.org/10.1136/pgmj.2003.013110.

Boelen, C. (2016). Why should social accountability be a benchmark for excellence in medical education. *Educación Médica, 17*(3), 101–105. https://doi.org/10.1016/j.edumed.2016.06.004.

Braithwaite, J., Herkes, J., Ludlow, K., Testa, L., & Lamprell, G. (2017). Association between organisational and workplace cultures, and patient outcomes: Systematic review. *BMJ Open, 2017,* e017708. https://doi.org/10.1136/bmjopen-2017-017708.

Britnell, M. (2015). *In search of the perfect health system*. Palgrave.

Britton, L., Rosenwax, L., & McNamara, B. (2015). Occupational therapy practice in acute physical hospital settings: Evidence from a scoping review. *Australian Occupational Therapy Journal, 62*(6), 370–377. https://doi.org/10.1111/1440-1630.12227.

Callahan, D. (2009). *Taming the beloved beast: How medical technology costs are destroying our health care system*. Princeton University Press.

Canadian Medical Association. (2022). *Health care funding in Canada*. Retrieved January 5, 2023, from https://www.cma.ca/news/health-care-funding-canada.

The Canadian Press. (2017). *Serial killer found guilty of professional misconduct by nursing college. National Post*. The Canadian Press. https://nationalpost.com/pmn/news-pmn/canada-news-pmn/convicted-serial-killer-faces-nurses-college-professional-misconduct-hearing/.

Carrier, A., Freeman, A. R., Levasseur, M., & Desrosiers, J. (2015). Standardised referral form: Restricting client-centred practice? *Scandinavian Journal of Occupational Therapy, 22*(4), 283–292. https://doi.org/10.3109/11038128.2015.1019922.

Carrier, A., Levasseur, M., Freeman, A. R., Mullins, G., Quénec'hdu, S., Lalonde, L., Gagnon, M., & Lacasse, F. (2013). Influence of societal and practice contexts on health professionals' clinical reasoning: A scoping study protocol. *BMJ Open, 3*(4), e002887. https://doi.org/10.1136/bmjopen-2013-002887.

Côté, N., & Freeman, A. R. (2023). L'évolution du travail professionnel dans le système de santé et de services sociaux: Enjeux et perspectives. In F. Gagnon, É. Martin, & M.-H. Morin (Eds.), *Le système de santé et de services sociaux au Québec: Territorialité et santé des populations* (pp. 135–156). Les Presses de l'Université du Québec.

Cronqvist, A., Burns, T., Theorell, T., & Lützén, K. (2001). Dissonant imperatives in nursing: A conceptualisation of stress in intensive care in Sweden. *Intensive and Critical Care Nursing, 17,* 228–236. https://doi.org/10.1054/iccn.2001.1588.

De Gaulejac, V. (2009). *La société malade de la gestion*. Points.

Drolet, M.-J. (2018). *Acting ethically? A theoretical framework and method designed to overcome ethical tensions in occupational therapy practice*. CAOT Publications ACE.

Durocher, E., Kinsella, E. A., McCorquodale, L., & Phelan, S. (2016). Ethical tensions related to systemic constraints: Occupational alienation in occupational therapy practice. *OTJR: Occupation, Participation & Health, 36*(4), 216–226. https://doi.org/10.1177/1539449216665117.

Egan, M., & Restall, G. (2022). The Canadian model of occupational participation. In M. Egan, & G. Restall (Eds.), *Promoting occupational participation: Collaborative relationship-focused occupational therapy* (pp. 73–95). CAOT Publications ACE.

Fisher, G., & Friesema, J. (2013). Implications of the affordable care act for occupational therapy practitioners providing services to Medicare recipients. *American Journal of Occupational Therapy, 67*(5), 502–506. https://doi.org/10.5014/ajot.2013.675002.

Flood, J. (2018). Professions and professional service firms in a global context: Reframing narratives. In M. Saks, & D. Muzio (Eds.), *Professions and professional service firms: Private and public sector enterprises in the global economy* (pp. 26–45). Routledge.

Fortune, T., Ryan, S., & Adamson, L. (2013). Transition to practice in supercomplex environments: Are occupational therapy graduates adequately prepared? *Australian Occupational Therapy Journal, 60*(3), 217–220. https://doi.org/10.1111/1440-1630.12010.

Freeman, A. R., & Jauvin, N. (2019). Analyzing the professional practice context using three lenses: An essential step for responding strategically. *Occupational Therapy in Health Care, 33*(2), 142–158. https://doi.org/10.1080/07380577.2018.1553086.

Freeman, A. R., Jauvin, N., Alain, V., & Marcoux, C. (2023). Analysing the context of professional practice: A conceptual framework for an effective response to maximise practice quality and meet professional obligations. *Occupational Therapy Now, 26*(1), 9–11.

Freeman, A. R., McKinstry, C., & Ledgerd, R. (2022). The context of occupational therapy internationally. In M. Egan, & G. Restall (Eds.), *Promoting occupational participation: Collaborative relationship-focused occupational therapy* (pp. 57–70). CAOT Publications ACE.

Freeman, A. R., McWilliam, C. L., MacKinnon, J. R., DeLuca, S., & Rappolt, S. G. (2009). Health professionals' enactment of their accountability obligations: Doing the best they can. *Social Science & Medicine, 69*, 1063–1071. https://doi.org/10.1016/j.socscimed.2009.07.025.

Freidson, E. (2001). *Professionalism: The third logic. On the practice of knowledge*. University of Chicago Press.

Gray, M., Clark, M., Penman, M., Smith, J., Bell, J., Thomas, Y., & Trevan-Hawke, J. (2012). New graduate occupational therapists' feelings of preparedness for practice in Australia and Aotearoa/New Zealand. *Australian Occupational Therapy Journal, 59*(6), 445–455. https://doi.org/10.1111/j.1440-1630.2012.01029.x.

Hughes, D., & Light, D. (Eds.). (2002). *Rationing: Constructed realities and professional practices*. Blackwell.

Jones, L., Fowler, D., Bialocerkowski, A., & Sheeran, N. (2022). Learning how to work in an interprofessional environment: How students transition to allied health professionals working interprofessionally. *Journal of Interprofessional Care, 36*(3), 419–427. https://doi.org/10.1080/13561820.2021.1950130.

Jongbloed, L., & Wendland, T. (2002). The impact of reimbursement systems on occupational therapy practice in Canada and the United States of America. *Canadian Journal of Occupational Therapy, 69*(3), 143–152. https://doi.org/10.1177/000841740206900304.

Klikauer, T. (2015). What is managerialism? *Critical Sociology, 41*(7–8), 1103–1119. https://doi.org/10.1177/0896920513501351.

Krusen, N. (2011). The influence of environment on clinical practice: Unspoken rules. *British Journal of Occupational Therapy, 74*(12), 546–553. https://doi.org/10.4276/030802211X13232584581335.

Law, M. (1991). 1991 Muriel driver lecture: The environment: A focus for occupational therapy. *Canadian Journal of Occupational Therapy, 58*(4), 171–179. https://doi.org/10.1177/000841749105800404.

Lencucha, R., & Shikako-Thomas, K. (2019). Examining the intersection of policy and occupational therapy: A scoping review. *Canadian Journal of Occupational Therapy, 86*(3), 185–195. https://doi.org/10.1177/0008417419833183.

Liu, L. (2018). Muriel Driver Memorial Lecture: Occupational therapy in the Fourth Industrial Revolution. *Canadian Journal of Occupational Therapy, 85*(4), 272–285. https://doi.org/10.1177/0008417418815179.

Mintzes, B. (2009). Should Canada allow direct-to-consumer advertising of prescription drugs? *Canadian Family Physician, 55*(2), 131–133.

Moir, E. M. A., Turpin, M. J., & Copley, J. A. (2021). The clinical challenges experienced by new graduate occupational therapists: A matrix review. *Canadian Journal of Occupational Therapy, 88*(3), 200–213. https://doi.org/10.1177/00084174211022880.

Morreim, E. H. (2001). *Holding health care accountable: Law and the new medical marketplace*. Oxford University Press.

Murray, C., Turpin, M., Edwards, I., & Jones, M. (2015). A qualitative meta-synthesis about challenges experienced in occupational therapy practice. *British Journal of Occupational Therapy, 78*(9), 534–546. https://doi.org/10.1177/0308022615586786.

Nancarrow, S., & Borthwick, A. (2021). *The allied health professions: A sociological perspective*. Policy Press.

Nelson, S., Turnbull, J., Bainbridge, L., Caulfield, T., Hudon, G., Kendel, D., Mowat, D., Nasmith, L., Postl, B., Shamian, J., & Sketris, I. (2014). Optimizing scopes of practice: New models of care for a new health care system. *Canadian Academy of Health Sciences*. https://cahs-acss.ca/optimizing-scopes-of-practice-new-models-of-care-for-a-new-health-care-system/.

Ng, S. K., Wright, S. R., & Kuper, A. M. (2019). The divergence and convergence of critical reflection and critical reflexivity: Implications for health professions education. *Academic Medicine, 94*(8), 1122–1128. https://doi.org/10.1097/ACM.0000000000002724.

Nixon, S. A., Yeung, E., Shaw, J. A., Kuper, A., & Gibson, B. E. (2017). Seven-step framework for critical analysis and its application in the field of physical therapy. *Physical Therapy, 97*(2), 249–257. https://doi.org/10.2522/ptj.20160149.

Noordegraaf, M. (2015). Hybrid professionalism and beyond: (New) forms of public professionalism in changing organizational and societal contexts. *Journal of Professions and Organization, 2*(2), 187–206. https://doi.org/10.1093/jpo/jov002.

Organisation for Economic Co-operation and Development. (2021). *Health at a glance: 2021 OECD indicators*. Author.

Parkhi, S. S. (2019). Lean management practices in the healthcare sector: A literature review. *Benchmarking: An International Journal, 26*(4), 1275–1289. https://doi.org/10.1108/BIJ-06-2018-0166.

Penny, N. H., Benjamin, T. M., Gonsalves, C. R., Gordon, A. L., Kinsley, E. N., & Markel, S. R. (2019). An investigation of the moral distress experienced by occupational therapy practitioners. *Annals of International Occupational Therapy, 2*(4), 161–170. https://doi.org/10.3928/24761222-20190625-02.

Restall, G., & Egan, M. (2022). Collaborative relationship-focused occupational therapy. In Egan, M., & Restall, G. (Eds.), *Promoting occupational participation: Collaborative relationship-focused occupational therapy* (pp. 97–117). CAOT Publications ACE.

Saks, M. (2021). *Professions: A key idea for business and society.* Routledge.

Shortell, S. M., Waters, T. M., Clarke, K. W. B., & Budetti, P. P. (1998). Physicians as double agents: Maintaining trust in an era of multiple accountabilities. *Journal of the American Medical Association, 280*, 1102–1108. https://doi.org/10.1001/jama.280.12.1102.

Susskind, R., & Susskind, D. (2015). *The future of the professions: How technology will transform the work of human experts.* Oxford University Press.

Swan, L., Boyes, H., Williams, K., Russell, D., & Campbell, S. (2010). Priority guideline development: A team building experience. *Occupational Therapy Now, 12*(2), 11–13.

Trentham, B., Laliberte Rudman, D., Smith, H., & Phenix, A. (2022). The socio-political and historical context of occupational therapy in Canada. In Egan, M., & Restall, G. (Eds.), *Promoting occupational participation: Collaborative relationship-focused occupational therapy* (pp. 31–55). CAOT Publications ACE.

Wennberg, J. E., & Thomson, P. Y. (2011). Time to tackle unwarranted variations in practice. *British Medical Journal, 342*, d1513. https://doi.org/10.1136/bmj.d1513.

World Health Organization. (2005). *Preparing a health care workforce for the 21st century: The challenge of chronic conditions.* World Health Organization.

World Health Organization. (2013). *Global action plan for the prevention and control of noncommunicable diseases 2013–2020.* World Health Organization.

World Health Organization. (2015). *World report on ageing and health.* World Health Organization.

World Health Organization. (2016). *Global strategy on human resources for health: Workforce 2030.* World Health Organization.

REFLECTION

1. What difficulties, if any, are experienced by occupational therapists in your region in meeting their professional obligations?

2. What trends exist in the context in which occupational therapists in your region are practising that might negatively impact their capacity to meet their professional obligations?

3. What examples can you think of in your region that illustrate managerialism and consumerism?

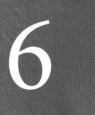

6 OCCUPATION

DEBBIE LALIBERTE RUDMAN ■ REBECCA M. ALDRICH

CHAPTER OUTLINE

Overview

Within this chapter, conceptualisations and assumptions related to the concept of occupation that guide occupational therapy practice and anchor occupational science research are outlined. Descriptions of an occupational perspective as well as occupation-based practice foreground deeper discussions of intertwined personal and environmental influences on occupational participation. Chapter themes include occupation as central to human living and occupational therapy practice; the evolution of knowledge about occupation; the importance of critical reflexivity and ongoing diversification of knowledge about occupation; occupation as situated, relational and political; and connections between occupational science knowledge and occupational therapy practice. Links to resources that can support continued learning about human occupation conclude this chapter.

KEY POINTS

- Occupation is central to human life at individual and collective levels.
- As professionals who are concerned with how human lives are lived, occupational therapists must remain informed about developments in knowledge about human occupation.
- Occupational science generates research about human occupation that complements, critiques, enhances and expands occupation-based occupational therapy practices.

■ Assumptions about occupation must be understood relative to the sociohistorical contexts in which they emerged.

■ Understandings about occupation must account for the multiplicity of factors that influence people's occupational participation.

■ Occupation has the potential to be a transformative force at individual, collective and societal levels.

INTRODUCTION

No understanding of occupational therapy or occupational science is complete without a definition of occupation; however, making sense of the myriad explanations of occupation can be a daunting task. Moreover, the global nature of occupational therapy and occupational science brings multiple linguistic and cultural elements into play when it comes to professional and disciplinary terminology. Yet, across the varied ways that occupation is conceived and conveyed, some core assumptions have emerged. This chapter addresses the centrality of occupation to occupational therapy, presents ideas about how occupation is experienced, organised and socially shaped, provides examples of how such knowledge about occupation informs occupational therapy practice, and points to the need for continued diversification of knowledge about the occupation. Taken together, the sections of this chapter demonstrate the ways in which occupation is fundamental to human life as well as to occupational therapy and occupational science, providing an entry point into the ever-growing knowledge base regarding occupation. A concluding list of selected resources offers readers additional pathways for lifelong learning about the occupation.

WHAT IS OCCUPATION?

Put in the simplest terms possible, occupations are the everyday actions and undertakings that define what it means to be a human being (Yerxa et al., 1990). Occupations can be so ordinary, such as getting dressed or completing homework (Clark et al., 1991), that people can 'do occupation all their lives, perhaps without ever knowing it' (Dickie, 2014, p. 2). Occupations also encompass extraordinary pursuits, such as preparing for a family holiday or running a marathon, that hold significance to a person or collective (Hocking, 2009; Molineux, 2010).

As illustrated in Table 6.1, many definitions of occupation inform research and practice around the world. Although some occupational scientists and occupational therapists are concerned by the lack of a standard definition of occupation, many authors suggest that a universal definition is neither desirable nor possible given the complex nature of occupation and people's diverse experiences (Galheigo, 2011; Laliberte Rudman et al., 2022; Magalhaes & Galheigo, 2010). In fact, some authors have argued that the ambiguity of occupation is a strength because the resulting malleability increases the concept's relevance across human experiences and contexts (Motimele & Peters, 2017). Such malleability helps explain the definitions in Table 6.1, which variably emphasise individual actors and social practices given their respective origins in individualist or collectivist worldviews.

Moreover, as will be further detailed in later sections of this chapter, contemporary understandings of occupation have expanded beyond a focus on occupations as determined and performed by individuals to seeing occupation as situated and relational (Laliberte Rudman et al., 2022). Situated understandings draw attention to contextual factors such as interpersonal dynamics, social norms, and even social policies that shape what people are expected to do, what they can do, and how they do occupations (Gappmayer, 2021; Laliberte Rudman, 2010). Relational understandings emphasise the ways in which occupations emerge through the interconnections among individuals, collectives and environmental features (Laliberte Rudman et al., 2022). Disruptions or barriers, such as individual health issues, socially produced inequities in opportunities for occupations, or changes in relationships, can unsettle the taken-for-granted nature of occupation and challenge individual and collective participation in desired and necessary occupations; addressing such challenges is a central focus of occupational therapy practice (Hammell, 2020).

Despite this variety and expansion, some key assumptions about occupation and its relationships to health and well-being underpin occupational therapy in many contexts. A primary assumption underlying the concept of occupation is that occupation matters to individuals and collectives (Cutchin & Dickie, 2012; Hammell, 2020). What people do, as individuals

TABLE 6.1	
Example Definitions of Occupation	
Source	Definition
Yerxa et al. (1990)	Specific chunks of activity within the ongoing stream of human behaviour which are named in the lexicon of the culture. (p. 1)
American Occupational Therapy Association (AOTA) (2020)	Occupations refer to the everyday activities that people do as individuals, in families, and with communities to occupy time and bring meaning and purpose to life. Occupations include things people need to, want to and are expected to do (WFOT, 2012a, p. 2). In the fourth edition of the Occupational Therapy Practice Framework: Domain and Process (OTPF–4), the term occupation denotes personalised and meaningful engagement in daily life events by a specific client. (AOTA, 2020, p. 7)
Frank (2013)	Actions that rearrange and reconstruct the world in which we live. (p. 233)
Kuo (2011)	Sociocultural practices and habits that originate from the social and express through the landscapes and places we live in. (p. 133)
Guajardo and Mondaca (2017)	Occupations are social practices and relationships, and within themselves constitute and produce subjects. (p. 104)
Laliberte Rudman et al. (2022)	The everyday and extraordinary doings of individuals and groups, which have implications for individuals, societies, and the Earth. (p. 310)

and collectives, is the core of occupational therapy practice because occupation is connected to health and well-being in a variety of ways. Scholars and practitioners also assume that occupation is transformative; in other words, participation in occupations can evoke changes in individuals and societies (Cunningham et al., 2022; Watson & Swartz, 2004). Likewise, occupations are complex: they occur over time, across spaces and places, through the context of daily experience, and through relations between people and environments (Christiansen & Townsend, 2010; Cutchin et al., 2008; Zemke 2004). Everyday occupations are associated with a multitude of meanings (Hasselkus & Dickie, 2021) that are shaped in relation to individual and collective worldviews and values (Laliberte Rudman, 2002). Taken together, these assumptions define occupations as what people do to live their lives as individuals and collective members (Wilcock & Hocking, 2015). As Virginia Dickie (2010) suggests, occupations are not 'processes too complicated to explain' (p. 195), but it is challenging to represent their complexity because they are often perceived as mundane.

OCCUPATION AS CORE TO OCCUPATIONAL THERAPY PRACTICE

Occupational therapy's founders argued that occupation is core to individual and collective health and well-being (Duncan, 2006; Reilly, 1962). The

profession is supported by research that demonstrates how occupation affects physical health, mental health, identity, social inclusion, collective functioning, well-being and group cohesion (Hammell, 2020). Although the increasing influence of biomedical and mechanistic health care models between the 1940s and 1970s challenged occupational therapy's focus on occupation, since the 1980s, there have been many initiatives to resituate occupation as the defining feature of occupational therapy practice (Duncan, 2006; Kielhofner, 2004). As articulated by Gustafsson et al. (2014), the contemporary overarching paradigm informing occupational therapy practice 'is focussed sharply on occupation and recognises that humans have an occupational nature and face occupational challenges' (p. 121).

One by-product of this renaissance of occupation is the diverse use of language tying the concept to practice. Fisher (2013) noted that the terms 'occupation-centred', 'occupation-based', and 'occupation-focused' are often used interchangeably without acknowledging their distinct meanings. Fisher wrote that 'if we think of being occupation-centred as a profession-specific perspective, and occupation-based as a method of evaluation and intervention that involves engaging a person in occupation', then the practice of occupational therapy must necessarily be 'occupation focused' (p. 166). As another example, within the Canadian Model of Occupational Participation (refer to Chapter 11), occupational therapy practice is focused on occupational participation in ways that involve supporting people to 'gain access to, initiate and sustain occupations they need or wish to pursue' (Egan & Restall, 2022, p. 76).

Occupation-focused practice entails using occupation in two primary ways: as a means and as an end (McLaughlin Gray, 1998; Trombly Latham, 2013). The idea of occupation as a means to skill development, functional recovery, relationship building, or social change implies that occupation is the mechanism through which health, well-being and transformation are achieved. Thus 'occupation as a means' involves using occupation as a medium of personal and social transformation. The idea of occupation as an end suggests that occupations – especially those associated with a person's roles and identities – are the goal of any occupational therapy process. Thus 'occupation as end' shifts the focus to occupations as outcomes, or as what people want to get back to doing so they can be and become who they want to be and belong to the collectives that mean most to them (Egan & Restall, 2022; Wilcock, 2006).

OCCUPATIONAL SCIENCE AS CORE TO EXPANDING KNOWLEDGE ABOUT THE OCCUPATION

Occupational science, a research-focused discipline committed to developing knowledge about occupation, arose in parallel with the resurgence of occupation-focused occupational therapy practice. Occupational science research poses a range of questions about the nature of occupation itself, determinants of occupations, how occupation is used to organise families and societies, how occupation can be a means for both oppression and resistance, and the consequences of inequities in possibilities for occupation (Calhoun, 2021; Hocking, 2009; Ramugondo, 2015).

Although the relationship between occupational science and occupational therapy has been the subject of some debate (Calhoun, 2021; Laliberte Rudman et al., 2008; Lunt, 1997), both the discipline and the profession are committed to understanding and applying an occupational perspective as a particular way of 'looking at and thinking about human doing' (Njelesani et al., 2014, p. 234). Given this perspective, occupational science has provided a powerful response to the need for knowledge that informs 'the

practice terrain of occupational therapy' (Molineux & Whiteford, 2011, p. 244). Occupational science knowledge has also helped expand and diversify occupational therapy practices by highlighting new areas of practice (Hocking & Wright-St. Clair, 2011) and by integrating critical and decolonising perspectives that can help disrupt oppressive power relations and generate new possibilities for understanding and supporting human doing (Galvaan, 2021; Mondaca, 2021).

As occupational science has developed, contributing scholars have increased not only in number but also in geographic, cultural, theoretical, and methodological locations and backgrounds (Calhoun, 2021; Hendricks et al., 2023). Continued efforts to make the knowledge base about occupation more pluralistic include generating knowledge that is relevant to diverse local contexts, disseminating knowledge in multiple languages, integrating diverse worldviews and epistemologies, and studying the occupations of collectives who are experiencing various forms of oppression and marginalisation (Magalhães et al., 2019; Ramugondo, 2015; Wijekoon & Peter, 2022). In recognition of occupational science's importance, the World Federation of Occupational Therapists (2012) issued a position statement in support of the discipline's growth, noting that occupational science's 'focus on occupation is what makes occupational therapy unique among the health professions' (p. 2). The remainder of this chapter outlines key aspects of the knowledge base regarding occupation, including evolving areas of exploration in occupational science, that show links between knowledge about occupation and occupational therapy practice.

OCCUPATION AS CORE TO HUMAN LIVING AND IDENTITY

In one of the most comprehensive published accounts of occupation, Ann Wilcock (2006) linked occupation to health, survival and well-being via the nexus of human biological capacities and environmental factors. Wilcock argued that many problems in modern society stem from occupations being 'out-of-step' with people's natural needs. By recognising that biological capacities and environmental characteristics can afford or constrain ways of doing, being, becoming, or belonging, Wilcock's work offers a foundation for understanding how the interplay of individual and environmental characteristics grounds occupational participation. Further scholarship built on this perspective has advanced discussions of justice and community development (Wilcock & Hocking, 2015), signalling that understandings about occupation can address both its presence and absence in people's lives.

Research from an occupational perspective has addressed the centrality of what people *do* in relation to their personal identities (or, how a person views the self), social identities (or, how a person wishes to be viewed and is viewed by others), and sense of being part of a collective (Christiansen, 2004; Kantartzis, 2016; Laliberte Rudman, 2002). Scholarship suggests a mutually informing relationship between occupation and identity; that is, the occupations of individuals or collectives influence individual or collective identity, and individual or collective identity influences what occupations individuals or collectives do (Christiansen, 2004; Ramugondo & Kronenberg, 2015). There is a similar relationship between occupational identity and context because engaging in identity-supporting occupations influences physical, social and other aspects of environments, just as environmental aspects can constrain or facilitate the types of occupations and occupational identities that are available to people (Laliberte Rudman, 2002, 2010; Phelan & Kinsella, 2009). Understanding the occupation-identity relationship sensitises occupational therapists to the challenge of occupational disruptions and losses by elucidating *why* particular occupations are vital to individuals and collectives. Such understandings inform how occupation can be used within occupational therapy practices to support identity management and reconstruction (Christiansen, 2004). Beyond applicability to the work that occupational therapists do with individuals and collectives, these ideas also have relevance for the ways that occupational therapists see themselves and are perceived as professionals. The structural aspects of practice settings can shape occupational therapists' perceptions about how their everyday 'doing' at work influences their ability to be the kind of occupational therapist they want to be (Durocher et al., 2016) and values implicit in the collective identity of occupational therapists can facilitate or hinder therapeutic relationships if they are perceived as being dismissive

of or at odds with the values of people receiving occupational therapy services (Hammell, 2020).

BEING REFLEXIVE AND EMBRACING THE ONGOING DIVERSIFICATION OF KNOWLEDGE REGARDING OCCUPATION

Although there is certainly evidence that supports the centrality of occupation to human life and societies, as well as knowledge about the occupation that provides directions for occupational therapy practices, occupational science and occupational therapy need to continue to diversify their knowledge base and practices. As practitioners and scholars seek evidence, they must be mindful of the perspectives through which they sort and interpret occupation-related understandings. Occupational therapy and occupational science have been critiqued for historically adopting a middle-class, Western, ableist and ethnocentric perspective that has constrained how occupation is studied and addressed in practice (Hammell, 2009b; Kiepek et al., 2014; Laliberte Rudman, 2021). Uncritical applications of this knowledge can perpetuate various forms of oppression, such as disablism, colonialism, or classism (Emery-Whittington, 2021; Galvaan, 2021; Hammell, 2020; Laliberte Rudman, 2021; Mondaca, 2021). Diversification of the knowledge base regarding occupation is ongoing and will continue to challenge taken-for-granted ways of understanding and addressing occupation. For example, critically oriented scholarship has destabilised assumptions that occupational choices are individually determined (Galvaan, 2014; Simaan, 2017) or that occupations have universal meanings, forms and purposes (Hendricks et al., 2023; Ramugondo & Kronenberg, 2015); such scholarship has also highlighted the need to understand historical and political forces that shape occupational possibilities (Emery-Whittington, 2021; Lavalley & Johnson, 2022) and marginalise ways of doing that exist outside approaches deemed normative within a sociopolitical context (Kiepek et al., 2019). Thus, as individuals and collectives, it is vital that occupational scientists and occupational therapists enact critical reflexivity regarding the knowledge they use and the practices they take up, and it is essential to commit to learning about and integrating the diversifying knowledge base generated through occupational science into occupational therapy education, scholarship and practices.

As one example of this critical reflexive approach, although research supports the long-standing assumption that occupation is connected to health and well-being, the belief that occupation is always health promoting or positive comes from particular religious and economic assumptions about the dangers of idleness and the inherent goodness of work (Kantartzis & Molineux, 2011). Accordingly, it is important to acknowledge that occupations can have negative effects at individual, collective and societal levels and that occupations cannot be simply categorised as positive or negative based on particular social norms (Durocher et al., 2014; Njelesani et al., 2014; Twinley & Addidle, 2012). Indeed, occupations can be health threatening: for instance, work-related stress has negative physical and psychological effects; dressing to reflect authentic gender identity can enhance risks of stigmatisation and violence if it is perceived to challenge the normative gender binary; and oppressive power relations can be imposed through restricting access to occupations on the basis of race, age and other social attributes of identity (Angell, 2014; Durocher et al., 2014; Lavelley & Johnson, 2022; Swenson et al., 2022). In addition, the dichotomous Western view of occupations as healthy or unhealthy fails to acknowledge that any occupation, including those socially viewed as risky, antisocial or bad, can have both positive and negative implications for health and well-being (Kantartzis & Molineux, 2011; Kiepek et al., 2019; Twinley & Addidle, 2012). For example, creating graffiti – which is often framed as deviant behaviour that negatively affects individual and community health – has been found to 'actually have health promoting benefits and [...] act as a potential pathway to engaging in health' (Russell, 2008, p. 95). Likewise, occupations that are ostensibly good, like automobile driving, can have detrimental environmental effects that can negatively affect human health and other occupational participation (Hudson & Aoyama, 2008). Given the variable nature of occupation as it is expressed and experienced across circumstances, and in light of the need to decolonise the knowledge base surrounding occupation, occupational therapists and occupational scientists must continue to be reflexive about the assumptions that underlie occupation-focused work

and generate knowledge regarding diverse occupations and ways of doing occupations (Galvaan, 2021; Njelesani et al., 2015).

Overall, within occupational therapy, it is important to guard against presumptions that certain occupations, or ways of doing the occupation, are negative and should be excluded from the domain of practice. Scholars have argued that occupational therapists and occupational scientists should generate and incorporate knowledge about the *situations* that promote participation in potentially harmful occupations (Aldrich & White, 2012) and the diverse contributions that a range of occupations make in peoples' lives (Kiepek et al., 2019).

OCCUPATION AS SITUATED, RELATIONAL AND POLITICAL

Given the historical dominance of Western perspectives, also sometimes referred to as a Global North worldview, occupational therapy practice and occupational science research have often taken an individualistic approach to occupation and the conditions that define people's participation in it. In other words, occupation has often been framed as determined by individuals and as separable from environments (Dickie et al., 2006; Laliberte Rudman & Huot, 2013; Whiteford, 2010). In response to this trend and in line with broader moves to expand beyond individually focused models of health and well-being (Raphael, 2016), scholars have refocused their attention on the situated and relational nature of occupation (Laliberte Rudman et al., 2022). These terms have drawn attention to how occupation is continuously 'shaped and negotiated within, as well as contributing to the shaping of, social systems and structures' (Laliberte Rudman, 2014, p. 4), and how occupations 'emerge through relationships that bind people with each other' (Laliberte Rudman et al., 2022, p. 18).

The transactional perspective (Dickie et al., 2006) is one key theoretical development that has helped foster such refocusing. The transactional perspective emphasises the situated and relational nature of occupation by applying the work of pragmatist philosophers such as John Dewey. The transactional perspective recognises that 'people and their environments coconstitute each other' (Cutchin & Dickie,

2012, p. 27); its application represents an attempt to provide a more balanced and complex account of occupational participation (Aldrich, 2008). Employing a transactional perspective challenges occupational therapists and occupational scientists to attend to occupation as a relational, in-process action through which individuals and collectives respond to situations (Cutchin et al., 2008; Lavalley, 2017). The recognition that 'occupation occurs at the level of the situation' (Dickie, 2014, p. 6) underscores the need to think about the individual, social, discursive and nonhuman elements that make situations and occupations what they are. For instance, in the situation of unemployment, the lack of a work occupation cannot only be explained by a person's individual history or national economic context: it is the nexus of governmental policies, a person's demographic characteristics and experiences, and the availability of financial and social resources that shape joblessness and its effects on nonwork occupations (Aldrich et al., 2020).

It has increasingly been recognised that 'no human action is independent of the social, cultural, political and economic contexts in which it occurs' (Whiteford et al., 2005, p. 10). Recent developments illuminate how practitioners and researchers can consider the complex intersection of individual, occupational and environmental aspects in human life. For example, occupational science research has highlighted how social constructions of gender, disability and age-based expectations can shape what occupations and identities are possible for people to take up in particular contexts (Laliberte Rudman, 2010; Phelan & Kinsella, 2009; Wicks & Whiteford, 2005). Such research demonstrates that social, physical, economic, political, cultural, ideological and geographic elements all affect whether, and in what way, people can participate in occupations. Taken-for-granted notions about gender, the physical layout of playgrounds and the structure of sports activities, for instance, are all seen as shaping the occupations and occupational identities of children (Angell, 2014). Likewise, although impairments can make it difficult to perform particular occupations, situated understandings of occupation reinforce that disability results from ableist assumptions and normative expectations that structure environments: a mobility impairment that reduces walking speed and a person's ability to navigate curbs only becomes problematic when traffic light durations and curb heights have been determined on the basis of assumptions about 'normal' mobility (McGrath, 2011). It is important to always situate occupational participation and understand its relational embeddedness so that occupational therapy practice addresses the complexity of intersecting elements that shape this participation (Egan & Restall, 2022; Wicks & Whiteford, 2005).

Ideas about the situated nature of occupation have prompted expanded attention to power relations and how they influence what types of occupations various groups of people can participate in, increasing awareness of the ways in which occupation is also politically situated and inequitably distributed (Kronenberg & Pollard, 2006; Molineux & Whiteford, 2011; Ramungondo, 2015). As highlighted by Galvaan and Peters (2017), given that 'hierarchies of power and privilege' (p. 285) are experienced and shaped through everyday occupation, it is crucial that occupational therapy practices attend to the 'politics of occupation' (p. 298). This involves addressing structural and systemic issues that shape and perpetuate occupational injustices and set limits on occupational possibilities. The concept of occupational justice, which was introduced in the 1990s by Elizabeth Townsend and Ann Wilcock, provides one means to understand how power affects occupation (Stadnyk et al., 2010; Wilcock & Townsend, 2009), although it is important to recognise that its foundations within a Eurocentric worldview set limits on the concept's universal applicability (Emery-Whittington, 2021). Scholarship addressing the concept of occupational justice has provided ways to think about how structures and systems produce disadvantage, oppression and exclusion, including occupational deprivation, which points to how external forces create extended exclusion from necessary and/or meaningful occupations; occupational imbalance, which encompasses being overoccupied and underoccupied; occupational marginalisation, which refers to individuals or collectives not having choices or opportunities to participate in valued and necessary occupations; and occupational alienation, which includes situations where individuals and collectives experience everyday occupations as lacking in meaning (Nilsson & Townsend, 2010; Stadnyk et al., 2010; Whiteford, 2000).

Aligned with the powerful premise that occupation is a human right (Galheigo, 2011; Hammell, 2008), research and practices that attend to occupational injustice seek to raise awareness of and alter situations in which 'some populations more than others are restricted from experiencing occupational rights, responsibilities and liberties, either deliberately or through taken-for-granted social exclusion from participation' (Nilsson & Townsend, 2010, p. 58). Within the everyday context of practice, applying an occupational justice lens means that occupational therapists work with people, as individuals and collectives, to understand, negotiate and alter social and structural factors that unfairly restrict occupational participation. Although the occupational justice-focused practice may appear different from traditional occupational therapy practice, it is becoming evident that most occupational therapy practices seek to promote justice and ensure occupational rights at some level (Bailliard & Aldrich, 2016; Bailliard et al., 2020).

Fuelled by the increasing integration of critical and decolonial frameworks into occupational science scholarship (refer to Chapters 1 and 2), a range of concepts for understanding the political, situated and relational nature of occupation have emerged and continue to be developed, such as occupational consciousness, occupational apartheid and occupational possibilities (Laliberte Rudman, 2010; Ramungondo, 2015; Simaan, 2017). Practice and conceptual frameworks informed by these evolving concepts, as well as critical and decolonial perspectives, are also emerging to support occupational therapists to continually enact culturally safer approaches to supporting occupational participation (Egan & Restall, 2022), such as the Capabilities, Opportunities, Resources and Environments (CORE) approach (Pereira & Whiteford, 2021), the Occupation, Capability and Well-Being Framework for Occupational Therapy (Hammell, 2020) (refer to Chapter 10), and the Occupation-Based Community Development Framework (Galvaan & Peters, 2017) (refer to Chapter 30).

INFORMING OCCUPATION-BASED PRACTICE: EXAMPLES RELATED TO THE EXPERIENCE AND ORGANISATION OF OCCUPATION

Integrating knowledge about occupation can '[inform] therapists' understandings of the meaning, demands and context of the occupations [people] aspire to' (Hocking, 2009, p. 140). This final section provides examples of developed and emerging concepts and insights to illustrate the applicability of such knowledge to occupational therapy practice.

Experiences of Occupation: Meaning, Purposes and Categories

Many scholars have focused on creating knowledge about occupation relative to three primary points: its forms, its functions and its meanings. The form of occupation includes aspects of occupation that elicit and guide performance. Knowledge about the form of occupation (Nelson, 1988) has grown as scholars have become better equipped to articulate the parameters of occupational participation (Hocking, 2009) that exist apart from people's experience of it (Dickie, 2010). For example, understanding that learning is a central part of quilt making (Dickie, 2003a) can help a therapist move beyond focusing on a particular person's physical impairment to seeing the social or intellectual experience of quilt making as an 'end' of intervention. Occupational science research has also endeavoured to clarify the purposes of occupation and the processes involved in its execution (Hocking, 2000). For instance, occupations related to spirituality may function as a way to connect people with a community (Beagan & Etowa, 2011), and the ways in which people participate in spiritual occupations can be understood in light of that particular purpose. Meaning, that the other part of this conceptual triad, has long been central to occupational therapists and occupational scientists' assumptions about occupation's influence on health and well-being (Christiansen, 1999). Research has shown that meaning is both individualised and socially influenced. For example, participants in a study examining the food-centred occupations of older women in New Zealand, Chiangmai and Kentucky experienced cooking as meaningful when it provided a means to maintain a role in a family structure, preserve cultural teachings or create new traditions (Hocking, 2009). Such research displays the importance of understanding people's perspectives on the meanings of various occupations and situating these meanings in various individual, familial and cultural contextual features, rather than assuming that meaning can be surmised by an outsider or inheres across similar occupations.

Researchers have also tried to understand the experience of occupation through the use of occupational categories. Although people may sometimes find it difficult to categorise their daily occupations (Aldrich et al., 2015) and the same occupation may be categorised differently by different individuals (Brooke et al., 2007), occupational therapists and occupational scientists often use categories to make sense of the ways in which occupation is central to human living. Such categories are often part of how occupation is defined (see Table 6.1), and they stem from foundational writings that propose work, play, rest and sleep as primary categories of occupational participation (Hammell, 2009a). Such categories have come to be seen as exclusionary because they were derived from and often assume a Western worldview that privileges individualistic and Judeo-Christian values over collectivist, Indigenous, and diverse spiritual and religious values (Emery-Whittington, 2021; Hammell, 2009b). These critiques have led scholars to question whether or not experience-based (rather than typology-based) categories are more informative and inclusive (Jonsson, 2008), whether or not occupational categories are dichotomous (Primeau, 1995), or whether or not there is a purpose in categorising occupations at all (Aldrich et al., 2015). Developing knowledge about occupational categories has redoubled some scholars' commitment to explicating the ways in which occupations are a core feature of human life (Hammell, 2004). Although the use of categories can provide an efficient way to inquire about each person's different occupations, occupational therapists need to be critically reflexive regarding how categories may exclude or silence occupations. Research points to the need to use categories cautiously and to talk with people using categories or experiences that are most relevant to their occupational participation (Aldrich et al., 2015; Laliberte Rudman et al., 2022).

Organising Occupation: Across the Lifespan, Through Routine and Habits, Transitions and Balance

Categories have also been used to conceptualise how occupations are organised across the lifespan. Human development has historically been broken down into stages using categories such as 'childhood', 'adolescence', 'adulthood' and 'older adulthood'. In looking at how occupation is organised across the lifespan (Humphry, 2002; Wiseman et al., 2005), scholars and practitioners have helped illuminate how play occupations are central to childhood (Parham, 1996) and work occupations are central to adulthood within particular national and geographic contexts (Dickie, 2003b). However, scholars have also recognised that play is culturally relative (Bazyk et al., 2003; Wiseman et al., 2005), that children can also work (Larson, 2004), and that adults also benefit from play and leisure (Suto, 1998). Such research illustrates that associations between categories of occupations and stages of life are not mutually exclusive; it also highlights the need to examine the diversity of occupations that comprise people's occupational repertoires at various ages and how these are situated within contextual elements. As Humphry and Wakeford (2006) articulated, research addressing the processes through which occupations are developed can inform practice that supports 'the acquisition of new occupation and transformations in occupational performance' (p. 265). That is, knowledge about how occupations develop throughout the lifespan can help occupational therapists assist people to learn or relearn occupations. At the same time, occupational therapists need to be wary of uncritically applying 'normative' ideas of development and occupation given that this can serve to reinforce oppressive power relations and marginalise ways of developing and doing that exist about those deemed ideal, appropriate and valued from a Western, ableist worldview (Hammell, 2020; White & Beagan, 2020).

Within understandings of development, scholars have examined how habits and routines mature, persist and decline across the lifespan and how changes in habits and routines affect occupational performance (Clark, 2000). Just as with assumptions about occupational categories, emerging knowledge suggests that viewing routine as a building block of occupation may not match people's experiences in situations like unemployment (Aldrich & Dickie, 2013) or retirement (Ludwig, 1998). Therefore occupational therapists whose practices emphasise routine may have to adjust their expectations of people whose situations defy routine-based descriptions.

Scholars and practitioners have also recognised that transitioning from one developmental stage to another often brings about changes in occupations. The concept of occupational transition – or a change in the occupations that a person or collective can, needs or wants to do – captures changes that occur for diverse reasons, such as progressive functional declines (Vrkljan & Polgar, 2006), age-related role changes (Wiseman & Whiteford, 2009), migrating from one country to another (Trimboli et al., 2019) or environmental degradation connected to climate change (Smith et al., 2020). Occupational therapists often intervene when people are experiencing an occupational transition, and occupational therapists can thus be viewed as supporting people in negotiating transitions. Research about occupational transitions provides insights into factors that can be addressed in practice to facilitate successful transitions, such as social support, an ability to link changes to the past and future, ensuring stable access to essential resources, and continued participation in familiar occupations (Kubina et al., 2013). Such research also reveals factors that can serve as barriers to the successful negotiation of transitions, such as a lack of recognition of work skills and credentials developed in a different context or having to deal with multiple transitions at the same time (Crider et al., 2014; Trimboli et al., 2019).

Whatever developmental stage a person occupies, the notion of a person's pursuits being occupationally balanced offers a way to think about the experience and organisation of occupation. The concept of balance has a long history in occupational therapy (Backman, 2004; Christiansen, 1996). Broadly speaking, people can either feel that they are experiencing appropriate or inappropriate variation and duration in their daily occupations (Wagman et al., 2012). The concept of occupational balance has been utilised to understand time use and qualities of experience (Jonsson & Persson, 2006) for a range of people, from those with health conditions (Bejerholm, 2010) to those entering new developmental stages (Pettican & Prior, 2011). Although this literature can provide occupational therapists with broad understandings about the types of experiences associated with health (Wilcock et al., 1997), understandings and experiences of occupational balance are also situated. As with assumptions about meaning, it is important to note that both individual and social views of balance influence the perceptions people have about their lives, and situated assessments of occupational balance require attention to the access that individuals and collectives have to the resources and living conditions that support achieving balance.

CONCLUSION

Occupation is occupational therapy's central construct, demonstrating how occupational science knowledge generation has both supported and challenged assumptions about occupation. This is an exciting time of growth and diversification for both the profession and the discipline, and the realisation of occupation-focused practice depends on increasing the number of people who use, and contribute to the ever-expanding knowledge base about occupation.

FURTHER RESOURCES TO SUPPORT CONTINUED LEARNING ABOUT OCCUPATION

- *Journal of Occupational Science* (http://www.tandfonline.com/loi/rocc)
- International Society for Occupational Science (https://www.international-society-for-occupational-science.org/)
- Canadian Society of Occupational Scientists (https://www.csoscanada.org/)
- Society for the Study of Occupation: USA (https://ssou.memberclicks.net/)
- Occupational Science Europe (https://os-europe.org/)

REFERENCES

Aldrich, R. M. (2008). From complexity theory to transactionalism: Moving occupational science forward in theorizing the complexities of behaviour. *Journal of Occupational Science, 15*(3), 147–156.

Aldrich, R. M., & Dickie, V. A. (2013). 'It's hard to plan your day when you have no money': Discouraged workers' occupational possibilities and the need to reconceptualize routine. *Work, A Journal of Prevention, Assessment, and Rehabilitation, 45*, 5–15.

Aldrich, R., Laliberte Rudman, D., Park, N. E., & Huot, S. (2020). Centering the complexity of long-term unemployment: Lessons learned from a critical occupational science inquiry. *Societies, 10*(3), 65. https://doi.org/10.3390/soc10030065.

Aldrich, R. M., McCarty, C., Boyd, B., Bunch, C., & Balentine, C. (2015). Empirical lessons about occupational categorization from case studies of unemployment. *Canadian Journal of Occupational Therapy, 81*(5), 289–297.

Aldrich, R. M., & White, N. (2012). Re-considering violence: A response to Twinley and Addidle (2012) and Morris (2012). *British Journal of Occupational Therapy, 75*(11), 527–529.

American Occupational Therapy Association. (2020). *Occupational therapy practice framework: Domain and process* (4th ed.). American Journal of Occupational Therapy, 74(Suppl. 2), 7412410010. https://doi.org/10.5014/ajot.2020.74S2001.

Angell, A. M. (2014). Occupation-centered analysis of social difference: Contributions to a socially responsive occupational science. *Journal of Occupational Science, 21*(2), 104–116.

Backman, C. L. (2004). Occupational balance: Exploring the relationships among daily occupations and their influence on well-being. *Canadian Journal of Occupational Therapy, 71*(4), 202–209.

Bailliard, A., & Aldrich, R. (2016). Occupational justice in everyday occupational therapy practice. In D. Sakellariou & N. Pollard (Eds.), *Occupational therapies without borders: Integrating justice with practice* (pp. 83–94). Elsevier.

Bailliard, A. L., Dallman, A. R., Carroll, A., Lee, B. D., & Szendrey, S. (2020). Doing occupational justice: A central dimension of everyday occupational therapy practice. *Canadian Journal of Occupational Therapy, 87*(2), 144–152. https://doi.org/10.1177/0008417419898930.

Bazyk, S., Stalnaker, D., Llerna, M., Ekelman, B., & Bayzk, J. (2003). Play in Mayan children. *The American Journal of Occupational Therapy, 57*(3), 273–283.

Beagan, B. L., & Etowa, J. B. (2011). The meanings and functions of occupations related to spirituality for African Nova Scotian women. *Journal of Occupational Science, 18*(3), 277–290.

Bejerholm, U. (2010). Occupational balance in people with schizophrenia. *Occupational Therapy in Mental Health, 26*(1), 1–17.

Brooke, K. E., Desmarais, C. D., & Forwell, S. J. (2007). Types and categories of personal projects: A revelatory means of understanding human occupation. *Occupational Therapy International, 14*, 281–296.

Calhoun, A. D. (2021). The development and future occupational science: A budding occupational scientist's reflections and assertions about the discipline. *Journal of Occupational Science, 28*(2), 193–207.

Christiansen, C. H. (1996). Three perspectives on balance in occupation. In R. Zemke & F. Clark (Eds.), *Occupational science: The evolving discipline* (pp. 431–452). F.A. Davis.

Christiansen, C. H. (1999). Defining lives: Occupation as identity: An essay on competence, coherence, and the creation of meaning. *American Journal of Occupational Therapy, 53*, 547–558.

Christiansen, C. H. (2004). Occupation and identity: Becoming who we are through what we do. In C. H. Christiansen & E. A. Townsend (Eds.), *Introduction to occupation: The art and science of living* (pp. 121–139). Prentice Hall.

Christiansen, C. H., & Townsend, E. A (2010). An introduction to occupation. In C. H. Christiansen & E. A. Townsend (Eds.), *Introduction to occupation: The art and science of living* (2nd ed., pp. 1–34). Prentice Hall.

Clark, F. (2000). The concepts of habit and routine: A preliminary theoretical synthesis. *Occupational Therapy Journal of Research, 20*(1 Suppl), 123S–137S.

Clark, F., Parham, D., Carlson, M. E., Frank, G., Jackson, J., Pierce, D., Wolfe, R. J., & Zemke, R. (1991). Occupational science: Academic innovation in the service of occupational therapy's future. *American Journal of Occupational Therapy, 45*(4), 300–310.

Crider, C., Calder, C. R., Bunting, K. L., & Forwell, S. (2014). An integrative review of occupational science and theoretical literature exploring transition. *Journal of Occupational Science, 22*(3), 304–319.

Cunningham, M., Warren, A., Pollard, N., & Abey, S. (2022). Enacting social transformation through occupation: A narrative literature review. *Scandinavian Journal of Occupational Therapy, 29*(8), 611–630. https://doi.org/10.1080/11038128.2020.1841287.

Cutchin, M. P., Aldrich, R., Bailliard, A., & Coppola, S. (2008). Action theories for occupational science: The contributions of Dewey and Bourdieu. *Journal of Occupational Science, 15*(3), 157–165.

Cutchin, M. P., & Dickie, V. A. (2012). Transactionalism: Occupational science and the pragmatic attitude. In G. E. Whiteford & C. Hocking (Eds.), *Occupational science: Society, inclusion and participation* (pp. 23–37). Wiley-Blackwell.

Dickie, V. A. (2003a). The role of learning in quilt making. *Journal of Occupational Science, 10*(3), 120–129.

Dickie, V. A. (2003b). Establishing worker identity: A study of people in craft work. *American Journal of Occupational Therapy, 57*(3), 250–261.

Dickie, V. A. (2010). Are occupations 'processes too complicated to explain'? What we can learn by trying. *Journal of Occupational Science, 17*(4), 195–203.

Dickie, V. A. (2014). What is occupation? In B. A. Boyt Schell, G. Gillen, & M. E. Scaffa (Eds.), *Willard & Spackman's occupational therapy* (12th ed., pp. 2–8). Lippincott Williams & Wilkins.

Dickie, V. A., Cutchin, M. P., & Humphry, R. (2006). Occupation as transactional experience: A critique of individualism in occupational science. *Journal of Occupational Science, 13*(1), 83–93.

Duncan, E. A. S. (2006). *Foundations for practice in occupational therapy* (4th ed.). Elsevier Churchill Livingstone.

Durocher, E., Kinsella, E. A., McCorquodale, L., & Phelan, S. (2016). Ethical tensions related to systemic constraints. *OTJR: Occupation, Participation, and Health, 36*(4), 216–226. https://doi.org/10.1177/1539449216665117.

Durocher, E., Rappolt, S., & Gibson, B. E. (2014). Occupational justice: Future directions. *Journal of Occupational Science, 21*(4), 431–442.

Egan, M. & Restall, G. (2022). The Canadian Model of Occupational Participation. In M. Egan & G. Restall (Eds.). Promoting occupational participation: Collaborative relationship-focused occupational therapy (pp. 74–95). Ottawa, Canada: Canadian Association of Occupational Therapists.

Emery-Whittington, I. G. (2021). Occupational justice – Colonial business as usual? Indigenous observations from Aotearoa New Zealand. *Canadian Journal of Occupational Therapy, 88*(2), 153–162. https://doi.org/10.1177/00084174211005891.

Fisher, A. G. (2013). Occupation-centered, occupation-based, occupation-focused: Same, or different? *Scandinavian Journal of Occupational Therapy, 20*, 162–173. https://doi.org/10.3109/11038128.2014.952912.

Frank, G. (2013). Twenty-first century pragmatism and social justice: Problematic situations and occupational reconstructions in post-civil war Guatemala. In M. P. Cutchin & V. A. Dickie (Eds.), *Transactional perspectives on occupation* (pp. 229–244). Springer.

Galheigo, S. M. (2011). What needs to be done? Occupational therapy responsibilities and challenges regarding human rights. *Australian Occupational Therapy Journal, 58*, 60–66.

Galvaan, R. (2014). The contextually situated nature of occupational choice: Marginalised young adolescents' experiences in South Africa. *Journal of Occupational Science, 22*(1), 39–53.

Galvaan, R. (2021). Generative disruption through occupational science: Enacting possibilities for deep human connection. *Journal of Occupational Science, 28*(1), 6–18. https://doi.org/10.1080/144 27591.2020.1818276.

Galvaan, R., & Peters, L. (2017). Occupation-based community development: Confronting the politics of occupation. In D. Sakellariou & N. Pollard (Eds.), *Occupational therapy without borders: Integrating justice with practice* (pp. 283–291). Elsevier.

Gappmayer, G. (2021). Disentangling disablism and ableism: The social norm of being able and its influence on social interactions with people with intellectual disabilities. *Journal of Occupational Science, 28*(1), 102–113. https://doi.org/10.1080/14427591.2020.1 814394.

Guajardo, A., & Mondaca, M. (2017). Human rights, occupational therapy and the centrality of social practices. In D. Sakellariou & N. Pollard (Eds.), *Occupational therapy without borders: Integrating justice with practice* (pp. 102–108). Elsevier.

Gustafsson, L., Molineux, M., & Bennett, S. (2014). Contemporary occupational therapy practice: The challenges of being evidence based and philosophically congruent. *Australian Occupational Therapy Journal, 61*(2), 121–123.

Hammell, K. W. (2004). Dimensions of meaning in the occupations of daily life. *Canadian Journal of Occupational Therapy, 71*(5), 296–303.

Hammell, K. W. (2008). Reflections on…wellbeing and occupational rights. *Canadian Journal of Occupational Therapy, 75*(1), 61–64.

Hammell, K. W. (2009a). Self-care, productivity, and leisure, or dimensions of occupational experience? Rethinking occupational 'categories'. *Canadian Journal of Occupational Therapy, 76*, 107–114.

Hammell, K. W. (2009b). Sacred texts: A skeptical exploration of the assumptions underpinning theories of occupation. *Canadian Journal of Occupational Therapy, 76*, 6–13. https://doi.org/10.1177/000841740907600105.

Hammell, K. W. (2020). *Engagement in living: Critical perspectives on occupation, rights and wellbeing.* CAOT Publications.

Hasselkus, B. R., & Dickie, V. (2021). *The meaning of everyday occupation* (3rd ed.). Slack.

Hendricks, F., Galvaan, R., & al-Ninowy, S. M. B. Y. (2023). Tensions in describing Muslim religious practices: Insights generated from an Islamic monotheist perspective. *Journal of Occupational Science, 30*(4), 673–683. https://doi.org/10.1080/14427591.2022.2 132997.

Hocking, C. (2000). Occupational science: A stock take of accumulated insights. *Journal of Occupational Science, 7*(2), 58–67.

Hocking, C. (2009). The challenge of occupation: Describing the things people do. *Journal of Occupational Science, 16*(3), 140–150.

Hocking, C., & Wright-St. Clair, V. (2011). Occupational science: Adding value to occupational therapy. *New Zealand Journal of Occupational Therapy, 58*(1), 29–35.

Hudson, M. J., & Aoyama, M. (2008). Occupational therapy and the current ecological crisis. *British Journal of Occupational Therapy, 71*(12), 545–548.

Humphry, R. (2002). Young children's occupations: Explicating the dynamics of developmental processes. *American Journal of Occupational Therapy, 56*(2), 171–179.

Humphry, R., & Wakeford, L. (2006). An occupation-centered discussion of development and implications for practice. *American Journal of Occupational Therapy, 60*, 258–267. https://doi.org/10.5014/ajot.60.3.258.

Jonsson, H. (2008). A new direction in the conceptualization and categorization of occupation. *Journal of Occupational Science, 15*, 3–8.

Jonsson, H., & Persson, D. (2006). Towards an experiential model of occupational balance: An alternative perspective on flow theory analysis. *Journal of Occupational Science, 13*(1), 62–73.

Kantartzis, S. (2016). Exploring occupation beyond the individual: Family and collective occupation. In D. Sakellariou, & N. Pollard (Eds.), *Occupational therapies without borders: Integrating justice with practice* (2nd ed., pp. 19–28). Elsevier.

Kantartzis, S., & Molineux, M. (2011). The influence of Western society's construction of a healthy daily life on the conceptualisation of occupation. *Journal of Occupational Science, 18*(1), 62–80.

Kielhofner, G. (2004). *Conceptual foundations of occupational therapy* (3rd ed.). F.A. Davis.

Kiepek, N., Beagan, B., Laliberte Rudman, D., & Phelan, S. (2019). Silences around occupations framed as unhealthy, illegal, and deviant. *Journal of Occupational Science, 26*(3), 341–353. https://doi.org/10.1080/14427591.2018.1499123.

Kiepek, N., Phelan, S., & Magalhaes, L. (2014). Introducing a critical analysis of the figured world of occupation. *Journal of Occupational Science, 21*(4), 403–417. https://doi.org/10.1080/14427591 .2018.1499123.

Kronenberg, F., & Pollard, N. (2006). Political dimensions of occupation and the roles of occupational therapy. *American Journal of Occupational Therapy, 60*(6), 617–626.

Kubina, L. A., Dubouloz, C. J., Davis, C. G., Kessler, D., & Egan, M. Y. (2013). The process of re-engagement in personally valued activities during the two years following stroke. *Disability and Rehabilitation, 35*(3), 236–243.

Kuo, A. (2011). A transactional view: Occupation as a means to create experiences that matter. *Journal of Occupational Science, 18*(2), 131–138.

Laliberte Rudman, D. (2002). Linking occupation and identity: Lessons learned through qualitative exploration. *Journal of Occupational Science, 9*(1), 12–19.

Laliberte Rudman, D. (2010). Occupational terminology: Occupational possibilities. *Journal of Occupational Science, 17*(1), 55–59.

Laliberte Rudman, D. (2014). Embracing and enacting an 'occupational imagination': Occupational science as transformative. *Journal of Occupational Science, 21*(4), 373–388.

Laliberte Rudman, D. (2021). Mobilizing occupation for social transformation: Radical resistance, disruption, and re-configuration. *Canadian Journal of Occupational Therapy, 88*(2), 96–107.

Laliberte Rudman, D., Aldrich, R., & Kiepek, N. (2022). Evolving understandings of occupation. In M. Egan & G. Restall (Eds.), *Promoting occupational participation: Collaborative relationship-focused occupational therapy* (pp. 11–30). CAOT Press.

Laliberte Rudman, D., Dennhardt, S., Fok, D., Huot, S., Molke, D., Park, A., & Zur, B. (2008). A vision for occupational science: Reflecting on our disciplinary culture. *Journal of Occupational Science, 15*(3), 136–146.

Laliberte Rudman, D., & Huot, S (2013). Conceptual insights for expanding thinking regarding the situated nature of occupation. In M. P. Cutchin & V. A. Dickie (Eds.), *Transactional perspectives on occupation* (pp. 51–64). Springer.

Larson, E. (2004). Children's work: The less considered childhood occupation. *American Journal of Occupational Therapy, 58*(4), 369–379.

Lavalley, R. (2017). Developing the transactional perspective of occupation for communities: 'How well are we doing together'? *Journal of Occupational Science, 24*(4), 458–469. https://doi.org/10.1080/14427591.2017.1367321.

Lavalley, R., & Robinson Johnson, K. (2022). Occupation, injustice, and anti-Black racism in the United States of America. *Journal of Occupational Science, 29*(4), 487–499. https://doi.org/10.1080/14427591.2020.1810111.

Ludwig, F. M. (1998). The unpackaging of routine in older women. *American Journal of Occupational Therapy, 52*(3), 168–175.

Lunt, A. (1997). Occupational science and occupational therapy: Negotiating the boundary between a discipline and a profession. *Journal of Occupational Science, 49*(2), 56–61.

Magalhães, L., Farias, L., Rivas-Quarneti, N., Alvarez, L., & Malfitano, A. P. S. (2019). The development of occupational science outside the Anglophone sphere: Enacting global collaboration. *Journal of Occupational Science, 26*(2), 181–192.

Magalhaes, L., & Galheigo, S. M. (2010). Enabling international communication among Brazilian occupational therapists: Seeking consensus on occupational terminology. *Occupational Therapy International, 17*(3), 113–124.

McGrath, C. (2011). Low vision and older adults: The role of occupational therapy. *Occupational Therapy Now, 13*(3), 26–28.

McLaughlin Gray, J. (1998). Putting occupation into practice: Occupation as ends, occupation as means. *American Journal of Occupational Therapy, 52*, 354–364.

Molineux, M. (2010). The nature of occupation. In M. Curtin, M. Molineux, & J. Supyk-Mellon (Eds.), Occupational therapy and physical dysfunction: Enabling occupation (6th ed., pp. 17–25). London: Churchill Livingstone.

Molineux, M., & Whiteford, G. E. (2011). Occupational science: Genesis, evolution and future contribution. In Duncan, E. A. S. (Ed.), *Foundations for practice in occupational therapy* (pp. 243–253). Elsevier.

Mondaca, M. (2021). 'Doing hope' as a possible way towards a responsive occupational science. *Journal of Occupational Science, 28*(1), 19–28.

Motimele, M., & Peters, L. (2017). Understanding human occupation. In S. A. Dsouza, R. Galvaan, & E. L. Ramugondo (Eds.), *Concepts in occupational therapy: Understanding Southern perspectives* (pp. 1–15). Manipal University Press.

Nelson, D. L. (1988). Occupation: Form and performance. *American Journal of Occupational Therapy, 42*(10), 633–641.

Nilsson, I., & Townsend, I. (2010). Occupational justice – Bridging theory and practice. *Scandinavian Journal of Occupational Therapy, 17*, 57–63.

Njelesani, J., Tang, A., Jonsson, H., & Polatajko, H. (2014). Articulating an occupational perspective. *Journal of Occupational Science, 21*(2), 226–235.

Njelesani, J., Teachman, G., Durocher, E., Hamdani, Y., & Phelan, S. K. (2015). Thinking critically about client-centred practice and occupational possibilities across the life-span. *Scandinavian Journal of Occupational Therapy, 22*(4), 252–259. https://doi.org/10.3109/11038128.2015.1049550.

Parham, L. D. (1996). Perspectives on play. In R. Zemke & F. Clark (Eds.), *Occupational science: The evolving discipline* (pp. 71–80). F.A. Davis.

Pereira, R. B., & Whiteford G. E. (2021) Enabling inclusive occupational therapy through the Capabilities, Opportunities, Resources, and Environments (CORE) Approach. In P. Liamputtong (Ed.) Handbook of Social Inclusion (pp. 1–18). Springer, Cham.

Pettican, A., & Prior, S. (2011). 'It's a new way of life' an exploration of the occupational transition of retirement. *British Journal of Occupational Therapy, 74*(1), 12–19.

Phelan, S., & Kinsella, E. A. (2009). Occupational identity: Engaging socio-cultural perspectives. *Journal of Occupational Science, 16*(2), 85–91.

Primeau, L. A. (1995). Work and leisure: Transcending the dichotomy. *American Journal of Occupational Therapy, 50*(7), 569–577.

Ramugondo, E. (2015). Occupational terminology: Occupational consciousness. *Journal of Occupational Science, 22*(4), 488–501. https://doi.org/10.1080/14427591.2015.1042516.

Ramugondo, E. L., & Kronenberg, F. (2015). Explaining collective occupations from a human relations perspective: Bridging the individual-collective dichotomy. *Journal of Occupational Science, 22*(1), 3–16. https://doi.org/10.1080/14427591.2013.781920.

Raphael, D. (2016). *Social determinants of health: Canadian perspectives* (3rd ed.). Canadian Scholars Press.

Reilly, M. (1962). Occupational therapy can be one of the great ideas of 20th century medicine. *American Journal of Occupational Therapy, 16*, 1–9.

Russell, E. (2008). Writing on the wall: The form, function and meaning of tagging. *Journal of Occupational Science, 15*(2), 87–97.

Simaan, J. (2017). Olive growing in Palestine: A decolonial ethnographic study of collective daily-forms-of-resistance. *Journal of Occupational Science, 24*(4), 510–523.

Smith, D. L., Fleming, K., Brown, L., Allen, A., Baker, J., & Gallagher, M. (2020). Occupational therapy and environmental sustainability: A scoping review. *Annals of International Occupational Therapy, 3*(3), 136–143.

Stadnyk, R., Townsend, E. A., & Wilcock, A. A (2010). Occupational justice. In C. H. Christiansen & E. A. Townsend (Eds.), *Introduction to occupation: The art and science of living* (2nd ed., pp. 329–358). Prentice Hall.

Suto, M. (1998). Leisure in occupational therapy. *Canadian Journal of Occupational Therapy, 65*(5), 271–278.

Swenson, R., Alldred, P., & Nicholls, L. (2022). Doing gender and being gendered through occupation: Transgender and nonbinary experiences. *British Journal of Occupational Therapy, 85*(6), 446–452.

Trimboli, C., Rivas-Quarneti, N., Blankvoort, N., Roosen, I., Simó Algado, S., & Whiteford, G. (2019). The current and future contribution of occupational therapy and occupational science to transforming the situation of forced migrants: Critical perspectives from a think tank. *Journal of Occupational Science, 26*(2), 323–328.

Trombly Latham, C. A. (2013). *Occupation: Philosophy and concepts.* In M. Radomski (Ed.), *Occupational therapy for physical dysfunction* (6th ed. pp. 339–357). Lippincott Williams & Wilkins.

Twinley, R., & Addidle, G. (2012). Considering violence: The dark side of occupation. *British Journal of Occupational Therapy, 75*(4), 202–204.

Vrkljan, B. H., & Polgar, J. M. (2006). Linking occupational participation and occupational identity: An exploratory study of the transition from driving to driving cessation in older adulthood. *Journal of Occupational Science, 14*(1), 1–10.

Wagman, P., Hakansson, C., & Bjorklund, A. (2012). Occupational balance as used in occupational therapy: A concept analysis. *Scandinavian Journal of Occupational Therapy, 19*, 322–327.

Watson, R., & Swartz, L. (Eds.). (2004). *Transformation through occupation.* Whurr.

White, T., & Beagan, B. L. (2020). Occupational therapy roles in an Indigenous context: An integrative review. *Canadian Journal of Occupational Therapy, 87*(3), 200–210.

Whiteford, G. E. (2000). Occupational deprivation: Global challenge in the new millennium. *British Journal of Occupational Therapy, 63*(5), 200–204. https://doi.org/10.1177/030802260006300503.

Whiteford, G. E. (2010). Occupation in context. In M. Curtin, M. Molineux, & J. Supyk-Mellon (Eds.), *Occupational therapy and physical dysfunction: Enabling occupation* (6th ed., pp. 136–148). Churchill Livingstone.

Whiteford, G. E., Klomp, N., & Wright-St. Clair, V. (2005). Complexity theory: Understanding occupation and practice in context. In G. Whiteford & V. Wright-St. Clair (Eds.), *Occupation & practice in context* (pp. 3–15). Churchill Livingstone.

Wicks, A., & Whiteford, G. E. (2005). Gender, occupation and participation. In G. Whiteford & V. Wright-St. Clair (Eds.), *Occupation & practice in context* (pp. 197–212). Elsevier.

Wilcock, A. A. (2006). *An occupational perspective of health* (2nd ed.). Slack.

Wilcock, A. A., Chelin, M., Hall, M., Hamley, N., Morrison, B., Scrivener, L., Townsend, M., & Treen, K. (1997). The relationship between occupational balance and health: A pilot study. *Occupational Therapy International, 4*(1), 17–30.

Wilcock, A. A., & Hocking, C. (2015). *An occupational perspective of health* (3rd ed.). Slack.

Wilcock, A. A., & Townsend, E. A. (2009). Occupational justice. In E. B. Crepeau, E. S. Cohn, & B. A. Boyt Schell (Eds.), *Willard and Spackman's occupational therapy* (11th ed., pp. 192–199). Lippincott Williams & Wilkins.

Wiseman, J. O., Davis, J. A., & Polatajko, H. P. (2005). Occupational development: Towards an understanding of children's doing. *Journal of Occupational Science, 12*(1), 26–35.

Wiseman, L., & Whiteford, G. (2009). Understanding occupational transitions: A study of older rural men's retirement experiences. *Journal of Occupational Science, 16*(2), 104–109.

Wijekoon, S., & Peter, N. (2022). Examining racial, ethnic, and cultural diversity in occupational science research: Perspectives of persons of color. *Journal of Occupational Science,* 1–20.

World Federation of Occupational Therapists. (2012). *Position statement: Occupational science (revised).* http://www.wfot.org/ResourceCentre.aspx.

Yerxa, E. J., Clark, F., & Frank, G. (1990). An introduction to occupational science, a foundation for occupational therapy in the 21st century. *Occupational Therapy in Health Care, 6*, 1–17.

Zemke, R. (2004). Time, space, and the kaleidoscopes of occupation. *American Journal of Occupational Therapy, 58*(6), 608–620.

REFLECTION

1. Explain how you would enact reflexivity about your occupation-related assumptions when meeting a person or group in practice for the first time.

2. Describe the ways in which knowledge about occupation has become more diverse.

3. Describe your occupational identity, the meaning of one of your occupations, and the ways in which that occupation reflects your broader habits, routines and life contexts.

7

REFLECTING ON THE CONTRIBUTION OF THE DIMENSIONS OF THE ENVIRONMENT TO OCCUPATIONAL PARTICIPATION

SALVADOR SIMÓ ALGADO

■ ■ ■ ■ ■ ■ ■ ■ ■ ■ ■ ■ ■ ■ ■ ■ ■

The human being is a being-in-the-World

(Heidegger, 1998).

CHAPTER OUTLINE

Overview

This chapter explores the concept of environment beginning with philosophical approaches, such as pragmatism and transactionalism, to establish an understanding of the relationship between human beings and the environment. Pragmatism promotes a deeper understanding of the different dimensions of the environment to develop intelligent action to improve human society. Transactionalism promotes understanding of the human being and the environment as co-constitutive elements rather than separate elements. Physical, virtual, social, cultural, economic and political dimensions of the environment are discussed. The alignment of these dimensions to the Canadian Model of Occupational Participation is demonstrated, and a practice story illustrates the application of these theoretical concepts.

KEY POINTS

- The environment is a complex concept.
- Understanding pragmatism and transactionalism can lead to a more informed understanding of the environment.
- People have the capacity to transform the environment.
- The person and environment are co-defining, co-constitutive and inseparable agents.
- The environment includes physical, virtual, social, cultural, economic, political and ecological dimensions.
- Considering the dimensions of the environment is key when promoting occupational participation.

INTRODUCTION

The environment has been defined as (Cambridge Dictionary, 2023):

1. The air, water and land in or on which people, animals and plants live.
2. The conditions that people live, work or spend time in and the way that they influence how they feel, behave or work.
3. The system in which a computer or computer program operates.

These definitions directly connect with the ecological, physical and virtual dimensions of the environment that will be explored in this chapter. The environment can also be referred to as nature, ecology, ecosystem, natural resources, the biosphere, home, town or context (Urdang, 2008).

Occupational therapy commenced with a reductionist understanding of the environment. Its mechanistic heritage, typical of the biomedical paradigm, created a disciplinary focus on the physical environment. Thus, aspects such as the width of a door or the inclination of a ramp or other physical adaptations to the home or workplace were considered, for example, in terms of accessibility for a person who used a wheelchair. Slowly, a broader understanding of the environment occurred, and occupational therapists began to consider other dimensions of the environment, such as social, political and cultural dimensions. For example:

- The development of a social occupational therapy in Brazil led by the Metuia group, introduced important concepts such as territory (Bianchi & Malfitano, 2020, 2022) (refer to Chapter 4).
- Iwama (2006) developed a culturally safe praxis, related to his Kawa model.
- Political aspects were introduced by authors such as Pollard et al. (2008).
- Ecological aspects of the environment have gained importance because of climate change and have been developed by authors such as Simó Algado (2012, 2023).

The World Federation of Occupational Therapists (WFOT) has also released several position papers related to the environment (2012, 2018) highlighting the significance of the environment to the occupational therapy profession.

Many of the points raised in this chapter, and the role occupational therapists can play, are illustrated in the practice story in Box 7.1.

THE RELATIONSHIP BETWEEN THE HUMAN BEING AND THE ENVIRONMENT

To better understand the environment, there needs to be a deeper understanding of the relationship between human beings and the environment, and of the dimensions of the environment. Pragmatism is a philosophical tradition that promotes the world as inseparable from agency within it (Goodman, 1995). It was promoted by philosophers such as John Dewey (1969) and William James (2022). Dewey (1969) stated that there is a need for intelligent action to improve human society, that is, action based on a profound understanding of the environment being in constant change. Action is a key element for pragmatism, and it has the same importance as theory; in fact, action and theory are considered co-dependent (Tostado, 2006).

Occupational therapy is underpinned by this need to deeply understand the environment and the call to action to improve it.

Transactionalism refers to the ongoing process of interaction between a person and the physical and social environment and was initially promoted by philosophers such as Pierce (2016), and Dewey and Bentley (1946). This theory emerged out of the idea that there is a continuous relationship between the person and environment, in which each person restructures their environment rather than adapts to it (Cutchin & Dickie, 2012). Conceptual models guiding occupational therapy practice emphasise the transactional relationships between individuals, the occupations they perform, and the environments in which they live (Law et al., 1997). Occupational science analyses the relationship between people, the environment, and adaptation to the environment. Individuals do not operate as separate entities, transactionalism considers the agents of person and environment to be co-defining and co-constitutive (Sullivan, 2001).

The relational perspective of transactionalism means that occupation is no longer seen as a thing or as

BOX 7.1
E GREEN SOCIAL DESIGN

E Green Social Design (EGSD) is a social entrepreneurship project that has been designed by the author and led by the University of Vic – Central University of Catalonia (UVic-UCC). The Fourth Industrial Revolution (Economy 4.0) involves technological innovations and presents new challenges and opportunities. Thousands of new jobs will appear, while thousands of traditional ones will disappear. As noted in Chapter 26, unemployment, and job precarity are two important occupational problems. They are directly connected to poverty, inequality and social exclusion, and have the potential to jeopardise health. In considering the ecological environment, a severe climate crisis looms. It is necessary to create a new economic paradigm based on a green economy.

EGSD will create a social enterprise that, through recycled materials and 3D printers, will produce interior design, urbanism and landscaping furniture that will be sold to the public and private sectors. Social enterprises are a real alternative to traditional capitalism. The mission of EGSD is to create meaningful employment for young people and to combat climate change through the creation of a green economy.

EGSD is committed to preparing the youth without occupational competencies for Economy 4.0. and to fight climate change through a green economy. During its first year of operation, EGSD plans to employ one occupational therapist who will train 12 young people for 6 months. They will be a multicultural group, as culture is a very important dimension of the project. After completing their training on how to recycle plastic materials into furniture and landscaping products using 3D printers and ICT, the young people will be supported by another occupational therapist to undertake a 3-month placement experience in different industries. Following these placements, it is expected that young people will be able to join the labour market. Two of the young people will remain in the social enterprise to train the next group of young people. The project aims to support the emotional and mental health needs of young people, as well as facilitate the development of their training, practice experience and entrepreneurship competencies.

EGSD is aligned with the United Nations Sustainable Developmental Goals (United Nations, 2015). Social media will be used to promote the project and consideration has been given to promoting the project in the metaverse in the future. Regarding the physical environment, the project is in an industrial warehouse with universal design and ergonomic principles informing the physical workspace.

Acknowledgement: The project is made possible thanks to a partnership led by UVic-UCC working collaboratively with local and national government and the private sector.

a type of self-action or inter-action arising from within individuals. Instead, occupation is an important mode through which human beings, as organisms-in-environment, function in their complex totality. As such, occupations become more central to the scientific understanding of person-context relations 'as extending beyond a single person's experience to encompass others and the social, physical, and cultural context [that] offers rich opportunities for study' (Dickie et al., 2006, p. 85).

THE DIFFERENT DIMENSIONS OF THE ENVIRONMENT

The environment is a reality as fascinating as it is complex. As Edgar Morin (2002) said, a complex reality can only be understood from a complex vision of its different dimensions. These dimensions are not watertight compartments, but rather interact with each other; they are communicating vessels. Occupational therapists need to understand the different dimensions of the environment and how these dimensions can both facilitate and impede a person's or collective's participation (Baum & Christiansen, 2005).

The Physical Dimension

The physical dimension of the environment can be understood as a human being-made environment. Occupational therapists recommend changes to the physical dimension to support occupational participation (American Occupational Therapy Association [AOTA], 2017). They address the occupational participation limitations of persons with illness, injury or impairment, and contribute to the design of the built environment to provide enriched contextual and occupational experiences (Larkin et al., 2015).

The occupational therapist's role can begin from the architectural design. For example, the design of residential accommodation for elderly people could include a community playground for children within it. In this way, intergenerational activities can be naturally integrated and considered within the built environment. The application of universal design principles is one method used by occupational therapists when considering environmental modification (AOTA, 2017). Universal design refers to the creation of products and environments that can be used by all people, to the greatest extent possible, without the need for adaptation (Mace, 1985), accommodating a wide range of users, regardless of age, ability, or preference. The seven principles of universal design (Table 7.1) assist with the evaluation of space, guidance in the design process, and education on features that provide increased usability of products, services, and environments (Center for Universal Design, 1997; Young et al., 2014) (refer to Chapters 29 and 31).

Occupational therapists often consider the adaptation of the home, workplace and/or leisure spaces (sports, culture, etc.) when working with people. However, occupational therapists must go beyond focusing

TABLE 7.1	
Principles of Universal Design	
Principles	**Guidelines**
1. **Equitable Use**. The design is useful and marketable to people with diverse abilities.	1a. Provide the same means of use for all users: identical whenever possible; equivalent when not.
	1b. Avoid segregating or stigmatising any users.
	1c. Provisions for privacy, security and safety should be equally available to all users.
	1d. Make the design appealing to all users.
2. **Flexibility in Use**. The design accommodates a wide range of individual preferences and abilities.	2a. Provide choice in methods of use.
	2b. Accommodate right- or left-handed access and use.
	2c. Facilitate the user's accuracy and precision.
	2d. Provide adaptability to the user's pace.
3. **Simple and Intuitive Use**. The use of the design is easy to understand, regardless of the user's experience, knowledge, language skills, or current concentration level.	3a. Eliminate unnecessary complexity.
	3b. Be consistent with user expectations and intuition.
	3c. Accommodate a wide range of literacy and language skills.
	3d. Arrange information consistent with its importance.
	3e. Provide effective prompting and feedback during and after task completion.
4. **Perceptible Information**. The design communicates necessary information effectively to the user, regardless of ambient conditions or the user's sensory abilities.	4a. Use different modes (pictorial, verbal, tactile) for the redundant presentation of essential information.
	4b. Provide adequate contrast between essential information and its surroundings.
	4c. Maximise the 'legibility' of essential information.
	4d. Differentiate elements in ways that can be described (i.e. make it easy to give instructions or directions).
	4e. Provide compatibility with a variety of techniques or devices used by people with sensory limitations.
5. **Tolerance for Error**. The design minimises hazards and the adverse consequences of accidental or unintended actions.	5a. Arrange elements to minimise hazards and errors: most used elements, most accessible; hazardous elements eliminated, isolated, or shielded.
	5b. Provide warnings of hazards and errors.
	5c. Provide fail-safe features.
	5d. Discourage unconscious action in tasks that require vigilance.
6. **Low Physical Effort**. The design can be used efficiently and comfortably and with a minimum of fatigue.	6a. Allow the user to maintain a neutral body position.
	6b. Use reasonable operating forces.
	6c. Minimise repetitive actions.
	6d. Minimise sustained physical effort.
7. **Size and Space for Approach and Use**. Appropriate size and space are provided for approach, reach, manipulation and use regardless of the user's body size, posture, or mobility.	7a. Provide a clear line of sight to important elements for any seated or standing user.
	7b. Make reach to all components comfortable for any seated or standing user.
	7c. Accommodate variations in hand and grip size.
	7d. Provide adequate space for the use of assistive devices or personal assistance.

From Center for Universal Design (1997). https://design.ncsu.edu/research/center-for-universal-design/.

only on physical alterations and adaptations, such as the width of a door or the inclination of a ramp and include other aspects of importance such as access to housing or transportation. Occupational therapists should be involved in both the adaptation of a home or workplace for an individual person, as well as bigger adaptations that impact collectives, such as the design of inclusive public housing, community spaces and the design of government access policies and procedures.

At a macro level, it is important that occupational therapists understand the relatively recent development of mega cities. This has brought with it the problem of de-population of rural areas and rapid urbanisation in many parts of the world. In 1800, only 2% of the world's population lived in urban areas. This percentage had risen to 15% in 1900, 30% in 1950, more than 50% in 2007, 54 % in 2014 and it is expected to increase by 72% percent by 2050, from 3.6 billion to 6.3 billion. There are currently 34 cities in the world with a population of 10 million or more. Large youth population and high growth rates indicate that most urban populations will come from within cities. Rapid global urbanisation will have tremendous positive and negative economic, social and environmental impacts (Quan, 2016) and directly influence the occupational patterns and participation of people and collectives.

The Cultural Dimension

Culture is a shared system of meanings that includes ideas, concepts, knowledge, beliefs, values and norms that form the standards and rules of behaviour undertaken by people in their daily lives (Dyck, 1998). Culture provides meaningful ways of living through a range of social, educational, recreational and economic human activities (Kymlicka, 1996). Cultures traditionally tended to be concentrated in a territory and based on a shared language, but information and communication technologies, such as social networks and virtual reality, are changing this perception.

For Bauman (1999) there are two ways of understanding culture:

1. As the activity of the free spirit. It is the seat of creativity, invention, self-criticism and self-transcendence, enabling a person to resist norms and set themselves above the ordinary. It is *poiesis*, art, *creatio ex* nihilo or creation from nothing in the divine style, the capacity to create that distinguishes the most daring spirits.
2. As an instrument at the service of the social order that acts as an instrument of continuity. This way of understanding culture is through regularity and pattern. Culture is an aggregate or coherent system of pressures supported by sanctions, internalised values and norms, which guarantees the preservation of tradition.

The two ways of understanding cultures stand one against the other; one denies what the other proclaims. In the second understanding, Adorno's (2003) reflections on mass culture cannot be ignored: a culture that does not emerge from the masses but is directed at the masses. Culture becomes a domesticating and social control element, a mere object of consumption typical of a capitalist society.

Sousa Santos (2011) proposed a diatopical hermeneutics based on the idea that all cultures are incomplete and that the *tópoi* or strong argumentative beliefs of each culture are also incomplete. *Topoi* makes it possible to create arguments and exchange them. These produce the illusion of wholeness. The goal of diatopical hermeneutics is to raise awareness of the reciprocal incompleteness of cultures through intercultural dialogue. One of the *topoi* of Western culture is the belief in independence, accompanied by each person for themself and, if necessary, against other people; a rude individualism based on the survival of the fittest. This belief in independence contrasts with the practice of many Asian and First Nations peoples, in which the interdependence between all human beings and with the natural environment is acknowledged.

These reflections are fundamental, due to the struggle between a cultural mix and an exclusive ethnonationalism. Globalisation has not implied a miscegenation at the cultural level, but rather the adoption or imposition of an American way of life on a planetary scale. In fact, so many world cultures are disappearing. Perhaps a better way to illustrate this adoption or imposition is with the depletion in the number of languages spoken in the world. From the estimated 10,000 ever existing languages, just 600 are considered secure at present (Davis, 2001). Davis (2001) spoke of the McDonaldisation of the world. According to Ritzer (2013), the McDonaldisation of society is a phenomenon that occurs when society, its institutions and organisations are adapted to have the same characteristics found within fast-food chains, such as McDonald's. These characteristics include cultural standardisation, efficiency, calculability, predictability and control. Iwama et al. (2009) explained how the Western cosmovision is based on a hierarchal narrative where God, men and nature are related in a hierarchal way. Men received nature as a possession from God. This narrative contrasts with Eastern and First Nations narratives where Gods, human beings and nature are interrelated and interdependent. There is much to be learnt about occupational patterns from Indigenous communities who live in harmony with their environment.

The Virtual Dimension

From social media to the metaverse people are progressing towards virtualisation of societies. Social media is the title used to refer to the set of sites and tools that have been born and developed in the space created by modern media, such as communication networks, the internet and mobile phones. It is argued that the ongoing virtualisation of societies urges people to conceive of virtual worlds as transforming the meaning of reality (Ollinaho, 2018). The metaphor of augmented reality becomes an effective tool of analysis in places where different social realities are mutually penetrating and where physical and digital, material and symbolic, private and public, and production and consumption components of human existence are mixed and integrated (Ivanov, 2020).

The metaverse has the potential to extend the physical world using augmented and virtual reality technologies allowing users to seamlessly interact within real and simulated environments using avatars and holograms. Virtual environments and immersive games, such as Second Life, Fortnite, Roblox and VRChat, have been described as antecedents of the metaverse. They have a huge impact on the way people interact with others and develop shared experiences that may be transformational. Sectors that will be significantly impacted include education, healthcare and business. In addition, there are potential negative societal effects relating to social interaction, and issues relating to trust, privacy, bias and disinformation as well as psychological aspects

linked to addiction and its impact on vulnerable people (Dwivedi et al., 2022; Garavand & Aslani, 2022).

Occupational therapists need to reflect on the impact social media will have on the wellbeing and occupational lives of individuals and collectives. Concerns about the effects of social media on mental health are often expressed. A press release from the American Association of Suicidology (2017) stated that social media can have a significant impact on mental health, especially for young people. The Royal Society for Public Health (2017) reported evidence demonstrating links between social media use and mental health issues. The American Academy of Pediatrics (AAP) (2011) claimed that Facebook Depression could develop among youth who used social media for prolonged periods of time. For example, a study related to student mental health around the years of Facebook's expansion found that the use of Facebook at a college had a negative impact on student mental health. Facebook use increased the likelihood with which students reported experiencing impairment in academic performance due to poor mental health (Braghieri et al., 2022). Negative consequences reported included anxiety, depression, loneliness, poor sleep quality, poor mental health indicators, thoughts of self-harm and suicide, increased levels of psychological distress, cyber bullying, body image dissatisfaction, fear of missing out and decreased life satisfaction. It is important to note that positive effects of using social media have also been reported, including accessing other people's health experiences and expert health information, managing depression, emotional support and community building, expanding and strengthening offline networks and interactions, improved self-expression and self-identity, and establishing and maintaining relationships (Sadagheyani & Tatari, 2021). It is necessary to consider how the virtual environment will impact occupational participation.

The Social Dimension

Consideration of the process of atomisation (Bauman, 2003) and individualisation (Beck & Beck-Gernsheim, 2002) that are impacting social life and breaking down traditional social ties is necessary. Added to this trend is the progressive virtualisation of life. New realities such as the appearance of the metaverse must be considered alongside the influence of social networks in the form of human socialisation.

People are living immersed in a liquid modernity (Bauman, 2000), where the social forms that were solid become liquid. For example, Bauman (2000) gave the example of having access to education to promote access to a permanent job. In the past, it was not uncommon for people to work for the same employer for their entire working life. This pattern of employment is now less common.

Change is a constant. The Greek philosopher, Heraclitus (Barnes, 1987), said that it was not possible to enter the same river twice. The current speed of change today has been unprecedented in human history. Experts speak of a VUCA context (Johansen & Euchner, 2013), marked by Volatility, Uncertainty, Complexity and Ambiguity. The VUCA context contributes to the perception that people are living in a society full of risk (Beck, 2006). This may be why problems related to mental health, such as stress, anxiety or depression are some of the most prevalent in contemporary society. According to the World Health Organization (WHO, 2023a) in 2019, 301 million people were living with an anxiety disorder including 58 million children and adolescents. Anxiety disorders are characterised by excessive fear and worry and related behavioural disturbances. Symptoms can be severe enough to result in significant distress or impairment. Depression is the number one health problem worldwide. Globally, it is estimated that 5% of adults experience depression. Depression is a leading cause of disability worldwide and is a major contributor to the overall global burden of disease, with evidence that depression can lead to suicide (WHO, 2023b). Based on these statistics, society is confronting a mental health challenge. This situation has worsened due to the COVID-19 pandemic.

One important feature has been the psychiatrisation of social unrest (Rendueles, 2006). The consequences of phenomena of social origin, such as poverty, unemployment, or job insecurity, may lead to a diagnosis of mental illness and be treated as such, ignoring their social causes. Thus, when a person loses their job and is unable to re-enter the labour market due to age, they may be diagnosed with depression. From then on, they are treated solely for the mental health problem, depression, with the basic social cause being ignored.

There is no question that depression must be treated from a mental health perspective, but the social cause must also be addressed, that is, it is essential to work on the social determinants of the resulting mental health issue. This approach is aligned with the social occupational therapy approach developed in Brazil (refer to Chapter 4), in which territory is considered the concrete ground of everyday life, public policies and the exercise of citizenship – 'the right to have rights is expressed, denied or claimed from concrete places: to live, to study, to work, to have fun, to live healthily, to transit, to opine, to participate' (Costa & Brasil, 2014, p. 438). Living in a community means being willing to experience identification with the territory, creating collective subjectivity, feeling safe and showing solidarity in the relationship with the actors of the social network (Silva et al., 2015, p. 147).

The Ecological Dimension

The term ecology, coined by biologist Kaeckel, combines two Greek words: *oikos* meaning house, and *logos* meaning study. Thus, ecology is the study of the global house. Ecology is the combination of abiotic and biotic elements that surround an organism (García, 2004), and the interaction and profound dialogue between all existing things, everything that exists and co-exists (Boff, 2001). Ecology is directly related to society and culture. It refers to the importance of caring for the Earth as a whole. A forward vision is required to avoid generational selfishness and to develop solidarity with all future generations.

Humanity stands at a historically defining moment. The Glasgow Climate Change Conference held in 2021 was a stage of a critical dialogue about the ecological challenge that started with the Club of Rome Report (Meadows, 1972). Agenda 21 (UN, 1993) states that the ecosystems on which the wellbeing of people depends are continuing to deteriorate; there is worsening poverty, hunger, literacy and health; and disparities within and between nations are ongoing. Global changes to the planet's ecosystem systems have been the most dramatic throughout human history. Societies are confronting an increase in the number of natural disasters. The Earth is confronting the sixth great extinction, with a species extinction rate estimated to be 100 times higher than before the First Industrial Revolution (Latouche, 2010).

A stable climate is directly connected to human health (Maibach et al., 2021). For a long time, Earth has been supporting an unsustainable ecological footprint (Latouche, 2010), that is, the amount of soil needed to produce our aliments and absorb our wastes, with humanity using more resources than the planet can renew. This reality is becoming increasingly critical, with overpopulation and climate change contributing to stress on freshwater supplies, food shortages, depletion of fisheries, loss of biodiversity and soil erosion. These global threats will harm health and human occupation. Thus, strategies are needed to mitigate the effects of climate change and to build individual and community resilience (Dennis et al., 2015).

Nature is considered a possession to be exploited by humans from the predominant Western culture, being considered a place of exteriority (Sousa Santos, 2011). People living in a Western culture have tended to become separated from nature. A deep belief in technological developments has made people ignore the law of entropy related to the nonreversibility of the exploitation of matter and energy (Latouche, 2010). Jonas (1995) wrote about the principle of responsibility, warning of the tremendous destructive power of human science and technology. There is much to be learned from other cultures, as culture has a significant impact on sustainable behaviours (Hocking, 2017). For example, Indigenous people have been observed to participate in sustainable and responsible occupations as their cultures valued stewardship (McNeil, 2016).

Human occupation has been a primary contributor to ecological degradation (Wilcock, 1998). Zemke (2004) encouraged reflection on how human occupation can contribute to planetary balance. The World Federation of Occupational Therapists (WFOT) (2012) recognised the repercussions of the global climate crisis as a great challenge to both human wellbeing and sustainable development. It clarified that it is vital that occupational therapists work towards environmental sustainability on two fronts: collaboratively with people and collectives, and within the profession. WFOT (2018) stated that unsustainable lifestyles are a major issue for occupational therapists and scientists. The adaptation of certain occupational patterns and lifestyles will determine the future health of humans and ecosystems (Lieb, 2020). Occupations must be understood from an ethical position in which the individual,

society and the species are considered as part of a planetary community (Méndez, 2011).

The ecological environment is the always present container of human occupations. Human occupations and the ecological environment mutually affect each other. Lack of access to meaningful occupations related to the ecological environment is a case of occupational deprivation and injustice. Occupational therapists and scientists need to write a new narrative for humanity connecting ecology with occupational justice (Simó Algado & Townsend, 2015). Occupational stewardship, a justice-based approach to promoting occupation for health without jeopardising the ecology, has also been advocated (Rushford & Thomas, 2016).

Occupational ecology is the study of the deep and inseparable connection between human occupation and the ecological environment (Simó Algado, 2012). It was originally referred to as a double moment of reflection and action; reflection about the serious ecological crisis provoked by human occupations that endangers the survival of the human beings followed by an urgent and proactive action for sustainability based on human occupation. This action-reflection continuous cycle was inspired by the French philosopher Mounier (2002) who compared it with the diastolic and systolic movements of the human heart. Occupational ecology has been further developed as a new emerging field for occupational science (Simó Algado, 2023). This can be connected to the critical occupational literacy proposed by Townsend (2015), a way to learn, think, write, make decisions, and make sense of occupational justice and ecological sustainability.

Occupational ecology can nourish an ecosocial occupational therapy that makes the transition between theory and practice. Ecosocial occupational therapy is based on the development of occupational therapy projects (preferably action research) that integrate the impact on wellbeing, social participation, and a positive ecological impact, from an occupational justice and human rights perspective. One of the purposes of such projects is 'to build healthy, inclusive, and sustainable communities. A human group that recognises its mutual interdependence in which everyone feels and participates as a citizen with full rights, regardless of any occupational problem. This community is evolving in harmony with the natural environment to meet the needs of the present without compromising those of future generations to meet their own needs' (Simó Algado, 2012, p. 13). Ecosocial occupational therapy is aligned with human rights, as defined in the United Nations' (1948) Universal Declaration of Human Rights, as foundational to the pursuit of occupational justice for all (WFOT, 2019), the Earth Charter, and the UN Sustainable Development Goals (Simó Algado, 2023).

The domain of ecology is essentially occupational (Simó Algado & Townsend, 2015). Two related concepts have appeared in recent years: ecopations and eco-occupations. *Ecopations* are occupations that promote wellbeing at individual and collective levels (Persson & Erlandsson, 2014). Ecopations are used as a tool to address sustainability issues in relation to future occupations for wellbeing. A core proposition is that doing, if guided by ecopations, could promote wellbeing at individual and collective levels if the personal, as well as the local and global, contexts are considered. *Eco-occupations* are occupations that are driven by the motivation of individuals and collectives to combine personal needs with protection of the ecosystem (Ung et al., 2020). Eco-occupations consider the environmental, economic, cultural and solidarity dimensions from a global perspective, that is a perspective that integrates the global with the local. Eco-occupations aim to maintain the balance of ecosystems, promote eco-occupations and support intergenerational occupational justice. They are rooted in eco-humanist values, being aware of the real role citizens of the world play.

The Economic Dimension

Global wealth inequalities are extremely pronounced. The poorest half of the global population barely owns any wealth at all, possessing just 2% of the total. In contrast, the richest 10% of the global population owns 76% of all wealth (Chancel et al., 2022). Occupational justice asserts that inequalities in participation are a breach of human rights (Wilcock & Townsend, 2000). Occupational justice emphasises equity and participation in relation to occupational choice, to enhance wellbeing and develop a more inclusive society (Hocking, 2017). It is based on the idea that humans have the right to engage in diverse occupations that are meaningful, support quality of life and promote health (Standyk et al., 2010).

Poverty, economy and ecological degradation are connected. Ecological resources are crucial to guarantee a wealthy future since they are key resources for reducing poverty and disease (Ewing et al., 2010). Land degradation and poverty are connected (Barbier & Hochard, 2018). Climate change provokes direct economic losses, such as crop failures and indirect losses such as mental illness (Pereira, 2009) thus increasing poverty and population health and social problems. Global change has a greater impact on poor countries, as they are directly exposed to ecological degradation (Tofeti & Dos Santos, 2020).

It is necessary to explore fairer and more sustainable economic alternatives to pursue occupational justice, which is understood as the promotion of a combined social and economic change that will allow access to meaningful occupations (Standyk et al., 2010). To do this, occupational therapists must understand the current economic framework as the economic environment is a determining environment. Few factors influence the occupational patterns of a person or community as much as the economic context in which they find themselves. Productivity has been considered a basic dimension of human occupation. For the most part, people live in a capitalist economic context, which although it has had important and positive contributions, is also linked to problems, such as unemployment, precariousness and climate change.[1]

Unemployment is one of the main problems of contemporary societies (refer to Chapter 26). As Bauman (2000, 2003) affirmed, the concept of unemployment went from being a temporary condition to being definitive for important sectors of the population. Beck also commented that the precariousness of the labour market is a global concern (Beck, 2000). Furthermore, it has been found that a job that jeopardises wellbeing and causes character corrosion negatively impacts health and wellbeing (Sennet, 2006).

Undoubtedly the current economic framework is marked by the emergence of the Fourth Industrial Revolution (4.0 Economy). This is based on new technologies, such as robotics, virtual reality, 3-dimensional printing and the internet. These technologies represent a drastic change in the labour market and this Fourth Industrial Revolution will mean the disappearance of thousands of jobs while creating new ones,

---

[1]Criticism of the capitalist system does not imply on the part of the author a position in favour of the traditional communist or socialist alternatives.

but only for those with the digital skills necessary to make the transition to this 4.0 Economy. At the same time, a green and circular economy is imposed in the face of the problems posed by climate change.

Given the prevailing economic model, which is a neoliberal capitalist model, interesting alternatives emerge that are of interest to occupational therapy to develop the proclaimed occupational justice, such as serene degrowth, the economy for the common good, the green economy, or social entrepreneurship, among others. The serene degrowth proposes reducing human consumption to a level that is sustainable (Latouche, 2010). The economy for the common good (Felber, 2019) is based, like a market economy, on private companies and individual initiatives. However, the difference with previous models is that companies do not strive to compete to obtain more economic benefit, but rather cooperate to achieve the greatest common good for society as a whole. The green economy is one that makes the transition from fossil sources to renewable energy; Rifkin (2019) predicted the collapse of the fossil economy by 2027. The green economy develops in parallel to a circular economy and a philosophy such as a cradle-to-cradle based on the elimination of waste. Social entrepreneurship seeks to provide innovative solutions to the main social, health and ecological problems of the planet. Social enterprises put benefits for the planet and people at the centre of their mission, transcending the mere accumulation of capital typical of traditional capitalism, and opening new opportunity scenarios for the development of projects related to the green economy.

The Political Dimension

The political sphere is where Arendt situates human action. For Arendt, a life without words and without action is literally dead (Arendt, 1997). People live in a time of proliferation of extremism. A frequent target of extremism is immigrants. Living with foreign people can provoke rejection and distrust. In many countries, there is a proliferation of walls. In recent years there have been movements such as Black Lives Matter in the United States. The war continues to be a perennial constant in the international political context. The wars in Syria and Yemen have been followed by the war in Ukraine; this reality has caused an unprecedented increase in refugees in the world, reaching figures not seen since the Second World War. The United Nations High Commission for Refugees (UNHCR) estimated that there are currently more than 100 million displaced people in the world, more than 1% of the world population. Eighty-six percent of refugees are hosted by developing countries (UNHCR, 2021). Considering the global challenges humanity faces, it is necessary to develop a cosmopolitan and multicultural citizenship, rather than try to solve these issues from a single State intervention.

Occupational therapists must contribute to the development of cosmopolitan and multicultural citizenship. The objective is the creation of healthy, inclusive and sustainable communities, where every person is recognised as a full citizen despite any occupational dysfunction, due to physical, psychological, social or environmental reasons. Occupational therapists must incorporate the language of human rights and sustainability in interventions (Simó Algado, 2012) as this is fundamental to ensuring individuals and collectives are aware of their rights and duties as citizens. It is essential to develop an occupational therapy practice that is based on human rights (Guajardo & Simó Algado, 2010), ensuring a powerful social and political activism, that leads to the development of a cosmopolitan and multicultural citizenship.

THE DIMENSIONS OF THE ENVIRONMENT AND PROMOTING OCCUPATIONAL PARTICIPATION

The Canadian Model of Occupational Participation (CanMOP) (Egan & Restall, 2022) (refer to Chapter 11) does not refer to the environment, but rather to context, which may be considered a synonym for environment. Participation in occupation takes place within the environment situated within a context. Context is defined as (Cambridge Dictionary, 2023):

1. The situation within which something exists or happens, and that can help explain it; and
2. The influences and events related to a particular event or situation.

Occupational participation, 'having access to, initiating, and sustaining valued occupations within meaningful relationships and contexts' (Egan & Restall, 2022, p. 76), cannot be promoted without a deep understanding of all the interconnected dimensions of the environment. The CanMOP emphasises the meaning of context through a focus on the micro, meso and macro dimensions of context. Micro context refers to 'interactions the individual has with people including family, friends, schoolmates, teachers, co-workers, and health and social service providers' (Egan & Restall, 2022, p. 81). Meso context refers to 'system structures, such as health care and social services organizations and their respective programs' (Egan & Restall, 2022, p. 81). Macro contexts refer to 'larger socioeconomic and political context grounded in international, national, provincial, and local governance' (Egan & Restall, 2022, p. 82); this macro context is aligned with the social, economic and political dimensions of the environment. All the dimensions of the environment are connected to these contexts. Meaning is considered from the perspective of the individual and/or collective and is 'derived from needs, relationships, and history' (Egan & Restall, 2022, p. 78). Reflecting on the different dimensions of the environment so many potential questions arise, such as:

- How to find meaning in the context of a liquid society?
- What is the meaning of developing restorative occupations in nature in the context of climate change?
- What is the meaning of practising a cultural ritual in the context of the disappearance of so many world cultures?
- What is the meaning of work when it provokes the corrosion of a person's character?
- What is going to be the meaning of occupations performed at the metaverse?

The CanMOP explores history 'through a life course perspective for persons and families, and through group or community history for larger collectives such as communities' (Egan & Restall, 2022, p. 79). Certainly, it is necessary to recover this broad perspective, transcending the contemporary individualisation process (Beck & Beck-Gernsheim, 2002) to confront challenges to humanity, such as inequality, declining democracy, poverty, unemployment and climate change.

Relationships refer to 'past, present, and hoped-for future relationships [and considers relating to others],

environments, histories, ancestors, cultures, knowledges, social, political, and economic structures, and the natural world' (Egan & Restall, 2022 p. 79). Therefore it has been argued that is necessary to develop an intra and intergenerational solidarity to confront the climatic crisis. The definition of ecology is the relation of everything with everything (Boff, 2014). Again, there is a need to consider the cultural, social, political and economic dimensions of the environment as they are part of these structures and part of our ancestors, knowledges and cultures.

The CanMOP affirms that, 'occupational therapists collaboratively consider access to and ways to initiate and sustain participation in valued occupations within meaningful contexts' (Egan & Restall, 2022, p. 81). Access refers to the availability of occupational possibilities. Initiate 'refers to commencing or recommencing a valued occupation in a meaningful context' (p. 83). Potential new questions arise: How can access to work be promoted instead of unemployment? To address this question there is a need to understand the job market. Otherwise, participants may be trained for obsolete professions in the new Economy 4.0. There is evidence that the green economy is opening amazing employment opportunities.

Collaborative relationship-focused therapy 'attends to, and concentrates on, the relational aspects of the therapist self and the individuals and collectives who use occupational therapy services' (Restall & Egan, 2022, p. 100) (refer to Chapter 12). This approach promotes rights-based self-determination; 'a rights-based definition of self-determination that acknowledges people's entitlement to make decisions that affect their lives and communities' (Restall & Egan, 2022, p. 107). 'Occupational therapy based on human rights, requires critical reflection on the contextual and relational elements of occupational therapy relationships […] with the therapist acknowledging that they themselves are an integral part of the relational context of therapy' (Restall & Egan, 2022, p. 101). 'Therapists must do the ongoing hard work of understanding how they are impacted by influences at the micro, meso and macro level as well as how these influences affect the individuals and collectives who use their services' (Restall & Egan, 2022, p. 104).

The Canadian Occupational Therapy Inter-Relational Practice Process (COTIPP) (Restall et al., 2022, p. 122) seeks to understand about context 'considered holistically and inter-relationally, appreciating that various aspects of context, influence, and are influenced by, other aspects' (Restall et al., 2022, p. 124) (refer to Chapter 12). The COTIPP promotes a critical reflection that 'challenges the therapist to consider more deeply how systems and structures may be supporting or creating barriers' for individuals and collectives and 'can identify new ways of thinking about and engaging in occupations' (Restall et al., 2022, pp. 130–131). Using justice, equity and rights-based lenses can enable occupational therapists to critically evaluate 'how practice contexts and their own practice processes promote or create barriers to justice, equity, and rights of the individuals and collectives they work with' and take 'action to reduce or remove barriers to occupational participation' (Restall, et al., 2022, p. 131). To remain critical and develop this justice-based approach, the profession of occupational therapy must transcend its original focus on the physical aspects of the environment, based on a biomedical mechanistic paradigm, and embrace the social, cultural, ecological, economic and political dimensions of the environment.

CONCLUSION

In a context of VUCA, it is important to understand the complex and interactive dimensions of the virtual, ecological, economic and political environment. Human occupation is the dialogue between the human being and the environment. Person and environment are co-defining and co-constitutive. Occupation is an important mode through which human beings, function in their complex totality. To be able to improve the occupational participation of individuals and collectives, occupational therapists require a deep understanding of the environment and all its interdependent dimensions: physical, cultural, virtual, social, ecological, economic and political.

Pragmatism invites occupational therapists to develop an intelligent action, that is, an action based on a profound understanding of the different dimensions of the environment to be able to improve human society. Transactionalism refers to a continuous relationship between a person and environment, in which people work towards restructuring their environment rather than adapting to it.

The Canadian Model of Occupational Participation (CanMOP) is a useful model to facilitate a deep understanding of the dimensions of the environment and is complemented by the concept of collaborative relationship-focused practice and the Canadian Occupational Therapy Inter-Relational Practice Process COTIPP).

REFERENCES

Adorno, T. (2003). *Obra completa*. Akal.

American Academy of Pediatrics. (2011). Clinical report – The impact of social media on children, adolescents, and families. *Pediatrics, 127*(4), 800–804. https://doi.org/10.1542/peds.2011-0054.

American Association for Suicidology. (2017). *Validity of the blue whale challenge is disputed, but social media's impact on young people's mental health is real*. https://www.einpresswire.com/article/393609296/validity-of-the-blue-whale-challenge-is-disputed-but-social-medias-impact-on-young-people-s-mental-health-is-real.

American Occupational Therapy Association. (2017). Occupational therapy practice framework: Domain and process. *The American Journal of Occupational Therapy, 68*(Supplement_1), S1–S48. https://doi.org/10.5014/ajot.2014.682006.

Arendt, H. (1997). *¿Qué es la política? (What is politic?)*. Paidos.

Barbier, E. B., & Hochard, J. P. (2018). Land degradation and poverty. *Nature Sustainability, 1*, 623–631. https://doi.org/10.1038/s41893-018-0155-4.

Barnes, J. (1987). *Early Greek philosophy*. Penguin Books.

Baum, C. M., & Christiansen, C. H. (2005). Person-environment-occupation-performance: An occupation-based framework for practice. In C. H. Christiansen, C. M. Baum, & J. Bass-Haugen (Eds.), *Occupational therapy: Performance, participation, and well-being* (pp. 243–259). SLACK.

Bauman, Z. (1999). *Culture as praxis*. Sage Publications.

Bauman, Z. (2000). *Trabajo, consumismo y nuevos pobres*. Gedisa.

Bauman, Z. (2000). *Liquid modernity*. Polity Press.

Bauman, Z. (2003). *Wasted lives: Modernity and its outcasts*. Polity Press.

Beck, U. (2000). *Un Nuevo mundo feliz : La precariedad del trabajo en la era de la globalización*. Paidós.

Beck, U., & Beck-Gernsheim, E. (2002). Individualization: institutionalized individualism and its social and political consequences. *Acta Sociologica, 13*, 221.

Beck, U. (2006). *La Sociedad del riesgo: Hacia una nueva modernidad*. Paidós.

Bianchi, P. C., & Malfitano, A. P. (2020). Território e comunidade na terapia ocupacional brasileira: Uma revisão conceitual. *Cadernos Brasileiros De Terapia Ocupacional, 28*(2), 621–639. https://doi.org/10.4322/2526-8910.ctoAR1772.

Bianchi, P. C., & Malfitano, A. P. (2022). Atuação profissional de terapeutas ocupacionais em países latino-americanos: O que caracteriza uma ação territorial-comunitária? *Cadernos Brasileiros De Terapia Ocupacional, 30*, e3053. https://doi.org/10.1590/2526-8910.ctoAO23163053.

Boff, L. (2001). *Ética planetaria desde el gran sur*. Trotta.

Boff, L. (2014). Ecology & liberation: A new paradigm. Orbis Books.

Braghieri, L., Levy, R., & Makarin, A. (2022). Social media and mental health. *American Economic Review, 112*(11), 3660–3693. https://doi.org/10.1257/aer.20211218.

Cambridge Dictionary. (2023). *Environment*. In Cambridge Dictionary, Cambridge University Press. https://dictionary.cambridge.org/.

Center for Universal Design. (1997). The principles of universal design. https://design.ncsu.edu/research/center-for-universal-design/.

Chancel, L., Piketty, T., Saez, E., & Zucman, G. (2022). World inequality report. https://wir2022.wid.world/www-site/uploads/2023/03/D_FINAL_WIL_RIM_RAPPORT_2303.pdf.

Costa, L. A., & Brasil, F. D. (2014). Cidade, territorialidade e redes na política de saúde mental. *Cadernos de Terapia Ocupacional da UFSCar, 22*(2), 435–442. https://doi.org/10.4322/cto.2014.065.

Cutchin, M. P., & Dickie, V. A. (2012). Transactionalism: Occupational science and the pragmatic attitude. In G. E. Whiteford & C. Hocking (Eds.), *Occupational science: Society, inclusion, participation* (pp. 23–38). Blackwell Publishing Ltd.

Davis, W. (2001). *Light at the edge of the world*. Douglas Mc.

Dennis, C. W., Dorsey, J. A., & Gitlow, L. (2015). A call for sustainable practice in occupational therapy. *Canadian Journal of Occupational Therapy, 82*(3), 160–168. https://doi.org/10.1177/0008417414566925.

Dewey, J., & Bentley, A. F. (1946). Interaction and transaction. *The Journal of Philosophy, 43*(19), 505–517. https://doi.org/10.2307/2019771.

Dewey, J. (1969). *The ethics of democracy*. Southern Illinois University Press.

Dickie, V., Cutchin, M. P., & Humphry, R. (2006). Occupation as transactional experience: A critique of individualism in occupational science. *Journal of Occupational Science, 13*(1), 83–93. https://doi.org/10.1080/14427591.2006.9686573.

Dwivedi, Y., Hughes, L., Baabdullah, A., Ribeiro, S., Giannakis, M., & Al-Debei, M. (2022). Metaverse beyond the hype. *International Journal of Information Management, 66*, 102542. https://doi.org/10.1016/j.ijinfomgt.2022.102542.

Dyck, I. (1998). Multicultural society. In D. Jones (Ed.), *Sociology and occupational therapy: An integrated approach* (pp. 67–80). Churchill Livingstone.

Egan, M., & Restall, G. (2022). The Canadian model of occupational participation. In M. Egan & G. Restall (Eds.), *Promoting occupational participation: Collaborative relationship-focused occupational therapy* (pp. 73–95). Canadian Association of Occupational Therapists.

Ewing, B., Moore, D., Goldfinger, S. H., Oursler, A., Reed, A., & Wackernagel, M. (2010). *Ecological footprint atlas 2010*. Global Footprint Network. http://www.footprintnetwork.org/images/uploads/Ecological_Footprint_Atlas_2010.pdf.

Felber, C. (2019). Change everything: Creating an economy for the common good. Zed Books.

Garavand, A., & Aslani, N. (2022). Metaverse phenomenon and its impact on health: A scoping review. *Informatics in Medicine Unlocked, 32*, 101029. https://doi.org/10.1016/j.imu.2022.101029.

García, E. (2004). *Medio ambiente y sociedad*. Alianza Editorial.

Goodman, R. (1995). *Pragmatism*. Routledge.

Guajardo, A., & Simó Algado, S. (2010). Occupational therapy based on human rights. *TOG (A Coruña), 12*, 1–25.

Hocking, C. (2017). Occupational justice as social justice: The moral claim for inclusion. *Journal of Occupational Science, 24*(1), 29–42. https://doi.org/10.1080/14427591.2017.1294016.

Ivanov, D. (2020). Augmented modernity: Effects of post-globalization and post virtualization. *Sotsiologicheskie Issledovaniya*, (5), 44–55. https://doi.org/10.31857/S013216250009397-9.

Iwama, M. K. (2006). *The Kawa model*. Elsevier Health Sciences. https://doi.org/10.1016/B978-0-443-10234-9.X5001-4.

Iwama, M. K., Thomson, N. A., & Macdonald, R. (2009). The Kawa model: The power of culturally responsive occupational therapy. *Disability and Rehabilitation, 31*(14), 1125–1135. https://doi.org/10.1080/09638280902773711.

James, W. (2022). *Pragmatism*. Longroad Classics.

Johansen, B., & Euchner, J. (2013). Navigating the VUCA World. *Research-Technology Management, 56*(1), 10–15.

Jonas, H. (1995). *El principio de responsabilidad*. Herder Editorial.

Kymlicka, W. (1996). *Ciudadanía multicultural*. Editorial Paidós.

Larkin, H., Hitch, D., Watchorn, V., & Ang, S. (2015). Working with policy and regulatory factors to implement universal design in the built environment: The Australian experience. *International Journal of Environmental Research and Public Health, 12*(7), 8157–8171. https://doi.org/10.3390/ijerph120708157.

Latouche, S. (2010). *Farewell to growth*. Polity.

Law, M., Polatajko, H., Baptiste, S., & Townsend, E. (1997). Core concepts of occupational therapy. In E. Townsend (Ed.), *Enabling occupation: An occupational therapy perspective* (pp. 29–56). CAOT Publications ACE.

Lieb, L. C. (2020). Occupation and environmental sustainability: A scoping review. *Journal of Occupational Science, 29*(4), 505–528. https://doi.org/10.1080/14427591.2020.1830840.

Mace, R. (1985). Universal design: Barrier free environments for everyone. *Designers West, 33*(1), 147–152.

Maibach, E., Miller, J., Armstrong, F., El Omrani, O., Zhang, Y., Philpott, N., Atkinson, S., Rudoph, L., Karliner, J., Wang, J., Pétrin-Desrosiers, C., Stauffer, A., & Jensen, G. K. (2021). Health professionals, the Paris agreement, and the fierce urgency of now. *Journal of Climate Change and Health, 1*, 100002. https://doi.org/10.1016/j.joclim.2020.100002.

McNeil, H. N. (2016). Māori and the natural environment from an occupational justice perspective. *Journal of Occupational Science, 24*(1), 19–28. https://doi.org/10.1080/14427591.2016.1245158.

Meadows, D. H., Meadows, D. L., Randers, J., & Beherens, W. (1972). *The limits of growth*. Universe Books.

Méndez, J. (2011). Ocupación como proceso ecológico [Occupation as an ecological process]. In J. Trujillo, A. Sanabria, L. Carrizosa, L. Parra, L. Rubio, S. Uribe, J. Rojas, C. Pérez, & L. Méndez (Eds.), *Ocupación: Sentido, realización y libertad* (pp. 129–147). Universidad Nacional de Colombia.

Morin, E. (2002). *Los siete saberes necesarios para la educación del futuro*. Paidós.

Mounier, E. (2002). *El personalismo*. Ediciones Sígueme.

Ollinaho, O. I. (2018). Virtualization of the life-world. *Human Studies, 41*(2), 193–209. https://doi.org/10.1007/s10746-017-9455-3.

Pereira, R. B. (2009). The climate change debate: Ageing and the impacts on participating in meaningful occupations. *Australian*

Occupational Therapy Journal, 56(5), 365–366. https://doi.org/10.1111/j.1440-1630.2009.00792.x.

Persson, D., & Erlandsson, L. (2014). Ecopation: Connecting sustainability, glocalisation and well-being. *Journal of Occupational Science, 21*(1), 12–24. https://doi.org/10.1080/14427591.2013.867561.

Pierce, C. (2016). *Charles peirce on pragmatism and pragmaticism*. Whealth of Nation.

Pollard, N., Sakellariou, D., & Kronenberg, F. (Eds.). (2008). *A political practice of occupational therapy*. Elsevier Science.

Quan, X. (2016). The trends, promises and challenges of urbanisation in the world. *Habitat International, 54*(3), 241–252. https://doi.org/10.1016/j.habitatint.2015.11.018-ç.

Rendueles, G. (2006). *Viejos y nuevos locos. La sociología crítica después de Foucalt*. Círculo de Bellas Artes.

Restall, G., & Egan, M. (2022). Collaborative relationship-focused practice occupational therapy. In M. Egan & G. Restall (Eds.), *Promoting occupational participation: Collaborative relationship-focused occupational therapy*. Canadian Association of Occupational Therapists (pp. 97–117).

Restall, G., Egan, M., Valavaara, K., Phenix, A., & Sack, C. (2022). Canadian occupational therapy inter-relational practice process. In M. Egan & G. Restall (Eds.), *Promoting occupational participation: Collaborative relationship-focused occupational therapy*. Canadian Association of Occupational Therapists (pp. 120–149).

Rifkin, J. (2019). *El new green dealt global*. Planeta.

Ritzer, G. (2013). *The McDonaldization of society: 20th Anniversary edition*. Sage.

Royal Society for Public Health. (2017). *Social media and young people's mental health and wellbeing*. https://www.rsph.org.uk/static/uploaded/d125b27c-0b62-41c5-a2c0155a8887cd01.pdf.

Rushford, N., & Thomas, K. (2016). Occupational steward-ship: Advancing a vision of occupational justice and sustainability. *Journal of Occupational Science, 23*(3), 295–307. https://doi.org/10.1080/14427591.2016.1174954P.

Sadagheyani, H. E., & Tatari, F. (2021). Investigating the role of social media on mental health. *Mental Health and Social Inclusion, 25*(1), 41–51. https://doi.org/10.1108/MHSI-06-2020-0039.

Sousa Santos, B. (2011). *El milenio huérfano: Ensayos para una nueva cultura política*. Editorial Trotta. World Federation of Occupational Therapists. http://trotta.es.

Silva, J. A., & Lima, E. M. F. A. L. (2015). Comunidades provisórias entre pessoas quaisquer: Encontros de delicadeza, criação artística e diferença. *Cadernos de Terapia Ocupacional da UFSCar, 23*(3), 673–681.

Simó Algado, S. (2012). Terapia ocupacional ecosocial: Hacia una ecología ocupacional. *Cadernos de Terapia Ocupacional da UFSCar, São Carlos, 20*(1), 7–16.

Simó Algado, S. (2023). Occupational ecology: An emerging field for occupational science. *Journal of Occupational Science, 30*(4), 684–696. https://doi.org/10.1080/14427591.2023.2185278.

Simó Algado, S., & Townsend, E. A. (2015). Eco-social occupational therapy. *British Journal of Occupational Therapy, 78*(3), 182–186. https://doi.org/10.1177/0308022614561239.

Standyk, R., Townsend, E., & Wilcock, A. (2010). Occupational justice. In C. H. Christiansen & E. A. Townsend (Eds.), Introduction to occupation: The art and science of living (2nd ed., pp. 329-358). Pearson Education.

Sullivan, S. (2001). *Living across and through skins: Transactional bodies, pragmatism and feminism*. Indiana University Press.

Tofeti, A. R., & Dos Santos, V. (2020). Sustainable occupational opportunities in protected areas in Brazil. *World Federation of Occupational Therapists Bulletin, 76*(1), 40–49. https://doi.org/10.1080/14473828.2020.1758398.

Tostado, M. G. (2006). El papel del académico en la construcción de la democracia. Reflexiones a partir del pensamiento de John Dewey. *Reencuentro. Análisis de Problemas Universitarios* (45), 0.

Townsend, E. (2015). Critical occupational literacy: Thinking about occupational justice, ecological sustainability, and aging in everyday life. *Journal of Occupational Science, 22*(4), 389–402. https://doi.org/10.1080/14427591.2015.1071691.

Ung, Y., Sarah, T. S., Drolet, M.-J., Simó Algado, S., & Soubeyran, M. (2020). Building occupational therapy practice ecological based occupations and ecosystem sustainability: Exploring the concept of eco-occupation to support intergenerational occupational justice. *World Federation of Occupational Therapists Bulletin, 76*(1), 15–21. https://doi.org/10.1080/14473828.2020.1727095.

United Nations. (1993). *Agenda 2: Programe of action for sustainable development: Declaration on environment and development; Statement of forest principles. June 1992*. United Nations Dept. of Public Information.

United Nations. (2015). *Sustainable development goals*. https://sdgs.un.org/goals.

United Nations. (2021). *Global report 2021*. https://reporting.unhcr.org/globalreport2021.

Urdang, L. (2008). *The MacMillan dictionary of synonyms and antonyms*. Palgrave Macmillan.

World Health Organization. (2023a). *Mental disorders*. https://www.who.int/news-room/fact-sheets/detail/mental-disorders.

World Health Organization. (2023b). *Depression*. https://www.who.int/news-room/fact-sheets/detail/depression.

Wilcock, A. (1998). *An occupational perspective of health*. Slack Incorporated.

Wilcock, A., & Townsend, E. (2000). Occupational terminology interactive dialogue. *Journal of Occupational Science, 7*(2), 84–86. https://doi.org/10.1080/14427591.2000.9686470.

World Federation of Occupational Therapists. (2012). *Position statement: Environmental sustainability, sustainable practice within occupational therapy*. Retrieved December 10, 2021, from https://wfot.org/resources/environmental-sustainability-sustainable-practice-within-occupational-therapy.

World Federation of Occupational Therapists. (2018). *Sustainability matters: Guiding principles for sustainability in occupational therapy practice, education and scholarship* (pp. 1–51). Retrieved December 10, 2021, from https://wfot.org/resources/wfot-sustainability-guiding-principles.

Young, D., Van Oss, T., & Wagenfeld, A. (2014). Universal design for a lifetime: Interprofessional collaboration and the role of occupational therapy in environmental modifications. *OT Practice, 19*(13), CE-1–CE-7.

Zemke, R. (2004). Time, space and the kaleidoscopes of occupation. *American Journal of Occupational Therapy, 58*(6), 608–620. https://doi.org/10.5014/ajot.58.6.608.

REFLECTION

1. Explain the contribution of pragmatism to our understanding of the environment.

2. Explain the contribution of transactionalism to our understanding of the environment.

3. Define ecology, occupational ecology and ecosocial occupational therapy.

8

THE CONTINUAL EVOLUTION OF THE OCCUPATIONAL THERAPY PROFESSION

MICHAEL CURTIN

CHAPTER OUTLINE

Overview

The occupational therapy profession began in the early 1900s at a time when the biomedical framework of health was dominant. Although the first occupational therapists were influenced by the moral treatment and arts and crafts movements, the profession soon became more aligned with the biomedical approach. The development of the biopsychosocial, International Classification of Functioning, Disability and Health (ICF), and socioecological health frameworks all had an impact on the evolution of the occupational therapy profession. This included a move away from the biomedical way of practice, to a stronger focus on the importance of occupation for people's health and well-being. This led to occupational therapists embracing occupation-focused strategies for working with collectives, in addition to working with individuals. Over recent years the profession has been critiqued for its colonising approach and neoliberal concepts, models

and practices that have not considered the global reach and diversity of the profession. These critiques challenge the profession to critically reflect, decolonise, embrace diversity, and accept that the continual evolution of the profession is important for its sustainability and relevance.

KEY POINTS

- The biomedical framework is based on the assumption that health is the absence of illness, injury or impairment in an individual.

- The biopsychosocial framework is underpinned by system theory in which a person's health is determined by the dynamic interaction of a person's body structures and functions, subjective behaviours, beliefs, thought processes, motivations and experiences, and culture, family, community and society.

- The International Classification of Functioning, Disability and Health framework integrates the biomedical and social models and recognises that health is multidimensional and affected by multiple factors.

■ The socioecological framework focuses on the prevention and social responsibility of illness, injury and impairment and the promotion of health and wellbeing, moving beyond the medical treatment of an individual and of medical conditions.

■ Each of these frameworks has affected the evolution of the profession.

■ Currently, the occupational therapy profession is being challenged to critically reflect on the Western-neoliberal aspects of the profession and to decolonise, embrace global diversity and continually evolve so that the profession remains sustainable and relevant in enhancing the health and wellbeing and occupational participation of individuals and collectives.

INTRODUCTION

The concept of health is dynamic and evolving, making it difficult to define (Taylor, 2008a). The multiplicity of meanings of health are specific to 'the unique individual, family, social and cultural context in which the term is used' (Liamputtong et al., 2012, p. 2). Even though health is difficult to define, the Australian Institute of Health and Welfare (AIHW) stated that, 'Health, or being in good health, is important to everyone […] [influencing] not just how we feel, but how we function and participate in the community' (Australian Institute of Health and Welfare, 2014, p. 3). Taylor (2008a, p. 4) stated that people understand that it is important to have 'good health and access to quality health care', both of which are considered basic human rights in the Universal Declaration of Human Rights (United Nations, 1948).

The nearest there is to having a universal definition of health is the one written in the Preamble to the Constitution of the World Health Organization (WHO) (World Health Organization, 1948, Preamble). Health is defined as 'a state of complete physical, mental and social wellbeing and not merely the absence of disease or infirmity'. In this definition health includes physical, mental and social factors, marking a significant shift from health being the absence of illness, injury or impairment to health being each person's subjective perception of, and satisfaction with, their life whether or not they had an illness, injury or impairment (King, 2014).

Taylor (2008b) proposed four health frameworks that were 'underpinned by differing conceptualisations of core constructs like health, illness and wellbeing, which become translated into health policy, service delivery and professional practice' (Taylor, 2008b, pp. 23–24):

■ Biomedical framework,
■ Biopsychosocial framework,
■ International Classification of Functioning, Disability and Health (ICF) framework, and
■ Socioecological framework.

Occupational therapy practice has been influenced by these frameworks. As different frameworks became more favoured or dominant, occupational therapy practice changed and the philosophy underpinning the profession evolved. Within this chapter, an overview of the four health frameworks proposed by Taylor will be described along with the associated evolution of the occupational therapy profession and practice.

BIOMEDICAL FRAMEWORK OF HEALTH

The biomedical framework is based on the premise that health is the absence of illness, injury or impairment in an individual, and the assumption that there are two states of being: a healthy state, in which there is no illness, injury or impairment, and a non-healthy state in which there is the presence of illness, injury or impairment (Taylor, 2008b). Germov (2018, p. 9) stated that this framework was

Based on the assumption that each disease or ailment has a specific cause that physically affects the human body in a uniform and predictable way, meaning that universal 'cures' for people are theoretically possible.

This framework emerged in the eighteenth and nineteenth centuries in line with the move towards rational and logical thinking, away from knowledge based on religious scriptures (Wilcock & Hocking, 2015). This was the period in which effective, more scientific, treatments for common diseases such as smallpox were being developed (Germov, 2018a; Wilcock & Hocking, 2015). The focus was on treating the disease, as it was believed that each disease had a single specific cause. Germov (2018) suggested that although public health measures, such as sanitation and hygiene, were introduced in the 1800s to prevent the transmission of disease among populations, these measures were 'cast aside for almost a century as the new science of biomedicine gained ascendancy' (p. 9).

This was also the period in which the mind and body were considered to be separate (Wilcock & Hocking, 2015). This was known as Cartesian mind-body dualism where issues of the body were the focus of medicine and issues of the mind were spiritual matters (Germov, 2018). This led to a detailed understanding of the anatomy and physiology of the human body and the impact of pathology (Germov, 2018). This in turn led to the creation of health experts who made clinical diagnoses based on a medical history and the use of tests and examination to identify signs of illness, injury or impairment and who prescribed drug and surgical treatments to cure disease and fix the body (Germov, 2018; Taylor, 2008b; Wilcock & Hocking, 2015).

The biomedical framework has come under robust criticism, particularly as different perspectives of health evolved from the mid-20th century. According to Taylor (2008b), Germov (2018a) and Wilcock and Hocking (2015) the main criticism is that the underpinning assumptions of this framework were reductionist and did not take into account other factors that affected health and the different ways of understanding health and illness. When using this approach the views and opinions of people experiencing the illness, injury or impairment were not sought, as the focus was on treating the condition, not the person. As a result, this reductionist approach could not provide a sound 'explanation of who becomes ill and who stays healthy, as it does not account for the complex interplay of personal, environmental, psychological, physiological and occupational factors that impact on health' (Wilcock & Hocking, 2015, p. 67). In addition, the separation of the mind and body, a result of the reductionist approach, contributed to a number of negative outcomes, such as the objectification of people who were referred to by their diagnosis and seen as 'patients' who were passive recipients of 'expert' health advice and treatment (Germov, 2018).

Even though the biomedical framework has received robust criticism, it still significantly influences current 'policies, service delivery, health-related research and professional healthcare practice' in Western countries (Taylor, 2008b). Partly this is because the scientific advances made under this framework have led to many beneficial treatments (Germov, 2018). Despite this, there has been a growing push for a broader approach to health, particularly since the 1970s, which led to the development of the biopsychosocial framework (Taylor, 2008b).

THE BEGINNING OF THE OCCUPATIONAL THERAPY PROFESSION

The occupational therapy profession started in the early 1900s when the biomedical framework was the primary way of understanding and improving health. Despite the dominance of the biomedical framework, the first occupational therapists were primarily influenced by a radically different approach. The first occupational therapists became focused on developing a more respectful and progressive way of working with people with mental illness that was informed by the moral treatment and the arts and crafts movements. They implemented approaches that focused on the importance of participating in valued daily activities as they believed this led to better health outcomes (Husman, 2014; Nastasi, 2014).

The moral treatment movement offered an alternative to treating people with mental health illness compared with the biomedical approach. The moral movement, which began in the early 1800s, was based on a humanistic philosophy that focused on treating people with a mental illness humanely and with respect. The focus was on providing opportunities for people with mental illness to be engaged in activities such as work, arts and crafts, and regular exercise, as an effective means of recovery from mental illness. Husman (2014, p. 34) stated that 'the implementation of the moral treatment paved the way for the use of occupation as a healing modality and set a course for the emerging profession of occupational therapy'.

The arts and crafts movement began in the 1800s in response to the disruption to the daily lives of people caused by the move from family farms into cities for work, mainly in factories, as a result of industrialisation. Proponents of the arts and crafts movement believed that the 'reliance on machines, poor working conditions, and displacement of human skill caused a deterioration of physical health as well as the common complaint of disease, anxiety, and fatigue' (Husman, 2014, p. 34). Engaging in activities that involved making arts and crafts products by hand, in a traditional manner, was seen as a way to prevent the perceived negative effects of factory work.

Based on these movements, the early pioneers of the occupational therapy profession instigated numerous approaches to engage people in art and craft activities. The integration of the two movements was believed 'to meet the rehabilitation goals of patients with both physical and mental disabilities' (Husman, 2014, p. 34) and was considered an effective means of maintaining and improving people's health (Ward et al., 2007).

Occupational Therapy Practice and the Biomedical Framework

With the advent of World War I and the increase in the number of people who developed physical and mental health illnesses, injuries and impairments, the work of the occupational therapy profession expanded. In addition to offering arts and crafts activities, occupational therapists began to construct and adapt equipment, and develop alternative ways for people to do everyday activities such as washing and dressing. This led to advances in the profession and to the adoption of the biomedical framework, as it was deemed that its rigorous scientific foundations were required for the profession to develop and to fit in with other health professionals. There was a move to create a more scientific basis for using activities to facilitate recovery.

Farias et al. (2019) suggested that the relatively early alignment of the profession with the biomedical framework and focus on rehabilitation meant the profession moved away from its initial intent of social reform and having a social focus. Pollard and Sakellariou (2012) supported this view writing that occupational therapy become more focused on medical conditions and less on social issues such as inequality, which contributed to the distribution of people who had an illness, injury or impairment. These authors noted that 'the prescription of interventions for specific conditions is different from the development of practices for social change' (Pollard & Sakellariou, 2012, p. 8). The close association that occupational therapists had with the

biomedical framework may have resulted in an uptake of deficit-based discourses as a dominant way of thinking about people who had an illness, injury or impairment (Reparon et al., 2024).

The biomedical focus of the profession continued during World War II as the rehabilitation movement developed in response to the injuries sustained by soldiers. In what is now recognised as an able-ist orientation, the rehabilitation movement 'began by recognizing that, with proper care and rehabilitation, individuals with disabilities could be independent and contributing members of the community' (Husman, 2014, p. 38). Occupational therapists embraced this movement by increasing their repertoire of technical skills, becoming experts in the training and fitting of orthotics, exercises and daily living activities, and expanding their scope of practice. More significantly occupational therapists became more aligned with the biomedical framework and focused primarily on treating and reducing 'deficits' and 'normalising' people who had an illness, injury or impairment (Husman, 2014).

As the rehabilitation movement expanded in the 1960s and medical knowledge became more advanced, medical fields became more specialised. Occupational therapists followed suit and became more specialised. The biomedical framework became even more influential and dominant, affecting the way occupational therapy was practised (Letts, 2011). The use of arts and crafts as a therapy intervention was reduced and occupational therapists began to integrate more 'scientific' approaches into their practice, incorporating theories and techniques from other professions, such as medicine, psychology and sociology, as a way of enhancing credibility (Turner, 2011). It has been suggested that occupational therapy became more mechanistic during this period (Gillen & Greber, 2014; Hocking, 2013) as assessments and interventions were primarily focused on body structures and functions, treating illness, injury or impairment, and using quantitative measures for monitoring improvement (e.g. muscle strength increase, increased range of motion).

A Brief Aside: The Expansion of the Occupational Therapy Profession

The World Federation of Occupational Therapists (WFOT) was established in 1952 and included

10 countries (Australia, Canada, Denmark, India, Israel, New Zealand, South Africa, Sweden, United Kingdom and the United States of America [https://wfot.org/about/history]). Following the establishment of WFOT the profession of occupational therapy spread to many other countries around the world. Hammell (2019, p. 13) stated that many of the first occupational therapists from countries from the Global South and East were educated in Western countries, such as the United States or United Kingdom. These occupational therapists were exposed to Western theories and practices developed within contexts that were different to their home countries. Hammell proposed that this education approach was a form of 'enculturation' that was 'coupled with the supremacy of the English language in occupational therapy journals and books', which, in turn, 'contributed to the global dominance of ideas originating in North America, Australasia and Britain' (Hammell, 2019, p. 13).

As an example of this, Murthi and Hammell (2021, p. 8) suggested that the development of the occupational therapy profession in India was 'steeped in values and ideologies that were not inherent to the cultural values of India' (p. 8). They stated that this education of early occupational therapists from India in Western countries – what they refer to as "Western colonisalism" – has had a lasting impact as there has been a 'tendency for [occupational therapy professionals] in [India] to adopt Western views without questioning their relevance in local contexts' (p. 8).

THE BIOPSYCHOSOCIAL FRAMEWORK OF HEALTH

Germov (2018) said that the biopsychosocial framework began to gain traction in the 1970s as an extension of the biomedical framework. The biopsychosocial framework was developed to be a multifactorial model of illness, injury or impairment that considered biological, psychological and social factors implicated in a person's condition. The biopsychosocial framework was underpinned by system theory, which was based on the premise that health was determined by the dynamic interaction of a person's body structures and functions, subjective behaviours, beliefs, thought processes, motivations and experiences, and culture, family, community and society.

The introduction of the biopsychosocial approach led to the development of the International Classification of Impairments, Disabilities, and Handicaps (ICIDH), a manual of disease consequences issued by WHO in 1980 (Peterson et al., 2010; WHO, 1980). The ICIDH was developed to categorise the consequences of disease according to three dimensions: structural and functional body impairments, disabilities and handicaps.

Within the ICIDH *impairment* was defined as a problem with a person's body function and structure, *disability* was defined as occurring as a result of the affected body function and structure, and *handicap* referred to the limitations experienced in the environment because of the affected body function and structure. Hence, the biopsychosocial framework focused on the individual's body function and structures being the sole cause of a person's disability and resulting handicap. This framework therefore led to a focus on treatments to make a person's body structure and function as 'normal' as possible. Alford et al. (2013, p. 2) stated that the ICIDH 'was developed to capture the overall health status of populations but […] focused more on disease and failed to capture the impact of the social and physical environment on functioning'.

A positive outcome of the adoption of the biopsychosocial framework was the introduction of the concept of *wellbeing*, which Taylor (2008a, pp. 11–12) described as 'a broader concept than health as it typically involves a person's sense of overall satisfaction with […] life'. Hence, health status began to include subjective experiences of quality of life (King, 2014), such as a fact that a person may have an illness, injury or impairment and feel healthy or, conversely, that a person may not have an illness, injury or impairment and feel unhealthy (Liamputtong et al., 2012). Taylor (2008a, p. 12) stated that 'subjective experiences of health are anchored in the complex sociocultural contexts of people's lives including their belief systems, life stage, past experiences, family context, perceived social responsibilities, cultural history and geographical locations'. Hammell and Iwama (2012) and Wilcock and Hocking (2015) considered wellbeing to be an interplay between different but interrelated factors leading to a state of contentment. These factors included a person's:

- Physical, emotional and spiritual health;
- Personal, economic, political and cultural safety;
- Sense of being valued by others and belonging to social groups and communities; and
- Ability to make choices and decisions and engage in personally valued activities.

Although the biopsychosocial framework of health was seen as a significant advance on the biomedical framework, it was eventually replaced by the ICF, a framework that proposed that health, illness and wellness are dynamic and exist along a continuum rather than a static state fixed in time (Alford et al., 2013; Taylor, 2008b).

THE INTERNATIONAL CLASSIFICATION OF FUNCTIONING, DISABILITY AND HEALTH (ICF) FRAMEWORK OF HEALTH

The realisation that medical conditions manifested differently across individuals and the increasing acknowledgement that the environment had a significant impact on a person's health led to the move away from the ICIDH to the International Classification of Functioning, Disability and Health (ICF). The ICF was a model of health that, while still individually focused, provided recognition of internal and external factors that influenced a person's health (Alford et al., 2013; Peterson et al., 2010). The ICF was described as

A framework for organising and documenting information on functioning and disability [...] It integrates the major models of disability – the medical model and the social model [and] recognises the role of environmental factors in the creation of disability, as well as the role of health conditions [and] provides a multiperspective, biopsychosocial approach which is reflected in the multidimensional model.

(World Health Organization, 2013, p. 5)

Taylor (2008b) saw the ICF as an extension of the biopsychosocial model, being based on the assumption that health existed along a continuum and resulted from dynamic interactions between the

person and the person's environment. The ICF is made up of two parts, each with two components (Peterson et al., 2010):

1. The individual: (i) a person's body functions and structures, and (ii) activities and participation; and
2. Contextual factors: (i) personal factors, and (ii) environmental factors. These contextual factors have an impact on a person's ability to participate and be involved in the activity and ultimately on a person's health.

Within the ICF *impairment* resulted from changes to a person's body functions and structures and leads to *activity limitations* (i.e. a person experiencing difficulty executing a task or action) and *participation restrictions* (i.e. the difficulty a person has doing things such as work, recreational and leisure activities, and personal care). However, contextual factors affect body functions and structures, activity limitations and participation restrictions.

A graphic illustration of the ICF is shown in Fig. 8.1.

Despite the broad acceptance of the ICF, there were a number of criticisms of this framework. Many criticisms revolved around the individual focus of the ICF and the categorisation of people based on their abilities, contributing to the oppression, stigmatisation and identification of differences of people who have an illness, injury or impairment (Hammell, 2015a, 2023). Conti-Becker (2009) suggested that, although the ICF was developed as an extension of the biopsychosocial model of health, it was still strongly influenced by the biomedical framework. She felt that many in the medical field used the ICF incorrectly, transposing biomedical concepts to fit the ICF framework, primarily by using the ICF language but not the essence of the ICF approach.

Hammell (2023) criticised the ICF as being based on assumptions of there being a 'normal' state, something she, and disability theorists, stated did not exist. Hammell (2023, p. 748) argued that

The ICF's underlying premise – that disabled bodies are inherently problematic and in need of remediation – privileges certain ways of being and doing over others, and produces and reinforces normal/

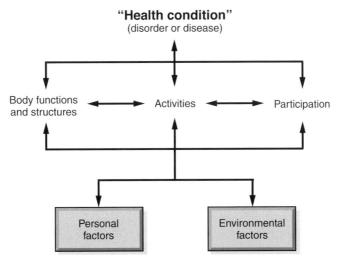

Fig. 8.1 ■ International Classification of Functioning, Disability and Health (ICF). (From World Health Organization. (2001). International classification of functioning, disability and health (ICF). World Health Organization).

abnormal, natural/unnatural, and abled/disabled binaries. Indeed, critical scholars contend that widespread adoption of the ICF within the rehabilitation sciences actively contributes to perpetuating a culture of ableism in both rehabilitation, and the wider society.

This focus on 'normality' created hierarchical experts who made judgements on what was considered normal and what was deviant, leading to exclusion, marginalisation and stigmatisation. These experts rarely, if ever, considered the views and opinions of people with an illness, injury or impairment, and the idea that these people could be considered partners in managing their health and wellbeing.

One of the claims of the ICF was that it could be used for all people and was applicable to all cultures (Australian Institute of Health and Welfare, 2014; World Health Organization, 2001). Gilroy et al. (2013, p. 43) contest this assertion, stating that the ICF did not pay 'enough attention to how the experience of colonisation influences the way that disability is conceptualised, understood and experienced in Indigenous communities'. For Indigenous communities, the consequences of colonisation – the trauma and loss of lands – are felt to be disabling; yet this aspect of disability is not captured by the ICF.

OCCUPATIONAL THERAPY PRACTICE AND THE BIOPSYCHOSOCIAL AND ICF FRAMEWORKS

In the 1980s there was a push in the occupational therapy profession to adopt a more holistic view of people who received occupational therapy services, and this led to the development of occupation-focused models of practice (Letts, 2011; Nastasi, 2014; Turner, 2011). These models assisted the occupational therapy profession in promoting the concept of occupation as core to the profession (Letts, 2011), leading to what Whiteford et al. (2000) referred to as the renaissance of occupation. Parnell and Wilding (2010) and Wilcock and Hocking (2015) argued that occupation, health and survival were inextricably linked and proposed that any negative impact on health and wellbeing could only be addressed by focusing on the occupational nature of people.

Embracing the term *occupation* was important for the occupational therapy profession (Fisher, 2013), as this started the move away from a professional identity based on a relationship with the medical profession. The renewed interest in the concept of occupation led to the recognition of the importance of the relationship between participating in occupation and a person's health and wellbeing (King, 2014). At this time, many in the occupational therapy profession were drawn to the ICF as they felt the concepts of 'activity' and 'participation' equated with the concepts of 'occupational engagement' and 'occupational performance' that were being used by occupational therapists.

However, occupational therapy's embrace of the ICF was contentious, in part because of the criticisms of this framework. Hammell (2023) argued that the uncritical acceptance of the ICF was evidence of the occupational therapy profession not acknowledging the critiques of the framework by disability theorists. In particular, she stated that

> *Occupational therapists collude with the ICF's classification as if this is a sophisticated form of needs-assessment and not a system specifically designed to code and classify individuals' deviations from assumed norms […] Yet the profession has rarely acknowledged that the classification of disabled people […] is not a neutral endeavour, but one that is both inherently political, and potentially fatal.*
>
> ***(Hammell, 2023, p. 748)***

Furthermore, it started becoming clear that both the ICF and occupation-focused concepts and models were too Western-centric to be relevant across the diverse range of cultural, political, economic and social contexts in which occupational therapy was being practised.

THE SOCIOECOLOGICAL FRAMEWORK OF HEALTH

According to Taylor (2008b, p. 41) the socioecological framework of health maximised 'health at all levels within society, from the individual to the whole community [and promoted] health rather than simply responding to illness after it has developed'. Germov (2018, p. 14) said that this framework linked, 'traditional public health concerns about physical aspects of the environment (clean air and water, safe food, occupational safety) with concerns about behavioural, social, and economic factors that affect peoples health'. The socioecological framework of health differed from the three previous frameworks because of its

focus on prevention, social responsibility for illness, injury and impairment, and promotion of health and wellbeing, moving beyond the medical treatment of an individual and medical conditions. Social health strategies are based on social justice principles (Hume Chambers & Walker, 2012) and focus on the health of collectives, taking into account the interaction between the multiple social determinants of health (Germov, 2018; Moll et al., 2013). This is in keeping with the right of people to have a high standard of health and health care (Taket, 2012; United Nations, 1948), regardless of their ethnicity, religious or political beliefs or economic or social condition (Wilcock & Hocking, 2015).

The move to improve the health of collectives with a focus on health promotion strategies is an outcome of the WHO (1978) Primary Health Care report of the International Conference at Alma Alta, underpinned by the WHO Ottawa Charter of Health Promotion (1986), a charter aimed at promoting good health of groups, communities, population and organisations. This charter was underpinned by an understanding of the social determinants of health (Jirojwong & Liamputtong, 2009), which WHO (2013) considered to be the main cause of health status inequalities seen among groups of people living within a country and also between countries.

The Australian Institute of Health and Welfare (AIHW, 2022) used a diagram to illustrate the impact of determinants of health (Fig. 8.2). Within this figure, it can be seen that the determinants are separated into four groups affecting a person's health and wellbeing over time, with the direction of determinants moving from left to right.

WHO (2023) stated that the social determinants of health had an important impact on health inequalities. WHO (2023, 2nd paragraph) stated that health inequalities referred to 'the unfair and avoidable differences in health status seen within and between countries. In countries at all levels of income, health and illness follow a social gradient: the lower the socioeconomic position, the worse the health'. AIHW (2022, p. 7) stressed that there is a clear relationship between the health of individuals 'and the circumstances in which they grow, live, work, play and age. Factors such as income, employment, education, housing, social connection and support, the environment, behaviours

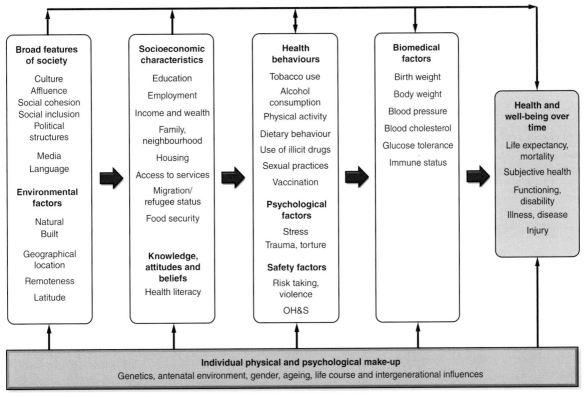

Fig. 8.2 ■ Determinants of health. (Reproduced with permission from Australian Institute of Health and Welfare (AIHW). (2014)).

and genetics influence health'. The inequitable distribution of social determinants of health contribute to health inequities throughout the lifespan and can be passed on from one generation to the next (Hammell, 2021).

One of the outcomes of the socioecological framework has been a growing understanding of the cultural influence on health. Culture has been defined as 'the knowledge, beliefs, values, assumptions, perspectives, attitudes, norms, and customs that people acquire through membership in a particular society or group' (Hammell, 2013, p. 225). A focus on population health, health equality and determinants of health highlights the disparity between the health of people from different cultures and also the inappropriateness of imposing a Western model of health (i.e. the biomedical, biopsychosocial and ICF frameworks) on people from non-Western backgrounds. Although culture is considered an environmental factor in the

ICF framework, a clearer understanding of culture has come from the development of population health. To illustrate this, a brief overview of the concept of health from the perspective of Aboriginal and Torres Strait Islander peoples of Australia is provided.

Duckett (2022) stated that the health of Aboriginal and Torres Strait Islander peoples was significantly worse than other Australians, as a result of the complex outcomes of colonisation, leading to spiritual harm caused by dispossession and alienation of the Aboriginal population from their lands. Land is considered fundamental to the wellbeing and core to the spirituality of Aboriginal and Torres Strait Islander peoples (McCalman et al., 2009). Their health and wellbeing are strongly associated with their identity, which is connected to their land, and their relationship with their community.

Gee et al. (2014) used the phrase 'social and emotional wellbeing' to capture the meaning of health for

BOX 8.1

NINE GUIDING PRINCIPLES THAT SHAPE ABORIGINAL AND TORRES STRAIT ISLANDER PEOPLES' CONCEPTUALISATION OF SOCIAL AND EMOTIONAL WELLBEING AND IDENTIFY CORE CULTURAL VALUES

1. Health as holistic
2. The right to self-determination
3. The need for cultural understanding
4. The impact of history in trauma and loss
5. Recognition of human rights
6. The impact of racism and stigma
7. Recognition of the centrality of kinship
8. Recognition of cultural diversity
9. Recognition of Aboriginal strengths

NB: Refer to the Social Health Reference Group (2004) reference for further explanation of these principles.

Modified from Gee, G., Dudgeon, P., Schultz, C., Hart, A., & Kelly, K. (2014). Aboriginal and Torres Strait Islander social and emotional wellbeing. In P. Dudgeon, H. Milroy & R. Walker (Eds.), *Working together: Aboriginal and Torres Strait Islander mental health and wellbeing principles and practice* (p. 57). Australian Government Department of the Prime Minister and Cabinet.

Aboriginal and Torres Strait Islander peoples. They indicated that this phrase signified 'a relatively distinct set of wellbeing domains and principles, and an increasingly documented set of culturally informed practices that differ in important ways with how the term is understood and used within Western health discourse' (Gee et al., 2014, pp. 56–57). These authors referred to the nine guiding principles presented in the Social and Emotional Wellbeing Framework document (Social Health Reference Group, 2004) that shape Aboriginal and Torres Strait Islander peoples' conceptualisation of social and emotional wellbeing and identify core cultural values (Box 8.1).

Gee et al. (2014) built on these principles to develop a model to conceptualise social and emotional wellbeing from the perspective of Aboriginal and Torres Strait Islander peoples (Fig. 8.3). This conceptualisation was 'grounded within a collectivist perspective that views the self as inseparable from, and embedded within, family and community' (Gee et al., 2014, p. 57). Within this illustration, the social and emotional wellbeing of Aboriginal and Torres Strait Islander individuals, families and communities is determined by connections to seven domains: body, mind and emotions, family and kinship, community, culture, land and spirituality.

Gee et al. (2014) suggested that disruption of these connections, particularly as a result of the historical and political impacts of colonisation, had negatively affected the social and emotional wellbeing of individuals, families and communities. It had been shown that the social determinants of health were evident among Aboriginal and Torres Strait Islander communities due to the common presence of determinants such as low socioeconomic status, poverty, poor education achievement and unemployment. However, these determinants were further complicated by the historical and political determinants related to the impacts of colonisation, in particular unresolved issues of land rights, self-determination and cultural security.

This insight into culture, and a greater understanding and acceptance of cultural ways of knowing, identifies an ideological conflict between Western perceptions of health and the perceptions of health by Indigenous people (Gibson et al., 2015). This has particular resonance when deciding the extent to which self-determination or assimilation should inform the guiding principles for deciding policies on Indigenous health (Gibson et al., 2015; Gibson 2020). The continuing strong influence of the biomedical, biopsychosocial and ICF frameworks on Western health practice, and the reliance on evidence-based principles with knowledge organised according to different health disciplines, is at odds with the holistic approach to health and wellbeing practised by many non-Western people (Emery-Whittington & Te Maru 2018; Emery-Whittington 2021; Gibson et al., 2015; Gibson 2020).

OCCUPATIONAL THERAPY AND THE SOCIOECOLOGICAL FRAMEWORK OF HEALTH

In line with the socioecological framework, during the late 1990s and early 2000s the occupational therapy profession in Western countries began to look beyond working with individuals who had an illness, injury or impairment (King, 2014). The profession saw the contributions it could make to population health and wellness (Wilcock & Hocking, 2015) by developing a

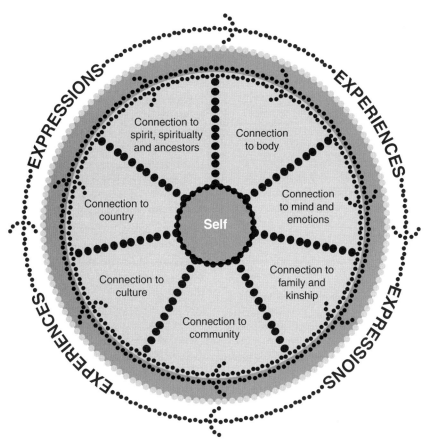

Fig. 8.3 ▪ Social and emotional wellbeing from the perspective of Aboriginal and Torres Strait Islander peoples. (Reproduced with permission from Gee, G., Dudgeon, P., Schultz, C., Hart, A., & Kelly, K. (2014). Aboriginal and Torres Strait Islander social and emotional wellbeing. In P. Dudgeon, H. Milroy & R. Walker (Eds.), *Working together: Aboriginal and Torres Strait Islander mental health and wellbeing principles and practice* (p. 57). Australian Government Department of the Prime Minister and Cabinet).

stronger social justice approach to practice. Occupational therapy as a profession expanded to address individuals *and* collectives, working in a variety of contexts and environments, focusing on wellness and wellbeing (Hocking, 2013; Nastasi, 2014).

Although occupational therapists in Western countries began to embrace the potential to work in population health and wellness, it must be noted that non-Western countries had been working this way since the 1970s. This is illustrated best by Brazil and the development of social occupational therapy (refer to Chapter 4). Frank and dos Santos (2020, p. 742) claim that among all the 'member countries in the World Federation of Occupational Therapist Brazil has been a leader in expanding the profession's scope of practice to address social inclusion and

social transformation'. According to Ambrosio et al. (2022), social occupational therapy and the Brazilian profession's focus on social justice, full citizenship and human rights, were a response to sociohistorical challenges and military rule in the country from the 1960s to the 1990s.

CONTEMPORARY AND FUTURE CHALLENGES FOR THE OCCUPATIONAL THERAPY PROFESSION

The contemporary nature of occupational therapy practice, with consideration of the socioecological framework of health, is evident in the current definition of the profession proposed by the World Federation of Occupational Therapists (WFOT):

Occupational therapy is a client-centred health profession concerned with promoting health and wellbeing through occupation. The primary goal of occupational therapy is to enable people to participate in the activities of everyday life. Occupational therapists achieve this outcome by working with people and communities to enhance their ability to engage in the occupations they want to, need to, or are expected to do, or by modifying the occupation or the environment to better support their occupational engagement.

(World Federation of Occupational Therapists, 2013, p. 3)

Within this definition, phrases such as 'promoting health and wellbeing', 'enable people to participate' and 'working with people and communities' are consistent with the socioecological framework. This is also evident in the release of a number of WFOT position papers on topics such as human displacement, community-based rehabilitation, disaster management, human rights, global health, diversity and culture (WFOT Resource Centre at www.wfot.org/Resource-Centre.aspx).

However, the alignment of the occupational therapy profession with the socioecological framework has also coincided with, and led to, significant critiques of the profession. One of the major critiques of the profession has been the global promotion of Western concepts and ideas. Hammell (2015c, pp. 718–720) argued that this is problematic for the profession because

Occupational therapy's leading theorists have almost exclusively been well-educated, urban, middle class, middle-aged, able-bodied, white Anglophones with Judeo-Christian backgrounds – thus representing a minority population, even within their minority region [of the world] [...] the uncritical promulgation of hegemonic Western ideas in non-Western cultures constitutes both ethnocentrism [...] and theoretical imperialism. [...] Colonialist practices are manifested when people of the South and East are encouraged to learn from those of the West or

North in a one-way flow of knowledge as if Western theories are inevitably valuable and universally relevant.

Gibson et al. (2015, p. 216) stated that the Western construction of the profession had impacted 'communication, understandings, world views and concepts and frameworks'. Ambrosio (2022) felt that the Western perspectives of the profession have resulted in the marginalisation and invisibility of non-Western groups. This view was supported by Murthi and Hammell (2021), who argued that the uncritical adoption of Western concepts and practices in non-Western countries has led to the development of services that are not relevant to the context and the oppression and alienation of the people the services are for. Hammell (2023) stated that it is imperative that the occupational therapy profession decolonises its theories, knowledge and practices. This process will,

Require the profession to disentangle its knowledge base from its deep colonial roots, contest its ableist assessments and obsession with classifying people; and resist practices that disempower, disable and oppress. [...] Decolonization is about dismantling white supremacy; but it is also about disputing and disassembling all the oppressions of coloniality. (p. 752)

Decolonising the occupational therapy profession (refer to Chapter 1) will involve cultural humility, engagement in 'a respectful exploration of the perspectives, priorities and values of cultural others, and thus a starting point for building respectful, culturally inclusive, relevant and effective occupational therapy theories and practices' (Hammell, 2019). This will allow the occupational therapy profession to embrace, celebrate and recognise the global nature of, and the diversity within, the profession and to genuinely learn from occupational therapists from all countries and backgrounds. Certainly there is a great deal to be learnt from the resistance to Western theories and models of occupation and practice in the evolution of occupational therapy in Brazil and other non-Western countries in the Global South, as well as from the critiques of the profession by First Nations occupational therapists in countries such as Australia, New Zealand

and Canada, who stress the need for the profession to decolonise and to authentically recognise cultural, historical and political contexts (Emery-Whittington, 2021; Emery-Whittington & Te Moro, 2018; Gibson et al., 2015; Gibson, 2020; Trentham et al., 2022).

Frank and dos Santos (2020, p. 741) argued that the occupational therapy profession will need to become more political as people, whether living in the Global South and Global North, are living in 'challenging times'. They argued that the 'alarming sweep of nationalism, populism, authoritarianism and racism threatens the health, wellbeing, rights and freedom of millions [of people]' (p. 741). They suggested that these global trends had a greater and disproportional impact on the most vulnerable people. They list the most at-risk as

Women, children, the unemployed, the structurally poor, people who are homeless, migrants, refugees, indigenous peoples, sexual and religious minorities, and people of African descent and cultures, as well as those with physical, developmental, psychological and cognitive disabilities, and chronic illnesses (p. 741).

In becoming more political, and 'promoting an agenda of social reform to address the socio-political process and conditions that contribute to maintaining occupational injustices' (Farias et al., 2019, p. 235), occupational therapists need to directly challenge 'oppressive social, legal, economic, political, institutional, cultural and religious barriers that uphold opportunities for some people and deny them to others' (Hammell 2015a, p. 78). Hocking (2019) suggested that to engage in community capacity building and society change the occupational therapy profession will need to work with vulnerable, at-risk collectives who have not been traditional recipients of occupational therapy services. Contemporary and future occupational therapy practice will involve expanding the field of practice beyond the health sphere and embracing aspects of community development to focus on justice, rights and social transformation – social and occupational justice – for collectives (Irvine-Brown et al., 2022).

Occupational therapists are being strongly encouraged to be critically reflective (refer to Chapter 2)

and 'question how theories and assumptions promote rather than challenge the status quo [...] to resist ways practice may be co-opted by the very structures and ideologies they aspire to challenge' (Irivine-Brown et al., 2022, p. 27). Of most concern is the 'prevailing neoliberal ideology that has become hegemonic as a mode of discourse and [that] has pervasive effects on ways of thought and political-economic practices to the point where it has become incorporated into the commonsense way [occupational therapists] interpret, live in and understand the world' (Murthi & Hammell, 2021, p. 2). Neo-liberalism is described as the,

Economic and political ideology that has dominated the Global North and been imposed on the Global South since the late 1970s, is regarded by scholars as being a form of covert colonialism; effectively entrenching the inequities of power created by colonialism. [...] Within a neoliberal ideology, people are valued according to their productivity and contribution to economic growth. To advance this agenda, neoliberalism promotes individualism, independence and self-reliance, values individuals who strive to improve their abilities and become more employable, and devalues states of dependency.

(Hammell, 2023, pp. 746–747)

It is proposed that many key concepts within occupational therapy, that have been developed in the Western world, are underpinned by neoliberal ideologies. As an example, occupational therapists in the West often promote the goal of *independence*. In doing this, Hammell (2023, p. 750) claimed that occupational therapists have not accounted for the assertion by disability theorists, Western ethicists and philosophers that autonomy is not about being

Physically independent, but to having the right, ability and opportunity to influence, choose, direct and manage one's life in accordance with one's values and priorities. [...] autonomy is about self-determination [...] [rather than physical independence] the aim of the most important occupations is interdependence.

Furthermore, neoliberalism ideologies have reshaped the social domain, linking a 'reduction in state services to the increasing call for personal responsibility' (Farias & Laliberte Rudman, 2019, p. 7). This focus on personal responsibility leads to the possibility of ignoring the sociopolitical cause of inequalities and injustices. Farias and Laliberte Rudman (2019) stated that critiquing and resisting the neoliberal underpinning of the occupational therapy profession is essential for the promotion of practices to support collective action for social change.

Neoliberal ideologies also have an impact on the context in which occupational therapy is practised. Farias and Laliberte Rudman (2019b) indicated that practice has been impacted by *healthism* and *managerialism*. *Healthism* 'is embraced within biomedical approaches in ways that discursively situate health problems at the level of the individual, obscuring social determinants of health' (p. 250). As indicated earlier, this approach to health can contribute to social and economic inequities as little consideration is given to the social determinants of health.

Managerialism refers to the development of policies, procedures and protocols to control costs and the quality of interventions; interventions that have outcomes aligned to personal responsibility, and the promotion of simplification, categorisation and reductionism (Farias & Laliberte Rudman, 2019a). Managerialism challenges the collaborative relationship-focused nature of occupational therapy practice, due to the increasing rationing of health services inherent in the contemporary managerial approach to health service provision, which is strongly influenced by government and organisational policies based on budgetary and staff restraints (Germov, 2018). This approach operates with a unitary purpose of work standardisation and can lead to allied health professionals losing their autonomy as their work becomes systematised and their practice constrained (Germov, 2018; Orton et al., 2022).

CONCLUSION

The occupational therapy profession and the practice of occupational therapists have continually evolved since it began in the early 1900s. This evolution has been influenced by the changing perception of health and health care, which has moved from the individualistic and treatment-focused biomedical, biopsychosocial and ICF frameworks, to the population- and health promotion–focused socioecological framework. It has also been influenced by the renewed interest in the importance of occupation to

the health and wellbeing of people. However, contemporary critiques of the profession state that it has been too Western-centric and has been influenced by neo-liberal ideologies. These critiques challenge occupational therapists and the profession to be critically reflective, and to embrace and learn from the profession's global diversity, seeing this as a strength. As well occupational therapists are encouraged to accept that the continual evolution of the profession, an evolution that is important for its sustainability and relevance. Hinojosa (2007) warns that the profession should not push for consistency and acceptance of one way of thinking, as this could stifle rather than enhance the evolution of the profession. He argues that

> *If we see the world as static, believing that occupational therapy is limited by what we currently can do, then we will act and respond consistently with those beliefs and views. But if we stretch our viewpoints and welcome change, realising interventions must be based on a [person's or collective's] problems or needs, we will act accordingly. We can shift our paradigms. Becoming innovators in adapting practices to meet the new realities of the world is essential to our profession's continuing development.*
> **(Hinojosa, 2007, p. 632)**

REFERENCES

Alford, V., Remedios, L., Webb, G., & Ewen, S. (2013). The use of the international classification of functioning, disability and health (ICF) in indigenous healthcare: A systematic literature review. *International Journal for Equity in Health, 12*(32), 1–10. https://doi.org/10.1186/1475-9276-12-32.

Australian Institute of Health and Welfare (2014). *Australia's health 2014: Australia's health series No. 14 Cat. No. AUS 178.* Australia's Health Series, Canberra: Australian Institute of Health and Welfare.

Australian Institute of Health and Welfare. (2022). *Australia's health 2022: In brief. Catalogue number. AUS 241.* In *Australia's Health Series number 18.* Canberra. Australian Institute of Health and Welfare.

Conti-Becker, A. (2009). Between the ideal and the real: Reconsidering the international classification of functioning, disability and health. *Disability and Rehabilitation, 31*(25), 2125–2129.

Duckett, S. (2022). *The Australian health care system* (6th ed.). Oxford University Press.

Emery-Whittington, I. (2021). Occupational justice – Colonial business as usual? Indigenous observations from Aotearoa New Zealand. *Canadian Journal of Occupational Therapy, 88*(2), 153–162. https://doi.org/10.1177/00084174211005891.

Emery-Whittington, I., & Te Maro, B. (2018). Decolonising occupation: Causing social change to help our ancestors rest and our descendants thrive. *New Zealand Journal of Occupational Therapy, 65*(1), 12–19.

Farias, L., & Laliberte Rudman, D. (2019a). Challenges in enacting occupation-based social transformative practices: A critical dialogical study. *Canadian Journal of Occupational Therapy, 86*(3), 243–252. https://doi.org/10.1177/0008417419828798.

Farias, L., & Laliberte Rudman, D. (2019b). Practice analysis: Critical reflexivity on discourses constraining socially transformative occupational therapy practices. *British Journal of Occupational Therapy, 82*(11), 693–697. https://doi.org/10.1177/0008417419828798.

Farias, L., Laliberte Rudman, D., Pollard, N., Schiller, S., Malfitano, A. P. S., Thomas, K., & van Bruggen, H. (2019). Critical dialogical approach: A methodological director for occupation-based social transformative work. *Scandinavian Journal of Occupational Therapy, 26*(4), 235–245. https://doi.org/10.1080/11038128.2018.1469666.

Fisher, A. (2013). Occupation-centred, occupation-based, occupation-focused: Same, same or different? *Scandinavian Journal of Occupational Therapy, 20*(3), 162–173.

Frank, G., & dos Santos, V. (2020). Occupational reconstruction: Resources for social transformation in challenging times. *Cadernos Brasileiros de Terapia Ocupacional, 28*(3), 741–745. https://doi.org/10.4322/2526-8910.ctoED2802.

Gee, G., Dudgeon, P., Schultz, C., Hart, A., & Kelly, K. (2014). Aboriginal and Torres Strait Islander social and emotional wellbeing. In Dudgeon, P., Milroy, H., & Walker, R. (Eds.), *Working together: Aboriginal and Torres Strait Islander mental health and wellbeing principles and practice*. Australian Government Department of the Prime Minister and Cabinet, 55–68.

Germov, J. (2018). Imagining health problems as social issues. In Germov, J. (Ed.), *Second opinion: An introduction to health sociology* (6th ed., pp. 2–23). Oxford University Press.

Gibson, C., Butler, C., Henaway, C., Dudgeon, P., & Curtin, M. (2015). Indigenous peoples and human rights: some considerations for the occupational therapy profession in Australia. *Australian Occupational Therapy Journal, 62*(3), 214–218. https://doi.org/10.1111/1440-1630.12185.

Gibson, C. (2020). When rives run dry: leadership, decolonisation and healing in occupational therapy. *New Zealand Journal of Occupational Therapy, 67*(1), 11–20.

Gillen, A., & Greber, C. (2014). Occupation-focused practice: Challenges and choices. *British Journal of Occupational Therapy, 77*(1), 39–41.

Gilroy, J., Donelly, M., Colmar, S., & Parmenter, T. (2013). Conceptual framework for policy and research development with Indigenous peoples with disabilities. *Australian Aboriginal Studies, 2*, 42–58.

Hammell, K. W. (2013). Occupation, wellbeing, and culture: Theory and cultural humility. *Canadian Journal of Occupational Therapy, 80*(4), 224–234.

Hammell, K. W. (2015a). Participation and occupation: The need for a human rights perspective. *Canadian Journal of Occupational Therapy, 82*(1), 4–5. https://doi.org/10.1177/0008417414567636.

Hammell, K. W. (2015b). Respecting global wisdom: Enhancing the cultural relevance of occupational therapy's theoretical base. *British Journal of Occupational Therapy, 78*(11), 718–721. https://doi.org/10.1177/0308022614564170.

Hammell, K. W. (2019). Building globally relevant occupational therapy from the strength of diversity. *World Federation of Occupational Therapists Bulletin, 75*(1), 13–26. https://doi.org/10.1080/14473828.2018.1529480.

Hammell, K. W. (2021). Building back better: Imagining an occupational therapy for a post-COVID-19 world. *Australian Occupational Therapy Journal, 68*(5), 444–453. https://doi.org/10.1111/1440-1630.12760.

Hammell, K. W. (2023). A call to resist occupational therapy's promotion of ableism. *Scandinavian Journal of Occupational Therapy, 30*(6), 745–757. https://doi.org/10.1080/11038128.2022.2130821.

Hammell, K. W., & Iwama, M. (2012). Wellbeing and occupational rights: An imperative for critical occupational therapy. *Scandinavian Journal of Occupational Therapy, 19*(5), 385–394.

Hinojosa, J. (2007). Becoming innovators in an era of hyperchange [Eleanor Clarke Slagle lecture]. *American Journal of Occupational Therapy, 61*, 629–637.

Hocking, C. (2013). Occupation for public health. *New Zealand Journal of Occupational Therapy, 60*(1), 33–37.

Hocking, C. (2019). A reflection on inclusion and human rights for occupational therapists. *New Zealand Journal of Occupational Therapy, 66*(2), 24–28.

Hume Chambers, A., & Walker, R. (2012). Introduction to health promotion. In Liamputtong, P., Fanany, R., & Verrinder, G. (Eds.), *Health, illness and wellbeing* (pp. 107–124). Oxford University Press.

Husman, C. B. (2014). History and philosophy. In K. Jacobs, N. MacRae, & K. Sladyk (Eds.), *Occupational therapy essentials for clinical competence* (pp. 33–42). Slack.

Irvine-Brown, L., Ware, V., & Malfitano, A. (2022). Exploring the praxis of occupational therapy community development practitioners. *Canadian Journal of Occupational Therapy, 89*(1), 26–35. https://doi.org/10.1177/00084174211066662.

Jirojwong, S., & Liamputtong, P. (2009). Primary health care and health promotion. In Jirojwong, S., & Liamputtong, P. (Eds.), *Population health, communities and health promotion* (pp. 26–42). Oxford University Press.

King, R. (2014). The experience of flow and meaningful occupation. In K. Jacobs, N. MacRae, & K. Sladyk (Eds.), *Occupational therapy essentials for clinical competence* (pp. 3–10). Slack.

Letts, L. (2011). Optimal positioning of occupational therapy. *Canadian Journal of Occupational Therapy, 78*(4), 209–219.

Liamputtong, P., Fanany, R., & Verrinder, G. (2012). Health, illness, and wellbeing: An introduction. In P. Liamputtong, R. Fanany, & G. Verrinder (Eds.), *Health, illness and wellbeing* (pp. 1–17). Oxford University Press.

McCalman, J., Tsey, K., Gibson, T., & Baird, B. (2009). Health of Indigenous Australians and health promotion. In S. Jirojwong, & P. Liamputtong (Eds.), *Population health, communities and health promotion* (pp. 69–91). Oxford University Press.

Moll, S., Gewurtz, R., Krupa, T., & Law, M. (2013). Promoting an occupational perspective in public health. *Canadian Journal of Occupational Therapy, 80*(2), 111–119.

Murthi, K., & Hammell, K. W. (2021). 'Choice' in occupational therapy: A critique from the situation of patriarchy in India. *Scandinavian Journal of Occupational Therapy, 28*(1), 1–12. https://doi.org/10.1080/11038128.2020.1769182.

Nastasi, J. (2014). Meaning and dynamic of occupation and activity. In K. Jacobs, N. MacRae, & K. Sladyk (Eds.), *Occupational therapy essentials for clinical competence* (pp. 57–70). Slack.

Orton, Y., Hocking, C., & Payne, D. (2022). Clinical governance of occupational therapy practice: Pinch-points and political action. *New Zealand Journal of Occupational Therapy, 69*(2), 34–40.

Parnell, T., & Wilding, C. (2010). Where can an occupation-focussed philosophy take occupational therapy? *Australian Occupational Therapy Journal, 57*(5), 345–348.

Peterson, D., Mpofu, E., & Oakland, T. (2010). Concepts and models in disability, functioning, and health. In E. Mpofu, & T. Oakland (Eds.), *Rehabilitation and health assessment: Applying ICF guidelines* (pp. 3–26). Springer.

Pollard, N., & Sakellariou, D. (2012). *Politics of occupation-centred practice: Reflections on occupational engagement across cultures.* Wiley-Blackwell.

Reparon, R., Block, P., Fudge Schormans, A., Laliberte Rudman, D., & Teachman, G. (2024). Critiquing representations of intellectual disability in occupation-based literature. *Scandinavian Journal of Occupational Therapy, 31*(1), 2289897. https://doi.org/10.1080/11038128.2023.2289897.

Social Health Reference Group. (2004). *Social and emotion well being framework: A national strategic framework for Aboriginal and Torres Strait Islander peoples' mental health and social and emotional well being 2004–2009.* National Aboriginal and Torres Strait Islander Health Council and National Mental Health Working Group.

Taket, A. (2012). Health and social justice. In P. Liamputtong, R. Fanany, & G. Verrinder (Eds.), *Health, illness and wellbeing* (pp. 278–301). Oxford University Press.

Taylor, S. (2008a). The concept of health. In S. Taylor, M. Foster, & J. Fleming (Eds.), *Health care practice in Australia: Policy, context and innovations* (pp. 3–21). Oxford University Press.

Taylor, S. (2008b). Contemporary frameworks of health care. In S. Taylor, M. Foster, & J. Fleming (Eds.), *Health care practice in Australia: Police, context and innovations* (pp. 22–45). Oxford University Press.

Trentham, B., Laliberte Rudman, D., Smith, H., & Phenix, A. (2022). The socio-political and historical context of occupational therapy in Canada. In I. M. Egan, & G. Restall (Eds.), *Promoting occupational participation: Collaborative relationship-focused occupational therapy* (pp. 31–56). Canadian Occupational Therapy Association.

Turner, A. (2011). The Elizabeth Casson memorial lecture 2011: Occupational therapy – A profession in adolescence? *British Journal of Occupational Therapy, 74*(7), 314–322.

United Nations. (1948). *Universal declaration of human rights.* United Nations. www.un.org/overview/rights.html.

Ward, K., Mitchell, J., & Price, P. (2007). Occupation-based practice and its relationship to social and occupational participation in adults with spinal cord injury. *OTJR: Occupation, Participation and Health, 27*(4), 149–156.

Whiteford, G., Townsend, E., & Hocking, C. (2000). Reflections on a renaissance of occupation. *Canadian Journal of Occupational Therapy, 67*(1), 61–69.

Wilcock, A., & Hocking, C. (2015). *An occupational perspective of health* (3rd ed.). Slack.

World Federation of Occupational Therapists. (2013). *Definition of occupational therapy from member organisations (revised 2013).* World Federation of Occupational Therapists. http://www.wfot.org/ResourceCentre.aspx.

World Health Organization. (1948). *Preamble to the constitution.* World Health Organization. www.who.int/hr/en.

World Health Organization. (1978). *Primary health care. Report of the international conference on primary health care.* World Health Organization.

World Health Organization. (1980). *International classification of impairments, disabilities, and handicaps: A manual of classification relating to the consequences of disease.* World Health Organization.

World Health Organization. (2001). *International classification of functioning, disability and health (ICF).* World Health Organization.

World Health Organization. (2013). *Health in all policies.* Paper presented at the 8th Global Conference on Health Promotion, Helsinki.

World Health Organization. (2023). *Social determinants of health.* World Health Organization. Retrieved November 23, 2023, from. https://www.who.int/health-topics/social-determinants-of-health#tab=tab_1.

World Health Organization, Health and Welfare Canada, & Canadian Public Health Association. (1986). *Ottawa charter for health promotion.* World Health Organization.

REFLECTION

1. Provide examples of the biomedical, biopsychosocial, International Classification of Functioning, Disability and Health (ICF), and socioecological frameworks being used in practice that you have observed during your placement/work experiences.

2. For each of the examples provided consider the impact the use of this framework may have had on the individuals and collectives receiving occupational therapy and other health/social services.

3. Considering the criticisms of the ICF should occupational therapists align themselves with this approch? Provide an explanation of your answer.

4. Embracing the socioecological health framework provides opportunities for occupatioanl therapists to expand their practice to work with collectives. One way to do this is to implement health promotion strategies. Provide one suggestion of how a health promotion approach could be used by an occupational therapist to achieve occupational participation outcomes for a collective.

5. What are your thoughts on how occupational therapist will evolve in the future and what will impact this evolution?

Section 2 — UNDERSTANDING AND EXPLORING OCCUPATIONAL PARTICIPATION

9

PROFESSIONAL REASONING

ROB BROOKS ▪ ELE GRIMWOOD

Overview

Professional reasoning is a key skill for occupational therapists to use throughout the occupational therapy process. It is an active thinking process where the occupational therapist integrates a broad range of information and knowledge to create decisions with the people they work with that are collaborative, evidence-informed, ethical and pragmatic. Developing proficiency and confidence in professional reasoning can seem complex for students and novice occupational therapists, with experienced occupational therapists seeming to just know what to do. Seminal and contemporary research is drawn on in this chapter to identify key types of professional reasoning with a focus on how to do and develop professional reasoning. The occupational therapy process and practice stories will be used to bring professional reasoning to life and to illustrate its application.

KEY POINTS

- Professional reasoning is an active thinking process.
- Current knowledge has emerged from occupational therapy practice in the Global North.
- Research into professional reasoning has continued to grow and knowledge is being summarised in literature reviews.
- There are classical, contemporary and emerging types of professional reasoning.
- Information processing and memory theory can help to explain the mental process of reasoning.
- There are a range of activities, such as reflection and interprofessional learning, that support the development of professional reasoning.

DEFINING PROFESSIONAL REASONING

Professional reasoning is an active iterative thinking activity that occupational therapists use throughout the occupational therapy process to make sense of a person's circumstances, formulate decisions about their interventions, and to communicate their practice with the multidisciplinary team and stakeholders. When using professional reasoning occupational therapists draw on their experience, knowledge, reflections on best practices, research and theory together with the perspectives of the individuals and collectives they are working with. Studies have shown that occupational therapists use different types of professional reasoning in different situations and that their ability to use professional reasoning develops over time (da Silva Araujo et al., 2022; Márquez-Álvarez et al., 2019; Unsworth & Baker, 2016). Sometimes students or novice occupational therapists will ask senior colleagues how they knew what to do next or how they made sense of what was going on – this is professional reasoning. This chapter aims to make explicit what can sometimes feel implicit, drawing on seminal and contemporary research to explain the language and types of professional reasoning as well as using three practice stories to bring ideas to life.

Professional reasoning is an essential skill for all healthcare professionals; it is not unique to occupational therapists, and it is used by, for example, physiotherapists (Huhn et al., 2019), medics (Koufidis et al., 2021), and nurses (Banning, 2008). In the literature, the term clinical reasoning and professional reasoning are often used interchangeably, usually referring to the same thing. It is proposed that the term professional reasoning better reflects the breadth of the work occupational therapists do and the broad range of settings they practice in, including nonmedical settings, such as schools, in communities, or in workplaces, that are not clinical in nature. As such, professional reasoning is used in this chapter, except where the studies referenced used a different term.

GLOBALISATION OF PROFESSIONAL REASONING

It is important from the outset to acknowledge that the foundations of professional reasoning evolved from the Global North, mostly North American and European occupational therapy practice and research. The cultural, political, economic, health and social contexts of these countries have shaped the way knowledge has been developed, understood and disseminated. A study conducted in South America (Garcia et al., 2021) has suggested that professional reasoning by occupational therapists in this context may be different to that commonly reported in other studies due to variances in language, lack of time and a scarcity of local research. This suggests that different contexts may result in different types of reasoning and there is a need to explore different ways of knowing professional reasoning, particularly from the Global South.

THE STUDY OF PROFESSIONAL REASONING

The roots of professional reasoning in occupational therapy are in the use of reflection. In the 1980s occupational therapists began to use reflection as a tool to consider how they were thinking in their practice (Schon, 1983). The first study of clinical reasoning in occupational therapy was published in 1982 (Rogers & Masagatani, 1982) and aimed to describe the reasoning process used by ten occupational therapists working in medical settings. The authors concluded that the participants found it difficult to outline their thought processes but focused on the medical diagnosis and the therapist-patient relationship. Interest in clinical reasoning grew in the profession and the American Occupational Therapy Association commissioned a Clinical Reasoning study. This seminal ethnographic study by Fleming (1991) led to the idea of the occupational therapist with the three-track mind and identified three types of clinical reasoning: procedural, interactive and conditional.

Research about professional reasoning has continued to grow over the last thirty years. It would not be possible to examine all studies in the scope of this chapter but the findings from three literature reviews provide a summary (da Silva Araujo et al., 2022; Márquez-Álvarez et al., 2019; Unsworth & Baker, 2016). All three reviews aimed to explore the nature of research related to professional reasoning in occupational therapy. Two were scoping reviews (da Silva Araujo et al., 2022; Márquez-Álvarez et al., 2019) and one was a systematic review (Unsworth &

Baker, 2016). Unsworth and Baker (2016) focused on describing literature relating to professional reasoning and found studies that examined ethics and reasoning, how professional reasoning develops in occupational therapy students and assistants, and how professional reasoning is used in specific areas of practice, such as working with people who have had a stroke and working in a paediatric setting. The authors concluded that many papers were descriptive and more rigorous replicable studies were needed.

Márquez-Álvarez et al. (2019) also sought to scope the history, nature and volume of research on professional reasoning. They found that research started in 1982 and has increased over time with publications in English predominating in the American Journal of Occupational Therapy and the British Journal of Occupational Therapy. Qualitative studies using ethnographic and phenomenological approaches have been more commonly used than quantitative studies and reviews. It is thought the use of qualitative methods is more suited to examining professional reasoning as it allows in-depth analysis of practice. Like Unsworth and Baker (2016), Márquez-Álvarez et al. (2019) also found articles that related to professional reasoning in specific fields of practice, they suggested that further work is needed to study information processing and develop professional reasoning models that could inform professional reasoning more broadly.

The review by da Silva Araujo et al. (2022) focused on mapping the outcomes of qualitative studies to describe how professional reasoning was being conceptualised and applied in occupational therapy. Through thematic analysis, four themes were identified. Firstly, professional reasoning is a process described in different types, such as procedural or narrative. Secondly, professional reasoning was found to be influenced by factors related to the occupational therapist, such as experience and self-confidence, the person, such as diagnosis and recovery rate, and the context, such as hospital or community settings. Thirdly, models or guides to professional reasoning were reported but these were often context-specific and nonlinear, suggesting that professional reasoning is iterative, dynamic and context driven. Finally, there were emerging perspectives on professional reasoning relating to metacognitive, narrative, intuitive, sustainable, and legal approaches that emphasise social justice, rights, political and environmental considerations.

TYPES OF PROFESSIONAL REASONING

The starting point for situating professional reasoning in occupational therapy practice is to place it within the worldview of the profession, that participation in occupation brings health and wellbeing. The models and theories that inform practice, such as the Canadian Model of Occupational Participation (Egan & Restall, 2022) (refer to Chapter 11) or the Model of Human Occupation (Taylor & Kielhofner, 2017) should also be a key component. It is from this starting point that the language of professional reasoning has developed to describe different types of reasoning, such as procedural and conditional. This language helps occupational therapist communicate with each other and with students and novice occupational therapists so that they can develop their own skills. The language of professional reasoning represents different layers of knowledge that occupational therapists might use as they transition from novice to expert. The names of the different types of professional reasoning are listed in Table 9.1.

In professional practice, occupational therapists refer to different types of professional reasoning. These types have been named after being observed in research studies. It is helpful for experienced occupational therapists to name the types of reasoning they are using in practice with students and novice occupational therapists; this makes explicit what has become implicit. It can then assist those developing professional reasoning skills to articulate their thinking using the types of professional reasoning as a structure.

A good starting point is the three classical types of reasoning: procedural, interactive and conditional (Fleming, 1991). These provide a foundational reasoning strategy for co-creating the conditions for how the occupational therapist and individual or collective will work together to understand the situation, make decisions about interventions, and consider the impact this might have on the future (Egan & Restall, 2022). Historically, procedural reasoning referred to reasoning about a person's illness, injury or impairment, reflecting the medical orientation of occupational therapy practice in the 1980s; now procedural reasoning is more about the individual's occupational participation, which reflects the focus on occupation in contemporary occupational therapy practice. Interactive

TABLE 9.1		
Types of Professional Reasoning		
Type of Professional Reasoning	Definition	Example
Procedural (Classical)	Reasoning about a person's illness, injury or impairment and/or an individual's occupational participation.	When an occupational therapist reviews medical notes or charts to collect information about a person's diagnosis.
Interactive (Classical)	Focuses occupational therapist's interaction with the person, with the goal of understanding them better.	During the occupational therapy process the occupational therapist uses open questions to develop a collaborative relationship.
Conditional (Classical)	Multidimensional reasoning that helps the occupational therapist and person think about their life within broader social and temporal contexts and what the future possibilities might be.	When setting meaningful occupational therapy goals the occupational therapist and person collaboratively consider where and when interventions might take place.
Narrative (Contemporary)	Using storytelling to understand the person's experience within a temporal context of the past, present and future.	The occupational therapist facilitates the person or collective to tell their story during an initial interview.
Pragmatic (Contemporary)	Considers pragmatic dimensions, such as the context of therapy and personal circumstances.	The occupational therapist and person consider what financial resources they have when deciding on an intervention.
Ethical (Contemporary)	The consideration of any ethical dilemmas, such as legislation, equity or occupational injustice.	Using a specific piece of legislation as rationale for why a person requires an adaptation to be made to their home environment.
Scientific (Contemporary)	Using logical methods, such as the use of theory, research or hypothesis testing. For example, using evidence-based practice.	Providing a splint for a person with a hand injury, based on research that has found this has been effective for this type of injury.
Generalisation (Emerging)	An occupational therapist reflecting on their own broader professional experience and integrating this into their thinking process	When an occupational therapist provides equipment for someone with a fractured hip because it worked well for someone with a similar condition before.

reasoning occurs when the occupational therapist and person or collective are together and through their interactions get to know and understand each other and develop a trusting and safe collaborative relationship. Conditional reasoning occurs when the occupational therapist brings together the person's story and their context with their own experiences and knowledge to provide a deeper interpretation and to imagine a new possible future (Fleming, 1991).

Since the inception of the classical types of reasoning studies have identified additional types of professional reasoning, including narrative, scientific, pragmatic, and ethical. It can be argued that narrative reasoning is an overarching reasoning approach that occupational therapists commonly use to understand a person's story and context. By listening to a person's story, the emphasis shifts from their diagnosis or condition and places their experience within their temporal-historical context. Scientific, pragmatic, and ethical reasoning represent more contemporary aspects of health and social care that require the occupational therapist to make decisions based on theory and research evidence (scientific reasoning), practicalities such as the practice environment of funding, time and space (pragmatic reasoning), as well as any ethical implications, such as legislation or occupational injustice (ethical reasoning). Generalisation has been identified as an emerging professional reasoning type (da Silva Araujo et al., 2022). Generalisation refers to the occupational therapist reflecting on their own broader professional experience and integrating this into their thinking process.

While a student or novice may find it helpful to label and break down thought processes and the types of professional reasoning, it is important to understand that more experienced occupational therapists use the different types of professional reasoning simultaneously. The next section details some of the cognitive strategies that might be helpful when doing professional reasoning.

DOING PROFESSIONAL REASONING

Unsworth (2016) explains that professional reasoning is underpinned by information processing theory and the related field of memory (Carr & Shotwell, 2008; Ericsson & Simon, 1993). The information gathered through the occupational therapist's senses, cognitive reasoning (thinking), theoretical knowledge and intuition (Chaffey et al., 2010) is 'chunked' and logically connected into 'scripts' or 'frames' that are mentally stored. It is generally understood that straightforward linear-style information about a particular issue or problem is stored in memory as a script. Frames are similar in that they are also a method of gathering information to be stored in an occupational therapist's long-term memory; however, they are generally perceived as more structured and complex (Carr & Shotwell, 2008). Frames are an approach for storing rich and complex knowledge in which there are many possible pathways and outcomes. Expert occupational therapists can rapidly (sometimes simultaneously) draw upon stored scripts or frames and use them to interact at the 'just right' level with each person and collective.

Although there are differing theories as to how professionals such as occupational therapists organise information in memory systems and access it when appropriate, the three most widely used are frame theory (Barsalou, 1992), the adaptive control of thought – rational (ACT-R) model (Anderson, 1983), and dual coding theory (Paivio, 1971). Each of these theories proposes a way to understand how people process, organise, and code information and store it for later use (Carr & Shotwell, 2008). Frame theory focuses on how people organise and connect information when multiple possibilities for relationships between this information exist. For example, frame theory helps provide an understanding of how an occupational therapist might choose a particular intervention from an available selection. The ACT-R model describes both a

person's memory for concepts and facts (declarative) and procedures of how to do things (procedural). To do something with a person, an occupational therapist needs to bring both procedural and declarative memories into the working memory and then generate the frame to engage in therapy. Finally, dual coding theory posits that knowledge is represented in memory using sensory-based coding (e.g. from sight, sound, touch, etc.). People are believed to have both verbal and nonverbal systems for encoding and storing information, and these systems interact to allow them to understand and respond (Carr & Shotwell, 2008). What all three theories have in common is that the key to recognising patterns and being able to construct and access scripts and frames is organisation of knowledge. An important role for educators is to enable occupational therapy students to organise their knowledge, as this will aid them in constructing more complete scripts and frames that can be accessed more quickly when needed.

There is some discussion in the literature about whether a model of professional reasoning can help to structure thinking or process; however, there is no consistent model reported (da Silva Araujo et al., 2022). To provide an example, the Matthews Model of Clinical Reasoning (Matthews et al., 2017) draws on the person-environment-occupation model constructs to guide professional reasoning (Baum et al., 2015). There is a strong emphasis in the reasoning model on being person centred, moving beyond diagnostic labels and focusing on a person's occupational life. The model suggests that the occupational therapist considers top-down and bottom-up assessments to understand the whole person within the context of their environment. The model also provides some practical application and may be useful for some students but there have been no further studies evaluating its use and further work is needed to map it to professional reasoning concepts.

USING PROFESSIONAL REASONING IN THE OCCUPATIONAL THERAPY PROCESS

To apply professional reasoning during the occupational therapy process it is recommended that a recognised process structure is used; in the literature there

BOX 9.1
MOHAMMED

Mohammed was a 40-year-old male, who transitioned to a secure inpatient hospital from prison. He had a diagnosis of schizophrenia and borderline learning disability. He was not eating well. He became angry when he could not complete his laundry. He was verbally and physically aggressive when he felt his needs were not met. It was unclear if he had occupational therapy input before; his previous contact with mental health services was in another city.

Information was gathered via an initial observation of Mohammed completing his laundry and a discussion with him about his occupational history and life. Mohammed completed the laundry task in a ritualistic manner and was distracted throughout the day by thoughts of cleanliness. He voiced that he felt everyone was dirty and noisy in hospital, which meant he avoided using the laundry room and main dining room when other people were there. Not being able to complete his laundry impacted his anxiety levels, resulting in heightened emotions, poor concentration, inability to focus on other activities of daily living and increased his risk of self-neglect. He also lost weight as he was missing mealtimes.

The occupational therapist created a visual laundry timetable with Mohammed, identifying when he could use the laundry room at set times without others present. He liked this idea and felt it would help to reduce his anxiety. He also agreed to engage in a graded plan with his occupational therapist to reduce the amount of time he spent in the laundry room and to learn anxiety management techniques, to enable him to engage more productively in other aspects of his day.

The occupational therapist used narrative reasoning when exploring Mohammed's occupational participation concerns and when co-designing priorities, goals, outcomes and plans. The occupational therapist 'heard' Mohammed's perspective of how the environment was preventing him from doing his laundry. They were able to use this to formulate a plan to enabled him to do his laundry. The occupational therapist 'heard' his values and goals and used a collaborative relationship-focused approach (refer to Chapter 12). Narrative reasoning allowed them to propose to the multidisciplinary team, that if barriers Mohammed identified were reduced/removed, e.g., other people being in the laundry room, this would enable him to engage in activities. Doing his laundry was a valued occupation for Mohammed and supporting him to do this allowed him and the occupational therapist to develop a rapport, which is interactive reasoning.

The occupational therapist used conditional reasoning during various stages of the practice process:

- To inform dynamic risk assessment, for example, what variables could contribute to an escalation in Mohammed's behaviour in relation to laundry, and how will these risks be managed effectively.
- In discharge planning, for example, considering how the interaction between Mohammed, the things he wants and needs to do, and the environment could influence his behaviour and engagement. If he moved into shared accommodation, how would he manage?
- Information gathering, for example, does Mohammed need information provided in a more accessible manner? Does he need the environment adapting to support his learning disability?
- Revision of intervention, for example, are there other aspects of his daily living which he needs support to overcome barriers, such as eating in main dining hall? Can a graded approach be utilised to improve his engagement with this part of ward life?

In addition, the occupational therapist used procedural reasoning to ascertain the most effective assessment and intervention methods and approach to meet Mohammed's needs. The ward routines were considered, and sessions organised with Mohammed when the ward was busy or in environments where fewer people were present.

With thanks to Frederique Lindh, senior occupational therapist with Bradford Foundation District Care Trust.

---

are several representations, including the Canadian Occupational Therapy Inter-relation Practice Process (Restall et al., 2022) (refer to Chapter 12) and the Occupational Therapy Practice Framework (OTPF; AOTA, 2020). Whilst each process may vary there are common places where professional reasoning is used as described in the following sections. The application of professional reasoning is illustrated in three practice stories presented in Boxes 9.1–9.3.

Gather Information to Understand and Seek Understanding About Context

At this early-stage occupational therapists know information but not the person or collective. Procedural and generalisation reasoning is used by the occupational therapist to recall scripts about individuals or collectives they have worked with before and what they know about similar health conditions or circumstances. Occupational therapists are encouraged to use

BOX 9.2
GEORGE

George was a 28-year-old male, who sustained an extensor tendon injury to his left hand, through a workplace injury at a factory. George was referred to occupational therapy via the hospital, for rehabilitation following surgical repair of the extensor tendons to his left middle, ring and little fingers. He lived with his parents and had no difficulties with day-to-day activities prior to his injury.

Medical notes were reviewed by the occupational therapist to gather information on his injury. An outpatient appointment was completed with George, which included subjective and objective assessments followed by an intervention. The subjective assessment ascertained his past medical history and the context and degree of participation in his daily occupations. George reported that he was getting married in three months and was feeling anxious, as he did not qualify for company sick pay. The objective assessment established his tendons were intact. Following this, a splint was fabricated to protect the repairs, targeted exercises given, precautions to protect the hand when doing everyday activities were advised, and a note was provided, listing suitable work activities and adaptations to his employer. A further out-patient occupational therapy appointment was arranged to review and progress his rehabilitation.

Narrative reasoning was used when exploring occupational participation, to understand George's injury and his current home and work situation. Conditional reasoning was used when co-designing priorities, goals, outcomes and plans, which included the need to protect his hand following the repair, otherwise he was at risk of rupture and long-term dysfunction of his left hand. However, he also needed to maintain his income to pay for his upcoming wedding and marriage. Although his left hand had been injured, he was right hand dominant so could do adapted work tasks.

Interactive reasoning was used when trialling the plan, exploring change and refining the plan, to work towards normal hand function within everyday occupations and continuing to work while recovering from his injury. Procedural reasoning was used when exploring occupational participation, when reviewing the medical notes and deciding which intervention regime might be suited to George. The regime selected should be evidence-based and take into consideration the surgery completed. Procedural reasoning was also utilised when reviewing the plan and planning for transition, to identify if the plan had been effective in reducing/resolving the occupational participation challenges posed by George's hand injury and when occupational therapy input was no longer required.

With thanks to Carolyn Macdonald, senior specialist occupational therapist (hand therapy) with Bradford Teaching Hospitals NHS Foundation Trust.

---

a collaborative relationship-focused approach (refer to Chapter 12) that promotes occupational participation, equity and justice. Ethical professional reasoning can help occupational therapist reflect on elements of collaborative relationship-focused therapy by considering their own identity, privileges, values, power and beliefs (Restall & Egan, 2021).

Connect With the Person or Collective and Explore Their Occupational Participation

Occupational therapists must first focus on a person or collective's occupational profile, with consideration of their patterns of occupational participation and their environment. This is an opportunity to engage with the person or collective, develop a collaborative relationship and listen to their story. Interactive and procedural reasoning are employed within a narrative reasoning framework. While narrative reasoning can seem straight forward it can often be the most difficult

for student and novice occupational therapists due to its lack of structure. The use of tools such as the Canadian Occupational Performance Measure (Law et al., 2014) (refer to Chapter 16) or the Occupational Circumstances Interview and Rating Scale (Forsyth et al., 2005) can help to provide this structure and guidance. The assessment of performance components that could hinder occupational participation is the second layer of assessment and could include evaluations of cognition or muscle strength; such testing reflects more procedural professional reasoning.

Co-design Occupational Formulation and Goals

This is the process of working with the person or collective to understand the occupational participation concerns and co-design goals, outcomes and plans (refer to Chapter 19). Brooks and Parkinson (2017) have advocated for the use of formulation and measurable

BOX 9.3
BRENDA

Brenda was a 70-year-old female, diagnosed with Bulbar Motor Neurone Disease, which is a progressive condition. Brenda was having difficulty with the stairs in her house and with bathing. She was very keen to maintain her independence. She lived with her husband in a small, rented property. Brenda made a self-referral to occupational therapy. This referral was screened, and she was placed on the waiting list for a home assessment.

The occupational therapist conducted a home visit to explore Brenda's occupational participation concerns. During the home visit, Brenda was observed doing several occupations in her own home and discussed the occupations she would like to continue to do. Brenda became extremely breathless and fatigued half-way up the stairs, making it difficult to complete other activities upstairs, such as transferring into the bath. The exploration of her occupational participation concerns identified safety issues on the stairs and in the bathroom. An assessment of her home environment was completed in which it was identified that there was one bathroom and toilet and that this was located upstairs.

Following the visit to Brenda, the occupational therapist worked with Brenda to co-design priorities, goals, outcomes and plans. Brenda wanted to continue to have a bath. Following discussion with Brenda, she was provided with a bath lift, as an interim measure to support her when she was transferring into the bath. She was also provided with a stair lift that enabled her to travel up and down the stairs without becoming too fatigued and breathless. This also enabled her to have easier access to her bathroom and toilet. As Brenda's condition will deteriorate, the occupational therapist explored long-term options of adapting the downstairs of her house to provide downstairs bathing facilities. This would require liaison with the housing provider and government grants for major environmental adaptations.

The occupational therapist utilised procedural reasoning when seeking to understand and define purpose, exploring occupational participation, co-designing priorities and trialling the plan. They considered how Brenda's condition would impact her abilities, the possible speed of the deterioration and how her occupational needs would change over time. This would impact on the co-designed plans, as certain procedures and funding may take longer to acquire. Due to this, the occupational therapist identified suitable interim measures that could be implemented quickly to reduce safety risks and maximise Brenda's abilities to remain independent.

Once the major adaptations had been completed, for example, downstairs bathing facilities, the occupational therapist utilised procedural reasoning to review the plan and outcomes, to ensure the adaptation met Brenda's need at that stage in her diagnosis.

The occupational therapist utilised narrative and interactive reasoning when seeking to understand and explore occupational participation, and when co-designing priorities, goals, outcomes and plans, to acknowledge Brenda's wishes about changes to her home environment, and how this would make her feel and be viewed by her husband with whom she shared her home. Initially, she did not want the bath lift, as she felt it was a big piece of equipment and would affect her husband's access to the bath. An interactive reasoning approach was then taken, to propose alternative ideas and suggestions based on the occupational therapist's knowledge and expertise. The occupational therapist ensured that Brenda's views and concerns were heard and taken into consideration when investigating the pros and cons of the various equipment options. Brenda was encouraged to trial this equipment to assist her to decide. This approach helped her progress to a point of acceptance.

With thanks to Laura Morton, Sumera Saboor, Samera Bi, Aneesah Afzal, Jodie Hartley, Tahmida Ali, Ngozi Omeje, Huda Sorathia, occupational therapists from City of Bradford Metropolitan District Council.

---

goal setting as a stage in the occupational therapy process. Formulation can be complex as it uses many types of professional reasoning to integrate information together to create a coherent whole. At its centre formulation uses conditional reasoning as the occupational therapist is considering the person within the context of their life – this is informed by narrative and interactive reasoning. In addition, procedural reasoning may be used to understand the impact of an illness, injury, impairment or circumstance on occupational participation. At this point, it is important that novice therapists do not rely on procedural reasoning and make sure they are being person centred and collaborative relationship focused. Emerging from formulation, goal setting brings the opportunity to use scientific reasoning (what is the evidence) pragmatic reasoning (what is practical based on time, space, funding and personal circumstances) and ethical reasoning (considering ethical dilemmas and solutions). Occupational participation goals should be negotiated with

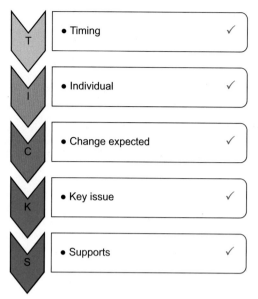

Fig. 9.1 ■ The TICKS (timeframe, individual, change expected, key issue, supports) goal-setting structure. (From Parkinson, S., & Brooks, R. (2020). *A guide to the formulation of plans and goals in occupational therapy*. Routledge).

the person or collective. The TICKS (timeframe, individual, change expected, key issue, supports) structure (Fig. 9.1) provides a format for writing them (Parkinson & Brooks, 2020).

Trial the Plan, Explore Change, Refine the Plan and Plan for Transition

This is when the occupational therapist works in collaboration with the person or collective to deliver plans and interventions that best address the identified occupational participation concerns. It is important the occupational therapist continues to use professional reasoning throughout the intervention, this may be a combination of all types of reasoning that feeds into a continual review of what is working and making a difference for the person and what might need to be modified or changed.

DEVELOPING PROFESSIONAL REASONING

Dreyfus and Dreyfus (1986) proposed that there are five stages a person passes through when learning a skill:

novice, advance beginner, competent, proficient, and expert. Applying this model to occupational therapy practice, novice occupational therapists are described as having very few experiences of the situations in which they are involved. Although novice occupational therapists know some of the rules, principles, and theories, they are often rigidly applied. An advanced beginner recognises recurring themes and patterns and begins to create scripts for practice. An advanced beginner occupational therapist still remembers theoretical information and as a result, may have limited flexibility in the application of theory. Competent occupational therapists are said to be consciously aware of the outcome of their actions; however, they lack the speed and flexibility of the proficient occupational therapist. Occupational therapists who are thought to be at the proficient level have a rapid and clear picture of a person or collective's whole situation and recognise recurring patterns. In the final level, an expert occupational therapist uses multiple frames to engage in a flexible and reflexive practice. Experts need less information when working on a problem and make better judgements, as they seem to have an intuitive grasp of the situation (Benner, 1984; Dreyfus & Dreyfus, 1986).

The idea that all healthcare professionals develop from novice to expert has been challenged as experience does not always lead to increasing expertise, with some never reaching expert status. Nevertheless, it is usual for occupational therapists to develop their professional reasoning and students and novice occupational therapists should integrate strategies to help development. There are a range of suggested activities that can promote professional reasoning:

■ Reflection on placement or in practice to know what went well and where it did not go as planned, thinking critically about a situation to develop learning and change practice (Jeffrey et al., 2021). The use of a reflective model, such as 'What? So what? Now what?' (Rolfe et al., 2001), in supervision may be helpful to the development of professional reasoning, particularly for occupational therapy students and those early in their careers (Guy et al., 2020).

■ Feedback from occupational therapy practice educators. This should include corrective elements with suggestions of how to improve (de Beer & Martensson, 2015).

■ A practice environment that encourages questioning and sharing of knowledge (Jeffrey et al., 2021).

■ Developing skills to understand and translate research evidence to practice which should be facilitated by expert occupational therapists (Jeffrey et al., 2021).

■ Use of practice stories (McCannon et al., 2004) with specific learning activities related to professional reasoning has been shown to improve occupational therapy students' professional reasoning. The use of videos enables an even greater consideration of a person and their context resulting in more inductive reasoning (Murphy & Stav, 2018).

■ Attending inter-professional learning. Evidence has suggested that being involved in interprofessional learning events as an occupational therapy student and graduate can enhance reflection and reasoning skills (Seif et al., 2014).

■ Consider the influence of professional values and local cultures. A study in stroke rehabilitation (Kristensen et al., 2012) found that personal values and clinical experience were a significant factor in influencing professional decision making.

■ Providing opportunities for occupational therapy students and graduates to talk through their reasoning with someone more experienced (Turpin et al., 2021).

TABLE 9.2
Questions to Guide Professional Reasoning
Where am I in the occupational therapy process?   Can I name the type of professional reasoning I am using?   Have I considered information from various sources to inform my reasoning?   Can I be informed by any research evidence or audit data?   What theory informs what I am doing?   What do I know about the person or collective's situation?   What intervention could work? What might the individual feel about this intervention?   Have I worked with any people with a similar presentation?   Am I being biased or taking any shortcuts to come to my conclusions?   Are there any local or national protocols?   Am I being person centred and using a collaborative approach?   Am I working within policies and legislation?   What are the person's own views and perspectives?   Am I being just and ethical?   What practicalities influence my reasoning?   Have I considered the person's goals and values?   Have I incorporated the person's cultural background?   Have I considered the person's financial means to engage in this intervention?   Am I working within my professional code of ethics and responsibilities?   What are alternative options?   In what ways have I drawn on my past experiences and outcomes of implementing this intervention?   Have I considered what other resources and support is available to the person to include during the intervention stage?   Have I appraised my own knowledge and skills?   Have I reflected on elements of collaborative relationship-focused therapy by considering my own identity, privileges, values, power and beliefs?

There are several other aspects of professional practice that have been found to influence professional reasoning. Some of these are situated with the person, including level of education, experience of professional reasoning, self-confidence, feelings towards the person, and professional habits (da Silva Araujo et al., 2022). Others are more context dependent, such as working in a hospital setting resulted in medical model perspectives in reasoning, while community rehabilitation was more person centred and focused on occupation. The context also impacts professional reasoning in terms of space, time, workload, resources, equipment, social attitudes, stigma, and carers' expectations. It is important that each occupational therapists is aware of the influence of themselves and their context on professional reasoning. A series of questions are presented in Table 9.2 to assist with the development of professional reasoning.

CONCLUSION

Professional reasoning is a complex activity. By understanding the different types and the cognitive processes used to support reasoning it is possible to elucidate the process. It is important that occupational therapists are aware of the intrinsic and extrinsic factors that may influence their professional reasoning. There is no current universal model for professional reasoning, but the classical, contemporary and emerging types do provide a framework to support how occupational therapists make decisions about how they work with the people receiving occupational therapy services. While not every occupational therapist may become an expert, professional reasoning does develop with time and experience. Occupational therapists should use the strategies presented to assist them to develop and apply their reasoning skills throughout the occupational therapy process.

Acknowledgement

The authors would like to thank the previous author of this chapter Carolyn Unsworth. The sections on information processing theory and memory, and novice to expert have used parts of her work.

REFERENCES

Anderson, J. R. (1983). *The architecture of cognition.* Harvard University Press.

AOTA. (2020). *Document, the occupational therapy practice framework: Domain and process* (4th ed.). AOTA.

Banning, M. (2008). Clinical reasoning and its application to nursing: Concepts and research studies. *Nurse Education in Practice, 8*(3), 177–183. https://doi.org/10.1016/j.nepr.2007.06.004.

Barsalou, L. W. (1992). Frames, concepts and conceptual fields. In A. Lehrer., & E. F. Kittay (Eds.), *Frames, fields and contrasts: New essays in semantic and lexical organisation* (pp. 21–74). Erlbaum.

Bass, J., Baum, C., & Christiansen, C. (2015). Interventions and outcomes: The person-environment-occupational performance (PEOP) occupational therapy process. In C. Christiansen, C. Baum, & J. Bass (Eds.), *Occupational therapy: Performance, participation, well-being* (4th ed.). Slack, 57–80.

Benner, P. (1984). *From novice to expert. Excellence and power in clinical nursing practice.* Addison–Wesley.

Brooks, R., & Parkinson, S. (2017). Occupational formulation: A three-part structure. *British Journal of Occupational Therapy, 81*(3), 177–179.

Carr, M., & Shotwell, M. (2008). Information processing theory and professional reasoning. In B. B. Schell & J. W. Schell (Eds.), *Clinical and professional reasoning in occupational therapy* (pp. 36–67). Lippincott Williams & Wilkins.

Chaffey, L., Unsworth, C. A., & Fossey, E. (2010). A grounded theory of intuition among occupational therapists in mental health practice. *British Journal of Occupational Therapy, 73*(7), 300–308.

da Silva Araujo, A., Anne Kinsella, E., Thomas, A., Demonari Gomes, L., & Quevedo Marcolino, T. (2022). Clinical reasoning in occupational therapy practice: A scoping review of qualitative and conceptual peer-reviewed literature. *The American Journal of Occupational Therapy, 76*(3), 7603205070. https://doi.org/10.5014/ajot.2022.048074.

de Beer, M., & Mårtensson, L. (2015). Feedback on students' clinical reasoning skills during fieldwork education. *Australian Occupational Therapy Journal, 62*(4), 255–264. https://doi.org/10.1111/1440-1630.12208.

Dreyfus, H. L., & Dreyfus, S. E. (1986). *Mind over machine: The power of human intuition and expertise in the era of the computer.* Free Press.

Egan, M., & Restall, G. (2022). Canadian model of occupational participation: Collaborative relationship-focused occupational therapy. In M. Egan, & G. Restall (Eds.), *Promoting occupational participation: Collaborative relationship-focused occupational therapy* (pp. 7). Canadian Association of Occupational Therapists.

Ericsson, K. A., & Simon, H. A. (1993). *Protocol analysis: Verbal reports as data.* MIT Press.

Fleming, M. H. (1991). The therapist with the three-track mind. *The American Journal of Occupational Therapy, 45*(11), 1007–1014. https://doi.org/10.5014/ajot.45.11.1007.

Forsyth, K., Deshpande, S., Kielhofner, G., Henriksson, C., Haglund, L., Olson, L., Skinner, S., Kulkarni, S., & Kielhofner, G. (2005). *The occupational circumstances assessment interview and rating scale (OCAIRS) version 4.0.* University of Illinois at Chicago.

Garcia, J., Copley, J., Turpin, M., Bennett, S., McBryde, C., & McCosker, J. L. (2021). Evidence-based practice and clinical reasoning in occupational therapy: A cross-sectional survey in Chile. *Australian Occupational Therapy Journal, 68*(2), 169–179. https://doi.org/10.1111/1440-1630.12713.

Guy, L., Cranwell, K., Hitch, D., & McKinstry, C. (2020). Reflective practice facilitation within occupational therapy supervision processes: A mixed method study. *Australian Occupational Therapy Journal, 67*(4), 320–329. https://doi.org/10.1111/1440-1630.12660.

Huhn, K., Gilliland, S. J., Black, L. L., Wainwright, S. F., & Christensen, N. (2019). Clinical reasoning in physical therapy: A concept analysis. *Physical Therapy, 99*(4), 440–456. https://doi.org/10.1093/ptj/pzy148.

Jeffery, H., Robertson, L., & Reay, K. L (2021). Sources of evidence for professional decision-making in novice occupational therapy practitioners: Clinicians' perspectives. *British Journal of Occupational Therapy, 84*(6), 346–354. https://doi.org/10.1177/0308022620941390.

Koufidis, C., Manninen, K., Nieminen, J., Wohlin, M., & Silén, C. (2021). Unravellingng the polyphony in clinical reasoning research in medical education. *Journal of Evaluation in Clinical Practice, 27*, 438–450. https://doi.org/10.1111/jep.13432.

Kristensen, H. K., Borg, T., & Hounsgaard, L. (2012). Aspects affecting occupational therapists' reasoning when implementing research-based evidence in stroke rehabilitation. *Scandinavian Journal of Occupational Therapy, 19*, 118–131. https://doi.org/10.3109/11038128.2011.556197.

Law, M., Baptiste, S., Carswell, A., McColl, M. A., Polatajko, H., & Pollock, N. (2014). *Canadian occupational performance measure* (5th ed.). CAOT Publications.

Márquez-Álvarez, L. J., Calvo-Arenillas, J. I., Talavera-Valverde, M.Á., & Moruno-Millares, P. (2019). Professional reasoning in occupational therapy: A scoping review. *Occupational Therapy International, 2019*(1), 6238245. https://doi.org/10.1155/2019/6238245.

Matthews, L. K., Mulry, C. M., & Richard, L. (2017). Matthews model of clinical reasoning: A systematic approach to conceptualize evaluation and intervention. *Occupational Therapy in Mental Health, 33*(4), 360–373. https://doi.org/10.1080/0164212X.2017.1303658.

McCannon, R., Robertson, D., Caldwell, J., Juwah, C., & Elfessi, A. (2004). Comparison of clinical reasoning skills in occupational therapy students in the USA and Scotland. *Occupational Therapy International, 11*(3), 160–176. https://doi.org/10.1002/oti.204.

Murphy, L. F., & Stav, W. B. (2018). The impact of online video cases on clinical reasoning in occupational therapy education: A quantitative analysis. *The Open Journal of Occupational Therapy,* Article 4, *6*(3). https://doi.org/10.15453/2168-6408.1494.

Paivio, A. (1971). *Imagery and visual processes.* Holt, Rinehart & Winston.

Parkinson, S., & Brooks, R. (2020). *A guide to the formulation of plans and goals in occupational therapy.* Routledge.

Restall, G., Egan, M., Valavaara, K., Phenix, A., & Sack, C. (2022). Canadian occupational therapy inter-relational practice process. In M. Egan, & G. Restall (Eds.), *Promoting occupational participation: Collaborative relationship-focused occupational therapy* (pp. 122). Canadian Association of Occupational Therapists.

Rogers, J. C., & Masagatani, G. (1982). Clinical reasoning of occupational therapists during initial assessment of physically disabled patients. *Occupational Therapy Journal of Research, 2,* 195–219.

Rolfe, G., Freshwater, D., & Jasper, M. (2001). *Critical reflection in nursing and the helping professions: A user's guide.* Palgrave Macmillan.

Schon, D. A. (1983). *The reflective practitioner: How professional think in action.* Basic Books Inc.

Seif, G., Coker-Bolt, P., Kraft, S., Gonsalves, W., Simpson, K., & Johnson, E. (2014). The development of clinical reasoning and interprofessional behaviors: Service-learning at a student-run free clinic. *Journal of Interprofessional Care, 28*(6), 559–564. https://doi.org/10.3109/13561820.2014.921899.

Taylor, R. R., & Kielhofner, G. (2017). Introduction to the model of human occupation. In Taylor, R. R. (Ed.), *Kielhofner's model of human occupation* (pp. 3–10). Lippincott, Williams and Wilkins.

Turpin, M., Fitzgerald, C., Copley, J., Laracy, S., & Lewis, B. (2021). Experiences of and support for the transition to practice of newly graduated occupational therapists undertaking a hospital graduate program. *Australian Occupational Therapy Journal, 68*(1), 12–20. https://doi.org/10.1111/1440-1630.12693.

Unsworth, C., & Baker, A. A. (2016). A systematic review of professional reasoning literature in occupational therapy. *British Journal of Occupational Therapy, 79*(1), 5–16. https://doi.org/10.1177/0308022615599994.

REFLECTION

1. Discuss the main types of professional reasoning.

2. Describe the use of professional reasoning in the occupational therapy process.

3. Identify a range of activities or strategies you could use to develop your professional reasoning.

4. Describe and reflect on four factors that can influence an occupational therapist's professional reasoning.

5. Consider how a person's or collective's cultural background may influence your professional reasoning.

6. Consider how a model of practice, for example, the Canadian Model of Occupational Participation, may influence your professional reasoning.

7. Reflect on how professional reasoning is incorporated into the occupational therapy process, and the importance of implementing professional reasoning.

10

AN OCCUPATION, CAPABILITY AND WELLBEING FRAMEWORK FOR OCCUPATIONAL THERAPY

KAREN WHALLEY HAMMELL

CHAPTER OUTLINE

Overview

The occupational therapy profession continues to evolve. Formerly preoccupied with promoting function and independence, and latterly, with 'enabling' individuals' performance of three occupations (self-care, productive, leisure), occupational therapy more recently committed to addressing 'occupational engagement (active, satisfying participation in occupations)' (Egan & Restall, 2022, p. 5). Such developments highlight the need for a new conceptual framework for occupational therapy; one firmly grounded in evidence derived from a diversity of disciplines, contexts and sources, and focused on the enhancement of human wellbeing through occupational engagement. Advancing rights- and strengths-based approach to practice, the *Occupation, Capability and Wellbeing Framework for Occupational Therapy* (OCWFOT) (Hammell, 2020) encourages consideration of individuals and collectives' abilities, resources and opportunities, promoting structurally competent practices that consider both the relational and contextual nature of engagement in occupations that 'matter'. Theoretically defensible, the OCWFOT provides a resource and structure around which future research and practice may be oriented.

KEY POINTS

- Occupational therapy requires a practice framework centred on the enhancement of wellbeing through occupation and rooted in evidence derived from multiple contexts and from a diversity of sources.
- The *Occupation, Capability and Wellbeing Framework for Occupational Therapy* (OCWFOT) promotes a rights-based and strengths-based approach to practice that requires structural competence and promotes cultural humility.

- The Framework focuses attention on the assessment and expansion of the capabilities of individuals and collectives to engage in valued occupations, promoting a relational approach in recognition that people are embedded and belong within collectives.

- The Framework eschews a neoliberal agenda promoting self-care, productivity, independence, individualism, and erasure of functional differences. The Framework employs an equity focus that promotes modes of practice responsive to the structural and social determinants of occupational engagement ('occupational engagement' refers to 'active, satisfying participation in occupations', Egan & Restall, 2022, p. 5).

- This chapter situates the OCWFOT within the ongoing evolution of occupational therapy.

INTRODUCTION

For many years, critical occupational therapy scholars in the Global North have sought to focus the profession's attention on the ableist, White, Western, middle-class norms and values that infuse its dominant models, and that have informed its international practices (Gerlach, 2015; Hammell, 2009a, 2009b, 2011, 2015; Iwama, 2003, 2006). Challenging the culturally specific and evidence-deficient assumptions that have underpinned occupational therapy, these critics have advocated for the profession to base its models, theories and practices on evidence and have called for this evidence to be derived from multiple contexts and from a diversity of sources. Their contentions have both mirrored and amplified critiques advanced by critical scholars in the Global South who have contested the colonial imposition of occupational therapy models and practices infused with specific Western values (e.g. Al Busaidy & Borthwick, 2012; Emery-Whittington, 2021; Galheigo, 2011; Gibson, 2020; Lim & Duqué, 2011; Malfitano, 2022; Malfitano & Lopes, 2018; Motimele & Peters, 2017; Ramugondo, 2018). Indeed, Grenier (2020) has articulated the need to 'radically dismantle and rebuild the "biased" frameworks and models on which the profession has relied for over a century' (p. 640).

These, and other challenges to the inadequacies of the profession's status quo pointed to the requirement for a new conceptual framework for occupational therapy; one grounded in evidence and explicitly focused on occupational therapy's unique domain of concern – the enhancement of human health, wellbeing, social participation, and quality of life through occupation. The impetus for, the evolution of, and potential for the *Occupation, Capability and Wellbeing Framework for Occupational Therapy* (OCWFOT, Hammell, 2020) are the focus of this chapter.

The author identifies as a White, temporarily non-disabled, straight cis-female holding citizenship status in two Anglophone nations within the Global North; currently living as a settler on the traditional, ancestral and unceded territory of Coast Salish people in Canada. She acknowledges the unearned benefits, advantages and privileges she has always derived from her White skin, able body and proximity to socially constructed and valued Western 'norms' of being and doing.

THE (EVOLVING) AIM OF OCCUPATIONAL THERAPY

This book draws from the Canadian Association of Occupational Therapists' recent publication – *Promoting occupational participation: Collaborative relationship-focused occupational therapy* (Egan & Restall, 2022) – in defining the aim of occupational therapy as 'helping people participate in valued occupations within meaningful relationships and contexts' (p. 5). Egan and Restall (2022) noted that this aim reflects an 'evolution' within the profession; an evolution they contend 'can be traced from promoting function (independently carrying out activities, particularly activities of daily living), to enabling occupational performance (accomplishing self-care, productivity, or leisure occupations), to occupational engagement (active, satisfying participation in occupations)' (p. 5). This evolution has been unevenly accomplished, with considerable professional attention remaining focused on promoting function, independence and occupational performance.

Underpinning this chapter is the understanding that individuals are relationally embedded – within partnerships, within genetic and chosen families, within friendship and tribal groups, within clans, communities and populations – and that occupational therapists' work should be undertaken both with collectives and with individuals. I refer, in this chapter, to 'individuals and collectives' to indicate the impossibility of viewing people as divisible from their relational contexts, and as a form of short-hand for the many possible manifestations of relationship configurations.

The Evolutionary Process: Aiming to Promote Function and Independence in Activities of Daily Living

Promoting Function

Occupational therapists' focus on 'promoting function' can be understood as an outcome of a hegemonic, ableist, neoliberal ideology that views typical (usual, 'normal') bodies, minds and abilities as superior, and those with bodily impairments as both inferior and flawed (Campbell, 2008; Hammell, 2023). Ableist values – which equate human worth with independence, productivity, and 'normal' (typical) abilities, functions, performances and appearances – inform occupational therapy practices focused on assessing, minimising or eliminating physical differences (for a review, see Hammell, 2023). Critical scholars have contested the assumption of 'normality' that underpins the rehabilitation industry (Gappmayer, 2021; Hammell, 2023). Furthermore, the self-appointed right of powerful 'experts' – such as occupational therapists – to judge 'normality' and the desirability of certain forms of performance has been challenged by disabled scholars for more than twenty years (Pfeiffer, 1999). Indeed, it has been suggested that the aim of 'normalising' functions may be less about enhancing the quality of disabled people's lives and more about inducing social conformity (Gappmayer, 2021; Gibson & Teachman, 2012; Hammell, 2023; Phelan, 2011; Phelan et al., 2014; Sandahl, 2003).

Promoting Independence in Activities of Daily Living

Occupational therapy has promoted the neoliberal ideology that independence is admirable, aspirational and universally valued (Hammell, 2020; Kristensen et al., 2017). In so doing, the profession has actively reinforced ableist stereotypes that demean and devalue those who are unable to achieve independence, who choose to accept the assistance extended by others (Hammell, 2006), who value occupational engagement that affords the opportunity for interdependence (Iwama, 2006), or who understand all humans to be embedded within relationships characterised by reciprocity and mutual support (Bryant et al., 2021; Hammell, 2019). Occupational therapy has ignored the assertion, advanced for several decades by disability theorists – that interdependence 'is an indispensable feature of the human condition' (Reindal, 1999, p. 354) – and has failed to heed the conclusion of its own scientists, that 'the aim of the most important occupations is interdependence' (Martín et al., 2015, p. 86).

The ideology that individuals are wholly responsible for their own health, wellbeing and social circumstances is central to a neoliberal political rationality (Gerlach et al., 2018). As Harris, Owen and Gould (2012, p. 826) have noted: 'Participation within a human rights framework seeks to address structural changes; but in a neoliberal climate, participation for citizens necessitates individual change'. Accordingly, occupational therapy's 'clients' are expected to comply with standardised treatment regimens, align their actions with an individualistic neoliberal agenda (Aldrich & Rudman, 2020), and strive to adhere to socially valued 'norms' of function and performance (Hammell, 2020). Collusion with neoliberalism's ableist norms, avowed aspirations to minimise bodily differences, 'normalise' occupational performances, and promote self-reliance, independence and productivity, have contributed to the perception – articulated by critical disability scholars – that occupational therapy is a disabling profession (for review, see Hammell, 2023).

By focusing on *individuals'* functional impairments and *in*-abilities occupational therapy has often overlooked people's abilities, skills, strengths, knowledge, social capital and resources. By placing the responsibility on each *individual* to strive for higher levels of function, occupational therapy failed to address the structural barriers that disable people with abilities differing from valued social 'norms' (Hammell, 2020). This focus exposes the profession's complicity in upholding the neoliberal structural arrangements that sustain, reproduce and compound injustices and inequities (Gerlach et al., 2018; Hayes et al., 2023).

The Evolutionary Process: Aiming to 'Enable' the Performance of Self-Care, Productive and Leisure Occupations

Neoliberalism's ableist premise – that people's value resides in their ability independently to perform self-care and productive occupations – is infused throughout occupational therapy's educational and clinical practices (Grenier, 2021). Thus, dominant Western occupational therapy has promoted three occupational categories: self-care, productivity and leisure (e.g. Townsend & Polatajko, 2013). These three specific categories betray the neoliberal-inspired values and priorities shared among privileged, able, employed White theorists in the Global North and were not informed by empirical evidence. To the contrary, research indicates that these three simplistic and individualistic categories do not encompass the rich range of forms, or purposes, of occupation that are meaningful to, and valued by human beings and of importance to their wellbeing. Indeed, researchers report that – if asked – people define their occupations according to experiential, geographical, temporal and role categories, and not according to categories they label self-care, productivity/work, or leisure/play (for review, see Hammell, 2020). A study that compared the ways in which people categorise their own occupations to those pre-established categories prioritised within occupational therapy's dominant models found that 40% of participants' chosen occupations fell outside the boundaries of the three categories promoted by the profession (Brooke et al., 2007).

Importantly, the tripartite framework obscures, ignores – and thus devalues – many of the occupations that are profoundly important to the quality of people's lives and essential to their wellbeing, such as those undertaken to facilitate, maintain and enrich relationships and sense of belonging; to contribute to, and care for others; to foster and facilitate creativity; to uphold, connect with, and transmit cultural and spiritual traditions; to care for the natural environment; to affirm, construct, and enact a gender identity; or to act in resistance to injustice (Hammell, 2020). Moreover, the specific Anglophone perspective that informed the three occupational categories effectively erases every occupation that cannot be directly translated into English (Magalhães et al., 2019). This is an injustice.

It has already been noted that by prioritising self-care and productive occupations, occupational therapy has uncritically embraced and advanced neoliberal values that equate personal worth with individualism, independence and productivity (Burgin, 2014; Gerlach et al., 2018), and that marginalise the very people occupational therapy services are ostensibly designed to help (Fadyl et al., 2020). Yet despite 'the ethical imperative to interrogate critically any suggestion that the profession promotes ableism and colludes in the disablement of people [with impairments]' (Hammell, 2023, p. 475), occupational therapy has largely failed to address the contention, levelled by disability scholars for more than a quarter century, that 'we need to argue against "productivity" […] as a measure of human value' (Finger, 1995, p. 15).

The inclusion of 'leisure' within the profession's privileged triad is equally contentious. Western ideas about what constitutes leisure do not adequately encompass the experiences, values, and perspectives of non-Western peoples (Stack & Iwasaki, 2009). Moreover, leisure is defined – even among the privileged Western minority whose values informed the categorical systems – according to specific situational factors, such as day of the week, time of day, location and the presence of others and who these others are, making a definitive categorisation of 'leisure' untenable. The reality that the languages of many global people do not have a word that means 'leisure' (Iwasaki et al., 2007; Kelly & Kelly, 1994) highlights the inappropriateness of its inclusion within occupational therapy models.

Adherence to the three privileged categories has effectively diverted occupational therapists' attention from the core concern of the profession: the relationship between occupation and human wellbeing (Jonsson, 2008). Clearly, it is more important to assess how people's wellbeing needs are being met through their occupational engagement than to assess their ability to 'perform' three forms of occupation valued by privileged Western occupational therapy theorists. It is also more important to focus on assessing and building the collective strengths, abilities, skills, knowledge, relationships and resources that will expand the opportunities for people to engage in the occupations that matter to them than to focus on 'norming non-standard' bodies and functions. Moreover, because a wealth of cross-cultural evidence demonstrates that occupation is a determinant of human health and wellbeing (Hammell, 2020), occupational therapy should focus primarily on addressing the capabilities of clients – as individuals and collectives – to engage in the occupations they value and that contribute positively to their wellbeing (Hammell, 2020).

The Evolutionary Process: Aiming for Occupational Engagement (Active, Satisfying Participation in Occupations)

The concerns that have been briefly outlined – and others – led to the search for a new conceptual framework for occupational therapy, one grounded in research evidence derived from a diversity of sources and explicitly focused on what 'matters' to people – the enhancement of wellbeing through occupational engagement. The development of this framework responded to evolutions within the occupational therapy profession in the early decades of the 21st century, when profound social injustices – such as sexism, racism, poverty and the ongoing impacts of colonialism – could no longer be ignored as significant determinants of occupational participation and individualistic approaches focused on modifying functions and enabling performances were recognised as inadequate responses to occupational injustices (Farias & Rudman, 2019; Gerlach, 2015; Gerlach et al., 2018; Hammell, 2019, 2020; Hammell & Beagan, 2017; Hammell & Iwama, 2012; Hocking, 2012; Rudman, 2013). During this period, occupational therapy theorists began to speak in terms of *occupational rights* (Hammell, 2008; Hammell & Iwama, 2012; Nilsson & Townsend, 2010; Townsend & Wilcock, 2004), defined as constituting 'the rights of all people to engage in meaningful occupations that contribute positively to their own well-being and the well-being of their communities' (Hammell, 2008, p. 62). Subsequently, the World Federation of Occupational Therapists (WFOT, 2019) declared that 'Occupational therapists around the world are obligated to promote occupational rights as the actualisation of human rights'.

Importantly, WFOT did not assert the occupational therapy profession's global contribution as being the enablement of self-care, productive and leisure occupations, nor as the maximisation of human function, performance and independence and elimination of physical difference, but as enablement of the *right* to occupational participation.

In recognition of the imperative for rights- and strengths-based approaches to practice, the current phase of occupational therapy's evolution has shifted the profession's attention to 'occupational engagement'; an approach 'focused clearly on expanding, not solely people's abilities, but their capabilities – their opportunities and equal rights – to engage in occupations that contribute positively to their health, well-being, participation and quality of life, and the health and wellbeing of their communities' (Hammell, 2020, p. 253). These values informed the development of the *Occupation, Capabilities and Wellbeing Framework for Occupational Therapy*, notably the emphasis on capabilities.

A Capabilities Approach

The WFOT (2019) *Position Statement on Human Rights* asserted that 'occupational rights are secured by identifying and addressing the capabilities (Sen, 2003), opportunities, and freedom of choice for individuals, communities and populations to participate in society'. By referencing *capabilities* in this important statement, WFOT recognised the significance of Amartya Sen's capabilities approach for the international occupational therapy profession.

Sen's Capabilities Approach (1999, 2005), which was developed as a framework to address wellbeing from a human rights perspective, is centrally concerned with people's abilities to do and be the things they value doing and being, *and* with their real opportunities to act on these wishes. The capabilities approach employs a multidimensional and contextualised view of human wellbeing; one that attends to the linkages between health, physical, mental, social and material wellbeing, and the physical, social, political, economic, religious and cultural dimensions of people's lives (Crocker & Robeyns, 2010). Embedded within Sen's conceptualisation of capabilities is a relational ontology (Robeyns, 2005; Terzi, 2005, 2011), in which capabilities are understood to be shaped – and partly constituted – by social circumstances (Entwistle & Watt, 2013), such that choices and actions reflect the outcome of interactions between individuals' abilities and their positions in society (Smith & Seward, 2009).

The capabilities approach's concern with both abilities *and* opportunities clearly aligns with occupational therapy's evolving attention to the contextual factors that promote or constrain people's opportunity to access, ability to initiate, and capability to sustain 'occupational engagement' in 'valued occupations within meaningful relationships and contexts' (Egan & Restall, 2022, p. 5; Hammell, 2022). Moreover, because the capabilities approach has been embraced by numerous other disciplines – such as public health, special needs education, social policy, disability studies and social medicine – it provides a shared language and perspective with others committed to advancing human wellbeing through assuring human rights, thus enhancing occupational therapy's own capabilities to accomplish its mandate and goals.

THE PRESENT MOMENT IN OCCUPATIONAL THERAPY'S EVOLUTION

From the arguments presented so far in this chapter, it is apparent that occupational therapists can no longer be preoccupied with identifying and cataloguing deficits, dysfunctions, and inabilities or with promoting functional independence to the exclusion of engagement in occupations valued by the individual. Moreover, it is apparent that focusing on *individuals* is inadequate for the work of enhancing occupational participation among people who are embedded within partnerships, families, friendship and tribal groups, clans, communities and populations, and whose occupations are both enabled and constrained by their environmental contexts. At this point in our profession's evolution, a new framework for practice is required; one focused on both abilities and opportunities and on occupation as a human right.

The occupational therapy profession's current phase of evolution supports a new framework for practice that reflects the following fundamental principles.

Principles Underpinning the Framework

■ The Framework is centred on the concept of *wellbeing*: 'a state of contentment – or harmony – with one's physical/mental health; emotional/spiritual health; personal and economic security; self-worth (sense of being capable, and of being valued by others); sense of belonging (which includes the ability to contribute to others and

to maintain valued roles and relationships, and which may include a sense of belonging and of connectedness to the land and nature); opportunities for self-determination (defined as the ability to enact choices and counteract powerlessness); opportunities to engage in meaningful and purposeful occupations; and sense of hope' (Hammell & Iwama, 2012, p. 387).

■ Occupation is a determinant of human health and wellbeing (refer to Chapter 6), and because having real opportunities to engage in occupations that contribute positively to wellbeing is a human right, the Framework promotes a *rights-based* approach to practice.

■ Environmental factors and systemic social forces sustain health inequities and determine occupational possibilities (Rudman, 2010) (refer to Chapter 7). The Framework therefore focuses attention on expanding people's *capabilities* (Sen, 1999, 2005) – their opportunities as well as their abilities – to engage in valued occupations. Integral to capabilities approach to practice is the consideration of

　a) The personal characteristics of service users (e.g. their ages, gender identities, impairments),

　b) Their assets, abilities and resources (as individuals and as members embedded within collectives), *and*

　c) The barriers – inequitable structures and unfair constraints – *and* facilitators that derive from their histories and environmental contexts (Mitra, 2006); that is, factors that impact the possibilities for expansion of their choices, conversion of their opportunities and resources into actions, actualisation of their values, and real capabilities to achieve wellbeing (Hammell, 2020).

The use of 'capabilities language' facilitates communication and collaboration with others working to advance human wellbeing and human rights (Hammell, 2022).

■ Occupational engagement and participation are dependent on both abilities and opportunities. Accordingly, the Framework advances a *strengths-based* approach (Bryant et al., 2021) that assesses and builds on individual and collective capacities, capabilities and resources (e.g. knowledges, skills, cultural and spiritual practices, material resources, social capital and sense of belonging within relationships and networks of support), and that eschews a deficit-saturated view of people – as 'dysfunctional' individuals and collectives.

■ Injustices, such as racism, colonialism, sexism, patriarchy, class and caste inequities, poverty, disablism, ageism, heteronormativity and gender binarism are determinants of occupational opportunity, engagement and participation (Hammell, 2021). The Framework therefore fosters an *equity focus*. To be equity-focused is to 'surface, challenge and, ultimately, change unjust social conditions' (Phipps & Masuda, 2018, p. 381), refusing to overlook, accept or collude with the injustices that unfairly disadvantage specific groups of people while unfairly advantaging others.

■ Occupational therapists need to be competent in analysing 'the forces that constrain decision making, frame choices, and limit life options' (Quesada et al., 2011, p. 342). Thus, the Framework promotes *structural competence*: the ability to discern, and the commitment to change the inequitable social and structural determinants of health and occupation (Metzl & Hansen, 2014). Structural competence has been identified as a core professional competency for occupational therapists (Hammell, 2021).

■ Occupational therapists are required to build, foster and sustain respectful, culturally safe, collaborative relationships with service users (Hammell, 2020; Restall et al., 2022). *Cultural humility* (Tervalon & Murray-Garcia, 1998) thus constitutes an important component of professional competence (Beagan, 2015; Hammell, 2013a), requiring occupational therapists to shed 'the protective mantle' of professional status and expertise (Phipps & Masuda, 2018). The Framework therefore focuses occupational therapists' attention on understanding and respecting the values and priorities of individuals and collectives with whom they are working. Cultural humility requires occupational therapists to hold a critical

consciousness of the effects of power inequalities that structure society and that accord unjust disadvantages and resources to some, while simultaneously awarding unjust and unearned advantages, resources, privileges and power to others (Feagin & Bennefield, 2014) (refer to Chapters 1 and 2). Cultural humility is not a set of skills but a way of being; one that incorporates both 'a life-long commitment to self-evaluation and self-critique' (Tervalon & Murray-García, 1998, p. 117), and attention to mitigating the imbalances of power that accompany different social positions (Fisher-Borne et al., 2015). Integral to self-critique is the conscious process of a person acknowledging their own privileged positionality (e.g. race, age, class, ability, gender identity, sexuality, education, economic and professional statuses), recognising and challenging their own beliefs and assumptions (e.g. concerning which occupations 'ought' to be priorities), reflecting on the ways these assumptions derive from social structures and hegemonic discourses, and considering the potential impact of these culturally specific values on the provision of safe professional practices.

■ People belong and are interconnected within interdependent relationships and communities that shape, support and constrain the options they consider and the choices they have the opportunity to make (Yap & Yu, 2016). The Framework, therefore, advances a *relational* approach to individual and collective (Donchin, 2001; Entwistle & Watt, 2013; Hunt & Ells, 2011; Smith & Seward, 2009), and is amenable to informing work at community and population levels (Crawford, 2017).

THE OCCUPATION, CAPABILITY AND WELLBEING FRAMEWORK FOR OCCUPATIONAL THERAPY

A conceptual framework is a network of linked concepts produced through a process of qualitative analysis that provides a comprehensive understanding of a phenomenon and an empirical structure for subsequent research and practice (Jabareen, 2009). The process of building the *Occupation, Capability and*

Identification of "what matters": Wellbeing aspirations and unmet needs (i.e. desired outcomes)
What matters to this person or collective?

This *might* include consideration of, for example: surviving and thriving, belonging and connecting; self-worth; purpose, meaning, and pleasure through occupational engagement; having the opportunity to enact choice; hope.

How might wellbeing and engagement in living for this individual/family/group/community be enlarged through occupation?

Process of assessing capabilities, by appraising:

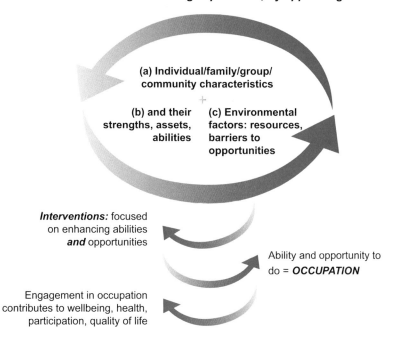

Level of occupational therapy outcome assessment

Appraising the achieved expansion of people's capabilities to achieve what matters most, their wellbeing aspirations, and self-identified needs.

Fig. 10.1 ■ Occupation, Capability and Wellbeing Framework for Occupational Therapy (OCWFOT) (Reproduced with permission from Hammell, K. W. (2020). An occupation, capability, and wellbeing framework for occupational therapy. In *Engagement in living: Critical perspectives on occupation, rights, and wellbeing* (p. 218). Ottawa, ON, CAOT Publications ACE).

Wellbeing Framework for Occupational Therapy comprised three phases:

1. An extensive review of multidisciplinary texts from the Global South and North addressing the phenomenon of interest;
2. Identification and naming of concepts; and
3. Synthesis of these concepts into a dynamic and flexible framework (Jabareen, 2009; Leamy et al.,

2011) and is fully described and supported in Hammell (2020).

Identification of 'What Matters'

A visual representation of the *Occupation, Capability, and Wellbeing Framework for Occupational Therapy* (OCWFOT) is provided in Fig. 10.1, in which the process of assessment begins, not with the detailed documentation of impairments, inabilities, performance deficits and dysfunctions, but with an appraisal of 'what matters most' to the individual or collective: the occupational outcomes desired following any occupational therapy intervention. This is the phase in which occupational therapists seek to understand what occupations individuals and collectives value, what motivates them in the occupational choices they aspire to make, within which relationships and in what places and spaces they wish to engage in these occupations, and how their wellbeing might be enhanced through participation in the occupations that matter to them. As Brown (2010) observed, 'asking what is important to the person inserts the person's values into the assessment situation, helping to set the direction of [interventions] and to avoid paths that are irrelevant to the service recipient's life' (p. S35).

As a guide for exploring 'what is important', reference is made in Fig. 10.1 to those contributors to wellbeing found to have cross-cultural and cross-developmental relevance (Hammell, 2020). This is not a comprehensive or mandatory list; rather, it is an *aide memoire*, a reminder of the scope and breadth of factors that individuals and collectives may find important. The inclusion of this 'list' is intended to suggest the range of possibilities and priorities that might be uncovered if occupational therapists refused to have their focus limited by diagnostic labels, normative judgements concerning how people 'ought' to live or what their priorities 'ought' to be, or by the categories of occupation that have traditionally dominated practice guidelines. The 'list' is a resource, not a prescription.

In striving to understand 'what matters' to people – what roles they most value, what forms of occupational engagement and participation they prioritise and with whom, and what unmet needs they wish most to address – occupational therapists will need to employ qualitative modes of inquiry, cultural humility, and a respectful approach to discerning the self-identified needs and wellbeing aspirations of service users, as individuals/collectives.

Process of Assessing Capabilities

Once the individual or collective and occupational therapists have identified desired outcomes, an assessment can be made of the elements that may contribute to transforming these needs and aspirations into an expansion of capabilities (refer to Chapter 13). If the occupational therapy profession is committed to a capabilities approach to practice, attention needs to be focused both on people's opportunities to engage in occupations 'that matter', as well as their abilities to engage in these occupations. This demands consideration of the personal characteristics of service users, for example, their ages, gender identities and impairments – as individuals or collectives: Who are these people? And in seeking to understand who these people are, occupational therapists will also appraise individual and collective capacities, capabilities, strengths, assets and resources: What abilities and resources support occupational engagement and participation?

For example, 'relational resources' derive from belonging to a social network (Gergen & Gergen, 2005), such that disabled people and those living in poverty may achieve higher levels of wellbeing and accomplish more of the occupations that matter to them if they are able to tap into the collective resources of their relationships and communities (Grech, 2011). Indeed, engagement in specific occupations may be valued, not for the ability to 'do' a specific occupation but for the opportunity to belong, contribute and connect with important others while occupationally engaged (Berger, 2011; Hancock et al., 2015; King et al., 2014). Researchers have demonstrated the possible interdependency of everyday occupations among couples; suggesting that the timing, balance, choice, and orchestration of occupations can be an interactive, co-occupational endeavour (Fallahpour et al., 2013, Van Nes et al., 2009). Collective capacities may be valuable resources for engagement in occupations that matter, yet the collective and relational dimensions of wellbeing (Yap & Yu, 2016), will be obscured and ignored if the profession's gaze remains focused on individuals.

The process of appraising people's strengths, assets and abilities therefore cannot focus solely on individuals' skills and knowledges but must encompass the assets and collective abilities derived from cultural traditions and lands, languages and material resources, and from belonging within networks of community support. And because people who have an illness, injury or impairment are connected and belong within families and broader collectives it is clearly inadequate (and can be demeaning) to focus on tallying the minutiae of ways in which their functions and abilities differ from social norms. Most occupational therapists will have worked with people whose financial resources and family support have enabled them to achieve high levels of occupational engagement and participation despite profound physical impairments; and others, with less significant physical impairments, whose occupational opportunities have been severely constrained by their marginal social statuses and dearth of resources and supports.

Occupational therapists treat what they have chosen to assess, so if the assessment process focuses primarily on individuals' deficits and dysfunctions, interventions are unlikely to focus on enhancing the person's wellbeing and occupational participation. The process of assessing capabilities therefore also needs to consider the barriers – inequitable structures and unfair constraints – and the facilitators that derive from people's histories and environmental contexts and that impact the possibilities for expansion of their choices, conversion of their opportunities into actions, actualisation of their values, and capabilities to engage in occupations that contribute to wellbeing.

Within Western occupational therapy scholarship, 'the environment' has been compartmentalised into four elements: social, cultural, physical and institutional (Townsend & Polatajko, 2013). Moreover, the environment is portrayed as something external to, and divisible from humanity, such that occupation is a 'bridge' connecting people and the environment (Townsend & Polatajko, 2013). This is a specific urban, minority world perception. Eastern modes of thought understand the individual and environment to be inseparable (Kupperman, 2001) such that people's skin is not what separates them *from* their environment, but what joins them *with* the environment (Watts, 1957). Indeed, the majority of the world's people perceive themselves to be seamlessly interrelated with nature, the cosmos, the air, land and oceans, and fundamentally interconnected with other people, including ancestors (e.g. Crichton-Hill et al., 2014; Mark & Lyons, 2010; Paluch et al., 2011; Sherry, 2010). To understand the indivisibility of people and environments – and the barriers and facilitators of occupational participation integral to this equation – demands an expanded vision of individuals' and collectives' situatedness within complex environments, and rejection of the

premise that occupations constitute a bridge between people and the world in which they are embedded.

The OCWFOT encourages consideration of service users' political, legal, policy and economic contexts; geopolitical contexts (e.g. territorial occupation); contexts of religious or spiritual traditions; ancestral and historical contexts (such as ongoing impacts of colonialism); the local context of safety and familiarity within home and community; the built environment; the local climate and impacts of climate change; and socially structured patterns of exclusion (e.g. racism, ableism, disablism, patriarchy, sexism, misogyny, heteronormativity, gender binarism, ageism) that lead to stigma, discrimination, inequitable access to employment, education, transportation, information, technology and other resources and opportunities. As an example, for many First Nations people, access to their land is a source of spiritual strength and a place where they can connect with ancestors, and engage in traditional cultural and collective occupations that contribute immeasurably to their wellbeing (Durkalec et al., 2015; MacDonald et al., 2015; McCubbin et al., 2013). Although specific lands and places may be valuable resources for engagement and participation in occupations 'that matter', access to these special places may be prohibited by colonial policies and practices.

Occupational therapists will need to develop and employ forms of assessment amenable to evaluating the relevant material and nonmaterial circumstances shaping people's lives, and the contextual factors that influence the occupational choices people can envision and realistically make (Hammell, 2020). Only then can appropriate intervention plans be formulated.

Interventions

Interventions will be co-designed by people and occupational therapists to enhance individual and collective abilities *and* opportunities to engage in occupations that 'matter'. Although occupational therapists and service users may draw from their combined knowledge of the idiosyncrasies of specific impairments, dysfunctions, and prognoses, interventions will not be impairment-specific. Informed by an understanding of the wellbeing aspirations and unmet needs (i.e. the desired outcomes) that have been identified through a conscious process of active and engaged listening, a critical awareness of power, privilege and positioning, a commitment to cultural humility, an attitude of kindness, caring, and respect for individuals and collectives' abilities, knowledge, experience and strengths, and their moral right to make choices concerning their lives (Hammell, 2013b), the occupational therapist and individuals and collectives will have co-created an assessment of available resources, structural barriers and constraints to achieving wellbeing through occupation (Hammell, 2013b). This provides the foundation for interventions that will focus both on enhancing the abilities of individuals and collectives, and on enhancing their real opportunities to use and expand their abilities and attain their occupational rights. This is not a linear process – thus there are no straight lines implying causality within the OCWFOT (Fig. 10.1). Together, service users and occupational therapists will continually re-evaluate what needs to change to accomplish the things that matter most; identifying new barriers, resources and required skills.

Assessment of Outcomes

The effectiveness of occupational therapy interventions cannot be gauged by simplistic measures, such as whether the range of motion of a joint has increased, whether self-care independence has been achieved, or whether wheelchair transfers have been mastered because these do not provide any insight into whether people's wellbeing or participation have increased (Hammell, 2020). It has long been recognised by occupational therapists that while some functionally independent people (e.g. with spinal cord injury) enjoy meaningful, socially active and fulfilling lives, others with similar impairments do not. This highlights the irrelevance of outcome measures focused on the attainment of physical skills that convey no information about the impact of interventions on people's lives. Moreover, because the notion that functional ability correlates positively with perceptions of high life satisfaction is contested by research evidence (Hammell, 2004; Pershouse et al., 2012; Savic et al., 2010), it is surely apparent that the outcome of occupational therapy interventions ought to be appraised through examination of 'the achieved expansion of people's capabilities to achieve their wellbeing aspirations and realise their unmet wellbeing needs through engagement in occupations that matter' (Hammell, 2020, p. 215).

The *Occupation, Capability, and Wellbeing Framework for Occupational Therapy* provides a basis for the development of measures of wellbeing. Although wellbeing is purported to be of central importance to occupational therapy, few efforts have been made to develop measures amenable to assessing people's wellbeing. The OCWFOT provides an incentive to develop measures that can identify dimensions of wellbeing that matter to individuals and collectives; measures that can assess strengths, assets, abilities, and resources in tandem with environmental barriers and resources (Hammell, 2020); and measures that can appraise the achieved expansion of people's capabilities 'to participate in valued occupations within meaningful relationships and contexts' (Egan & Restall, 2022, p. 5).

FEASIBILITY

Occupational therapy is situated within a hegemonic neoliberal political environment that advances specific modes of governance, such that the profession demonstrates an adherence to 'standardised' assessments, an allegiance to quantitative outcome measurement (Kristensen et al., 2017), and a commitment to modifying individuals (Aldrich & Rudman, 2020; Hammell, 2023; Hayes et al., 2023). McColl (2021) recently noted that within Western occupational therapy, 'Occupational performance problems are mostly viewed as personal and family issues, to be addressed on an individual basis' (p. 5), and that, 'Despite increased attention in recent years to the role of the environment in occupational therapy, the emphasis is still on understanding the components of the individual responsible for occupational problems, and where possible, remediating those; or where not possible, compensating or re-framing' (p. 5). By viewing occupational problems as individual issues, and by locating these problems in individuals' 'components' occupational therapy colludes in advancing neoliberalism's aim of inducing individuals to 'overcome' their impairments (Hammell, 2020), thereby obscuring the socio-political roots of inequities (Farias & Rudman, 2019). This prompts consideration of the feasibility of the OCWFOT for occupational therapists employed within neoliberal institutions preoccupied with economics, managerialism, and the modification of individuals, and not with the advancement of human wellbeing.

Few rehabilitation researchers have chosen to explore the adverse effects of rehabilitation (Wade, 2009). However, evidence from those who have indicated that considerable resources and time are wasted when rehabilitation professionals strive to induce individuals to achieve goals they do not value (Brown, 2010; Fischer et al., 1999; Towle & Godolphin, 1999). This suggests that working collaboratively towards goals that 'matter' for individuals is likely to be both a more accountable and efficient use of time and resources, in addition to being a more ethical approach to practice.

But more importantly, occupational therapy cannot silently uphold institutional practices that perpetuate inequities and injustices. Clearly, when occupational therapists strive to resist or transform elements of the structural environment that perpetuate unfairness and injustice, this is a political act. But it is important to understand that when occupational therapists choose to remain silent – complying with practices that support an ableist, neoliberal agenda – this is also a political act (Hammell, 2006).

Aldrich and Rudman (2020, p. 138) noted that 'Globally, occupational therapy scholars and practitioners are acknowledging the need to recognise, navigate, and transform the power relations through which they work'. This may require occupational therapy practitioners to contest organisational protocols that clash with their own professional values in seeking to provide the services appropriate to users' needs. This, in turn, requires the profession's associations to support and defend their members for actions taken to identify and address 'the capabilities, opportunities, and freedom of choice for individuals, communities and populations to participate in society' (WFOT, 2019), as *required* by our World Federation.

CONCLUSION

The factors motivating the development of the *Occupational, Capability and Wellbeing Framework for Occupational Therapy* (Hammell, 2020) have been outlined in this chapter. This conceptual framework focuses explicitly on assessing and enhancing abilities rather than on documenting deficits and on 'normalising' functions. The OCWFOT deliberately considers structural and other environmental factors that enable or constrain the availability of occupational

opportunities, capabilities, and the realisation of wellbeing. The Framework encourages consideration both of the collective nature of occupational engagement and participation and of the contextual nature of occupational engagement. Moreover, the Framework, which helps to foreground and organise existing knowledge, 'is theoretically defensible, provides conceptual clarity and may be used as a resource and structure around which future research, practice and outcome strategies may be oriented' (Hammell, 2020, p. 214). Importantly, it provides the flexibility necessary for application in a diversity of global contexts and contributes to focusing occupational therapy practices on 'helping people to participate in valued occupations within meaningful relationships and contexts' (Egan & Restall, 2022, p. 5).

REFERENCES

Al Busaidy, N. S. M., & Borthwick, A. (2012). Occupational therapy in Oman: The impact of cultural dissonance. *Occupational Therapy International, 19*, 154–164.

Aldrich, R. M., & Rudman, D. L. (2020). Occupational therapists as street-level bureaucrats: Leveraging the political nature of everyday practice. *Canadian Journal of Occupational Therapy, 87*(2), 137–143.

Beagan, B. L. (2015). Approaches to culture and diversity: A critical synthesis of occupational therapy literature. *Canadian Journal of Occupational Therapy, 82*, 272–282.

Berger, S. (2011). The meaning of leisure for older adults living with vision loss. *OTJR: Occupation, Participation and Health, 31*, 193–199.

Brooke, K. E., Desmarais, C. D., & Forwell, S. J. (2007). Types and categories of personal projects: A revelatory means of understanding human occupation. *Occupational Therapy International, 14*, 281–296.

Brown, M. (2010). Participation: The insider's perspective. *Archives of Physical Medicine and Rehabilitation, 91*, S34–S37.

Bryant, J., Bolt, R., Botfield, J. R., Martin, K., Doyle, M., Murphy, D., Graham, S., Newman, C. E., Bell, S., Treloar, C., Browne, A. J., & Aggleton, P. (2021). Beyond deficit: 'Strengths-based approaches' in Indigenous health research. *Sociology of Health and Illness, 43*, 1405–1421.

Burgin, E. R. (2014). Liberation health and LGBT communities. In D. B. Martinez, & A. Fleck-Henderson (Eds.), *Social justice in clinical practice: A liberation health framework for social work* (pp. 44–57). Routledge.

Campbell, F. A. K. (2008). Exploring internalized ableism using critical race theory. *Disability and Society, 23*(2), 151–162.

Crawford, E. (2017). Continuing the dialogue: A rights-approach in occupational therapy. *Australian Occupational Therapy Journal, 64*, 505–509.

Crichton-Hill, Y., McCall, T., & Togiaso, G. (2014). Pacific health. In L. Beddoe, & J. Maidment (Eds.), *Social work practice for promoting health and wellbeing: Critical issues* (pp. 122–132). Routledge.

Crocker, D. A., & Robeyns, I. (2010). Capability and agency. In C. Morris (Ed.), *Amartya Sen* (pp. 60–90). Cambridge University Press.

Donchin, A. (2001). Understanding autonomy relationally: Toward a reconfiguration of bioethical principles. *Journal of Medical Philosophy, 26,* 365–386.

Durkalec, A., Furgal, C., Skinner, M. W., & Sheldon, T. (2015). Climate change influences on environment as a determinant of Indigenous health: Relationships to place, sea ice, and health in an Inuit community. *Social Science and Medicine, 136-137,* 17–26.

Egan, M., & Restall, G. (Eds.) (2022). *Promoting occupational participation: Collaborative relationship-focused occupational therapy.* CAOT.

Emery-Whittington, I. (2021). Occupational justice – Colonial business as usual? Indigenous observations from Aotearoa New Zealand. *Canadian Journal of Occupational Therapy, 88*(2), 153–162.

Entwistle, V. A., & Watt, I. S. (2013). Treating patients as persons: A capabilities approach to support delivery of person-centred care. *American Journal of Bioethics, 13*(8), 29–39.

Fadyl, J. K., Teachman, G., & Hamdani, Y. (2020). Problematizing 'productive citizenship' within rehabilitation services: Insights from three studies. *Disability and Rehabilitation, 42*(20), 2959–2966.

Fallahpour, M., Jonsson, H., Joghataei, M. T., Nasrabadi, A. N., & Tham, K. (2013). 'I am not living my life': Lived experience of participation in everyday occupations after stroke in Tehran. *Journal of Rehabilitation Medicine, 45,* 528–534.

Farias, L., & Rudman, D. L. (2019). Challenges in enacting occupation-based social transformative practices: A critical dialogical study. *Canadian Journal of Occupational Therapy, 86*(3), 243–252.

Feagin, J., & Bennefield, Z. (2014). Systemic racism and U.S. health care. *Social Science and Medicine, 103,* 7–14.

Finger, A. (1995). 'Welfare reform' and us. *Ragged Edge.* Nov/Dec:15&36.

Fischer, D., Stewart, A., Bloch, D., Lorig, K., Laurent, D., & Holman, H. (1999). Capturing the patient's view of change as a clinical outcome measure. *Journal of the American Medical Association, 282,* 1157–1162.

Fisher-Borne, M., Cain, J. M., & Martin, S. L. (2015). From mastery to accountability: Cultural humility as an alternative to cultural competence. *Social Work Education, 34,* 165–181.

Galheigo, S. M. (2011). What needs to be done? Occupational therapy responsibilities and challenges regarding human rights. *Australian Occupational Therapy Journal, 58,* 60–66.

Gappmayer, G. (2021). Disentangling disablism and ableism: The social norm of being able and its influence on social interactions with people with intellectual disabilities. *Journal of Occupational Science, 28*(1), 102–113.

Gergen, M. M., & Gergen, K. J. (2005). Positive aging: Reconstructing the life course. In J. Worell, & C. Goodheart (Eds.), *Handbook of girls' and women's psychological health: Gender and well-being across the life span* (pp. 416–424). Oxford University Press.

Gerlach, A. J. (2015). Sharpening our critical edge: Occupational therapy in the context of marginalized populations. *Canadian Journal of Occupational Therapy, 82,* 245–253.

Gerlach, A. J., Teachman, G., Laliberte-Rudman, D., Aldrich, R. M., & Huot, S. (2018). Expanding beyond individualism: Engaging critical perspectives on occupation. *Scandinavian Journal of Occupational Therapy, 25*(1), 35–43.

Gibson, B. E., & Teachman, G. (2012). Critical approaches in physical therapy research: Investigating the symbolic value of walking. *Physiotherapy Theory and Practice, 28*(6), 474–484.

Gibson, C. (2020). When the river runs dry: Leadership, decolonisation and healing in occupational therapy. *New Zealand Journal of Occupational Therapy, 67,* 11–20.

Grech, S. (2011). Recolonising debates or perpetuated coloniality? Decentring the spaces of disability, development and community in the global South. *International Journal of Inclusive Education, 15,* 87–100.

Grenier, M.-L. (2020). Cultural competency and the reproduction of White supremacy in occupational therapy education. *Health Education Journal, 79*(6), 633–644.

Grenier, M.-L. (2021). Patient case formulations and oppressive disability discourses in occupational therapy education. *Canadian Journal of Occupational Therapy, 88*(3), 226–272.

Hammell, K. W. (2004). Exploring quality of life following high spinal cord injury: A review and critique. *Spinal Cord, 42,* 491–502.

Hammell, K. W. (2006). *Perspectives on disability and rehabilitation: Contesting assumptions; Challenging practice.* Churchill Livingstone Elsevier.

Hammell, K. W. (2008). Reflections on…well-being and occupational rights. *Canadian Journal of Occupational Therapy, 75,* 61–64.

Hammell, K. W. (2009a). Sacred texts: A sceptical exploration of the assumptions underpinning theories of occupation. *Canadian Journal of Occupational Therapy, 76,* 6–13.

Hammell, K. W. (2009b). Self-care, productivity and leisure, or dimensions of occupational experience? Rethinking occupational 'categories'. *Canadian Journal of Occupational Therapy, 76,* 107–114.

Hammell, K. W. (2011). Resisting theoretical imperialism in the disciplines of occupational science and occupational therapy. *British Journal of Occupational Therapy, 74*(1), 27–33.

Hammell, K. W. (2013a). Occupation, well-being and culture: Theory and cultural humility. *Canadian Journal of Occupational Therapy, 80,* 224–234.

Hammell, K. W. (2013b). Client-centred occupational therapy in Canada: Refocusing on core values. *Canadian Journal of Occupational Therapy, 80*(3), 141–149.

Hammell, K. W. (2015). Respecting global wisdom: Enhancing the cultural relevance of occupational therapy's theoretical base. *British Journal of Occupational Therapy, 78*(11), 718–721.

Hammell, K. W. (2019). Building globally relevant occupational therapy from the strength of our diversity. *World Federation of Occupational Therapists' Bulletin, 75,* 13–26.

Hammell, K. W. (2020). *Engagement in living: Critical perspectives on occupation, rights and wellbeing.* Ottawa, ON, CAOT Publications ACE.

Hammell, K. W. (2021). Social and structural determinants of health: Exploring occupational therapy's structural (in)competence. *Canadian Journal of Occupational Therapy, 88*(4), 365–374.

Hammell, K. W. (2022). Securing occupational rights by addressing capabilities: A professional obligation. *Scandinavian Journal of Occupational Therapy, 29*(1), 1–12.

Hammell, K. W. (2023). A call to resist occupational therapy's promotion of ableism. *Scandinavian Journal of Occupational Therapy, 30*(6), 745–757.

Hammell, K. W., & Beagan, B. (2017). Occupational injustice: A critique. *Canadian Journal of Occupational Therapy, 84*, 58–68.

Hammell, K. W., & Iwama, M. K. (2012). Well-being and occupational rights: An imperative for critical occupational therapy. *Scandinavian Journal of Occupational Therapy, 19*, 385–394.

Hancock, N., Honey, A., & Bundy, A. C. (2015). Sources of meaning derived from occupational engagement for people recovering from mental illness. *British Journal of Occupational Therapy, 78*, 508–515.

Harris, S. P., Owen, R., & Gould, R. (2012). Parity of participation in liberal welfare states: Human rights, neoliberalism, disability and employment. *Disability and Society, 27*, 823–836.

Hayes, K., Santos, V. D., Costigan, M., & Morante, D. (2023). Extension, austerity, and emergence: Themes identified from a global scoping review of non-urban occupational therapy services. *Australian Occupational Therapy Journal, 70*, 142–156.

Hocking, C. (2012). Occupations through the looking glass: Reflecting on occupational scientists' ontological assumptions. In G. E. Whiteford, & C. Hocking (Eds.), *Occupational science: Society, inclusion, participation* (pp. 54–66). Wiley Blackwell.

Hunt, M. R., & Ells, C. (2011). Partners towards autonomy: Risky choices and relational autonomy in rehabilitation care. *Disability and Rehabilitation, 33*, 961–967.

Iwama, M. (2003). Toward culturally relevant epistemologies in occupational therapy. *American Journal of Occupational Therapy, 57*(5), 582–588.

Iwama, M. K. (2006). *The Kawa model: Culturally relevant occupational therapy.* Churchill Livingstone Elsevier.

Iwasaki, Y., Nishino, H., Onda, T., & Bowling, C. (2007). Leisure research in a global world: Time to reverse the Western domination in leisure research? *Leisure Sciences, 29*, 113–117.

Jabareen, Y. (2009). Building a conceptual framework: Philosophy, definitions and procedure. *International Journal of Qualitative Methods, 8*, 49–62.

Jonsson, H. (2008). A new direction in the conceptualization and categorization of occupation. *Journal of Occupational Science, 15*, 3–8.

Kelly, J. R., & Kelly, J. R. (1994). Multiple dimensions of meaning in the domains of work, family and leisure. *Journal of Leisure Research, 26*, 250–274.

King, G., Gibson, B. E., Mistry, B., Pinto, M., Goh, F., Teachman, G., & Thompson, L. (2014). An integrated methods study of the experiences of youth with severe disabilities in leisure activity settings: The importance of belonging, fun, and choice and control. *Disability and Rehabilitation, 36*, 1626–1635.

Kristensen, H. K., Præstegaard, J., & Ytterberg, C. (2017). Discourses in stroke rehabilitation as they present themselves in current physiotherapy and occupational therapy. *Disability and Rehabilitation, 39*, 223–235.

Kupperman, J. J. (2001). *Classic Asian philosophy.* Oxford University Press.

Leamy, M., Bird, V., Le Boutillier, C., Williams, J., & Slade, M. (2011). Conceptual framework for personal recovery in mental health: Systematic review and narrative synthesis. *The British Journal of Psychiatry, 199*, 445–452.

Lim, K. H., & Duque, R. L. (2011). The challenge for occupational therapy in Asia becoming an inclusive, relevant, and progressive profession. In F. Kronenberg, N. Pollard, & D. Sakellariou (Eds.), *Occupational therapies without borders (Vol. 2). Towards an ecology of occupation-based practices* (pp. 103–112). Churchill Livingstone Elsevier.

MacDonald, J. P., Willox, A. C., Ford, J. D., Shiwak, I., Wood, M., IMHACC Team, & Rigolet Inuit Community Government. (2015). Protective factors for mental health and well-being in a changing climate: Perspectives from Inuit youth in Nunatsiavut, Labrador. *Social Science and Medicine, 141*, 133–141.

Magalhães, L., Farias, L., Rivas-Quarneti, N., Alvarez, L., & Malfitano, A. P. S. (2019). The development of occupational science outside the Anglophone sphere: Enacting global collaboration. *Journal of Occupational Science, 26*, 181–192.

Malfitano, A. P. S. (2022). An anthropophagic proposition in occupational therapy knowledge: Driving our actions towards social life. *World Federation of Occupational Therapists' Bulletin. 78*(2), 70–82. https://doi.org/10.1080/14473828.2022.2135065.

Malfitano, A. P. S., & Lopes, R. E. (2018). Social occupational therapy: Committing to social change. *New Zealand Journal of Occupational Therapy, 65*(1), 20–26.

Mark, G. T., & Lyons, A. C. (2010). Maori healers' views on wellbeing: The importance of mind, body, spirit, family and land. *Social Science and Medicine, 70*, 1756–1764.

Martín, I. Z., Martos, J. A. F., Millares, P. M., & Björklund, A. (2015). Occupational therapy culture seen through the multifocal lens of fieldwork in diverse rural areas. *Scandinavian Journal of Occupational Therapy, 22*, 82–94.

McColl, M. A. (2021). What can occupational therapy & disability studies contribute to one another? *Canadian Journal of Occupational Therapy, 88*(1), 4–11.

McCubbin, L. D., McCubbin, H. I., Zhang, W., Lisa, K., & Strom, I. (2013). Relational well-being: An indigenous perspective and measure. *Family Relations, 62*, 354–365.

Metzl, J. M., & Hansen, H. (2014). Structural competency: Theorizing a new medical engagement with stigma and inequality. *Social Science and Medicine, 103*, 126–133.

Mitra, S. (2006). The capability approach and disability. *Journal of Disability Policy Studies, 16*, 236–247.

Motimele, M., & Peters, L. (2017). Understanding human occupation. In S. A. Dsousa, R. Galvaan, & E. L. Ramugondo (Eds.), *Concepts in occupational therapy. Understanding Southern perspectives* (pp. 1–15). Manipal University Press.

Nilsson, I., & Townsend, E. (2010). Occupational justice – Bridging theory and practice. *Scandinavian Journal of Occupational Therapy, 17*, 57–63.

Paluch, T., Allen, R., McIntosh, K., & Oke, L. (2011). Koori occupational therapy scheme: Contributing to first Australian health through professional reflection, advocacy and action. *Australian Occupational Therapy Journal, 58*, 50–53.

Pershouse, K. J., Barker, R. N., Kendall, M. B., Buettner, P. G., Kuipers, P., Schuurs, S. B., & Amsters, D. I. (2012). Investigating changes in quality of life and function along the lifespan for people with spinal cord injury. *Archives of Physical Medicine and Rehabilitation, 93*(3), 413–419.

Pfeiffer, D. (1999). The categorisation and control of people with disabilities. *Disability and Society, 21*(3), 106–107.

Phelan, S. K. (2011). Constructions of disability: A call for critical reflexivity in occupational therapy. *Canadian Journal of Occupational Therapy, 78*(3), 164–172.

Phelan, S. K., Wright, V., & Gibson, B. E. (2014). Representations of disability and normality in rehabilitation technology promotional materials. *Disability and Rehabilitation, 36*, 2072–2079.

Phipps, E., & Masuda, J. R. (2018). Towards equity-focused intersectoral practice (EquIP) in children's environmental health and housing: The transformational story of RentSafe. *Canadian Journal of Public Health, 109*, 379–385.

Quesada, J., Hart, L. K., & Bourgois, P. (2011). Structural vulnerability and health: Latino migrant laborers in the United States. *Medical Anthropology, 30*(4), 339–362.

Ramugondo, E. (2018). Healing work: Intersections for decoloniality. *World Federation of Occupational Therapists' Bulletin, 74*, 83–91.

Reindal, S. M. (1999). Independence, dependence, interdependence: Some reflections on the subject and personal autonomy. *Disability and Society, 14*, 353–367.

Restall, G., Egan, M., Valavaara, K., Phenix, A., & Sack, C. (2022). Canadian occupational therapy inter-relational practice framework. In M. Egan, & G. Restall (Eds.), *Promoting occupational participation: Collaborative relationship-focused occupational therapy* (pp. 119–150). CAOT.

Robeyns, I. (2005). The capability approach: A theoretical survey. *Journal of Human Development, 6*, 93–114.

Rudman, D. L. (2010). Occupational terminology – Occupational possibilities. *Journal of Occupational Science, 17*(1), 55–59.

Rudman, D. L. (2013). Enacting the critical potential of occupational science: Problematizing the 'individualizing of occupation'. *Journal of Occupational Science, 20*(4), 298–313.

Sandahl, C. (2003). Queering the crip or cripping the queer? In R. McRuer, & A. L. Wilkerson (Eds.), *Desiring disability: Queer theory meets disability studies* (pp. 25–56). Duke University Press.

Savic, G., Charlifue, S., Glass, C., Soni, B. M., Gerhart, K. A., & Ali Jamous, M. (2010). British ageing with SCI study: Changes in physical and psychological outcomes over time. *Topics in Spinal Cord Injury Rehabilitation, 15*(1), 41–53.

Sen, A. (1999). *Development as freedom*. Oxford University Press.

Sen, A. (2003). Development as capability expansion. In S. Fukuda-Parr, & A. K. S. Kumar (Eds.), *Readings in human development* (pp. 41–58). Oxford University Press.

Sen, A. (2005). Human rights and capabilities. *Journal of Human Development, 6*, 151–166.

Sherry, K. (2010). Culture and cultural competence for occupational therapists. In V. Alers, & R. Crouch (Eds.), *Occupational therapy: An African perspective* (pp. 60–77). Sarah Shorten.

Smith, M. L., & Seward, C. (2009). The relational ontology of Amartya Sen's capability approach: Incorporating social and individual causes. *Journal of Human Development and Capabilities, 10*, 213–235.

Stack, J. A. C., & Iwasaki, Y. (2009). The role of leisure pursuits in adaptation processes among Afghan refugees who have immigrated to Winnipeg, Canada. *Leisure Studies, 28*, 239–259.

Tervalon, M., & Murray-Garcia, J. (1998). Cultural humility versus cultural competence: A critical distinction in defining physician training outcomes in multicultural education. *Journal of Health Care for the Poor and Underserved, 9*(2), 117–125.

Terzi, L. (2005). Beyond the dilemma of difference: The capability approach to disability and special educational needs. *Journal of Philosophy of Education, 39*, 443–459.

Terzi, L. (2011). Vagaries of the natural lottery? Human diversity, disability, and justice: A capability perspective. In K. Brownlee, & A. Cureton (Eds.), *Disability and disadvantage* (pp. 86–111). Oxford University Press.

Towle, A., & Godolphin, W. (1999). Framework for teaching and learning informed shared decision making. *British Medical Journal, 319*, 766–769.

Townsend, E. A., & Polatajko, H. (2013). *Enabling occupation II: Advancing an occupational therapy vision for health, well-being & justice through occupation* (2nd ed.). CAOT Publications ACE.

Townsend, E., & Wilcock, A. (2004). Occupational justice and client-centred practice: A dialogue in progress. *Canadian Journal of Occupational Therapy, 71*, 75–87.

Van Nes, F., Runge, U., & Jonsson, H. (2009). One body, three hands and two minds: A case study of the intertwined occupations of an older couple after a stroke. *Journal of Occupational Science, 16*, 194–202.

Wade, D. (2009). Adverse effects of rehabilitation – An opportunity to increase quality and effectiveness of rehabilitation. *Clinical Rehabilitation, 23*, 387–393.

Watts, A. W. (1957). *The way of Zen*. Random House.

World Federation of Occupational Therapists. (2019). *Position statement: Occupational therapy and human rights (revised)*. World Federation of Occupational Therapists. www.wfot.org.

Yap, M., & Yu, E. (2016). Operationalising the capability approach: Developing culturally relevant indicators of Indigenous wellbeing – An Australian example. *Oxford Development Studies, 44*(3), 315–331.

REFLECTION

1. Explain why the occupational therapy profession require a practice framework centred on the enhancement of wellbeing through occupation.

2. Provides reasons why the occupational therapy profession should avoid a neoliberal agenda that promotes self-care, productivity, independence, individualism, and erasure of functional differences.

3. Review and critique each of the principles underpinning the *Occupation, Capability and Wellbeing Framework for Occupational Therapy*.

4. Describe the *Occupation, Capability and Wellbeing Framework for Occupational Therapy*.

11

THE CANADIAN MODEL OF OCCUPATIONAL PARTICIPATION (CanMOP)

MARY EGAN ■ GAYLE RESTALL

CHAPTER OUTLINE

Overview

The Canadian Model of Occupational Participation (CanMOP) is the most recent evolution of the occupation models endorsed by the Canadian Association of Occupational Therapists. The CanMOP centres occupational participation as the essential focus of occupational therapy with individuals and collectives. Occupational participation is defined as having access to and initiating and sustaining valued occupations within meaningful relationships and contexts. The CanMOP supports collaborative exploration of the meaning and purpose of the valued occupations of individuals and collectives. Occupational therapists explore the meaning and purpose of specific occupations by considering how the individual's or collective's needs are met by the occupation as influenced by their history and relationships, and their micro, mesa and macro contexts. The CanMOP recognises the influence of micro, meso and macro contexts on occupational possibilities and supports collaborative change to create the best conditions for expanding possibilities for accessing, initiating and sustaining valued occupations.

KEY POINTS

- The Canadian Model of Occupational Participation (CanMOP) identifies the focus of occupational therapy as promoting occupational participation with individuals or collectives.

- Occupational participation is defined as having access to, initiating and sustaining valued occupations within meaningful relationships and contexts.

- The purpose of an occupation for an individual or collective is considered according to the needs they are attempting to meet; the meaning of an occupation is explored through a life course or community history lens and considering associated relationships.

- The micro, meso and macro contexts expand or limit occupational possibilities by affecting access to, and initiation and sustaining of, valued occupations.

- Collaborative relationship-focused occupational therapy is the approach used in promoting occupational participation.

- The CanMOP is the latest in a series of models of occupation developed with or for the Canadian Association of Occupational Therapists.

INTRODUCTION

Occupational therapists use models to think about how individuals and collectives do valued occupations within meaningful contexts. These models help occupational therapists determine where to focus their attention when they are learning about the occupations of an individual or a collective. The models foster the collaborative development of plans that promote participation in valued occupations in meaningful contexts.

Occupational therapy models are made up of concepts and relationships between these concepts. They also include explicit and implicit ideas about people, occupations, and how people come to do the things they do. Occupational therapists refer to these concepts and relationships as they speak about what occupational therapy can contribute to health, social care and community development. These important discussions are carried out with individuals and collectives receiving occupational therapy. They are also carried out among occupational therapists and with interprofessional colleagues, administrators, funders, community groups and others.

Occupational therapy models evolve over time based on practice experience, research into various aspects of the model, advances in knowledge in areas related to occupational therapy and the perspectives of people who receive occupational therapy services. The Canadian Model of Occupational Participation, or CanMOP, is the current version of the model of occupation endorsed by the Canadian Association of Occupational Therapists (Fig. 11.1).

The CanMOP explicitly recognises the primary goal of occupational therapy as *promoting occupational participation among individuals and collectives.* Collectives include families, groups, communities and populations. Occupational participation is at the centre of the model because it is the primary focus of the work of occupational therapists. Occupational participation is defined as 'having access to, initiating, and sustaining valued occupations within meaningful relationships and contexts' (Egan & Restall, 2022, p. 75).

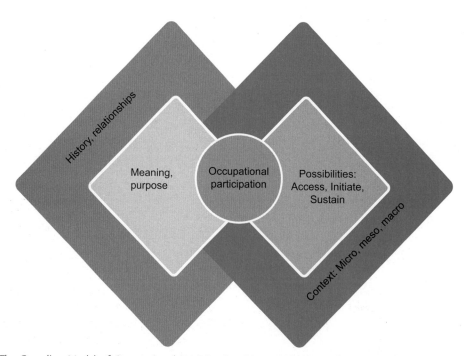

Fig. 11.1 ■ The Canadian Model of Occupational Participation (CanMOP). (Reproduced with permission from M. Egan & G. Restall (Eds.). (2022). The Canadian model of occupational participation (CanMOP). In *Promoting occupational participation: Collaborative relationship-focused occupational therapy* (p. 77). Canadian Association of Occupational Therapists).

On either side of occupational participation are two sets of overlapping major conceptual elements. On the left-hand side are conceptual elements that help occupational therapists work collaboratively with an individual or collective to understand *their valued occupations within meaningful relationships and contexts.* The key underlying assumption is that understanding the how, where, what, with whom and why of individual and collective occupations is essential when occupational therapists work with people to help them build or rebuild satisfying occupational lives. On the right-hand side are major conceptual elements that help occupational therapists work collaboratively with an individual or collective to understand and improve *access to* and expand possibilities for *initiating and sustaining valued occupations within meaningful relationships and contexts.* The key underlying assumption is that access to, initiation of and sustained occupational participation are affected by multilayered micro, meso and macro contexts. These major conceptual elements associated with the CanMOP are described below.

UNDERSTANDING VALUED OCCUPATIONS WITHIN MEANINGFUL RELATIONSHIPS AND CONTEXTS

Meaning and Purpose, History and Relationships

To better understand the valued occupations of individuals or collectives, occupational therapists collaboratively explore the meaning and purpose of these occupations for them. Purpose relates to what the individual or collective is hoping to achieve by doing the occupation. Purpose is intimately connected with meeting essential human needs. These needs include promoting survival and safety (Maslow, 1967; Rasskazova et al., 2016), as well as connection, autonomy and competency (Ryan & Deci, 2019). For example, an individual wishing to return to work following an injury or illness may be hoping to earn enough money for food and housing, accrue additional years required to obtain a pension, spend time with people outside the home, resume work on a highly valued project, or some combination of these or other goals or priorities. A neighbourhood developing a community garden may be hoping to increase sources of food for community

members experiencing food insecurity, teach skills to underemployed young people, create opportunities for neighbours to get to know each other or several other possible objectives. Occupational therapists collaboratively explore the purpose of the occupation with the individual or collective. This helps occupational therapists avoid making assumptions about the purpose of the occupation based on their personal experiences, values or beliefs.

The meaning of participating in an occupation also needs to be considered along with the purpose of the occupation, to fully understand what the occupation looks like when it is done in a context that is significant to the individual or collective. The meaning of doing the occupation is influenced by the individual's or collective's history and relationships. Within CanMOP, for individuals, history is considered using a life course framework (Elder, 1994). Rather than simply referring to normative life stages, life course considers historical events and unique life circumstances that have influenced the purpose and meaning of valued occupations for the individual. For example, the meaning of higher education for young people who experienced long periods of their high school education virtually, separated from peers due to the COVID-19 pandemic, may be very different from the meaning for people who completed high school in person before this period.

The meaning of valued occupations is also shaped by past, present and future hoped-for relationships. Among individuals, occupations are rarely done alone; and, even when they are, how a person came to do these things typically starts within relationships to other people, as well as to animals and the natural world. For example, certain aspects of food preparation essential to an individual or group may come from family traditions, cultural norms, or religious observances. These aspects came to be important in the context of relationships with family and community as well as relationships with the land. When these relationships and the meanings they bring are not considered, food preparation occupations become less relevant to the individual or collective. Additionally, the meaning of valued individual or collective occupations may require consideration of hoped-for relationships. For example, an individual may wish to make a friend or find a partner; a family or community may wish to develop ties with neighbours or ancestors. That is to be valued, the occupation may need to include others with whom the individual or collective is hoping to develop or deepen a relationship.

Expanding Occupational Possibilities Through Work At the Appropriate Context Level

The right side of the model helps the occupational therapist consider micro, meso and macro levels of context to collaboratively explore with the individual or collective how aspects of each context interact with characteristics of the individual or collective to promote or limit occupational possibilities. This becomes a catalyst for the occupational therapist and the individual or collective to collaboratively explore and expand occupational possibilities. The CanMOP highlights three aspects of occupational participation that are essential to consider:

1. Access to participation in the occupation;
2. Initiation of the occupation; and
3. Sustained participation in the occupation.

Access to Participation in the Occupation

Access to participation in occupations is often considered to be related to individual problems rather than contextual factors. However, occupational therapists have long been aware that not all people have the same level of access to valued occupations within meaningful relationships and contexts. Taking their cue from disability rights advocates, occupational therapists have often led the way in pointing out that such broad access issues are questions of justice. Occupational therapists have identified where implicit and explicit institutional policies (meso context) restrict occupational participation for many individuals and collectives (Bailliard et al., 2020; Townsend, 1993). They also point out how societal attitudes (macro context) have created and sustained such policies (Kirsh et al., 2012). Addressing these meso and macro contextual barriers to access to occupations must be addressed collectively to adequately deal with structural and systemic barriers to occupational participation.

Using the CanMOP, occupational therapists remain attentive to issues of access to valued occupations among individuals and collectives. For example, access to sports occupations can be restricted among

adolescents who experience racism (Box 11.1). Limited access may be related to overt restrictions to spaces or activities but may also be related to the unwelcoming nature of teams or leagues known for racist attitudes or behaviour (Baker-Lewton et al., 2017). These types

---

BOX 11.1

IMPACT OF RACISM ON ACCESS TO RECREATION AND LEISURE IN A CANADIAN TOWN

Meso and macro context issues often lead to a lack of access to valued occupations, particularly for racialised individuals. In August 2017, five racialised boys were involved in a fight at a community centre in a small town in Ontario, Canada. The fight was quickly broken up, and there were no injuries, but the police were called in. The administration of the community centre banned the youths from entering the centre for at least a year. Further, on the advice of the police, the youths were also banned from the public library. This ban far exceeded any sanction experienced by nonracialised youths, even those who had been in repeated fights. The boys essentially lost their access to a valued basketball program, other leisure programs and library services.

Parents of the youths filed a complaint with the Ontario Human Rights Tribunal. The case was investigated, and the ruling revealed discriminatory behaviour on the part of the community centre staff. Interviews with the boys, their parents and additional racialised community members revealed a pattern of racist behaviour among community centre staff members that typically made it uncomfortable for racialised youth to participate in valued occupations there. Given the biases of centre staff members, the Tribunal recommended that the town hire racialised staff members (Bascaramurty, 2020).

The meso context issues that cut off access to basketball for the youths included a lack of organisational guidelines for determining, documenting and reviewing the consequences of particular behaviours, allowing racist patterns to go unidentified. For example, there were no guidelines for when and how to involve the police. The macro context issues included racism on the part of staff members who implemented the ban and administrators who did not see it as problematic when contacted by parents.

The CanMOP helps occupational therapists recognise the multilayered factors that influence inequitable access to valued occupations in meaningful contexts. In this way, CanMOP supports occupational therapists in advocating for individuals but also working in solidarity with antiracist advocacy groups to advocate for system changes.

of structural barriers to access to occupations require collective efforts from occupational therapists working with others, such as other members of the health, education or social care teams, families and advocacy groups, to ensure that all people have access to their valued occupations within meaningful relationships and contexts. An example of such action is described in Box 11.2.

Initiating Participation in Valued Occupations

Occupational therapists also work to help individuals and collectives initiate or re-initiate valued occupations when these occupations are difficult due to illness, injury, impairment, or other concerns. This is perhaps the best known of the three aspects of promoting occupational participation. It typically involves exploring interacting factors in closest contact with the individual or collective and collaboratively determining which changes could lead to improved participation in an effective and timely manner.

For individuals, this includes consideration of the current physical, cognitive and affective characteristics of the person (often referred to as performance components) and how these interact to facilitate or impede the performance of the occupation. Aspects of the micro context also include, among others, characteristics of the physical space, time of day and activities of others. The occupational therapist collaboratively considers how these factors can be modified to promote the performance of the occupation.

The occupational therapist also considers aspects of the meso and macro contexts that determine how characteristics of the micro context have been shaped and maintained and affect the initiation of occupational participation. The meso context can include implicit and explicit rules and policies of organisations such as the explicit or implicit rules of an assisted living facility that may limit residents' abilities to continue with valued occupations. These rules and policies are influenced by social norms and expectations. Occupational therapists' efforts to foster occupational possibilities must consider aspects of the meso and macro contexts and influence them when necessary. Lamarre and colleagues (2020) describe the facilitation of a meaningful occupation of a resident of an assisted living facility that demonstrates the importance of considerations of meso contexts as facilitators of occupational participation (Box 11.3).

The macro context includes assumptions, attitudes and values that lead to the construction of the micro and meso contexts in particular ways. For example, Kirsh and colleagues described attitudes of stigma against injured workers (Kirsh et al., 2012). Societal attitudes such as stigma contribute to micro context issues detrimental to returning to work, including unfriendliness of co-workers. Notably, these attitudes also contribute to meso context issues such as punitive workers' compensation policies that require injured workers to navigate through complex benefits procedures and deal with skeptical healthcare providers. Kirsh and colleagues worked collaboratively with injured workers and the provincial Workers' Compensation Board to develop a better understanding of stigma and its negative impacts, and develop plans towards changing both attitudes and related policies and practices (Kirsh, 2015). Other examples of the

BOX 11.3
MESO CONTEXT ASPECTS OF ENGAGING IN A MEANINGFUL OCCUPATION

After moving to an assisted living facility, Mrs Helen Quinn (a pseudonym) told occupational therapy student Julie that the thing she would most like to do was to start painting again. Julie asked Mrs Quinn about the history and meaning of painting to her. Mrs Quinn related that she had spent a big part of her adult life raising a large family and travelling all over Canada with them. She always loved to paint but had little time for this. Together Mrs Quinn and Julie explored what 'painting' would look like to be most satisfying. Mrs Quinn began to consider enrolling in a painting course in the community with other adults run by a painting instructor who was open to supporting her given her balance, mobility and memory problems.

Julie knew that facilitating this occupation was going to be challenging. She enlisted the help of the residence well-being director, Amanda, and Mrs Quinn's son, Bob. At first, Amanda wanted have someone come into the residence to do a painting class, but she soon came to understand the value for Mrs Quinn going out to a community class. Amanda arranged for Mrs Quinn to be reminded of the painting class and organised an earlier lunch for her on the day of the class. Bob arranged adapted public transportation for his mother to attend the class, and Julie and Mrs Quinn asked for the instructor to meet her at the entrance to the centre where the class was taking place.

Mrs Quinn and Amanda collectively developed several strategies to help facilitate this important occupation. Many important facilitators were meso context considerations. These included residence policies that allowed the wellbeing director to help facilitate participation in 'outside' programs, flexibility in the dining schedule and among the personal support staff who were able to include reminders in their routine care, and an adapted transportation service that was not restricted to transportation to medical appointments and was available to people living in assisted living (Lamarre et al., 2020).

BOX 11.4
STIGMA AND OCCUPATIONAL PARTICIPATION

For many people, participating in valued occupations within meaningful contexts is affected by stigma. For example, Nossum and colleagues (2018) asked people experiencing obesity about the challenges they face in their valued occupations. Several participants reported that the glances from other people restricted their participation in swimming and other sports activities, and reduced their use of public transportation, further limiting participation in valued occupations.

Krupa and colleagues (2009) documented the impact of stigma on employment among people diagnosed with mental illness. Stigma affected employers' ideas about people in terms of competence and potential for dangerousness. Also, stigma was linked to people questioning the legitimacy of mental health as an illness, believing that work should be avoided to limit any negative impact on health, and feelings that employing people who have experienced mental illness is a charitable act, rather than a business transaction.

Stigma is an aspect of the macro context that affects policies (meso context) and the behaviour of others (micro context). Occupational therapists need to be aware of how stigma may limit people's possibilities for access to, and initiation and sustaining of, valued occupations within meaningful contexts and relationships. Occupational therapists must address stigma, and work collectively to counter stigma, both within the profession as well as in the wider community (Krupa, 2008).

impact of stigma on occupational participation are described in Box 11.4.

Sustaining Participation in Valued Occupations

Once valued occupations are accessed and initiated, it is also extremely important that they be sustained. For example, although an individual may be able to carry out an occupation in a clinic setting, or at home with the occupational therapist present, it is important to identify what is needed to ensure that they will be able to continue with the occupation after therapy ends. This might include considering whether the individual or the collective has the resources (e.g. time, energy and funds) necessary to support continuing the occupation within the context of other demands of everyday life. It may also involve how prepared or open others, such as work and social groups, are in ensuring the continued involvement of the individual or collective in the occupation. Meso context factors may be particularly important, as these considerations determine whether micro changes will continue to be supported. As well, macro context factors will be critical to whether others believe that the individual or collective can or should be doing the occupation.

DISTINCTIVE FEATURES OF THE CanMOP

The CanMOP builds on previous Canadian occupation models and related occupational therapy models but is distinct in a variety of ways. Previous versions of the Canadian model have depicted an individual person at the centre of the model, with physical, cognitive and affective performance components highlighted. However, the CanMOP places occupational participation at the centre. This has several advantages. First, it clarifies that the primary focus of occupational therapy is occupational participation. This makes it evident that occupational therapy involves promoting occupational participation, not repairing or improving aspects of an individual's body or mind. It also makes it clear that while occupational therapists work with individuals, they also work with collectives, such as families, groups, communities and populations.

Another distinctive feature of the CanMOP is that it emphasises the complexity and interrelatedness of the individual or collective and their environments in promoting occupational participation. The emphasis is less on 'normalising' an individual or collective and more on examining the ways that valued occupations can be facilitated (Hammell, 2006). When working with individuals, physical, cognitive and affective performance components are considered in the model in relationship to micro, meso and macro contexts. This allows for an analysis that is more explicitly holistic (McColl, 1994) and that appreciates the transactional nature of occupation (Aldrich & Cutchin, 2013).

Previous versions of the Canadian model have categorised occupation as productivity, self-care and leisure. This categorisation has been removed from the CanMOP. The categorisation of occupations has been challenged for many years. Critiques include that the categories do not comprehensively cover all the things people do (Hammell, 2009; Magasi, 2012), and that categorisation can be different for different people or for the same people under different conditions (Brooke et al., 2007). Also, the removal of categorisation responds to the critique that such categorisation may promote only white Eurocentric images of occupations (Hammell, 2019). Free of categorisation, occupational therapists are more able to explore what individuals and collectives want to do and need to do to enjoy a life of satisfying occupations, without consciously or unconsciously defining what these occupations might look like. In this way, the use of the CanMOP helps ensure that occupational therapists' understanding pays close attention to individuals' and collectives' values, and cultural and historical contexts by collaboratively exploring the meaning and purpose of the things they need to do and want to do.

Finally, the CanMOP explicitly considers occupational possibilities. This helps ensure that occupational therapists do not assume that all people have the same possibilities for accessing, initiating and sustaining valued occupations. Again, it makes it clear that the primary objective of occupational therapy is to expand occupational possibilities through addressing barriers and incorporating facilitators in context.

CONCLUSION

An overview of the CanMOP, the current evolution of the occupation model endorsed by the Canadian Association of Occupational Therapists, has been presented in this chapter. Occupational therapists can use the CanMOP to guide their practice as they collaboratively explore what people need to do and want to do. Occupational therapists can also use the CanMOP to collaboratively explore and expand occupational possibilities through examining and addressing barriers and facilitators in micro, meso and macro contexts.

REFERENCES

Aldrich, R. M., & Cutchin, M. P. (2013). Dewey's concepts of embodiment, growth, and occupation: Extended bases for a transactional perspective. In M. P. Cutchin & V. A. Dickie (Eds.), Transactional perspectives on occupation (pp. 13–23). Springer. https://doi.org/10.1007/978-94-007-4429-5_2.

Bailliard, A. L., Dallman, A. R., Carroll, A., Lee, B. D., & Szendrey, S. (2020). Doing occupational justice: A central dimension of everyday occupational therapy practice. *Canadian Journal of Occupational Therapy, 87*(2), 144–152. https://doi.org/10.1177/0008417419889930.

Baker-Lewton, A., Sonn, C. C., Vincent, D. N., & Curnow, F. (2017). 'I haven't lost hope of reaching out … ': Exposing racism in sport by elevating counternarratives. *International Journal of Inclusive Education, 21*(11), 1097–1112. https://doi.org/10.1080/13603116.2017.1350316.

Bascaramurty, D. (2020). *Off the court: How drama at a rec centre led to an Ontario town's reckoning with race.* The Globe and Mail. https://www.theglobeandmail.com/canada/article-off-the-court-how-drama-at-a-rec-centre-led-to-an-ontario-towns/.

Brooke, K. E., Desmarais, C. D., & Forwell, S. J. (2007). Types and categories of personal projects: A revelatory means of understanding human occupation. *Occupational Therapy International, 14*(4), 281–296.

Egan, M., & Restall, G. (2022). *The Canadian model of occupational participation*. In M. Egan & G. Restall (Eds). *Promoting occupational participation: Collaborative relationship-focused occupational therapy* (pp. 73–95). Canadian Association of Occupational Therapists.

Elder, G. H. (1994). Time, human agency, and social change: Perspectives on the life course. *Social Psychology Quarterly, 57*(1), 4. https://doi.org/10.2307/2786971.

Hammell, K. W. (2006). *Perspectives on disability and rehabilitation.* Elsevier.

Hammell, K. W. (2009). Sacred texts: A sceptical exploration of the assumptions underpinning theories of occupation. *Canadian Journal of Occupational Therapy, 76*(1), 6–13. https://doi.org/10.1177/000841740907600105.

Hammell, K. (2019). Building globally relevant occupational therapy from the strength of our diversity. *World Federation of Occupational Therapists Bulletin, 75*(1), 13–26.

Kirsh, B. (2015). Transforming values into action: Advocacy as a professional imperative. *Canadian Journal of Occupational Therapy, 82*(4), 212–223. https://doi.org/10.1177/0008417415601395.

Kirsh, B., Slack, T., & King, C. A. (2012). The nature and impact of stigma towards injured workers. *Journal of Occupational Rehabilitation, 22*(2), 143–154. https://doi.org/10.1007/s10926-011-9335-z.

Krupa, T. (2008). Part of the solution … Or part of the problem? Addressing the stigma of mental illness in our midst. *Canadian Journal of Occupational Therapy, 75*(4), 198–205. https://doi.org/10.1177/000841740807500404.

Krupa, T., Kirsh, B., Cockburn, L., Gewurtz, R. (2009). Understanding the stigma of mental illness in employment. *Work, 33*(4), 413–425. https://doi.org/10.3233/WOR-2009-0890.

Lamarre, J., Egan, M., Kessler, D., & Sauvé-Schenk, K. (2020). Occupational performance coaching in assisted living. *Physical & Occupational Therapy in Geriatrics, 38*(1), 1–7.

Magasi, S. (2012). Negotiating the social service systems: A vital yet frequently invisible occupation. *OTJR: Occupation, Participation and Health, 32*(1_suppl), S25–S33. https://doi.org/10.3928/15394492-20110906-03.

Maslow, A. H. (1967). *Toward a psychology of being.* Van Norstrand.

McColl, M. A. (1994). Holistic occupational therapy: Historical meaning and contemporary implications. *Canadian Journal of Occupational Therapy, 61*(2), 72–77. https://doi.org/10.1177/000841749406100202.

Nossum, R., Johansen, A. E., Kjeken, I. (2018). Occupational problems and barriers reported by individuals with obesity. *Scandinavian Journal of Occupational Therapy, 25*(2), 136–144.

Rasskazova, E., Ivanova, T., & Sheldon, K. (2016). Comparing the effects of low-level and high-level worker need-satisfaction: A synthesis of the self-determination and Maslow need theories. *Motivation and Emotion, 40*(4), 541–555. https://doi.org/10.1007/s11031-016-9557-7.

Ryan, R. M., & Deci, E. L. (2019). Brick by brick: The origins, development, and future of self-determination theory. In A. J. Elliot (Ed.). *Advances in Motivation Science,* (Vol. 6 pp. 111–156). Elsevier. https://doi.org/10.1016/bs.adms.2019.01.001.

Townsend, E. (1993). Occupational therapy's social vision. *Canadian Journal of Occupational Therapy, 60*(4), 174–184.

Whiteford, G., Jones, K., Rahal, C., & Suleman, A. (2018). The participatory occupational justice framework as a tool for change: Three contrasting case narratives. *Journal of Occupational Science, 25*(4), 497–508. https://doi.org/10.1080/14427591.2018.1504607.

REFLECTION

1. Ask a friend to identify an occupation that is very important to them. Develop questions to help you better understand what this occupation looks like when it is done in a way that is meaningful to your friend. For example, where are they, who is with them? Develop questions to help you understand the purpose and meaning of this occupation within the context of their history and relationships.

2. Think of a group in your community who do not have good access to a particular occupation. How might an occupational therapist work at the community level with members of this group to explore what satisfying occupational participation would look like and improve access.

3. Imagine that you are an occupational therapist working in a day hospital program with older adults who are experiencing frailty due to complex medical conditions. Your service includes a group program where participants identify valued occupations and begin to work towards re-engaging in these activities. One of the participants, Mrs Marchand, is experiencing decreased mobility (she uses a walker for short distances) and has a mild cognitive impairment. She has recently moved to be closer to her family. She has identified gardening as a highly valued occupation she would like to return to and has located a small plot within a community garden. Using the CanMop as a guide, what questions might you ask to better understand how Mrs Marchand can sustain occupational participation in gardening.

12

THE COLLABORATIVE RELATIONSHIP-FOCUSED PRACTICE AND THE CANADIAN OCCUPATIONAL THERAPY PRACTICE PROCESS FRAMEWORK

GAYLE RESTALL ■ MARY EGAN ■ KAARINA VALAVAARA ■ ANGELA PHENIX

CHAPTER OUTLINE

Overview

Growing awareness of factors that influence equitable and just opportunities to engage in occupational therapy and to participate in occupations that are valued and meaningful has spurred consideration about new processes of doing occupational therapy. In this chapter, the *collaborative relationship-focused occupational therapy* approach is presented. The approach builds on traditional understandings of client-centred practice and adds new concepts to help address the complexity of building and sustaining equitable and just therapy relationships in a variety of contexts. The approach complements and is embedded in the *Canadian Occupational Therapy Practice Process* (COTIPP) framework. The COTIPP guides occupational therapists to attend to three foundational processes and six action domains as they consider their intentions and engage in reasoning to promote occupational participation. Along with the Canadian Model of Occupational Participation (CanMOP), collaborative

relationship-focused occupational therapy and the COTIPP provide guidance for occupational therapists working with individuals and collectives to promote just and equitable opportunities for occupational participation.

KEY POINTS

- Growing awareness of contextual factors have influenced the need for evolving occupational therapy approaches and practice processes toward addressing equity and justice.

- Collaborative relationship-focused occupational therapy is an approach that centres occupational therapist's relationships with the individuals and collectives they work with.

- The Canadian Occupational Therapy Inter-Relational Practice Process Framework guides occupational therapists as they create the conditions for building and sustaining relationships with the people they work with and act to promote occupational participation in the context of equity and justice.

INTRODUCTION

Occupational therapists work with people as they engage or re-engage in valued occupations within meaningful contexts and relationships. Occupational therapists have long recognised that occupational therapy is not something that one does *to* people. Rather it is a skillful collaborative process that occurs within relationships. Similarly, they recognise that occupational therapy expertise does not rely on a set of standardised procedures that relies on 'if x is the problem, then y is the solution' type of reasoning. Rather, occupational therapy expertise is characterised by the ability to enter into and maintain collaborative relationships with individuals and collectives that promote rights-based self-determination. Occupational therapy expertise includes complex reasoning to understand the contexts and valued occupations of the individual or collective they work with, as well as the contexts of the occupational therapist and their practice. Collectives include families, groups, communities and populations. Occupational therapists incorporate complex reasoning grounded by justice, equity and rights-based lenses. Occupational therapy expertise encompasses an understanding of the complexity of promoting occupational participation with the ability to move fluidly through and between interrelated actions.

In this chapter collaborative relationship-focused occupational therapy (Restall & Egan, 2021, 2022) and the Canadian Occupational Therapy Inter-relational Practice Process (COTIPP) framework (Restall et al., 2022) are described. Along with the Canadian Model of Occupational Participation (CanMOP) (Egan & Restall, 2022) (refer to Chapter 11), collaborative relationship-focused occupational therapy and the COTIPP are used by occupational therapists as they apply their expertise to collaborate with individuals and collectives as they enact their vision of a good life that includes valued occupations in meaningful relationships and contexts.

The approaches described in this chapter build upon, but are also fundamentally different from, many of the approaches that have guided occupational therapy to date. Occupational therapists have become increasingly aware of how previous approaches are limited in the ability to facilitate human rights such as equitable access to healthcare and occupational justice. Research, program evaluations, clinical practice, and the voices of people requiring and accessing occupational therapy have demonstrated a need to reconsider how occupational therapy is done. Pressures from practice settings can often guide the occupational therapist to prioritise biomedical concerns while ignoring or minimising the social structures and systems that may be leading to occupational disruption. This narrow focus influences how people requiring occupational therapy are prioritised and who can access services. Additionally, individualistic, biomedical approaches are a particularly poor fit when occupational therapists promote occupational participation with collectives.

The approach and practice framework described in this chapter have emerged from, and build upon, previous scholarship that has influenced an evolving critical understanding of occupational therapy practice. The scholarship related to client-centred and person-centred approaches has contributed to guiding occupational therapy relationships by describing the importance of:

- occupational therapist's trustworthiness (Gerlach et al., 2017; Lauckner et al., 2019; Prescott et al., 2019; Wimpenny et al., 2014);
- attention to power structures in the relationship (Sumsion & Law, 2006; Townsend et al., 2013);
- respect for people's rights to make choices and informed decisions about their lives (Law et al., 1995; Sumsion, 2000; Sumsion & Law, 2006), and
- collaboration with individuals and collectives using occupational therapy services (Corcoran, 1993; Townsend et al., 2013).

The practice approach and framework presented here builds on these concepts by explicitly recognising expectations for occupational therapists to engage in critical analysis of their own positionalities and worldviews, and those of the systems and contexts in which they work. Occupational therapists are not 'outside' or 'neutral' but integral to the unfolding of the process and relationship with individuals and collectives. Previous practice models, while sometimes acknowledging meso and macro contexts, have not forefronted the need for occupational therapists to critically reflect on the influence of systems and structures, such as colonialism and climate change, on practice and occupational participation. In addition, occupational therapists from underrepresented groups have valuable worldviews and lived experiences that enhance understanding of occupation and occupational therapy through challenging predominant occupational therapy values and approaches in a variety of practice situations. Collaborative relationship-focused occupational therapy and the COTIPP build on previous scholarship to more explicitly consider multi-level contexts and the justice, equity and rights influences on the individuals and collectives that occupational therapists work with.

COLLABORATIVE RELATIONSHIP-FOCUSED OCCUPATIONAL THERAPY

Collaborative relationship-focused occupational therapy is an overarching approach to working with individuals and collectives. Collaborative relationship-focused occupational therapy is defined as 'an approach to occupational therapy that attends to, and concentrates on, the relational aspects of the occupational therapist self and the individuals and collectives (i.e. families, groups, communities and populations) who use occupational therapy services. These relationships are embedded within the multilayered historical and contemporary contexts in which people live and occupational therapy occurs. The occupational therapist continuously strives to develop a collaborative relationship with the individual or collective to jointly work toward priorities and goals that are meaningful to the individual or collective' (Restall & Egan, 2022, p. 100).

There are four major aspects of collaborative relationship-focused occupational therapy: contextually relevant, nuanced, strives for safety and promotes rights-based self-determination.

Contextually Relevant Practice

Contextually relevant practice requires a critically reflexive and critically reflective stance (White & Beagan, 2020). Through critical reflexivity, each occupational therapist gains awareness of how their own social identities and positionalities, implicit and explicit biases, histories and their own worldviews and that of the dominant culture interact with the

worldviews of the individuals and collectives they work with. Without this self-awareness oppression is inevitable. An occupational therapist's implicit or explicit biases originating from their own worldview, life experiences and ideologies can shape how they relate to an individual or collective, what services they may offer, or the duration of this service. For example, an occupational therapist may interpret difficulty attending appointments as a lack of engagement in therapy on the part of a racialised family with limited education and low income and may prematurely discontinue therapy with their child. They may fail to explore the possibility that the family is having difficulty attending appointments due to inflexible work schedules and lengthy travel times due to their reliance on public transportation. Oppressive documentation may result when the occupational therapist misinterprets reasons for discharge citing organisational policies about missed appointments rather than implicating the policies themselves as discriminatory toward people with limited resources (MacLachlan & Grenier, 2022). Occupational therapists must be vigilant in understanding their own biases and how these biases, as well as the potentially discriminatory biases of the organisations in which they work, may be influencing their interpretations and actions.

Collaborative relationship-focused practice requires that occupational therapists seek to understand micro-, meso- and macro-level influences on themselves and the individuals and collectives who use their services. Contextually relevant relationships require occupational therapists to critically reflect on how stigmas, ableism, racism, sexism, ageism and additional discriminatory behaviours are created and maintained in systems, structures and by their own behaviours (Tam, 2019). They must recognise oppression and discrimination when they occur and take action to mitigate their effects (Rudman, 2021). This extends to critically reflecting on how taken-for-granted ways of doing assessments or interventions commonly used in occupational therapy can be oppressive. A list of critically reflective questions that can help occupational therapists to determine whether an assessment or intervention might be oppressive or discriminatory in context is presented in Box 12.1.

BOX 12.1

REFLECTIVE QUESTIONS TO SUPPORT ANTIOPPRESSIVE ASSESSMENTS AND INTERVENTIONS

When considering standardised assessments and interventions, some critical reflection questions an occupational therapist might ask themself to support anti-oppressive and anti-discriminatory practices are:

1. What assumptions does this assessment or intervention make?
2. Whose agenda does this assessment or intervention align with?
3. Whose knowledge and values does this assessment align with?
4. Am I upholding the rights of self-determination? For example, Can the person say no to this assessment or intervention and what happens if they do?
5. Do I understand how I uphold Indigenous self-determination and rights with my decisions and actions?
6. Have I allowed room for collaboration and partnership?
7. What is the status of my relationship with this person? Do I have a sense of their beliefs and values?
8. What can I do to reduce the power differential between me and the person I am working with?
9. How does current evidence about particular interventions match with the context (e.g. presence of family/friend, timing and location, full informed and ongoing consent) in which I am working?

Adapted from MacLachlan, J., Phenix, A., & Valavaara, K. (2019). *Can occupational therapists assessments be culturally safe?* Presented at the Canadian Association of Occupational Therapists Annual Conference.

Nuanced Relationships

Contextually relevant collaborative relationships are nuanced. This means that occupational therapists adapt their relationship approaches to the context of promoting occupational participation and the unique needs, desires and vulnerabilities of the individuals or collectives they work with. Their relationship approaches respond to the micro-, meso- and macro-level environmental contexts that shape the development of collaborative relationships. Occupational therapists recognise that relationships with individuals will be different than relationships with communities (Janse van Rensburg, 2018). As well, they recognise that communities have traditions, values and processes that must be recognised and acknowledged. For example, community protocols for access

and obtaining consent may be essential guides for how the occupational therapist respectfully engages with the community and will shape ongoing relationships. Occupational therapists may need to co-create processes that respect culture and community standards and traditions, while ensuring that regulations and laws regarding confidentiality and individual autonomy are respected. A practice example of critically reflective questions that an occupational therapist needs to consider when developing collaborative relationships is provided in Box 12.2.

Occupational therapists recognise that therapy relationships are dynamic and, thus, nuanced over time. As the contexts, the purpose of therapy, and people's needs, desires and vulnerabilities change, so will the relationship. For example, an occupational therapist will always inquire about people's goals for occupational participation and work collaboratively to develop and evaluate plans. However, in some situations, such as the onset of a traumatic brain injury or severe illness, some people may express the need for more direction from the occupational therapist to explore and take action to promote occupational participation. Over time, as the individual or collective becomes more autonomous in their decisions about their own lives, the occupational therapist will need to adjust their expectations and role in the relationship.

Strives for Safety in Relationships

The occupational therapist continuously strives to build and sustain safer collaborative relationships. In health care settings, safety is often considered only with regards to potential physical injury. Collaborative relationship-focused occupational therapy considers safety and risk in a much broader and more nuanced sense. Safety in this context has physical, emotional, cultural, and spiritual dimensions and can only be evaluated by the individual or collective with whom the occupational therapist is working (First Nations Health Authority, n.d.; Baba, 2013; Curtis et al., 2019). Furthermore, the occupational therapist striving for safety within collaborative relationship-focused practice must always keep in mind their responsibility to minimise the risks for which they are directly responsible. Examples of actions that occupational therapists take to strive for safety in therapy relationships include:

■ Remain up to date with the evidence related to the effectiveness of assessments and interventions in

---

BOX 12.2

PRACTICE EXAMPLE WITH CRITICALLY REFLECTIVE QUESTIONS TO PROMOTE COLLABORATIVE THERAPEUTIC RELATIONSHIPS IN NEW, UNFAMILIAR CONTEXTS

Entering into collaborative relationships can be challenging and requires skills that occupational therapists will need to cultivate throughout their careers. Building authentic, collaborative therapeutic relationships requires active learning and reflection on the part of the occupational therapist regarding the people involved and multilayered contexts. Consider an occupational therapist who is asked to work as a school-based occupational therapist in a community with which they are not familiar. Some questions they might critically reflect on are:

- What are the multiple overlapping contexts I must consider? For example:
  - immediate social, physical, cultural and institutional environments of the classroom and school?
- Do I understand what events might be occurring outside of the school, in the broader community, that are informing current occupational participation of students? For example:
  - community losses?
  - collective celebrations?
  - seasonal and familial responsibilities?
  - teacher and staff wellness?

- Do I understand guardianship and kinship in the community to know who will provide consent for the student? If this differs from dominant legal expectations, how will I navigate consent?
- Do I understand relationships within the community? For example,
  - parenting practices?
  - peer relationships?
  - family relationships within the school?
- What is the history of professionals doing assessments in this community? What has been the relevance of these assessment to the community?
- What are the expectations of parents, teachers, school administrators and community leaders about the services I can provide? What is my scope of practice within the community in terms of the model of care I am working within (consultation vs direct therapy) and how does that fit with the expectations of the community?

Courtesy Angela Phenix and Kaarinna Valavarra.

---

their area of practice to ensure that they offer the best options relevant to the context and discontinue any interventions that have been shown to be ineffective or cause harm;

- Maintain healthy interpersonal boundaries with the individuals and collectives they work with;
- Disrupt all forms of oppression in therapy practices (Pooley & Beagan, 2021);
- Be transparent by sharing information about the therapy process (Ranner et al., 2019);
- Apply universal precautions including those that are trauma informed (Edgelow & Cramm, 2020; Tam, 2019);
- Follow the guidance of equity-deserving groups for establishing culturally safer relationships (e.g. Baba, 2013)

Promotion of Rights-Based Self-Determination

Collaborative relationship-focused occupational therapy rests on the recognition of the individual's and collective's right to self-determination. Occupational

therapists have an obligation to promote rights-based self-determination by practising in ways that facilitate an individual's or collective's agency to make choices and decisions that affect their health, wellbeing, survival, and participation in occupations. Occupational therapists recognise that people's choices are made in the context of their relationships (Durocher et al., 2015; Hunt & Ells, 2011) and embedded within the rights and responsibilities of people to themselves, their families, their communities and the natural environment. Importantly, social and structural factors facilitate or constrain people's choices highlighting the ways that people's choices for occupational participation are inequitably distributed among groups in society (Hammell, 2020). Occupational therapists promote rights-based self-determination by:

- affirming the rights of individuals and communities for self-determination within their relational contexts;
- recognising the individual and socially constructed constraints to people's choices about occupational participation;

- acknowledging that risk is required for growth; and
- critically reflecting on their own worldviews when people's choices may be generated from worldviews that diverge from their own or those of the dominant culture.

Occupational therapists must respect people's rights to make choices that are risky or in opposition to Western ways of doing things, without labelling the person as nonadherent or unwilling to engage in therapy. Choices are influenced by contextual factors that are often not understood or recognised by the occupational therapist. In collaborative relationship-focused practice, occupational therapists have a responsibility to promote rights-based self-determination of individuals and collectives through facilitating informed decisions about occupational participation and addressing the contextual factors that limit people's choices.

The overall approach that occupational therapists take when working with individuals or collectives has been presented. This approach guides occupational therapists to ensure that their work is underpinned by relationships that are contextually relevant, nuanced, strives for safety and promotes rights-based self-determination. Keeping this approach in mind, the Canadian Occupational Therapy Inter-Relational Practice Process Framework (COTIPP) is now described.

CANADIAN OCCUPATIONAL THERAPY INTER-RELATIONAL PRACTICE PROCESS FRAMEWORK

The COTIPP (Fig. 12.1) affirms the importance of occupational therapists continuously building and sustaining relationships through collaborative relationship-focused occupational therapy. Relationships form the essential underlying process for quality, ethical and justice-oriented practice. As occupational therapists engage in the three foundational processes and six action domains of the COTIPP, building and sustaining relationship remains central to the ability of occupational therapists to promote occupational participation.

COTIPP Foundational Processes

The COTIPP presents three foundational processes that are critical for occupational therapy practice.

These foundational processes are considered throughout practice. Each foundational process is described separately with the recognition that all are interrelated and dynamic. The three foundational processes are: seek to understand the context; reflect, critically reflect and reason; and use justice-, equity- and rights-based lenses.

Seek to Understand Context

Understanding the contextual factors that influence occupational participation is essential and includes dimensions of the occupational therapist's context, the practice context, and the context of the individuals and collectives that access occupational therapy services. Seeking to understand context begins with the occupational therapist considering their own social identities, histories and experiences, including the unearned privileges and oppressions that are associated with their identities (Nixon, 2019). Ongoing reflection begins prior to the first connection with an individual or collective and continues throughout practice and through the occupational therapist's career. It includes critical reflexivity about the ways that the occupational therapist's own social identities related to sex, gender, sexual orientation, race, age, disability, social class, ethnicity, history, religion and additional identities may affect their relationships with people whose social identities are similar or different from their own.

Occupational therapists also seek to understand their practice context beginning as soon as they enter a practice setting. Using socio-ecological (Bronfenbrenner, 1977) and determinants of health and wellbeing perspectives (Greenwood & de Leeuw, 2012; Marmot, 2005) assists them in examining the origins and implications of context as factors influencing occupational participation, health and wellbeing. These perspectives facilitate a critical examination of how macro-level structures, both historical and contemporary, perpetuate and entrench racism, ableism, ageism, sexism, heteronormativism, classism, and additional sources of oppression. In seeking to understand context, occupational therapists examine how their practice environment's policies, procedures, values and beliefs are influenced by macro-level structures. They gain an understanding of how Global North worldviews have created and sustained systems of oppression in health, education and social services

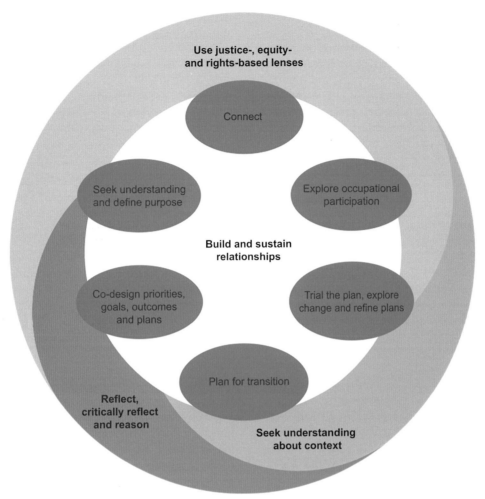

Fig. 12.1 ■ Canadian Occupational Therapy Inter-Relational Practice Process (COTIPP). (Reproduced with permission from Restall, G., Egan, M., Valavarra, K. Phenix, A., & Sack, C. (2022). The Canadian occupational therapy inter-relational practice process (COTIPP) framework. In M. Egan, & G. Restall (Eds.), *Promoting occupational participation: Collaborative relationship-focused occupational therapy* (p. 122). Canadian Association of Occupational Therapists.)

and how they continue to influence the everyday practices of occupational therapists (Grenier, 2020; Lavalley & Johnson, 2020). Importantly, occupational therapists recognise the strengths and resources of the practice environment that can be leveraged to disrupt barriers to quality occupational therapy services and promote people's choices and opportunities for occupational participation.

Occupational therapists seek to understand the contexts of the individuals and collectives who access occupational therapy services. They learn about the communities in which people live and work. They explore the effects of history and contemporary social structures on occupational possibilities. As they seek to understand these contexts, they humbly recognise that these contexts can never be fully known.

Reflect, Critically Reflect and Reason

The second foundational process provides guidance for occupational therapists thinking and reasoning while doing occupational therapy. Reflection is a cornerstone of occupational therapy practice (Kinsella, 2001). It involves processes of reflecting both in-practice and on-practice (Schön, 1983). Reflecting in-practice assists the occupational therapist in adapting their approaches to the people they are working with during therapy moments. Reflecting on-practice assists the occupational therapist to reflect after an interaction to consider what went well and what they need to change to their approach with a particular individual or collective or to their practice in general. Finally, through critical reflection, the occupational therapist not only examines their own practice but also calls into question oppressive systems and considers alternatives (Brookfield, 2009). Critical reflection requires action to change oppressive systems. This includes everyday acts to disrupt oppressions as well as well-planned actions done in collaboration with colleagues and advocates.

Occupational therapists engage in practice reasoning to make decisions about what they do in practice. Ethical decision-making is an integral part of good practice reasoning (Rogers, 1983; VanderKaay et al., 2020). Practice reasoning is a complex and context-dependent process (Unsworth & Baker, 2015). Making high-quality and ethical decisions is dependent on many factors including the skills with which the occupational therapist accesses and understands empirical, experiential, and theoretical knowledge and integrates it with additional knowledge of the people with whom they work. Contextually, practice reasoning relies on the occupational therapist's understanding of the contexts of the people they work and their practice setting. Importantly, high-quality and ethical reasoning that results in practice improvement is facilitated by an occupational therapist's understanding and critical reflexivity on their own beliefs and assumptions and how these influence their decision-making (Schell & Benfield, 2018).

Use Justice-, Equity- and Rights-Based Lenses

The third foundational process is using justice-, equity- and rights-based lenses throughout practice. Occupational therapy scholars have recognised occupational therapists' responsibility to uphold people's rights and facilitate their equitable access to occupational participation (Polatajko et al., 2013). Using justice-, equity- and rights-based lenses helps occupational therapists to meet their moral and ethical responsibility to promote justice and equity within society and the programs and services they offer (Restall et al., 2018). These lens

can guide actions to address justice, equity and rights at macro, meso and micro levels of practice (Bailliard et al., 2020).

Action Domains

Using the COTIPP framework Occupational therapists engage in six action domains as they work with individuals and collectives, while ensuring practices are based on collaborative relationships and keeping in mind the three foundational processes. The COTIPP's six action domains are: (1) connect; (2) seek understanding and define purpose; (3) explore occupational participation; (4) co-design priorities, goals, outcomes and plan; (5) trial the plan, explore change, and refine the plan; and (6) plan for transition.

These action domains are conceptualised as dynamic interrelated processes that often blend into one another. The nonlinear nature of the COTIPP may represent a challenge to occupational therapists because it diverges significantly from typical algorithm styles of depicting professional reasoning. These interrelated processes closely reflect the complexity of occupational therapy reasoning. Importantly, rejecting linear thinking is necessary for rights-based, relationship-focused occupational therapy. An occupational therapist *may* follow a specific path through the domains but, typically, the practice situation will require a more fluid and iterative approach in which the occupational therapist moves in multiple directions depending on an individual's or collective's needs, priorities, goals, desires and responses to actions within the domains. Not all domains will be appropriate in every situation. The occupational therapist will collaborate with the individual or collective as they make shared decisions and journey through the domains. A description of each action domain, a summary of intentions within the domain, and critically reflective questions to promote practice reasoning within that domain are provided in Table 12.1.

CONCLUSION

An approach to practice, the collaborative relationship-focused occupational therapy, and a framework for practice, the Canadian Occupational Therapy Inter-Relational Practice Process Framework have been presented in this chapter. This approach and framework

	TABLE 12.1	
	Action Domains of the COTIPP	
Action Domain	**Description and Intentions**	**Reflective Questions for Practice Reasoning**
Connect	Start to build a collaborative relationship. Create an equitable first point of connection with the individual or collective. Determine the equity barriers to accessing occupational therapy and address the barriers. Learn the expectations for occupational therapy from multiple perspectives as appropriate and applicable to the individual or collective, referral source and other important people in the environment (respecting privacy and confidentiality). Have a mutual dialogue with the individual or collective about perspectives on the reasons for occupational therapy. Obtain consent as appropriate to the situation, considering individual rights to be informed, meaningful consent and community protocols for consent.	What practices, processes, organisational rules, or structural factors create barriers to accessing and using occupational therapy services for individuals or collectives? What is the occupational therapist's scope of practice, that is, what does the occupational therapist have the knowledge and skills to do? Has the occupational therapist adequately explained their scope of practice to the individual or collective? What are the constraints and possibilities for occupational therapy within the practice setting and what are the ethical considerations in that situation? Does the occupational therapist have a conflict of interest that could negatively impact the individual or collective? What behaviours are consistent with individual cultural and normative protocols and avoid oppression, traumatisation or retraumatisation? What are the conditions under which the individual or collective wishes to engage with occupational therapy?
Seek understanding and define the purpose	Continue to build and sustain a collaborative relationship. Create the conditions for the individual or collective to share their stories, desires and priorities regarding occupational participation. Learn about occupations in the context of the individual's or collective's life including their identities, strengths, resources, challenges, contexts, history and cultural importance. Co-identify initial ideas for occupational therapy and, based on those ideas, explain what the occupational therapy process could involve. Provide information as applicable about how much time the process is expected to take and whether there are constraints to the available time. Listen deeply to the individual's or collective's thoughts and feelings about this vision of the process and determine any necessary modifications. Meet legal, moral and ethical obligations related to relationship, transparency and informed meaningful consent.	What does the individual or collective hope their occupational participation will look like? What approaches will maximise the occupational therapist's understanding of the individual's or collective's story? How can the occupational therapist create the conditions for interpersonal and physical safety to prevent trauma for the individual or collective? Are the occupational therapy models of practice and frameworks that are typically used appropriate to this situation? If not, is there an alternative? What approaches are most appropriate in this context to facilitate collaborative shared decision-making? What are the potential barriers to continued access to occupational therapy, and what are ways to mitigate them?
Explore occupational participation	Co-create the conditions for exploring the individual's or collective's occupational participation concerns, aspirations, and possibilities, desire for change, and important relationships. Co-assess and co-evaluate occupational participation, including the personal or collective factors *along with contextual* factors that can influence occupational possibilities. Co-analyse with the individual or collective occupational participation concerns and develop priorities for addressing the concerns. Document the findings mindfully and with transparency, avoiding oppressive language and interpretations.	Throughout the therapy encounter, what formal and informal exploratory approaches will maximise understanding of the individual's or collective's story while promoting and supporting conditions for interpersonal, cultural, spiritual and physical safety? What are the most appropriate communication approaches for sharing observations, findings and perspectives? What potential ongoing strategies can address structural and systemic barriers to occupations?

Continued

TABLE 12.1		
Action Domains of the COTIPP—cont'd		
Action Domain	**Description and Intentions**	**Reflective Questions for Practice Reasoning**
Co-design priorities, goals, outcomes and plans	Co-create the conditions for collaboratively developing priorities, goals and outcomes through mutual sharing of perspectives about occupational participation concerns. Co-design plans with the individual or collective, while carefully supporting autonomy and rights-based self-determination. Co-create the conditions for collaborative and mutual sharing of perspectives about perceived risks and benefits of the plan. Explore justice and equity barriers to achieving the individual's or collective's goals and plans. Document the findings mindfully and with transparency, avoiding oppressive language and interpretations.	What communication approaches will encourage rights-based self-determination? What empirical, experiential and theoretical knowledge might be important to consider? What are the most effective and appropriate occupational therapy strategies that are acceptable to the individual or collective and are likely to have maximum benefit for the individual or collective, considering the constraints and possibilities within the practice environment? What justice and equity barriers to therapy and occupational participation need to be addressed?
Trial the plan, explore change and refine the plan	Collaborate with the individual or collective to trial the plan for promoting or sustaining occupational participation. Obtain the individual's or collective's perspectives of their experiences working with the plan, particularly how it did or did not promote occupational participation. Continuously monitor shared understanding and perspectives of progress and safety in therapy, and collaboratively adjust the plan when needed. Co-create the conditions for sharing perspectives about outcomes of occupational therapy. Co-design new plans as needed. Document changes and adjustments to the plan. Examine barriers to equitable access and quality of therapy.	How does the occupational therapist's role and relationship with the individual or collective need to evolve as therapy progresses? What are the most appropriate methods to collaboratively monitor progress and the individual's or collective's personal, relational and contextual factors that may be affecting progress? Is there a need to adjust the therapy plan including objectives, models, frameworks and strategies? What are the most appropriate timing and approaches to discussing potential changes in the plan with the individual or collective and collaboratively deciding on changes? What are the most appropriate methods for exploring outcomes in collaboration with the individual or collective? What was the quality and effectiveness of therapy including unintended consequences, both positive and negative?
Plan for transition	Elicit, listen to and seek to understand the individual's or collective's perspectives on the transition from occupational therapy. Intentionally co-create a transition plan with the individual or collective. Share occupational therapy-related information with the individual or collective and additional key people with appropriate and meaningful consent. Document transition plans.	What are the best ways to share therapy-related information in collaboration with the individual or collective? What are the implications of transition for the individual or collective? How can occupational participation gains be sustained? What additional resources can the individual or collective access?

Adapted with permission from Restall, G., Egan, M., Valavarra, K. Phenix, A., & Sack, C. (2022). Canadian occupational therapy inter-relational practice process framework. In M. Egan, & G. Restall (Eds.), *Promoting occupational participation: Collaborative relationship-focused occupational therapy* (pp. 139–143). Canadian Association of Occupational Therapists.

centres on the essential nature of the building and sustaining therapy relationships through collaborative relationship-focused practice that is contextually relevant, nuanced, strives for safety, and promotes rights-based self-determination. The three foundational processes of the COTIPP – seek to understand context, reflect and reason, and use justice-, equity- and rights-based lenses – are necessary throughout an occupational therapist's career. The six action domains of the COTIPP are intended to be flexible enough to guide practice with individuals, families, communities and populations in a variety of occupational therapy practice contexts.

REFERENCES

Baba, L. (2013). *Cultural safety in first nations, inuit and métis public health: Environmental scan of cultural competency and safety in education, training and health services*. National Collaborating Centre for Aboriginal Health.

Bailliard, A. L., Dallman, A. R., Carroll, A., Lee, B. D., & Szendrey, S. (2020). Doing occupational justice: A central dimension of everyday occupational therapy practice. *Canadian Journal of Occupational Therapy, 87*(2), 144–152. https://doi.org/10.1177/0008417419898930.

Bronfenbrenner, U. (1977). Toward an experimental ecology of human development. *American Psychologist, 32*(7), 513–531.

Brookfield, S. (2009). The concept of critical reflection: Promises and contradictions [Article]. *European Journal of Social Work, 12*(3), 293–304. https://doi.org/10.1080/13691450902945215.

Corcoran, M. A. (1993). Collaboration: An ethical approach to effective therapeutic relationships [Article]. *Topics in Geriatric Rehabilitation, 9*(1), 21–29. https://doi.org/10.1097/00013614-199309000-00005.

Curtis, E., Jones, R., Tipene-Leach, D., Walker, C., Loring, B., Paine, S.-J., & Reid, P. (2019). Why cultural safety rather than cultural competency is required to achieve health equity: A literature review and recommended definition. *International Journal for Equity in Health, 18*(1), 174. https://doi.org/10.1186/s12939-019-1082-3.

Durocher, E., Kinsella, E. A., Ells, C., & Hunt, M. (2015). Contradictions in client-centred discharge planning: Through the lens of relational autonomy [Article]. *Scandinavian Journal of Occupational Therapy, 22*(4), 293–301. https://doi.org/10.3109/11038128.2015.1017531.

Edgelow, M., & Cramm, H. (2020). Developing an occupation-centred framework for trauma intervention. *Occupational Therapy in Mental Health, 36*(3), 270–290. https://doi.org/10.1080/0164212X.2020.1808148.

Egan, M., & Restall, G. (2022). Canadian model of occupational participation (CanMOP). In M. Egan, & G. Restall (Eds.), *Promoting occupational participation: Collaborative relationship-focused occupational therapy*. Canadian Association of Occupational Therapists, 73–95.

First Nations Health Authority. (n.d.). *Creating a climate for change: Cultural safety and humility in health services for first Nations and Aboriginal peoples in British Columbia*. https://www.fnha.ca/Documents/FNHA-Creating-a-Climate-For-Change-Cultural-Humility-Resource-Booklet.pdf.

Gerlach, A. J., Browne, A. J., & Greenwood, M. (2017). Engaging Indigenous families in a community-based Indigenous early childhood programme in British Columbia, Canada: A cultural safety perspective. *Health & Social Care in the Community, 25*(6), 1763–1773. https://doi.org/10.1111/hsc.12450.

Greenwood, M. L., & de Leeuw, S. N. (2012). Social determinants of health and the future well-being of aboriginal children in Canada. *Paediatrics & Child Health, 17*(7), 381–384.

Grenier, M.-L. (2020). Cultural competency and the reproduction of White supremacy in occupational therapy education. *Health Education Journal, 79*(6), 633–644. https://doi.org/10.1177/0017896920902515.

Hammell, K. W. (2020). Making choices from the choices we have: The contextual-embeddedness of occupational choice. *Canadian Journal of Occupational Therapy, 87*(5), 400–411. https://doi.org/10.1177/0008417420965741.

Hunt, M. R., & Ells, C. (2011). Partners towards autonomy: Risky choices and relational autonomy in rehabilitation care. *Disability & Rehabilitation, 33*(11), 961–967. https://doi.org/10.3109/09638288.2010.515703.

Janse van Rensburg, E. (2018). A framework for occupational enablement to facilitate social change in community practice. *Canadian Journal of Occupational Therapy, 85*(4), 318–329. https://doi.org/10.1177/0008417418805784.

Kinsella, E. A. (2001). Reflections on reflective practice. *Canadian Journal of Occupational Therapy, 68*(3), 195–198. https://doi.org/10.1177/000841740106800308.

Lauckner, H., Leclair, L., & Yamamoto, C. (2019). Moving beyond the individual: Occupational therapists' multi-layered work with communities [Article]. *British Journal of Occupational Therapy, 82*(2), 101–111. https://doi.org/10.1177/0308022618797249.

Lavalley, R., & Johnson, K. R. (2020). Occupation, injustice, and anti-black racism in the United States of America. *Journal of Occupational Science, 29*(4), 487–499. https://doi.org/10.1080/14427591.2020.1810111.

Law, M., Baptiste, S., & Mills, J. (1995). Client-centred practice: What does it mean and does it make a difference? *Canadian Journal of Occupational Therapy, 62*(5), 250–257. https://doi.org/10.1177/000841749506200504.

MacLachlan, J., & Grenier, M.-L. (2022). Accounting for our words: Anti-oppressive documentation in occupational therapy practice. *Occupational Therapy Now, 25*, 27.

Marmot, M. (2005). Social determinants of health inequalities. *Lancet, 365*(9464), 1099–1104. https://doi.org/10.1016/s0140-6736(05)71146-6.

Nixon, S. A. (2019). The coin model of privilege and critical allyship: Implications for health. *BMC Public Health, 19*(1), 1637. https://doi.org/10.1186/s12889-019-7884-9.

Polatajko, H., Davis, J., Stewart, D., Cantin, N., Amoroso, B., Purdie, L., & Zimmerman, D. (2013). Specifying the domain of concern: Occupation as core. In E. Townsend, & E. A. Polatajko (Eds.), *Enabling occupation II: Advancing an occupational therapy vision for health, well-being, & justice through occupation* (2nd ed., pp. 13–36). CAOT Publication ACE.

Pooley, E. A., & Beagan, B. L. (2021). The concept of oppression and occupational therapy: A critical interpretive synthesis. *Canadian Journal of Occupational Therapy, 88*(4), 407–417. https://doi.org/10.1177/00084174211051168.

Prescott, S., Fleming, J., & Doig, E. (2019). Refining a clinical practice framework to engage clients with brain injury in goal setting. *Australian Occupational Therapy Journal, 66*(3), 313–325. https://doi.org/10.1111/1440-1630.12556.

Ranner, M., Guidetti, S., von Koch, L., & Tham, K. (2019). Experiences of participating in a client-centred ADL intervention after stroke. *Disability & Rehabilitation, 41*(25), 3025–3033. https://doi.org/10.1080/09638288.2018.1483434.

Restall, G. J., & Egan, M. Y. (2021). Collaborative relationship-focused occupational therapy: Evolving lexicon and practice. *Canadian Journal of Occupational Therapy, 88*(3), 220–230. https://doi.org/10.1177/00084174211022889.

Restall, G., & Egan, M. (2022). Collaborative relationship-focused occupational therapy. In M. Egan, & G. Restall (Eds.), *Promoting occupational participation: Collaborative relationship-focused occupational therapy* (pp. 98–117). Canadian Association of Occupational Therapists.

Restall, G., Egan, M., Valavaara, K., Phenix, A., & Sack, C. (2022). Canadian occupational therapy inter-relational practice process framework. In M. Egan, & G. Restall (Eds.), *Promoting occupational participation: Collaborative relationship-focused occupational therapy* (pp. 120–149). Canadian Association of Occupational Therapists.

Restall, G. J., MacLeod Schroeder, N. J., & Dubé, C. D. (2018). The equity lens for occupational therapy: A program development and evaluation tool: L'Equity lens for occupational therapy: Un outil pour le développement et l'évaluation de programme [Article]. *Canadian Journal of Occupational Therapy, 85*(3), 185–195. https://doi.org/10.1177/0008417418756421.

Rogers, J. C. (1983). Eleanor Clarke Slagle lectureship—1983; Clinical reasoning: The ethics, science, and art. *AJOT: American Journal of Occupational Therapy, 37*(9), 601–616. http://uml.idm.oclc.org/login?url=https://search.ebscohost.com/login.aspx?direct=true&db=c8h&AN=107615152&site=ehost-live.

Rudman, D. L. (2021). Mobilizing occupation for social transformation: Radical resistance, disruption, and re-configuration: Mobiliser l'occupation pour une transformation sociale: Résistance radicale, perturbation et reconfiguration. *Canadian Journal of Occupational Therapy, 88*(2), 96–107. https://doi.org/10.1177/00084174211020836.

Schell, B. A. B., & Benfield, A. (2018). Aspects of professional reasoning. In B. A. B. Schell, & J. W. Schell (Eds.), *Clinical and professional reasoning in occupational therapy* (2nd ed., pp. 127–144). Wolters Kluwer.

Schön, D. (1983). *The reflective practitioner: How professionals think in action*. Basic Books.

Sumsion, T. (2000). A revised occupational therapy definition of client-centred practice. *British Journal of Occupational Therapy, 63*(7), 304–309. https://doi.org/10.1177/030802260006300702.

Sumsion, T., & Law, M. (2006). A review of evidence on the conceptual elements informing client-centred practice. *The Canadian Journal of Occupational Therapy, 73*(3), 153–162. http://uml.idm.oclc.org/login?url=https://search.proquest.com/docview/212995209?accountid=14569.

Tam, T. (2019). *Addressing stigma: Toward a more inclusive health system*. Public Health Agency of Canada. https://www.canada.ca/en/public-health/corporate/publications/chief-public-health-officer-reports-state-public-health-canada/addressing-stigma-toward-more-inclusive-health-system.html.

Townsend, E. A., Beagan, B., Kumas-Tan, Z., Versnel, J., Iwama, M., Landry, J., Stewart, D., & Brown, J. (2013). Enabling: Occupational therapy's core competency. In E. Townsend, & H. J. Polatajko (Eds.), *Enabling occupation: Advancing an occupational therapy vision for health, well-being and justice through occupation* (2nd ed.). CAOT Publication ACE, 87–133.

Unsworth, C., & Baker, A. (2015). A systematic review of professional reasoning literature in occupational therapy. *British Journal of Occupational Therapy, 79*(1), 5–16. https://doi.org/10.1177/0308022615599994.

VanderKaay, S., Letts, L., Jung, B., & Moll, S. E. (2020). Doing what's right: A grounded theory of ethical decision-making in occupational therapy. *Scandinavian Journal of Occupational Therapy, 27*(2), 98–111. https://doi.org/10.1080/11038128.2018.1464060.

White, T., & Beagan, B. L. (2020). Occupational therapy roles in an indigenous context: An integrative review. *Canadian Journal of Occupational Therapy, 87*(3), 200–210. https://doi.org/10.1177/0008417420924933.

Wimpenny, K., Savin-Baden, M., & Cook, C. (2014). A qualitative research synthesis examining the effectiveness of interventions used by occupational therapists in mental health. *British Journal of Occupational Therapy, 77*(6), 276–288. https://doi.org/10.4276/030802214X14018723137959.

REFLECTION

1. You are working for a home care program in a region that is new to you. This region includes a large Indigenous population. Outline how you will reflect on your own context, including positionality and worldviews, as well as how you will learn about the context of this community.

2. How do you define collaboration? Describe possible opportunities for collaboration with individuals or collectives at four or more of the action domains of the COTIPP.

3. Describe what is meant by rights-based self-determination and how it applies to collaborative relationship-based practice with individuals and collectives.

13

PROCESS OF EXPLORING OCCUPATIONAL PARTICIPATION

CLARE HOCKING ■ KAREN WHALLEY HAMMELL

Overview

Explorations of occupational participation are undertaken to identify and document the wellbeing aspirations, skills, strengths, meanings, relationships, assets, resources and abilities of individuals and collectives. The process is collaborative, strengths-based and occupation-focused. Congruent with the social determinants of health, it encompasses aspects of the broader context – social, political, policy, economic – that determine the occupational opportunities available to people. The purpose is to collect, synthesise and interpret information needed to address people's occupational participation needs. Screening to assure the suitability of an occupation-focused approach, planning strategies for action, monitoring progress and evaluating outcomes are all part of the process. Professional and ethical considerations include consent, documentation and reporting processes, gathering and interpreting information in a culturally safe, decolonising manner, and ongoing review of progress towards outcomes.

KEY POINTS

■ Exploring people's occupational participation is a considered and collaborative process of collecting, synthesising and interpreting the information necessary to take appropriate actions to address their occupational needs.

■ Parallel with the profession's conceptual shifts, explorations of participation focus on what really matters to people, identifying their occupational participation aspirations and needs rather than focusing predominantly on measuring impairments and dysfunctions.

■ The occupational focus of assessment may pertain to orchestration (the organisation and balance of occupations within everyday life), or to analysis of people's access to, performance of, and engagement in specific occupations.

■ Congruent with an understanding of the social determinants of health and with occupational therapists' commitment to human rights, the opportunities available to people to exercise their abilities and participate in the occupations they need, want, or are required to do are explored.

157

- The process encompasses screening, assembling necessary information, monitoring progress and evaluation of outcomes, and continues throughout the occupational therapy process.

- Occupational therapists respond to people rather than their 'conditions'. This means that assessments must be appropriate to their age, gender roles and cultural background; a requirement that demands attention to cultural safety and decolonisation.

- Standardised assessments are of limited utility within an evolved, occupation-focused practice, but might be employed if there is compelling evidence of their validity with people of the same age group, demographic profile, cultural background, language and geographic location (urban/rural, Global South/North), and where the findings generated directly inform participation in occupations people have reason to value. Moreover, information derived from standardised assessments may be required by those acting as gatekeepers to the services disabled people need. However, other forms of exploration are available that are more appropriate to the identification of individuals' and collectives' priorities, and information of relevance to the enlargement of their occupational engagement. These methods will be highlighted.

- Occupational therapists must ensure information-gathering processes are conducted professionally and ethically, with particular attention to transparency in obtaining informed consent on an ongoing basis.

INTRODUCTION

> *'The social construction of a problem shapes our social and institutional responses to its resolution'*
> **(Priestley, 2005)**

The 'central concern' addressed by this book is how to best respond to the occupational participation aspirations and needs of individuals and collectives experiencing illness, injury, or impairment. This chapter addresses one aspect of that response: the process of exploring opportunities to participate in occupations and evaluating the outcomes of occupational therapy interventions. Occupational therapists' efforts to understand and resolve problems with occupational participation have changed over the decades in line with profound shifts in thinking, notably the increasing focus on valued occupations, wellbeing and human rights. It is important to understand those conceptual

shifts because traces of earlier assumptions persist, continuing to shape practice despite the profession's espoused commitment to newer ways of thinking and working. In the following section, the changing paradigms characterising occupational therapy's worldview are outlined, from the perspective of exploring people's occupational aspirations and opportunities.

To situate the discussion, we offer a brief note on our positionality. Clare has English heritage and identifies as Pākehā, that is, a settler on the traditional lands of Māori people in Aotearoa (New Zealand). She is deeply steeped in occupational science and has actively influenced the incorporation of human rights, occupational justice and inclusion in the World Federation of Occupational Therapists' documents. Karen identifies as a White, temporarily nondisabled, straight cisfemale, currently living as a settler on the traditional, ancestral and unceded territory of Coast Salish people in Canada. Both authors acknowledge the unearned benefits, advantages and privileges they have always derived from having white skin, able bodies, and proximity to socially constructed and valued Western 'norms' of being and doing.

SHIFTING THE FOCUS OF ASSESSMENT

Occupational therapy's roots are firmly embedded in observations of the therapeutic power of occupation. The profession's early alliance with medicine and increasing identification with the medical model stimulated a turn towards mechanistic rationale (Psillas & Stav, 2021) informed by measured deficits in physical, cognitive, perceptual and social functions. From the 1970s, the resultant loss of professional identity spurred a renaissance of occupation (Whiteford et al., 2000) and stimulated discussion of 'top-down' assessment, meaning assessment processes that start by enquiring about the occupations people consider important, rather than by measuring and classifying their differences from socially valued norms and developmental milestones. Aligning with that commitment, it is now recognised that assessments designed to identify or quantify impairments and dysfunction are only relevant if the score generated is required for institutional reasons, such as gaining access to services and support (Fisher, 2009). This philosophical shift paralleled the

World Health Organization's move from an impairment focus to emphasising participation and the role environments play in creating disability (WHO, 2001).

However, the legacy of occupational therapy's mechanistic era persists in the continued development and use of assessment tools to measure the status of specific functions. While such tests can confirm the extent and nature of suspected dysfunction, they have limited value in informing interventions because they do not identify occupations people value or their experience of participating in them. In addition, they cannot be used to monitor improvement in people's experience of doing the things they aspire to do. At worst, measures of dysfunction and the interventions that follow can be experienced as pathologising people (Taylor, 2023), discounting the skills and strategies they develop for themselves, imposing value judgements that privilege 'normal function' and independence over diverse ways of being human, including accepting help, and as reinforcing an ableist ideology that seeks to identify and classify 'flawed' bodies, eradicate 'abnormal' ways of being and doing, and induce social conformity (Hammell, 2023).

Viewed critically, both restoration of discrete functions and insisting on carrying out occupations in ways the occupational therapist deems 'normal' are underpinned by ableist values, which view disabled people as falling short, in terms of their productivity, fitness, intelligence and desirability (Yao et al., 2022). Such discriminatory and oppressive assumptions are visible in assessment processes that measure people against population norms in order, as far as possible, to intervene to minimise differences. The emerging paradigm of promoting participation in valued occupations within meaningful contexts and relationships ensures more just and respectful service (Egan & Restall, 2022), especially for those who do not aspire to ableist values (Hammell, 2023). That shift is in tune with international recognition of disability as a human rights issue, with equitable opportunities for participation (on their own terms) being central to that assertion. Acknowledgement of the interrelationship of health, disability and rights brings the fact that disabled people 'do not have equal access to health care, education, and employment opportunities [...] and experience exclusion from everyday life activities' (WHO & World Bank, 2011, p. xxi) fully into view.

It directs attention to societal influences on people's opportunities to meet their basic needs, engage in diverse, meaningful occupations, and enjoy the same life chances and opportunities as people who do not experience impairment, illness or injury.

The World Federation of Occupational Therapists (2019) position statement on occupational therapy and human rights asserts that occupational therapists around the world 'are obligated to promote occupational rights as the actualisation of human rights' (p. 1). It goes on to identify 'persistent poverty, economic restrictions, disease, social discrimination, displacement, natural and man-made disasters, armed conflict, [and] historic disadvantage' (p. 1) as key societal issues giving rise to occupational injustices. Bringing an occupational justice perspective to the assessment process necessitates identifying people's opportunities and freedom to participate in society, and their capabilities to do so. That demands attention to the ways in which occupational therapists gather information about people's occupational participation needs and aspirations, given that 'our assessments establish the boundaries of our vision, within which we shall only find what we are looking for' (Hammell, 2015a). Accordingly, occupational therapy assessments of structural barriers to health and wellbeing must become the 'new normal'; an accepted and essential component of the assessment and evaluation process.

Importantly, given the long histories of human rights violations that Indigenous peoples continue to endure as a consequence of colonisation, occupational therapists also have a professional obligation to ensure that their exploration of peoples' occupational participation needs and aspirations is not just culturally safe but decolonising (refer to Chapter 1). The process of decolonising occupational therapy requires the profession to challenge the assumed universality and supremacy of Western knowledge and values, contest the Eurocentric White norms that have informed our assessments and preoccupation with classifying people according to their perceived physical differences, and end racist, ableist and heteronormative practices that disempower, disable and oppress service users, students and colleagues (Hammell, 2024). Decolonising occupational therapy requires, for example, the unstated assumption that 'everyone' values, performs and experiences occupations the same way must be exposed and disrupted. It also requires recognition of 'White privilege', the inherent and unearned advantages that accrue to White people in a world structured by racial injustice and inequality, and of White supremacy – the dominance, centrality and assumed superiority of people perceived as White (Hammell, 2024). These toxic ideologies inform the false presumption that Western civilisations are superior, such that 'other' ways of knowing, doing, being, belonging and of relating to the earth and other lifeforms are overlooked, ignored, disparaged, or silenced (Gibson & Farias, 2020). The way forward, Ryall and colleagues (2021) explain, involves listening respectfully to peoples' experiences of health, wellbeing and occupation from a strengths-based, human rights perspective.

OPENING UP THE ASSESSMENT PROCESS

Broadly speaking, occupational therapy practice proceeds through a series of stages, each influencing the next. The process gives order and predictability, keeping the practice on track even when new insights indicate a need to circle back to revisit an earlier stage. At three points in the process – screening, assessment and evaluation – attention is given to gathering information to inform the next step. Simply put, assessment is designed to generate an accurate understanding of what is going on, what outcomes are sought, appropriate ways of working towards those outcomes, and what was achieved. But assessment is complex because there will be multiple perspectives on what is happening.

Occupational therapists' commitment to collaborative practice directs attention to the people with the occupational need as a critical source of information because they have experiential evidence of the quality, circumstances and outcomes of their occupations; moreover, only they can decide which occupations matter most in the context of their lives and values. They also make judgements about what they wish to change and how high they are aiming, have expectations about the way intervention decisions will be made, and have opinions about which courses of action are acceptable and preferable. The profession's knowledge of evidence-based practice brings another strand to the collaborative process of assessment, informing choices about the parameters of information needed to inform subsequent interventions.

Bringing a strengths-based perspective into the assessment process shifts attention from impairments, inabilities, and problems to wellbeing aspirations, abilities (e.g. aptitudes, skills, knowledge), strengths (e.g. experience, interests, values, commitments) and resources (e.g. assets, income, supportive relationships and networks). Assessment processes that fail to attend to strengths generate partial understandings, risk being distressing and demoralising, and at best, lead to inadequate, partial interventions. A primary focus on assessing strengths, skills, assets and opportunities, supplemented with exploration of specific deficits as necessary to understand what might help promote occupational participation, provides a more nuanced, hopeful and complete picture.

A human rights perspective further opens thinking about the assessment process. Hammell (2015a) reminded occupational therapists of the substantial evidence showing that environmental barriers and social inequities, rather than physical impairments, account for much of the diminished quality of life experienced by disabled people. Thus, occupational therapists must acknowledge that people need more than determination, skills, knowledge, volition, the right genes, and a measure of good luck to be healthy and to participate in their society; they need opportunities to gain and apply their abilities, skills and knowledge. Recognising this fact reveals that the assessment process needs to draw in information about social attitudes, policies, and economic, and political realities, and other aspects of the meso and macro contexts of occupation that impede or support people's opportunities to engage in valued occupations in a way they find meaningful. For example, many forced migrants living in Canada identified their primary goal as securing meaningful employment. Thus, in addition to exploring the migrants' previous work experience, the alignment between their skills and the kind of work they were seeking, and their work readiness, the occupational therapists working with them drew in information about their real opportunities to engage with the community and build community capacity and about how to navigate the health, education and employment systems with which migrants engage (Krishnakumaran et al., 2022).

Amartya Sen's capabilities approach usefully informs a human rights perspective (Hammell, 2015b; Pereira, 2012; Whiteford & Pereira, 2012). The capabilities approach recognises that social inequities and structural barriers unfairly constrain the opportunities available for some members of society to develop and use their knowledge, skills and abilities; limiting their alternatives and the choices they can make. Viewed from a capabilities perspective, disability is recognised to be the denial of choices and opportunities to be and to do. Thus informed, issues of health and occupational justice can be considered in light of the opportunities afforded or denied by the environment, irrespective of whether the occupational participation need sits with an individual, family, selected community members and the agencies that serve them, or an entire community (Pizzi et al., 2010). Building on this perspective, more culturally inclusive modes of assessment might be employed to encompass the collective capabilities of marginalised groups and communities, such as self-help networks or the self-determination expertise of Indigenous peoples.

CRITICALLY INFORMED ASSESSMENT PROCESSES

As the discussion above reveals, the occupational therapy profession's declared commitment to human rights demands critical reflection on the assessment process, encompassing what information is needed, where to get it, and the appropriate focus for action. For example, knowledge of the association between low income and stroke alerts us to the value of attending to the social determinants of health (e.g. poverty, discrimination) as indicators of the differential health risks and the widely varying prognoses experienced by advantaged and disadvantaged people, and majority and minority groups (Bernard et al., 2019). In this way, the assessment process becomes somewhat less centred on specific individuals and collectives, and situations, because this information is demographic rather than diagnostic. As such, assessment of environmental barriers and social inequities is ongoing, as occupational therapists continue to build and update both their understandings and channels of information about the social, economic and political forces that deliver differential health outcomes to different

sectors of society. The results of such assessments will augment information learned through an assessment of the occupational participation needs of individuals or collectives. Combined, these assessments are used to determine which referrals to accept, how occupational therapists' time is apportioned across the various people they are working with, and the balance of interventions targeting change in the socio-political environment, the social and economic resources available to support participation, and people's skills, knowledge and impairments. Insights gained from an appraisal of the social determinants impacting service users might also usefully be shared among other members of the therapy team.

To illustrate those ideas, stimulating change in the socio-political environment might incorporate lobbying for legislative changes to enforce access to sports clubs for disabled adults, to equalise their activity choices with those of other adults and assure equality of opportunity for community participation, as is their human right. Another example might be legislation to enforce appropriate workplace accommodations for people with enduring mental illness, on a par with environmental modifications for people with physical impairments. While these examples are limited, in both being disability focused, their achievement would be supported by occupational therapists assessing and documenting discrepancies between health-promoting occupations people and communities want and are able to do versus what they can gain access to (their opportunities to do). An example of a resource-focused intervention might be promoting the provision of comfortable seating in shopping malls to encourage older adults to socialise and be physically active in a relatively safe environment. Such initiatives would be supported by asking about and documenting the community-based exercise opportunities preferred by older adults, alongside evidence of managerial efforts to displace them in favour of a more fashion-conscious consumer demographic with more disposable income (Hart & Heatwole Shank, 2015).

The capabilities of disabled people to function might most usefully be understood by assessing their practical opportunities rather than their personal attributes. The problem of unemployment among disabled women, for example, might be due to poverty, lack of access to public transport, or misogyny rather than to having musculoskeletal impairments. Consider the following account, reported by the Canadian Broadcasting Corporation (CBC, 2015). A 9-storey building in Vancouver's most economically deprived neighbourhood houses some of the city's most marginalised citizens. In the spring of 2015, the only elevator in the building broke down. More than a week later it had still not been repaired, leaving 'John', a man with a spinal cord injury stranded on an upper floor. This had repercussions for his occupational participation opportunities: he was unable to shower because the only wheelchair-accessible shower was on the ground floor, he lost money because he could not travel to his job, and he was unable to move outside to enjoy the sunshine. John discovered that his options, and his abilities to shower, to work and to participate in the life of his community, were of little use without opportunity. Clearly, his capabilities – abilities and opportunities – were constrained due to socially structured barriers to his full participation in society.

Adopting a mode of assessment that permits consideration of both abilities and opportunities will reveal appropriate targets for intervention. For example, an assessment of workers with diabetes, HIV infection, dyslexia or other invisible impairments, who experience excessively demanding work requirements and fear the consequences of revealing their diagnoses, might expose a need to equip employers with strategies for creating inclusive and accessible workplaces. This is a human right, as described in the United Nations Convention on the Rights of Persons with Disabilities (2006), which asserts the right to equality of opportunity, to full and effective participation and inclusion in society, and access to facilities and services on an equal basis with others. Regrettably, these rights to equality of opportunity are frequently violated, even in resource-rich countries such as Canada, where it has been reported that almost 90% of employers have no provisions in place for people challenged by inadequate access (Reeve & Gottselig, 2011). While time spent accessing and assessing demographic data, documenting, and reporting barriers to health-giving occupations, educating others and lobbying will inevitably take time from interventions targeting people's impairments and immediate context, the societal impact would be more far reaching. Further, occupational therapists would be freed from the self-perpetuating

cycle of solving the same problem over and over again, with each person individually (Hocking et al., 2014).

A critical rethinking of assessment practices also brings into focus that the choices people make are dependent upon the choices available to them. Structural barriers may constrain the choices of entire communities, effectively limiting their life options and opportunities (Quesada et al., 2011). Their apparent 'choices' may be tainted by histories of state oppression, systemic racism, experiences of over-surveillance, and confounded by chronic poverty and housing insecurity. For example, against the backdrop of colonialism, how could Indigenous families engage with government-sponsored intervention programmes? Any assessment process that did not seek to understand the history and socio-political context would likely misconstrue the agency exhibited by Indigenous people when they choose not to engage with professionals. Perpetuation of racialised labels such as 'noncompliant' or 'disinterested' are real risks in situations where individuals' actions or inaction are decontextualised and thus reduced to expressions of personal volition (Gerlach et al., 2018). Confronting the limitations of assessing community-embedded individuals in isolation means that occupational therapists are responsible for identifying situations in which it is more useful to assess and reinforce the collective capabilities (opportunities) of a family or community than to target assessments and interventions at the abilities of an individual disabled person (Dubois & Trani, 2009).

AN OCCUPATIONAL FOCUS

Having argued the need for assessment processes infused with an occupational justice perspective, we now consider the centrality of occupation in the selection and design of information-gathering strategies. An occupational focus means exploring occupational aspirations, levels of participation in preferred and necessary occupations, the quality or ease of performing occupations that matter, plus the barriers encountered and their effect. Assessments that focus directly on occupation make both the relevance and intended outcome of occupational therapy evident (Hocking, 2001; Molineux, 2004), revealing problems such as not knowing how to do something (Polatajko et al., 1999), not wanting to do it, or not having opportunities to engage in the occupations of concern. Both the way occupations come together into a pattern or lifestyle and the quality of performing specific occupations are important. Depending on people's occupational aspirations and needs, the assessment process might focus on one or both of these. When people's pattern of occupations is the focus, attention is given to aspects such as coordinating occupations with other people, competing role demands and time use. Systemic barriers to occupation are identified, such as the absence of safe places to walk in lower socio-economic neighbourhoods, discriminatory practices of employers, sporting, recreation, religious, arts, cultural and social organisations, or appointments with health services that impinge on the working day.

Occupational performance refers to the way people carry out an occupation. Consistent with the idea that participation in occupation is a transactional process, people's performance is viewed as an interaction with the demands of the occupation in which they participate, the performance environment, and the socio-political and cultural context (Cutchin & Dickie, 2012a). The focus of the assessment is on exploring what people aspire to do, how they experience occupations of concern, and how skilfully they perform them, as demonstrated by how the occupation proceeds and the barriers to effective performance that become apparent. Commonly cited categorisations of performance skills are motor, process and social interaction skills, which direct attention to actions such as gripping objects, positioning oneself in relation to the task, initiating steps in a task, gathering necessary tools and materials, and gesturing and approaching people in a manner appropriate to the situation.

Two important considerations must be front of mind during assessment processes. First, bodily impairments do not preclude skilful occupational performance. Second, the cause of ineffective performance may be environmental, such as unexpectedly heavy loads or unreasonable expectations, rather than performers' diminished capacity (Fisher & Griswold, 2019). Thus, people with impairments may be significantly disabled in some physical or social environments and not disabled at all in others (Koca-Atabey, 2013). Additional assessment considerations are people's capacity to take up alternative ways of performing or changing their environment, and their right to reject offered solutions.

Such decisions might be informed, for example, by a reluctance to incorporate assistive technologies into their identity, anxiety about changing their habitual and familiar performance and environment, or the low value of the occupation to the person being assessed.

Assessment of occupational performance can be highly personalised, but that does not necessarily equate to homing in on an individual, given that people often support each other's performance in acknowledged and unacknowledged ways. This fact reinforces the legitimacy and importance of assessments that seek input from all those engaged in co-operative, collaborative, or communal occupational participation.

ENACTING ASSESSMENT PROCESSES

To fulfil occupational therapy's commitment to occupational justice (WFOT, 2019), responsiveness to the social determinants of health must be a primary concern, as discussed earlier. A culturally safe practice, which requires health professionals to attend, for example, to inequities of power, social mores, hygiene practices and spiritual beliefs in their interactions, is also imperative. That includes respecting and actively responding to diverse occupations, languages, and health beliefs, working inclusively, and confronting institutional and personal racism and heterosexism (WFOT, 2009). A useful concept in this regard is cultural humility, which requires therapists to embrace attitudes of openness, develop self-awareness and be self-critical, and commit to ongoing learning about power dynamics, and about the communities with which they interact (Singh et al., 2022).

The assessment process is usually depicted as beginning with an initial screening, to decide whether input from an occupational therapist is indicated and whether beneficial outcomes are likely. This is followed by more detailed exploration to inform decisions about what to do, and then evaluation of the outcomes to determine if the intentions were achieved. Based on that evaluation, the process is concluded or further goals and/or the need to refer to other services are identified. In community development contexts, which might involve engagement with diverse individuals and issues, the initial steps in the process are more elaborated. For example, the International Mental Health

Collaborating Network (n.d.) specifies a stepwise process of learning about the community, listening to community members, bringing people together to develop a shared vision, assessing community assets, resources, needs and issues, and helping community members to recognise and articulate areas of concern and what causes them; a model that might usefully inform practices with people who experience physical illnesses, injuries or impairments, and the communities in which they belong and are embedded.

While exploration of occupational participation aspirations and needs is described as occurring at specific points in the occupational therapy process, this is an ongoing process in which the implementation of planned actions is monitored and progress towards anticipated outcomes is appraised. Judgements about what information to gather and how, who will do that, and when there is sufficient information to agree on a course of action are also ongoing (Table 13.1). Recognising that assessment continues throughout occupational therapy interventions suggests that this is a dynamic process, with therapists exploring aspects of participation in occupation as the need to do so becomes evident. The literature describes a lamentable failure of ongoing review of assessment results concerning a woman who told her therapists that she wanted to walk after sustaining a stroke, but later worried about whether 'my arm got neglected' (Brown et al., 2014, p. 1023). If the assessment had been dynamic and ongoing, initial assumptions and findings may have come into question and new areas for exploration opened.

Screening

The purpose of screening is to obtain a sense of people's aspirations, current occupational status, context, issues and capacity to learn and change and to look for indicators that occupational therapy intervention is likely to prove beneficial (Shotwell, 2019). It is necessary to take a capabilities approach to screening that attends to people in context, appraising their opportunities as well as their abilities (Fig. 13.1). A strengths-based approach that acknowledges people as experts in their own occupations (Egan & Restall, 2022) and circumstances is also essential (and congruent with occupational therapy's espoused collaborative approach). Careful screening avoids wasting the time and resources of both service recipients and

TABLE 13.1

Questions Addressed by Assessment Findings at Each Step of the Occupational Therapy Process

Step in the Occupational Therapy Process	Questions Assessment Findings Address
Screening	■ Does occupational therapy have anything to offer? ■ Is what occupational therapy has to offer welcome? ■ Is intervention likely to be beneficial? (evidence)
Assessing	■ What is the occupational issue? ■ What is the context? (social determinants, cultural and physical context) ■ What is their perspective? How might that perspective be shaped/restricted by the context? ■ What might help? ■ What abilities, resources and opportunities do people have? Are there additional collective capabilities? ■ What is the nature of the problem? (if this needs to be clarified to determine how to intervene)
Identifying needs	■ What occupational needs are apparent? ■ Do they warrant intervention? ■ Is this the best service to address those needs? ■ Is referral to another service warranted?
Negotiating goals	■ What does the community/group/family/person want? ■ What do others want? ■ What has priority? ■ Should the focus for change be the people, the physical or social environment, at an institutional or policy level (or a combination of these)? ■ Can the goals be legally and ethically supported?
Planning and implementing intervention	■ Are things progressing as expected? ■ Are observations consistent with previous understandings? ■ If not, why not?
Evaluating outcomes	■ What was achieved? ■ Was that enough?
Renegotiating goals or discharge	■ Are further needs apparent? ■ If so, can occupational therapy address them?

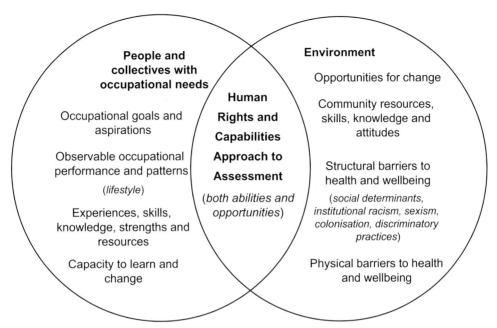

People and collectives with occupational needs

Occupational goals and aspirations

Observable occupational performance and patterns
(*lifestyle*)

Experiences, skills, knowledge, strengths and resources

Capacity to learn and change

Human Rights and Capabilities Approach to Assessment

(*both abilities and opportunities*)

Environment

Opportunities for change

Community resources, skills, knowledge and attitudes

Structural barriers to health and wellbeing
(*social determinants, institutional racism, sexism, colonisation, discriminatory practices*)

Physical barriers to health and wellbeing

Fig. 13.1 ▪ Assessment of people and their contextual capabilities.

providers. It is the first step in collaborating to set the parameters for further assessment and the broad goals of intervention, and as such it gives people a sense of what occupational therapy can realistically offer. Put another way, this is the consultation and contracting phase of the occupational therapy process, where therapists and the people they work with identify whether occupational therapy has anything relevant to offer and thus whether to continue. It is also an opportunity to start to get to know people and establish a collaborative relationship. In medical or rehabilitation contexts, screening is often also about prioritising therapists' workloads and, as discussed earlier, that judgement should include consideration of occupational justice issues, such that priority is given to communities enduring the greatest injustices.

Assessing

Having determined that occupational therapy is indicated, a more extensive exploratory process begins. Assessment of the context to identify possibilities for and barriers to occupational participation may involve exploration and interpretation of the determinants of health, collection of demographic data, and becoming familiar with characteristics of the micro,

meso and macro contexts. Environmental scanning includes identifying services that are already in place, both because replicating existing services is inefficient and, in the case of community development initiatives, because diverting resources or income away from existing services can inadvertently jeopardise the livelihood of the local people (Thibeault, 2013).

Considerations in relation to the intended recipients of occupational therapy include the nature of the assessment itself – what it would be like to 'be assessed' (Hocking, 2001). Is it a collaborative experience of discovery and problem solving or an oppressive exercise wherein the assessor strives to achieve a detached and objective stance? Is it a confidence-building exercise focused on identifying strengths, knowledge, resources and abilities, or a depressing and demeaning experience highlighting inabilities, dysfunctions and deficits? Does it involve self-chosen, familiar occupations in a familiar context or simulated activities and unfamiliar tasks in an unfamiliar context? Are the assessment activities and the way they are administered consistent with people's background, status, and worldviews, or foreign and irrelevant? To address cultural safety and avoid perpetuating the harms of colonisation, assessment tasks and materials should incorporate people's language and familiar occupations, concepts, and images, because failure to do so risks subtly (or blatantly) conveying disrespect, undermining their performance (Ryall et al., 2021) and reproducing colonialism. Consistent with cultural practices, thought must also be given to welcoming support people and including them as active participants where they have a culturally sanctioned role in providing assistance with whatever is being assessed, in speaking for or making decisions on behalf of family members, or when they are collaborative members of co-occupations. Clearly, these concerns will, at most times, eliminate the use of standardised assessments developed on a different population or in a different time and place, or designed to be administered on a one-on-one basis and/or in a 'controlled' environment. Implicit assumptions that discussion of the results will immediately lead to decisions about intervention, without reflection and collaborative problem-solving or allowing time for the people being assessed to consult significant others or pray, are also challenged.

Further considerations include whether the same assessment can be used as a reassessment once intervention is completed and where assessments should be conducted. Few standardised assessments have established ecological validity – which refers to the correspondence of people's occupational performance in an unfamiliar context, such as a clinic, compared to their natural environment – rendering them useless outside the artificial parameters of a clinic. There is a real risk of disadvantaging people by assessing them anywhere but their real-life contexts, leading to inaccurate understandings of their capability to realise their occupational participation aspirations (Crist, 2015). Clearly, because people are inseparable from their environments, and because environments are integral to occupational participation, a relevant assessment of occupational participation will need to be undertaken within the relevant environment. The picture gained of the people being assessed, the context, and occupational participation concern sets the stage for establishing relevant goals addressing valued occupational participation outcomes, and selection of those interventions people perceive to be appropriate, achievable and tolerable. Intervention planning based on flawed assessments may result, for example, in intervention

for things that are not perceived as problems or concerns by the person experiencing illness, injury or impairment, and that fail to account for factors that *are* critically important, or that lead to imposition of 'solutions' that are either irrelevant or unnecessarily restrictive or prescriptive.

Evaluating

To evaluate something means to appraise it, and often, to find out how much of it there is. In this context, 'it' refers to the outcomes of intervention and the extent to which they were achieved. Service users often value this information because it summarises what has been accomplished, helping them both to realise how far they have progressed and to feel satisfied with their efforts. Evaluation results also assist occupational therapists and others to determine whether intervention is complete, and if not, whether new goals or different ways of intervening need to be explored.

There are a number of additional reasons for ascertaining what was accomplished. Recording evaluation results is part of concluding the written record, showing the progression from presenting issues to outcomes. Occupational therapists also report evaluation results to others, such as referral sources and health insurers, services that people are referred on to, a community that will decide whether occupational therapy input helps move things forward and so on. Whatever the audience, occupational therapists must carefully consider how to present evaluation findings. In many cases, specific observations of enhanced occupational participation and the means by which that was achieved will suffice.

ASSESSMENT STRATEGIES

Occupational therapists have a wide variety of assessment strategies available to them. Information about the social determinants of health or systemic barriers to occupation may be gleaned from health statistics, demographic data and reports. More nuanced information about the presence and impact of human rights issues will be available through engagement, for example, with Indigenous peoples, minority groups, disability rights activists and cultural advisors. Strategies employed to gather information directly from people include observation, evaluation, dialogue and interviews, and self-reporting. Assessments can be nonstandardised or standardised.

Selecting and Using Nonstandardised Assessments

Nonstandardised assessments have advantages in being implicitly occupation-focused and flexible, and thus able to encompass the complexities of diverse peoples, situations and occupations. That flexibility also means that occupational therapists can design their assessment processes to address their ethical responsibilities for culturally safe, decolonising practices. In addition, nonstandardised assessments can accommodate the exploration of people doing things together, as well as the practices, resources and aspirations of groups of people. These may include locally developed checklists, report formats, 'standard' interview questions, tasks that therapists use repeatedly and hand on to each other, as well as one-off interviews, observations and group discussions. A crucial requirement is that the therapist and those being assessed or providing data have a shared understanding of the purpose of the assessment, and what will be required of each person.

Nonstandardised assessments make it possible to intermingle assessment with problem solving and trialling of solutions. Dynamic performance analysis (refer to Chapter 18), is a prime example of this. Using nonstandardised methods to explore occupation means that the findings are highly dependent on the occupational therapist's expertise, while the repeatability of an assessment depends on detailed documentation of the assessment process. Occupational therapists, therefore, have a professional responsibility for having a clear rationale for what is included and what is left out, informed by evidence of the things disabled people and carers are concerned about. Partnering with the people with whom nonstandardised assessments will be used – whether disabled, Indigenous, elderly, a minority cultural group, or vulnerable population – to think through the focus and process of the assessment is obviously essential.

The decision to opt for nonstandardised assessments can also be driven by occupational therapists' discomfort with the outdated premise that objectivity and neutrality are either desirable or possible within therapist/service user relationships (Hammell, 2021); and by oppressive administration protocols that require occupational therapists to suspend their efforts to engage with and encourage people, to wait and watch while people struggle with tasks and fail, and to resist their intuitions about ways to modify tasks, instructions, or questions to elicit a more adaptive response (Managh & Cook, 1993).

Selecting and Using Standardised Assessments

Standardised assessments are informed by positivism; reflecting the premise that human actions are unaffected by environmental context and that human activity can be understood by observation alone (and without also understanding the person's mood, motivation or meanings). This premise is contested by occupational therapy's contention that 'humans' physical, social and cultural milieus are always part of who they are, how they think, and what they do' (Cutchin & Dickie, 2012b, p. 25). Inevitably grounded in the issues deemed important to their developers, standardised assessments generally require an individual to respond to predetermined questions, be interviewed about predetermined topics, rate their experiences on a set scale, or engage in a set task, sometimes within a set timeframe and in a set location. Assessors are generally required to administer the assessment and record and score the findings in a prescribed way; one that precludes documentation of valuable qualitative data arising from service users during the assessment process. The objects used to undertake the assessment and how these are arranged may be predetermined. There may or may not be normative data, which enable the person's results to be compared with the population representative of the context in which the assessment was developed. Such assessments are almost exclusively focused on documenting individualistic flaws or skills. In addition, there are no standardised assessments applicable to groups of people.

As with any form of assessment, there are important ethical responsibilities inherent to the selection and use of standardised assessments. Because standardised assessments are developed and tested in a specific historical, socio-political context, with people of a particular age, gender identity, demographic profile, cultural background and language, there is a clear imperative to consider cultural safety and to act in ways consistent with a commitment to decolonisation.

The worldview of the developers is inevitably built into the assessment itself, reflecting their understandings of people's capacities based on their morphology, normative experiences over their lifetime, their perceptions of what people do and how they ought to do it, how they think, what they value and so on. The importance of independence, for example, is implicit in the Western activities of daily living assessments that have been used extensively within the occupational therapy profession for generations. These assessments were explicitly designed to appraise a skill that occupational therapists in the Global North valued highly, but that people encultured with different values might not value at all. Thus, using standardised assessments with people other than the groups with which they were developed risks creating a misleadingly negative portrayal of the abilities of members of minority groups, who may have cultivated a different skill set, informed by different values and opportunities.

If occupational therapists are compelled by institutional pressures to employ standardised assessments, they must make a careful judgement about the specific test based on information about its developers, its development and the demographic characteristics of the participants in the studies undertaken to establish its psychometric properties, the population from which normative data were derived, and so on. It is inappropriate and unethical, for example, to use standardised life satisfaction scales developed for elderly people (who are predominantly female) to assess the perspectives of people with recent spinal cord injuries, who are primarily young and predominantly male. Use of standardised assessments can be discriminatory, racist, sexist and experienced as demeaning and colonising. Because many standardised assessments have proven unsuitable for use among Indigenous people (White & Beagan, 2020), Phenix and Valavaara (2016) assert that occupational therapists should be encouraged to examine critically the suitability of all assessments being used with Indigenous service users. Clearly, such critical interrogation of the suitability of specific assessments is demanded of occupational therapists working with all people. Ensuring the cultural safety of all recipients of occupational therapy is irreconcilable with generating a standard data set across the population served.

Occupational therapists who are required to employ standardised measures and who are looking for assistance in identifying or choosing appropriate standardised assessments might usefully consider published reviews or, if none are available, use evidence-based approaches to critically evaluate the research behind them. On occasion, significant safety concerns, for both the occupational therapist and the person being assessed, may constitute a legitimate reason to opt for a standardised assessment, such as choosing a virtual driving assessment over an on-road test (Lee, 2006).

At a service level, standardised assessments have often been viewed as generating scientifically strong evidence of occupational therapy outcomes that can be collated to demonstrate the overall efficacy of services provided; hence, their prevalence within institutional settings. However, occupational therapists must guard against using data derived from standardised assessments primarily – or solely – to benefit the profession, by demonstrating its contribution to health outcomes or its cost-effectiveness. Clearly, this would violate the ethical obligation to engage in practices – and to use time – to the benefit of service users. Furthermore, the results of occupational therapy's standardised assessments can be used to inform triage decisions, making disabled people ineligible for government-funded housing modifications (Cox, 2023), medical interventions (Thorneycroft & Asquith, 2021), access to fertility services, and so on.

From a human rights perspective, it has been suggested that outcome measures used to gauge the effectiveness of occupational therapy services should assess the degree to which disabled people are able to transcend a marginalised status and assume the occupational rights and opportunities accorded to other citizens (Hammell, 2006). This might be accomplished through assessments of capabilities (abilities and opportunities) and of community participation, which will require new, nonstandardised forms of assessment.

PROFESSIONAL AND ETHICAL COMMITMENTS

Skill in exploring occupational concerns, synthesising information from multiple sources, and professional reasoning are vital, affecting the accuracy of information gained and the meanings and interpretations that therapists and service recipients derive from and attribute to this information. Occupational therapy's commitment to addressing what matters demands skilfully collaborating with people, and tailoring the explorative process to their needs. It also means recognising that people may have extensive or life-long experience of the issue and its context, such as people who have lived with an impairment for many years, or at the other extreme, very limited knowledge of it, such as people facing a situation they have not previously encountered or who have a newly acquired impairment. Occupational therapists must vary their approach accordingly, acknowledging some people as experts and guiding others in their role as 'co-investigators' of issues of which they may only vaguely be aware. Additionally, regardless of how careful or comprehensive the assessment process has been, occupational therapists must not conflate having sufficient information to make an informed judgement with fully understanding people's life experience (Duncan & Creek, 2014).

Occupational therapists are required to build, foster and sustain respectful, culturally safe, collaborative relationships with service users (Restall & Egan, 2022). The kindness and compassion demonstrated by occupational therapists will impact the degree to which people share important information that may impact the therapeutic process; information that may be sensitive or embarrassing. The sensitivity occupational therapists employ in gathering information will also influence people's preparedness to coach the occupational therapist through cultural practices that may influence how occupations are carried out, how decisions are made, and agreements or disagreements conveyed, how the occupational therapist ought to behave as a visitor, ought to convey respect for elders, ought to negotiate gender boundaries, and so on.

Occupational therapists' professional responsibilities include ensuring that they clearly document the assessment of need and that assessment methods and findings are comprehensively and accurately reported (Royal College of Occupational Therapists, 2021). Care must be taken to represent people's views accurately and fairly, and to provide an interpretation of results in a form that can be understood by others – both within and outside the profession. Careful consideration must

also be given to who has a right to know the assessment results and any recommendations arising from them, and how best to convey that information.

The assessment process incorporates multiple ethical demands. Primary amongst these is the issue of informed consent, which means recognising that people have a legitimate choice about engaging in assessment. Consent is only 'informed' if people have been given all the relevant information about the purpose of the assessment, what it will involve and how the results will be used, in a way that they understand. Consent is not a 'one-off', but ongoing, such that service users must know they can refuse to participate at any stage of the assessment process. Despite its importance, little attention has been given to the complexities of eliciting consent from people whose capacity to give consent is compromised or who might be disadvantaged by the outcome. One small-scale study in New Zealand revealed that therapists in both mental and physical health services used various strategies to entice people with cognitive impairments into cooperating with assessments. These included being friendly, providing rewards (such as cooking tasks), eliciting their help with providing information 'the doctors' want, skimping on information about what the assessment would involve or how the results would be used, and modifying standardised assessments if they anticipated that people would resist completing some assessment tasks, thereby nullifying their psychometric properties and rendering the results meaningless and useless. That is, they prioritised fulfilling their professional role, by gathering information to inform rehabilitation decisions, and preserving harmonious relationships with the person to be assessed (through deception) over their right to give or withhold consent (White et al., 2014). Exerting professional dominance through such strategies as persuasion and coercion (Moats, 2007) is incompatible with ethical practices.

Ethical considerations also include determining the appropriateness of offering an occupational therapy service and only gathering information that will be used to inform occupational therapy interventions. As with all aspects of occupational therapy, therapists must recognise the limitations of their knowledge and expertise. That includes their capacity to design informal assessments and proficiency in administering standardised assessments in a manner that preserves their validity and reliability in instances where these are deemed to be appropriate. A final consideration, in relation to both informal and standardised assessment processes, is not overstating the significance or trustworthiness of findings, given that they potentially inform life-changing decisions such as discharge destination or the focus for community development.

CONCLUSION

Occupational therapy assessments are conducted in a professional context that increasingly demands responsiveness to human rights, occupational justice and decolonisation, cultural safety, occupation and evidence-focused practice, and to collaborative ways of working. Their purpose is to generate information about what occupations matter to people, the functions those occupations serve in their lives, what happens when occupational participation is disrupted or dysfunctional (and why occupational participation is sub-optimal), and the impact of opportunities on the ability to participate in occupation: opportunities that are not equally distributed across society.

Assessment processes are complex. They span the most intimate to the most public occupations, the mundane requirements of everyday living to spiritual expression, and every occupational setting people might create or enter, alone or in cooperation with others. Running through this diversity is a consistent demand for high levels of ethical and professional behaviour, which requires constant updating of occupational therapists' knowledge of and skill in implementing assessment processes and devising trustworthy, culturally safe, nonstandardised assessment processes. The imperative for the best possible assessment practices lies in the consequences for people and communities with an occupational concern as well as the societal messages occupational therapists reinforce, about human rights, the value of occupation, and the meaning of living if occupational performance is compromised.

REFERENCES

Bernard, S., Sauvé-Schenk, K., & Egan, M. (2019). Low income and stroke rehabilitation: A tale of two clients. *The Open Journal of Occupational Therapy, 7*(2). https://doi.org/10.15453/2168-6408.1487.

Brown, M., Levack, W., McPherson, K. M., Dean, S. G., Reed, K., Weatherall, M., & Taylor, W. J. (2014). Survival, momentum, and things that make me 'me': Patients' perceptions of goal setting after stroke. *Disability and Rehabilitation, 36*(12), 1020–1026.

Canadian Broadcasting Corporation. (2015). *Disabled Portland Hotel residents left stranded without elevator.* Canadian Broadcasting Corporation. http://www.cbc.ca/news/canada/british-columbia/disabled-portland-hotel-residents-left-stranded .09.03.2015.

Cox, S. C. (2023). *Showers: Discourse, disability and the state.* Auckland University of Technology. https://hdl.handle.net/10292/16203.

Crist, P. A. (2015). Framing ecological validity in occupational therapy practice. *The Open Journal of Occupational Therapy, 3*(3), 11. https://doi.org/10.15453/2168-6408.1181.

Cutchin, M., & Dickie, V. (Eds.). (2012a). *Transactional perspectives on occupation.* Springer.

Cutchin, M. P., & Dickie, V. A. (2012b). Transactionalism: Occupational science and the pragmatic attitude. In G. E. Whiteford, & C. Hocking (Eds.), *Occupational science: Society, inclusion, participation* (pp. 23–37). Blackwell.

Dubois, J.-L., & Trani, J.-F. (2009). Extending the capability paradigm to address the complexity of disability. *ALTER: European Journal of Disability Research, 3*, 192–218.

Duncan, E. M., & Creek, J. (2014). Working on the margins: Occupational therapy and social inclusion. In W. Bryant, J. Fieldhouse, & K. Bannigan (Eds.), *Creek's occupational therapy and mental health* (5th ed., pp. 457–473). Churchill Livingstone.

Egan, M., & Restall, G. (Eds.). (2022). *Promoting occupational participation: Collaborative relationship-focused occupational therapy.* Canadian Occupational Therapy Association.

Fisher, A. G. (2009). *Occupational therapy intervention process model: A model for planning and implementing top-down, client-centred, and occupation-based interventions.* Three Star Press.

Fisher, A. G., & Griswold, L. A. (2019). Performance skills. In B. A. Boyt Schell, & G. Gillen (Eds.), *Willard and Spackman's occupational therapy* (13th ed., pp. 335–350). Wolters Kluwer.

Gerlach, A. J., Teachman, G., Laliberte Rudman, D., Aldrich, R. M., & Huot, S. (2018). Expanding beyond individualism: Engaging critical perspectives on occupation. *Scandinavian Journal of Occupational Therapy, 25*(1), 35–43. https://doi.org/10.1080/11038128.2017.1327616.

Gibson, C., & Farias, L. (2020). Deepening our collective understanding of decolonising education: A commentary on Simaan's learning activity based on a Global South community. *Journal of Occupational Science, 27*(3), 445–448. https://doi.org/10.1080/14427591.2020.1790408.

Hammell, K. W. (2006). *Perspectives on disability and rehabilitation: Contesting assumptions; Challenging practice.* Churchill Livingstone Elsevier.

Hammell, K. W. (2015a). Occupational rights and critical occupational therapy: Rising to the challenge. *Australian Occupational Therapy Journal, 62*(6), 449–451. https://doi.org/10.1111/1440-1630.12195.

Hammell, K. W. (2015b). Quality of life, participation and occupational rights: A capabilities perspective. *Australian Occupational Therapy Journal, 62*(2), 78–85. https://doi.org/10.1111/1440-1630.12183.

Hammell, K. W. (2021). Social and structural determinants of health: Exploring occupational therapy's structural (in)competence. *Canadian Journal of Occupational Therapy, 88*(4), 365–374. https://doi.org/10.1177/00084174211046797.

Hammell, K. W. (2023). A call to resist occupational therapy's promotion of ableism. *Scandinavian Journal of Occupational Therapy, 30*(6), 745–757. https://doi.org/10.1080/11038128.2022.2130821.

Hammell, K. W. (2024). 'Time's up' for White occupational therapy: Toward decolonizing, anti-oppressive, structurally-competent and globally-relevant theories and practices. In S. Baptiste, & S. Shann (Eds.), *Routledge international handbook of occupational therapy*. Routledge.

Hart, E. C., & Heatwole Shank, K. (2015). Participating at the mall: Possibilities and tensions that shape older adults' occupations. *Journal of Occupational Science, 22*(3), 1–15. https://doi.org/10.1080/14427591.2015.1020851.

Hocking, C. (2001). The issue is: Implementing occupation based assessment. *American Journal of Occupational Therapy, 55*(4), 463–469. https://doi.org/10.5014/ajot.55.4.463.

Hocking, C., Townsend, E., Galheigo, S. M., Erlandsson, L.-K., & de Mesquita Chagas, J. N. (2014). *Driving societal change: Occupational therapy, health and human rights*. 16th International Congress of the World Federation of Occupational Therapists: Sharing Traditions, Creating Futures.

International Mental Health Collaborating Network. (n.d.). *Community development*. https://imhcn.org/bibliography/transforming-services/community-development/#:~:text=Steps%20in%20Community%20Development%20Work.

Koca-Atabey, M. (2013). A personal validation of the social nature of disability: Different environments, different experiences. *Disability and Society, 28*(7), 1027–1031. https://doi.org/10.1080/09687599.2013.820535.

Krishnakumaran, T., Bhatt, M., Kiriazis, K., & Giddings, C. E. (2022). Exploring the role of occupational therapy and forced migration in Canada. *Canadian Journal of Occupational Therapy, 89*(3), 238–248. https://doi.org/10.1177/00084174221084463.

Lee, H. C. (2006). Virtual driving tests for older adult drivers? *British Journal of Occupational Therapy, 69*(3), 138–141.

Managh, M. F., & Cook, J. V. (1993). The use of standardized assessment in occupational therapy: The BAFPE-R. *American Journal of Occupational Therapy, 47*(10), 877–884. https://doi.org/10.5014/ajot.47.10.877.

Moats, G. (2007). Discharge decision-making, enabling occupations and client-centered practice. *Canadian Journal of Occupational Therapy, 74*, 91–101.

Molineux, M. (2004). Occupation in occupational therapy: A labour in vain? In M. Molineux (Ed.), *Occupation for occupational therapists* (pp. 1–14). Blackwell.

Pereira, R. B. (2012). Viewpoint: The potential of occupational therapy services for students with disabilities within tertiary education settings. *Australian Occupational Therapy Journal, 59*, 393–396.

Phenix, A., & Valavaara, K. (2016). Reflections on the truth and reconciliation commission: Calls to action in occupational therapy. *Occupational Therapy Now, 18*(6), 17–18.

Pizzi, M. A., Reitz, M., & Scaffa, M. E. (2010). Assessments for health promotion practice. In M. E. Scaffa, S. M. Reitz, & M. A. Pizzi (Eds.), *Occupational therapy in the promotion of health and wellness* (pp. 173–194). F. A. Davis.

Polatajko, H., Mandich, A., & Martini, R. (1999). Dynamic performance analysis: A framework for understanding occupational performance. *American Journal of Occupational Therapy, 54*, 65–72. https://doi.org/10.5014/ajot.54.1.65.

Priestley, M. (2005). Disability and social inequalities. In M. Romero, & E. Margolis (Eds.), *The Blackwell companion to social inequalities (Chapter 16)*. Blackwell. https://doi.org/10.1111/b.9780631231547.2005.00021.x.

Psillas, S. M., & Stav, W. B. (2021). Development of the dynamic model of occupation-based practice. *The Open Journal of Occupational Therapy, 9*(4), 1–14. https://doi.org/10.15453/2168-6408.1807.

Quesada, J., Hart, L. K., & Bourgois, P. (2011). Structural vulnerability and health: Latino migrant laborers in the United States. *Medical Anthropology, 30*, 339–362.

Reeve, T., & Gottselig, N. (2011). *Investigating workplace accommodation for people with invisible disabilities*. BC Coalition of People with Disabilities. http://www.disabilityalliancebc.org/docs/employmentinvisibledis.pdf.

Restall, G., Egan, M., Valavaara, K., Phenix, A., & Sack, C. (2022). Canadian occupational therapy inter-relational practice framework. In M. Egan, & G. Restall (Eds.), *Promoting occupational participation: Collaborative relationship-focused occupational therapy* (pp. 119–150). CAOT.

Royal College of Occupational Therapists. (2021). *Professional standards for occupational therapy practice, conduct and ethics*. Royal College of Occupational Therapists. https://www.rcot.co.uk/publications/professional-standards-occupational-therapy-practice-conduct-and-ethics.

Ryall, J., Ritchie, T., Butler, C., Ryan, A., & Gibson, C. (2021). Decolonising occupational therapy through a strengths-based approach. In T. Brown, H. M. Bourke-Taylor, S. Isbel, R. Cordier, & L. Gustafsson (Eds.), *Occupational therapy in Australia: Professional and practice issues* (2nd ed., Chapter 11 pp. 130–142). Routledge. https://doi.org/10.4324/9781003150732-13.

Shotwell, M. P. (2019). Evaluating clients. In B. A. Boyt Schell, & G. Gillen (Eds.), *Willard and Spackman's occupational therapy* (13th ed., pp. 369–389). Wolters Kluwer.

Singh, H., Sangrar, R., Wijekoon, S., Nekolaichuk, E., Kokorelias, K. M., Nelson, M. L. A., Mirzazada, S., Nguyen, T., Assaf, H., & Colquhoun, H. (2022). Applying 'cultural humility' to occupational therapy practice: A scoping review protocol. *BMJ Open, 12*, e063655. https://doi.org/10.1136/bmjopen-2022-063655.

Taylor, E. (2023). Beyond 'bad' behaviors: A call for occupational scientists to rethink autism. *Journal of Occupational Science, 30*(4), 575–590. https://doi.org/10.1080/14427591.2022.2136231.

Thibeault, R (2013). Occupational justice's intents and impacts: From personal choices to community consequences. In M. P. Cutchin, & V. A. Dickie (Eds.), *Transactional perspectives on occupation* (pp. 245–256). Springer.

Thorneycroft, R., & Asquith, N. L. (2021). Unexceptional violence in exceptional times: Disablist and ableist violence during the

COVID-19 pandemic. *International Journal for Crime, Justice and Social Democracy, 10*(2), 140–155.

United Nations. (2006). *Convention on the rights of persons with disabilities.* United Nations.

White, T., & Beagan, B. L. (2020). Occupational therapy roles in an Indigenous context: An integrative review. *Canadian Journal of Occupational Therapy, 87*(3), 200–210. https://doi.org/10.1177/0008417420924933.

White, A., Hocking, C., & Reid, H. (2014). How occupational therapists engage adults with cognitive impairments in assessments. *British Journal of Occupational Therapy, 77*(1), 2–9. https://doi.org/10.4276/030802214X13887685335427.

Whiteford, G. E., & Pereira, R. B. (2012). Occupation, inclusion and participation. In G. E. Whiteford, & C. Hocking (Eds.), *Occupational science: Society, inclusion and participation* (pp. 187–207). Wiley-Blackwell.

Whiteford, G., Townsend, E., & Hocking, C. (2000). Reflections on a renaissance of occupation. *Canadian Journal of Occupational Therapy, 67*(1), 61–69.

World Federation of Occupational Therapists. (2009). *Diversity matters: Guiding principles on diversity and culture.* World Federation of Occupational Therapists. http://www.wfot.org/ResourceCentre/tabid/132/did/306/Default.aspx.

World Federation of Occupational Therapists. (2019). *Position statement: Occupational therapy and human rights.* World Federation of Occupational Therapists. https://www.wfot.org/resources/occupational-therapy-and-human-rights.

World Health Organization. (2001). *International classification of functioning, disability and health.* World Health Organization. http://www.who.int/classifications/icf/en/.

World Health Organization and The World Bank. (2011). *World report on disability.* WHO Press. http://www.who.int/disabilities/world_report/2011/report.pdf.

Yao, D. P. G., Sy, M. P., Martinez, P. G. V., & Laboy, E. C. (2022). Is occupational therapy an ableist health profession? A critical reflection on ableism and occupational therapy. *Cadernos Brasileiros de Terapia Ocupacional, 30*, e3303. https://doi.org/10.1590/2526-8910.ctoRE252733032.

REFLECTION

1. Explain why the process of exploring occupational participation must be collaborative, strengths-based and occupation-focused.

2. Why does the occupational therapy's profession to human rights demand a critical reflection on the occupational therapy assessment process.

3. Identify benefits and limitations of using non-standardised assessments to identify occupational participation needs.

4. Identify benefits and limitation of using standardised assessments to identify occupational participation needs.

5. Discuss with peers the professional and ethical considerations and responsibilities of occupational therapists when exploring the occupational participation of individuals and collectives.

EXPLORING OCCUPATIONAL NEEDS AND EXPANDING OCCUPATIONAL POSSIBILITIES OF COLLECTIVES

MARIE GRANDISSON ■ CATHERINE VALLÉE

Overview

More and more occupational therapists are expanding their scope of practice by engaging with communities in social action or community development initiatives. Occupational therapists are invited to adopt community-centred and community-driven stance, while grounding their interventions in key concepts and values such as empowerment, critical reflexivity, occupational possibilities, collective occupations, capabilities and equity. This chapter not only introduces these concepts but also proposes a practical and iterative approach to guide occupational therapists in exploring and strengthening communities' capacity to expand their occupational possibilities, and by doing so, help them meet valued occupational needs. As occupational therapists engage in collaborative processes with communities, they need to exercise reflexivity to obtain results that will be sustainable, culturally relevant and that will lead to greater equity. Two practice stories illustrate how occupational therapists can support communities to expand occupational possibilities by strengthening their capacities to access, initiate or sustain occupational participation.

KEY POINTS

- Occupational therapists can support communities as they strive to increase their capacity to meet valued occupational needs.

- A relationship-focused approach is needed to partner with communities.

- Reflexivity is necessary throughout the process.

- Five principles to guide processes aimed at expanding the occupational possibilities of a community are proposed: relationship-focused, empowerment, cultural humility, equity, and sustainability.

- An iterative three-step process is proposed: getting to know each other, planning together, and doing and learning together.

- Occupational therapists can support communities to access, initiate or maintain occupational participation through community development initiatives while nurturing an occupational perspective.

INTRODUCTION

In the last decade, occupational therapy guidelines called for a shift in the way occupational therapists view the people they provide services to; occupational therapists are now encouraged to shift their focus from an individualistic perspective to embrace a perspective where they provide services to groups, communities, organisations and populations (Casto et al., 2021; Christiansen et al., 2015; Restall & Egan, 2022; Townsend et al., 2013). Such a change is needed to counter a prevalent perspective where problems of social origin, such as barriers to social and occupational participation are viewed as the result of individual limitations that can be resolved through person-oriented interventions (Restall & Egan, 2022; Wilcock & Hocking, 2015). Other perspectives of occupational therapy practice, coming from South America and South Africa, advocate for and promote a social practice of occupational therapy, done for and with communities (Lopes & Serrata Malfitano, 2021; Ramugundo & Kronenberg, 2015, Sakellariou & Pollard, 2017).

Engaging with population and communities is critical, as occupational therapists strive to reduce social inequalities and influence positively, through occupation, the social determinants of health. As Hammell points out 'if disabled people have the right to equality of occupational opportunity and for full societal participation on an equal basis with others, then occupational therapists do not have the right to focus solely on trying to change individuals' (2015, p. 3).

In this chapter, key concepts associated with community-centred and community-driven practices are defined, occupational therapists' roles in this area are explored and a practical approach assisting occupational therapists to engage with communities in accessing, initiating and sustaining occupational participation is proposed.

DEFINING A COMMUNITY

There is no universal definition of 'community'. It is generally accepted that a community is a group of people sharing an occupational engagement, an interest, an identity, an issue, circumstances or a geographical location in which to work, play or carry out other roles (Hyett et al., 2016; Labonté, 2022; Leclair, 2010; Restall et al., 2005; Townsend et al., 2013). The members of a community may live within a neighbourhood and share common services, or they may be engaged in a virtual community interacting online. A community is often organic, with moving or permeable contours. Beyond the physical features of a community, communities also have a spiritual dimension such as personal or symbolic affiliations and a sense of belonging (Hyett et al., 2016). The community as a place of belonging and affiliation offers leverage for mobilisation and social change. This largely echoes the recent writings on the pan-occupational paradigm which suggests that being, doing and becoming (Wilcock, 1998) constitute a dynamic assemblage, strongly contextualised in belonging (Hitch & Pépin, 2020; Hitch et al., 2018). These authors suggest that belonging remains the strongest determinant of health, wellbeing and justice.

DEFINING COMMUNITY DEVELOPMENT

Community practice generally refers to interventions based in and carried out for a community. It is not a synonym for community development. Rather, community development is one stream of community practice in which interventions are carried out with community members, at every stage of the process (Leclair et al., 2019; Scaffa & Reitz, 2020). It is a collaborative process aimed at building a community's capacity, to help 'people to help themselves' (Rothman et al., 1995, p. 29). Community representatives are considered experts regarding their own situations and are invited to reflect and make decisions on how to address their difficulties (Lauckner et al., 2011). The practitioner generally acts as a facilitator in a process focused on supporting community members to define and solve their problems and on building the community's capacity to develop and implement actions (Labonté, 2022; Leclair, 2010; Leclair et al., 2019). In other words, community development is a community-centred and community-driven process aimed at providing greater opportunities for all to participate actively in their communities, including disadvantaged groups (Lauckner et al., 2007).

Rothman and colleagues (1995) propose three levels of community intervention: locality development, social planning/policy and social action. While locality development is more often associated with community development, adding social planning and social action can be at times more effective (Rothman et al., 1995). These levels can help occupational therapists see a continuum of community development initiatives (Lauckner et al., 2011) and draw on the approach or approaches that best suit their situation. Social action initiatives, which emphasise advocacy to change social structures and redistribute decision-making power and resources, are also compatible with community development, especially when community members are actively involved throughout the process. Thus, a community development practitioner may work with community groups to define their priorities and explore potential action plans, locate empirical data to choose a target group or to facilitate group decisions, build local capacity and/or foster change by transferring knowledge and skills, referring to other resources, or advocating.

OCCUPATIONAL THERAPY AND COMMUNITY DEVELOPMENT

Community development in occupational therapy is a powerful and sustainable way of engaging with a community to strengthen its capacity to freely expand its occupational possibilities and, by doing so, facilitate participation in valued occupations. Occupational possibilities refer to the ways and types of doing that come to be viewed as ideal and possible and that are promoted and made available within that context (Laliberte Rudman, 2005). Occupational possibilities are often created, shaped, limited or perceived through the influence of everyday power structures. Structural and environmental factors such as socio-political and sociohistorical contexts, culture, public discourses, institutions and laws greatly impact occupational possibilities (Laliberte Rudman, 2005, 2010, 2013). Such influences may dissuade participation in occupations tacitly framed as nonideal or unhealthy, thus limiting one's occupational possibilities (Njelesani et al., 2015) or perpetuating occupational injustices (Laliberte Rudman, 2010). Expanding occupational possibilities may be done by questioning what is taken for granted and by facilitating change in the micro, meso or macro contexts to facilitate access to, initiation of

or maintenance of occupational participation (Egan & Restall, 2022).

Strengthening the capacity of a community to expand its occupational possibilities to meet valued goals is not efficient if opportunities are limited and constrained or if power dynamics prevent community members from engaging freely in occupations that are in accordance with what they value. The capability approach is the relevant approach to use when exploring occupational needs and possibilities (refer to Chapter 10). This strength-based and rights-focused approach allows the exploration of the real opportunities available to individuals within their environments and how they can freely (or not) enact their valued choices. Capabilities are not just a set of abilities or capacities expressed by a person or a group. There are shaped, in various life domains, by three interrelated elements (Bailliard, 2016; Hammell, 2015, 2016, 2021):

1. Functioning: what people are able to achieve, what they are able to do and who they are able to be;
2. Opportunities: the real alternatives that are available and
3. Agency: the freedom to choose and the power to accomplish what is valued.

Through a community-centred and community-driven process, occupational therapists can assist communities in defining their occupational needs and expand opportunities for occupational participation by fostering the development of communities' capabilities (Peters & Galvaan, 2021), building supportive environments or modifying occupational demands. While some occupational therapists have positions in which their main role is to strengthen the capacity of a community or an organisation, many work with individuals experiencing disruptions in their occupations. These occupational therapists often come to see patterns or trends of occupational needs or common barriers faced by the people they work with (Lauckner et al., 2019). These patterns can be opportunities to propose a different focus, an opportunity to explore communities' occupational needs and engage in actions that will empower community members or that will remove barriers for many people. Table 14.1 presents examples from the literature on how occupational therapists can be involved to strengthen a community's capacity to meet its occupational needs.

TABLE 14.1
Examples of Occupational Therapy Implications to Strengthen a Community's Capacity to Meet Their Occupational Needs

- Engage with women in a residential area to help them advocate for resources to develop their daily living skills (Restall et al., 2005).
- Educate tenants of a seniors' apartment building to enable them to respond to peers' health and quality of life needs (Cockburn & Trentham, 2002).
- Collaborate with individuals with physical impairments and municipal recreation facilities' staff to identify barriers to participation for all. Use universal design principles to remove barriers (Restall et al., 2005).
- Design a user-friendly tool for improving environmental accessibility in recreational programs (Banks & Head, 2004).
- Design age-friendly environments considering the entire bus transport chain, the consequences of aging on skills and on assistive device use and environmental factors. Act as a consultant and advocate for environmental changes (Broome et al., 2009).
- Collaborate with youth, community leaders and interested residents of a neighbourhood to create opportunities for youth to engage in healthier occupations by helping them identify a new occupation (i.e. creating art) and find the place and resources to carry it out (Restall et al., 2005).
- Collaborate with people who have had a stroke, rehabilitation centre staff and a community partner to design a pilot peer-mentoring project and help them develop the skills needed to implement it (Lauckner et al., 2011).
- Coordinate services by linking seniors with volunteer opportunities in a community garden and a neighbourhood project (Lauckner et al., 2011).
- Collaborate with community members in identifying a shared occupation and engage them in developing opportunities for all to participate in it. Engage them in developing the community garden. Coordinate with organisations to obtain land, plants, benches or other resources (Leclair, 2010).
- Coach a group of outpatients to create meaningful work for themselves (Cockburn & Trentham, 2002).
- Supporting an advocacy group that aimed at making the neighbourhood more accessible and supportive for seniors through several actions/projects leading to the creation of a grocery delivery guide for homebound seniors; improvements in the urban planning/safety and increased sidewalks adaptations (Trentham et al., 2007)
- Advocate for playgrounds facilitating access and use by all children and caregivers, including those with disabilities (Ripat & Becker, 2012).

Five Principles to Expand Occupational Possibilities

Five principles to guide processes aimed at expanding occupational possibilities of a community are proposed: relationship-focused, empowerment, cultural humility, equity, and sustainability.

Relationship-Focused

Occupational therapists should always keep in mind that nurturing relationships with the community should be their priority, as no projects will really be successful if community members do not feel valued or listened to. As Thibeault (personal communications, 2011) says, occupational therapists should focus on: 'Partners before projects'. Community development requires the development of authentic partnerships with organisations or stakeholders belonging to the targeted community, partnerships in which everyone's contributions and opinions are valued (Doll, 2009; Labonté, 2022; Letts et al., 2022). It requires a commitment to collaborate (Labonté, 2022). Expanding

occupational possibilities should be done for, but most importantly, with communities (Letts et al., 2022). Occupational therapists should focus on developing and nurturing their relationships with communities (Restall et al., 2022). Having knowledge of collaborative practices and being able to develop community partnerships are therefore necessary when working with communities (Leclair et al., 2019).

Empowerment

Empowerment is the process by which individuals are given a voice and a place to participate in decisions that affect them or their daily lives (Braveman et al., 2009). It can be defined as 'an intentional, ongoing process centered in the local community, involving mutual respect, critical reflection, caring and group participation, through which people lacking an equal share of valued resources gain greater access to and control over those resources' (Salzer, 1997, pp. 426–427). For some, occupational engagement is perceived as the first step toward empowerment. In sharing responsibilities and supporting self-determination of community members, occupational therapists must grant others and themselves the right to make mistakes, optimise access to information and offer meaningful alternatives. Moreover, occupational therapists must consider that empowerment is always context-specific; therefore, occupational therapists must continually consider the evolution and shifts of power dynamics throughout their work. In essence, they support local leaders and champions in making their voices heard and act as facilitators rather than as experts (Galvaan & Peters, 2017; Leclair et al., 2019).

Cultural Humility

To remain relevant and respectful of the community members they engage with, occupational therapists must establish culturally nuanced relationships (Restall & Egan, 2022) by cultivating cultural humility. Cultural humility translates into being open-minded, endorsing the perspective that each person is a lifelong learner while maintaining constant reflexivity on the potential influence of biases and preconceptions (Agner, 2020; Foronda et al., 2016). Additionally, cultural humility requires practitioners to recognise the impact of power differences that may exist between providers and people receiving health services (Agner, 2020; Foronda, 2020; Kools et al., 2015). In community development, this applies to all the relationships between occupational therapists and citizens. Occupational therapists must also recognise their privileges, the 'colonialist' aspects that underlie professional knowledge and the value of local and experiential knowledge (Auger et al., 2019; Beagan, 2015; Curtis et al., 2019; Gerlach, 2012; Hammell, 2013; Jasmin et al., 2019).

Equity

Occupational therapists engaged with a community should be mindful of subgroups within the community that may have greater occupational needs and should be careful not to create larger inequities within the community. They should focus on providing more equitable occupational opportunities so that all people, regardless of their individual profiles, can have their occupational needs met (Hammell, 2020). Restall et al. (2018) propose the application of an equity lens to evaluate whether programs and services create inequities. It calls for considerations of diverse elements in the process, including the identification of groups experiencing inequities, of the cause of the inequities and of whether the issue is related to access, utilisation or quality. Health inequities are preventable, systematic and socially produced differences in health between and within populations (Jull & Giles, 2012; World Health Organization, 2018). Individuals and groups may experience inequities in relation to different characteristics they have or who they happen to be (Nixon, 2019). This includes, for example, people's gender, their socioeconomic status, their abilities or neurological profiles, the colour of their skin, their language or the place where they live. One potential way to make sure initiatives do not further disadvantage some subgroups is to think of the different elements known to influence access to services. These include, for example, the acceptability and affordability of the services, as well as the ability to reach them and to engage in them (Davy et al., 2016).

Sustainability

Community development is a strength-based intervention, building on existing strengths and resources. Instead of fixing a 'what is wrong', such initiatives strive for consolidating what is strong within the community and creating sustainable options. One of the ongoing challenges is to seek and secure ongoing funding or support. Although community development requires a long-term commitment from practitioners (and community members), occupational therapists should carefully plan a transitional phase that will allow them to phase out and let community members take full control of their initiative (Dhillion et al., 2015; Leclair et al., 2019; Restall & Egan, 2022).

PRACTICAL APPLICATION TO OCCUPATIONAL THERAPY

In this section, a practical approach to guide occupational therapists in strengthening a community's capacity to meet its meaningful occupational needs is presented. This approach aligns with key principles of community development as well as recent occupational therapy models and processes. It is intended to offer guidance to facilitate occupational therapists' involvement in community development or social action initiatives. However, flexibility and sensitivity to local characteristics are essential; this approach should not be rigidly followed since other models may also be relevant.

The proposed approach is grounded in the five steps for community development practice (Leclair et al., 2019), while it attempts to further articulate the notion that the occupational therapist and the community are engaged in the process together, as they get to know each other, as they plan and as they do and learn together. This is aligned with the recent Canadian guidelines for occupational therapy practice recognising the critical place that relationships and contexts play in service delivery (Restall & Egan, 2022). As recommended in these guidelines, the proposed process

emphasises that learning occurs while implementing the plan and that occupational therapists need to be open to modifying the plan as it evolves. It involves three steps:

1. Getting to know each other;
2. Planning together and
3. Doing and learning together.

It is expected to be iterative and to be done with the community, in a manner that makes sense to that community. The three-step process is illustrated in two practice stories in Box 14.1 and 14.2.

The three-step process is anchored in reflexivity, following Irvine-Brown et al. (2022) work on praxis and the call for critical reflection in a collaborative

---

BOX 14.1
PARTNERING WITH A REGIONAL ASSOCIATION FOR PEOPLE WITH TRAUMATIC BRAIN INJURY

BACKGROUND

A regional association provides services to people with moderate to severe traumatic brain injury (TBI) who have severe cognitive and motor limitations. The goal of the services provided is to enable people with TBI to participate in meaningful occupations through adapted work, support meetings, board games, scrapbooking, cooking, painting, hockey and a monthly journal publication. Three staff members and ten volunteers deliver most of the services.

Ann is an occupational therapist who frequently refers individuals to this association following rehabilitation. She contacted the manager of this association to determine whether and how two occupational therapy students could be involved in the association during an 8-week fieldwork placement focused on community development, which she would supervise.

STEP 1 GETTING TO KNOW EACH OTHER

Upon acceptance, the occupational therapy students, Sarah and Jason, started their placement by getting to know the organisation's staff members and volunteers, participating in the organisation's activities and becoming familiar with the organisation's mission, services, target population and culture. The students then explained their vision of what they could contribute to the association. However, the students and the association's representatives struggled to understand occupational therapy's potential contribution to community development, as they were more familiar with occupational therapy's traditional roles in rehabilitation centres. Support from the students' supervisor was key to clarifying each other's expectations.

STEP 2 PLANNING TOGETHER

The students then facilitated a discussion with community representatives using the Tree of Occupational Needs and Possibilities. After considering different options, a consensus emerged that it was critical to improve access to the different activities in the centre for all members, staff and volunteers, whatever equipment they use to move around and whatever their capacities are.

STEP 3 DOING AND LEARNING TOGETHER

To achieve this, the students facilitated two workshops with interested staff, volunteers and members with TBI who had a variety of profiles (e.g. using a wheelchair or a cane, with or without cognitive limitations). Together, they designed a reconfiguration of the facilities taking into consideration how the rooms are used, the abilities of the people with TBI and feasibility of implementing change. At the end of the students' fieldwork, the association had a detailed plan of the improved facilities in their hands. Ann, the occupational therapy supervisor, supported the organisation in implementing the plan, including looking for funding for small renovations, moving furniture around and making accessible signs to clarify activities held in each room.

Six months later, the organisation was satisfied with the changes and felt that the occupational need had been addressed. While Ann could leave at this point, organisation representatives mentioned that they would like to have her support to improve the perseverance of members with TBI in the adapted work program provided by the organisation. A new cycle had begun.

BOX 14.2

STARTING FROM A COMMON ISSUE EXPERIENCED BY INDIVIDUALS SEEN IN A CLINIC

BACKGROUND

An occupational therapist working in a community centre realised that many of the people she saw in her one-on-one services faced the same issue: they were refused access to adapted transportation. This issue hindered progress towards their occupational goals as they were limited in the places they could go on their own and many of them were frustrated by the situation. The occupational therapist talked to her manager to propose a different way of responding to this situation – to move away from her traditional role to invest some of her time into a special project to facilitate access to adapted transportation services. Coming to her manager with convincing arguments (e.g. number of people facing the issue, impact of the issue on the most vulnerable, importance of doing something, time spent in advocacy actions with and for each individual), she received the needed support from her manager to invest up to one day a week on this project.

STEP 1 GETTING TO KNOW EACH OTHER

She reviewed information from her records and asked her colleagues whether some of the people they saw experienced similar issues. She also involved the individuals who had been refused access to participate in the small social action initiative to raise awareness about the issue and influence decision-makers. Together, they realised that whenever the primary diagnosis was related to mental health, even though many also had mobility issues, individuals were denied access to the adapted transportation services.

STEP 2 PLANNING TOGETHER

They developed an action plan that would allow them to raise awareness about the issue and document barriers. They decided to hop on the bus in various neighbourhoods to go along different bus routes at different times of the day. The occupational therapist provided transportation to the different neighbourhoods, organised data collection and accompanied a few volunteers in their actions.

STEP 3 DOING AND LEARNING TOGETHER

As a bus stopped, they tried to access it – but buses could not accommodate their scooters or their wheelchairs, the floor could not be lowered, etc. Every time, they noted the name of the bus driver and asked the driver to confirm that they could not access the bus independently. Meanwhile, other group members wrote a letter and requested a meeting with stakeholders perceived to hold power over the situation, including the local transportation agency and municipal decision-makers.

The occupational therapist and a person with lived experience of the issue went to the transportation service office to deliver the letter and they requested a meeting with a manager. When that meeting happened, the person with lived experience presented most of the information and explained how decisions like that had a very negative impact on their lives and their social participation. The occupational therapist was also there to explain how this issue affected many of the individuals she saw in different ways and to answer questions.

The manager was already aware of how this directive was arbitrary and how it impacted services, having heard from bus drivers encountered by the group. The manager asked what the group's recommendations would be.

STEP 2: PLANNING TOGETHER

A second wave of activities was initiated – as the group decided to plan how they would develop the recommendations. They decided to run focus groups with those who were experiencing the services or denied access to the services and with professionals working with them. The occupational therapist was one of the professionals invited to participate in the focus groups.

STEP 3: DOING AND LEARNING TOGETHER

The group ran the focus groups and then shared the lessons learned in each group together. They drafted the recommendations together and then met the manager to share them. One of the individuals with lived experience shared the group's recommendations. The occupational therapist was present to answer questions specific to the therapist's expertise but was not the designated spokesperson.

---

relationship-focused approach (Restall & Egan, 2022). This is meant to highlight that occupational therapists should reflect on themselves, reflect on actions, take a step back to try to understand why certain practices are effective or not, exchange with community members on this matter and draw on the evidence available (Irvine-Brown et al., 2022). While such reflexivity is encouraged throughout the process, planning specific times to reflect, write and have a dialogue with community representatives may help bring the reflections further (Irvine-Brown et al., 2022).

As presented in Fig. 14.1, this reflexivity can be guided by the key principles of empowerment, cultural humility, equity and sustainability. Reflective questions are provided in the Table 14.2 to support this critical reflexivity.

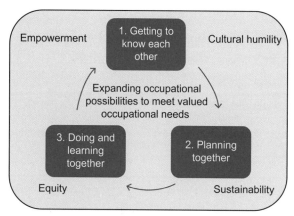

Fig. 14.1 ■ Process proposed to strengthen communities' capacities to expand their occupational possibilities to meet valued occupational needs.

TABLE 14.2
Examples of Questions That Can Be Reflected on During the Process

- What biases do I have regarding this community?
- How can power and privilege be considered in our relationship?
- Do we focus enough on developing and nurturing our partnership?
- How can we value the perspectives of all the people involved?
- How can I make sure community members have the freedom to choose what they value the most?
- How can I present myself as a facilitator?
- How can we improve the likelihood that the subgroups experiencing inequities be reached?
- How can we share power and responsibilities in the plan?
- How can we plan something that will be sustainable, even if I leave?
- Does our plan include actions at all meaningful context levels?
- Do we build from the strengths of community members and from the community assets?
- Do we foster belonging?
- Which changes are needed to our initial plan?
- How can I amplify the voice of the most concerned individuals?
- Are my actions still needed or should I gradually hand over responsibilities?

Step 1: Getting to Know Each Other

Step 1 emphasises the need for occupational therapists and community members to develop or consolidate their partnership. While getting to know each other is particularly important when occupational therapists and communities engage for the first time, occupational therapists should not take for granted what they have learned about a community in previous experiences or in other contexts. Occupational therapists should devote time, before trying to do formal evaluations, to get to know the community's identity, culture, strengths, leaders, safe spaces, occupations, resources and barriers. This includes listening to the language used by community members to talk about occupations, health, disability, equity and their situations. While getting to know the community, occupational therapists should keep in mind the situated nature of occupations, namely the dynamic and transactional interactions between the occupations and the context in which they are situated (Aldrich & Laliberte Rudman, 2016; Cutchin & Dickie, 2013; Lavalley, 2017).

Occupational therapists should strive to identify the existing assets, strengths and resources of the community rather than focusing mainly on occupational issues, which are often more obvious. Occupational therapists should also consider how the physical, social, cultural, political and economic context shape occupational possibilities within the community. Collective occupations should also be explored, as they are critical in meeting belonging needs, cocreating meaning, building shared goods and resources or re-writing community history (Kantartzis, 2017; Kantartzis & Molineux, 2017; Ramugondo & Kronenberg, 2015).

In this step, community members also need to gain an understanding of who the occupational therapist is, what their role can be and what is their practice context. Both parties should recognise the historical, political and societal context of their relationship, including notions of power and privilege (Restall & Egan, 2022). Guidance regarding the elements that can be documented in the occupational therapy process during the first step is provided in Table 14.3.

An informal, collaborative relationship-focused approach (refer to Chapter 12) is used to get to know the community (Leclair et al., 2019) and for the community to get to know the occupational therapist. This may include walking in the community, attending meaningful activities or events, spending time in community places and observing and having conversations with various community members, including local leaders. Care should be given to making sure the methods chosen to get to know each other are appropriate

TABLE 14.3

Guidance Regarding Step 1: Getting to Know Each Other

Key questions or what you both need to better understand

Who is this community?

- What is important for me to know regarding the culture of this community (identity, values, history, relationships, daily habits, meaning, language, patterns of occupational needs, sense of belonging)?
- What are the main strengths of this community?
- Who are the communities' leaders and the social actors?
- What are the safe spaces or meaningful projects in this community?
- What subgroups experience iniquities regarding occupational participation?
- What occupations or collective occupations are important?
- How does change happen in this community?
- What are the main resources and barriers in the community?

What does the community know about occupational therapy in community development?

- What are the expectations of community members and leaders?
- How does my practice context influence our relationship?
- What is important regarding the historical, political and societal context of our relationship?

to the context, that they are not imposed by the occupational therapist and that they make sense for the people involved. While occupational therapists can also review important documents, websites or social media of this community to learn about the community, they should focus on listening to the stories of the community and observing their ways of doing.

Step 2. Planning Together

Step 2 involves understanding the community's priorities regarding the occupational need they would most like to see change happening for and for which they would like the occupational therapist to be involved. Occupational therapists should be mindful that even if an occupational need exists and is often expressed, it does not mean that community members wish to engage in a process with the occupational therapist. Other options may be preferred, sometimes without professional intervention. Once an occupational need has been selected, the main barriers can be examined and possible facilitators identified. Occupational therapists and community members then work together

to plan actions to expand occupational possibilities. This may involve facilitating access to, initiation of or maintenance of occupational participation for the larger community or for one or more subgroups (Egan & Restall, 2022).

This plan is designed together, making sure that the actions chosen align with the culture of the community and do not further disadvantage an already disadvantaged subgroup (Restall et al., 2018). Occupational therapists should have in mind the importance of creating safe spaces within the community (Leclair et al., 2019), spaces in which everyone feels comfortable sharing their thoughts and wishes, even when they disagree with the majority, spaces in which everyone feels respected and valued. Occupational therapists should also attempt to provide opportunities for social connectedness (Leclair et al., 2019). As they support the community in making decisions regarding the plan, they can strategically use their position, skills and resources to build community members' capacity (e.g. as peer-mentors), to strengthen existing resources or programs, to link sectors and resources or to influence health care (Lauckner et al., 2011). Social actions can also be considered and planned to remove contextual barriers to occupational participation not only with senior managers but also with political actors at different levels (Carrier et al., 2021; Dhillion et al., 2015; Leclair et al., 2019). Guidance regarding what needs to be documented in Step 2 is provided in Table 14.4.

Occupational therapists act as facilitators, sharing information regarding occupational possibilities or potential political actions that might help expand occupational possibilities. The occupational therapist can use formal and informal methods to develop the plan with community members. The *Tree of Occupational Needs and Possibilities* and the *Occupational Priority Scale* might be used and adapted to facilitate conversations with community members. The *Tree of Occupational Needs and Possibilities* (Fig. 14.2) may be used to structure the process of exploring occupational needs and generating ideas regarding barriers, facilitators and actions that could be done to expand occupational possibilities. This tool was inspired by the *Problem Tree* proposed by Chevalier and Buckles (2021). A step-by-step approach to using this tool is presented in Table 14.5.

TABLE 14.4

Guidance Regarding Step 2: Planning Together

Key questions or what you both need to better understand

Which occupational need(s) would the community most like to see change?

- For whom is it a need?
- Which one is most important to them?
- Why is that a priority?
- What would mobilise them??
- Whether the priority is to improve access, to initiate or to sustain participation?
- What would be most meaningful to work on with the occupational therapist?
- What would the situation look like if this need was addressed?

What are the main barriers and facilitators with regard to this occupational need?

- What are the main strengths and resources that are in place or that can be used to address this need (within the community, the health system, politics or natural support systems)?
- What are the characteristics of the occupation (e.g. demands, flexibility, context)?
- Who holds power regarding the situation?
- What resistance might there be?
- Is there political support?

How can prioritised occupational needs be met building on the community's strengths and resources?

- How can we facilitate links with existing resources in the health system or in the community to expand occupational possibilities?
- How can community members' capacity be strengthened (e.g. leadership)?
- How can we develop further occupational opportunities or safe spaces?
- How can we build upon occupational opportunities that already exist?
- How can the occupation be modified to facilitate participation?
- How can we promote social connectedness?
- How can we remove barriers or influence the system?
- How can we advocate or support self-advocacy?
- How can local leaders or champions be involved?
- How can social media be used to mobilise the community?
- At which context level(s) should actions be done?
- How can funding be mobilised and sustained?
- What are the priorities for action?

The *Occupational Priority Scale* (Fig. 14.3), inspired by the *Contribution and Feasibility* tool proposed by Chevalier and Buckles (2021), can be useful to support communities in their decision-making regarding which occupational need should be prioritised and which action(s) are most critical among different options. For each occupational need or potential action, the occupational therapist asks community members to position it on the vertical line, representing the value given by the community to this occupational need or potential action. They may consider the urgency of doing something, how meaningful it would be for community members and how the impact would be distributed among community members. Then, the occupational therapist asks community members to position the same occupational need or potential

action on the horizontal line, representing feasibility or the likeliness to yield sustainable change in occupational possibilities.

Step 3. Doing and Learning Together

Step 3 emphasises the need for occupational therapists not only to collaboratively plan actions that would be implemented by community actors but also to support the community in implementing these actions. The occupational therapist should share power and responsibilities with community leaders and members (Lauckner et al., 2011) in a manner that is acceptable to all the parties involved and that fosters sustainability (Hyett et al., 2019; Lauckner et al., 2019). The use of multiple methods simultaneously, the importance of having good leaders and of

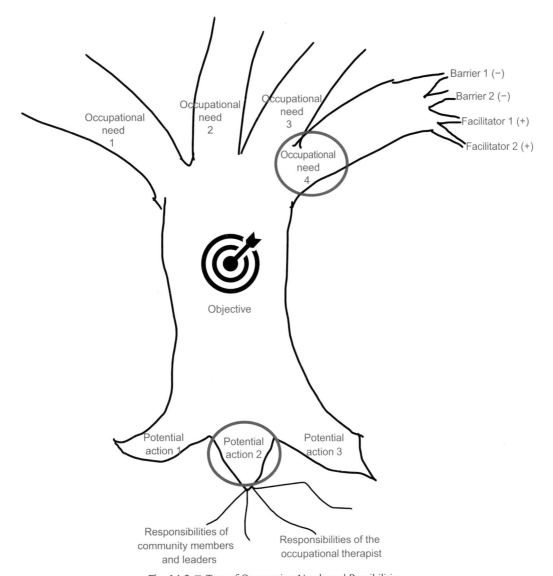

Fig. 14.2 ■ Tree of Occupation Needs and Possibilities.

growing participation through social media is suggested by Hyett et al. (2019). This step also centres on the importance of learning in action, of checking in regularly to verify whether the needs are met, adjustments or further support are required and new needs emerged. Dhillion and colleagues (2015) highlight the importance of knowing when to step back, of being able to identify when to hand over responsibility or when the community does not need the occupational therapist's input anymore. Learning is intentionally emphasised in this step to invite occupational therapists and community members to use reflexivity and keep a humble and open mind to make necessary changes while the process evolves. Guidance regarding what needs to be documented in Step 3 is presented in Table 14.6.

TABLE 14.5
A Step-by-Step Approach to Using the Tree of Occupational Needs and Possibilities Tool

1) **Write the main occupational needs on the tree branches:** Discuss the occupational need(s) for which the community would most like to see change and what the situation would look like if it was addressed.

2) **Circle the prioritised occupational need:** Which one is most important for them? Why is that a priority? Whether the priority is to improve access, to initiate or to sustain participation? For whom is it a priority? The Occupational Priority Scale may be used.

3) **Write the main barriers (–) and facilitators (+) with regards to this prioritised occupational need on the smaller branches:** Make sure to focus on strengths and resources in place and to consider potential resistance.

4) **Write objectives on the tree trunk:** Focus on occupational participation and changes that need to happen in the context.

5) **Write potential actions to expand occupational possibilities on the tree roots:** Make sure to consider actions at diverse levels and to be congruent with your analysis of the barriers and facilitators.

6) **Circle the prioritised actions:** Focus on actions that are valued and likely to yield sustainable change. The Occupational Priority Scale may be used.

7) **Write how you plan to share responsibilities on the smaller roots:** Make sure to foster empowerment and sustainability and to consider how local champions and social media can play a role.

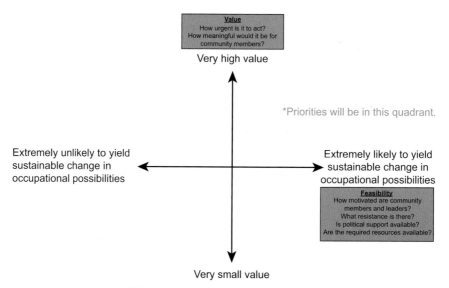

Fig. 14.3 ■ Occupational Priority Scale.

TABLE 14.6
Guidance Regarding Step 3: Doing and Learning Together

Key questions or what you both need to better understand

How can we share responsibilities in implementing the plan to expand occupational possibilities?
■ What has been done? What has not?
■ Who is mobilised? Who is not?

What can we learn from the action or from the result of our actions?
■ Has change happened? In what direction? For whom?
■ Are some community members left behind? Why?
■ What can we learn from the challenges encountered?
■ How can we do better?
■ What further trainings or reflections do we need to undertake?

CONCLUSION

Occupational therapists can play an important role in strengthening communities' capacity to fulfil their most important occupational needs. By focusing on developing and nurturing relationships with community members and leaders, they can help expand occupational possibilities in a sustainable way. A practical approach to achieve this has been presented in this chapter. It is hoped that this will contribute to enhancing occupational therapists' desire and confidence to be engaged with communities, whatever their practice context is. Research evaluating occupational therapy initiatives to strengthen communities' capacities is needed to help build the evidence base in this area, encourage others to take on this challenge and convince decision-makers that it is more than time to invest in community development using an occupational lens.

REFERENCES

Agner, J. (2020). Moving from cultural competence to cultural humility in occupational therapy: A paradigm shift. *The American Journal of Occupational Therapy, 74*(4), 7404347010p1–7404347010p7. https://doi.org/10.5014/ajot.2020.038067.

Aldrich, R., & Laliberte Rudman, D. (2016). Situational analysis: A visual analytic approach that unpacks the complexity of occupation. *Journal of Occupational Science, 23*(1), 51–66. https://doi.org/10.1080/14427591.2015.1045014.

Auger, M., Crooks, C. V., Lapp, A., Tsuruda, S., Caron, C., Rogers, B. J., & van der Woerd, K. (2019). The essential role of cultural safety in developing culturally-relevant prevention programming in First Nations Communities: Lessons learned from a national evaluation of Mental Health First Aid First Nations. *Evaluation and Program Planning, 72*, 188–196. https://doi.org/10.1016/j.evalprogplan.2018.10.016.

Bailliard, A. (2016). Justice, difference, and the capability to function. *Journal of Occupational Science, 23*(1), 3–16. https://doi.org/10.1080/14427591.2014.957886.

Banks, S., & Head, B. (2004). Partnering occupational therapy and community development. *Canadian Journal of Occupational Therapy, 71*(1), 5–8. https://doi.org/10.1177/000841740407100104.

Beagan, B. L. (2015). Approaches to culture and diversity: A critical synthesis of occupational therapy literature. *Canadian Journal of Occupational Therapy, 82*(5), 272–282. https://doi.org/10.1177/0008417414567530.

Braveman, B., & Suarez-Balcazar, Y. (2009). Social justice and resource utilization in a community-based organization: A case illustration of the role of the occupational therapist. *American Journal of Occupational Therapy, 63*(1), 13–23.

Broome, K., McKenna, K., Fleming, J., & Worrall, L. (2009). Bus use and older people: A literature review applying the Person-Environment-Occupational model in macro practice.

Scandinavian Journal of Occupational Therapy, 16, 3–12. https://doi.org/10.1080/11038120802326222.

Carrier, A., Éthier, A., Beaudoin, M., Hudon, A., Bédard, D., Jasmin, E., & Verville, F. (2021). Acting as change agents: Insights into Québec occupational therapists' current practice. *Canadian Journal of Occupational Therapy, 88*(2), 173–181. https://doi.org/10.1177/0008417421994367.

Casto, S. C., Davis, C., Dorsey, J., Lannigan, E. L. G., Metzger, L., Miller, J., Owens, A., Rives, K., Synovec, C., Winistorfer, W. L., Lieberman, D., & Revised by the Commission on Practice, 2020. (2021). Standards of practice for occupational therapy. *The American Journal of Occupational Therapy, 75*(Supplement_3), 7513410030. https://doi.org/10.5014/ajot.2021.75S3004.

Chevalier, J. M., & Buckles, D. J. (2021). *Handbook for participatory action research, planning and evaluation*. SAS² Dialogue.

Christiansen, C., Baum, C. M., & Bass, J. D. (2015). *Occupational therapy: Performance, participation, and well-being* (4th ed.). SLACK Incorporated.

Cockburn, L., & Trentham, B. (2002). Participatory action research: Integrating community occupational therapy practice and research. *Canadian Journal of Occupational Therapy, 69*, 20–30. https://doi.org/10.1177/000841740206900102.

Curtis, E., Jones, R., Tipene-Leach, D., Walker, C., Loring, B., Paine, S. J., & Reid, P. (2019). Why cultural safety rather than cultural competency is required to achieve health equity: A literature review and recommended definition. *International Journal for Equity in Health, 18*(1), 174. https://doi.org/10.1186/s12939-019-1082-3.

Cutchin, M. P., & Dickie, V. A. (2013). *Transactional perspectives on occupation*. Springer. https://doi.org/10.1007/978-94-007-4429-5.

Davy, C., Harfield, S., McArthur, A., Munn, Z., & Brown, A. (2016). Access to primary health care services for Indigenous peoples: A framework synthesis. *International Journal for Equity in Health, 15*, 163. https://doi.org/10.1186/s12939-016-0450-5.

Dhillion, S., Wilkins, S., Stewart, D., & Law, M. (2015). Understanding advocacy in action: A qualitative study. *British Journal of Occupational Therapy, 79*(6), 345–352. https://doi.org/10.1177/0308022615583305.

Doll, J. (2009). *Program development and grant writing in occupational therapy: Making the connection*. Jones & Bartlett Learning.

Egan, M., & Restall, G. (2022). Chapitre 4: Modèle Canadien de la participation occupationnelle. In G. Restall, & M. Egan (Eds.), *Promoting occupational participation: Collaborative relationship-focused occupational therapy* (4th ed., pp. 81–106). Canadian Association of Occupational Therapists.

Finlayson, M. (2007). Community-based practice: Assessing community needs and strengths. *OT Practice, 12*(5), 29–31.

Foronda, C. (2020). A theory of cultural humility. *Journal of Transcultural Nursing, 31*(1), 7–12. https://doi.org/10.1177/1043659619875184.

Foronda, C., Baptiste, D. L., Reinholdt, M. M., & Ousman, K. (2016). Cultural humility: A concept analysis. *J Transcult Nurs, 27*(3), 210–217. https://doi.org/10.1177/1043659615592677.

Galvaan, R., & Peters, L. (2017). Occupation-based community development: Confronting the politics of occupation. In D. Sakellariou, & N. Pollard (Eds.), *Occupational Therapies without borders: Integrating justice with practice* (pp. 283–291). Elsevier press.

Gerlach, A. J. (2012). A critical reflection on the concept of cultural safety. *Canadian Journal of Occupational Therapy, 79*(3), 151–158. https://doi.org/10.2182/cjot.2012.79.3.4.

Hammell, K. W. (2013). Occupation, well-being, and culture: Theory and cultural humility. *Canadian Journal of Occupational Therapy, 80*(4), 224–234. https://doi.org/10.1177/0008417413500465.

Hammell, K. W. (2015). Occupational rights and critical occupational therapy: Rising to the challenge. *Australian Occupational Therapy Journal, 62*, 449–451. https://doi.org/10.1111/1440-1630.12195.

Hammell, K. W. (2016). Empowerment and occupation: A new perspective. *Canadian Journal of Occupational Therapy, 83*(5), 281–287. https://doi.org/10.1177/0008417416652910.

Hammell, K. W. (2020). Action on the social determinants of health: Advancing occupational equity and occupational rights. *Cadernos Brasileiros de Terapia Ocupacional, 28*(1), 378–400. https://doi.org/10.4322/2526-8910.ctoARF2052.

Hammell, K. W. (2021). Securing occupational rights by addressing capabilities: A professional obligation. *Scandinavian Journal of Occupational Therapy, 29*(1), 1–12. https://doi.org/10.1080/11038128.2021.1895308.

Hitch, D., & Pepin, G. (2020). Doing, being, becoming and belonging at the heart of occupational therapy: An analysis of theoretical ways of knowing. *Scandinavian Journal of Occupational Therapy*, 1–13. 1–13. https://doi.org/10.1080/11038128.2020.1726454.

Hitch, D., Pepin, G., & Stagnitti, K. (2018). The pan occupational paradigm: Development and key concepts. *Scandinavian Journal of Occupational Therapy, 25*(1), 27–34.

Hyett, N., Kenny, A., & Dickson-Swift, V. (2019). Re-imagining occupational therapy clients as communities: Presenting the community-centred practice framework. *Scandinavian Journal of Occupational Therapy, 26*(4), 246–260. https://doi.org/10.1080/11038128.2017.1423374.

Hyett, N., McKinstry, C. E., Kenny, A., & Dickson-Swift, V. (2016). Community-centred practice: Occupational therapists improving the health and wellbeing of populations. *Australian Occupational Therapy Journal, 63*(1), 5–8. https://doi.org/10.1111/1440-1630.12222.

Irvine-Brown, L., Ware, V. A., & Serrata-Malfitano, A. P. (2022). Exploring the praxis of occupational therapy-community development practitioners. *Canadian Journal of Occupational Therapy, 89*(1), 26–35. https://doi.org/10.1177/00084174211066662.

Jasmin, E., Masse, J., & Stucki, V. (2019). La diversité culturelle. In E. Jasmin (Ed.), *Des sciences sociales à l'ergothérapie: Mieux comprendre la société et la culture pour mieux agir comme spécialiste en habilitation à l'occupation* (1st ed., pp. 214–249). Presses de l'Université du Québec.

Jull, J. E. G., & Giles, A. R. (2012). Health equity, Aboriginal peoples and occupational therapy. *Canadian Journal of Occupational Therapy, 79*(2), 70–76. https://doi.org/10.2182/cjot.2012.79.2.2.

Kantartzis, S. (2017). Exploring occupation beyond the individual: Family and collective occupations. In D. Sakellariou, N. Pollard, D. Laliberté Rudman, & A. Guajardo (Eds.), *Occupational therapies without borders: Integrating justice with practice* (2nd ed., pp. 19–28). Elsevier.

Kantartzis, S., & Molineux, M. (2017). Collective occupation in public spaces and the construction of the social fabric. *Canadian Journal of Occupational Therapy, 84*(3), 168–177. https://doi.org/10.1177/0008417417701936.

Kools, S., Chimwaza, A., & Macha, S. (2015). Cultural humility and working with marginalized populations in developing countries. *Glob Health Promot, 22*(1), 52–59. https://doi.org/10.1177/1757975914528728.

Labonte, R. (2022). Community, community organizing, and the forming of authentic partnerships: Looking back, looking ahead. In M. Minkler, & P. Wakimoto (Eds.), *Community organizing and community building for health* (4th ed., pp. 91–128). Rutgers University Press. https://doi.org/10.36019/9781978824775.

Laliberte Rudman, D. (2005). Understanding political influences on occupational possibilities: An analysis of newspaper constructions of retirement. *Journal of Occupational Science, 12*(3), 149–160. https://doi.org/10.1080/14427591.2005.9686558.

Laliberte Rudman, D. (2010). Occupational terminology: Occupational possibilities. *Journal of Occupational Science, 17*(1), 55–59.

Laliberte Rudman, D. (2013). Enacting the critical potential of occupational science: Problematizing the 'individualizing of occupation'. *Journal of Occupational Science, 20*(4), 298–313. https://doi.org/10.1080/14427591.2013.803434.

Lauckner, H., Leclair, L., & Yamamoto, C. (2019). Moving beyond the individual: Occupational therapists' multi-layered work with communities. *British Journal of Occupational Therapy, 82*(2), 101–111. https://doi.org/10.1177/0308022618797249.

Lauckner, H., Pentland, W., & Paterson, M. (2007). Exploring Canadian occupational therapists' understanding of and experiences in community development. *Canadian Journal of Occupational Therapy, 74*, 314–325. https://doi.org/10.2182/cjot.07.005.

Lauckner, H. M., Krupa, T. M., & Paterson, M. L. (2011). Conceptualizing community development: Occupational therapy at the intersection of health services and community. *Canadian Journal of Occupational Therapy, 78*, 260–268. https://doi.org/10.2182/cjot.2011.78.4.8.

Lavalley, R. (2017). Developing the transactional perspective of occupation for communities: 'How well are we doing together?'. *Journal of Occupational Science, 24*(4), 458–469. https://doi.org/10.1080/14427591.2017.1367321.

Leclair, L. (2010). Re-examining concepts of occupation and occupation-based models: Occupational therapy and community development. *Canadian Journal of Occupational Therapy, 77*, 15–21. https://doi.org/10.2182/cjot.2010.77.1.3.

Leclair, L. L., Lauckner, H., & Yamamoto, C. (2019). An occupational therapy community development practice process. *Canadian Journal of Occupational Therapy, 86*(5), 345–356. https://doi.org/10.1177/0008417419832457.

Letts, L., Donnelly, C., Hand, C., Leclair, L., & Wener, P. (2022). Chapitre 9: Promouvoir la participation occupationnelle auprès des communautés. In G. Restall, & M., Egan (Eds.), *Promoting occupational participation: Collaborative relationship-focused occupational therapy* (4th ed., pp. 219–238). Canadian Association of Occupational Therapists.

Lopes, R. E., & Serrata Malfitano, A. P. (2021). *Social occupational therapy: Theoretical and practical designs*. Elsevier.

Njelesani, J., Teachman, G., Hamdani, Y., Durocher, E., & Phelan, S. K. (2015). Thinking critically about client-centred practice and occupational possibilities across the life-span. *Scandinavian Journal of Occupational Therapy, 22*(4), 252–259. https://doi.org/10.3109/11038128.2015.1049550.

Nixon, S. A. (2019). The coin model of privilege and critical allyship: Implications for health. *BMC Public Health, 19*, 1637. https://doi.org/10.1186/s12889-019-7884-9.

Peters, L., & Galvaan, R. (2021). A scoping review exploring 'opportunity' in occupational science: Possibilities for conceptual development. *Journal of Occupational Science, 28*(2), 249–261. https://doi.org/10.1080/14427591.2020.1832906.

Ramugondo, E. L., & Kronenberg, F. (2015). Explaining collective occupations from a human relations perspective: Bridging the individual-collective dichotomy. *Journal of Occupational Science, 22*(1), 3–16. https://doi.org/10.1080/14427591.2013.781920.

Restall, G., & Egan, M. (2022). *Promoting occupational participation: Collaborative relationship-focused occupational therapy. Canadian Association of Occupational Therapists.*

Restall, G., Egan, M., Valavaara, K., Phenix, A., & Sack, C. (2022). Chapitre 6: Cadre Canadien pour un processus ergothérapique axé sur les relations collaboratives. In G. Restall, & M. Egan (Eds.), *Promoting occupational participation: Collaborative relationship-focused occupational therapy* (4th ed., pp. 131–166). Canadian Association of Occupational Therapists.

Restall, G., Leclair, L., & Banks, S. (2005). Inclusiveness through community development. *Occupational Therapy Now, 7*(5), 7–9. http://www.caot.ca/default.asp?pageid=7.

Restall, G. J., MacLeod-Schroeder, N. J., & Dubé, C. D. (2018). The equity lens for occupational therapy: A program development and evaluation tool. *Canadian Journal of Occupational Therapy, 85*(3), 185–195. https://doi.org/10.1177/0008417418756421.

Ripat, J., & Becker, P. (2012). Playground usability: What do playground users say? *Occupational Therapy International, 19*, 144–153. https://doi.org/10.1002/oti.1331.

Rothman, J., Erlich, J. L., & Tropman, J. E. (1995). *Strategies of community intervention: Macro practice* (5th ed.). F.E. Peacock Publishers, Inc.

Sakellariou, D., & Pollard, N. (2017). *Occupational therapies without borders: Integrating justice with practice (Second, Ser. Occupational therapy essentials).* Elsevier.

Salzer, M. S. (1997). Consumer empowerment in mental health organizations: Concept, benefits, and impediments. *Administration and Policy in Mental Health, 24*(5), 425–434.

Scaffa, M. E., & Reitz, S. M. (2020). *Occupational therapy in community and population health practice* (3rd ed.). F.A. Davis.

Townsend, E. A., Cockburn, L., Thibeault, R., & Trentham, B. (2013). Chapter 6: Enabling social change. In E. A. Townsend, & H. J. Polatajko (Eds.), *Enabling occupation II: Advancing an occupational therapy vision for health, well-being, & justice through occupation* (2nd ed., pp. 153–171). 9th Canadian Occupational Therapy Guidelines. CAOT Publications ACE.

Trentham, B., Cockburn, L., & Shin, J. (2007). Health promotion and community development: An application of occupational therapy in primary care. *Canadian Journal of Community Mental Health, 26*(2), 53–70.

Wilcock, A. A., & Hocking, C. (2015). *An occupational perspective of health* (3rd ed.). SLACK Incorporated.

Wilcock, A. A. (1998). Reflections on doing, being and becoming. *Canadian Journal of Occupational Therapy, 65*, 248–257.

World Health Organization. (2018). Health inequities and their causes. https://www.who.int/news-room/facts-in-pictures/detail/health-inequities-and-their-causes.

REFLECTION

1. What are the three main steps proposed to explore a community's occupational needs and to strengthen its capacity to address them?

2. What are the five key principles proposed to guide processes aimed at expanding the occupational possibilities of a community? What do they mean to you?

3. What are some strategies that can be used to reflect as the process evolves?

4. An occupational therapist developed an 8-week program to help manual wheelchair users develop the skills they need to further explore their community. The program is offered on the premises of a community organisation. It has been offered for 15 years by the occupational therapist. Why do you think this is not a good example of a process aimed at building the community's capacity to fulfil their occupational needs? What could be done differently?

EXPLORING THE IMPACT OF THE ENVIRONMENT ON OCCUPATIONAL PARTICIPATION

15

GUNILLA CARLSSON ■ AGNETA MALMGREN FÄNGE

Overview

The environment provides opportunities for occupational participation, but sometimes the physical design, people's attitudes and other environmental issues prevent people from participating in necessary and desired occupations, such as employment, shopping and social and cultural events. A person's participation and experience of an occupation are affected by individual factors, such as functional capacity, values, and history, but also contextual factors at micro, meso and macro levels. In this chapter, aspects of the environment impacting occupational participation are elucidated, with particular focus on the physical environment. If diversity in the population is considered in the planning stage, the occupational possibilities will increase. Occupational therapists can provide some environmental interventions, but many must be implemented at meso and macro level. Thus the complexity and impact of the environment need to be considered by occupational therapists together with other professions when co-designing and implementing interventions to promote occupational participation.

KEY POINTS

- A person's participation in occupation is influenced by personal factors, such as functional capacity, values and history and by contextual factors.

- The environment is part of the context.

- The context or the environment can be classified in many ways, for example, in terms of micro, meso and macro contexts; immediate, local and global contexts; or physical, social, cultural and institutional environments.

- Issues at meso and macro levels impact the micro context, and thereby, a person's occupational participation.

- The micro level has been a prevailing focus within occupational therapy, but a wider understanding of the impact of the meso and macro contexts on occupational participation is necessary.

- To determine the impact of the environment on occupational participation, quantitative as well as qualitative data are needed.

- Due to the complexity of the environment, several perspectives are necessary in each situation to support people's participation.

THEORETICAL ASPECTS OF THE CONTEXT AND THE ENVIRONMENT

To understand the impact of the environment on occupational participation, theory and models have been developed to support occupational therapists' reasoning and intervention planning. As the impact of the environment on occupational participation is complex, it is essential to be systematic in gaining an understanding of this impact. In some models, the concept of context describes what impacts occupational participation, whereas in other models, the focus is on the concept of environment. In the Canadian Model of Occupational Participation (CanMOP), the context is defined in terms of micro, meso and macro levels (refer to Chapter 11). The micro context focuses on the person's or collective's interactions with the immediate surroundings, including people and the physical environment. Communities can also be considered as micro contexts, as they can include the interrelationships between the community members. The meso context encompasses system structures, and the macro context is the larger socioeconomic and political context (Egan & Restall, 2022). In the Model of Human Occupation (Taylor, 2017) three contexts at different levels are described: immediate, local and global context levels. On all three levels, the physical and social environments create occupational environments for individuals and collectives (Prior et al., 2020).

In the International Classification of Functioning, Disability and Health, ICF (WHO, 2001), the levels in focus are labelled individual and societal levels, but environmental factors are also classified as products and technology; natural environments and human-made changes to the environment; support and relationships; attitudes and services and systems and policies. The 17 United Nation's Sustainable Development Goals, UNSDG (United Nations, 2015), is another way of addressing environmental dimensions together with economic and social dimensions. For example, UNSDG #1 addresses sustainable cities and communities, which include access for all to adequate, safe and affordable housing, to basic services and to the upgrade of slums.

In some models, assistive devices are classified as an environmental factor, as in the ICF[2] (WHO, 2001), while in other models, for example, the Human Activity Assistive Technology, (HAAT) model (Cook & Polgar, 2008), such devices are considered as a separate unit. According to the HAAT model, assistive technology is interacting with the human and the activity in the context in which these three factors exist. In a recent scoping review (Kirschner et al., 2023), a typology of environmental and contextual factors affecting occupational participation is suggested. Fifty-three terms are structured into four main areas: physical factors, social factors, societal and organisational factors and support and relationship factors. The terms cover a broad range of environmental factors, such as contrast, speed-timing, weather, clutter and availability of transportation. The value of classifying the environment is not that complexity is reduced; instead, the different perspectives that should be considered are articulated in the dynamic relationship between the person, environment and occupation. Examples of different perspectives of these dynamic relationships are performance focusing on the ability to choose, organise and satisfactorily perform meaningful occupations (Townsend & Polatajko, 2007); what a person actually does in their daily environment (WHO, 2001); participation as involvement in a life situation (WHO, 2001); and occupational participation as having access to, initiating and sustaining valued occupations withing meaningful relationships and contexts (Egan & Restall, 2022, p. 76). From some perspectives, professional judgments can be made, while in other situations only the individuals themselves make the final judgement, such as for occupational participation.

In the ecological model (Lawton & Nahemow, 1973), further developed in the Ecological Model of Aging (Scheidt & Norris-Baker, 2003), the dynamic relationships between person and environment are described and used to highlight the balance between competence in the person and environmental demands. This overall perspective is useful to describe how medium and high demands might be inspiring and challenging for people with higher levels of functioning, whereas too high or too low environmental demands might have a negative impact on the occupational participation of a person. People with lower functional capacity may be more sensitive to the demands of the environment than people with higher functional capacity (Box 15.1).

To initiate and sustain occupations, a basic prerequisite is access to the environments in which those

---

BOX 15.1
AMANDA

Amanda is 45 years old and has a spinal cord injury after a riding accident. She is a teacher at the university in the city where she lives. She uses a wheelchair and the physical environment at the campus is built according to the national building regulations and standards. This includes the ramp to the entrance door. Despite this, Amanda has severe difficulties using the ramp due to her limited physical capacity. In fact the demands of the environment are too high for her even though the university has adhered to all regulations. Subsequently, doing the same occupations as her colleagues is very difficult and her work is at risk.

---

occupations are performed (Egan & Restall, 2022). Regarding the physical environment, the concepts of accessibility and usability are often used. In many countries, accessibility and usability are anchored in the planning and building legislation, and accordingly, buildings are meant to fulfil such requirements. The definition of accessibility used in this chapter is based on the Ecological Model of Ageing (Iwarsson & Ståhl, 2003) and defined as a relative concept denoting the relationship between a person's functional capacity and the prevalence of environmental barriers (Iwarsson & Slaug, 2010). Usability targets the possibility that the environment offers for being able to perform specific occupations (Oswald & Kaspar, 2012). According to the International Standardization Organization, ISO, usability is defined as 'the extent to which a product can be used by specified users to achieve specified goals with effectiveness, efficiency and satisfaction in a specified context of use' (ISO 9241-210:2019), which reflects the relationship between the person, the environment and the task. The environmental component of the person-environment interaction in accessibility is based on regulations, whereas usability addresses the subjective aspects of interaction with the environment (Iwarsson & Ståhl, 2003). The qualitative aspect of usability is how easy and comfortable a person finds the environment, including human-made objects, to perform occupations and different tasks. The quantitative aspect of usability is demonstrated by the frequency and consistency with which the person participates in different kinds of occupations (Arthanat et al., 2007).

OCCUPATIONS ARE CONTEXTUALLY SITUATED

Eating or focusing more specifically on one meal, such as having lunch, is a daily occupation, but experience and participation differ depending on the context. Besides a person's individual values (Erlandsson et al., 2011), needs, relationships and experiences (Egan & Restall, 2022), the context has an impact on occupational choices and the way occupations are performed. Occupational choices therefore have a contextually situated nature (Galvaan, 2015; Hammell, 2020).

Past experiences and habits guide participation in occupations. A meal might differ depending on whether a person is at home, in a forest or in a restaurant, together with colleagues, friends or alone. It matters if the person can enter the restaurant independently or with assistance and if the restaurant serves food that the person can eat based on their values, food habits, dietary requirements, etc. To be able to choose and participate in occupations, a basic requirement is to have access to them, and that the environmental preconditions to carry them out are available. Environmental cues guide the continuation of the occupation, and the environment thus provides different occupational possibilities (Rudman, 2010). Engagement in one situation constitutes the precondition for what is done next (Madsen & Josephsson, 2017), and the value of an occupation can vary from person to person. For example, if a person is thirsty or hungry, they make something to drink or eat, which requires tools, a place to make the dish and a place to eat. Eating can also on the other hand be a way of meeting friends and socialising (Box 15.2).

Physical, social, cultural and institutional aspects of the environment as well as different context levels, such as the micro, meso and macro levels (Bronfenbrenner, 2004; Egan & Restall, 2022), can be identified when participating in occupations (Canadian Association of Occupational Therapists [CAOT], 2007). For example, physical, social, cultural and institutional aspects of the environment can be identified in Galvaan's (2015) description[3] of how young adolescents in South Africa scouted around in the physical environment at a local rubbish dump. By doing so, they repeated prevailing social positions in their community, and they seized the opportunities that occurred against their cultural background. With regard to how different contextual

---

BOX 15.2
ANNE

On a Friday, after planning the next year's budget, Anne and her colleagues have lunch in the restaurant together with the head of the department. She works some more hours and, in the evening, before she goes to bed, she has a cup of tea at home in front of the daily news. On Saturday, she is hiking with her friends in the forest. They are physically active, enjoying each other's company and for lunch, they build a fire and make soup.

---

levels interact with each other, another example is that high levels of crime at the meso level, may impact the micro level in terms of access to safe spaces for recreational activities (D'Anna et al., 2018), or residents' strategies to actively engage with the community (Taei et al., 2023). At the macro level, legislation and political decisions impact, for example, the planning of health care funding schemes and thus affect a person's access to affordable healthcare.

Both the past and future are present in occupational participation as environmental aspects such as laws, regulations and social support. From a societal perspective, several aspects are important to address to promote occupational participation and to provide occupational justice and equity for all citizens (Egan & Restall, 2022). Occupational possibilities derive not only from the overall planning of society, such as the built environment and the planning of welfare systems but also from social as well as cultural contexts in which people live (D'Anna et al., 2018).

Occupational therapist may be more focused on interventions that target the person rather than the society. However, it has become increasingly recognised that interventions to improve a person's occupational participation at the micro level require interventions at meso and macro levels. Occupational therapists are experts on occupation, but they need to draw on knowledge from a range of sciences, including occupational, medical, technical, psychological and social sciences, to increase their understanding of the environmental impact and contribute with knowledge about prerequisites for occupational participation. This knowledge might also influence how occupational therapists assess the impact of the environment on occupational participation.

INCLUDING AND EXCLUDING ENVIRONMENTS

All environments, whether physical or social, should enable equitable participation for all people. Therefore, features and conditions that include and exclude people from occupational participation must be considered. For example, an inclusive building allows all people to enter it comfortably, through the same entrance. The building is on the other hand exclusive when a person using a wheelchair is prevented from entering it due to steps at the entrance. Physical exclusion might lead to social exclusion, but social exclusion can also occur because of social interactions and attitudes in society. For example, at bars and clubs that are physically inclusive, adults with impairments may face exclusion due to invisible social barriers and the perception of 'we and them'. Specific environmental solutions implemented with the intention of including people with impairments can also be stigmatising and exclusive, such as when a person who uses a wheelchair cannot sit together with his or her friends in the cinema and instead is directed to the space allocated for wheelchair users. Further, as is the case for Amanda (Box 15.1), the lack of an environment adapted to her functional capacity may lead to stigmatisation and exclusion.

Inclusive environments also acknowledge the need to ensure the safety and security of the people using them. It is essential to avoid danger or unnecessary risks for people (Khalili et al., 2023). There are many examples, including the need for homes and sheltered housing to be friendly and accommodating for people with dementia (Struckmeyer & Pickens, 2016)· For example, to enhance orientation, good lightning and easily interpreted signs are important design features. When it comes to public environments, it is important to reduce the risk of people falling (Clemson et al., 2019). Measures to reduce this risk relate very much to surface (tarmac, paving stones) and the lightning during dark hours.

Universal design (UD) has become a worldwide movement that aims to create physical environments, products, services and technology that are usable, accessible, safe and convenient for the vast majority of people (Mace, 1985) (refer to Chapters 29 and 31). The principles of universal design, such as equitable use, simple and intuitive use and tolerance for error, elucidate important aspects of the design process, but the wide range of people who use and experience a specific environment at a specific time makes it difficult to develop valid and reliable assessments. As a result, there are no reliable and valid criteria for evaluating 'universally designed' buildings and devices. Instead, Erdtman and colleagues (2022) suggested the following strategies for inclusive practices and implementation of UD:

i)   Communicate the reasons for UD,
ii) Consider human diversity and individual needs and
iii) Integrate access needs in learning processes.

COMPLEX ENVIRONMENTS AS THE BASIS FOR OCCUPATIONAL PARTICIPATION

People organise their lives through their daily occupations, and thereby, there are a multitude of environmental arenas for participation; these are difficult to illustrate in theoretical terms and models. The complexity applies partly to all environments that can be included in an entire occupation and partly to specific environments that are complex in themselves. In addition, the environment is dynamic and can change quickly or slowly over the course of time. The weather, for example, can change the environmental conditions for occupational participation, as can events such as pandemics, wars and natural disasters (e.g. bushfires, floods, storms and earthquakes).

To illustrate the complexity of all environments included in everyday occupation, a concept from public transport planning can be considered. The expression 'travel chain perspective' has been introduced to emphasise the complexity of a person's travel and used as an approach for the exploration of travels. A travel chain is defined as the actual chain of events that occurs while moving from origin to destination (Risser et al., 2015). Irrespective of whether the occupation includes travelling or not, several environmental arenas are linked to each other when a person participates in an occupation. This perspective is also in line with the fact that single tasks are situated in larger situations (Madsen & Josephsson, 2017). To illustrate the complexity of defining the environment for everyday

---

BOX 15.3
JOHN

John, 77 years old, has decided to go grocery shopping. He walks through the entrance to his home and goes down three steps. He then walks along the pedestrian path to the bus stop near his house. He catches the bus and disembarks at the bus stop closest to the grocery shop, where he meets a friend and talks for a while. After entering the shop, he walks around the numerous aisles pushing a shopping trolley and collecting his groceries from the shelves. He purchases his groceries with a credit card, packs them in his backpack and walks to the bus stop to catch a bus back to his home. He steps off the bus at the stop closest to his home and then walks on the pedestrian path towards his home. When he reaches his home, he walks along his garden path and up the three steps to his front door and then enters his house.

John may do this trip by himself or with his partner. He feels comfortable enough to make this trip as he is very familiar with the environment and with the occupation of grocery shopping. Thus the current meso and macro environments facilitate John's occupation of going grocery shopping, as does his familiarity with the occupation, and his physical and cognitive capacities. However, changes within the environment or the occupation or in John's physical and cognitive capability could impact his ability to do grocery shopping.

---

occupations, an example of John going grocery shopping is presented (Box 15.3).

For John to be able to participate in the occupation of shopping access to the public environment is required. In fact, meso and macro contexts impact on John's micro context. That is, when designing public environments, the diversity of the population needs to be considered; the design process must focus on the usefulness and usability of the environment for as many as possible (Erdtman et al., 2022).

When it comes to the complexity of specific environments, public environments often present more challenges than the home environment and, thereby, potentially have a greater negative impact on occupational participation among people with reduced functional capacity (Brorsson et al., 2013; Gaber et al., 2019; Wenger et al., 2021). Individual needs such as tailored adaptations are difficult to accommodate in public environments, and decisions at macro and meso levels, such as decisions to digitalise services, can create risks of exclusion. For example, the implementation

---

BOX 15.4
LIZA

Liza is an 86-year-old woman who lives alone. Over the last few years, she has faced increasing problems in daily life due to macular degeneration and age-related declining health, resulting in a need for daily physical assistance by homecare staff. Liza's home is small and challenges the physical work environment requirements of the staff. The staff have made a few adaptations based on their individual ergonomic needs and up to now it has worked well also for Liza. However, in the past two months, the staff have noticed changes in Liza's behaviour, and she seems to have problems with her memory. In particular, she is having difficulty remembering the placement of things around the house. It turns out that adaptations made to accommodate the needs of the staff increasingly challenge Liza's independence and possibilities for her to participate in occupations.

BOX 15.5
CARLOS

Carlos, 18 years old, lived with his family in a small, two-bedroom apartment during the COVID-19 pandemic. On one particular day, he had a digital math class requiring him to have a discussion with his teachers and classmates online. At the same time, his mother had a digital meeting with international customers, and his father, a university teacher in English, led an online seminar with students. Carlos' younger sister was playing in the hall. Due to the curfew, their possibilities for physical activity were limited, and Carlos, who used to play football four times a week, found it increasingly difficult to focus on his studies over time. In turn, his results declined. The members of his family also became irritated with each other and did not feel the usual joy of being together. Every situation easily escalated to a family conflict, and their routines were disrupted. For example, usually Carlos' father took pride in cooking healthy and tasty meals, but over time, the family started to eat whatever they had at home, without paying notice to the quality of the food.

---

of digital ticket machines in public transportation can create difficulties for people with reduced cognitive capacity to enact their citizenship (Gaber et al., 2019). Such technology is often used for the safety of drivers but creates problems for people with reduced cognitive capacity. Common complex environments among frail older people are care homes. Moving to a care home is intended to increase the opportunities to be active and participating even when facing major care needs. However, given the fact that both care homes and private homes are not only the homes of the people living there but also the workplace for the staff, conflicts can arise as to who makes the final decision on how to use the environment. When the needs of the staff are prioritised above the needs and preferences of the people living there, the environmental demands on the people living there increase and vice versa (Pettersson et al., 2021). That is, to a large extent moving to a care home can constrain the possibilities for occupational participation (Box 15.4).

A specific physical environment might hinder occupational participation, but this is also the case of more extensive changes in the environment, such as the changes that took place in most countries during the COVID-19 pandemic. In a study among older people in Sweden, 3 months into the pandemic, participants expressed how they initially stopped all visits to shops, either having family or friends do their shopping for them or shopping online; however, they eventually went back to shopping themselves. Mostly the reason was that they did not want to bother relatives, which has a social dimension, but also because they were disappointed with the digitally ordered deliveries (Carlsson et al., 2022). This means that the environment did not support their occupational participation as they expected. All generations had to adapt in different ways during the pandemic, and in many countries, the education system became digital and outdoor visits among children were restricted. Among others, these restrictions would have impacted the occupational participation of families from lower socio-economic backgrounds (López-Bueno et al., 2021) and those living in small apartments (Box 15.5).

The environmental impact on occupational participation can be slow, as for people with deteriorating neurological impairment allowing them to adjust to declining functional capacity (Andersson et al., 2021). Changes can also be very dramatic, as, for example, people who have become asylum seekers as a result of war and may have to travel in unsafe conditions and live in places that are physically, socially, culturally and institutionally different from their homes (Morville et al., 2015). In such situations, their health and wellbeing may be negatively impacted, as will their occupational identity and roles be. That is, since their living environments have changed dramatically, new strategies to live their lives need to be developed. Thus disasters, natural or created by a war, for example, may result in enormous damage to a person's life and social roles. Occupational therapists can be involved in preparations for, responses to and recovery from natural disasters (Jeong et al., 2016) or other dramatic situations (Morville et al., 2015).

ASSESSING THE ENVIRONMENT

The environment plays an important role in promoting occupational participation, and the environment is complex in different ways. However, the evaluation of the impact of the environment is not always obvious in occupational therapists' assessments of occupational participation, despite the central role it plays in the theory and models guiding the profession. The aim of assessing the environment is to determine how it influences occupational participation and how to best design or adapt the environment to make it more accessible and usable for all. Different assessments of personal experiences and systematic inquiries are needed to capture different perspectives and serve as a basis for interventions. Subjective data, such as experiences of using apps or of barriers to participation can be collected and analysed by means of quantitative as well as qualitative methods. Objective data, such as frequency of using devices or the number of barriers, is mostly collected and analysed by means of quantitative methods.

Quantitative data can be collected by means of psychometrically tested and validated instruments, and commonly in occupational therapy, occupational performance or participation are in focus. However, often with these types of assessments, the impact of the environment is at best indirectly targeted. For example, in the Activities of Daily Living (ADL) taxonomy, transportation is defined as getting to, in and out of public or private transport (Törnquist & Sonn, 2014). This means that the environmental conditions for this activity can vary from one situation to another and thus need to be considered in the assessment of transportation. However, the environmental condition is not the focus of this assessment item.

Focusing on everyday technology and assistive devices, the Everyday Technology Use Questionnaire (ETUQ) (Hällgren et al., 2011) aims to investigate the perceived relevance and difficulty in using everyday technology such as smartphone, computer, tablet, etc. In ETUQ devices can be considered part of the environment, but the specific devices are not identified. Another assessment instrument developed by occupational therapists is the Participation in Activities and Places Outside Home (ACT-OUT) (Margot-Cattin et al., 2019), targeting older adults with cognitive impairments. This instrument focuses on places outside home and comprises questions about certain places, for instance, if the individual went there in the past and if they see themselves going there in the future. Further, there are questions about what kind of activity they do in a certain place, why, when and how often they go there and how well they know the place. The Craig Hospital Inventory of Environmental Factors (CHIEF) focuses on perceived environmental demands, the majority outside home (Whiteneck et al., 2004). In this instrument, perceived environmental barriers reported are based on questions of how often, in the past 12 months, environmental features have been barriers to participation in activities that matter to each person within five areas: attitudes/support; service/assistance; physical/structural; work/school; and policies. However, most of the questions are posed at a general level, and the specific geographical area is not defined. For all these instruments, supplementary information is necessary for intervention planning, and the results of the assessments cannot be used to improve specific issues in the macro, societal level environment.

Assessment instruments explicitly focusing on different aspects of the environment are predominantly based on concepts relating to accessibility, usability and safety. However, to be able to serve as a basis for societal interventions, specific information about the environment is needed. For example, information collected by means of the Housing Enabler instrument (Iwarsson & Slaug, 2010) is related to a specific apartment or house. Information about the presence/absence of physical barriers in the housing environment is collected and defined according to national standards and guidelines for housing design. What constitutes an environmental barrier can thus differ depending on the national, legislative context. In the next step, the environmental barrier is related to the functional capacity of the individual. With this type of assessment, the results reported can demonstrate that accessibility problems are considerable and can be present even in newer dwellings (Slaug et al., 2020). Also, accessibility problems are related to the individual depending on their functional capacity. However, this instrument focuses on person-environment fit in general only and does not assess the impact it has on occupational participation. For this purpose, other instruments or data collection methods are necessary.

An assessment instrument in which specific geographical information is collected is the Stakeholders Walkability/Wheelability Audit in Neighbourhoods (SWAN) (Mahmood et al., 2020). Using this assessment, specific neighborhood environments can be defined and assessed both with objective and subjective items. The results can then serve as the basis for discussion about environmental improvements. Environmental features are essential parts of the design of restorative environments and are mainly used in architecture and landscape architecture. The environmental qualities for different groups of individuals are focused on in terms of proximity, closeness, safety and social opportunities, for example, the study by Bengtsson and Grahn (2014). Despite the availability of different assessment instruments that may have a focus on the environment, it is important to note that all necessary information for intervention planning cannot be collected by one single instrument, and collaboration with the individual or collective is essential.

Standardised or unstandardised self-reporting during an interview or in a diary is commonly used. For example, using interviews followed by a content analysis, Andersson and colleagues (2021) investigated sensory input and strategies used in daily occupations among people with serious mental illness. The results demonstrated how people who participated in this study enabled daily life through strategies clearly involving changes to and/or adaptation of the environment, such as creating a home that provides rest, finding a safe place and using nature and animals for relaxation. Another method that can be used to collect self-reported data is the think-aloud method. Vergouw and colleagues (2020) identified needs, barriers and facilitators among community-dwelling older adults

with one or more chronic health conditions, in using online eHealth applications to support general practice services. Besides the subthemes derived from the think-aloud data, they showed how think-aloud data complemented the interview data.

By applying mixed methods approaches (Creswell & Plano Clark, 2017), both quantitative and qualitative data can be integrated. For example, in a study by Simpson and colleagues (Simpson et al., 2022), psychosocial and quality of life outcomes among people who sustained spinal cord injury earlier versus later in life were explored, together with their post-injury experiences. They used the CHIEF instrument (Whitneck et al., 2004), combined with demographic information to assess environmental factors and interviews and thematic content analyses to explore the qualitative dimensions of the outcomes. Tse and colleagues (2022) applied a mixed methods design to understand occupational participation three months following a stroke. Quantitative data were collected by means of the Activity Card Sort-Australia (Packer et al., 2008) concurrent with qualitative semi-structured interviews about activity limitations. The results illustrated how personal, environmental and temporal dimensions could explain reasons and changes in reasons for activity participation.

ADAPTING AND REDESIGNING THE ENVIRONMENT TO ENHANCE OCCUPATIONAL PARTICIPATION

When co-designing interventions, it is fundamental that they focus on occupations valued by the person (Erlandsson et al., 2011), accounting for their needs, relationships and history (Egan & Restall, 2022). That is, participating in an occupation might have a concrete, symbolic or self-rewarded value for the person and contribute to the overarching experience of meaning and wellbeing. For example, Kallhed and Mårtensson (2018) argue that occupational value seems to determine the choice of strategy used to enhance occupational performance after a pain rehabilitation program and achieving an acceptable balance of activities embracing personal resources, specific activities and environmental factors that fit together. Having a restorative home environment might be the key to a highly valued social life in case of, for example, fatigue after brain injury (Box 15.6).

BOX 15.6
STEINAR

Steinar is 32 years old. A few years ago he had a brain injury after a bicycle accident. He participated in a rehabilitation program after the injury, and his friends were happy that he recovered so well. He returned to work as a plumber but experienced fatigue and could not cope with all the daily demands. With the help of an occupational therapist, he joined a fatigue self-management program. Steinar found the program very supportive and helpful. Above all, he better understood the reasons why he experienced fatigue. He developed strategies to reduce fatigue in everyday life, such as pacing and energy conservation strategies. He re-arranged the layout of his house to reduce unnecessary stimuli and provide a calm and restorative environment. He reflected upon the importance of his social life and prioritise time to meet his friends.

BOX 15.7
HAMID

Hamid, 25 years old, lives together with his parents in an apartment on the ground floor. Since he was born with spina bifida, he uses a wheelchair. Previously, there were two steps to the entrance door which made it difficult for Hamid to go outdoors. Hamid and his family live in a country where all adaptations to the housing need to be paid by the families themselves. Hamid's father is a handyman and he managed to remove the steps and install a ramp between the patio and door. Thus nowadays Hamid can independently go outdoors and meet friends, even if there are more barriers in his neighborhood. It gives him opportunities to socialise with his friends.

These kinds of environmental arrangements that support social participation and leisure engagement are important for many people who experience illness, injury or impairment and such interventions are, to a large extent, health promoting. And for community-dwelling older adults, health promotion interventions might constitute community-based group interventions, self-management of diseases and/or leisure education (Smallfield & Lucas Molitor, 2018). No matter the intervention, the environmental foci vary.

Interventions in the physical environment may include the provision of assistive devices and home modifications (Bolt et al., 2019; Ekstam et al., 2016; Liu et al., 2018; Lynn et al., 2019; Novak & Honan, 2019). These types of interventions are often based on a person's individual needs and risks (Lynn et al., 2019; Wellecke et al., 2022) and include adaptations at home, at school or at work. For most individuals, the home has a symbolic meaning and therefore home modifications that occupational therapists sometimes suggest can affect the perception of the home negatively (Liu et al., 2018), even if it is individually tailored and aims to increase occupational participation. Thus an individual's values must be considered when a home modification is suggested (Box 15.7). Often, it is the individual's own responsibility to finance assistive devices and home modifications, but this varies between countries.

Digital technology is becoming increasingly common, and its implementation in all societal sectors challenges people's occupational routines and habits. Therefore it is of relevance to occupational therapy practice on micro, meso and macro levels (Gaber et al., 2019; Gaber et al., 2023; Lindberg et al., 2023; Olivier et al., 2020). Digital technology is commonly used to book appointments and buy tickets and has replaced cash and cash cards when paying for goods. Such technology saves time and increases accessibility to societal services for many people but can be a challenge to others with difficulties learning how to use it (Box 15.8).

If the diversity in the population had already been considered in the planning stage, the occupational possibilities would have increased. That is, if differences between individuals had been considered prior to building the house, then Hamid (Box 15.7) might have been able to go out and socialise with his friends much earlier; and Barbara (Box 15.8) would have been able to travel if an alternative to electronic tickets had been available.

Digital technology can enable and facilitate occupational participation. For example, people with sensorimotor disorders may have difficulties writing or moving around, and to them, the availability of digital technology may compensate for reduced physical capacity. Digital access to voice-recorded lectures may increase the possibility of a university student with visual impairment to complete their studies (Lintangsari & Emaliana, 2020) (Box 15.9).

BOX 15.8
BARBARA

Barbara, 73 years old, goes to a club each Wednesday to socialise with her friends. She generally uses public transportation and buys the bus ticket using a mobile phone app. Lately, she has developed a mild cognitive impairment which makes it difficult for her to use the app. Barbara is physically capable of moving around easily but since the only way of buying tickets is by using the app she is now dependent on a friend to drive her to the club when there is time. Barbara cannot visit the club on her own terms anymore.

BOX 15.9
CHARLIE

Charlie is in the third semester at the university and was born blind. The university program is organised around lectures and seminars but also a significant amount of practical, professional training. Digital assistive technology enables Charlie to study at the university as documents can be listened to, webpages read using voice-to-text, and lectures can be recorded and listened to at a time convenient to Charlie. This technology is essential for Charlie, enabling him to complete his theoretical subjects. However, the practical, professional training is challenging and dependent on personal support. The lecturers are very open to Charlie's needs and frequently discuss with Charlie how to ensure they can meet his learning needs.

The occupational therapy profession has always considered the health promotion and restorative potential of environments for people (Patil et al., 2019; Smallfield & Lucas Molitor, 2018). For example, therapeutic gardens have been shown to be beneficial for people with illnesses or impairments (Murroni et al., 2021; Son et al., 2022), and allotment gardening can positively contribute to health and wellbeing (Genter et al., 2015). The presence of natural spaces in care homes has also been considered important for recreation and recovery (Berg et al., 2020; Olszewska-Guizzo et al., 2022).

Occupational therapists have an essential role in the development of environments designed to facilitate and expand occupational participation. For example, during the COVID-19 pandemic, older people and people with illness, injury or impairments experienced restrictions regarding who could visit their homes as well as their ability to meet people outside their homes. During the pandemic, occupational therapists could guide people, relatives and healthcare staff to find environmental support such as the creation of adapted outdoor visit spaces in care homes, ordering groceries online and connecting with people via online meeting software.

Even if the individual, micro context has been a prevailing focus within occupational therapy, occupational therapists have contributed to interdisciplinary work on meso and macro context levels. For example, by supporting employers of people with autism with a specific workplace tool, the chances of success for the individual increases (Scott et al., 2018). Another example is that occupational therapists' knowledge and understanding of the dynamic relationships between person, environment and occupation, as well as experience in occupational analysis, has been used in fire safety contributing to the needs of people with impairments being considered (Bukvic et al., 2021). To give input at the societal level on environments supporting occupational participation and to contribute in an efficient way with knowledge of other disciplines, it is also important for occupational therapists to understand the complexity of implementing environments that give access to occupations (Carlsson et al., 2023).

The world is rapidly changing, and new technology is being designed and used. Communication between individuals and groups of people is increasingly digitalised, posing challenges to people with different kinds of impairments. In general, technological developments are putting higher demands on individuals; however, the picture is complex. While digital technology can be easy to use for people with a low spinal cord injury, for example, it can be very difficult for people with high-level tetraplegia or people with upper limb coordination difficulties as it often requires manipulation and grip ability. The rapid development and implementation of new technology also impacts what is considered an ordinary device and what is considered an assistive device prescribed for a specific person.

CONCLUSION

Occupations are situated in a context, and thereby, the environment provides different opportunities for occupational participation. Participation in one task may constitute the precondition for what is done next, which means that mostly, it is important to apply a chain perspective to support occupational participation. This also applies to the environment. Occupational therapists may be more focused on interventions that target individual people rather than the broader society. However, it has become increasingly recognised that interventions to improve a person's occupational participation at the micro level require interventions of the environment at the meso and macro levels as well. Thus occupational therapists need to consider the environment when implementing interventions. They need to assess the environment using qualitative, quantitative and mixed methods to identify the impact of the environment on occupational participation. They also need to clarify at which level interventions are needed and contribute with systematically gained knowledge to adapt and redesign the environment to support occupational participation.

REFERENCES

Andersson, H., Sutton, D., Bejerholm, U., & Argentzell, E. (2021). Experiences of sensory input in daily occupations for people with serious mental illness. *Scandinavian Journal of Occupational Therapy, 28*(6), 446–456. https://doi.org/10.1080/11038128.2020.1778784.

Arthanat, S., Bauer, S. M., Lenker, J. A., Nochajskia, S. M., & Wub, Y. W. B. (2007). Conceptualization and measurement of assistive technology usability. *Disability and Rehabilitation: Assistive Technology, 2*(4), 235–248. https://doi.org/10.1080/17483100701343665.

Bengtsson, A., & Grahn, P. (2014). Outdoor environments in healthcare settings: A quality evaluation tool for use in designing healthcare gardens. *Urban Forestry & Urban Greening, 13*(4), 878–891. https://doi.org/10.1016/j.ufug.2014.09.007.

Bolt, M., Ikking, T., Baaijen, R., & Saenger, S. (2019). Scoping review: Occupational therapy interventions in primary care. *Primary Health Care Research & Development, 20,* e28. https://doi.org/10.1017/S146342361800049X.

Bronfenbrenner, U. (2004). *Making human beings human: Bioecological perspectives on human development.* Sage.

Brorsson, A., Öhman, A., Cutchin, M., & Nygård, L. (2013). Managing critical incidents in grocery shopping by community-living people with Alzheimer's disease. *Scandinavian Journal of Occupational Therapy, 20*(4), 292–301. https://doi.org/10.3109/11038128.2012.752031.

Bukvic, O., Carlsson, G., Gefenaite, G., Slaug, B., Schmidt, S. M., & Ronchi, E. (2021). A review on the role of functional limitations on evacuation performance using the International Classification of Functioning, Disability and Health. *Fire Technology, 57,* 507–528. https://doi.org/10.1007/s10694-020-01034-5.

Carlsson, G., Granbom, M., Fristedt, S., Jonsson, O., Hägg, L., Ericsson, J., & Kylén, M. (2022). A hundred days in confinement:
Doing, being, becoming, and belonging among older people in Sweden during the COVID-19 pandemic. *Journal of Occupational Science, 29*(3), 402–416. https://doi.org/10.1080/14427591.2022.2057572.

Carlsson, G., Jonsson, O., Olander, S., Salén, M., Månsson Lexell, E., & Slaug, B. (2023). Exploration of a web-based accessibility tool for public facilities. *Facilities, 41*(15–16), 66–84. https://doi.org/10.1108/F-10-2022-0132.

Clemson, L., Stark, S., Pighills, A. C., Torgerson, D. J., Sherrington, C., & Lamb, S. E. (2019). Environmental interventions for preventing falls in older people living in the community. *Cochrane Database of Systematic Reviews, 2019*(2), CD013258. https://doi.org/10.1002/14651858.CD013258.

Cook, A. M., & Polgar, J. M. (2008). *Cook & Hussey's assistive technologies principles and practice.* Mosby Elsevier.

Creswell, J. W., & Plano Clark, V. L. (2017). *Designing and conducting mixed methods research* (3rd ed.). SAGE Publications Inc.

D'Anna, L. H., Sabado, P., Valdez-Dadia, A., Canjura, C., Peong, V., Hansen, M. C., & Hong, M. (2018). Barriers to physical and mental health: Understanding the intersecting needs of Cambodian and Latino residents in urban communities. *Journal of Immigrant and Minority Health, 20*(5), 1243–1260. https://doi.org/10.1007/s10903-017-0677-2.

Egan, M., & Restall, G. (2022). *Promoting occupational participation: Collaborative relationship-focused occupational therapy.* CAOT.

Ekstam, L., Malmgren Fänge, A., & Carlsson, G. (2016). Negotiating control: From recognizing a need to making a decision to apply for a housing Adaptation. *Journal of Housing for the Elderly, 30*(4), 345–359. https://doi.org/10.1080/02763893.2016.1224788.

Erdtman, E., Rassmus-Gröhn, K., & Hedvall, P.-O. (2022). Let us move beyond word battles and separatism: Strategies and concerns regarding universal design in Sweden. *Equality, Diversity and Inclusion, 41*(9), 15–29. https://doi.org/10.1108/EDI-04-2021-0108.

Erlandsson, L.-K, Eklund, M., & Persson, M. (2011). Occupational value and relationships to meaning and health: Elaborations of the ValMO-model. *Scandinavian Journal of Occupational Therapy, 18*(1), 72–80. https://doi.org/10.3109/11038121003671619.

Gaber, S. N., Nygård, L., Brorsson, A., Kottorp, A., & Malinowsky, C. (2019). Everyday technologies and public space participation among people with and without dementia. *Canadian Journal of Occupational Therapy, 86*(5), 400–411. https://doi.org/10.1177/0008417419837764.

Gaber, S. N., Nygård, L., Malinowsky, C., Brorsson, A., Kottorp, A., & Hedman, A. (2023). Enacting citizenship through participation in a technological society: A longitudinal three-year study among people with dementia in Sweden. *Ageing & Society, 43*(2), 276–297. https://doi.org/10.1017/S0144686X21000544.

Galvaan, R. (2015). The contextually situated nature of occupational choice: Marginalised young adolescents' experiences in South Africa. *Journal of Occupational Science, 22*(1), 39–53. https://doi.org/10.1080/14427591.2014.912124.

Genter, C., Roberts, A., Richardson, J., & Sheaff, M. (2015). The contribution of allotment gardening to health and wellbeing: A systematic review of the literature. *British Journal of Occupational Therapy, 78*(10), 593–605. https://doi.org/10.1177/0308022615599408.

Hällgren, M., Nygård, L., & Kottorp, A. (2011). Technology and everyday functioning in people with intellectual disabilities: A rasch analysis of the everyday technology use questionnaire (ETUQ). *Journal of Intellectual Disability Research, 55*(6), 610–620. https://doi.org/10.1111/j.1365-2788.2011.01419.x.

Hammell, J. (2020). Making choices from the choices we have: The contextual-embeddedness of occupational choice. *Canadian Journal of Occupational Therapy, 87*(5), 400–411. https://doi.org/10.1177/000841742096574.

ISO 9241-210. (2019). Ergonomics of human-system interaction — Part 210: Human-centred design for interactive systems.

Iwarsson, S., & Slaug, B. (2010). *The housing enabler: An instrument for assessing and analysing accessibility problems in housing.* Veten & Skapen HB & Slaug Enabling Development.

Iwarsson, S., & Ståhl, A. (2003). Accessibility, usability and universal design – positioning and definition of concepts describing person-environment relationships. *Disability and Rehabilitation, 25*(2), 57–66. https://doi.org/10.1080/0963828021000007969.

Jeong, Y., Law, M., DeMatteo, C., Stratford, P., & Kim, H. (2016). The role of occupational therapists in the contexts of a natural disaster: A scoping review. *Disability and Rehabilitation, 38*(16), 1620–1631. https://doi.org/10.3109/09638288.2015.1106597.

Kallhed, C., & Mårtensson, L. (2018). Strategies to manage activities in everyday life after a pain rehabilitation program. *Scandinavian Journal of Occupational Therapy, 25*(2), 145–152. https://doi.org/10.1080/11038128.2017.1283442.

Khalili, M., Jonathan, C., Hocking, N., Van der Loos, M., Mortenson, W. B., & Borisoff, J. (2023). Perception of autonomy among people who use wheeled mobility assistive devices: Dependence on environment and contextual factors. *Disability and Rehabilitation: Assistive Technology, 18*(7), 1066–1073. https://doi.org/10.1080/17483107.2021.1978565.

Kirschner, L., Doyle, N. W., & Desport, B. C. (2023). Uncovering the obstacles—A typology of environmental and contextual factors affecting occupational participation: A scoping review. *The American Journal of Occupational Therapy, 77*, 7701205040. https://doi.org/10.5014/ajot.2023.050043.

Lawton, M. P., & Nahemow, L. (1973). Ecology and the aging process. In C. Eisdorfer, & M. P. Lawton (Eds.), *The psychology of adult development and aging.* America Psychological Association.

Lindberg, M., Månsson Lexell, E., Ranner, M., & Larsson Lund, M. (2023). Self-initiated management strategies in digitalized work and everyday life – experiences of people with cognitive difficulties due to neurological disorders. *Scandinavian Journal of Occupational Therapy, 30*(4), 559–571. https://doi.org/10.1080/11038128.2023.2175724.

Lintangsari, A. P., & Emaliana, I. (2020). Inclusive education services for the blind: Values, roles, and challenges of university EFL teachers. *International Journal of Evaluation and Research in Education, 9*(2), 439–447. https://doi.org/10.11591/ijere.v9i2.20436.

Liu, C.-J., Chang, W.-P., & Chang, M. C. (2018). Occupational therapy interventions to improve activities of daily living for community-dwelling older adults: A systematic review. *The American Journal of Occupational Therapy, 72*(4), 7204190060p1–7204190060p11. https://doi.org/10.5014/ajot.2018.031252.

López-Bueno, R., López-Sánchez, G. F., Casajús, J. A., Calatayud, J., Tully, M. A., & Smith, L. (2021). Potential health-related behaviors for pre-school and school-aged children during COVID-19 lockdown: A narrative review. *Preventive Medicine, 143*, 106349. https://doi.org/10.1016/j.ypmed.2020.106349.

Lynn, J. D., Rondón-Sulbarán, J., Quinn, E., Ryan, A., McCormack, B., & Martin, S. (2019). A systematic review of electronic assistive technology within supporting living environments for people with dementia. *Dementia, 18*(7–8), 2371–2435. https://doi.org/10.1177/1471301217733649.

Mace, R. (1985). *Universal design: Barrier free environments for everyone.* Designers West.

Madsen, M., & Josephsson, S. (2017). Engagement in occupation as an inquiring process: Exploring the situatedness of occupation. *Journal of Occupational Science, 24*(4), 412–424. https://doi.org/10.1080/14427591.2017.1308266.

Mahmood, A., O'Dea, E., Bigonnesse, C., Labbe, D., Mahal, T., Qureshi, M., & Mortenson, W. B. (2020). Stakeholders walkability/wheelability audit in neighbourhoods (SWAN): User-led audit and photographic documentation in Canada. *Disability & Society, 35*(6), 902–925. https://doi.org/10.1080/09687599.2019.1649127.

Margot-Cattin, I., Kuhne, N., Kottorp, A., Cutchin, M., Öhman, A., & Nygård, L. (2019). Development of a questionnaire to evaluate out-of-home participation for people with dementia. *The American Journal of Occupational Therapy, 73*(1), 7301205030p1–7301205030p10. https://doi.org/10.5014/ajot.2019.027144.

Morville, A.-L., Amris, K., Eklund, M., Danneskiold-Samsøe, B., & Erlandsson, L.-K. (2015). A longitudinal study of changes in asylum seekers ability regarding activities of daily living during their stay in the asylum center. *Journal of Immigrant and Minority Health, 17*(3), 852–859.

Murroni, V., Cavalli, R., Basso, A., Borella, E., Meneghetti, C., Melendugno, A., & Pazzaglia, F. (2021). Effectiveness of therapeutic gardens for people with dementia: A systematic review. *International Journal of Environmental Research and Public Health, 18*(18), 9595. https://doi.org/10.3390/ijerph18189595.

Novak, I., & Honan, I. (2019). Effectiveness of paediatric occupational therapy for children with disabilities: A systematic review. *Australian Occupational Therapy Journal, 66*(3), 258–273. https://doi.org/10.1111/1440-1630.12573.

Olivier, B., Verdonck, M., & Caseleijn, D. (2020). Digital technologies in undergraduate and postgraduate education in occupational therapy and physiotherapy: A scoping review. *JBI Evidence Synthesis, 18*(5), 863–892. https://doi.org/10.11124/JBISRIR-D-19-00210.

Olszewska-Guizzo, A., Fogel, A., Escoffier, N., Sia, A., Nakazawa, K., Kumagai, A., Dan, I., & Ho, R. (2022). Therapeutic garden with contemplative features induces desirable changes in mood and brain activity in depressed adults. *Frontiers in Psychiatry, 7*(13), 757056. https://doi.org/10.3389/fpsyt.2022.757056.

Oswald, F., & Kaspar, R. (2012). On the quantitative assessment of perceived housing in later life. *Journal of Housing for the Elderly, 26*(1–3), 72–93. https://doi.org/10.1080/02763893.2012.673391.

Packer, T. L., Boshoff, K., & DeJonge, D. (2008). Development of the activity card sort - Australia. *Australian Occupational Therapy Journal, 55*(3), 199–206. https://doi.org/10.1111/j.1440-1630.2007.00686.x.

Patil, G., Asbjørnslett, M., Aurlien, K., & Levin, N. (2019). Gardening as a meaningful occupation in initial stroke rehabilitation: An occupational therapist perspective. *The Open Journal of Occupational Therapy, 7*(3), 1–15. https://doi.org/10.15453/2168-6408.1561.

Pettersson, C., Nilsson, M., Andersson, M., & Wijk, H. (2021). The impact of the physical environment for caregiving in ordinary housing: Experiences of staff in home- and health-care services. *Applied ergonomics, 92*, 103352. https://doi.org/10.1016/j.apergo.2020.103352.

Prior, S., Maciver, D., Aas, R. W., Kirsh, B., Lexen, A., van Niekerk, L., Fitzpatrick, L. I., & Forsyth, K. (2020). An enhanced individual placement and support (IPS) intervention based on the model of human occupation (MOHO); a prospective cohort study. *BMC Psychiatry, 20*, 361. https://doi.org/10.1186/s12888-020-02745-3.

Risser, R., Månsson Lexell, E., Bell, D., Iwarsson, S., & Ståhl, A. (2015). Use of local public transport among people with cognitive impairments – a literature review. *Transportation Research Part F: Traffic Psychology and Behaviour, 29*, 83–97. https://doi.org/10.1016/j.trf.2015.01.002.

Rudman, D. L. (2010). Occupational terminology. Occupational possibilities. *Journal of Occupational Science, 17*(1), 55–59. https://doi.org/10.1080/14427591.2010.9686673.

Scheidt, R. J., & Norris-Baker, C. (2003). The general ecological model revisited: Evolution, current status and continuing challenges. *Annual Review of Gerontology and Geriatrics, 23*, 34–58.

Scott, M., Falkmer, M., Falkmer, T., & Girdler, S. (2018). Evaluating the effectiveness of an autism-specific workplace tool for employers: A randomised controlled trial. *Journal of Autism and Developmental Disorders, 48*, 3377–3392. https://doi.org/10.1007/s10803-018-3611-0.

Simpson, E., Sawatzky, B., Forwell, S., Backman, C. L., Symington, D., Vu, M., & Mortenson, B. W. (2022). A mixed-methods study exploring and comparing the experiences of people who sustained a spinal cord injury earlier versus later in life. *Spinal Cord, 60*(8), 706–711. https://doi.org/10.1038/s41393-022-00767-0.

Slaug, B., Granbom, M., & Iwarsson, S. (2020). An aging population and an aging housing stock – housing accessibility problems in typical Swedish dwellings. *Journal of Aging and Environment, 34*(2), 156–174. https://doi.org/10.1080/26892618.2020.1743515.

Smallfield, S., & Lucas Molitor, W. (2018). Occupational therapy interventions supporting social participation and leisure engagement for community-dwelling older adults: A systematic review. *The American Journal of Occupational Therapy, 72*(4), 7204190020. https://doi.org/10.5014/ajot.2018.030627.

Son, H.-J., Kim, D.-S., & Park, S.-A. (2022). Horticultural therapy for improving the work performance and interpersonal relationships of persons with intellectual disabilities. *International Journal of Environmental Research and Public Health, 19*, 13874. https://doi.org/10.3390/ijerph192113874.

Struckmeyer, L. R., & Pickens, N. D. (2016). Home modifications for people with Alzheimer's disease: A scoping review. *The American Journal of Occupational Therapy, 70*(1). 7001270020p1-9. https://doi.org/10.5014/ajot.2015.016089.

Taei, A., Jönson, H., & Granbom, M. (2023). Crime, disorder, and territorial stigmatization: Older adults living in deprived neighborhoods. *The Gerontologist, 63*(5), 910–919. https://doi.org/10.1093/geront/gnac159.

Taylor, R. (2017). *Kielhofner's model of human occupation*. Lippincott Williams and Wilkins.

Törnquist, K., & Sonn, U. (2014). Towards an ADL taxonomy for occupational therapists. *Scandinavian Journal of Occupational Therapy, 21*(Supp 1), 20–27. https://doi.org/10.3109/11038128.2014.952885.

Townsend, E., & Polatajko, H. (2007). *Enabling occupation II – Advancing an occupational therapy vision for health, well-being & justice through occupation*. CAOT.

Tse, T., Lentin, P., Douglas, J., & Carey, L. M. (2022). Understanding activity participation 3-months after stroke: A mixed methodology study. *Disability and Rehabilitation, 44*(12), 2868–2878. https://doi.org/10.1080/09638288.2020.1849429.

United Nations, UN. (2015). Agenda 2030. Retrieved March 21, 2023, from https://sdgs.un.org/goals.

van den Berg, M. E. L., Winsall, M., Dyer, S. M., Breen, F., Gresham, M., & Crotty, M. (2020). Understanding the barriers and enablers to using outdoor spaces in nursing homes: A systematic review. *Gerontologist, 60*(4), e254–e269. https://doi.org/10.1093/geront/gnz055.

Vergouw, J. W., Smits-Pelser, H., Kars, M. C., van Houwelingen, T., van Os-Medendorp, H., Kort, H., & Bleijenberg, N. (2020). Needs, barriers and facilitators of older adults towards eHealth in general practice: a qualitative study. *Primary health care research & development, 2*, 21:e54. doi: 10.1017/S1463423620000547. PMID: 33263272; PMCID: PMC7737136.

Wellecke, C, D'Cruz, K., Winkler, Di., Douglas, J., Goodwin, I., Davis, E., & Mulherin, P. (2022). Accessible design features and home modifications to improve physical housing accessibility: A mixed-methods survey of occupational therapists. *Disability and Health Journal, 15*(3), 101281. https://doi.org/10.1016/j.dhjo.2022.101281.

Wenger, I., Schulzeb, C., Lundström, U., & Prellwitz, M. (2021). Children's perceptions of playing on inclusive playgrounds: A qualitative study. *Scandinavian Journal of Occupational Therapy, 28*(2), 136–146. https://doi.org/10.1080/11038128.2020.181076.

Whiteneck, G. G., Harrison-Felix, C. L., Mellick, D. C., Brooks, C. A., Charliefue, S. B., & Gerhart, K. A. (2004). Quantifying environmental factors: A measure of physical, attitudinal, service, productivity, and policy barriers. *Archives of Physical Medicine and Rehabilitation, 85*(8), 1324–1335. https://doi.org/10.1016/j.apmr.2003.09.027.

World Health Organization, WHO. (2001). International Classification of Functioning, Disability and Health (ICF). Retrieved March 21, 2023, from http://www.who.int/classifications/icf/en/.

REFLECTION

1. Choose a situation and focus on one occupation in that situation. Describe how the micro, meso and macro contexts may impact occupational participation.

2. To evaluate environmental impact on occupational participation, different approaches and methods must be used. Suggest one qualitative and one quantitative method to assess the environmental impact on occupational participation. Describe how the environment is addressed using these methods.

3. What kind of data is needed to make environmental interventions on societal levels?

16

EXPLORING OCCUPATIONAL PARTICIPATION USING THE CANADIAN OCCUPATIONAL PERFORMANCE MEASURE

HEATHER COLQUHOUN ■ ANNE W. HUNT ■ JANET F. MURCHISON

CHAPTER OUTLINE

Overview

The Canadian Occupational Performance Measure (COPM) and how it is used to determine a person's self-identified issues with their occupational performance and measure improvements over the course of occupational therapy intervention are described in this chapter. A historical review of the COPM is provided followed by a description of current resources for incorporating it into practice. Theoretical considerations with emphasis on the strong alignment between the COPM and the Canadian Model of Occupational Participation (CanMOP) and essential characteristics and key administration issues are presented. Focus is placed on common communication pitfalls that hinder occupational performance issue identification and professional considerations or 'tips' for each of the steps undertaken to administer the tool. A general overview of the tool's psychometric characteristics is provided.

KEY POINTS

- The Canadian Occupational Performance Measure (COPM) is a semistandardised assessment to identify occupational performance issues and measure individuals' perceptions of change in occupational performance and satisfaction.

- The COPM encourages practice that is based on a collaborative relationship between the person and the occupational therapist and is person-centred, occupation-focused and outcome-oriented.

- The COPM consists of a semistructured interview to identify occupational performance issues, followed by a rating of these issues for importance and current performance and satisfaction regarding this performance.

- The COPM aligns with the Canadian Model of Occupational Participation.

- Common COPM pitfalls include a disconnect between what an individual expresses and what an occupational therapist perceives as important, questions that include too many occupational performance issues and insufficient time given for the individual to fully clarify their issues.

■ The COPM is reliable and valid with good clinical utility.

INTRODUCTION

The Canadian Occupational Performance Measure (COPM) is a semistandardised assessment designed to be used by occupational therapists (Law et al., 2019). Considered a gold standard for identifying occupational performance[1] issues and measuring individuals' perceptions of change in the performance and satisfaction of doing occupations (McColl et al., 2005; Parker & Sykes, 2006; Wressle et al., 2002), the COPM encourages practice that is based on a collaborative relationship and is person-centred, occupation-focused and outcome-oriented. It is applicable for use with people who have a wide range of occupational performance concerns that may be impacted by their illness, injury or impairment. The COPM is also applicable to use in a broad range of practice settings.

In the following sections, the history of the COPM is presented, along with the relationship between the COPM and the Canadian Model of Occupational Participation (CanMOP) (Egan & Restall, 2022). The measure is then described. Throughout this description, advice is provided and some potential barriers are discussed regarding the administration of the tool. A general overview of the tool's psychometric characteristics is provided.

THE CANADIAN OCCUPATIONAL PERFORMANCE MEASURE

The COPM was developed by Canadian occupational therapy leaders Mary Law, Sue Baptiste, Anne Carswell, Mary Ann McColl, Helene Polatajko and Nancy Pollock and was first published in 1990 (Law et al., 1990). It is now in its fifth (revised) edition (Law et al., 2019).

---

[1]'Occupational performance' is currently the concept assessed and the terminology used by the COPM. While the term 'occupational participation' is used as a preferred term in this book in order to align with the introduction of the Canadian Model of Occupational Participation, we have used the term 'occupational performance' in this chapter to maintain alignment with the COPM.

In addition to complete administration and scoring instructions, the latest COPM administration manual provides an excellent up-to-date summary of the related research. The COPM has been used in practice with a diverse range of people and age spans. It has been translated into at least 36 languages and includes an aphasia-friendly version (Coates et al., 2015).

The COPM is valuable both as an individual assessment and as a tool for demonstrating the effectiveness of occupational therapy interventions. Individual results of the COPM demonstrate the extent to which individuals feel they have improved over the course of receiving occupational therapy in valued occupations that they identified as ones with which they were having difficulty. The COPM is an individualised outcome measure in that the issues to be addressed and measured are unique to the individual (Donnelly & Carswell, 2002).

Theoretical Considerations and Alignment With the Canadian Model of Occupational Participation

The COPM was originally developed for use in practice guided by the Canadian Model of Occupational Performance (Law et al., 1997), by extension the Canadian Model of Occupational Performance and Engagement (CMOP-E; Townsend & Polatajko, 2007) and more recently the CanMOP (Egan & Restall, 2022) (refer to Chapter 11). There are numerous examples of how the key concepts that underpin the COPM are aligned to the CanMOP and its associated process framework, The Canadian Occupational Therapy Inter-Relational Practice Process (COTIPP) (refer to Chapter 12). At its core, the COPM requires that the therapist values the person as an expert in their occupational participation within their own contexts and values the relationship that is built and the resulting engagement as a critical part of the assessment process.

The COPM was developed to be a person-centred tool predicated on the recognition that people are both experts about their occupational performance and partners in their own care. The concept of person-centred is in alignment with the CanMOP concept of collaborative relationship-focused practice, as it acknowledges the contextual relevance to the lived experience of the person. One of the six action domains in the COTIPP is 'Exploring Occupational Participation'. At its core, the COPM requires that the therapist sees the person as an expert in their occupational participation within their own contexts and values the relationship that is built and the resulting engagement as a critical part of the process. Another of the CanMOP six action domains is 'codesign priorities, goals, outcomes and plans'. The use of the COPM facilitates collaboration between the person and the occupational therapist that supports codesigning of occupational goals and measuring outcomes in a person and relationship-centric manner. The issue identification process inherent in the COPM includes a discussion of the importance the person places on each issue. This is a further example of exploring and understanding occupational participation. The COPM's format as a self-report measure is in keeping with a strong commitment to the inclusion of a person's perspective in all steps of the occupational therapy process, from identification of priorities to evaluation of outcomes.

The CanMOP outlines eight important questions to consider when choosing an assessment, all of which support the use of the COPM. For example, answering the questions *What are the assumptions upon which the assessment is based?' (Question #1)* or *'Whose knowledge and values does the assessment align with'* (Question #3) or *'Does the assessment allow room for collaboration and partnership'* (Question #6) becomes straightforward when using the COPM. The COPM places the person at the centre of the assessment and encourages them to identify contextually meaningful occupational performance issues and to self-rank importance and self-evaluate performance and satisfaction with these issues. The COPM is an ideal tool for collaboratively exploring occupational concerns, identifying priorities and examining change following the development and implementation of an intervention.

THE COPM PROCESS

The COPM is carried out using a semistructured interview in which the person is guided to identify occupational performance issues. The occupational therapist guides the person to rate how important the identified issues are and leads the person to select up to five key issues that can be the focus of therapy. Then, the person rates their current performance and satisfaction with each of the occupational performance issues that have been prioritised.

Care should be taken to ensure that the person understands what occupational therapy is and why the COPM is being used. That is, the person should appreciate that the COPM results will guide which occupations will be the focus of occupational therapy. Additionally, care must be taken to allow for the interaction necessary to develop the therapeutic relationship while carrying out this assessment.

The COPM manual provides detailed instructions. Scoring sheets allow for efficient recording of the person's responses, as well as performance and satisfaction scores during the initial administration and reevaluation. The manual and scoring sheets are necessary for administering the COPM.

The COPM is considered a semistandardised assessment, as there are specific steps that need to be included in the process and specific results that are gathered. However, there is no prescribed script for the semistructured interview. Each interview is unique. Exactly what will be said during the interview depends on a combination of the interpersonal styles of the therapist and the person being interviewed.

It is common to complete the COPM as part of an initial assessment. The COPM interview is an opportunity to facilitate the development of the therapeutic relationship and to set an initial standard of individual engagement in the therapeutic process. However, there may be times when it is beneficial to develop the therapeutic relationship in other ways before introducing the COPM.

Once a therapist is experienced with the process, administering the COPM takes approximately 20 to 40 minutes, although it has been shown to take as little as 9 minutes (McKittrick et al., 2022). People who are familiar with occupational therapy services and their own occupational performance and participation priorities may complete the process relatively quickly. Those who are less knowledgeable regarding occupational therapy or who have little experience working in a collaborative relationship with a health-care provider, may require more time. In addition, if there are communication challenges between the occupational therapist and the person, as for example when the occupational therapist does not speak the person's first language or when the person has expressive or receptive language problems, additional administration time may be needed.

Implementing the COPM in practice may be challenging for a number of reasons. It can be difficult to listen to and acknowledge an individual's occupational performance issues, knowing that these may be quite different from what the occupational therapist thinks should be the focus of therapy. Also, it does take time, something that always seems to be in short supply in a busy practice (McColl et al., 2005). However, the overall therapeutic experience is enhanced when time is taken at the outset of therapy to identify meaningful occupational performance issues using the COPM.

There are five steps to administering the COPM. In the descriptions of each step that follows, administration suggestions are provided along with recommendations for handling potentially challenging situations. Each step concludes with a set of key professional considerations. For specific instructions regarding COPM administration, readers should refer to the most recent COPM manual (Law et al., 2019) or the COPM website (www.thecopm.ca).

Step 1: Identify Occupational Performance Issues

The COPM begins with the identification of the occupational performance issues the person is experiencing. To assist a person to identify these issues the occupational therapist may ask them what they need to do, want to do and are expected to do in their daily lives. The occupational therapist may ask the person to describe a typical day or provide examples of occupations that are often identified by others with similar health challenges. The occupational therapist records all of the important occupational performance issues that the individual identifies.

Identification of priority occupational performance issues is central to the initiation of effective, collaborative relationship-focused, person-centred occupational therapy. Key facilitators of this step include reflective listening, acknowledgement and affirmation and open-ended questioning. Reflective listening means providing each person with the time they need to respond, listening carefully to what has been said and responding in a way that promotes additional information and clarification.

Simple acknowledgements (such as, 'Okay' or 'hmm') and affirmations (such as, 'That seems really important for you') have been shown to facilitate occupational

performance issue identification (Hunt et al., 2015). In interviews, these types of statements are typically followed by a natural pause in conversation. These pauses provide people with opportunities to talk more about their specific concerns and priorities. This in turn facilitates the identification of key occupational performance issues.

Open-ended questions are used to learn more about occupational performance issues in general. They may also be used to prompt people to talk about issues that they may not have considered. For example, 'How are you managing your grocery shopping?' may prompt a person who is having difficulty moving around the community to consider this as a potential occupational performance issue. Such prompts may be particularly helpful for people experiencing cognitive impairment.

A number of common communication pitfalls that hinder the identification of issues have been highlighted (Hunt et al., 2015). These tend to reflect a disconnection between what a person has said and what the occupational therapist has heard or judged important. This can happen when occupational therapists do not obtain enough detail about an issue to properly define it. This can also occur when occupational therapists prematurely form a picture in their minds of the issue or dismiss some issues as not achievable and therefore not worthy of discussion (Kessler et al., 2019).

Posing a question that includes multiple occupational performance issues can also inhibit the identification of important issues. For many people, a question that includes a list of multiple issues may be confusing. People experiencing cognitive or communication difficulties may still be processing the first issue raised after the occupational therapist has moved on to other potential issues. Specific questions that encourage a person to reflect on everyday occupations may be more useful than a long list of items. For example, rather than saying, 'Tell me about your showering, dressing and meal preparation', the occupational therapist could say, 'Tell me about your morning routine'.

Moving abruptly from one occupational performance issue to another is also a common cause of inadequate occupational therapist understanding of the issues. Sudden changes of topic may signal to the person that their responses are not important or are to be kept short. This not only limits the amount of information the person is able to provide; it may also make the person reluctant to share important concerns. In addition to listening carefully, leaving space for details and confirming that the occupational therapist's understanding of the issue is accurate, it is suggested that occupational therapists make a concluding statement or question before moving on to the next section – for example, 'Before we finish with our discussion of your morning routine, is there anything else you would like to discuss?' Key professional considerations for Step 1 are listed in Box 16.1.

Step 2: Rate and Choose the Five Occupational Performance Issues That Are Most Important to the Person

In this step, the occupational therapist works together with the person to choose up to five most important occupational performance issues. This begins with numerically rating all of the identified occupational performance issues. For some people, this is easy; for others, it is not. It is acceptable and even encouraged to try different approaches to rating importance; there is no 'one way' to complete this task. The COPM manual contains a visual rating scale that can be used to facilitate this rating of importance.

Once the rating is done, the occupational therapist confirms with the person their five most highly rated issues. This is done by reviewing these issues in light of the other highly rated issues and asking the person to confirm that these are in fact the issues they want to focus on. Five key occupational performance issues are generally considered the maximum number of issues that can be worked on at one time (Law et al., 2019). A person may choose fewer issues and additional issues can be considered later. Key professional considerations for Step 2 are listed in Box 16.2.

Step 3: Score Performance and Satisfaction with Performance

For each selected occupational performance issue each person is asked to rate: (1) their perception of their current performance and (2) how satisfied they are with the current performance. A visual rating scale is provided in the COPM manual to facilitate this task. People may find it easier to first consider how well they feel they perform an occupational performance issue and then think about how satisfied they are with this

> **BOX 16.1**
> **KEY PROFESSIONAL CONSIDERATIONS FOR STEP 1**
>
> **SET THE STAGE FOR USING THE COPM**
> Ensure the person understands that the therapist wants to engage in a collaborative relationship in which the person's occupational needs and desires are of critical importance. Situate the COPM within the overall assessment process. For example, if other assessments will be used, the occupational therapist should explain that the COPM is one of the assessments that will be conducted to gain an overview of the difficulties the person is experiencing in their daily life. The person should be informed that the COPM will help determine the focus of therapy.
>
> Be ready to assist the person in speaking in terms of occupational performance issues. If instead of occupational performance issues, the person identifies issues relating to performance components (such as strength or pain), the occupational therapist should assist the person in identifying how these problems are affecting what the person needs to do and wants to do. For example, 'What does your fatigue mean for your morning routine?'
>
> **PHRASE THE ISSUE IN A WAY THAT IS SHORT BUT CLEAR**
> Ensure that the wording clearly reflects the performance issue. For example, 'swimming' could be more clearly stated as 'knowing how to swim' or 'going swimming regularly' depending on the person's concern.
>
> **AVOID CENSORING THE PERSON'S OCCUPATIONAL PERFORMANCE CONCERNS**
> Occupational therapists need to be aware of their own thoughts about the feasibility of a particular occupation, the potential to work on the occupation within the practice setting or other issues related to their feelings about the occupation, as these can cause the occupational therapist to consciously or unconsciously dismiss particular concerns raised by the person. Write down all of the person's concerns to ensure that this does not happen.

performance. That is, it is usually easiest for the person to rate performance and satisfaction of each issue in turn. Key professional considerations for Step 3 are listed in Box 16.3.

Step 4: Reassessment

Reassessment consists simply of returning to Step 3 and asking the person to rate their current performance and satisfaction with each of the selected occupational performance issues.

BOX 16.2
KEY PROFESSIONAL CONSIDERATIONS FOR STEP 2

USE THE VISUAL RATING SCALE AS NEEDED

The visual rating scale may be helpful for people who might benefit from the use of a prompt (such as people experiencing cognitive impairments).

CONSIDER ADAPTING RATING SCALES

Some people have difficulty making decisions and feel anxious about committing to a number. Feel free to use descriptors instead of numbers if this seems to be the case (e.g. very important, somewhat important, not that important, very unimportant).

HELP THE PERSON TO PRIORITISE AREAS OF EQUAL IMPORTANCE

If the person rates more than five areas of equal importance, ask, 'Which is more important to you, this problem or that problem?' or 'Which issues are most important for you to work on in therapy?' or 'Which issues are the ones that you would like to start working on today, knowing that if we have time, we could go back to some of the other ones?'

EXPLAIN HOW IDENTIFYING THE MOST IMPORTANT OCCUPATIONAL PERFORMANCE ISSUES WILL BE USED

Ensure that the person understands that the occupational performance issues identified as most important will guide the discussion to collaboratively determine the goals that will be addressed in occupational therapy.

REMEMBER THAT IDENTIFYING OCCUPATIONAL PERFORMANCE ISSUES IS NOT GOAL SETTING

Although the priority occupational performance issues will indicate what the person wants to work on in therapy, typically it will not provide an indication of the goal (i.e. what the person wants the performance to look like after intervention). Working with the person to develop a clear description of the goal for each occupational performance issue is an important step that must take place after the completion of the COPM and before the intervention begins.

BOX 16.3
KEY PROFESSIONAL CONSIDERATIONS FOR STEP 3

COMPLETE BOTH RATINGS FOR AN OCCUPATIONAL PERFORMANCE ISSUE AT THE SAME TIME

Have the person complete the performance and satisfaction ratings for each problem before rating the next occupational performance issue.

USE THE VISUAL RATING SCALE AS NEEDED

The visual rating scale may be helpful for people who benefit from the use of a prompt (such as those experiencing cognitive impairment).

PROVIDE EXAMPLES

Use examples of numeric rating systems that may be familiar to the person (e.g. rating an Olympic performance).

OFFER REASSURANCE

For people who are anxious about committing to a number, emphasise that their rating is only a general way of gaining an understanding of how they feel about their performance at this time. That there is no right or wrong answer.

MODIFY THE LANGUAGE USED

Experiment with different ways of simply explaining performance and satisfaction.

---

a descriptive measure to identify priority occupational performance issues and related current rating of performance and satisfaction.

There have been many studies of the COPM's psychometric properties. Summaries of these can be found in an annotated bibliography (CAOT, 2006) and the COPM manual (Law et al., 2019). The COPM website (www.thecopm.ca) also provides references of studies using or testing the COPM. Brief highlights of these studies are discussed below.

Clinical Utility

The clinical utility, specifically the ease of administration and usefulness of an instrument, is critical to its value in practice (Law, 1987). The COPM is easily accessible to occupational therapists through the Canadian Occupational Performance Measure website (www.thecopm.ca/). No specific qualifications are required to conduct the COPM; however, using the measure requires that the occupational therapist be

---

Key professional considerations for Step 4 are listed in Box 16.4.

PSYCHOMETRIC PROPERTIES OF THE COPM

The COPM was primarily designed for use as an evaluative measure of changes in occupational performance and satisfaction. The COPM can also simply be used as

BOX 16.4
KEY PROFESSIONAL
CONSIDERATIONS FOR STEP 4

INTERPRETATION OF RESULTS SHOULD INCLUDE THE PERSON

Therapists should work in partnership with the person to appropriately interpret the person's scores.

APPRECIATE THAT EACH INDIVIDUAL'S CONCERNS AND STANDARDS MAY SHIFT

Sometimes, people rate their performance and satisfaction differently as they progress in therapy. During the course of therapy people may become more aware of their current occupational performance. They may find that they are having more difficulty than they thought they would with a particular occupation or that they are able to carry out this occupation more easily than they had imagined. Either situation may lead them to alter the way they approach their performance or satisfaction ratings. It may also lead them to alter their goals. Such changes may lead to smaller change scores than the therapist had anticipated based on the changes the therapist observed in the person's performance.

REMEMBER THAT THE COPM IS NOT A GOAL ATTAINMENT SCALE

COPM scores may not always reflect the degree to which goals have been met but rather reflect each individual's perspective on how well they currently perform the occupational performance issues and their satisfaction with that performance. In addition to COPM change scores, occupational therapy reports should include an indication of the attainment of goals that were set at the beginning of therapy.

comfortable with a collaborative relationship-focused, person-centred and occupation-based approach to both assessment and intervention (Law et al., 2019).

Occupational therapists have indicated that the COPM is useful in the occupational therapy process. Studies suggest that using the COPM assists with goal setting and intervention planning, provides useful feedback on the performance improvements of people receiving occupational therapy and facilitates communication (Wressle et al., 2002). Use of the COPM has been found to increase the person-centred nature of practice (Colquhoun et al., 2012; Donnelly & Carswell, 2002; McColl et al., 2005), to improve goal-setting (Chen et al., 2002) and to assist in defining the work of occupational therapy (Fedden et al., 1999).

Occupational therapists state that using the COPM allows them to work more holistically with people and assists with developing realistic and person-centred goals (Chen et al., 2002). Using the COPM as a routine part of practice improved the quality of occupational therapy service on a number of important practice dimensions, such as occupational therapist knowledge of the person's perspective, professional decision-making and documentation (Colquhoun et al., 2012). Occupational therapists indicate that their priorities are often different from the priorities of people receiving occupational therapy (Law et al., 1990), suggesting that the COPM provides an important window into these people's perspectives.

Reliability

Test-retest reliability refers to the level of consistency between scores across two administrations of the tool over a period when scores would not be expected to change. Test-retest reliability provides an indication as to whether a change in a score measured using the same instrument between the initial assessment and the reassessment is a real change. Test-retest reliability has been found to be between $r = .65$ and $r = .85$ (Law et al., 2019), meaning that the COPM demonstrates moderate to high reliability (Portney & Watkins, 2000).

Validity

A valid tool measures what it is designed to measure (Portney & Watkins, 2000). Overall, the COPM demonstrates good validity across multiple studies and validity types. Content validity is generally viewed as good, as it explicitly addresses core dimensions of occupation (Law et al., 2019).

The COPM has been shown to have good convergent and divergent validity. That is, its scores correlate with scores of related measures rather than with scores of measures to which its results should be unrelated. For example, the COPM correlates well with other self-report measures of occupation such as the Return to Normal Living Index (Chen et al., 2002) but correlates poorly with measures of functional status and performance components, such as the Functional Independence Measure (Chan & Lee, 1997), the Disability of the Arm, Shoulder and Hand scale and the Michigan Hand Outcomes Questionnaire (van de Ven-Stevens et al., 2015).

The COPM is responsive to change in an individual's performance and satisfaction with their occupational performance (Carpenter et al., 2001; Eyssen et al., 2011). A two-point change in performance and satisfaction is generally considered clinically significant (Law et al., 2019).

Over three decades since the development and initial publication of the COPM, research on its psychometric properties continues. Some of these more recent papers focus on the value of the COPM in specific health conditions such as spinal cord injury (Berardi et al., 2019), populations such home-dwelling older adults (Tuntland et al., 2016), practice settings such as primary care (Donnelly et al., 2017) and varying country or language diversities such as Denmark (Enemark et al., 2021) and Turkey (Torpil et al., 2021).

Two systematic reviews have recently been published that synthesised studies of COPM measurement properties in general (Ohno et al., 2021) and specifically to geriatric rehabilitation (de Waal et al., 2022). There is also a scoping review that synthesises how the COPM is being used with children with impairments, how it contributes to family-centred practice and how it is used in combination with development assessments (Mathews et al., 2020).

The COPM has also received the attention of knowledge translation researchers who have conducted a theoretical domains framework study on the COPM that profiles behaviour change and reports theory-derived barriers to the use of the COPM (Colquhoun et al., 2020).

CONCLUSION

The COPM is an individualised outcome measure that provides the occupational therapist and the person receiving occupational therapy services with prioritised occupational performance issues and pre-intervention and postintervention measures of their performance and satisfaction with this performance. It is aligned with the CanMOP, and it is applicable for use with a very broad range of people receiving occupational therapy services and is available in many languages. In addition to providing an excellent indication of how well occupational therapy has addressed an individual's occupational performance

issues, it can also be used to demonstrate the overall effectiveness of occupational therapy within a caseload or service.

REFERENCES

Berardi, A., Galeoto, G., Guarino, D., Marquez, M. A., De Santis, R., Valente, D., Caporale, G., & Tofani, M. (2019). Construct validity, test-retest reliability, and the ability to detect change of the Canadian Occupational Performance Measure in a spinal cord injury population. *Spinal Cord Series and Cases, 5*(1), 52.

Canadian Association of Occupational Therapists. (2006). *Research on the Canadian occupational performance measure: An annotated resource.* CAOT Publications ACE.

Carpenter, L., Baker, G. A., & Tyldesley, B. (2001). The use of the Canadian occupational performance measure as an outcome of a pain management program. *Canadian Journal of Occupational Therapy, 68,* 16–22.

Chan, C. C., & Lee, T. (1997). Validity of the Canadian occupational performance measure. *Occupational Therapy International, 4,* 231–249.

Chen, Y. H., Rodger, S., & Polatajko, H. (2002). Experiences with the COPM and client-centred practice in adult neurorehabilitation in Taiwan. *Occupational Therapy International, 9,* 167–184.

Coates, R., Irvine, C., & Sutherland, C. (2015). Development of an aphasia-friendly Canadian occupational performance measure. *British Journal of Occupational Therapy, 78,* 196–199.

Colquhoun, H. L., Letts, L. J., Law, M. C., Macdermid, J. C., & Missiuna, C. A. (2012). Administration of the Canadian occupational performance measure: Effect on practice. *Canadian Journal of Occupational Therapy, 79,* 120–128.

Colquhoun, H. L., Islam, R., Sullivan, K. J., Sandercock, J., Steinwender, S., & Grimshaw, J. M. (2020). Behaviour change domains likely to influence occupational therapist use of the Canadian Occupational Performance Measure. *Occupational Therapy International, 2020*(1), 3549835.

de Waal, M. W. M., Haaksma, M. L., Doornebosch, A. J., Meijs, R., & Achterberg, W. P. (2022). Systematic review of measurement properties of the Canadian Occupational Performance Measure in geriatric rehabilitation. *European Geriatric Medicine, 13*(6), 1281–1298.

Donnelly, C., & Carswell, A. (2002). Individualized outcome measures: A review of the literature. *Canadian Journal of Occupational Therapy, 69,* 84–94.

Donnelly, C., O'Neill, C., Bauer, M., & Letts, L. (2017). Canadian Occupational Performance Measure (COPM) in primary care: A profile of practice. *The American Journal of Occupational Therapy, 71*(6), 7106265010p1–7106265010p8.

Egan, M., & Restall, G. (Eds.). (2022). *Promoting occupational participation: Collaborative relationship-focused occupational therapy.* CAOT Publication ACE.

Enemark Larsen, A., Jessen Winge, C., & Christensen, J. R. (2021). Clinical utility of the Danish version of the Canadian Occupational Performance Measure. *Scandinavian Journal of Occupational Therapy, 28*(3), 239–250.

Eyssen, I., Steultjens, M., Oud, T., Bolt, E. M., Maasdam, A., & Dekker, J. (2011). Responsiveness of the Canadian Occupational

Performance Measure. *Journal of Rehabilitation Research & Development, 48,* 517–528.

Fedden, T., Green, A., & Hill, T. (1999). Out of the woods: The Canadian Occupational Performance Measure, from the manual into practice. *British Journal of Occupational Therapy, 62,* 318–320.

Hunt, A. W., Le Dorze, G., Polatajko, H., Bottari, C., & Dawson, D. R. (2015). Communication during goal-setting in brain injury rehabilitation: What helps and what hinders? *British Journal of Occupational Therapy, 78,* 488–498.

Kessler, D., Walker, I., Sauvé-Schenk, K., & Egan, M. (2019). Goal setting dynamics that facilitate or impede a client-centered approach. *Scandinavian Journal of Occupational Therapy, 26*(5), 315–324.

Law, M. (1987). Measurement in occupational therapy: Scientific criteria for evaluation. *Canadian Journal of Occupational Therapy, 54,* 133–138.

Law, M., Baptiste, S., Carswell, A., Mccoll, M., Polatajko, H., & Pollock, N. (2019). *Canadian occupational performance measure* (5th ed.-revised). COPM Inc.

Law, M., Baptiste, S., Mccoll, M., Opzoomer, A., Polatajko, H., & Pollock, N. (1990). The Canadian Occupational Performance Measure: An outcome measure for occupational therapy. *Canadian Journal of Occupational Therapy, 57,* 82–87.

Law, M., Polatajko, H., Baptiste, S., & Townsend, E. (1997). Core concepts of occupational therapy. In E. Townsend, S. Stanton, & M. Law (Eds.), *Enabling occupation: An occupational therapy perspective* (pp. 29–56). CAOT Publications.

Mathews, S. B., Mozolic-Staunton, B., & Salehi, N. (2020). Canadian Occupational Performance Measure and early intervention: A scoping review. *Journal of Occupational Therapy, Schools, & Early Intervention, 13*(4), 353–373.

McColl, M. A., Law, M., Baptiste, S., Pollock, N., Carswell, A., & Polatajko, H. J. (2005). Targeted applications of the Canadian Occupational Performance Measure. *Canadian Journal of Occupational Therapy, 72,* 298–300.

McKittrick, A., Jones, A., Lam, H., & Biggin, E. (2022). A feasibility study of the Canadian Occupational Performance Measure (COPM) in the burn cohort in an acute tertiary facility. *Burns, 48*(5), 1183–1189.

Ohno, K., Tomori, K., Sawada, T., Seike, Y., Yaguchi, A., & Kobayashi, R. (2021). Measurement properties of the Canadian Occupational Performance Measure: A systematic review. *The American Journal of Occupational Therapy, 75*(6), 1–15.

Parker, D. M., & Sykes, C. H. (2006). A systematic review of the Canadian Occupational Performance Measure: A clinical practice perspective. *British Journal of Occupational Therapy, 69,* 150–160.

Portney, L. G., & Watkins, M. P. (2000). *Foundations of clinical research: Applications to practice.* Prentice Hall.

Torpil, B., Ekici Çağlar, G., Bumin, G., & Pekçetin, S. (2021). Validity and reliability of the Turkish Canadian Occupational Performance Measure (COPM-TR) for people with multiple sclerosis. *Occupational Therapy In Health Care, 35*(3), 306–317.

Townsend, E. A., & Polatajko, H. J. (2007). *Advancing an occupational therapy vision for health, well-being, and justice through occupation.* CAOT Publications.

Tuntland, H., Aaslund, M. K., Langeland, E., Espehaug, B., & Kjeken, I. (2016). Psychometric properties of the Canadian Occupational Performance Measure in home-dwelling older adults. *Journal of multidisciplinary healthcare, 9,* 411–423.

van de Ven-Stevens, L. A., Graff, M. J., Peters, M. A., Van Der Linde, H., & Geurts, A. C. (2015). Construct validity of the Canadian Occupational Performance Measure in participants with tendon injury and Dupuytren disease. *Physical Therapy, 95,* 750–757.

Wressle, E., Eeg-Olofsson, A.-M., Marcusson, J., & Henriksson, C. (2002). Improved client participation in the rehabilitation process using a client-centred goal formulation structure. *Journal of Rehabilitation Medicine, 34,* 5–11.

REFLECTION

1. Briefly describe how using the COPM facilitates person-centred practice.

2. You are about to try using the COPM at your workplace or fieldwork setting. What might be important to include in a presentation to your colleagues or supervisor describing how this will improve your practice?

3. Identify three challenges you might face administering the COPM with a person who is having problems with memory and concentration. State what you might do to overcome these challenges.

4. The COPM is often carried out during the initial interview with a person. Describe a situation where you might decide to do the COPM a little later in therapy process.

5. If you are working on a team who might be interested in the results of the COPM, how might you share information with them?

17

EXPLORING OCCUPATIONAL PARTICIPATION USING TASK, ACTIVITY AND OCCUPATIONAL ANALYSES

CYNTHIA PERLMAN ■ CHRISTINE GUPTILL

CHAPTER OUTLINE

Overview

Occupational analysis, a perspective unique to the profession of occupational therapy, is explored as a continuum beginning with task analysis, followed by activity analysis and culminating in occupational analysis itself. The analysis process begins with understanding the sequential components of and inherent skills needed for specific activities and then builds towards participation in occupations of personal and social significance. An activity becomes an occupation when it is personally meaningful and when participation is reinforced through the process of grading and adapting. This chapter highlights the conceptual frameworks and models needed for a successful occupational analysis, including the Person-Environment-Occupation (PEO) Model, the Canadian Model of Occupational

Performance and Engagement (CMOP-E), the Model of Human Occupation (MOHO) and the new Canadian Model of Occupational Participation (CanMOP). Examples of each type of analysis and the subsequent grading and adapting of the activity/occupation, including discussion of the environmental contexts, are provided through a practice story in which grocery shopping is analysed.

KEY POINTS

- The analysis process is viewed as a continuum beginning from a task analysis to an activity analysis, leading to an occupational analysis.
- An activity becomes an occupation when its personal meaning is acknowledged and pursued, the goals are personally set, the required skills to perform are

considered and the environmental context is acknowledged.

- Occupational analysis is a perspective unique to the profession of occupational therapy, enabling the occupational therapist to evaluate and validate the meaning of the occupation for a person or collective when participating within a chosen environmental context at the micro, meso and macro levels (physical, social, cultural and institutional).

- Occupational analysis is supported by the philosophical foundations of occupational therapy and occupational science, which point to the role of meaningful occupation and occupational participation in health and wellbeing (Rush Dunton, 1931; Yerxa, 1990; 2000).

- The Person-Environment-Occupation Model (Law et al., 1996), an open systems theory-based approach, can be used as a foundational support and preanalysis tool for occupational analysis to further build upon the value of purposeful, meaningful occupations, as well as to promote further understanding of the occupation-based contexts.

- Using the results of an occupational analysis, occupational therapists can grade or adapt the activity/occupation to lead to optimal participation, engagement and competence for people, groups and communities receiving occupational therapy.

THE MEANING OF OCCUPATION FOR ANALYSIS OF ACTIVITIES AND OCCUPATIONS

A historical shift in the paradigm of occupational therapy occurred in the 1970s when there was a transition from a mechanistic/reductionist perspective of a task or activity to an occupation-focused perspective, which allowed the development of occupation-centred intervention (Aiken et al., 2011; Bauerschmidt & Nelson, 2011; Kielhofner, 2008; Wilding & Whiteford, 2007). This shift addressed the personal values and meaning attributed to occupations by a person or collective performing the occupation, whereas previously the focus was on skill-based competency and attributes, regardless of values, meaning or specific context.

Occupations are personalised activities chosen and performed by individuals or collectives because they hold meaning and purpose to them including the context in which they are performed (Reed et al., 2011; Thomas, 2023; Townsend & Polatajko, 2013). The meaning of

occupations is constructed and interpreted by the people who engage in them. People participate in occupations that have meaning and value to them, in unique, person-specific ways (Blesedell Crepeau et al., 2013; Hasselkus & Dickie, 2021; Taylor, 2017). Occupation offers experiences of creativity, cultural and spiritual expression and connection to individuals and collectives (Hasselkus & Dickie, 2021; Wilcock & Hocking, 2015), and 'Meaning is created in spaces and places in which we live' (Hasselkus & Dickie, 2021, p. xiv). Occupational therapists understand the impact of occupations on participation and engagement. They use fundamental analysis frameworks to analyse either a nonspecific contextual activity and the skills required to perform it or an occupation as a whole considering its inherent component parts and the specific environments or contexts in which it is performed. The focus of this chapter explains the concepts of task analysis, activity analysis and occupational analysis as a continuum of an analysis process. To understand this continuum, it is first important to differentiate the terms *task*, *activity* and *occupation*. These are described in Table 17.1.

When Does an Activity Become an Occupation?

Therapeutic and meaningful activities and occupations remain core professional concepts that are valued as both a *means and an end* or outcome from the intervention process. An activity becomes an occupation when the personal meaning of it is acknowledged and pursued, the goals are set, the required skills to perform it are considered and the environmental context is acknowledged.

The Influence of Meaningful Occupation on Practice

The practice of occupational therapy is *occupation-focused* and founded on a belief that humans are occupational in nature and that emphasis should be placed on the value and meaning personally attributed to the particular occupations. Nelson (1997) reiterated that pride and professional confidence result from full identification and adoption of the term *occupation,* a definitive domain of occupational therapy.

Fisher (2013) posited that a worldview and appreciation of occupation to guide professional reasoning is termed *occupation-centred*. The actual therapeutic process of engaging a person in meaningful occupations

TABLE 17.1 Differentiating Among Task, Activity and Occupation	
A task	A task comprises the general procedural steps or actions required to complete it without consideration of a context or environmental space. It refers to the conventional sequence and timing of actions or list of steps required to complete an activity (Thomas, 2015).
An activity	The actual concrete doing or completion, without a context, of the list of actions or steps that involve skills, materials and interaction with the environment. Activities comprise components and parts that can be analysed (Mosey, 1986).
An occupation	The contextual, meaningful, goal-directed everyday activities that people choose to do to occupy themselves, including caring for oneself (self-care), enjoying and participating in life outside of work (leisure) and contributing to society (productivity/work) (CAOT, 2002). Occupations are shaped by culture and evolve through the lifespan as they are reflective of personal goals, skills, roles, habits and values (Kielhofner, 2008; Taylor, 2017; Thomas, 2023).

that foster choice-making, satisfaction and restoration can be termed *occupation-based* (Fisher, 2013; Polatajko & Davis, 2012). Occupation-focused perspectives foster goals that address meaningful occupational participation that is not necessarily performance-driven. Occupation-focused occupational therapy promotes occupational participation with potential for sustainability, rather than a focus on altering body structures and functions or reducing the impairment (Martini et al., 2022). When occupational therapists are grounded by the occupation-focused paradigm, they acknowledge their expertise in maintaining the occupational perspective and focus throughout the therapeutic process (Aiken et al., 2011; Egan & Restall, 2022; Fisher, 2013; Letts, 2011).

Townsend and Polatajko (2013) identified the following attributes of occupation:

■ Basic human drive to do and to participate.
■ Source of meaning and purpose as it reflects personal interests, values and pursuits.

■ Source of control over own life through intentional choice-making.
■ Source of self-expression leading to self-identity and a trueness of self across the lifespan.
■ Source of satisfaction and self-fulfilment through participation.
■ Means for interaction with the environment (physical, social, cultural, institutional).
■ Means of organising time, behaviour, space and materials.
■ Means of skill development and competence.

Underlying these attributes is the influence of occupational participation. Occupational participation includes having access to, initiating and sustaining occupations of personal and social significance within supportive environmental contexts (Egan & Restall, 2022; Larssen-Lund & Nyman, 2017). Laws (2002, p. 640) suggests that it is 'Through participation, we acquire skills and competencies, connect with others and our communities and find purpose and meaning in life'. Participation is also expressed within the International Classification of Functioning, Disability and Health (ICF; WHO, 2001) and implies the importance of contributing and receiving through doing with others in supportive environments, thereby appreciating the health benefits of occupation beyond the execution of a task or action to one of agency, authenticity and shared purpose.

CONTINUUM OF ANALYSES: TASK, ACTIVITY AND OCCUPATION

A search of the literature reveals minimal consensus on how to define and properly differentiate between the terms *task analysis*, *activity analysis* and *occupational analysis*. Results from a Brazilian scoping review on the use and meaning of the term activity versus occupation inferred that definitions of occupation internationally are outlined and agreed upon; however, due to plurality of perspectives and diversity in fields of practice or areas of expertise, each country may also adapt its use and definition (Figueiredo et al., 2020). The delineations between activity and occupational analyses are more evident than those between task and activity analyses as they are based on occupation-focused philosophy and terminology. Blesedell Crepeau et al. (2013) advocated for using both activity and occupational analyses

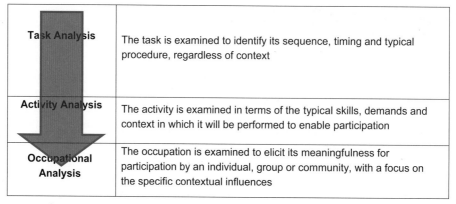

Fig. 17.1 ■ The task analysis–activity analysis–occupational analysis continuum.

to gain a deeper understanding of how people relate to their occupations. 'Practitioners must be able to analyse both the general idea of how an activity occurs within culture, as well as, the actual occupations as they are performed by the particular individuals' (Blesedell Crepeau et al., 2013, p. 237). The task analysis–activity analysis–occupational analysis can be placed on a continuum. See Fig. 17.1.

This continuum begins with the task analysis, which describes an activity's sequence and timing of steps and its typical procedure regardless of context (Allen, 1982; Thomas, 2015). For example, the task of brushing one's teeth first comprises a sequence of retrieving the toothbrush and toothpaste, opening the toothpaste tube by rotating the cap and then squeezing the toothpaste and placing a small amount along the bristles of the toothbrush.

Activity analysis, the next stage in the continuum, starts with task analysis of the sequence and timing of steps and then further examines the skills and general content required to perform the activity. 'Activity analysis is a clinical practice tool which must be learned and applied by all occupational therapy students in order to meet and fulfil the occupational performance needs of their clients, at any point within the lifespan' (Perlman et al., 2005, p. 154). As a result of an activity analysis, the inherent skills and abilities needed to perform the activity are identified; however, they are not specific to a particular individual. This analysis acknowledges or considers the context in which the activity is being performed, how it is normally done and the required body structures or functions (but

not specific to an individual's skill capacity (Polatajko et al., 2000). Hersch et al. (2005) stated that an activity analysis involves a step-by-step dissection of an activity and the skills required to perform the activity in order to enable participation.

The final stage in the continuum is the occupational analysis. Through occupation-focused activity analysis, and subsequent grading and adapting, the activity's or occupation's participatory potential is identified (Thomas, 2023). This analysis combines the results of task and activity analyses with an additional focus on the specific challenges, interests and lifestyle, relationships, as well as the environmental contexts of the individual or collective (Thomas, 2023).

To demonstrate this continuum, the occupation of grocery shopping will be explored from the perspective of a young mother, Bernice (Practice Story 17.1).

Activity Analysis of Grocery Shopping

With regards to Bernice's grocery shopping, the occupational therapist may anticipate the following expected demands of the activity:

- Position of the person in relation to the activity as well as the location of the activity in relation to environmental space;
- Tools/utensils/objects/materials used to participate in the activity;
- Environmental opportunities, demands and/or constraints of the large grocery store;
- Contextual opportunities and demands to enable the meaning of activity for the person (space;

Bernice

Bernice is a 34-year-old woman with a recent diagnosis of multiple sclerosis. Bernice was referred to occupational therapy to address her symptoms of decreased upper extremity strength, fatigue and decreased endurance. She lives with her husband and her 18-month-old son in a two-bedroom apartment. Bernice recently returned to work part time (3 days a week) as a receptionist at her community recreation centre after an extended maternity leave.

An initial evaluation using the Canadian Occupational Performance Measure (Law et al., 2019) was implemented (see Chapter 16). Bernice identified the following occupations as challenging: work-related activities that required endurance (e.g. greeting and directing clients, answering phone and email correspondences, keeping record of visitors and patrons) and self-care activities of grocery shopping and house cleaning. Bernice expressed significant satisfaction with her roles as wife, mother and homemaker and stated that she hoped to maintain her capacity to fulfil these roles. She expressed strong, foundational values on relationships with her immediate and extended family including her parents, in-laws, two siblings and her maternal grandparents, who all live within the same city.

Bernice looked forward to her weekly trips to the grocery store with her son as it enabled her to stimulate her child with the sights, smells and tastes while grocery shopping and to participate in an activity within the community. She often asked her mother to join them for the activity to optimise the social experience, and they often followed up this activity with a coffee and snack at a local coffee shop.

The environmental context comprised a large general grocery store with outdoor parking situated within Bernice's local urban neighbourhood. Her mother drove Bernice and her son to the grocery store. They parked close to the entrance, often finding a reserved spot for families. Bernice has not yet applied to the government for an accessible parking permit.

TASK ANALYSIS OF GROCERY SHOPPING

Bernice's grocery shopping activity can be broken down into the following parts or tasks to determine the required skills and abilities. The task analysis simply breaks down grocery shopping into a sequence of steps that could be completed by anyone in any generic store.

1. Retrieve re-usable bags from the back seat of the car: pull door handle and pull the door open, bend and reach to grasp bags, push door closed.
2. Retrieve cart from the exterior cart depot: Pull cart to separate from rack of carts, turn and push cart through doorway into store.
3. Lift and place son in cart and enter store.
4. Walk through aisles to targeted destination while pushing cart; start and stop.
5. Item One – Apples:
    a. Retrieve produce bag.
    b. Select and grasp apple.
    c. Release apple in bag; repeat for desired number of apples.
    d. Twist or tighten bag to close.
    e. Release bag of apples into cart.
6. Walk through aisles to targeted destination while pushing cart; start and stop.
7. Item Two – Bread:
    a. Select and grasp bread from shelf.
    b. Read label on bag for freshness date.
    c. Release bread into cart.
8. Walk through aisles for targeted destination while pushing cart; start and stop.
9. Repeat previous steps for additional items:
    a. Reach, hold, and release 2 L carton of orange juice.
    b. Reach and grasp aluminium foil package and release into cart.
10. At checkout, bend, reach, grasp, lift and place each item and re-usable bags onto conveyor belt.
11. Retrieve wallet and take out required amount of money or credit card for purchase.
12. Hand money or credit card to cashier and obtain receipt.
13. Shopping items are bagged and placed into cart by a store employee.
14. Push cart out of store to car.
15. Open trunk of car, lift and release each bag into trunk of car.
16. Replace cart.

TABLE 17.2

Activity Analysis of Selecting Apples: Sensory Performance Skill Domain

Visual	Visually scanning the environment to locate produce bags and to determine where apples are located and which specific type is desired. Visual awareness of potential obstacles or people in path. Visual assessment of apple to ensure it is blemish free, lacking bruises or holes. Visually checking the price above the apple bin.
Auditory	Tuning out/habituating to background noise of store (other shoppers, music playing, announcements, etc.)
Gustatory	Not utilised at this time unless samples are offered; possible activation of salivary glands when thinking about taste of apple.
Olfactory	Smelling apples to help determine freshness. Tuning out other odours in the store (odours of meat, fish, other vegetables, cleaning products).
Tactile	Tactile discrimination is utilised through handling of each apple to verify the appropriate firmness, smooth texture and lack of any spots. Temperature of apple is noted, as well as overall weight. Secured grasp may be adapted according to size and weight of an apple.
Vestibular	Maintaining balance while retrieving apples and visually scanning the environment.
Proprioceptive	Awareness of position in space relative to the cart, apple display, location of bag in hand and the distance to other shoppers or store displays.

objects; tools; equipment, including virtual or electronic forms; sequence and temporal patterns; social interactions); and

■ Requisite skills and abilities needed for successful completion of the activity (motor, sensory-perceptual, cognitive, emotional, social/communicative).

Breaking down each larger activity and determining the expected outcomes for success is strongly suggested for an activity analysis (Thomas, 2023). To illustrate, an activity analysis of the sensory performance skill domain, as well as the environmental domain for an activity of selecting apples, is described in Tables 17.2 and 17.3, respectively. In Table 17.2, the activity of retrieving apples from a fruit bin in the grocery store is analysed through the sensory domain. The expected skills within this domain are described. Success for this task would be defined as physically collecting a set number of fresh, unblemished red apples from the bin and placing them in a plastic or reusable bag.

In Table 17.3, the activity of retrieving apples from a fruit bin in the grocery store is analysed through the domains of the environmental context: physical, social, cultural and institutional as expressed within the Canadian Model of Occupational Performance and Engagement (CMOP-E) (Canadian Association of Occupational Therapists [CAOT], 2002; Townsend & Polatajko, 2013). The expected opportunities and demands or expected behaviours within the domain are described. Success for this task would be defined as easily finding the apple bins and choosing preferred produce.

OCCUPATIONAL ANALYSIS: A CORNERSTONE OF OCCUPATIONAL THERAPY PRACTICE

Philosophical Influences on Occupational Analysis

An appreciation of the influence of occupation on health and self-efficacy promotes a thorough occupational analysis that identifies the meaning and purpose of chosen occupations for the individual or collective. Three philosophical influences that support current practices of occupational analysis are an occupational perspective on health, value-based approaches and strengths-based approaches.

Participation in occupation is strongly linked to the social determinants of health and the drive to meet not only survival needs but also the desire for dignity, self-identity, self-determination and competence (Hammell, 2017; Hasselkus & Dickie, 2021; Taylor, 2017). The outcome is health and wellbeing through agency, meaning, balance, satisfaction, opportunity and self-actualisation (Wilcock, 1998, 2006). As social beings, healthy participation in occupations often involves others (Martini, et al., 2022). Meaning is drawn from the community and culture in places and spaces and

TABLE 17.3
Environmental Context for Selecting Apples

Domain	Opportunities	Demands (Expected Behaviours)

Physical setting:
  Natural/built
  Space
  Objects
	■ Choice making
	■ Sensorial experience with food items (taste, touch, smell, visual)
		■ Access to area and equipment
		■ Location of objects
		■ Availability of fresh items
		■ Ease of navigation, way-finding

Social:
  Groups
  Roles
	■ Interact with employees, other shoppers, accompanying participants (mother, son)
	■ Fulfil roles (i.e. homemaker)
		■ Respect of others
		■ Social and conversational skills
		■ Social pragmatics (i.e. turn taking)

Cultural:
  Temporal concepts
  Values
  Life situations
  Experiences
	■ Choice making for health promotion
	■ Choice making of culturally preferred apples
	■ Support meal planning
		■ Temporal availabilities (store hours)
		■ Budget constraints (organic versus nonorganic, local versus imported)
		■ Availability of apple variety

Institutional:
  Physical spaces
  Policies and procedures
  Rules and regulations
	■ Variety of apple selection to choose from
	■ Purchasing power for discounted items at large commercial institution
	■ Ease of navigation in larger stores
		■ Access to scale to weigh produce
		■ Self-serve policies
		■ Provisions for taste testing

relationships in which people interact. Martini et al. (2022) related the importance and challenge of considering alternative ways of doing and 'not dismissing a valued occupation as impossible' (p. 181). Acknowledging the effects of the pandemic, changes in the physical and social environments have impacted ways of doing and knowing occupations. There is a need to appreciate not only the individual lived experience but also the involvement and influence of the broader social community and its accessibility on meaningful doing.

An occupational perspective on health (promotion) leads to wellbeing and supports the opportunity to do, to be true to self and to strive to become (Wilcock, 2006). Doing, being, becoming (Fidler & Fidler, 1978; Wilcock, 1998) and belonging (Hitch et al., 2014; Wilcock & Hocking, 2015) lead to outcomes of improved health. *Doing* is living and participating individually or with others in meaningful occupations. Doing is synonymous with function and occupational participation. *Being* is a philosophical state: being true to self while engaging in meaningful occupations (spirituality). *Becoming* is a process leading to self-actualisation, to augmenting one's full potential, to being constantly in development (Wilcock, 1998). *Belonging* is a socially driven connection to others within a social network. The social context may be collaborative or competitive but is always relational,

acknowledging the existing diversity of interactions, expectations and role scripts (Hitch et al., 2014). This philosophical perspective highlights the significance of rights-based occupational participation for health, wellbeing and self-determination (Hammell, 2017).

Value-based approaches, as a theory of philosophical values, promote the integration of person-centred practice in professional skills development. Fulford (2004) postulated that person-perspective values are at the top of a values hierarchy, signifying the importance of the person's narrative in collaborative decision making. Embracing differences and diversity in values, beliefs and decisions certainly supports ethical reasoning in daily occupational therapy practice. Values and beliefs are significantly correlated with a sense of being through occupational participation. In addition, scientific and evidence-based practices are linked with value-based philosophies. As Fulford notes, 'scientific progress increasingly opens up choices and with choices goes values' (Fulford, 2004, p. 59). When the people receiving occupational therapy services are given volitional power to enable choice making, their values and interests are acknowledged and integrated. The recognition and transparency of values and choices inherent in practice-based decision making facilitates ethical reasoning in occupational therapy practice (Clair & Newcombe, 2014; Hammell, 2020). Ethical reasoning also necessitates advocacy when choice is limited by socio-political and systemic inequities (Hammell, 2020).

These value-based philosophies are evident within the Model of Human Occupation (MOHO) (Kielhofner, 2008; Taylor, 2017). For example, personal causation drives the volitional process for choice making and motivation, which are reflective of the human experience and human behaviour in which human values are particularly diverse and personal.

In sustaining occupational participation that a person or collective needs to do, wants to do and optimally chooses to do, a collaborative relationship-focused occupational therapy practice is considered. Collaborative relationship-focused practice within CanMOP (Restall & Egan, 2022) reflects the tenets of person-centred practice yet 'shifts to an approach in which people feel safer, that promotes rights-based self-determination of individuals and collectives' (Restall & Egan, 2022, p. 99). Acknowledging diversity of values, agency and power relations with respect to meaningful occupational participation requires an occupational therapist to critically reflect on the influence of social, economic and political systems (Beagan, 2015; Gerlach, 2015) on people's abilities to 'access, initiate and sustain occupations' (Restall & Egan, 2022, p. 76). Inherent in this is the right to engage and participate in occupations that contribute positively to their own wellbeing and the wellbeing of their communities (Hammell, 2017). Through occupational analysis, the details of the chosen or required occupations, access to opportunities for participation and engagement (Restall & Egan, 2022), and the benchmarks for personal success are examined to determine their therapeutic benefit. If the chosen or required occupations are responsive to people's strengths and address their occupational participation goals, skills and values, then health, wellbeing and social participation can be promoted (Reitz & Scaffa, 2020).

Strengths-based approaches reflect the humanistic shift from focusing on a disability to focusing on the whole person, looking at current and potential functioning. Understanding what types of supports may enable participation requires an analysis of the needs, goals and values of a person or collective and also an analysis of the environmental resources and barriers (Bantinx, 2013). This is integrated within an occupational analysis. Strengths-based approaches enable personal authenticity, agency and potentially a more positive collaboration in occupational therapy interventions as the focus is placed on the person's or collectives' strengths and assets.

THEORETICAL INFLUENCES ON OCCUPATIONAL ANALYSIS

The Person-Environment-Occupation Model as a Foundational Framework for Occupational Analysis

Occupational therapy embraces a dynamic systems approach to the interaction among person, environment and occupation. This is described as an open system in which there is constant interplay among these domains. A change in one domain will affect change in the other two domains and change necessitates adaptation for performance, participation and even survival. For example, a change in a person's motor capacity (e.g. proximal humeral fracture) will affect the way the person performs or engages in occupations (e.g. washing hair), thereby affecting the environmental demands (e.g. assistance from a family member). Environmental demands will influence the need for adaptation or adaptive aids, for social support or for institutional advocacy. Occupational performance is an outcome from the dynamic interaction of the person, environment and occupation that continues to evolve throughout a person's life; as a result occupational performance is flexible and variable. Meaning in occupations is derived from dynamic interactions and personal experiences and therefore is critical to self-identity, self-determination and wellbeing.

The Person-Environment-Occupation (PEO) Model (Law et al., 1996) may be seen as a foundational conceptual framework for occupational analyses as it facilitates an understanding of how an individual or collective may choose meaningful occupations. It also facilitates communication within and outside the profession through a common language of occupation-focused domains (Strong et al., 1999). Within the PEO, occupational performance comprises experiences and interpretations by the individual so that the personal meaning of the occupation is acknowledged. It can shape self-identity and adaptability to changing priorities (Law et al., 1996). It enables choice making, occupational organisation and satisfaction from participating in occupations that have value, thereby fostering meaning (CAOT, 2002; Townsend & Polatajko, 2013).

The model assumes that the three major domains (person, environment, occupation) continually interact across time and space in ways that increase or decrease their support for occupational performance. Across time occupation is positioned as dynamic and never static. Law et al. (1996) posited that a person is active, determined and perpetual in building skills and attributes, across the lifespan, while interacting with various occupations and environments. If the interaction and overlap of domains is greater, it is assumed that the occupational performance is better supported and therefore more satisfying and meaningful for the person (Law et al., 1996). In meaningful occupation, the human skills and capacities (of the person) are acknowledged and the environmental context is explored and accounted for through collaborative relationship-focused practices. When the interaction between domains is optimal, the person will pursue occupational choices that are meaningful and satisfying.

In-depth understanding of the person-environment-occupation dynamic supports the occupational analysis as it recognises what is required for full participation (person: skills, attributes, roles, habits, spiritual capacity) and how and where the activity/occupation is performed (environments: physical, social, cultural, institutional). In addition, the personal meaning behind the chosen occupations (tasks and activities comprising necessary functions of daily life) is acknowledged and pursued in order to maintain participation and engagement (Moll et al., 2015).

A thorough analysis of the environmental contexts must also be implemented to fully enable participation at the micro, macro and community levels (Leclair, 2010). Environmental contexts can accommodate or constrain adaptation as they are never static. These contexts function as a feedback loop: for example, the context can affect behaviour, but in turn, behaviour influences the environmental context. Intervention planning comprises activity and occupational analyses, thereby supporting the inclusion of the PEO Model as an appropriate theoretical framework to guide occupational therapy practice applications (Strong et al., 1999). The occupational therapist enables this pursuit and supports meaningful choice through occupational analysis.

The Person-Environment-Occupation Model for Preanalysis

The PEO Model as a framework (Law et al., 1996) may be chosen to support a *preanalysis* step to set the context of the activity leading to occupational analysis. A preanalysis builds on values of purposeful, meaningful activity and occupation-based frameworks and promotes an understanding of the person-based and occupation-based contexts (Perlman et al., 2010; Perlman & Gisel, 2000). By first reflecting on the domains of the PEO Model, the occupational therapist gains an appreciation and understanding of the specific contexts of the person, environment and occupation so that the occupational analysis remains aligned with the tenets of occupation-based and value-based perspectives. The preanalysis (Perlman & Gisel, 2000) format presented in Table 17.4 allows the occupational therapist to do the following:

- Build on prior knowledge of occupation-based models and meaningful activities through the sequence of steps.
- Review the domains of occupation-based models and appreciate the dynamic relationship between each domain and the impact on performance and participation.
- Recognise the components of two models of occupation: CMOP-E (Townsend & Polatajko, 2013) and MOHO (Kielhofner, 2008; Taylor, 2017); these two models provide a comprehensive framework for an occupational analysis
- Analyse more complex situations and occupations and focus on salient issues for enablement of occupation relevant to specific individuals.

Essential Domains for Occupational Analysis

The PEO framework provides a scaffold for an occupational analysis comprising the specific domains that should be included in the analysis. A generic list of characteristics under each domain of the person, environment and occupation that should be included in an occupational analysis are listed in Table 17.5. This PEO framework aligns well with the two evidence-based models of occupation: CMOP-E (Townsend & Polatajko, 2013) and MOHO (Kielhofner, 2008; Taylor, 2017). These two models focus on domains reflective

TABLE 17.4
Preanalysis Step to Set the Context of the Activity Leading to Occupational Analysis (Perlman & Gisel, 2000)

Activity: _____

OCCUPATION: Identify area(s)

PERSON: Identify predominant skill components:

☐ motor	☐ sensory	☐ cognitive
☐ perceptual	☐ social	☐ affective/emotional

ENVIRONMENT:

☐ physical	☐ social	☐ cultural	☐ institutional

Preanalysis, person

Physical:

	☐ trunk stability	☐ balance	☐ U/E strength (including hands)
			☐ hand dexterity
☐ L/E strength		☐ coordination	☐ endurance
☐ mobility			

Identify characteristics:

Sensory processing:

	☐ visual	☐ tactile	☐ vestibular
☐ auditory		☐ proprioceptive	☐ kinesthetic

Affective:

	☐ satisfied	☐ optimistic	☐ pessimistic
☐ introverted	☐ extroverted		

Cognitive:

☐ memory for this activity	☐ oriented to time and place
	☐ attention span for this activity
☐ concentration for this activity	☐ problem-solving skills

Spiritual:

☐ values quality of life	☐ expresses choices
	☐ positive attitude towards autonomy
☐ is motivated to perform this activity	☐ activity is meaningful to the individual

Physical   Setting:

Objects/items:	☐ natural	☐ built
	☐ required	☐ not necessary

Preanalysis, environment Identify characteristics:

Rules of physical accessibility	Orientation and wayfinding:	☐ observe safety	☐ general accessibility

Social

	Group size:	☐ small	☐ large	☐ N/A
	Individual:	☐ in isolation	☐ alone but within a social milieu	☐ N/A
	Roles:	☐ leader	☐ follower ☐ participant	☐ N/A
	Task:	☐ serious	☐ playful	☐ competitive
			☐ educational	
			☐ collaborative	

Cultural:

☐ ethnicity	☐ age	☐ religion
☐ gender	☐ life situations and experiences	

Rules of social conduct:

☐ code of conduct in this environment	☐ observe safety	☐ respect for others

TABLE 17.5

Generic Subdomains Listed Under the Domains of the Person, Environment and Occupation for Occupational Analysis

Person	Environment	Occupation
■ Motor	Physical	■ Work
■ Sensory/perceptual	■ Natural or built setting	■ Play
■ Cognitive	■ Objects and tools	■ Volunteer work
■ Affective	■ Space management	■ Retirement preparation or adjustment
■ Social communication	■ Accessibility	■ Sports
■ Spiritual	Social	■ Social participation
	■ Social groups	■ Community participation
	■ Socially constructed tasks	■ Rest and sleep
	Culture	■ Dressing
	■ Values and beliefs	■ Bathing
	■ Generational transmission of knowledge	■ Feeding
	■ Rituals; customs; rite of passage	■ Toileting
	■ Temporal significance	■ Transfers
	■ Institutional	■ Community mobility
	■ Policies and procedures	■ Health management
	■ Rules and regulations	■ Banking
	■ Accessibility	■ Meal preparation
	■ Integration	■ Grocery shopping

of human occupation (performance skills and choice making), the person's attributes and skills and their dynamic interactions with the physical, social, cultural, institutional environments. The CMOP-E (Townsend & Polatajko, 2013) comprises the domains of the person (motor, cognitive, affective and spiritual), the occupation (productivity, leisure and self-care) and the environment (physical, social, cultural and institutional). It embraces person-centred occupational participation across the lifespan and supports a vision for health, wellbeing and occupational justice. The model postulates that engagement in meaningful occupations leads to occupational development, competence and identity, which are linked to spirituality (a source of agency comprising self-determination and personal control through occupational choices).

The MOHO (Kielhofner, 2008; Taylor, 2017) advances an understanding that human occupation is chosen (volition), organised and patterned through habits and roles (habituation) and performed (performance capacity) within an environmental context (physical, social, occupational). Occupation is described through a person's participation, occupational capacity and skills (motor, process, social and communication skills) while doing (subjective experience through the lived body) within an environmental context (Kielhofner, 2008; Taylor,

2017). Each environmental context affords opportunities, resources, demands and constraints, thereby dynamically influencing the person and occupation. This model also embraces person-centred enablement of occupation (person's unique attributes and values) across the lifespan and supports occupational competence and self-identity through purposeful, meaningful doing.

The assumptions to support each model's proximity to occupation-based practice through person-centred enablement and its influence on health and wellbeing, as well as a comparison of the domains of the CMOP-E (Townsend & Polatajko, 2013) and the MOHO (Kielhofner, 2008; Taylor, 2017) with the PEO domains (to highlight their association with occupation-focused concepts that support an occupational analysis) are presented in Table 17.6.

APPLICATION OF OCCUPATIONAL ANALYSES

Application of an Occupational Analysis: Examples Using the CMOP-E, MOHO & CanMOP

An example of the occupational analysis of environment domain of the CMOP-E (Townsend & Polatajko,

		TABLE 17.6	
		Comparison of Domains of Two Models of Occupation, the CMOP-E and the MOHO, with the Domains of the PEO Model	
Model	**PEO (Law et al., 1996)**	**CMOP-E (Townsend & Polatajko, 2013)**	**MOHO (Kielhofner, 2008; Taylor, 2017)**
Assumption	Explains person-centred enablement through the dynamic relationship of the person, environment and occupation. Changes in one domain will influence the others and will affect occupational performance and satisfaction	Explains person-centred occupational therapy enablement of occupation to ensure occupational engagement, participation and adaptation. The model envisions health, wellbeing and justice as attainable through occupation and embraces the dynamic relationship among the person, environment and occupation	Explains how human occupations are motivated (volition), patterned through doing (habituation – habits and roles) and performed (performance capacity) within everyday environmental contexts. These occupations influence the capacity for occupational identity, competence and adaptation through the dynamic relationship among the person, environment and occupation
Domains	Person	■ Physical ■ Cognitive ■ Affective ■ Spiritual	■ Volition ■ Habituation ■ Performance capacity
	Environment	■ Physical ■ Social ■ Cultural ■ Institutional	Physical Social Occupational
	Occupation	■ Productivity ■ Leisure ■ Self-care	Performance capacity Lived body (subjective) Impact of Performance capacity o occupations (objective) Motor; sensory motor Process Communication

CMOP-E, Canadian Model of Occupational Performance and Engagement; MOHO, Model of Human Occupation; PEO, Person-Environment-Occupation Model.

2013) as Bernice participates in the occupation of grocery shopping is provided in Table 17.7. The analysis remains specific to the environmental context of the large community-based grocery store. The subdomains of the environment are identified as physical (settings natural or built; objects and space), social (social groups and interactions at the micro [personal], meso [families or work groups] and macro [societal] levels), cultural (values, beliefs, life experiences) and institutional (economic, political and societal influences). These environmental domains may offer facilitators or barriers to participation, engagement and performance.

An example of the occupational analysis of the domain of volition of the MOHO (Kielhofner, 2008; Taylor, 2017) as Bernice participates in the occupation of grocery shopping is provided in Table 17.8.

The MOHO explicitly identifies occupational participation as the broadest dimension of people's doing, 'above occupational performance (doing an occupational task) and occupational skills (goal directed actions)' (Larsson-Lund & Nyman, 2017; p. 394). The analysis remains specific to Bernice's skills, attributes, roles, habits and lived experience capacity as she participates in the activity within the environmental context of the large community-based grocery store. The subdomains of volition are identified as *personal causation* (knowledge of skill capacity and self-efficacy), *values* (personal values/beliefs, sense of obligation) and *interests* (attraction and preferences of a given activity). The volitional domain can be used to explain how Bernice anticipates, chooses, experiences and interprets the grocery shopping activity in its entirety, thereby influencing her occupational participation and ability to sustain

TABLE 17.7

Application of CMOP-E for Grocery Shopping: Domain of Environment

Physical	Social	Cultural	Institutional
■ Built space ■ Objects and equipment required (cart, bags, money, credit cards, purse) ■ Aisles to navigate ■ Obstacles to navigate ■ Food items ■ Nonfood items	■ Interaction with staff to request items or ask for assistance ■ Interaction with child and/or family member ■ Interaction with cashier and employee	■ Value activity as a leisure occupation (mother/child outing) ■ Value the productivity role as homemaker, wife, mother ■ Choose culturally specific, meaningful food items ■ Perform activity at own pace, be respectful of personal preferences	■ Follow rules and regulations of public space including not eating food without paying ■ Respect other shoppers ■ Pay for all items ■ Bring recyclable shopping bags ■ Expectation to load bags into car and to return cart

CMOP-E, Canadian Model of Occupational Performance and Engagement

TABLE 17.8

Application of the MOHO Occupational Analysis for Grocery Shopping: Domain of Volition

PERSONAL CAUSATION		VALUES		INTERESTS	
Knowledge of Capacity	Sense of Efficacy	Personal Convictions	Sense of Obligation	Attraction	Interests
■ Organisational skills for planned outing: shopping list, materials, child and transportation by car ■ Drive car to grocery store ■ Choose food and nonfood items according to list ■ Restriction of navigation of whole store due to fatigue and decreased endurance ■ May choose lighter items	■ Appropriate control of organisational and choice-making skills ■ Decreased control of physical endurance and strength to complete activity and carry heavy bags – may affect choice of items on a given day	■ Values activity to fulfil roles as homemaker, wife, mother and daughter ■ Values choice making and selection of culturally preferred items ■ Values activity for social participation in her community ■ Values choice making for health promotion	■ To fulfil role as homemaker, wife, mother and daughter ■ To complete this instrumental activity of daily living with success, leading to food preparation for family	■ Social participation and social outing in community ■ Fulfilment of roles as wife, mother, daughter and homemaker	■ Grocery shopping as a weekly pleasurable activity ■ Social outing with child and mother ■ Choice making of culturally preferred food items

MOHO, Model of Human Occupation.

it. Success in participation will be determined by her thoughts and feelings about her own capacity for mastery, her values and her enjoyment and satisfaction attributed to the tasks of grocery shopping.

The new Canadian Model of Occupational Participation (CanMOP) (Egan & Restall, 2022) supports

reflection on occupational participation. This model comprises two essential components to support occupational participation: (1) the purpose and meaning of the occupational participation and (2) the occupational possibilities to access, initiate and sustain participation as supported by meaningful relationships and environmental contexts (Egan & Restall, 2022). Grocery shopping is meaningful to Bernice as it allows her to fulfil her roles as mother, wife and homemaker while also providing a social experience with her mother. Her mother drives Bernice and her son to the grocery store and accompanies them, thereby providing physical and social supports for Bernice to access, initiate and complete the grocery shopping. Her mother can help push the carriage, gather items and attend to her son, as needed. This occupation is also meaningful and enjoyable because afterwards, Bernice and her mother always spend time together at a local coffee shop.

Grocery shopping would require more adaptation if these physical and social environmental supports were not provided. For example, if Bernice needed to take public transport to the grocery store, she may have additional physical or financial challenges with access and ease to travel, including the physical, cognitive and emotional demands of attending to her son and buying the groceries, then carrying the grocery bags and returning home. Adaptations could include having her husband drive her during off-peak hours, park within close proximity in a reserved parking space for mothers or those with mobility issues (with use of a accessible parking permit) and assist with the grocery shopping tasks including paying for and packing and loading the items into the car. As a result of the adaptations, Bernice would also not have the opportunity to share coffee time with her mother.

Grading and Adapting an Occupation

Once an occupational analysis is complete, the occupational therapist will then grade or adapt the activity components or environmental factors to understand its meaning and value to an individual. Both grading and adapting foster change and adaptation that potentially leads to greater participation and engagement, as well as increased competence.

Grading is a modification of the occupational challenge (either increased or decreased) for a person performing the activity (Perlman et al., 2010; Thomas, 2015). Hersch et al. (2005) posited that the grading process integrates the results of the occupational analysis and then works backwards to determine how best to change the activity to facilitate successful participation. This can be achieved by progressively changing the task complexity, the steps, the physical assistance,

the social interaction and relational or the environmental demands. In addition, the demands of the sequence of steps and temporal variables should be considered, including timing or scheduling of the activity during specific times of the day, week or month and the duration of the whole activity. To grade the occupation for success, consider the most challenging activity demands for the person and the impact of these demands on performance, participation and satisfaction.

Some examples of grading an occupation include the following:

- Reducing steps or repetitions of movements to promote completion.
- Providing preprepared materials to eliminate task components.
- Providing lighter weight materials to facilitate grasp or increase endurance.
- Pairing up two individuals to complete one activity,
- Positioning all materials on the functional side for easy access.

Adapting is explained as modifying or changing an aspect of the occupation or environment with the goal of allowing participation or increased independence (Thomas, 2015). Although adapting shares similarities to grading, the objective is not to increase or decrease the demands of the activity on the person. An occupational therapist can creatively adapt the task, activity or the environment to improve the individual's ability to perform and succeed at the chosen activity. This can involve changing components of the environment such as physical space, tools and equipment, lighting and sensory input or may involve the provision of adaptive technologies. Technologies are comprised of technical aids, adaptive supports and virtual or simulated environments that enable participation. Technology in its simple (low) or complex (high) forms supports an adaptive intervention approach that promotes acquisition or restoration of compensatory skills, habits and routines and is often integrated when grading and adapting activities or occupations. An example of a simple low-technology adaptation is the application of a built-up handle of a spoon to facilitate self-feeding. An example of more complex, high-technology grading application is the use of motion capture sensors through a virtual program, such as *Jintronix,* to stimulate range of motion of the upper extremity and provide biofeedback to the person who will use the technology.

Some examples of adapting an occupation include the following:

- Providing a tool that allows for a modified grasp (i.e. replace a conventional computer mouse with a joystick mouse for easier grasp and manipulation).
- Providing prompting or personal assistance with the activity (i.e. verbal prompting to guide actions to complete a puzzle; hand-over-hand support to brush teeth).
- Providing online support to ensure participation (i.e. online shopping with home delivery).
- Choosing a time of day when a location is likely to be less occupied and overstimulating (i.e. playing in a park early in the morning rather than midmorning).
- Reading a book with an enlarged font (for visual impairments) or with a condensed story line (for attention difficulties).

TABLE 17.9		
Grading and Adapting of Grocery Shopping for Bernice		
Activity Demands (Challenges)	**Grade**	**Adapt**
Complete navigation of circumference of grocery store	Preplan route to minimise backtracking Decrease the time allowance per shopping trip by scheduling a second trip to grocery store within the week to complete shopping list	Use a scooter provided by store to reduce walking and to conserve energy Use an online shopping/delivery service
Manoeuvre cart through stops and starts	Reduce selection of number of weighted items to reduce cart weight Minimise starts and stops of cart by reducing items for purchase on a given visit	Use smallest cart available to reduce weight Ensure chosen cart is easy to manoeuver
Reach and grasp objects from shelf or produce bin	Use bilateral grasp for heavier objects Select items within reach on shelf Ensure cart is within close proximity to minimise distance object is carried	Ask for assistance from her mother or employees for items that are too high or too heavy
Hold objects and release into grocery cart	Use bilateral grasp for heavier objects and hold closer to body Limit number of items in bags to decrease weight Ensure cart is within close proximity to minimise length of time object is grasped and released	Ask for assistance from mother (or staff) for heavier items Use online services for heavier items and personally shop for lighter, more manageable items
Release apples in bag and twisting bag to close	Secure placement of produce bag on top of apples or in cart to minimise weight of bag as apples are released Buy preselected bag of apples	Use plastic reusable clips to close bag rather than twisting or knotting
Attend to active child in child seat of cart	Ensure child is fastened into cart seat Actively engage child in shopping experience (provide pictures of items to be purchased; play 'I Spy' game). Reduce time of shopping trips to habituate child to the routine of grocery shopping	Find childcare for child Ask her mother to assist in keeping child safely seated in cart while she shops Ask her mother gather items while she engages her child in other shopping experiences Ask her husband to accompany as an alternative
Complete grocery shopping activity within 45-minute time frame	Shop for items only itemised on shopping list Set watch or phone timer to monitor time frame Follow preplanned route	Shop during early morning or evening hours when store is less occupied Wear comfortable shoes and clothing to facilitate efficiency of movements Acquire a reserved parking permit for easier access and proximity

- Engaging in a simplified version of a board game to promote successful participation.

A number of possible ways that the occupation of grocery shopping can be graded or adapted for Bernice are presented in Table 17.9. The activity demands reflect Bernice's challenges with decreased upper extremity strength, fatigue and decreased endurance.

CONCLUSION

This chapter provides an overview of the concepts of task analysis, activity analysis and occupational analysis within occupation-focused frameworks. These analyses are recognised to form a continuum of the analysis process and are appreciated from an occupation-focused lens, in which valued occupations within meaningful relationships and contexts are essential to occupational therapy intervention. The continuum of the analysis process begins with a task analysis describing the sequence and timing of actions or list of steps within an activity. An activity analysis then examines the skills and context of the activity in the environment. Finally, an occupational analysis, the perspective most unique to the profession of occupational therapy, validates the value of the activity for the specific person performing it within an environmental context. An activity becomes an occupation when it is meaningful and valued to the person, group or community performing and participating in it.

Theoretical practice models are useful to occupational therapists as a tool to enable analysis of occupations to help guide their understanding of the personal, occupational and relational demands in preparation for interventions. The PEO Model (Law et al., 1996) provides foundational support for occupation-focused application of activity/occupational analyses and highlights the dynamic and influential relationship among the person, environment and occupation. The CMOP-E (Townsend & Polatajko, 2013), the MOHO (Kielhofner, 2008; Taylor, 2017) and the CanMOP (Restall & Egan, 2022) occupation-focused models of practice are applied to the occupational analyses. They each focus on domains reflective of human occupation (performance skills, attributes, agency and relational experiences) and their interactions with the physical, social, cultural and institutional environments.

Occupational therapists have the expertise to assess the environment and systems at the micro, meso and macro levels, the inherent sequence and timing of occupations, as well as the required skills and capacities needed for participation in an activity or occupation. Participation in personal and socially meaningful occupations is strongly linked to the social determinants of health. When occupations are justly accessible, they are initiated and sustained within supportive environments. By grading and adapting activities or occupations, personal meaning is reinforced, potentially leading to greater participation, engagement and competence. This outcome further fosters health and wellbeing and quality of life for people, groups or communities receiving occupational therapy services.

REFERENCES

Aiken, F. E., Fourt, A. M., Cheng, I. K. S., & Polatajko, H. J. (2011). The meaning gap in occupational therapy: Finding meaning in our own occupation. *Canadian Journal of Occupational Therapy, 78*(5), 294–302.

Allen, C. K. (1982). Independence through activity: The practice of occupational therapy (psychiatry). *American Journal of Occupational Therapy, 36*(11), 731–739.

Bantinx, W. H. E. (2013). Ch. 2: Understanding disability: A strengths based approach. In M. L. Wehmeyer (Ed.), *The Oxford handbook of positive psychology and disability* (pp. 7–18). Oxford University Press.

Bauerschmidt, B., & Nelson, D. L. (2011). The terms occupation and activity over the history of official occupational therapy publications. *American Journal of Occupational Therapy, 65*(3), 338–345.

Beagan, B. L. (2015). Approaches to culture and diversity: A critical synthesis of occupational therapy literature. *Canadian Journal of Occupational Therapy, 82*(5), 272–282.

Blesedell Crepeau, E., Gillen, G., & Scaffa, M. E. (2013). Analyzing occupations and activity. In B. A. Schell, G. Gillen, M. E. Scaffa, & E. S. Cohn (Eds.), *Willard and Spackman's occupational therapy* (12th, pp. 234–248). Lippincott Williams & Wilkins.

Canadian Association of Occupational Therapists. (2002). *Enabling occupation: An occupational therapy perspective.* CAOT Publications ACE.

Clair, V. A., & Newcombe, D. B. (2014). Values and ethics in practice-based decision making. *Canadian Journal of Occupational Therapy, 81*(3), 154–162.

Egan, M., & Restall, G. (2022). Ch. 4: The Canadian model of occupational participation. In M. Egan, & G. Restall (Eds.), *Promoting occupational participation: Collaborative relationship-focused occupational therapy, 10th Canadian Occupational Therapy Guidelines.* CAOT.

Fidler, G. S., & Fidler, J. W. (1978). Doing and becoming: Purposeful action and self-actualization. *American Journal of Occupational Therapy, 32*(5), 305–310.

Figueiredo, M. O., Gomes, L. D., Silva, C. R., & Martinez, C. M. S. (2020). Human occupation and activity in occupational therapy: Scoping review in the national literature. *Cadernos Brasileiros de Terapia Ocupacional, 28*(3), 967–982. https://doi.org/10.4322/2526-8910.ctoAR1858.

Fisher, A. G. (2013). Occupation-centred, occupation-based, occupation-focused: Same, same or different? *Scandinavian Journal of Occupational Therapy, 20*(3), 162–173.

Fulford, K. L. M. (2004). Ten principles of values-based medicine (VBM). In T. Schramme, & J. Thome (Eds.), *Philosophy and psychiatry* (pp. 50–82). Walter de Gruyter.

Gerlach, A. J. (2015). Sharpening our critical edge: Occupational therapy in the context of marginalized populations. *Canadian Journal of Occupational Therapy, 82*(4), 245–253.

Hammell, K. W. (2017). Critical reflections on occupational justice: Toward a rights-based approach to occupational opportunities. *Canadian Journal of Occupational Therapy, 84*(1), 47–57.

Hammell, W. H. (2020). Making choices from the choices we have: The contextual-embeddedness of occupational choice. *Canadian Journal of Occupational Therapy, 87*(5), 400–411.

Hasselkus, B. R., & Dickie, V. A. (2021). *The meaning of everyday occupation* (3rd ed.). Slack Incorporated.

Hersch, G. I., Lamport, N. K., & Coffey, M. S. (2005). *Activity analysis: Application to occupation* (5th ed.). Slack.

Hitch, D., Pepin, G., & Stagnitti, K. (2014). In the footsteps of Wilcock, part one: The evolution of doing, being, becoming, and belonging. *Occupational Therapy in Health Care, 28*(3), 231–246.

Kielhofner, G. (2008). *Model of human occupation: Theory and application* (4th ed.). Lippincott Williams & Wilkins.

Larsson-Lund, M., & Nyman, A. (2017). Participation and occupation in occupational therapy models of practice: A discussion of possibilities and challenges. *Scandinavian Journal of Occupational Therapy, 24*(6), 393–397.

Law, M. (2002). Participation in the occupations of everyday life; 2002 Distinguished Scholar Lecture. *America Journal of Occupational Therapy, 56*(6), 640–649.

Law, M., Baptiste, S., Carswell, A., McColl, M. A., Polatajko, H. J., & Pollock, N. (2019). *Canadian occupational performance measure* (5th ed.-revised). COPM Inc.

Law, M., Cooper, B., Strong, S., Stewart, D., Rigby, P., & Letts, L. (1996). The person- environment-occupation model: A transactive approach to occupational performance. *Canadian Journal of Occupational Therapy, 63*(1), 9–23.

Leclair, L. L. (2010). Re-examining concepts of occupation and occupation-based models: Occupational therapy and community development. *Canadian Journal of Occupational Therapy, 77*(1), 15–21.

Letts, L. J. (2011). Muriel Driver Memorial Lecture 2011: Optimal positioning of occupational therapy. *Canadian Journal of Occupational Therapy, 78*(4), 209–217.

Martini, R., Egan, M., & Cantin, N. (2022). Ch. 7: Promoting occupational participation with individuals and families. In M. Egan, & G. Restall (Eds.), *Promoting occupational participation: Collaborative relationship-focused occupational therapy, 10th Canadian Occupational Therapy Guidelines*. CAOT.

Moll, S. E., Gewurtz, R. E., Krupa, T. M., Law, M. C., Larivière, N., & Levasseur, M. (2015). 'Do- Live-Well': A Canadian framework for promoting occupation, health, and well-being. *Canadian Journal of Occupational Therapy, 82*(1), 9–23.

Mosey, A. C. (1986). *Psychological components of occupational therapy*. Raven Press.

Nelson, D. L. (1997). The 1997 eleanor clarke slagle lecture: Why the profession of occupational therapy will flourish in the 21st century. *American Journal of Occupational Therapy, 51*(1), 11–24.

Perlman, C., & Gisel, E. (2000). *Pre-analysis: Web-based tutorial for activity analysis*. In *OCC1 550-002 Enabling Human Occupation (myCourses, 2000courses)*. McGill University.

Perlman, C., Weston, C., & Gisel, E. (2005). A web-based tutorial to enhance student learning of activity analysis. *Canadian Journal of Occupational Therapy, 72*(3), 153–163.

Perlman, C., Weston, C., & Gisel, E. (2010). Enabling meaningful learning through web-based instruction with occupational therapy students. *Educational Technology Research & Development, 58*(2), 191–210.

Polatajko, H. J., & Davis, J. A. (2012). Advancing occupation-based practice: Interpreting the rhetoric. *Canadian Journal of Occupational Therapy, 79*(5), 259–263.

Polatajko, H. J., Mandich, A., & Martini, R. (2000). Dynamic performance analysis: A framework for understanding occupational performance. *American Journal of Occupational Therapy, 54*(1), 65–72.

Reed, K. D., Hocking, C. S., & Smythe, L. A. (2011). Exploring the meaning of occupation: The case for phenomenology. *Canadian Journal of Occupational Therapy, 78*(5), 303–309.

Reitz, S. M., & Scaffa, M. E. (2020). Occupational therapy in the promotion of health and well-being. *American Journal of Occupational Therapy, 74*(3), 1–14.

Restall, G., & Egan, M. (2022). Ch. 5: Collaborative relationship-focused occupational therapy. In M. Egan, & G. Restall (Eds.), *Promoting occupational participation: Collaborative relationship-focused occupational therapy. 10th Canadian Occupational Therapy Guidelines*. CAOT.

Rush Dunton, W. (1931). Occupational therapy 1. *Occupational Therapy & Rehabilitation, 10*(2), 113–121.

Strong, S., Rigby, P., Stewart, D., Law, M., Letts, L., & Cooper, B. (1999). Application of the person-environment-occupation model: A practical tool. *Canadian Journal of Occupational Therapy, 65*(3), 122–133.

Taylor, R. R. (2017). *Kielhofner's model of human occupation: Theory and application* (5th ed.) pp. 91–106. Wolters Kluwer.

Thomas, H. (2015). *Occupation-based activity analysis* (2nd ed.). Slack.

Thomas, H. (2023). *Occupation-based activity analysis* (3rd ed.). Slack.

Townsend, E. A., & Polatajko, H. J. (2013). *Enabling occupation II: Advancing an occupational therapy vision for health, well-being & justice through occupation* (2nd ed.). CAOT Publications ACE.

Wilcock, A. A. (1998). International perspective: Reflections on doing, being and becoming. *Canadian Journal of Occupational Therapy, 65*(5), 248–256.

Wilcock, A. A. (2006). *An occupational perspective of health* (2nd ed.). Slack.

Wilcock, A. A., & Hocking, C. (2015). *An occupational perspective of health* (3rd ed.). Slack.

Wilding, C., & Whiteford, G. (2007). Occupation and occupational therapy: Knowledge paradigms and everyday practice. *Australian Occupational Therapy Journal, 54*(3), 185–193.

World Health Organization. (2001). *International classification of functioning, disability and health.* WHO.

Yerxa, E. J. (1990). An introduction to occupational science, a foundation for occupational therapy in the 21st century. *Occupational Therapy In Health Care, 6*(4), 1–17.

Yerxa, E. (2000). Occupational Science: A renaissance of service to humankind through knowledge, *Occupational Therapy International, 7*(2), 87–98. doi: https://doi.org/10.1002/oti.109.

REFLECTION

1. Explain the difference between an activity and an occupation.

2. Identify key features of occupation through participation by reflecting on a personally meaningful everyday occupation that you do. Describe how this occupation supports your participation by reflecting on the following six key features of occupation:
   i) Reflects my personal values and interests
   ii) Offers a sense of control through choice making
   iii) Promotes my self-identity
   iv) Promotes my competence and skill development
   v) Enables interaction with my social environment
   vi) Provides structure and organisation to my day

3. Choose an everyday activity that you do (e.g. brushing teeth, dressing, making coffee).
   i) Briefly identify the objects, tools, and equipment that are needed to complete the activity.
   ii) Complete a task analysis by breaking down the activity into a sequence of steps.

4. Create a table, similar to Table 17.7 and 17.8, applying the Canadian Model of Occupational Participation to the occupation of grocery shopping.

18

DYNAMIC PERFORMANCE ANALYSIS

ROSE MARTINI ■ JENNIFER BERTONI ■ DOROTHY KESSLER

CHAPTER OUTLINE

Overview

Dynamic performance analysis (DPA) is a task-oriented, performance-based approach to occupational performance analysis that is centred on the person's actual performance of an occupation, activity, task, action and/or movement (occupation and/or its sublevels). The purpose of DPA is to identify a person's performance issues or breakdowns. The analysis process focuses on the dynamic transaction of the occupation and/or its sublevels, person and environment relative to the person's performance of the activity and not on the components necessary for that performance. The DPA process (depicted by a decision tree) begins by observing the person perform the occupation and identifying whether the performance is competent or not, taking note of the omissions/errors or breakdowns. For each performance breakdown, an iterative analysis process is undertaken that considers the person, the occupation and/or its sublevels and the environmental context. Two practice stories with illustrated decision trees are presented as a guide through this iterative analysis process. Two scenarios are also provided to guide the occupational therapist when undertaking a DPA with an occupation they may not be familiar with.

KEY POINTS

- Dynamic performance analysis (DPA) is an analysis process that focuses on the actual performance of an occupation, activity, task, action and/or movement (occupation and/or its sublevels) so as to be able to identify performance issues or breakdowns (Polatajko et al., 2000).

- Although activity analysis is usually done without a particular person in mind, DPA requires the observation of the person performing the occupation and/or its sublevels.

- DPA is a nonstandardised performance analysis process that can be used with any occupation and/or its sublevels and anyone receiving occupational therapy.

- DPA is a task-oriented assessment process that is continuous and iterative and can be applied not only at the beginning and end of the intervention but also continuously throughout the intervention sessions.

- In addition to being a tool for occupational therapists to use, DPA may be considered an ability that can be developed by people receiving occupational therapy services, which may be key for improving skill performance and intertask transfer.

INTRODUCTION

As occupational therapists, our mission is to aid people to participate in valued occupations that are meaningful to them (Egan & Restall, 2022). This includes accessing, initiating and sustaining their desired occupations within the relationships and contexts they value (Egan & Restall, 2022). The occupational performance (i.e. the accomplishment of a specific activity or task) may be a factor that contributes to occupational participation. A person's performance proficiency is the result of a dynamic interaction among the occupation, person and environment. Dynamic performance analysis and activity analysis are tools that occupational therapists use to understand occupational performance.

The process of activity analysis provides the occupational therapist with an understanding of what is needed to perform an activity and is a fundamental skill to develop. Activity analysis is useful to identify potential activity demands and required performance skills. However, activity analysis does not always allow for consideration of the individualised, interactive and dynamic components of real-time task performance by a specific individual, nor does it acknowledge the role of context as a possible influence on the activity. Dynamic Performance Analysis (DPA) was developed to meet this need.

DPA is a performance-based approach to occupational performance analysis. The analysis process focuses on the actual performance of an occupation, activity, task, action and /or movement (occupation and/or its sublevels) and the identification of performance problems or breakdowns (Polatajko et al., 2000). DPA evolved in the context of the development of a person-centred, top-down or task-oriented[1] intervention approach called Cognitive Orientation to Daily Occupational Performance (CO-OP) Approach (Polatajko et al., 2000) (refer to Chapter 28). The CO-OP Approach is a metacognitive[2] problem-solving approach in which an occupational therapist guides

individuals to identify their task performance breakdowns and discover strategies that will enable them to overcome or solve the issues they identified (Polatajko & Mandich, 2004). To be able to guide a person through this metacognitive problem-solving process, the occupational therapist needs to first identify where, during task performance, the performance breaks down. Such analysis requires the observation of actual occupational performance.

THE HIERARCHY OF OCCUPATIONAL PERFORMANCE

Occupational performance can be understood as having different levels of complexity (Polatajko et al., 2012). In DPA, it is important to understand the hierarchical structure of occupational performance (Polatajko et al., 2007), whereby the occupation is comprised of a set of activities and activities are comprised of a set of tasks, which are comprised of a set of actions. These actions, in turn, are comprised of voluntary movements or mental processes (Polatajko et al., 2007). In this chapter, hierarchical structure of occupational performance is captured in the phrase occupations and/or its sublevels. It is important to note that each higher level of this hierarchical structure subsumes the characteristics of those below it, permitting an occupational therapist to focus on a particular level of performance at a time (Polatajko et al., 2000). For instance, when considering the occupation of *self-care* (Fig. 18.1), the activities may include *dressing, bathing, toileting* and so on. Each of these activities consists of different tasks; *dressing*, for example, can involve *putting on a shirt, putting on pants, putting on shoes* and so on. Similarly, each of these tasks will consist of actions; *putting on a shirt*, for example, may require *holding the shirt, orienting the shirt, raising the arm* and so on. Finally, each of these actions is composed of individual voluntary movements or mental processes; when *holding a shirt*, for example, one needs to *flex fingers, oppose thumb* and so on.

PERFORMANCE ANALYSIS

When occupational therapists talk about *performance*, they tend to refer to an accomplishment or an execution of an occupation, activity, task or action. For each of these levels, a person's performance proficiency is

---

[1]Top-down, task-specific or task-oriented approaches focus on functional tasks and not remediating underlying processes presumed to be required to perform a task (Sugden & Chambers, 2005).

[2]Metacognition is the process of thinking about one's thinking and learning (Flavell, 1979). A metacognitive approach encourages individuals to think explicitly about their learning, oftentimes by teaching them specific strategies for planning, monitoring and evaluating their learning.

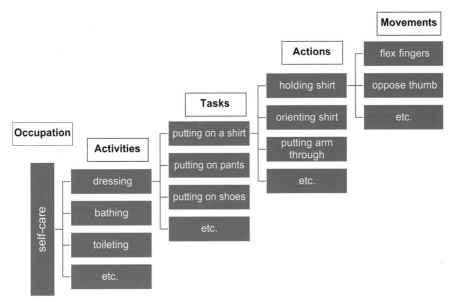

Fig. 18.1 ■ Occupational hierarchy of dressing. (Inspired from Fig. 1 in Polatajko et al., 2000, p. 67.)

the result of a dynamic interaction among the occupation, person and environment (or context). An activity analysis process recognises the interaction among person, occupation and environment factors, the focus of the analyses remains targeted on the underlying components from each of these dimensions and not the result of their interaction. When an occupational therapist carries out an activity analysis, the activity is analysed as it is typically done, usually without a particular person or context in mind (Thomas, 2012). To understand the intricacies of a particular person's performance breakdown, activity analysis is not enough; a performance analysis must be done.

Performance analysis is embedded in a top-down, task-oriented framework and is based on the direct observation of a person performing a desired, needed or expected occupation and/or its sublevels (Fisher, 1997, 2013; Fisher & Griswold, 2014; Polatajko et al., 2000). The focus is on the quality of the dynamic transaction among the elements (of occupation and/or its sublevels, person and environment) with respect to the person's performance of the activity or task, rather than the components necessary for performance (Fisher, 2013; Fisher & Griswold, 2014). In this type of analysis, the units of observation are the actions and movements required for accomplishing the occupation. For

example, the actions and movement required for the activity of putting on socks include grasping sock, orienting sock to foot and pulling sock onto foot. Each action and movement itself is a result of a goal-directed transaction among the person, the occupation and the environment (Fisher & Griswold, 2014).

Standardised performance analysis procedures exist. For instance, the Assessment of Motor and Process Skills (Fisher, 1997) is a standardised, observational assessment that is used to assess the quality of a person's performance in real-life tasks, and the Activities of Daily Living Profile (Dutil et al., 2005). It was developed to assess everyday activities of people with traumatic brain injury (TBI). Fisher and Griswold (2014) describe several advantages of using a standardised performance analysis including the objectivity of analysis, consistency in evaluation practices and facilitated interpretation of results by virtue of established criterion measures and normative values (likely based on Western cultures). On the other hand, these authors also identify limitations such as (1) the formal training needed to be able to administer these standardised assessments; (2) the lack of flexibility these instruments provide with respect to the tasks and activities encompassed and (3) lack of generalisability to other populations.

A significant advantage of a nonstandardised performance analysis process, such as DPA, is that it does not require costly occupational therapist training, it affords unlimited flexibility with respect to the activities and tasks that can be analysed, and it can be conducted with people experiencing a broad range of challenges. Furthermore, this dynamic assessment process permits a continuous and iterative assessment process, not only at the beginning and end of the intervention but also throughout the intervention sessions.

DYNAMIC PERFORMANCE ANALYSIS

DPA is a top-down, task-oriented framework for analysing occupational performance applicable to all occupations, activities and tasks. Although its development began with the analysis of task performance of children with developmental coordination disorder, it is not limited to use with people of any particular age or diagnosis. Unlike activity analysis, in DPA, the reference point is not the typical way a task is done. There is a recognition that there is no set or predetermined way of 'doing' an occupation and/or its sublevels. Rather, the occupational therapist bases their analysis on the person's own way of doing the occupation and/or its sublevels, taking into consideration the person's characteristics, the occupation and the environment, all in interaction with each other (Polatajko et al., 2000). Furthermore, it is the person themself who defines apriori what competent or successful performance is. The occupational therapist should verify the person's expectations rather than assume or impose their (or society's) notion of successful performance. Thus DPA aligns with a collaborative relationship-focused practice.

When undertaking a DPA, it is helpful to keep in mind this top-down, task-oriented perspective in concert with the hierarchical nature of occupational performance, as this is the central aspect of the DPA. However, two other elements need to be considered before proceeding with the dynamic analysis: the occupational therapist and the person doing the occupation, activity, task, action or movement (the performer).

Occupational Therapist Prerequisites

To successfully carry out a DPA, it is helpful if the occupational therapist enters the process with the following four prerequisites.

1. It is important for the occupational therapist to begin the process with a task-orientation or top-down mindset. The focus in DPA is on the activity and sublevels of activity, rather than on the person's impairment (e.g. strength, coordination and balance) in relation to the occupation and/or its sublevels demands and performance skills (as is the case in activity analysis). When the focus is on the person's impairment and activity demands, the tendency is to identify problems with respect to how a person should typically do an occupation and/or its sublevels, rather than pay attention to the fit between the occupation and environment and the person's abilities, skills and actions (Polatajko & Mandich, 2004). The aim with DPA is to identify at what point in the occupation and/or its sublevels, a person's performance breaks down. Only after the activity performance breakdown is identified can the occupational therapist then examine the person–occupation–environment interaction to determine how to overcome this breakdown.

2. The occupational therapist needs to have a certain level of knowledge with respect to the occupation and/or its sublevels at hand. It is difficult to identify where a performance is breaking down if the occupational therapist does not know or understand the occupation and/or its sublevels. When this knowledge is lacking, the occupational therapist should actively seek to understand the essentials of the occupation. This can be done in collaboration with the person, with others or by searching online sources. For instance, if undertaking the DPA of a beginner karate kata (a detailed pattern of movements practiced in martial arts), consultation with a Sensei (martial arts teacher) may be helpful to review the series of movement patterns and elements for a successful kata performance for the person's beginner level. Detailed examples of the occupational therapist's preparation process when faced with an unfamiliar task can be found in Box 18.1 and Fig. 18.2 and Box 18.2 and Fig. 18.3.

3. The occupational therapist appreciates that *there is usually more than one way to do things.* Unlike activity analysis, where a specific manner of doing an activity forms the template for

the analysis, DPA recognises that there is more than one way to achieve an occupation and/or its sublevels. For the activity of dressing, for instance, the task of putting on a pair of pants requires putting both legs into the pant legs. This can be done by: (a) standing and putting one leg into a pant leg at a time, (b) sitting on a chair and putting one leg into a pant leg at a time or (c) sitting on a chair and putting both legs into both pant legs at the same time. Any one of these three methods will accomplish the task of putting both legs into the pant legs (other methods may also exist). Although one method may be the more 'typical' method or the more 'preferred' by the occupational therapist, this may or may not be the method used or selected by the person receiving occupational therapy services.

4. To undertake a DPA, the occupational therapist needs to actually observe the person doing the occupation and/or its sublevels, to identify where the performance breakdown occurs. This is because the actions or methods to achieve an occupation and/or its sublevels are contingent on the person and the context in which the occupational performance actually takes place. While observation in the context is not always possible, there needs to be a recognition that the more similar the context of the occupational performance is to that of the occupational participation, the more authentic will be the identification of the breakdowns.

Performer Prerequisites

From the person's perspective, two prerequisites are required to engage in the occupational performance: *motivation* and *task knowledge* (Polatajko et al., 2000).

1. *Motivation* is what provides the impetus to do. It not only predicts learning (Pintrich, 2003), but also a person's readiness to learn (Shonkoff & Phillips, 2000). Motivation is necessary for the acquisition and performance of occupations and subsumed activities, tasks, actions and movements. Researchers have shown that motivation is an important factor in the ability to use existing knowledge and skills, as well as to persist when an occupation and/or its sublevels becomes extremely challenging (Anshel et al., 1992; Deci & Ryan, 1992; Dweck, 1986; Miller et al., 2014). A person must have a minimum level of motivation for an occupation and/or its sublevels to be initiated (Polatajko et al., 2000). As such, before embarking on a DPA, the occupational therapist needs to determine whether the person is motivated or willing to perform the occupation and/or its sublevels being considered. If the person is not motivated or willing to perform the occupation and/or its sublevels, it will not be possible to do a proper DPA.

2. *Task knowledge* refers to the level of understanding the person has about the occupation and/or its sublevels being performed (Polatajko & Mandich, 2004). At least a minimum or basic level of knowledge about the occupation and/

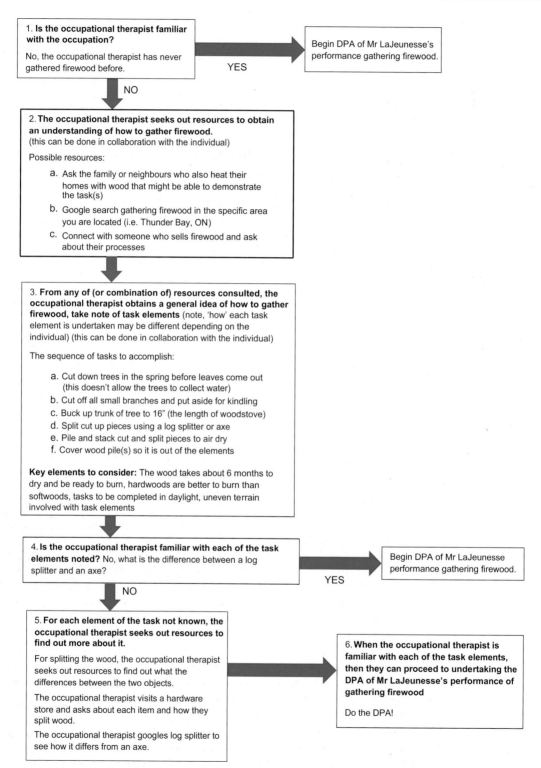

1. Is the occupational therapist familiar with the occupation?

No, the occupational therapist has never gathered firewood before.

YES → Begin DPA of Mr LaJeunesse's performance gathering firewood.

NO ↓

2. The occupational therapist seeks out resources to obtain an understanding of how to gather firewood. (this can be done in collaboration with the individual)

Possible resources:

a. Ask the family or neighbours who also heat their homes with wood that might be able to demonstrate the task(s)

b. Google search gathering firewood in the specific area you are located (i.e. Thunder Bay, ON)

c. Connect with someone who sells firewood and ask about their processes

3. From any of (or combination of) resources consulted, the occupational therapist obtains a general idea of how to gather firewood, take note of task elements (note, 'how' each task element is undertaken may be different depending on the individual) (this can be done in collaboration with the individual)

The sequence of tasks to accomplish:

a. Cut down trees in the spring before leaves come out (this doesn't allow the trees to collect water)

b. Cut off all small branches and put aside for kindling

c. Buck up trunk of tree to 16" (the length of woodstove)

d. Split cut up pieces using a log splitter or axe

e. Pile and stack cut and split pieces to air dry

f. Cover wood pile(s) so it is out of the elements

Key elements to consider: The wood takes about 6 months to dry and be ready to burn, hardwoods are better to burn than softwoods, tasks to be completed in daylight, uneven terrain involved with task elements

4. Is the occupational therapist familiar with each of the task elements noted? No, what is the difference between a log splitter and an axe?

YES → Begin DPA of Mr LaJeunesse performance gathering firewood.

NO ↓

5. For each element of the task not known, the occupational therapist seeks out resources to find out more about it.

For splitting the wood, the occupational therapist seeks out resources to find out what the differences between the two objects.

The occupational therapist visits a hardware store and asks about each item and how they split wood.

The occupational therapist googles log splitter to see how it differs from an axe.

→ **6. When the occupational therapist is familiar with each of the task elements, then they can proceed to undertaking the DPA of Mr LaJeunesse's performance of gathering firewood**

Do the DPA!

Fig. 18.2 ■ Preparation process to understand unfamiliar occupation before commencing DPA: Collecting firewood.

After their head injury, Fede exhibits several difficulties in executive functioning skills (e.g. planning, organising and time management) that are impacting on their occupational performance in several daily activities. One daily activity that is particularly important for Fede is making potato gnocchi, a dish they learned from their Nonna (grandmother). Fede finds making gnocchi relaxing and makes them feel close to their Nonna and Italian origins.

The occupational therapist and Fede agree on the goal of making potato gnocchi. As the occupational therapist has never made gnocchi before, she discusses with Fede about the ingredients, equipment and steps to make gnocchi. Fede says they do not seem to properly remember the details. Fede and the occupational therapist discuss that it would be helpful for Fede to use a recipe to help them remember the details for making gnocchi. For the next therapy session, the occupational therapist asks Fede to find a gnocchi recipe that they can follow.

In the meantime, the occupational therapist seeks out resources to obtain an understanding of how to make gnocchi so that she can undertake a proper DPA. There are several possible resources; the occupational therapist has an Italian recipe book at home and finds a gnocchi recipe. While reading the recipe, she takes note of the activity elements (ingredients, sequence of tasks and key elements to consider). One of the steps in the recipe refers to using a potato ricer, something she has never heard of, so she Google searches what it is. In her search, she finds that it is possible to make gnocchi without a potato ricer and finds a video that demonstrates the steps for making potato gnocchi without it. The occupational therapist is now familiar with each of the task elements of making gnocchi and is ready to undertake the DPA of Fede's performance of making potato gnocchi. The preparation process that the occupational therapist follows prior to commencing DPA is illustrated in Fig. 18.3.

or its sublevels is necessary for performance. For instance, to put on a pair of pants, one must have an idea of what pants are and that the two legs go into the pant legs individually. Without basic task knowledge, it will not be possible for the person to initiate task performance and so not possible to undertake a DPA.

DPA Decision Tree

The DPA process is guided by the DPA decision tree (Fig. 18.4). This decision tree provides the occupational therapist with a framework for structuring observations. There are two sets of questions that the occupational therapist will ask: *performer prerequisites* and *performance requisites*.

Performer Prerequisites Questions

As described earlier, the purpose of the first set of questions is to determine whether the person has the prerequisites for engaging in the occupational performance. If the person is not motivated or willing to perform the occupation and/or its sublevels,[3] then the DPA process cannot continue. The occupational therapist exits the decision tree and explores the person's motivational issues with respect to the activity. For instance, if when undertaking a DPA of riding a bicycle the person is unwilling to sit on the bicycle, the occupational therapist needs to explore why. For example, is it perhaps because of a fear of falling or angst around making a mistake or looking silly? The occupational therapist must address these with the person before continuing with the DPA.

Once motivation is addressed, the person is asked to try the occupation and/or its sublevels, and the occupational therapist then determines the person's general level of task knowledge. The occupational therapist does this by questioning or observing the person attempting the occupation and/or its sublevels. If the person does not demonstrate a rudimentary level of task knowledge, the occupational therapist cannot proceed with the DPA. The occupational therapist needs to exit the decision tree and address the lack of knowledge through providing information, demonstration or other means. If the person has basic task knowledge, then they can attempt the occupation and/or its sublevels and enter the performance requisites part of the decision tree. As mentioned, DPA is an interactive process. The occupational therapist repeats this line of questioning considering each level of the occupational performance (i.e. occupation, activity, task and action).

---

[3]For the purpose of simplicity, the *activity* level of the occupational hierarchy is being used; however, please note that this can be replaced by any other level (e.g. occupation and task or action).

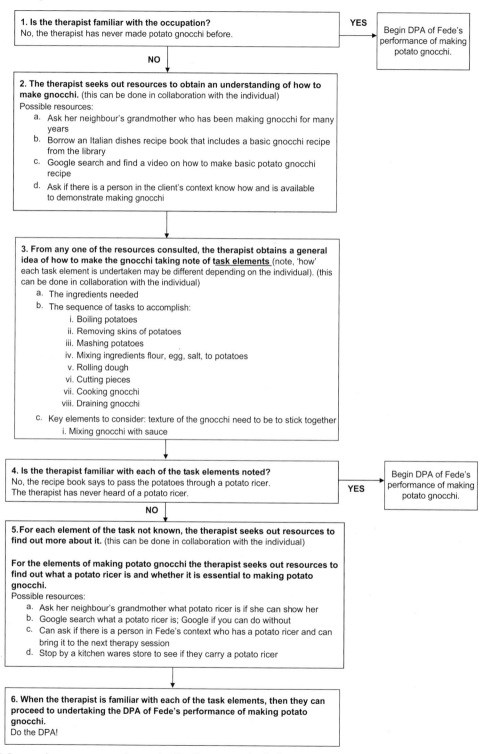

1. Is the therapist familiar with the occupation?
No, the therapist has never made potato gnocchi before.

YES → Begin DPA of Fede's performance of making potato gnocchi.

NO ↓

2. The therapist seeks out resources to obtain an understanding of how to make gnocchi. (this can be done in collaboration with the individual)
Possible resources:
- a. Ask her neighbour's grandmother who has been making gnocchi for many years
- b. Borrow an Italian dishes recipe book that includes a basic gnocchi recipe from the library
- c. Google search and find a video on how to make basic potato gnocchi recipe
- d. Ask if there is a person in the client's context know how and is available to demonstrate making gnocchi

3. From any one of the resources consulted, the therapist obtains a general idea of how to make the gnocchi taking note of <u>task elements</u> (note, 'how' each task element is undertaken may be different depending on the individual). (this can be done in collaboration with the individual)
- a. The ingredients needed
- b. The sequence of tasks to accomplish:
    - i. Boiling potatoes
    - ii. Removing skins of potatoes
    - iii. Mashing potatoes
    - iv. Mixing ingredients flour, egg, salt, to potatoes
    - v. Rolling dough
    - vi. Cutting pieces
    - vii. Cooking gnocchi
    - viii. Draining gnocchi
- c. Key elements to consider: texture of the gnocchi need to be to stick together
    - i. Mixing gnocchi with sauce

4. Is the therapist familiar with each of the task elements noted?
No, the recipe book says to pass the potatoes through a potato ricer.
The therapist has never heard of a potato ricer.

YES → Begin DPA of Fede's performance of making potato gnocchi.

NO ↓

5. For each element of the task not known, the therapist seeks out resources to find out more about it. (this can be done in collaboration with the individual)

For the elements of making potato gnocchi the therapist seeks out resources to find out what a potato ricer is and whether it is essential to making potato gnocchi.
Possible resources:
- a. Ask her neighbour's grandmother what potato ricer is if she can show her
- b. Google search what a potato ricer is; Google if you can do without
- c. Can ask if there is a person in Fede's context who has a potato ricer and can bring it to the next therapy session
- d. Stop by a kitchen wares store to see if they carry a potato ricer

6. When the therapist is familiar with each of the task elements, then they can proceed to undertaking the DPA of Fede's performance of making potato gnocchi.
Do the DPA!

Fig. 18.3 ■ Preparation process to understand unfamiliar occupation before commencing DPA: Making Nonna's potato gnocchi.

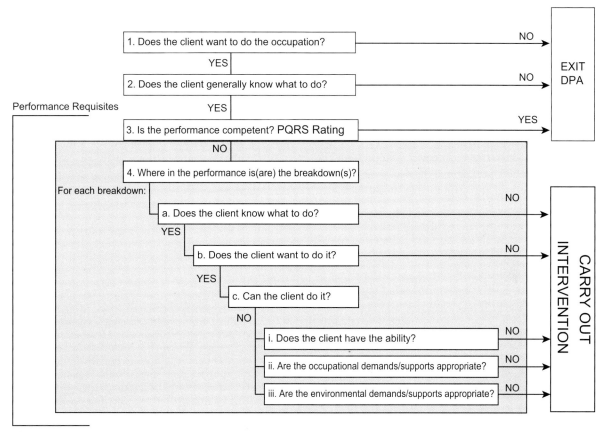

Fig. 18.4 ■ DPA decision tree. (From Polatajko, H. J., Mandich, A., & Martini, R. (2000). Dynamic performance analysis: A framework for understanding occupational performance. *American Journal of Occupational Therapy, 54,* 65–72.)

Performance Requisites Questions

Once the person possesses the necessary motivation and sufficient general task knowledge to attempt the task in question, the occupational therapist can begin analysing the actual performance. At this point, the person is asked to perform the occupation and/or its sublevels while the occupational therapist observes. The occupational therapist uses task knowledge and observation skills to identify whether the performance is competent or not, taking note of errors or breakdowns. Once the occupational therapist identifies a breakdown, the next series of questions in the decision tree are asked to ascertain the possible source(s) of the difficulties.

For each breakdown, the occupational therapist verifies (a) motivation, (b) knowledge and (c) competence

(depicting the embedded, iterative process of DPA). The person's competence is explored by considering his or her (1) abilities relative to the (2) occupational or activity demands and (3) environmental demands and supports. Once the sources of the person–occupation–environment imbalance are identified, the occupational therapist can then begin intervention to address these imbalances. This process is undertaken for each identified breakdown as depicted in Figs. 18.5 and 18.6.

It should be noted that there is a certain hierarchy of breakdowns. In some instances, a breakdown can be identified that does not impede the person from continuing with the activity (Box 18.3 and Fig. 18.5). In such an instance, subsequent breakdowns in performance can be identified, resulting in a series of breakdowns that can be addressed. However, there are times when a breakdown does not permit the ongoing performance of the activity (Box 18.4 and Fig. 18.6). In such cases, the occupational therapist needs to address this breakdown before the DPA process can continue for the rest of the occupation and/or its sublevels. In this way, intervention can be closely tied to the DPA process. DPA does not just occur before intervention; it is a process that continues throughout the intervention process. Once the breakdown is addressed, the person will be able to continue the occupation and/or its sublevel performance and further breakdowns can be identified if that is the case.

Collaborative DPA

One of the prerequisites for DPA is that the occupational therapist be able to observe the person participate in the occupation and/or its sublevels. However, there are times that the nature of the occupation and/or its sublevels undertaken makes it impractical for observation. Elements such as (1) the time the activity occurs (e.g. getting ready for bed at night), (2) the duration of the activity (e.g. preparing a holiday dinner), (3) the location of the activity (e.g. at a work site) or (4) the social construct of the activity (e.g. a job interview) render it impractical for an occupational therapist to be present to observe the person in

---

BOX 18.3
MAKING TEA

Marie was referred to community occupational therapy because her family reported that her memory was decreasing, and they were concerned about her ability to cook safely. They had found a stove burner left turned on a few times when visiting her.

The occupational therapist visited Marie in her home and began speaking to Marie. When talking about her cooking habits, Marie reported that she did not make big meals, just simple meals like soup, a sandwich and tea. She also reported that her children had arranged for one meal a day to be delivered to her, and this was usually enough food for the whole day. Marie acknowledged that her children had noticed a stove burner left on when visiting and had made quite a fuss about it. With a bit of probing, Marie admitted that this was a concern for her as well. She did not want to start a fire but wanted to remain in her apartment.

The occupational therapist asked if she could observe Marie making tea to see how she managed and determine whether there was anything that could be done to address her and her family's concerns. Marie agreed stating that she enjoyed having a quiet cup of tea and had been making tea since she was a young girl. To make tea, she had always used a kettle that was boiled on the stove (Steps 1 and 2, Fig. 18.5).

While observing Marie making tea, Beth noted two areas of performance breakdown. First, when Marie poured the water into the cup, she poured more water on the table than in the teacup. Second, Marie left the stove burner on after the kettle had boiled and replaced the kettle on the burner (Steps 3 and 4, Fig. 18.5).

In analysing the first breakdown, the occupational therapist determined that Marie knew what to do – that is, that water should be poured into the cup instead of on

the table (Step 4 Breakdown i-a, Fig. 18.5) and that she did not want to pour the water onto the table and make a mess (Step 4 Breakdown i-b, Fig. 18.5). However, although Marie was physically able to fill the kettle, the kettle shook in her hand when pouring it. On further analysis, the occupational therapist determined that Marie was not able to hold the full kettle still with one hand while pouring (Step 4 Breakdown i-c-i, Fig. 18.5) and that the occupational demands were not appropriate because the kettle was too heavy (Step 4 Breakdown i-c-ii, Fig. 18.5). Keeping this analysis in mind, the occupational therapist considered intervention options.

Similarly, when analysing the second breakdown, during which Marie left the stove burner on after the kettle had boiled and replaced the kettle on the burner, the occupational therapist determined that Marie knew that she should turn the stove burner off when she was finished with it and that Marie wanted to remember to turn it off, recognising the fire risk. Despite her physical ability to turn off the burner, during the task, Marie did not realise that she had left the burner on. During the performance analysis, the occupational therapist determined that (1) Marie did not appear to have the memory ability to consistently remember to turn off the stove burner; (2) the occupational demands or supports were not adequate – that is, the task provided insufficient cues to help Marie notice that the stove burner was still on; and (3) the environmental demands or supports were not appropriate to facilitate competent task completion that is, there were not enough cues in the environment to help Marie notice that the burner is still on. The occupational therapist considered all of these factors when determining an intervention with Marie to enable her make tea in a safe manner.

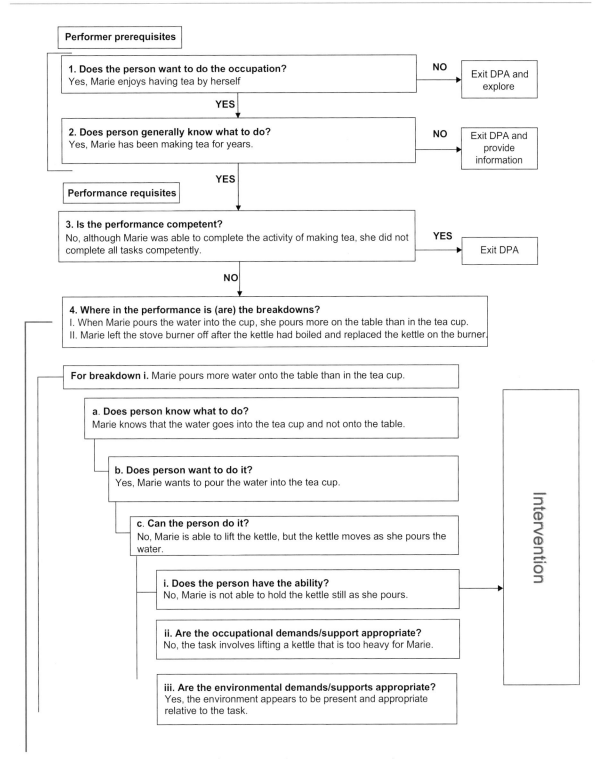

Performer prerequisites

1. Does the person want to do the occupation?
Yes, Marie enjoys having tea by herself

NO → Exit DPA and explore

YES

2. Does person generally know what to do?
Yes, Marie has been making tea for years.

NO → Exit DPA and provide information

YES

Performance requisites

3. Is the performance competent?
No, although Marie was able to complete the activity of making tea, she did not complete all tasks competently.

YES → Exit DPA

NO

4. Where in the performance is (are) the breakdowns?
I. When Marie pours the water into the cup, she pours more on the table than in the tea cup.
II. Marie left the stove burner off after the kettle had boiled and replaced the kettle on the burner.

For breakdown i. Marie pours more water onto the table than in the tea cup.

a. Does person know what to do?
Marie knows that the water goes into the tea cup and not onto the table.

b. Does person want to do it?
Yes, Marie wants to pour the water into the tea cup.

c. Can the person do it?
No, Marie is able to lift the kettle, but the kettle moves as she pours the water.

i. Does the person have the ability?
No, Marie is not able to hold the kettle still as she pours.

ii. Are the occupational demands/support appropriate?
No, the task involves lifting a kettle that is too heavy for Marie.

iii. Are the environmental demands/supports appropriate?
Yes, the environment appears to be present and appropriate relative to the task.

Intervention

Fig. 18.5 ■ Making tea. (see next page)

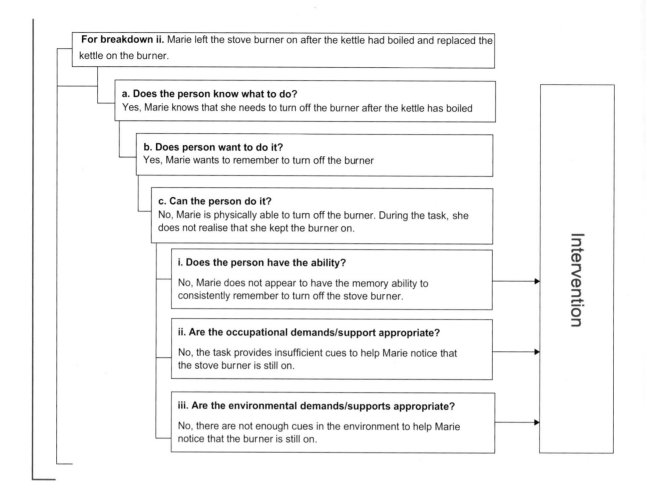

For breakdown ii. Marie left the stove burner on after the kettle had boiled and replaced the kettle on the burner.

a. Does the person know what to do?
Yes, Marie knows that she needs to turn off the burner after the kettle has boiled

b. Does person want to do it?
Yes, Marie wants to remember to turn off the burner

c. Can the person do it?
No, Marie is physically able to turn off the burner. During the task, she does not realise that she kept the burner on.

i. Does the person have the ability?
No, Marie does not appear to have the memory ability to consistently remember to turn off the stove burner.

ii. Are the occupational demands/support appropriate?
No, the task provides insufficient cues to help Marie notice that the stove burner is still on.

iii. Are the environmental demands/supports appropriate?
No, there are not enough cues in the environment to help Marie notice that the burner is still on.

Intervention

action. At such times, other techniques can be used to initiate DPA, such as talking the person through the occupation and/or its sublevels, as used with adults after a traumatic brain injury by Dawson et al. (2009) or talking through and roleplaying, as used with children diagnosed with high functioning autism spectrum disorder by Rodger et al. (2008) and Rodger and Vishram (2010). Through these strategies, the occupational therapist seeks to obtain as much information as possible about how a person does an occupation and/or its sublevels so as to understand how it is actually performed by the person. To ensure proper detailed understanding of the person's performance, a collaborative relationship-focused practice approach is critical, whereby the therapist asks questions to ascertain details or obtain clarity.

A SKILL FOR DEVELOPMENT

Besides being a tool for occupational therapists, DPA may also be considered a skill that the people receiving occupational therapy services can develop. Martini et al. (2004) showed that during their attempt to evaluate their own performance, children (with and without developmental coordination disorder – DCD) recognised that something in their performance was not working. Unlike their non-DCD peers, the children with DCD evaluated their performance inappropriately or inaccurately, leading to ineffective strategy selection. Hyland and Polatajko (2012) reviewed videos and examined statements of children who received a CO-OP Approach intervention and those who did not receive CO-OP

Approach. They found that children who received CO-OP Approach demonstrated a greater number and quality of statements that reflected a DPA, and they were able to spontaneously apply DPA to the performance of another child. This finding indicated that DPA may be considered as an ability that can be improved.

Furthermore, Polatajko et al. (2012) suggest that the process of learning DPA plays a role in enabling people to *transfer strategies* and skills to new situations. Indeed, two randomised controlled trials on the effectiveness of the CO-OP Approach with adults who had experienced cerebrovascular accident found significant improvements in the skill performance of trained skills as well as transfer to untrained skills based on perceived performance and satisfaction with performance using the Canadian Occupational Performance Measure (Ahn et al., 2017) (refer to Chapter 16) and evaluator ratings of skill using the Performance Quality Rating Scale (Ahn et al., 2017; McEwen et al., 2015). These positive findings are thought to be due to the combination of learning DPA and problem-solving strategies within the context of meaningful skill acquisition (Polatajko et al., 2012).

BOX 18.4
PUTTING ON A BUTTONED SHIRT

Mr Hassan experienced a right hemispheric cerebrovascular accident (CVA) one week ago and was recently admitted to an inpatient stroke rehabilitation program. As a result of the CVA, he had left hemiparesis with a flaccid left upper extremity. He was beginning to have some movement in this arm (e.g. minimal movement at his shoulder and slight finger flexion).

During the initial interview with the occupational therapist, Mr Hassan commented that he was not able to get dressed by himself and that he was tired of wearing a hospital gown. On further inquiry, the occupational therapist learned that Mr Hassan worked in a bank and always wore a buttoned dress shirt. When it was suggested that they could explore ways for Mr Hassan to put a buttoned shirt on by himself, Mr Hassan sat up straighter and immediately agreed. The occupational therapist arranged to see Mr Hassan the following morning.

The occupational therapist had determined that Mr Hassan had the performance prerequisites (Steps 1 and 2, Fig. 18.6) of wanting to be able to put on a buttoned shirt and knowing what was involved in putting one on. During the assessment, he examined whether Mr Hassan's performance was competent (Step 3, Fig. 18.6). The occupational therapist noted that Mr Hassan began dressing by putting his right arm into the shirt sleeve. After he had his right arm in the sleeve and the shirt pulled around to his left side, he could not get his left arm into the sleeve. At this point, the occupational therapist knew that Mr Hassan's performance was not competent and that he had to address this performance breakdown before continuing with the DPA. In analysing this performance breakdown (Step 4, Fig. 18.6) where Mr Hassan was not able to reach with his left arm to find the sleeve and push his arm through the sleeve, the occupational therapist determined that Mr Hassan knew that both arms needed to go into the shirt sleeves (Step 4 Breakdown i-a, Fig. 18.6) and that he wanted to be able to get both arms into the sleeves (Step 4 Breakdown i-b, Fig. 18.6). However, Mr Hassan was not capable of lifting his left arm to position his hand to go into the sleeve (Step 4 Breakdown i-c-i, Fig. 18.6). In addition, the demands of the task based on Mr Hassan's usual sequence of putting his right arm into the sleeve first did not allow successful performance (Step 4 Breakdown i-c-ii, Fig. 18.6). The occupational therapist implemented an intervention to enable Mr Hassan to put both arms into the shirt sleeves and continued with the DPA.

The occupational therapist observed that after putting both arms into the sleeves, Mr Hassan straightened his shirt and aligned the buttons. He started to do up the buttons starting with the top button. Mr Hassan was able to grasp the button but was not able to get it completely through the buttonhole (Step 4 Breakdown ii, Fig. 18.6). In examining Mr Hassan's performance, the occupational therapist determined that Mr Hassan knew what was required to fasten a button and that he wanted to be able to do it (Steps 4 Breakdown ii-a & b, Fig. 18.6). He observed that Mr Hassan was able to hold the button of the shirt but was not holding the buttonhole part of the shirt in a way that enabled him to manipulate the button through the hole so that he could grasp it and pull it all the way through (Step 4 Breakdown ii-c, Fig. 18.6). Mr Hassan did not have the motor ability in his left hand to assist his right hand by either stabilising the shirt or manipulating the button (Steps 4 Breakdown ii-c-i, Fig. 18.6). In addition, the shirt that Mr Hassan had was smooth and a bit slippery and the buttons were small, making the demands of the task more challenging (Step 4 Breakdown ii-c-ii, Fig. 18.6). The occupational therapist discussed intervention options with Mr Hassan and together they decided on an intervention approach to enable Mr Hassan to be able to do up his buttons.

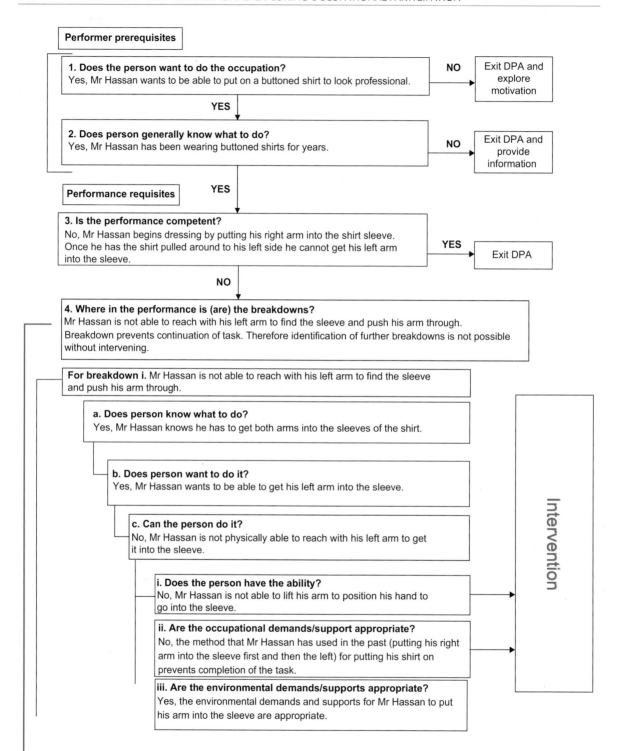

Performer prerequisites

1. Does the person want to do the occupation?
Yes, Mr Hassan wants to be able to put on a buttoned shirt to look professional.

NO → Exit DPA and explore motivation

YES

2. Does person generally know what to do?
Yes, Mr Hassan has been wearing buttoned shirts for years.

NO → Exit DPA and provide information

YES

Performance requisites

3. Is the performance competent?
No, Mr Hassan begins dressing by putting his right arm into the shirt sleeve. Once he has the shirt pulled around to his left side he cannot get his left arm into the sleeve.

YES → Exit DPA

NO

4. Where in the performance is (are) the breakdowns?
Mr Hassan is not able to reach with his left arm to find the sleeve and push his arm through. Breakdown prevents continuation of task. Therefore identification of further breakdowns is not possible without intervening.

For breakdown i. Mr Hassan is not able to reach with his left arm to find the sleeve and push his arm through.

a. Does person know what to do?
Yes, Mr Hassan knows he has to get both arms into the sleeves of the shirt.

b. Does person want to do it?
Yes, Mr Hassan wants to be able to get his left arm into the sleeve.

c. Can the person do it?
No, Mr Hassan is not physically able to reach with his left arm to get it into the sleeve.

i. Does the person have the ability?
No, Mr Hassan is not able to lift his arm to position his hand to go into the sleeve.

ii. Are the occupational demands/support appropriate?
No, the method that Mr Hassan has used in the past (putting his right arm into the sleeve first and then the left) for putting his shirt on prevents completion of the task.

iii. Are the environmental demands/supports appropriate?
Yes, the environmental demands and supports for Mr Hassan to put his arm into the sleeve are appropriate.

Intervention

Fig. 18.6 ■ Putting on a buttoned shirt. (see next page)

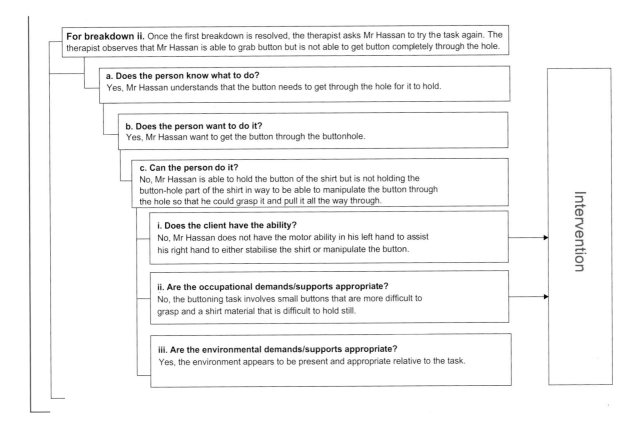

For breakdown ii. Once the first breakdown is resolved, the therapist asks Mr Hassan to try the task again. The therapist observes that Mr Hassan is able to grab button but is not able to get button completely through the hole.

a. Does the person know what to do?
Yes, Mr Hassan understands that the button needs to get through the hole for it to hold.

b. Does the person want to do it?
Yes, Mr Hassan want to get the button through the buttonhole.

c. Can the person do it?
No, Mr Hassan is able to hold the button of the shirt but is not holding the button-hole part of the shirt in way to be able to manipulate the button through the hole so that he could grasp it and pull it all the way through.

i. Does the client have the ability?
No, Mr Hassan does not have the motor ability in his left hand to assist his right hand to either stabilise the shirt or manipulate the button.

ii. Are the occupational demands/supports appropriate?
No, the buttoning task involves small buttons that are more difficult to grasp and a shirt material that is difficult to hold still.

iii. Are the environmental demands/supports appropriate?
Yes, the environment appears to be present and appropriate relative to the task.

Intervention

CONCLUSION

DPA is a performance-based, top-down, task-oriented approach to occupational performance analysis. This analysis process takes into consideration the dynamic interaction between a person's characteristics, the occupation and the environment. As such, unlike activity analysis, where the analysis may be based on the typical way a task is done, DPA is based on the *person's* way of doing the occupation and/or its sublevels. Its focus is on the actual performance of an occupation and its sublevels and identifying performance problems or breakdowns (Polatajko et al., 2000). DPA is a flexible analysis process that can be applied with any and at all levels of the hierarchical structure of occupational performance as well as any and all populations of people receiving occupational therapy services. Finally, although DPA was developed as a tool for occupational therapists to use, there are early indications that DPA may be considered an ability that can be developed and that it may be key for improving skill performance and intertask transfer.

REFERENCES

Ahn, S. N., Yoo, E. Y., Jung, M. Y., Park, H. Y., Lee, J. Y., & Choi, Y. I. (2017). Comparison of cognitive orientation to daily occupational performance and conventional occupational therapy on occupational performance in individuals with stroke: A randomized controlled trial. *NeuroRehabilitation, 40*(3), 285–292.

Anshel, M. H., Weinberg, R., & Jackson, A. (1992). The effects of goal difficulty and task complexity on intrinsic motivation and motor performance. *Journal of Sport Behavior, 15,* 159–176.

Dawson, D. R., Gaya, A., Hunt, A., Levine, B., Lemsky, C., & Polatajko, H. J. (2009). Using the cognitive orientation to occupational performance with adults with traumatic brain injury. *Canadian Journal of Occupational Therapy, 76,* 115–127.

Deci, E. L., & Ryan, R. M. (1992). The initiation and regulation of intrinsically motivated learning and achievement. In A. K. Boggiano, & T. S. Pittman (Eds.), *Achievement and motivation: A social-developmental perspective* (pp. 9–36). Cambridge University Press.

Dutil, E., Bottari, C., Vanier, M., & Gaudreault, C. (2005). *ADL profile: Description of the instrument* (4th ed.). Les Editions Emersion.

Dweck, C. S. (1986). Motivational processes affecting learning. *American Psychologist, 41,* 1040–1048.

Egan, M., & Restall, G. (Eds.). (2022). Promoting occupational participation: Collaborative relationship-focused occupational therapy. Canadian Association of Occupational Therapists.

Fisher, A. G. (1997). Multifaceted measurement of daily life task performance: Conceptualizing a test of instrumental ADL and validating the addition of personal ADL tasks. *Physical Medicine and Rehabilitation: State of the Art Reviews, 11*, 289–303.

Fisher, A. G. (2013). Occupation-centred, occupation-based, occupation-focused: Same, same or different? *Scandinavian Journal of Occupational Therapy, 20*, 162–173.

Fisher, A. G., & Griswold, L. A. (2014). Performance skills: Implementing performance analyses to evaluate quality of occupational performance. In B. A. B. Schell, G. Gillen, M. E. Scaffa, & E. S. Cohn (Eds.), *Willard & Spackman's occupational therapy* (12th ed., pp. 249–264). Wolters Kluwer Lippincott Williams & Wilkins.

Flavell, J. H. (1979). Metacognition and cognitive monitoring: A new area of cognitive-developmental inquiry. *American Psychologist, 34*(10), 906–911.

Hyland, M., & Polatajko, H. J. (2012). Enabling children with developmental coordination disorder to self-regulate through the use of dynamic performance analysis: Evidence from the CO-OP approach. *Human Movement Science, 31*, 987–998.

Martini, R., Wall, A. E., & Shore, B. M. (2004). Metacognitive processes underlying psychomotor performance in children with differing psychomotor abilities. *Adapted Physical Activity Quarterly, 21*, 248–268.

McEwen, S., Polatajko, H., Baum, C., Rios, J., Cirone, D., Doherty, M., & Wolf, T. (2015). Combined cognitive-strategy and task-specific training improve transfer to untrained activities in subacute stroke: An exploratory randomized controlled trial. *Neurorehabilitation and Neural Repair, 29*(6), 526–536.

Miller, L., Ziviani, J., Ware, R., & Boyd, R. N. (2014). Mastery motivation in children with congenital hemiplegia: Individual and environmental associations. *Developmental Medicine & Child Neurology, 56*, 267–274.

Pintrich, P. R. (2003). A motivational science perspective on the role of student motivation in learning and teaching contexts. *Journal of Educational Psychology, 95*, 667–686.

Polatajko, H. J., & Mandich, A. (2004). *Enabling occupation in children: The cognitive orientation to daily occupational performance (CO-OP) approach.* CAOT Publications ACE.

Polatajko, H. J., Mandich, A., & Martini, R. (2000). Dynamic performance analysis: A framework for understanding occupational performance. *American Journal of Occupational Therapy, 54*, 65–72.

Polatajko, H. J., McEwen, S. E., Ryan, J. D., & Baum, C. M. (2012). Brief report – pilot randomized controlled trial investigating cognitive strategy use to improve goal performance after stroke. *American Journal of Occupational Therapy, 66*, 104–109.

Polatajko, H., Davis, J., Stewart, D., Cantin, N., Amoroso, B., Purdie, L., & Zimmerman, D. (2007). Specifying the domain of concern: Occupation as core. In E. A. Townsend, & H. J. Polatajko (Eds.), *Enabling occupation II: Advancing an occupational therapy vision for health, well-being, & justice through occupation* (pp. 9–36). CAOT Publications ACE.

Rodger, S., & Vishram, A. (2010). Mastering social and organizational goals: Strategy use by two children with Asperger's syndrome during cognitive orientation to daily occupational performance. *Physical and Occupational Therapy in Pediatrics, 30*(4), 264–276.

Rodger, S., Ireland, S., & Vun, M. (2008). Can cognitive orientation to daily occupational performance (CO-OP) help children with Asperger's syndrome to master social and organizational goals? *British Journal of Occupational Therapy, 71*(1), 23–32.

Shonkoff, J. P., & Phillips, A. J. (2000). *From Neurons to neighbourhoods: The science of early childhood development.* The National Academies Press.

Sugden, D. A., & Chambers, M. E (2005). Models of intervention: Towards an eco-developmental approach. In D. A. Sugden, & M. E. Chambers (Eds.), *Children with developmental coordination disorder* (pp. 189–211). Whurr.

Thomas, H. (2012). *Occupation-based activity analysis.* Slack.

REFLECTION

1. Provide examples of the hierarchy of occupational performance using a range of occupations that you do everyday (refer to Figure 18.1).

2. Mr C is a 30-year-old man with a right hemiplegia. He wants to be able to open his own water bottle and not have to rely on his wife for this task. You ask him to show you how he opens the water bottle. You observe Mr C as he stands, places the bottle on the table and places his right (affected) hand on the table next to the bottle (not holding the bottle as he is not able to supinate his hand into a neutral position or attempt to grasp the bottle with his right hand). He takes hold of the bottle cap with his left (unaffected) hand and begins to turn it towards the left to unscrew it. As he begins to turn the bottle cap, the bottle moves on the table, and when Mr C exerts more effort to unscrew the cap, the bottle topples over onto the table.

   Use the dynamic performance analysis (DPA) decision tree (Fig. 18.2) to do the following:
   a) Identify Mr C's breakdown points in opening his own soft drink bottle. Remember to describe the breakdown points with respect to the task itself and not with respect to Mr C's impairments.
   b) Examine the identified breakdowns.

3. Do you possess the occupational therapist prerequisites to successfully carry out a DPA? Keeping Mr C in mind, identify the occupational therapist's prerequisites, reflect on these and explain how you meet each of them.

CO-DESIGNING PLANS TO ACCESS, INITIATE AND SUSTAIN OCCUPATIONAL PARTICIPATION

KATE D'CRUZ ■ EMMA ELIZABETH GEE

CHAPTER OUTLINE

Overview

Co-design is a critical approach that occupational therapists use when supporting people to access, initiate and sustain occupational participation. Co-design is a human-centred approach that *values* and *leverages* the lived experience of people experiencing illness, injury or impairment to better meet their needs. Aligned with the Canadian Model of Occupational Participation (CanMOP) and the key characteristics of Collaborative Relationship-Focused Occupational Therapy, co-design is a collaborative relational process. Drawing upon the Canadian Occupational Therapy Inter-Relational Practice Process (COTIPP) Framework, this chapter outlines a guide for co-designing in occupational therapy, identifying barriers and enablers as well as strategies to optimise the participation of people experiencing illness, injury or impairment. Lived experience examples are used throughout the chapter to illustrate co-design. The chapter concludes with a reflection on the value of co-design, as well as the potential for transformational growth afforded through participating in co-design.

KEY POINTS

■ Occupational participation and its relationship with health and wellbeing underpin the practice and focus of occupational therapy.

■ The overall goal of occupational therapy is to enable people to participate in meaningful occupations of choice.

■ Co-design is a collaborative process that supports shared understanding between people experiencing illness, injury or impairment and occupational therapists.

■ Collaborative relationship-focused practice is foundational to occupational therapy and co-design.

■ The Canadian Occupational Therapy Inter-Relational Practice Process (COTIPP) Framework is a useful guide for using co-design in occupational therapy practice.

■ Embracing lived experience and partnering with people experiencing illness, injury or impairment fosters empowerment and opportunities for transformational growth.

INTRODUCTION

The focus of this chapter is to provide an overview of co-design of occupational therapy intervention plans and implementation for people experiencing illness, injury or impairment. More specifically, the chapter will include an exploration of co-designing plans to access, initiate and sustain occupational participation, within meaningful relationships and contexts. Initially, a justification will be given as to why occupational therapists

245

need to focus on occupation when working with people, with consideration of valued occupations within meaningful relationships. The concept of co-design is then presented as a foundational process for promoting occupational participation, with reference to the Canadian Occupational Therapy Inter-Relational Practice Process (COTIPP) (refer to Chapter 12). Barriers and enablers to co-design are outlined, along with strategies to optimise participation. The chapter concludes with a reflection on the value of co-design, as well as the potential for transformational growth afforded through participating in co-design.

Throughout the chapter, lived experience examples from Emma Gee provide insights into the perspective of individuals experiencing illness, injury or impairment. Emma is an occupational therapist and stroke survivor, as well as a published author of 'Reinventing Emma' and lived experience consultant. Emma attributes her experience as a stroke survivor as transformational to her worldview and understanding of occupational therapy and healthcare practice. Emma brings this unique perspective to illustrate the importance of valuing the experiences and insights of people experiencing illness, injury or impairment and integrating this perspective into occupational therapy practice.

FOCUS ON OCCUPATION

Occupation is the unique concern, expertise and contribution of occupational therapy. Foundational to occupational therapy is the recognition of humans as occupational beings, with an underlying assumption that occupational participation influences our health and wellbeing (Wilcock, 2006). In the third edition of *An Occupational Perspective of Health*, Wilcock and Hocking (2015) provide a detailed analysis of the importance of occupation to the health and wellbeing of individuals, groups and communities, contesting that a lack of participation in occupation contributes to ill health. In accordance with the view that humans are occupational beings, occupation is essential for the fulfilment of basic biological and safety needs, in addition to the need for autonomy, relationships and a sense of competence (Egan & Restall, 2022). A substantial body of evidence, generated by occupational scientists and occupational therapists attest to the ways

in which participation in occupations of choice, meaning and purpose, contributes to personal and social identity, wellbeing, social inclusion and the expression of occupational justice (Rudman et al., 2022).

While occupation is important to our wellbeing (Christiansen, 1999; Christiansen & Townsend, 2010; Doble & Santha, 2008; Townsend & Polatajko, 2013; Wilcock, 2006; Wilcock & Hocking, 2015), the meaning attributed to occupation is uniquely defined. Indeed, the new Canadian Model of Occupational Participation (CanMOP) (refer to Chapter 11) resists the urge to define or categorise occupations, rather emphasising the complexity of occupational participation. Occupational participation is dependent on the dynamic and complex interaction among the type of occupation, the abilities, habits, skills and experience of the person and the physical, geographical, cultural, attitudinal and social aspects of the environment (Christiansen et al., 2015; Doble & Santha, 2008). Hence, the occupations people engage in are not static; they are dynamic, influenced by positive and negative experiences and factors throughout the lifespan and contribute to the sense of 'doing', 'being', 'belonging' and 'becoming' (Doble & Santha, 2008; Wilcock & Hocking, 2015). To account for the complexity of occupation, Wilcock and Hocking (2015) use the terms 'doing, being, belonging and becoming as a way to discuss the meaning given to occupation in relation to health' (p. 134).

Doing refers to 'action, getting something done, carrying out, achieving, making, executing, performing, acting, completing, fixing, preparing, organising and undertaking […] exploits, deeds and accomplishments and seeing to, sorting out or looking after' (pp. 134–135). Doing includes what people want to do and what they need to do (Hammell, 2004; Wilcock, 1998, 1999) and is recognised as contributing to experiences of 'competence', 'self-worth' and 'being valuable'(Hammell, 2004).

Being encompasses how each person feels about what they do, the sense of who they understand themselves to be and has also been used to describe a state of existing in the moment (Hitch et al., 2014; Wilcock, 1998, 1999). Wilcock and Hocking (2015) noted that individually 'it is often a period of quiet contemplation about the self and about personal past, present and future pleasures, difficulties and achievements' and for collectives it refers to 'support and reflection, such as in prayer or grief or in times of great joy or celebration that affect a community at large' (p. 135). Being was originally identified as a process of connecting with the inner life (Wilcock, 1998, 1999), while Hammell (2004) made the connection between the construct of being and lived experience. Doble and Santha (2008) summarise this by stating that 'occupation does not simply refer to what is done but to the process of doing or the here and now of individuals' occupational experiences' (p. 185).

Belonging accounts for the social nature of people and their need to affiliate with other people, places and things that have meaning to them (Wilcock & Hocking, 2015). Belonging addresses the importance of social connectedness experienced through meaningful occupational engagement (Wilcock, 2007). Having a sense of belonging can contribute to a person feeling accepted, valued, secure and happy and can facilitate engagement in occupations. The concept of belonging has been described as the experience of being part of something bigger than oneself (Shank & Cutchin, 2010), while others have recognised the importance of reciprocity to the concept of belonging, emphasising giving, sharing and contributing (Molineux & Baptiste, 2011).

Becoming refers to the potential of people, the 'possibility, growth and the ongoing evolution of individuals' occupational identities' (Doble & Santha, 2008, p. 185). Wilcock and Hocking (2015) state that 'the word "becoming" is linked with the idea of undergoing change, transformation, or development [...] coming to be, changing to, emerging as, or to metamorphose (turning or growing into something or becoming somehow different, more knowledgeable, or mature)' (p. 137). Becoming as a concept embraces temporality by looking to future selves and lives, considered in relation to the present and past (Hammell, 2004; Hitch et al., 2014; Wilcock, 1999).

The importance of occupation and its relationship with health and wellbeing underpin the practice and focus of occupational therapy. Occupational therapists consider, 'the unique meanings of necessary and desired occupations for people and collectives and how these meanings define what people need to do, wish to do, and how they wish to do these occupations, with whom, where, when and to what ends' (Egan & Restall, p. 76). The CanMOP (Egan & Restall)

LIVED EXPERIENCE REFLECTION

The Meaning and Purpose of Occupation

The following excerpt from Emma's book captures her experience of why meaning and purpose matter in occupational participation.

During community-based rehabilitation following her stroke, Emma was relearning to walk independently without her walking frame. She was motivated to achieve this goal so that she could fulfil her role as Maid of Honour at her twin sister's wedding and walk down the aisle. For nine months, she practised walking back and forth on the cricket pitch at her local park. Once this goal was achieved and she walked down the aisle at her sister's wedding, she continued to practice her walking on the cricket pitch. However, Emma realised that the walking no longer held purpose.

The big day was over. My twin sister departed on her honeymoon adventure, and I felt left behind. I'd worked so hard towards that day, and I now felt as if I had no direction, no purpose. I kept going with my rigorous routine, but without a specific goal the effort didn't seem worthwhile.

(GEE, 2016, P. 191)

---

describes occupational participation as, 'having access to, initiating and sustaining valued occupations with meaningful relationships and contexts' (p. 76). This definition brings into focus not just someone's ability to perform occupations or the experience of their occupational engagement but the purpose and meaning of occupational participation and occupational possibilities afforded by the broader social, political, cultural and environmental context.

RELATIONSHIP-FOCUSED OCCUPATIONAL THERAPY

Collaborative relationship-focused practice is foundational to occupational therapy (Restall et al., 2022) (refer to Chapter 12). Building upon the central tenets of client or person-centred practice (D'Cruz et al., 2016; Law et al., 1995; Sumsion & Law, 2006) relationship-focussed practice emphasises the role of the relationship in delivering a humanised approach to occupational therapy. Restall et al. (2022) describe collaborative relationship-focused practice as comprising four key characteristics: (1) contextually relevant, (2) contextually and temporally nuanced,

(3) strives for safety and (4) promotes rights-based self-determination (p. 100).

Depending upon the identified needs and context, collaborative relationships may be formed with individuals and collectives, as well as with health professionals and funders or service providers. Investment is needed both in the development and in the maintenance of these relationships, forming the basis for authentic partnerships from which to explore and support meaningful occupations. Opportunities to build and sustain these relationships must be prioritised within practice, including consideration of the impact of incidental interactions upon relationships.

In addition to the role of the occupational therapist in building and sustaining their relationship with the person experiencing illness, injury or impairment, it is important to be aware of the individual's broader relationship experiences. For some individuals experiencing injury, illness or impairment, especially those with an acquired injury, the maintenance of existing relationships and the development of new relationships can be challenging. The occupational therapist can play an important role in enabling individuals to

LIVED EXPERIENCE REFLECTION

The Supporter Relationship

In this passage, Emma shares her experience of navigating changed relationships and the importance of being able to contribute and reciprocate in these relationships.

Throughout my recovery, I have grappled with establishing a good balance in relationships with both informal and formal support. Feeling such a burden on my informal family support was so prevalent, especially earlier on in my recovery when I was a lot more reliant on their care. I hated being a hindrance and that my disability encroached so negatively on all my relationships. I longed to be the 'Old Em' that they loved. I'd cringe when I would hear my Mum exclaim, 'I just saw a glimpse of the old Em'. To me, she was gone. Trying to build a new identity and establish a different dynamic in our relationship was so challenging. I became so reliant on my existing support's acceptance that the old Em had gone. New relationships I have formed since acquiring my disability are somewhat easier as they have no comparison to make between who I was and who I am now. Those existing relationships that have lasted have accepted the new dynamic in our relationship, enable me to reciprocate and always have an immense belief in me. They also really value my input and support my contribution.

(EMMA GEE, PERSONAL REFLECTION, 2023)

LIVED EXPERIENCE REFLECTION

Relationships in Rehabilitation

This quote from Emma's book shows the personal impact of an incidental interaction between her and her doctor during rehabilitation.

I remember in about my second week of rehab the first time I really tried to communicate with one of my doctors. He was walking down the corridor on my ward at the end of the day, carrying a pile of notes. I couldn't call out or wave my arms about to get his attention, so I fixed my eyes in his direction. I knew he could see me, but he was busy reading the notes, so he kept looking down and continued walking. I know I have done the same myself as a therapist, but the impact his behaviour had on me that day, when I already felt so stripped of all other means of communicating, was huge. I felt so forgotten, like an odd sock. Powerless. If he'd said 'Em, I'll see you tomorrow' that would've been fine. The disregard that I received that day really made me see how powerful communication is, and how simple things like eye contact and body language can really impact your relationships and recovery.

(GEE, 2016, P. 129)

build on their existing relationships, to support continued connection and to assist in preventing the loss of relationships. Indeed, a relationship-focused approach to practice emphasises the importance of considering the individual within their broader family, social and cultural context, understanding the impact of changed relationships and helping individuals to navigate these relationships in everyday life.

WHAT IS CO-DESIGN?

Informed by participatory design, co-design is a human-centred approach that values and leverages lived experience knowledge to improve outcomes (Dobe et al., 2022). Participatory design asserts the right of people to participate in research that is about them or impacts them, doing so through a relationship of doing 'with' rather than 'to' (Minkler & Wallerstein, 2008). Co-designing with people experiencing illness, injury or impairment is increasingly an expectation of healthcare service development, research and practice (Lindblom et al., 2021). For the purpose of this book, co-design is best defined as a collaborative partnership between the individuals or collectives experiencing illness, injury or impairment and occupational therapists with the shared aim of creating improved outcomes. In the context of occupational therapy practice, the shared aim is for successful occupational participation that reflects the needs, preferences and hopes of individuals or collectives. Co-design supports 'better design' of treatment plans and interventions based on a richer, deeper understanding of what service users know, feel and want. Critical to this 'deeper understanding' is a collaborative process of exploring and identifying needs and solutions in partnership between the person or collective and the occupational therapist (Masterson et al., 2022).

Key features of co-design include:

- Values lived experience wisdom and knowledge.
- Appreciates the uniqueness of human experience.
- Invests in a collaborative partnership that is non-hierarchical.
- Seeks shared understanding.
- Follows an iterative process of sharing, listening, brainstorming, problem solving, designing, planning, implementing, reviewing and changing.

While co-design is increasingly recognised as imperative to ensuring best practice in healthcare (Dobe et al., 2022; Masterson et al., 2022), concerns have been raised about the risks associated with poorly executed co-design. For example, studies have shown that tokenistic involvement can result in individuals feeling undervalued, underappreciated and frustrated (Slattery et al., 2020), thus undermining the value of co-design. Examples of tokenism might include when people have little or no influence in a project, despite the external appearance of user involvement or when the use of co-design is a tick-the-box exercise to be perceived as doing the 'right thing', rather than reflecting a genuine participatory approach.

Furthermore, poorly executed co-design may perpetuate the power dynamics between healthcare professionals and individuals or communities co-designing together, rather than minimising the power differential. Studies by Dobe et al., 2022 and Lindblom et al. (2021) found that this was the experience of people who had experienced a stroke who felt inferior in their skills and knowledge compared to the health professionals with whom they were co-designing. It is critical that co-design is implemented authentically and is tailored

to the skills and experiences of individuals, especially those who experience changed or impaired cognitive or communication skills. While people experiencing illness, injury or impairment are likely to offer valuable insights into their needs and preferences to support participation, it should be the responsibility of the occupational therapist and not the 'person' to ensure that accessibility considerations are integrated into the design and planning of co-design.

Accessibility considerations for co-design include:

- Tailor complexity, format and amount of information to the skills and cognitive or communication needs of individuals and collectives.
- Use of multimedia communication tools such as visual-analogue scales, ranking tasks, illustrations and photo diaries.
- Provide role clarity; co-design is a new and unfamiliar experience for many people.
- Flexibility and tailoring to individual needs.
- Be mindful of fatigue; limit the length of sessions.
- Provide session plans and summaries to assist with planning and recall of content.

LIVED EXPERIENCE REFLECTION

Creating Opportunities to Share Experiences

In this blog post, Emma advocates the importance of people experiencing illness, injury or impairment having the opportunity to share their story. Rather than limiting these opportunities for fear of emotional overwhelm or exhaustion, Emma encourages use of proactive strategies and encouragement to support people to share.

*Having the opportunity to relay your story can be gruelling but also so cathartic and empowering. It makes what you've been through worthwhile. Rather than **not** giving those you advocate for the opportunity, or assuming their needs, what is it that you can do to support them to voice their thoughts? Perhaps, it's helping them process, articulate and write their thoughts to find out what matters to them. Maybe it's educating others about their needs. It could be just organising the logistics, such as arranging a meeting, or identifying access barriers or simply encouraging them. There are so many aspects to consider when enabling another to share their lived experience. Importantly, advocate WITH them not FOR them.*

(EMMA GEE, EDITED BLOG POST, OCTOBER 21, 2022)

Using Co-Design to Support Occupational Participation

There are various approaches to using co-design in practice; however, the COTIPP Framework provides a useful guide (Egan & Restall, 2022) (refer to Chapter 12). Embedded within the CanMOP (refer to Chapter 11), the COTIPP has been developed to guide the practice of occupational therapy with individuals and collectives. The COTIPP has three underlying assumptions about occupational therapy: (1) Occupational therapy is different in every context; (2) Occupational therapy often has a defined beginning and end, but sometimes does not and (3) Occupational therapy can follow a step-by-step process but, more often, is an iterative process that influences and responds to context and relationships (Egan & Restall, p. 123). These three assumptions, perfectly align with the 'lived experience' lens of co-design, reinforcing the importance of embracing and adapting to the uniqueness of each occupational therapy interaction.

At the centre of COTIPP is what is described as, 'the essential underlying process of occupational therapy practice, which is to build and sustain relationships' (Restall et al., 2022, p. 123). As outlined earlier in this chapter, building and sustaining relationships is informed by the four characteristics of Collaborative Relationship-Focused Occupational Therapy. Building upon this central relationship focus, the framework presents three foundational processes: (1) seek to understand context; (2) critically reflect and reason and (3) use justice-, equity-, and rights-based lenses. These interrelated and dynamic processes guide occupational therapists to critically reflect throughout their practice, in partnerships with the people with whom they are collaborating.

Within the COTIPP, there are six action domains that capture what occupational therapists do to promote occupational participation. These domains include: (1) Connect; (2) Explore occupational participation; (3) Seek understanding and define purpose; (4) Co-design priorities, goals, outcomes and plan; (5) Trial plan, explore change and refine plan and (6) Plan for transition. While the COTIPP defines each of these action domains individually, the processes are not mutually exclusive; indeed they flow into and across each other (Restall et al., 2022). Similarly, while co-design is noted

TABLE 19.1
A Summary of Co-Design Considerations for Each Action Step of the COTIPP

1. Connect
- Being empathic, open-minded and encouraging
- Planning for and allowing time for building a connection
- Use of accessible format to share information about roles and expectation

2. Seek understanding and define purpose
- Sharing stories and listening to the lived experience

3. Explore occupational participation
- Personal narratives give precedence to the lived experience
- Strength-based approach, embedded with hope and possibility

4. Co-design priorities, goals, outcomes and plans
- Address power structures and hierarchies
- Continued investment in relationship and trust building
- Value lived experience wisdom

5. Trial the plan, explore change and refine the plan
- Iterative process of reflection and learning
- Creating a safe space

6. Plan for transition
- Acknowledge outcome achievement
- Transparency in shared decisions

as one of the action domains, it is suggested that the six domains, considered in context with the three foundational processes and the essential underlying process of building and sustaining relationships, reflect the entirety of co-design.

A summary of key co-design considerations for each action step of the COTIPP is provided in Table 19.1.

Connect

Investing in the development of a trusting and comfortable collaborative relationship is a crucial first step in building a healthy dynamic in co-design (Kearns et al., 2020; Lindblom et al., 2021) This involves adopting a humanised approach to getting to know the person or collective as unique people experiencing illness, injury or impairment but not defined by this experience. This is particularly relevant for people with an acquired illness, injury or impairment who may be experiencing a disconnect with their pre-post illness, injury or impairment identity. For some, this might also include recognising and understanding current or past trauma or negative experiences that might impact the development of the relationship. A key part of this process involves developing a shared understanding of roles and expectations and gaining consent for participation. While this involves bi-directional sharing and listening, it is the responsibility of the occupational therapist to facilitate the process, ensuring accessibility of information for people with cognitive and/or communication difficulties.

Seek Understanding and Define Purpose

This process builds on the initial connection that is formed to create a shared understanding of what occupational therapy could involve. At this point in the process, it is important to consider the person or collective within their context, such as 'identities, strengths, resources, challenges, history and cultural importance' (Restall et al., 2022, p. 136). Central to this process is seeking to understand occupational participation hopes and concerns and discussing the process of collaboratively co-designing goals and plans. The role of the occupational therapist at this stage is to actively listen to the person or collective, showing curiosity and interest in their lived experience, thereby demonstrating care and commitment. Achieving a shared purpose is critical at this stage of the process.

Explore Occupational Participation

This process involves a variety of approaches for co-analysing the factors that influence occupational participation (Restall et al., 2022). Examples of such approaches include interviews, questionnaires, observations in people's environments, formal assessment tools, sharing circles and community forums. An important factor in this process is the iterative nature of the 'data' collection and analysis, informing the understanding of occupational participation, from the perspective of both the occupational therapist and the person or collective working in partnership with the occupational therapist. This may also include collaboration with other practitioners from the multidisciplinary team to inform a holistic understanding of occupational participation possibilities. Underpinning this process is the valuing of lived experience, recognition of strengths and commitment to a rights-based understanding of occupational participation.

Co-Design Priorities, Goals, Outcomes and Plans

Building upon the shared understanding created through the earlier phases, 'in this action domain, the therapist and the individual or collective co-create the conditions for co-designing priorities, goals, outcomes and plans' (Restall et al., p. 137). This involves taking the time to fully understand the value and meaning of occupational participation and translating this into the design of a treatment plan or intervention. Central to this process and aligned with the core tenets of co-design is the coming together of the unique wisdom and experience of the person experiencing illness, injury or impairment with the practice wisdom and experience of the occupational therapist. It is through this coming together that there is alignment of perspectives within the social, institutional or environmental context. This may include involvement of family and friends, other people in the community or community organisations to ensure cultural relevance and accessibility.

Trial the Plan, Explore Change and Refine the Plan

Consistent with the iterative nature of the co-design process, in this action domain, there is an emphasis on learning and refinement of the intervention through the 'doing' of the intervention. This involves constant evaluation of, and investing in, the collaborative relationship, as well as adjustment to goals, hopes and plans. Central to this phase is the notion of change and growth, informed by reflection and an openness to learning. Incumbent upon the occupational therapists is the creation of a safe space for making mistakes and learning through the process of trial and error. Within this process, the potentiality of occupational participation is realised.

Plan for Transition

This final phase of the process recognises achievement and plans for transition into everyday living. It is a time of reflection in which the perspectives and experiences of the occupational therapist and the person or collective are shared, informing the development of an intentional transition plan. Depending upon the context, goals and needs, this next phase may or may not include ongoing occupational therapy or consideration of changing needs over time, such as is the case with progressive conditions. Critical to the success of this final phase is a shared understanding of outcomes achieved and plans for the future, as well as confirmation of the closure of therapy and the relationship between the person or collective and the occupational therapist.

The Value of Co-Design

The COTIPP framework presents occupational therapists with a helpful guide for the implementation of co-design in practice. Aligned with the principles of co-design, the COTIPP framework recognises the importance of building and sustaining relationships with people experiencing illness, injury or impairment in occupational therapy practice. It is through this relationship and listening that occupational therapists best understand the priorities and needs of those with whom they work.

Co-designing together also builds capacity. A collaborative relationship between an occupational therapist and a person or collective shifts the power differential and communicates to the individual or collective that they are respected and valued. This belief in capacity and safety in a supportive and trusted relationship fosters autonomy and a confidence to embrace opportunities for occupational participation. Underpinning both occupational therapy and co-design is a strengths-based approach to working with people experiencing illness, injury or impairment and a belief in the possibility of transformational growth.

LIVED EXPERIENCE REFLECTION

Co-Design Partnerships Build Capacity.

The following reflections capture Emma's views on the importance of a collaborative approach to recovery.

The importance of adopting a collaborative approach throughout my recovery has been phenomenal. Not only to ensure that I was included or involved and had a role but also that I was proactive in my recovery. Feeling appreciated and valued is essential to building and sustaining good relationships. It also ensures our self-worth remains intact. When I was cast as the 'victim' in relationships throughout my recovery, I lost my autonomy, became reactive to my predicament and reliant on others to act on my behalf. They became the drivers of my recovery, rather than me.

(EMMA GEE, PERSONAL REFLECTION, 2023)

CONCLUSION

This chapter provides an overview of a co-design partnership approach to occupational therapy practice. Lived experience examples from Emma Gee, stroke survivor and occupational therapist, have been incorporated into the chapter to illustrate the value of co-design. Drawing upon the COTIPP Framework as well as key characteristics of Collaborative Relationship-Focused Occupational Therapy, this chapter has outlined a process of using co-design in occupational therapy, identifying barriers and enablers, as well as strategies to optimise the participation of people experiencing illness, injury or impairment. Co-design is a valuable tool when used in occupational therapy practice, supporting the development of productive and collaborative partnerships that value and use lived experience wisdom to inform interventions that work towards achieving meaningful occupational participation.

REFERENCES

Christiansen, C. H. (1999). Defining lives: Occupation as identity: An essay on competence, coherence, and the creation of meaning. *American Journal of Occupational Therapy, 53*, 547–558.

Christiansen, C., Baum, C., & Bass, J. (2015). The Person-Environment-Occupation-Performance (PEOP) model. In C. Christiansen, C. Baum, & J. Bass (Eds.), *Occupational therapy: Performance, participation and well-being* (4th ed., pp. 23–47). Slack.

Christiansen, C., & Townsend, E (2010). An introduction to occupation. In C. Christiansen, & E. Townsend (Eds.), *Introduction to occupation: The art of science and living* (pp. 2–34). Prentice Hall.

D'Cruz, K., Howie, L., & Lentin, P. (2016). Client-centred practice: Perspectives of persons with a traumatic brain injury. *Scandinavian Journal of Occupational Therapy, 23*(1), 30–38. https://doi.org/10.3109/11038128.2015.1057521.

Dobe, J., Gustafsson, L., & Walder, K. (2022). Co-creation and stroke rehabilitation: A scoping review. *Disability and Rehabilitation, 45*(3), 562–574. https://doi.org/10.1080/09638288.2022.2032411.

Doble, S., & Santha, J. (2008). Occupational well-being: Rethinking occupational therapy outcomes. *Canadian Journal of Occupational Therapy, 75*(3), 184–190.

Egan, M., & Restall, G. (2022). *Promoting occupational participation: Collaborative relationship-focused occupational therapy.* CAOT.

Gee, E. (2016). *Reinventing Emma.* Author.

Hammell, K. W. (2004). Dimensions of meaning in the occupations of daily life. *Canadian Journal of Occupational Therapy - Revue Canadienne d'Ergotherapie, 71*(5), 296–305.

Hitch, D., Pepin, G., & Stagnatti, K. (2014). In the footsteps of Wilcock, part one: The evolution of doing, being, becoming and belonging. *Occupational therapy in health care, 28*(3), 231–246. https://doi.org/10.3109/07380577.2014.898114.

Kearns, Á., Kelly, H., & Pitt, I. (2020). Rating experience of ICT-delivered aphasia rehabilitation: Co-design of a feedback questionnaire. *Aphasiology, 34*(3), 319–342. https://doi.org/10.1080/02687038.2019.1649913.

Law, M., Baptiste, S., & Mills, J. (1995). Client-centred practice: What does it mean and does it make a difference? *Canadian Journal of Occupational Therapy, 162*(5), 250–257. https://doi.org/10.1177/000841749506200504.

Lindblom, S., Flink, M., Elf, M., Laska, A. C., von Koch, L., & Ytterberg, C. (2021). The manifestation of participation within a co-design process involving patients, significant others and health-care professionals. *Health Expectations, 24*, 905–916. https://doi.org/10.1111/hex.13233.

Masterson, D., Areskoug Josefsson, K., Robert, G., Nylander, E., & Kjellström, S. (2022). Mapping definitions of co-production and co-design in health and social care: A systematic scoping review providing lessons for the future. *Health Expectations, 25*(3), 902–913. https://doi.org/10.1111/hex.13470.

Minkler, M., & Wallerstein, N. (2008). *Community-based participatory research for health: From process to outcome.* Jossey-Bass.

Molineux, M., & Baptiste, S. (2011). Emerging occupational therapy practice: Building on the foundations and seizing the opportunities. In M. Thew, M. Edwards, S. Baptiste, & M. Molineux (Eds.), *Role emerging occupational therapy* (pp. 3–14). Wiley-Blackwell.

Restall, G., Egan, M., Valavaara, K., Phenix, A., & Sack, C. (2022). Canadian occupational therapy inter-relational practice process framework. In M. Egan, & G. Restall (Eds.), *Promoting occupational participation: Collaborative relationship-focused occupational therapy* (pp. 11–30). CAOT.

Rudman, L., Aldrich, R. M., & Kiepek, N. (2022). Evolving understandings of occupation. In M. Egan, & G. Restall (Eds.), *Promoting occupational participation: Collaborative relationship-focused occupational therapy* (pp. 119–150). CAOT.

Shank, K. H., & Cutchin, M. P. (2010). Transactional occupations of older women aging-in-place: Negotiating change and meaning. *Journal of Occupational Science, 17*(1), 4–13.

Slattery, P., Saeri, A. K., & Bragge, P. (2020). Research co-design in health: A rapid overview of reviews. *Health Research, Policy and Systems*, 18, 17. https://doi.org/10.1186/s12961-020-0528-9.

Sumsion, T., & Law, M. (2006). A review of evidence on the conceptual elements informing client-centred practice. *Canadian Journal of Occupational Therapy, 73*(3), 153–162. https://doi.org/10.1177/000841740607300303.

Townsend, E., & Polatajko, H. (Eds.). (2013). *Enabling occupation II: Advancing an occupational therapy vision for health, well-being, and justice through occupation.* CAOT Publications ACE.

Wilcock, A. A. (1998). Doing, being, becoming. *Canadian Journal of Occupational Therapy - Revue Canadienne d Ergotherapie, 65*, 248–257.

Wilcock, A. A. (1999). Reflections on doing, being and becoming. *Australian Occupational Therapy Journal, 46*, 1–11.

Wilcock, A. A. (2006). *An occupational perspective of health* (2nd ed.). Slack.

Wilcock, A. A. (2007). Occupation and health: Are they one and the same? *Journal of Occupational Science, 14*(1), 3–8.

Wilcock, A., & Hocking, C. (2015). *An occupational perspective of health* (3rd ed.). Slack.

REFLECTION

1. Explain why co-design is a critical approach for occupational therapists to use when working with individuals and collectives.

2. Provide an overview of six action steps of the Canadian Occupational Therapy Inter-Profession. Explain what this framework is a useful guide for using co-design in occupational therapy practice.

3. Consider you practical experiences. Identify where you observed good examples of occupational therapists co-designing intervention plans with the people and collectives they were working with. Why were these good examples?

4. Consider your practical experiences. Identify where you observed examples of occupational therapists *not* co-designing intervention plans with the people and collectives they were working with. What impact did this have on the plans.

20

EXPLORING SAFETY AND RISK TO PROMOTE OCCUPATIONAL PARTICIPATION

HEATHER MACLEOD ■ MONIA D'AMOURS ■ VÉRONIQUE PROVENCHER

CHAPTER OUTLINE

Overview

Occupational participation in everyday life may inherently involve risks for negative consequences, but it can equally result in positive outcomes. Balancing the benefits and the potential harm in everyday occupations is where occupational therapists can utilise their expertise in co-creating plans that assist people to realise their goals. This can be done by leveraging the skills and resilience people have developed over a lifetime of occupational participation and utilising a systematic approach to risk assessment and management. The physical, social and psychological safety concerns that may occur in everyday life at home are introduced in this chapter. The Living with Risk: Decision Support Approach (LwR:DSA) is then reviewed as a collaborative relationship-focused approach to examine risk. The chapter concludes with how the LwR:DSA can be used as a way to co-create plans that mitigate potential home-safety-related injuries for people who have experienced illness, injury or impairment. While the LwR:DSA is discussed in the specific context of occupational participation of older people and home safety, the LwR:DSA is a broad enough approach that may be helpful to explore safety and risk in the occupational participation of other people and collectives.

KEY POINTS

- Safety at home is multi-faceted.

- Learning and growth require risk.

- What is considered 'safe' or necessary for safety in a situation may vary from different perspectives, including those of the individual, family care partners and occupational therapists.

- The Living with Risk: Decision Support Approach can assist in developing a fuller understanding of potential risks for harms and effective strategies for the prevention of undesirable outcomes.

INTRODUCTION

Occupational therapists are often called on to provide an opinion regarding people's risk for injury at home. This most frequently happens in the context of providing service to older adults who are often seen as less capable of making decisions regarding their health and safety than younger adults. Older people's adult children and occupational therapists may view them as dangerously hindered by sudden or cumulative health issues associated with aging. Older people themselves, on the other hand, may feel that they have successfully dealt with multiple challenges throughout their lives and through this experience have developed the knowledge and skills to safely adapt. This chapter introduces a reflection process that will assist occupational therapists to discuss and co-evaluate concerns regarding physical harms and collaboratively develop plans to promote safety. First, however, it is important to consider essential concepts and issues relevant to safety when supporting older people in their homes.

SAFETY AT HOME

People purposely participate in occupations to fulfil four basic needs: relatedness, competence, autonomy and survival and safety (Maslow, 1967; Ryan & Deci, 2019). Home is one place where these basic needs can be fulfilled, making it an important context for older people and occupational therapists. For instance, home is where relationships exist, where a person can build or maintain skills and abilities and where they can live their life and have choice and control over what they do. In this chapter, the focus is on how a person can fulfil the fourth basic need, survival and maintenance of physical safety at home. This is specifically important to address for older people because they identify that safety is a barrier to remaining at home (Brim et al., 2021). Additionally, not only is safety a basic need but feeling safe at home is also important for a person's wellbeing (Dahlin-Ivanoff et al., 2007; Swedberg et al., 2012). The early co-identification of potential safety concerns by both the older person and the occupational therapist can result in safety measures being put in place to circumvent harmful consequences that could lead to unwelcomed relocation.

Safety is the 'ability to live without unintentional harm or injury' (Douglas et al., 2012, p. 1); therefore, health-related home safety focuses on reducing preventable, unintended harm that could threaten a person's ability to live safely at home (Lau et al., 2007; Lette et al., 2020). Older people identify both objective and subjective meanings of home safety. For instance, the objective physical hazards that might impair the older person's ability to safely move about their home (Brim et al., 2021) and the subjective emotions of feeling safe by being in a familiar place where risks are known (Kivimäki et al., 2020). Home safety can further be broken down into three dimensions: physical, social and psychological (Clarke & Mantle, 2016; Jones, 2016; Kivimäki et al., 2020). Each dimension can either support or threaten home safety.

Three Dimensions of Home Safety

Physical, social and psychological safety are three dimensions of home safety that older people strive for as they aim to remain autonomous and injury free in their homes. Categorising safety is important as it ensures that occupational therapists endorse a comprehensive overview of all types of safety pertaining to community-dwelling older people. Additionally, each dimension of safety can be a focus of occupational therapy interventions aimed at promoting home safety or addressed to avoid negative outcomes (Jones, 2016; Kivimáki et al., 2020). Deconstructing home safety into these three dimensions supports a broadened review of potential safety concerns. It is also important to be aware of concerns that may affect all three dimensions of safety, such as elder abuse. While the dimensions of home safety are described next, it is important to acknowledge that any person-focused safety initiatives must be co-created with the person, as safety is personally defined. For this reason, it is important for occupational therapists to consider how home safety is perceived by the older person as part of the process of co-designing interventions.

Physical Safety

Physical safety pertains to all things related to the person's physical wellbeing within their home (Kivimáki et al., 2020). Older people acknowledge the importance of the physical environment of their home in contributing to home safety (Brim et al., 2021). Older people worry about safety concerns stemming from their physical environment such as fire safety or fall hazards, and safety can be maintained if these hazards are addressed (Brim et al., 2021). For instance, improvements in a home's physical environment (e.g. railings in stairwells, grab bars in the bathroom) and use of technology (e.g. fall monitoring systems) can be introduced to promote a person's physical safety, whereas unaddressed failing health or accidents from home hazards (e.g. falls) could threaten their safety (Kivimäki et al., 2020). By co-identifying potential physical safety concerns and co-creating intervention plans with the older person, occupational therapists can assist in preventing potential physical harm and make it easier for people to live safely at home.

Social Safety

Social safety pertains to older people having relationships with other people on their terms (Bigonnesse et al., 2014). Social safety can be maintained with access to quality relationships but can be threatened when people are socially isolated (Kivimäki et al., 2020). Promoting social safety can have positive impacts on physical and mental wellbeing as social isolation has been linked to significant negative mental and physical health consequences such as increased risk of dementia, cardiovascular disease, depression, elder abuse, increased alcohol consumption and physical inactivity (National Institute on Ageing, 2022). Occupational therapists can help people initiate or maintain contact with others important to them through co-developed plans for social engagement.

Psychological Safety

Psychological safety (also called 'emotional safety') relates to an older person feeling safe and secure in their home (Kivimäki et al., 2020). Furthermore, feelings of enjoyment of living at home are associated with greater safety in the home. However, psychological home safety is threatened when there are feelings of general unhappiness or when the older person fears for their personal safety, such as being taken advantage of (i.e. abuse) (Kivimäki et al., 2020). Not feeling safe has a negative impact on health as it is associated with higher stress and lower health-related quality of life (Milberg et al., 2014). Psychological safety is threatened when one is fearful at home, such as having a fear of falling or burglary or other heightened risks in

a neighbourhood that feels unsafe (Bigonnesse et al., 2014; Cott & Tierney, 2013). Occupational therapists can work with older people to co-identify areas negatively impacting their emotional safety and co-develop ways to improve these.

SAFETY AND RISK: EMBRACING UNCERTAINTY AND BOTH POSITIVE AND NEGATIVE OUTCOMES

Safety is often discussed parallel to the concept of risk as occupational therapists may see risk as almost always negatively impacting a person's life and safety. For instance, occupational therapists may label older people as 'living at risk' when they have concerns about the person's physical, social or psychological safety and make judgements about an older person's cognitive abilities when they suggest changes and the older person does not agree. Safety is a state or outcome, whereas risk is the probability of an outcome, either negative or positive.

Risk is a complex concept with multiple definitions but the common understanding in health care is described in the following similar definitions: '*possibility of loss or injury*' (Merriam-Webster Dictionary, n.d.); '*the possibility of something bad happening*' (Cambridge Dictionary, n.d.) and '*a situation that could be dangerous or have a bad result*' (Oxford Learners Dictionary, n.d.). All these definitions have two concepts in common: the outcome is uncertain (there is no absolute certainty it will happen) and believed to be completely negative. Both concepts make it difficult for occupational therapists to embrace risk taking for two reasons. First, occupational therapists may be uncomfortable working in uncertain situations (Ilgen et al., 2019), and second, the bioethics principles of 'do no harm' (nonmaleficence) and 'do good' (beneficence) make it difficult for occupational therapists to support activities that may lead to negative consequences. However, risk assessment skewed towards negative outcomes can lead to hidden harms for the older person. For example, occupational therapists can promote decisions that lead to unintended physical, emotional and social consequences, such as deconditioning, anxiety and isolation, by recommending that people limit their activities to prevent potential physical injuries (Egan et al., 2017; Rush et al., 2016).

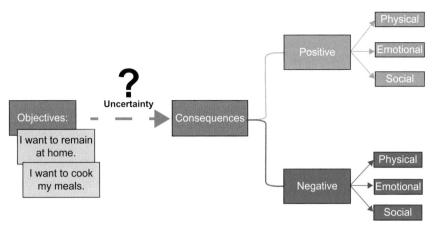

Fig. 20.1 ■ Definition of risk. From Purdy, G. (2010). ISO 31000:2009—setting a new standard for risk management. *Risk Analysis*, *30*(6), 881–892. https://doi.org/10.1111/j.1539-6924.2010.01442.x.

To avoid such unintended outcomes, occupational therapists are better able to support risk taking when they broaden their definition to acknowledge that there are both negative and positive consequences of risk (Titterton, 2005). This is reflected in Purdy's (2010, p. 882) definition stating that 'risk is the effect of uncertainty on objectives where the consequences could vary from loss and detriment to gain and benefit'. This definition is illustrated in Fig. 20.1.

While this broadened definition still embraces the concept of uncertainty, acknowledging the positive aspects of risk taking allows for a more comprehensive understanding of risk. It is important to note that people typically focus on positive outcomes when choosing to do something considered risky. For instance, climbing a ladder to clear off the roof, skydiving for the thrill of the adrenaline, eating fries because they taste good or riding a bike for exercise. That is, people engage in activities with risks because of their benefits. Yet the benefits of risk taking are rarely part of the exploration of risk discussions in healthcare settings. Occupational therapists may primarily focus on the negative consequences of taking risks, without considering the positive benefits. Embracing the concept of therapeutic risk-taking in occupational therapy practice ensures that occupational therapists acknowledge the positive health and wellbeing outcomes that can arise from risk taking (Marsh & Kelly, 2018). For instance, personal growth and resiliency develop by taking risks

and overcoming adversity and challenges (MacLeod et al., 2016). Preventing this opportunity for learning and development goes against people's rights to self-determination, as illustrated by the term dignity of risk. Dignity of risk highlights people's right to make decisions (risky or not) and their right to succeed or fail as a result of these decisions (Ibrahim & Davis, 2013; Woolford et al., 2020).

The need to balance the negative and positive consequences of risk taking with the potential negative and positive consequences is well illustrated in the example provided in the risk enablement practice guidelines from the United Kingdom's Department of Health [UK] (2010, p. 8) '*the risk of getting lost if a person with dementia goes out unaccompanied needs to be set against the possible risks of boredom and frustration from remaining inside*'.

A thorough review of risk requires an understanding of uncertainty. Uncertainty means that the probability of both positive and negative outcomes is unknown. That is, the likelihood of either negative or positive outcomes of a certain action for a given person cannot be accurately predicted as the factors contributing to the harms and benefits are too varied and too difficult to measure (Stevenson et al., 2018). Occupational therapists can manage uncertainty and be more tolerant of decisions they consider illogical when they acknowledge that risk is inherent in all aspects of living and that everyone makes decisions that could be considered risky by someone else.

RELATIONAL CONSIDERATIONS

In addition to the risk of harm, there are also relational factors that influence decision making. For instance, when there is a dissonance between perceptions of risk and the value of maintenance of autonomy, there can be an impact on relationships between older persons and their care partners (Anderson et al., 2022). This can result in the need to negotiate new boundaries due to changing power dynamics between child and parent (Anderson et al., 2022). It might be necessary to have difficult conversations regarding how much care an adult child is able to provide. Additionally, goals of care may often differ between the older person, their care partner and the occupational therapist when there are safety concerns (Kuluski et al., 2013). Again, difficult dialogues regarding acceptance of self-determination may need to occur.

Additionally, when older adults are at risk of adverse outcomes, the tension between supporting autonomy and preventing harm can cause moral distress and anxiety for the occupational therapist (Atwal et al., 2012). Occupational therapists may also worry that failure to convince people to accept recommendations could result in legal retributions (Egan et al., 2017). In an attempt to resolve their moral distress and fear, occupational therapists may engage in decision making that is not person-centred. They may push older adults to accept relocation or unwanted or unaffordable services through subtle or overt means (Durocher et al., 2015). Engaging in a collaborative relationship-focused approach and implementing a broadened risk assessment and management process can ensure that the positive outcomes for the older person are prioritised.

A COLLABORATIVE RELATIONSHIP-FOCUSED APPROACH TO EXAMINING RISK

Being collaborative, risk tolerant and systematic can result in a more balanced and broadened approach to risk assessment and management. Risk-tolerant approaches are grounded in person-centered, rights-based ideologies and are a result of significant knowledge of the individual (Stevenson et al., 2018). These important concepts are key features to collaborative relationship-focused occupational therapy (Restall & Egan, 2022) (refer to Chapter 12). More specifically, they form the foundation of *the Living with Risk: Decision Support Approach* (LwR:DSA: https://lwrdsa-viv-reaveclesrisques.recherche.usherbrooke.ca/#).

The LwR:DSA (Fig. 20.2) is a four-step approach that systematically guides a holistic and comprehensive risk assessment and management process in the clinical context of home-related safety concerns (MacLeod et al., 2023). It improves clinical thinking, decision making and communication by engaging the older person and their care partner in a balanced and broadened approach to the exploration of safety concerns. It is helpful to use the LwR:DSA when the clinical situation is complex and when there are differences of opinion about the treatment plan or recommendations. The LwR:DSA guides the occupational therapist through four key steps within the risk assessment and management process. These steps are discussed below. While the LwR:DSA was developed based on home-related safety concerns and older people, this approach is generic enough that it may be helpful for risk and safety concerns related to the occupational participation of other people and collectives.

Step 1a: What Is the Client at Risk of?

What Are the Safety Concerns?

Starting the risk assessment process by clearly identifying the concern ensures that everyone is beginning the process on the same page. Examples of concerns that threaten a person's physical, social or psychological safety are multiple. For instance, physical safety concerns could include falls, medication mismanagement, wayfinding problems, decreased house maintenance, decreased health maintenance, physical abuse or malnourishment. Social safety concerns could be emotional abuse or social isolation. Psychological safety concerns could encompass the risk of suicide, fear of falling, a fear of personal safety within their neighbourhood or feeling overprotected or constrained. It is recommended to list all the main significant safety concerns and work through all steps separately for each concern, starting with the most concerning.

The safety concern is further understood by identifying the contexts in which the concern occurs, the potential causes and all the possible positive and negative consequences (Fig. 20.3). Acknowledging these

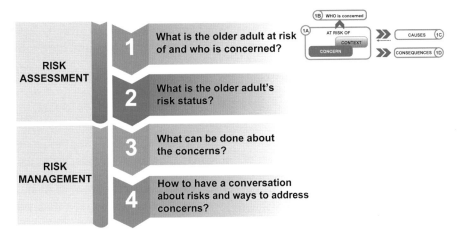

Fig. 20.2 ■ The Living with Risk: Decision Support Approach (LwR:DSA).

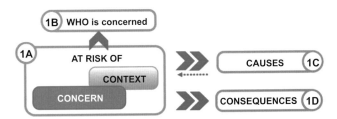

Fig. 20.3 ■ Step 1 of the Living with Risk: Decision Support Approach (LwR:DSA).

three aspects (context, causes and consequences) facilitates a comprehensive understanding of all possible factors related to the safety concern. Once the concern has been identified, it is helpful to determine if it is a new and different concern or whether it has been a concern in the past that has become heightened. If this concern has been identified and addressed before, it is important to consider what new factors led to its re-emergence.

In What Contexts Does the Concern Occur?

Many safety concerns occur in specific contexts. It is helpful to understand the context in which the concern is occurring as this information can lead to specific ways to mitigate risk. Are there activity-specific, temporal, or spatial triggers? Are they related to changes in the person's physical environment or social support (formal or informal)? For instance, in the case of falls, do falls only occur when getting dressed (activity) or

when the person is getting up in the middle of the night to urinate (temporal) or when walking outside on uneven pavement (spatial)? Understanding the type of contributing contextual factors for the safety concern helps point to very different potential solutions. For example, an occupational therapists could collaboratively problem-solve solutions with the person receiving occupational therapy services; the solutions may include sitting down while getting dressed, decreasing evening fluid intake or using a mobility aid when walking outside on uneven pavement.

What Are the Causes?

If the identified concern is new or changed, then the potential causes could be related to changes in the person's physical, medical, cognitive or mental health. For instance, for falling, is the cause related to the person's poor balance caused by a recent stroke (physical health), particular medications or combinations of medications, declining vision, or peripheral neuropathy caused by diabetes (medical), changes in the person's short-term memory impacting on remembering to use a mobility aid (cognitive health), or new onset of apathy from low mood (mental health)? Understanding all the possible causes of the concern and to what extent they could be changed or modified can assist with the collaborative problem-solving process.

It is important to acknowledge that there are also system-related causes that increase a person's risk for negative outcomes. For instance, equipment costs and eligibility, wait lists, service costs, or rigidness of service rules can all impact home safety (Macdonald et al., 2013; Warren, 2016). Changes to system-level factors are difficult and generally can only be addressed through group actions. It is important for occupational therapists to work together to advocate for changes in their own organisations' policies that increase unnecessary risk.

What Are the Consequences?

Once the specific safety concern, the context(s) in which it occurs and the possible causal factors are identified, the last consideration for a fulsome understanding is to acknowledge the potential health and life-related consequences of taking the risk. While the occupational therapist might have a solid understanding of the potential negative consequences of the concern, it is only the person themselves who fully appreciates the positive consequences. In this way, the LwR:DSA requires a collaborative, shared decision-making process with the older person.

Step 1b: Who Is Concerned?

While determining aspects of the safety concern, its context, causes and consequences, it is also important to identify who is concerned. Occupational therapists, other healthcare providers, older people, and their care partners may all perceive the concern differently due to the multiple meanings of risk (Clarke et al., 2011; Stevenson et al., 2018). These multiple meanings can often lead to conflicting perspectives (Stevenson, et al., 2018). The goal of this step is to understand and elicit how everyone views the concern. This can help work through disagreements and clarify who else needs to be involved in the co-creation of plans. It is important to note that, even within a group, people may

differ in their beliefs and understanding about risk. For instance, each healthcare provider may define risk differently dependent on where they work, years of experience and beliefs about risk (MacLeod & Stadnyk, 2015).

Older People's Perspectives on Risk

Older people rarely identify as being at risk, as they are making decisions that are typically in line with their values, beliefs, goals, preferences, personal identity or activities that are important to them (Bedin et al., 2020; Stevenson et al., 2019). Furthermore, older people are often more concerned about maintaining their autonomy rather than focusing on risks (Stevenson et al., 2019). Additionally, older people identify risk, health and autonomy as more important than safety and supervision (Huby et al., 2004; MacCourt & Tuokko, 2010).

Older people's conceptualisations of risk and safety at home are tied to their personal meaning of home and the positive consequences of remaining at home. To support an individual's occupational participation at home, it is not only important to understand the context of home (type of home and living arrangements); it is imperative that the occupational therapist understands the meaning of home to this individual.

Meaning of Home

Home has multiple meanings to people. For instance, home is a place of identity, where the person feels known, where they recognise themselves and where they feel seen by others (Saarnio et al., 2018). Home is a place of belonging where one is connected to people (Board & McCormack, 2018; Saarnio et al., 2018), pets, places, cherished possessions, symbols and values (Molony, 2010). Home is a place where a person can be autonomous and exert choice and control (Board & McCormack, 2018; Molony, 2010) and a place where they engage in purposeful and meaningful activities supporting feelings of competency. Home may also be a place of refuge and comfort (Molony, 2010) full of olfactory, auditory, tactile and visual sensory stimuli (Board & McCormack, 2018). As home can contribute to so many different aspects of a person, it is not surprising that people are attached to their homes. As such, attachment to place combines social, environmental, functional, emotional and psychological meanings of home (Butcher & Breheny, 2016). Furthermore, this attachment could be related further to the person's neighbourhood (Stones & Gullifer, 2016). Part of the exploration of the context of home is listening for which aspects of the home are important to the person and what factors drive the person's attachment to their home. This information is crucial so that this can either be supported in the current home environment or recreated in a new home environment if the person moves.

Benefits of Home

Living at home is not only a preference for most older persons, but it has tangible health benefits. For instance, quality of life is higher among older people who live and are active in their community compared to individuals living in long-term care facilities (Castillo et al., 2020). Additionally, older people who live at home experience other benefits such as increased autonomy, wellbeing (Stones & Gullifer, 2016), belonging (Wiles et al., 2012) and decreased health costs (U.S. Department of Housing and Urban Development, 2020). Living in a familiar home environment also contributes to positive experiences in later life (Van Dijk et al., 2015). While the many benefits of aging at home have been described, there are also numerous internal and external factors that facilitate or restrict safety at home (Benefield & Holtzclaw, 2014).

Importantly, each occupational therapist must reflect on their own values and beliefs about older people and risk to ensure that these are not keeping them from co-creating possibilities for occupational participation. For instance, how does the appearance of a home affect the occupational therapist's beliefs about a person's ability to manage risk? How do relative wealth and education influence the occupational therapist's feelings about an older person's judgment about risk? While working with a person who has often been inadequately housed for much of their lives, is the occupational therapist more likely to question their ability to collaboratively develop risk management strategies?

Occupational Therapists and Other Healthcare Providers' Perspectives on Risk

Occupational therapists and other healthcare providers' meaning and understanding of risk tend to be shaped by their medical knowledge and prior experience (Stevenson et al., 2018). When clinical situations are considered risky, healthcare providers tend to be risk averse (Ibrahim & Davis, 2013) due to a focus on the negative physical consequences (Titterton, 2005) and concerns regarding potential extreme harms (Felton et al., 2017). Healthcare providers tend to overestimate risk (Marsh & Kelly, 2018), focus on potential future rather than immediate impacts (Cott & Tierney, 2013) and act paternalistically (Felton et al., 2017). These protectionist approaches may be influenced by perceived legal requirements and a fear of litigation should something go wrong (Stevenson et al., 2018). Healthcare providers have a high alertness to risk in their practice resulting in the prioritisation of the reduction of physical risk (Woolford et al., 2020) and a tendency to recommend avoiding activities rather than promoting active living (Egan et al., 2017; Rush et al., 2016). In the context of discharge planning, healthcare providers tend to prioritise physical safety over client concerns (Durocher, 2015).

Additionally, individual healthcare providers have different understandings and tolerances for risk (MacLeod & Stadnyk, 2015). Therefore, healthcare providers need to ensure clear communication with other healthcare providers about what they feel the person is at risk of. It is equally important for occupational therapists to reflect on their beliefs about risk and whether these help or hinder safety. For instance, some occupational therapists may assume that all people with cognitive impairment are unable to evaluate risk, but this is not true. Some healthcare providers may privilege their own judgment based on professional knowledge over the lived experience of the older person (Dickins et al., 2018); however, the person may have coped all their life with similar risks. These examples highlight how a risk assessment needs to be individualised for the occupational therapist to support collaborative relationship-focused occupational therapy.

A collaborative relationship with the older person also requires the occupational therapist to consider their position of power in the therapeutic relationship, especially when addressing safety concerns. For instance, the occupational therapist needs to understand how their recommendations might overtly or covertly influence or possibly coerce a person to accept unwanted recommendations.

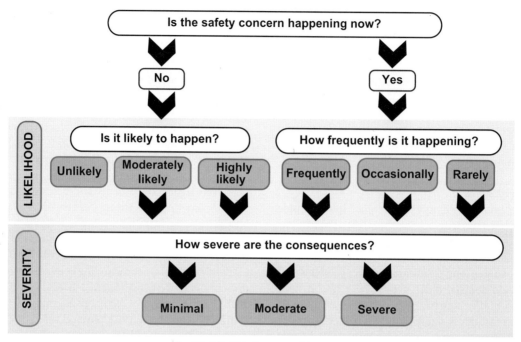

Fig. 20.4 ■ Risk Status Decision Tree.

Step 2: What Is the Client's Potential Physical Risk Status?

Once the concern has been ascertained and clarified and the people who are concerned identified, the next step is to determine the level of risk. This helps prevent the occupational therapist from either underestimating or overestimating the concern. Occupational therapists describe low risk as being safe or tolerable risk versus a higher risk situation may be suggestive of an unsafe situation. The occupational therapist considers the likelihood of the concern occurring and the severity of the consequences to determine if this is a low, medium or high potential risk by first asking if the safety concern is occurring now (Fig. 20.4). If the concern is happening now, then it is important to determine if the frequency is rare (low risk), occasional (medium risk) or frequent (high risk). If the safety concern is not occurring now, the occupational therapist determines how likely it is that the safety concern would happen. If it is unlikely to happen, then the risk is considered low and no further action is needed. If the older person has risk factors or elements that make it possible that the safety concern would happen. this would be considered moderately likely (medium risk). Lastly, if the safety

concern is considered highly likely to occur, then this would be considered high risk. For all situations but the unlikely to occur, the occupational therapist would determine how severe the consequences would be. The consequences may be minimal (low risk), moderate (medium risk) or severe (high risk).

The occupational therapist then puts the likelihood and severity rating into the risk status matrix (Fig. 20.5) to determine the overall risk status. For medium- and high-risk situations, additional factors should be considered as they could either heighten or lower the level of risk. First, the occupational therapist considers if the immediacy of the consequences either raises or diminishes the level of risk. For instance, it takes time for the consequences of malnourishment to occur (lower risk) versus the more immediate consequences of falls or fires (higher risk). Second, a person who is capable of making their healthcare decisions related to the safety concern needs to have their decisions respected. Third, a person can lower the level of risk by having reliable and consistent support in place. Last, when multiple safety concerns are occurring, an occupational therapist may suggest that the situation might be a high level of risk.

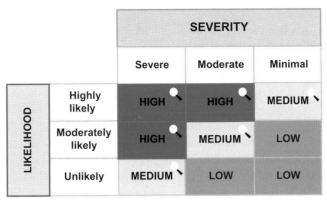

Fig. 20.5 ■ Risk Status Matrix.

Establishing the risk status helps prioritise safety concerns as occupational therapists focus on investing time in addressing the concerns that correspond to a medium (yellow) or high (red) level of risk. In prioritising concerns, it is also helpful to consider the likelihood of harm occurring against the likelihood that the intervention could negatively affect quality of life (Clarke & Mantle, 2016). Understanding the risk status also helps the occupational therapist focus the cocreation of plans that could reduce risk levels.

Step 3: What Can Be Done About the Concerns?

The focus of Step 3 of the LwR:DSA is to consider the factors elicited in Step 1 and 2 to generate ways to mitigate the risk of harm. This step focuses on codesigning priorities, goals, outcomes and plans (refer to Chapter 19). Co-design and shared decision making are imperative for the risk assessment and management process to ensure that the person's perspective and priorities are taken into consideration and the developed plans are appropriate, useful and sustainable (Leape et al., 2009; Martini et al., 2022). Co-creation also ensures that the plans leverage the person's strengths. This step focuses on potential recommendations that can (1) prevent or minimise the frequency of the concern, (2) adapt or modify the context, (3) address, optimise and adapt the causes of the concern, (4) minimise the negative consequences and increase the positive consequences and (5) reduce the overall level of risk.

The intervention plan must be co-created with the person so that it is individualised, person-centered, focused on the person's goals and in line with their values, preferences and what matters most to them. It is the older adult who gets to define what are the acceptable and unacceptable risks for themselves (Egan et al., 2017). It is also important at this step to acknowledge the positive physical, emotional and social consequences associated with the decisions that the person is making.

After an initial assessment, the occupational therapist would collaboratively consider ways to address the causes of the safety concern. For instance, would the person who is at risk for falls benefit from and be interested in a strength and balance exercise program? How can the person's strengths be leveraged? Are there ways the person's physical environment can be adapted to improve mobility and reduce fall risk? Can the person's social environment be adapted or leveraged to reduce the risk of falls or consequences from falls such as an increase in formal or informal in-home support? Can the activities associated with higher fall risk be adapted in any way? Or are there alternative activities that are less risky for the safety concerns but still meet the psychosocial needs of the individual (i.e., identity) (Lee et al., 2019)? To reduce the negative consequences such as physical injuries, can the person learn to fall in a way that minimises injury; can they learn to stand up from a fall? Would the person benefit from an emergency alert button to summon help?

It is also important for the occupational therapist to challenge their assumptions that may be limiting the co-creation of intervention plans that support occupational participation in the context of home safety concerns. For instance, do they believe that risk is an acceptable part of everyday life when pursuing engagement in meaningful activity (Dickens et al., 2018)? Do they believe that risk is necessary for quality of life and should be embraced or mitigated rather than avoided (Clarke & Mantle, 2016)? Do they believe that older people have strengths that can be leveraged rather than weaknesses that they need to be protected from (Clarke & Mantle, 2016; Egan et al., 2017)? Do they believe that risk can lead to new opportunities rather than only negative harm (Egan et al., 2017)? Do they focus on protecting older people from harm to reduce their own anxiety (Woolford et al., 2020)?

Step 4: Ways to Have a Conversation About Risks and Address Concerns.

It is important to support intentional and productive conversations between the person, care partners (where present) and the occupational therapist about risks and ways to address concerns. The occupational therapist needs to support the older adult's priorities and focus on what matters most for the person. When there are differences of opinion, the occupational therapist should initiate and support discussions in which people can speak openly about the difficult topic of risk (Rush et al., 2016).

The occupational therapist can create a safe space to have these conversations. Where the person is capable of making decisions related to their health care, the occupational therapist must accept these decisions. Older persons have asked that quality of life be prioritised over safety, that healthcare providers focus on what can be done not on what cannot be done, involve them in decision making and provide rationales for impressions and decisions (MacLeod et al., 2023). Framing conversations about risk around abilities and strengths rather than losses helps ensure that older people do not feel the need to hide or minimise risk and that they feel comfortable engaging in fulsome discussions about safety concerns (Rush et al., 2016).

A key outcome for risk communication is to focus on reaching a shared understanding rather than a shared agreement (Department of Health [UK], 2010). Additionally, it is important to provide time for the person and the care partners to process the information, make choices and adapt to the changes requested. This is important as typically these conversations occur during a time of crisis such as changes in health or functional skills, changes in behaviour or a situation,

changes in tolerability, loss of support or an accumulation of risk factors (Stevenson et al., 2018).

Additional Interventions

Occupational therapists can also support home safety by intervening at both the organisation (meso) or community (macro) levels. For instance, at the meso level, the occupational therapist can review their organisation's or profession's culture and policies that are creating a risk-averse environment and advocate for changes that acknowledge and support the benefits of risk taking (Clarke et al., 2011).

As older people's abilities to safely live in their homes are influenced by policies, occupational therapists can lead changes at the meso level (Means, 2007). Occupational therapists can advocate for supportive home and community care policies and services. They can lend their expertise to community groups (i.e. Councils on Aging) to support their advocacy for better systems and policies that promote safe aging in place. They can apply their occupational lens within other systems to promote home safety for all. For instance, influencing future building codes, architecture and legislation, working with emergency support services or volunteering with local business improvement associations to ensure that local businesses meet the needs of older persons. Community organisations are well positioned to help build a safety net to support quality of life, while people are aging in place.

Policies (meso context) determine many elements of the macro context. Both are influenced by the micro context, that is implicit values and beliefs. Ageism and neoliberalism are prominent features of many Western societies. These systems of belief lead to policies that disregard the needs of older adults and deny societal responsibility for policies and interventions that help older people live satisfying lives in the community or in care settings. Occupational therapists can help people move towards a less ageist and individualistic society by working with others interested in questioning these values and beliefs.

CONCLUSION

Supporting occupational participation in the home often triggers a conversation about safety and risk of harm after people experience illness, injuries or impairment. Three dimensions of home safety (physical, cognitive and psychological) can be leveraged to support safety or remove threats to safety. It is important to note that risk is inherent in everyday living and that interfering with this right is ageist and paternalistic and may itself lead to harm. Generally, older people want to remain at home even if their health changes (Canadian Mortgage and Housing Corporation, 2008), and they have asked that occupational therapists and other healthcare providers focus on quality of life and on what can be done to enable them to remain at home even when there are safety concerns (MacLeod et al., 2023). Risk has both positive and negative consequences. Acknowledging the positive consequences during a risk assessment recognises that personal growth and the development of resiliency can occur from risk taking.

The Living with Risk: Decision Support Approach (LwR:DSA) was reviewed as a tool to support a broadened and balanced process of risk assessment and management. The LwR:DSA's four steps guide the occupational therapist through a systematic examination of safety concerns to facilitate a thorough discussion with the older person leading to co-creating plans for safe and satisfying occupational participation in the home environment. While the use of the LwR:DSA was demonstrated in the context of older people's occupational participation in their home environment, the LwR:DSA is currently used in other contexts (long-term care) and with other healthcare providers (physiotherapists, nurses, physicians, social workers). The LwR:DSA is a broad enough approach that may be helpful to explore safety and risk in the occupational participation of other people and collectives.

Occupational therapy's collaborative relationship-focused approach that focuses on occupational possibilities aligns well with a broadened and balanced approach to risk assessment and management when safety concerns may be a barrier to living safely at home.

REFERENCES

Anderson, H., Stocker, R., Russell, S., Robinson, L., Hanratty, B., Robinson, L., & Adamson, J. (2022). Identity construction in the very old: A qualitative narrative study. *PLoS One, 17*(12), e0279098. https://doi.org/10.1371/journal.pone.0279098.

Atwal, A., McIntyre, A., & Wiggett, C. (2012). Risks with older adults in acute care settings: UK occupational therapists' and physiotherapists' perceptions of risks associated with discharge and professional practice. *Scandinavian Journal of Caring Sciences, 26*(2), 381–393. https://doi.org/10.1111/j.1471-6712.2011.00946.x.

Bedin, M. G., Kuhne, N., & Droz Mendelzweig, M. (2020). Volition to risk taking in the ordinary activities of daily life of older people living at home alone. A study using explicitation interviews. *Health, Risk & Society, 22*(7–8), 421–436. https://doi.org/10.1080/13698575.2020.1861223.

Benefield, L. E., & Holtzclaw, B. J. (2014). Aging in place: Merging desire with reality. *The Nursing Clinics of North America, 49*(2), 123–131. https://doi.org/10.1016/j.cnur.2014.02.001.

Bigonnesse, C., Beaulieu, M., & Garon, S. (2014). Meaning of home in later life as a concept to understand older adults' housing needs: Results from the 7 age-friendly cities pilot project in Québec. *Journal of Housing for the Elderly, 28*(4), 357–382.

Board, M., & McCormack, B. (2018). Exploring the meaning of home and its implications for the care of older people. *Journal of Clinical Nursing, 27*(15–16), 3070–3080. https://doi.org/10.1111/jocn.14495.

Brim, B., Fromhold, S., & Blaney, S. (2021). Older adults' self-reported barriers to aging in place. *Journal of Applied Gerontology, 40*(12), 1678–1686. https://doi.org/10.1177/0733464820988800.

Butcher, E., & Breheny, M. (2016). Dependence on place: A source of autonomy in later life for older Māori. *Journal of Aging Studies, 37*, 48–58. https://doi.org/10.1016/j.jaging.2016.02.004.

Cambridge Dictionary. (n.d.). The definition of risk. Retrieved December 11, 2022, from https://dictionary.cambridge.org/us/dictionary/english/risk.

Canadian Mortgage and Housing Corporation. (2008). *Impacts of the aging of the Canadian population on housing and communities.* CMHC.

Castillo, D., Trevino, L., Suarez, R., Arreola-Castaneda, G., Fierro, C., & Lin, M.-L. (2020). Aging in place: Measuring quality of life of the aging population. *The American Journal of Occupational Therapy, 74*(4_Supplement_1), 7411505098p1. https://doi.org/10.5014/ajot.2020.74S1-PO1610.

Clarke, C., & Mantle, R. (2016). Using risk management to promote person-centred dementia care. *Nursing Standard, 30*(28), 41–46.

Clarke, C., Wilcockson, J., Gibb, C. E., Keady, J., Wilkinson, H., & Luce, A. (2011). Reframing risk management in dementia care through collaborative learning. *Health & Social Care in the Community, 19*(1), 23–32.

Cott, C. A., & Tierney, M. C. (2013). Acceptable and unacceptable risk: Balancing everyday risk by family members of older cognitively impaired adults who live alone. *Health, Risk & Society, 15*(5), 402–415.

Dahlin-Ivanoff, S., Haak, M., Fänge, A., & Iwarsson, S. (2007). The multiple meaning of home as experienced by very old Swedish people. *Scandinavian Journal of Occupational Therapy, 14*(1), 25–32. https://doi.org/10.1080/11038120601151714.

Department of Health [UK]. (2010). *'Nothing ventured, nothing gained': Risk guidance for people with dementia.* Department of Health.

Dickins, M., Goeman, D., O'Keefe, F., Iliffe, S., & Pond, D. (2018). Understanding the conceptualisation of risk in the context of community dementia care. *Social Science & Medicine, 208*, 72–79. https://doi.org/10.1016/j.socscimed.2018.05.018.

Douglas, A., Letts, L., Eva, K., & Richardson, J. (2012). Measurement of harm outcomes in older adults after hospital discharge: Reliability and validity. *Journal of Aging Research, 2012*, 150473–150477. https://doi.org/10.1155/2012/150473.

Durocher, E., Kinsella, E. A., Ells, C., & Hunt, M. (2015). Contradictions in client-centred discharge planning: Through the lens of relational autonomy. *Scandinavian Journal of Occupational Therapy, 22*(4), 293–301. https://doi.org/10.3109/11038128.2015.1017531.

Egan, M. Y., Laliberte Rudman, D., Ceci, C., Kessler, D., McGrath, C., Gardner, P., King, J., Lanoix, M., & Malhotra, R. (2017). Seniors, risk and rehabilitation: Broadening our thinking. *Disability and Rehabilitation, 39*(13), 1348–1355. https://doi.org/10.1080/09638288.2016.1192227.

Felton, A., Wright, N., & Stacey, G. (2017). Therapeutic risk-taking: A justifiable choice. *BJPsych Advances, 23*(2), 81–88. https://doi.org/10.1192/apt.bp.115.015701.

Huby, G., Stewart, J., Tierney, A., & Rogers, W. (2004). Planning older people's discharge from acute hospital care: Linking risk management and patient participation in decision-making. *Health. Risk & Society, 6*(2), 115–132. https://doi.org/10.1080/1369857042000219797.

Ibrahim, J. E., & Davis, M.-C. (2013). Impediments to applying the 'dignity of risk' principle in residential aged care services. *Australasian Journal on Ageing, 32*(3), 188–193. https://doi.org/10.1111/ajag.12014.

Ilgen, J. S., Eva, K. W., de Bruin, A., Cook, D. A., & Regehr, G. (2019). Comfort with uncertainty: Reframing our conceptions of how clinicians navigate complex clinical situations. *Advances in Health Sciences Education: Theory and Practice, 24*(4), 797–809. https://doi.org/10.1007/s10459-018-9859-5.

Jones, S. (2016). Alternative perspectives of safety in home delivered health care: A sequential exploratory mixed method study. *Journal of Advanced Nursing, 72*(10), 2536–2546. https://doi.org/10.1111/jan.13006.

Kivimäki, T., Stolt, M., Charalambous, A., & Suhonen, R. (2020). Safety of older people at home: An integrative literature review. *International Journal of Older People Nursing, 15*(1), e12285. https://doi.org/10.1111/opn.12285.

Kuluski, K., Gill, A., Naganathan, G., Upshur, R., Jaakimainen, R. L., & Wodchis, W. P. (2013). A qualitative descriptive study on the alignment of care goals between older persons with multi-morbidities, their family physicians and informal caregivers. *BMC Family Practice, 14*, 133.

Lau, D. T., Scandrett, K. G., Jarzebowski, M., Holman, K., & Emanuel, L. (2007). Health-related safety: A framework to address barriers to aging in place. *The Gerontologist, 47*(6), 830–837. https://doi.org/10.1093/geront/47.6.830.

Leape, L., Berwick, D., Clancy, C., Conway, J., Gluck, P., Guest, J., Lawrence, D., Morath, J., O'Leary, D., O'Neill, P., Pinakiewicz, D., & Isaac, T. (2009). Transforming healthcare: a safety imperative, *Quality and Safety in Health Care 18*(239) 424–428. https://doi.org/10.1136/qshc.2009.036954.

Lee, L., Hillier, L., Lu, S., Martin, S., Pritchard, S., Janzen, J., & Slonim, K. (2019). Person-centered risk assessment framework: Assessing and managing risk in older adults living with dementia.

Neurodegenerative Disease Management, 9(1), 47–57. https://doi.org/10.2217/nmt-2018-0031.

Lette, M., Ambugo, E. A., Hagen, T. P., Nijpels, G., Baan, C. A., & de Bruin, S. R. (2020). Addressing safety risks in integrated care programs for older people living at home: A scoping review. *BMC Geriatr, 20*, 81. https://doi.org/10.1186/s12877-020-1482-7.

MacCourt, P., & Tuokko, H. (2010). Marginal competence, risk assessment, and care decisions: A comparison of values of health care professionals and older adults. *Canadian Journal on Aging/La Revue Canadienne du Vieillissement, 29*(2), 173–183.

Macdonald, M., Lang, A., Storch, J., Stevenson, L., Donaldson, S., Barber, T., & Iaboni, K. (2013). Home care safety markers: A scoping review. *Home Health Care Services Quarterly, 32*(2), 126–148. https://doi.org/10.1080/01621424.2013.783523.

MacLeod, H., & Stadnyk, R. L. (2015). Risk: 'I know it when I see it': How health and social practitioners defined and evaluated living at risk among community-dwelling older adults. *Health, Risk & Society, 17*(1), 46–63. https://doi.org/10.1080/13698575.2014.999749.

MacLeod, H., Veillette, N., Klein, J., Delli-Colli, N., Egan, M., Giroux, D., Kergoat, M. J., Gingrich, S., & Provencher, V. (2023). Shifting the narrative from living at risk to living with risk: Validating and pilot-testing a clinical decision support tool: A mixed methods study. *BMC Geriatr, 23*, 338. https://doi.org/10.1186/s12877-023-04068-w.

MacLeod, S., Musich, S., Hawkins, K., Alsgaard, K., & Wicker, E. R. (2016). The impact of resilience among older adults. *Geriatric Nursing, 37*(4), 266–272.

Marsh, P., & Kelly, L. (2018). Dignity of risk in the community: A review of and reflections on the literature. *Health, Risk & Society, 20*(5–6), 297–311.

Martini, R., Egan, M., & Cantin, N. (2022). *Chapter 7: Promoting occupational participation with individuals and families*. In M. Egan & G. Restall. *Promoting occupational participation: Collaborative relationship-focused occupational therapy*. Ottawa: Canadian Association of Occupational Therapists, 978-1-989900-01-7.

Maslow, A. H. (1967). A theory of metamotivation: The biological rooting of the value-life. *Journal of Humanistic Psychology, 7*(2), 93–127.

Means, R. (2007). Safe as Houses? Ageing in place and vulnerable older people in the UK. *Social Policy & Administration, 41*(1), 65–85. https://doi.org/10.1111/j.1467-9515.2007.00539.x.

Merriam-Webster Dictionary. (n.d.). Definition of risk. Retrieved December 11, 2022, from https://www.merriam-webster.com/dictionary/risk.

Milberg, A., Friedrichsen, M., Jakobsson, M., Nilsson, E.-C., Niskala, B., Olsson, M., Wåhlberg, R., & Krevers, B. (2014). Patients' sense of security during palliative care—What are the influencing factors? *Journal of Pain and Symptom Management, 48*(1), 45–55. https://doi.org/10.1016/j.jpainsymman.2013.08.021.

Molony, S. L. (2010). The meaning of home: a qualitative meta-synthesis. *Research in Gerontological Nursing, 3*(4), 291–307. https://doi.org/10.3928/19404921-20100302-02.

National Institute on Ageing. (2022). *Understanding social isolation and loneliness among older Canadians and how to address it*. National Institute on Ageing, Toronto Metropolitan University.

Oxford Learners Dictionary. (n.d.). The definition of risk. Retrieved December 11, 2022, from https://www.oxfordlearnersdictionaries.com/definition/english/risk_1.

Purdy, G. (2010). ISO 31000:2009—setting a new standard for risk management. *Risk Analysis, 30*(6), 881–892. https://doi.org/10.1111/j.1539-6924.2010.01442.x.

Restall, G., & Egan, M. (2022). Chapter 5: Collaborative relationship-focused occupational therapy. In M. Egan & G. Restall (Eds.), *Promoting occupational participation: Collaborative relationship-focused occupational therapy* (pp. 99–117). Canadian Association of Occupational Therapists.

Rush, K. L., Kjorven, M., & Hole, R. (2016). Older adults' risk practices from hospital to home: A discourse analysis. *The Gerontologist, 56*(3), 494–503. https://doi.org/10.1093/geront/gnu092.

Ryan, R. M., & Deci, E. L. (2019). Brick by brick: The origins, development, and future of self-determination theory. *Advances in Motivation Science, 6*, 111–156.

Saarnio, L., Boström, A., Gustavsson, P., Hedman, R., & Öhlén, J. (2018). Temporally and spatially shaped meanings of at-homeness among people 85 years and over with severe illness. *International Journal of Older People Nursing, 13*(1), e12165. https://doi.org/10.1111/opn.12165.

Stevenson, M., Savage, B., & Taylor, B. J. (2019). Perception and communication of risk in decision making by persons with dementia. *Dementia (London, England), 18*(3), 1108–1127.

Stevenson, M., McDowell, M. E., & Taylor, B. J. (2018). Concepts for communication about risk in dementia care: A review of the literature. *Dementia (London, England), 17*(3), 359–390. https://doi.org/10.1177/1471301216647542.

Stones, D., & Gullifer, J. (2016). 'At home it's just so much easier to be yourself': Older adults' perceptions of ageing in place. *Ageing and Society, 36*(3), 449–481. https://doi.org/10.1017/S0144686X14001214.

Swedberg, L., Chiriac, E. H., Törnkvist, L., & Hylander, I. (2012). Patients in 24-hour home care striving for control and safety. *BMC Nursing, 11*(1), 9. https://doi.org/10.1186/1472-6955-11-9.

Titterton, M. (2005). *Risk and risk taking in health and social welfare.* Jessica Kingsley Publishers.

U.S. Department of Housing and Urban Development. (2020). Measuring the costs and savings of aging in place. Retrieved May 28, 2023, from https://www.huduser.gov/portal/periodicals/em/fall13/highlight2.html.

Van Dijk, H. M., Cramm, J. M., van Exel, J., & Nieboer, A. P. (2015). The ideal neighbourhood for ageing in place as perceived by frail and non-frail community-dwelling older people. *Ageing and Society, 35*(8), 1771–1795. https://doi.org/10.1017/S0144686X14000622.

Warren, M. (2016). Shaping risky choices: Ethics and the effects of organizational decisions. *Healthcare Management Forum, 29*(4), 165–167. https://doi.org/10.1177/0840470416644384.

Wiles, J. L., Leibing, A., Guberman, N., Reeve, J., & Allen, R. E. S. (2012). The meaning of 'Aging in Place' to older people. *The Gerontologist, 52*(3), 357–366. https://doi.org/10.1093/geront/gnr098.

Woolford, M. H., Lacy-Vawdon, C., Bugeja, L., Weller, C., & Ibrahim, J. E. (2020). Applying dignity of risk principles to improve quality of life for vulnerable persons. *International Journal of Geriatric Psychiatry, 35*(1), 122–130. https://doi.org/10.1002/gps.5228.

REFLECTION

1. How does the LwR:DSA directly support the development of satisfying occupational participation of importance to the person?

2. How does the use of the LwR:DSA allow an occupational therapist to appreciate and incorporate the knowledge and strengths of the individual and or family?

3. How does the use of the LwR:DSA create opportunities to address key contextual elements that if addressed would lead to more satisfying occupational participation?

SKILLS AND STRATEGIES TO PROMOTE OCCUPATIONAL PARTICIPATION

21 ADVOCACY

MONICA VILLAÇA GONÇALVES ■ DIEGO EUGÊNIO ROQUETE
GODOY DE ALMEIDA ■ GIOVANNA BARDI

CHAPTER OUTLINE

Overview

The concept of advocacy and its relationship to occupational therapy professional practice are presented in this chapter. Theoretical frameworks about these concepts and real-world examples of how occupational therapists can advocate for and with the different people and collectives they work with, such as those who are experiencing illness, injury or impairment. Advocacy is an important skill and strategy for occupational therapists to use to promote the social and occupational rights of the people with whom they work. There are limitations to advocacy practices, and occupational therapists must be aware of them.

KEY POINTS

- One of the objectives of occupational therapy practice is to foster the social and occupational participation of people and collectives whose participation has been affected.
- Although the literature suggests that advocacy is a traditional role of occupational therapists, definitions are still nonspecific and inconsistent.

- Advocacy refers to speaking up publicly about issues of interest, arguing to support a cause or idea and using communication and persuasive actions to impact policies, positions and programs. Lobbying can be a form of advocacy.
- Advocacy can occur in micro and macro contexts.
- Principles and different technologies and resources can be used by occupational therapists to support advocacy practice.
- Occupational therapists must be aware of the limitations of advocacy practice and continue to seek social transformations for the people and collectives with whom they work.

INTRODUCTION

The populations assisted by occupational therapists – regardless of their area of expertise – are historically vulnerable populations that are having and/or have had their social and occupational rights violated. This may include people with impairments or chronic illnesses, older people and socially vulnerable populations such as homeless people, immigrants, refugees and residents of areas of conflict and environmental disasters, among others.

This violation of rights hinders the occupational participation of people in everyday life. Therefore, one of the objectives of occupational therapy practice is to co-develop interventions that foster the social and occupational participation[1] of people and collectives[2] (Malfitano, 2021; da Silva & Oliver, 2019). When these populations have their rights violated, occupational therapists must advocate with and for them.

CONCEPTS

What is Advocacy?

Advocacy is studied and practised by various disciplines such as law, social work, political science, medicine, nursing and occupational therapy, as well as by not-for-profit organisations. Generally advocacy refers to speaking up publicly about issues that are of interest to oneself or to others (Arnold, 2016).

Although the literature suggests that advocacy is a traditional role of occupational therapists (American Occupational Therapy Association [AOTA], 2020; Stover, 2016), definitions are still nonspecific and inconsistent (Dhillon et al., 2016). According to the 4th edition of the Occupational Therapy Practice Framework: Domain and Process, advocacy involves 'Efforts directed toward promoting occupational justice and empowering clients to seek and obtain resources to support health, well-being and occupational participation' (AOTA, 2020, p. 61). Examples of this focus on advocacy include (AOTA, 2020):

- funding to train a service animal for an individual;
- ensuring there is a suitable meeting space in the community to support transgender young adults;
- contributing to the development of policies to improve transportation for older citizens and

services for people with impairment to support them in their lives and work in the community;
- creating or expanding policies that reduce inequalities in access to health care.

Advocacy can address the needs of both individuals and collectives (Dhillon et al., 2016). A framework for advocacy developed by Hubinette et al. (2017) is presented in Box 21.1.

What Is Lobbying?

Lobbying can be a form of advocacy. Lobbying is practised when an organised group attempts to influence legislation, a political decision or a policy in favour of its interests. Considering the social, economic and cultural inequalities that have an impact on the social and occupational participation of populations with whom occupational therapists work, advocating with policymakers is an efficient way to ensure rights and promote social and occupational justice.

Despite being closely associated with corruption and illegality, lobbying is not necessarily negative or a crime (Willson, 2020). In modern democratic societies, the term refers to representative politics through which it is possible to exert influence in favour of the interests of an institution, sector or group. Negotiating with and trying to influence those in power is part of the political game, as civil society has the right to participate in decision-making processes, and organised movements and actors with social prestige are more likely to gain the attention and support of public agents.

It is worth mentioning that lobbying is regulated in some countries but not in others. In the United States, for example, lobbying is a legal and regulated activity, whereas in Brazil, although not illegal, it is not regulated. The absence of a legal framework opens room for distortions; for example, when advantages are offered to buy support from political agents. On the other hand, professionals and academics lobby 'positively' when they actively engage with government policymakers based on research and records of their practice, participating in a complex environment of legal requirements and institutional policies that are not always comfortable and familiar (Fernandez Lynch et al., 2020). For that reason, there are texts that use other terms to describe this tense work with elected representatives

---

[1]For a more comprehensive discussion on social and occupational participation and its relationship to social and occupational justice, see da Silva & Oliver (2019).

[2]The expression 'individuals and collectives' will be used because we understand that occupational therapy practice occurs in contexts other than the health context and therefore the terms 'patient/client/service user' would not be adequate to exemplify what is presented here.

BOX 21.1
ADVOCACY FRAMEWORK

According to Hubinette et al. (2017), advocacy activities (vertical axis) are divided into two types: agency and activism, whereas advocacy participation (horizontal axis) presents two approaches: shared and directed (Fig. 21.1).

Agency: Activities that involve accessing and browsing the public system, such as providing individuals and collectives with information and education on their rights; making connections to community and territorial resources, promoting complete and co-responsible care; making intersectoral referrals to ensure rights, for example, to supportive housing, school inclusion, social income protection and food. In this sense, advocacy works with the constraints of the system to help gather resources for individuals and collectives.

Activism: Actions aimed at raising awareness of an issue, including scientific-lay knowledge translation; engaging, supporting and mediating community and social issues; intervening in institutional dynamics and local or regional policies. Activism aims to institutionalise persistent economic, political and social change.

Shared advocacy (with): Needs, objectives, strategies and forms of evaluation in a given claim are determined collaboratively with people and groups, that is, advocacy *with* is a participatory process in which there is no role of guardianship or dependency. Occupational therapists should position their expertise 'alongside' the interpretations and perspectives of the individuals and collectives with whom they work, valuing nonscientific knowledge, life experiences,

questions and solutions emerging from the context under analysis.

Directed advocacy (for): Needs are determined from the professional perspective and experience of the occupational therapist or other professionals. This involves representation or expert guidance on an issue, resulting in advocacy *for* individuals and collectives. This type of advocacy is discouraged when the leading role of specialists is disconnected from the guidelines and collective action determined by social movements and other civil organisations. The absence of a real representation, which mobilises the engagement of interested people, can incur paternalism – a strong enemy of deliberative democracy. Thus, to increase the autonomy and participation of individuals and collectives in society, the advocacy process should be within the scope of action of occupational therapists.

Para-advocacy: Routine practices that are an integral part of advocacy (Petri et al., 2020). For example, for people to go to a conference to stand up for their rights, advocates need to prepare for the trip, correspond with organisers and fellow participants, plan interventions, learn about the debate, valued agendas etc. All these practices are carried out routinely, and occupational therapists must be aware of the complexity of the personal and contextual factors required in advocacy when considering people with motor, sensory or cognitive impairments, with mental disorders or even children and young people. It is not just a matter of acquiring skills for political participation but mostly of understanding how everyday occupations have political meanings (Petri et al., 2020).

Self-advocacy: Assertiveness and willingness to represent one's interests. It is about increasing the interest of people and groups from more individual dimensions towards a collective dimension and vice versa. It is assumed that for self-advocacy to occur, people need to be aware of their own needs, desires, potentialities and vulnerabilities so that they can gather essential elements to communicate and make their claims heard (Test et al., 2005). However, the opposite is also a possibility; collectives and social movements can help people become aware of their needs and start advocating for themselves based on what they have learned from their peers.

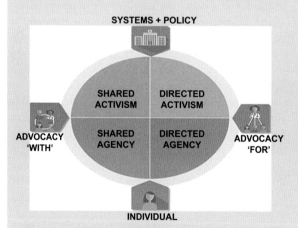

Fig. 21.1 ■ The four quadrants of the University of British Columbia (UBC) Health Advocacy framework. (From Hubinette, M., Dobson, S., Scott, I., & Sherbino, J. (2017). Health advocacy. *Medical Teacher*, 39(2), 128–135. https://doi.org/10.1080/0142159X.2017.1245853.)

Note: It is important to emphasise that this framework is a proposal for a didactic 'division/classification' of the types/modes of advocacy. Nevertheless, there are other possibilities, and in occupational therapy practice, they are often mixed as in the examples presented throughout the text.

and legislators in the defence of the rights of some groups. In Brazil, for instance, it is common to use the term 'technician's political role' (Lopes & Malfitano, 2021).

ADVOCACY PRACTICE PRINCIPLES

There are six principles of advocacy:

1. Base advocacy practice on evidence.

In public policy work, evidence-based advocacy is particularly valuable in comparison with other forms of advocacy, such as that based only on personal values. Evidence refers to knowledge derived from qualitative and quantitative research used to support decision making. Thus scientific evidence would be the starting point in advocacy because it is difficult to support any policy without the support of evidence (Farrer et al., 2015).

Social reality is complex, and it is unlikely that scientific evidence will be conclusive in decision making. However, syntheses of studies suggests some useful strategies (Farrer et al., 2015), such as:

- Use qualitative, interdisciplinary research that employs mixed methods, as they can be especially valuable in advocacy efforts.
- Translate scientific knowledge into language accessible to those on the front line of care. Different types of advocacy messages can accompany the evidence, but they should be strategically adapted for the target population;
- Recognise the leading role of care professionals and civil society in experiences of deprivation and suffering as these actors tend to be particularly persuasive in advocacy efforts. Even so, researchers can be active in advocacy by improving the acceptance of scientific rationality in political processes.

2. Do not establish a guardianship relation – understand the importance of the real participation of people and collectives.

Advocacy practice should be carried out with the people and groups assisted, not for them. In addition to understanding the need to promote social justice, autonomy and emancipation, advocating without the participation of people and collectives can lead to political actions that do not respond to the real demands of the population. For example, Parnell and Wilding (2010) evaluated pedestrian paths and bicycle lane pathways in regional communities in Australia. The paths/lanes built by the authorities were considered of limited benefit to the community as they did not connect to existing paths/lanes or community resources and facilities. As a result, the population was not interested in financial investment in this proposal. According to these authors, this reaction was in part, due to the fact that these paths and lanes were built without community consultation. They argued that because occupational therapists work directly with the everyday activities and occupations of people and groups, they can be present with them and assist with the advocacy process for their real needs in the implementation of policies, such as the construction of highways, roads and paths/lanes.

3. Do not individualise collective issues and work to combine territory and community.

Advocacy cannot be carried out to respond to any personal demands, without an ethical, political or scientific filter. Some people claim unsatisfactory political privileges or responses that are sometimes antidemocratic. A very common example of this in the work of occupational therapists in the Brazilian school context is when problems related to the use of psychoactive substances arise within the school: teachers, students and families usually demand individualised, psychological or even psychiatric therapy for students, unconsciously rejecting other collective strategies involving the community and the school. In this case, demanding greater health care at school would not respond to the complexity of the situation.

Therefore territorial and community approaches should be considered in advocacy practices, as they provide important information about local and collective demands.

4. Advocate in different sectors.

Although the advocacy role within the field of health is more traditional in occupational therapy, it is important to understand that advocacy should also occur in other fields, including in the proposal of policies in other sectors.

In the case of health policies, effective advocacy must include persistent efforts to raise awareness and understanding of the social determinants of health – the social, economic, cultural, ethnic/racial, psychological and behavioural factors that influence the occurrence of health problems and risk factors for the population, such as housing, food, schooling, income, employment and conditions under which people live and work (Farrer et al., 2015; Hubinette et al., 2017). These factors contribute significantly to an individual's and a collective's health outcomes. Thus health advocacy, equity and social determinants of health go hand in hand, unfolding in activities that guarantee access to care, navigation in the system, mobilisation of resources, improvement in living and housing conditions, influence on health policies and changes in the system (Hubinette et al., 2017). Advocacy in the health field plays a central role in promoting equity, given the challenges that unite the worlds of civil society, research and politics.

However, the social and occupational participation of people and groups does not depend solely on their health conditions. People require access to education, leisure, culture, work, transportation, social support networks and information, among other aspects of everyday life; therefore occupational therapists should advocate in a broad range of sectors.

5. Understand advocacy work as a continuous practice.

Claiming rights that are not yet ensured is especially necessary, and advocacy should not be limited to what is already institutionally guaranteed by the government. In many countries and locations, human rights are far from being realised, even if they are present in many of their constitutions. The rights to freedom and individual and collective equality go far beyond palliative or compensatory measures offered by neoliberal policies. For example, in Brazil, the right to the social name of transgender people is recent, as is the right to adoption by same-sex couples and punishment for homophobic crime. This right was only guaranteed by judicial measures after a considerable struggle by socially organised groups regarding this agenda. However, the observed advances proved insufficient to adequately protect the LGBTQIA+

population[3]. Judicial decisions are emblematic, given that the Supreme Court has acted precisely due to the lack of a federal law that deals exclusively with this population, specifically addressing the effects of heterocisnormativity. Even with recent legal and legislative advances, the situation of the LGBTQIA+ community in Brazil is far from ideal. The high number of deaths of these individuals means Brazil has the highest rate of transgender murders in the world (Transgender Europe, 2023). For this reason, social movements are constantly claiming the rights of this population and denouncing violations, as well as running awareness campaigns on the theme.

6. Work towards social justice and advocate for the rights that do not yet exist.

There is no consensus in the literature that advocacy is an action aimed at social justice, although some academics defend the expansion of rights and equity. In this regard, it should be considered that any need must become defensible and legitimate in the light of a debate on justice so that particularisms are not incurred or oppression is perpetuated.

Advocacy should focus on social justice from a two-dimensional view: redistribution and recognition (Fraser, 2002). In the redistribution dimension, injustice reflects the ills of capitalism. The heart of injustice involves income inequality as much as exploitation, deprivation and marginalisation or exclusion from labour markets. Consequently, the radical response to injustice encompasses not only the transfer of income but also the reorganisation of labour division, the transformation of the property ownership structure and the democratisation of decision-making processes. In the recognition dimension, injustice involves cultural domination, stigmatisation and disrespect. Thus the solution is to transform the symbolic order that underlies racism, phobia against the LGBTQIA+ population, ableism, misogyny and other forms of oppression. Therefore critical advocacy should always base its actions on a theoretical framework capable of identifying the cause of injustices and providing truly emancipatory solutions, despite the structural limits imposed on the action.

---

[3]The acronym LGBTQIA+ stands for lesbian, gay, bi+, trans, gender diverse, non-binary, intersex, queer, asexual and aromantic (ace and aro) people (The Equality Project, 2020).

Social justice should be the purpose of advocacy. Equity and social or occupational participation are means to this end, and occupational therapists are important allies in overcoming the relationships of dependence and exploitation that affect individuals and groups on a local and global scale.

INTERVENTION TECHNOLOGIES USED BY OCCUPATIONAL THERAPISTS IN ADVOCACY

Micro and Macro Social Sphere

Advocacy should happen at the intersection between the micro and macro social spheres. Everyday life is indeed a key concept in occupational therapy advocacy (Galheigo, 2003, 2020) because it defines a specific way of analysing social participation based on a social totality. However, it does not mean simply adding fragments of occupations in a holistic approach where everything is important. The analysis of everyday life emphasises social determinants based on social theory. This is because every society has specific organisations and structures that are directly related to certain social intentions, conditioned by class interests. Therefore, the analytical key of everyday life in occupational therapy: (1) prompts an adjustment of analytical scale, focusing on the relationship between the particular and the generic, the micro and the macro social; (2) recognises the primacy of everyday life over historical frameworks; (3) recognises occupations based on a totality (nonadditive whole) because of the relational nature established between individual experience, politics, culture and economy (Almeida, 2020).

In the microsocial sphere, advocacy refers to the defence of social and occupational rights in community and territorial problems.

The community and territorial approaches are based on the concept that the territory is 'a space of possibilities for concrete expressions of life [...] One of the main places of knowledge production regarding life, problems and possibilities for creating solutions' (Malfitano & Bianchi, 2013, p. 564). Therefore the real demands for which one needs to advocate can be identified in community and territorial practices. Territorial and community practices are also a way to avoid advocacy for an individual demand since not every personal demand is a necessity.

The macro social sphere encompasses the role of occupational therapists in the scope of public policies. This action should occur in the different policies that promote greater occupational participation of people in social life, that is, not only in health but also in social assistance, social security, work, education, culture, sports, leisure and urban planning, among others that are configured according to the reality of each country. Studies addressing the involvement and participation of occupational therapists in public policies are evident in the literature, demonstrating the relevance of knowing and working with them.

Considering that occupational therapists are professionals who work in this society seeking means to facilitate the social inclusion of people, participation in public spaces to determine those needs is required. Facing up to social inequality is imperative because it is mainly through public policies that occupational therapists can act in the everyday lives of people to foster social participation and inclusion (Malfitano, 2021, p. 62).

Advocacy Resources, Methods and Strategies Used by Occupational Therapists

Occupational therapists can use a range of resources, methods and strategies when involved in advocacy. These include workshops on activities, dynamics and projects; individual territorial follow-ups; articulation of resources in the social field; dynamisation of the support network; deliberative dialogues; communicative actions; internet activism and communities of practice.

It should be noted that occupational therapists practice *advocacy* to promote autonomy, participation and access to social and occupational rights, as well as occupational participation in desired activities. Occupational therapists should not establish a relationship of authoritarianism or guardianship but one of mediation between individuals and collectives, their occupations and territories. In Brazil, social occupational therapy[4] (refer to Chapter 4) has developed

---

[4]Subarea of occupational therapy that advocates 'social practices that focus on vulnerable populations demand reflection and action based on sociological analyses and should be based outside the illness-health axis to confront the conflicting power dynamics in encounters between biomedical and transformative models of practice'.

some social intervention technologies that can be used in territorial and community advocacy (Lopes et al., 2021). These technologies can also be used in other contexts and with different populations.

Workshops of Activities, Dynamics and Projects

According to Silva (2007), workshops of activities, dynamics and projects are 'spaces consisting of social grouping in which proposals associated with doing and human activities promote shared learning. The active character of the individual and the dynamic character of these relational experiences are highlighted in this process: between participants, space, materials, memory, and sensations' (p. 213).

Workshops of activities, dynamics and projects can be used in different spaces where occupational therapists work, including health services such as hospitals, outpatient clinics, social assistance and community centres, schools and workplaces. They can also be applied to different populations and adapted according to their needs and cultural, social and territorial contexts.

Figs. 21.2 and 21.3 show two different moments of an experience that took place in Brazil: the first was a workshop in which we discussed with young students a change in an education policy that would result in major changes in teaching and schools (called High School Reform). Many of the changes were considered harmful by scholars and experts on the subject but were being publicised through official government communication as beneficial, despite limited consultation. Through participating in the workshops,

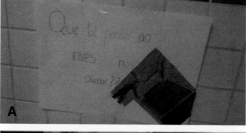

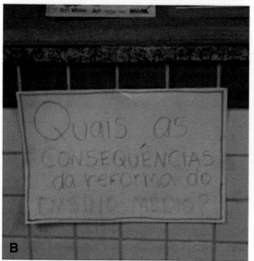

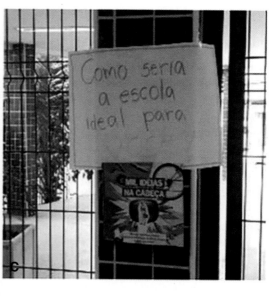

Fig. 21.2 ■ Advocacy in school. Posters spread around the school in an activity about political reform in education, with phrases such as:
(A) 'How about thinking instead of alienating us?'
(B) 'What are the consequences of the High School Reform'
(C) 'What would the ideal school be like for you?'
(From 'Youth Project: Urban Art-Culture Interventions in the Territory'; published with permission.)

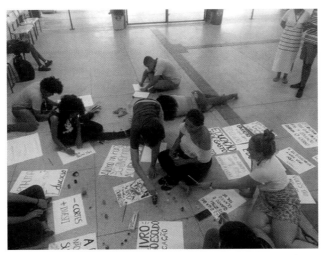

Fig. 21.3 ■ Advocacy in the school context. Description: Young people making posters to take to a demonstration against government budget cuts. (From 'Youth Project: Urban Art-Culture Interventions in the Territory'; published with permission.)

students' opinions were heard, and they made posters to indicate what type of school they wanted (Takeiti et al., 2020).

The second experience happened 2 years later at the same school. The Brazilian Government cut funding for education policies and the students at this school wanted to go to a large demonstration organised by social movements to claim their rights. A workshop was held to enable students to make posters they could take to the street demonstration (Fig. 21.3).

These workshops supported the high school students to express their desires and rights to advocate for themselves, thereby contributing to a collective and social movement to change education policy and funding.

Individual Territorial Follow-Ups

Individual territorial follow-ups are defined as 'intervention strategies that enable real perception of and interaction with the everyday lives and life contexts of people, interconnecting their histories and pathways and their current situations and social networks' (Lopes et al., 2021, p. 173). Individual territorial follow-ups may occur concurrently with other collective interventions but with a focus on individual needs related to the contexts and territories of those being followed up. This is illustrated in Box 21.2.

Articulation of Resources in the Social Field

Articulation of resources in the social field is a strategy for managing practices at different levels of care around common objectives and using available financial, material, relational and affective resources, whether in the micro or macro social spheres. It comprises actions conducted from the individual level from groups and collectives to policy and management levels. Therefore intervention methodologies that are also included in these different levels are needed to enable the identification, negotiation and effective contribution of these resources (Lopes et al., 2021).

Dynamisation of the Support Network

Dynamisation of the support network aims to map, disseminate and consolidate all programs, projects and actions directed to a particular population group and/or its community to foster integration between them, combining the different sectors and intervention levels, facilitating the effectiveness and direction of strategies (Lopes et al., 2021).

An example of using the combination of resources in the social field and dynamisation of the support network is the identification of these actors and resources as shown in Fig. 21.4. This figure shows a meeting with a nongovernment organisation (NGO) that was a partner in a project that sought to ensure the social

---

BOX 21.2
A HISTORY OF AGENCY AND ADVOCACY (WITH) IN OCCUPATIONAL THERAPY PRACTICE

The story of Luiz, a young man aged 21 at the time, who lived in a favela in Brazil, can exemplify the shift in advocacy from working with, to the person making their own decisions and following their own direction. Luiz attended a nongovernmental organisation (NGO) the objective of which was to promote actions to ensure human rights for the population of this favela. A university developed a project in partnership with this NGO focused on young adults. In this project, most of the interventions were in groups, and the resource of workshops on activities, dynamics and projects was used. At the time, the focus was on the theme of everyday urban mobility and the right to the city, and one of the activities conducted was the construction of the 'City of Youth' (Gonçalves & Malfitano, 2020), in which young adults represented on paper, through drawings, cuttings and collages, how they imagined this ideal city.

Luiz commented that he did not have much to say about himself or the city he lived in, so an individual territorial follow-up was started with him in which the places he visited around the city were mapped using a printed map and photographs he took with his cell phone (Gonçalves et al., 2020). From this, he was able to reflect and become aware of his urban mobility around the city, the public spaces which he accessed, and consequently, of his rights. He also reflected on the feeling of belonging to each of these spaces in the city, given the stigma of being a young favela dweller.

This work provided the opportunity for him to understand the factors that affected his urban mobility and his right to the city: access to public higher education through social inclusion policies and participation in social projects linked to the area of culture and cultural production.

Today, Luiz participates and works with projects to support his community, providing visibility to the favela culture, especially among young people. He produces content for virtual social networks showing his everyday life and these projects, takes a political stance and strengthens groups of young people who fight for their rights. It is important to emphasise that it was not only the occupational therapy follow-up in the individual sphere that made advocacy with Luiz possible. Nor was it imposed that he advocated for himself or others. However, occupational therapy provided an opportunity to raise awareness of his reality, apprehend the context and awaken the desire to follow his path. We started *with* Luiz, but today he follows his path by himself.

- Instagram @luizrafs: https://www.instagram.com/luizrafs/
- TikTok @luizrafs: https://www.tiktok.com/@luizrafs

---

and occupational rights of young favela dwellers were not violated (Takeiti & Gonçalves, 2021). At this meeting, spaces and institutions that also offered activities or resources for young adults aiming to promote joint actions between them were mapped. In this mapping, a technique called *Ecomap was used*, an instrument proposed by Ann Hartman in 1975 (Hartman, 1978) that uses a solar diagram to identify social networks and relationships between people, places and activities. The relationships are indicated by symbols (Correia, 2017). Other social organisations and NGOs, schools, health, social assistance, culture devices and public spaces related to the everyday lives of these young people were identified.

After this identification, places were visited, professionals and young adults were engaged in discussions and additional information and contacts were collected. A communication group was created through mobile/cell phone messaging application programs. Monthly meetings were scheduled to discuss what each place could offer the young adults and what demands had not yet been met to collectively seek the missing resources. In this example, the occupational therapist advocated *with* the young adults to enable them to advocate *for* their interests in the future.

Deliberative Dialogues

Deliberate dialogues are a type of group process, which occurs in meetings between people interested in a particular issue. Deliberate dialogues evaluate, complement and/or question key factors that influence the use of research evidence in policymaking. In general, deliberate dialogues are organised around an evidence summary document that will be discussed according to contextual aspects of the problem to find options/answers based on the scientific literature. The document is analysed by guest participants from their experiences and knowledge. At this point, specialists in the field, people who experience the reality and/or policymakers are encouraged to respond to an identified need (Lavis et al., 2014).

Deliberative dialogues can be a useful resource to bridge the gap between scientific knowledge production and advocacy. Engaging civil society alongside

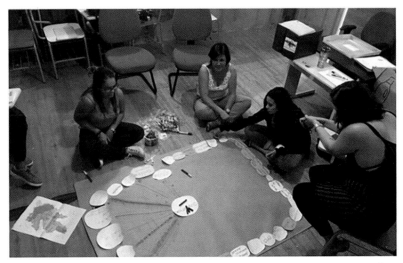

Fig. 21.4 ■ Mapping of the territorial support network. Mapping activity held in a non-governmental organisation in a favela complex in Brazil. (From 'Youth Project: Urban Art-Culture Interventions in the Territory'; published with permission.)

policymakers and researchers reinforces essential values of democracy and citizenship, which may result in greater co-responsibility by the interested parties, qualification of advocated demands and more effective political decisions (Scurr et al., 2022). An example of deliberate dialogues is presented in Box 21.3.

Communicative Actions

Communication is essential for people and groups to have access to information related to political events, health care, research results, their social rights and how to enjoy them. Thus communication is important for advocacy, and it should be accessible to the population. Therefore communicative actions need to be creatively synthesised to be used as an advocacy tool.

Farrer and collaborators (2015) suggested that using summaries of evidence accumulated around a theme holds more promise when advocating for health equity than simply relying on highly focused systematic reviews. This approach addresses the lack of familiarity with scientific language that may be an issue for some parts of the population. Other suggestions to enhance the clarity of messaging in advocacy materials or presentations include:

- presenting simple and brief texts;
- avoiding jargon;
- using precise, powerful language and active verbs;

- balancing stories of common interest with scientific discoveries;
- using facts and figures in a clear accessible way ('1 in 4 women' instead of '25% of women');
- using metaphors for laypeople;
- telling stories, photos and 'good news' is suggested because these materials are more likely to persuade people, groups and policymakers that social and health outcomes can be changed;
- avoiding negative stereotypes when presenting research to avoid blaming individuals for their living conditions and leading to lack of political action.

The instruments accessible to people with impairments should be considered when developing advocacy materials. These instruments may include:

- easy-to-read fonts with contrast or application programs that read the text for people with a visual impairment;
- alternative communication symbols for those who use this communication tool;
- application programs that allow reading for blind people, such as QR codes;
- translating information into sign language for people with hearing impairments.

BOX 21.3
DELIBERATE DIALOGUES

While participating in a community project, occupational therapy academics at a public university encountered several problems faced by health professionals during the COVID-19 pandemic. Among these problems was the difficulty of community health agents (CHA)[1] in creating health education strategies during the peak of the pandemic.

Faced with this situation, occupational therapy students collected information from health managers, physicians, nurses and community residents. The problems identified were related to the ways of carrying out health education in the pandemic context, the working conditions of the CHA and the existence of standards, guiding documents or guiding instruments.

It was a challenging context because the people who assisted at the service resisted the vaccine or did not adopt safety measures such as social distancing. At the same time, the CHA reported exhaustion, fear of contamination and a feeling of impotence at work. Thus the project aimed to understand the work processes of the CHA and find ways to advocate for better working conditions.

The first cycle consisted of holding meetings to accommodate personal and institutional demands to find an initial intervention focus. After that occupational therapy students conducted a review in search of materials addressing health education in the context of the pandemic. Next, a series of deliberate dialogues were conducted to analyse the purpose, types of resources and language used, as well as the quality of knowledge provided to the readers of these materials.

Finally, a report of all the contents produced in the deliberate dialogues was prepared in an attempt to influence health managers and policymakers of the municipality regarding the need to invest in continuing education, emotional support to the CHS and the production of contextualised and effective documents and forms.

---

[1]Community Health Agents are professionals in the Brazilian health system who have the role of integrating Primary Health Care (preventive) services into the community. Their attributions include health prevention and promotion through home or community, individual or collective actions.

Internet Activism

Another important issue in communication in relation to advocacy is the consideration of using virtual social media as a tool. An increasing number of people are connected to the Internet through tablets and smartphones, and many people have profiles on social networks like Facebook, Instagram, X (formerly known as Twitter), TikTok and commonly watch videos on YouTube and listen to podcasts as a form of entertainment and information.

Internet Activism, the use of information and communication technologies to expand forms of virtual interactivity and the composition of activism and social movements, is increasing in popularity. Collectives and movements use the Internet to make calls, activate relationships and communication networks, build new relationships between media and production processes and share information and knowledge (Ferigato et al., 2017). Many social movements use social networks to denounce violations of rights and abuses and tell their own version of a story. Hashtags such as #OccupyWallStreet, #MeToo and #BlackLivesMatter are examples that have reached global projection, but there are others more focused on local territorial demands that are also important.

Occupational therapists can and should be aware of these tools and use them in their advocacy efforts. They can work by assisting the government in communicating with the population, making healthcare information and social rights accessible to all, helping collectives and social movements to use social networks in their favour and by using these tools to publicise the profession for those who, for some reason, have remained unfamiliar with it.

In Brazil, Instagram is commonly used to communicate and engage in advocacy. An Instagram page (@metuia_ufes: https://www.instagram.com/metuia.ufes/) was used in a university project that aimed to enhance social participation through territorial and community actions with socially vulnerable populations. On this page, which complements the actions of researchers involved in the project in the field, a range of content was published such as disclosure of actions carried out by the project, occupational therapy frameworks in accessible and simplified language for laypeople, dissemination of events, information and cultural tips that are of interest to the population involved (Fig. 21.5).

An outcome of this page is that occupational therapy actions have become accessible to professionals and managers of public services. Professionals in education, social assistance and human rights can understand, through the posts, what the goals and interventions of the services are.

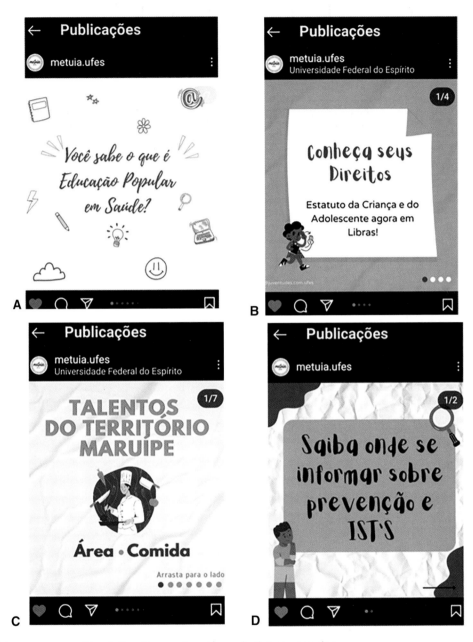

Fig. 21.5 ■ Instagram posts. Description: Four posts on the project's Instagram site:
(A) 'Do you know what Popular Education and Health are?' and presents a carousel of images that inform this approach that can be performed by occupational therapists.
(B) 'Know your Rights! Child and Adolescent Statute in Libras (Brazilian Sign Language)' and the post features a video made by the Government that presents the law that deals with the rights and duties of children and adolescents in Libras.
(C) 'Talents of the Maruípe Territory-Area-Food' and discloses people who work with food, formally or informally, in the neighborhood where the project is carried out as a way to strengthen the local economy and solidarity network.
(D) 'Know where to inform yourself about STD (sexually transmitted diseases)' and gives tips on reliable and accessible information channels on the subject.
(From Instagram @metuia.ufes: https://www.instagram.com/metuia.ufes/)

Communities of Practice

Communities of practice are groups of people who share a concern about or interest in something they are dedicated to, learning and exchanging strategies to qualify their actions as long as they interact regularly (Wenger-Trayner & Wenger-Trayner, 2015). The relational dimensions that support a community of practice are the participants' commitment capable of sustaining mutual engagement; the constant observation of the reality–possibility relationship that leads to joint actions; the shared repertoire, verified using expressions, anecdotes, symbols, jargon and any other elements that indicate integration. An example of a community of practice is presented in Box 21.4.

CONCLUSION

Advocacy – especially that of advocacy with – is a necessary skill and strategy of occupational therapy practices. Advocacy is an action that simultaneously combines political and technical knowledge and is directly linked to what is understood as a need or right of people, groups and populations. Advocacy presupposes a worldview and therefore needs a social theory capable of elucidating the roots of oppression and inequalities that affect the lives of the assisted people. Many topics on this theme require further exploration.

There are six principles that guide advocacy, and it is important for occupational therapists to be familiar with them. They are: (1) base your advocacy practice on evidence; (2) do not establish a guardianship relation – understand the importance of authentic participation of people and collectives; (3) do not individualise collective issues, and work to combine territory and community; (4) advocate in a broad range of sectors; (5) understand advocacy work as a continuous practice; and (6) work towards social justice and advocate also for the rights that do not yet exist.

Professional practice encompasses various occupational therapy resources and technologies that can be used by occupational therapists in advocacy work. These are workshops on activities, dynamics and projects; individual territorial follow-ups; articulation of resources in the social field; dynamisation of the support network; deliberative dialogues, communicative actions; internet activism and community of practices.

BOX 21.4
COMMUNITY OF PRACTICE

A project coordinated by academics from different Brazilian universities created a community of practice to bring together occupational therapists who work in the services of the Unified Social Assistance System (SUAS)[1] to exchange knowledge, strengthen the understanding of their professional role in this sector and disseminate information about their work (Bardi et al., 2023).

In the first cycle of this project, professionals exchanged experiences and knowledge and discussed and identified demands, readings and theories about their work in social assistance. These meetings provided access to theoretical information to support the daily practice of occupational therapists working in the SUAS, making it possible to advocate for the space of professionals in their workplaces (Borges & Bardi, 2022).

In the second cycle of this project, two strategies were implemented: (1) a study group to discuss topics related to occupational therapy professional practice at SUAS and (2) a group to produce and disseminate information about the work of occupational therapists at SUAS. From the information production and dissemination group, a blog (https://to-nosuas.blogspot.com/) and an Instagram page (@to.no.suas: https://www.instagram.com/to.no.suas/) were created to regularly share information about the work of occupational therapists at SUAS (Borges & Bardi, 2022). The two strategies aimed to advocate for the occupational therapy professional role beyond the typical work expected of occupational therapists, providing greater media reach so that other occupational therapists who did not participate in the community of practice could strengthen their practice in the SUAS.

In addition, the community of practice held an online event, broadcast on YouTube, with the participation of representatives of federal and regional entities that act in the regulation of occupational therapy in the country. The debates at this table emphasised the demand for continual professional development of occupational therapists so that they can work in social assistance. The debates also highlighted the need to insert content about working in social assistance in the curricula of undergraduate courses, as well as the need to improve working conditions in policy. This action demonstrates how a group can advocate for their role in the services of the SUAS through political representation.

---

[1]In Brazil, social assistance services are organised by the SUAS system, which is regulated by a public policy.

Advocacy is the first step in the search for change. Occupational therapists are encouraged to develop practices – and develop theories based on them in dialogue with different areas of knowledge – that are revolutionary to build an effectively transformative occupational therapy.

To close this chapter, a quote by Paulo Freire (2011) about utopia is presented:

I never speak of utopia as an impossibility that sometimes works out. I never speak of utopia as a refuge for those who do not act or [as] an unattainable assertion of those who only daydream. On the contrary, I speak of utopia as a fundamental necessity of human beings. It is part of their nature, constructing itself historically and socially. Under normal conditions, men and women cannot do without dreams and without utopias (Freire, 2011, p. 85).

Just like Freire, utopia as a possibility of fulfilling dreams to plan a future based on a critical awareness of the relationships between the individuals and collectives with whom occupational therapists work and the world before the historical-social context (Freire, 1987, 2011). Being aware of the limitations of occupational therapy in advocacy is part of a critical and reflective professional education process that enables the development of actions that seek real social transformations and the construction of other futures and then the desired social justice.

REFERENCES

Almeida, D. E. R. G. (2020). Policy and resistance in the homosexual nightlife. *Cadernos Brasileiros De Terapia Ocupacional, 28*(4), 1251–1267. https://doi.org/10.4322/2526-8910.ctoAO2102

American Association of Occupational Therapy – AOTA. (2020). Occupational therapy practice framework: Domain and process—fourth edition. *The American Journal of Occupational Therapy, 74*(Supplement_2). 7412410010p1–7412410010p87. https://doi.org/10.5014/ajot.2020.74S2001.

Arnold, K. C. (2016). Impact of one training session on improving advocacy, knowledge, and empowerment in medical students. *Education in Medicine Journal, 8*(2), 76–82. https://doi.org/10.5959/eimj.v8i2.412.

Bardi, G., Oliveira, M. L. de, Coelho, F. dos S., Zanoti, L. F., Soares, C. R. S., Malfitano, A. P. S., & Almeida, M. C. de (2023). Community of Practice in Occupational Therapy in the Unified Social Assistance System: Articulating meetings and promoting debates in social occupational therapy. *Cadernos Brasileiros De Terapia Ocupacional, 31*(spe), 1–23, e3389. https://doi.org/10.1590/2526-8910.ctoAO260133891.

Borges, L. S., & Bardi, G. (2022). Produção e divulgação de conteúdos sobre a terapia ocupacional no Sistema Único de Assistência Social. *Scientific Initiation Final Report. Federal University of Espírito Santo [Relatório Final de Iniciação Científica. Universidade Federal do Espírito Santo] Vitória* (p. 14).

Correia, R. L. (2017). O ecomapa na prática terapêutica ocupacional: Uma ferramenta para o mapeamento das percepções sobre a participação nas redes sociais de suporte. *Revista Interinstitucional Brasileira de Terapia Ocupacional – REVISBRATO, 1*(1), 67–87. https://doi.org/10.4777/2526-3544.rbto4263.

da Silva, A. C. C., & Oliver, F. C. (2019). Social participation in occupational therapy: What are we talking about? *Brazilian Journal of Occupational Therapy, 27*(4), 858–872. https://doi.org/10.4322/2526-8910.ctoAR1883.

Dhillon, S., Wilkins, S., Stewart, D., & Law, M. (2016). Understanding advocacy in action: A qualitative study. *British Journal of Occupational Therapy, 79*(6), 345–352. https://doi.org/10.1177/0308022615583305.

Farrer, L., Marinetti, C., Cavaco, Y. K., & Costongs, C. (2015). Advocacy for health equity: A synthesis review. *The Milbank Quarterly, 93*(2), 392–437. https://doi.org/10.1111/1468-0009.12112.

Ferigato, S. H., Silva, C. R., & Gozzi, A. P. N. F. (2017). O advendo da cibercultura e das cibercidades e a produção de novas estéticas e a reconfiguração dos processos de inclusão e exclusão social. In G. B. Bertelli & G. Feltran (Eds.), *Vozes à margem: Periferias, estética e política* (pp. 215–231). EDUFSCar.

Fernandez Lynch, H., Bateman-House, A., & Rivera, S. M. (2020). Academic advocacy: Opportunities to influence health and science policy under U.S. lobbying law. *Academic Medicine, 95*(1), 44–51. https://doi.org/10.1097/ACM.0000000000003037.

Fraser, N. (2002). A justiça social na globalização: Redistribuição, reconhecimento e participação. *Revista Crítica de Ciências Sociais, 63*, 7–20.

Freire, P. (1987). *Pedagogia do oprimido* (17a). Paz e Terra. http://www.dhnet.org.br/direitos/militantes/paulofreire/paulo_freire_pedagogia_do_oprimido.pdf.

Freire, P. (2011). *Pedagogia dos sonhos possíveis*. In A. M. A. Freire (Ed.). UNESP.

Galheigo, S. M. (2003). O cotidiano na terapia ocupacional: Cultura, subjetividade e contexto histórico-social. *Revista de Terapia Ocupacional da Universidade de São Paulo, 14*(3), 104–109. http://doi.org/10.11606/issn.2238-6149.v14i3p104-109.

Galheigo, S. M. (2020). Occupational therapy, everyday life and the fabric of life: Theoretical-conceptual contributions for the construction of critical and emancipatory perspectives. *Cadernos Brasileiros de Terapia Ocupacional, 28*(1), 5–25. http://dx.doi.org/10.4322/2526-8910.ctoAO2590.

Gonçalves, M. V., & Malfitano, A. P. S. (2020). Brazilian youth experiencing poverty: Everyday life in the favela. *Journal of Occupational Science, 27*(3), 311–326. https://doi.org/10.1080/14427591.2020.1757495.

Gonçalves, M. V., Bezerra Neto, L. R., & Malfitano, A. P. S. (2020). O cotidiano revelado por imagens da cidade. *Interface – Comunicação, Saúde, Educação, 24*, 1–14. https://doi.org/10.1590/interface.190418.

Hartman, A. (1978). Diagrammatic assessment of family relationships. *Social Casework, 59*, 465–476.

Hubinette, M., Dobson, S., Scott, I., & Sherbino, J. (2017). Health advocacy. *Medical Teacher, 39*(2), 128–135. https://doi.org/10.1080/0142159X.2017.1245853.

Lavis, J. N., Boyko, J. A., & Gauvin, F.-P. (2014). Evaluating deliberative dialogues focussed on healthy public policy. *BMC Public Health, 14*(1), 1287. https://doi.org/10.1186/1471-2458-14-1287.

Lopes, R. E., & Malfitano, A. P. S. (Eds.) (2021). *Social occupational therapy – theoretical and practical designs.* Elsevier. https://shop.elsevier.com/books/social-occupational-therapy/lopes/978-0-323-69549-7.

Lopes, R. E., Malfitano, A. P. S., Silva, C. R., & de O Borba, P. L. (2021). Resources and technologies in social occupational therapy: Actions with Poor Urban Youth. In R. E. Lopes & A. P. S. Malfitano (Eds.), *Social occupational therapy – Theoretical and practical designs* (pp. 169–176). Elsevier.

Malfitano, A. P. S. (2021). Social context and social action: Generalizations and specificities in occupational therapy. In R. E. Lopes & A. P. S. Malfitano (Eds.), *Social occupational therapy- Theoretical and practical designs.* Elsevier.

Malfitano, A. P. S., & Bianchi, P. C. (2013). Terapia ocupacional e atuação em contextos de vulnerabilidade social: Distinções e proximidades entre a área social e o campo de atenção básica em saúde. *Cadernos de Terapia Ocupacional Da UFSCar, 21*(3), 563–574. https://doi.org/10.4322/cto.2013.058.

Parnell, T., & Wilding, C. (2010). Where can an occupation-focussed philosophy take occupational therapy? *Australian Occupational Therapy Journal, 57*(5), 345–348. https://doi.org/10.1111/j.1440-1630.2010.00860.x.

Petri, G., Beadle-Brown, J., & Bradshaw, J. (2020). Redefining self-advocacy: A practice theory-based approach. *Journal of Policy and Practice in Intellectual Disabilities, 17*(3), 207–218. https://doi.org/10.1111/jppi.12343.

Scurr, T., Ganann, R., Sibbald, S. L., Valaitis, R., & Kothari, A. (2022). Evaluating public participation in a deliberative dialogue: A single case study. *International Journal of Health Policy and Management, 11*(11), 2638–2650. https://doi.org/10.34172/ijhpm.2022.6588.

Silva, C. R. (2007). Oficinas. In M. B. Park, R. S. Fernandes, & A. Carnicel (Eds.), *Palavras-chave da educação não formal* (pp. 213–214). Editora Setembro/Centro de Memória da Unicamp.

Stover, A. D. (2016). Client-centered advocacy: Every occupational therapy practitioner's responsibility to understand medical necessity. *The American Journal of Occupational Therapy, 70*(5). 7005090010p1–70 05090010p6. https://doi.org/10.5014/ajot.2016.705003.

Takeiti, B. A., & Gonçalves, M. V. (2021). *Juventude(s) e arte-cultura no Complexo do Alemão: Narrativas de uma experiência em extensão* (1st ed.). Brazil Publishing. https://doi.org/10.31012/978-65-5861-732-7.

Takeiti, B. A., Gonçalves, M. V., Macedo, J. C., & Maturano, R. G. (2020). Experiências sensíveis com as juventudes no contexto da escola pública: Um debate sobre a Reforma do Ensino Médio no Rio de Janeiro. *Educação Em Foco, 23*(41), 168–189. https://revista.uemg.br/index.php/educacaoemfoco/article/view/4931/3148.

Test, D. W., Fowler, C. H., Brewer, D. M., & Wood, W. M. (2005). A content and methodological review of self-advocacy intervention studies. *Exceptional Children, 72*(1), 101–125. https://doi.org/10.1177/001440290507200106.

The Equality Project. (2020). *Australian LGBTQIA+ Policy Guide 2020.* https://www.theequalityproject.org.au/policy?gad=1&gcli d=CjwKCAjwvdajBhBEEiwAeMh1UwU_vZN1efizFbOuNkqD-sNk3Shdq9IOFrltmyUz2vDscaSgnOz74lBoCaFcQAvD_BwE.

Transgender Europe. (2023). *Trans murder monitoring update.* https://transrespect.org/en/map/trans-murder-monitoring/?submap=tmm_relative_numbers.

Wenger-Trayner, E., & Wenger-Trayner, B. (2015). Comunidades de práctica: Una breve introducción. *Proyecto Educación y Nuevas Tecnologías–Área Educación, 5.* http://www.pent.org.ar/sites/default/files/institucional/publicaciones/Breve%20introduccio%CC%81n%20 a%20las%20comunidades%20de%20pra%CC%81ctica.pdf.

Willson, P. D. (2020). The importance of lobbying to advance health and science policy. *Academic Medicine, 95*(1), 13–15. https://doi.org/10.1097/ACM.0000000000003036.

REFLECTION

1. Find examples from the text that fit each of the items below regarding the proposition presented for advocacy framework?
   a. Agency
   b. Activism
   c. Advocacy with
   d. Advocacy for
   e. Para-advocacy
   f. Self-advocacy

2. What concerns should an occupational therapist have when identifying advocacy demands?

3. Traditionally occupational therapists work in health services, thus many studies have addressed the relationship between advocacy and health demands; however, several examples of occupational therapy practice in other sectors were presented in this chapter. According to your geographic reality, in which places do you believe you could work as an occupational therapist and advocate with people and/or collectives?

22

EDUCATION

YELIZ PRIOR ■ ALAN MATHEW

Change is the result of all true learning
Leo Buscaglia

CHAPTER OUTLINE

Overview

This chapter highlights the role of education in occupational therapy practice, aiming to facilitate occupational participation for people facing injury, illness or impairment. To achieve this, various educational theories and models are presented, providing a foundation for the development, implementation and assessment of education interventions. While the chapter integrates broader models and theories to enhance education provision in occupational therapy, at its core, a collaborative and relationship-focused approach serves as the foundation for advocating shared decision making,

cultural sensitivity, equity and social justice in practice. Various formats of education interventions, including audio, audio-visual, written, verbal, online and group-based activities, are explored, alongside considerations of health literacy, digital poverty and universal design principles. Additionally, the significance of formal and informal evaluations is stressed to ensure meaningful impact and effectiveness of education interventions. Armed with these insights, occupational therapists can offer high-quality education interventions, ultimately improving health and wellbeing outcomes for individuals.

KEY POINTS

■ Occupational therapy education interventions should be grounded in a collaborative, relationship-focused approach. Building trust and rapport between occupational therapists and learners is crucial for effective learning and growth.

■ Creating a compassionate and empathetic learning environment is essential. This environment fosters a sense of safety, enabling learners to engage fully in the educational process.

■ Education interventions should be carefully tailored to meet the unique goals, preferences and needs of learners. One-size-fits-all approaches are less effective in promoting meaningful outcomes.

■ Occupational therapists should actively involve learners in the decision-making process regarding their education plans. This promotes shared ownership and co-creation of educational goals.

■ Recognising and addressing power and privilege dynamics within the therapeutic relationship is important. Creating an inclusive and equitable learning environment empowers individuals and collectives to actively participate in their own education and decision making, leading to more sustainable outcomes.

INTRODUCTION

The healthcare landscape has experienced significant shifts in recent years, characterised by a strong emphasis on empowering individuals to actively participate in their own care and decision-making processes (Krist et al., 2017; NICE, 2022; Vahdat et al., 2014). This shift reflects a broader recognition of the importance of person-centred care, where people's values, preferences and goals are at the forefront of healthcare delivery (Greene et al., 2012; Waldman & Terzic, 2019). One notable change in the healthcare landscape is the increased focus on prevention through education (The NHS Long Term Plan, 2019; Schiavone & Ferretti, 2021). There is a growing recognition that proactive measures, such as health education and promotion, can help prevent the onset or progression of health conditions through early detection and lifestyle modifications (Parliamentary Under Secretary of State for Public Health and Primary Care, 2019). This preventive approach aims to optimise health and wellbeing by addressing risk factors, promoting self-management education and healthy behaviours and

encouraging individuals to take proactive steps in maintaining their health (Birkeland et al., 2022; Jones et al., 2019; Kuruvilla et al., 2018).

Community-based care has also gained prominence as a key aspect of the healthcare landscape. It recognises that health and wellbeing are influenced by various social determinants and environmental factors within communities (O'Mara-Eves et al., 2015; OHID, 2022). Community-based care involves providing healthcare services, including education interventions, in community settings to ensure accessibility and relevance to the local population (Bonsaksen et al., 2020; Tuntland et al., 2015).

Additionally, self-management has become a central component of healthcare delivery as the number of people living with chronic conditions continue to increase (Dineen-Griffin et al., 2019). Recognising that individuals are experts in their own lives, self-management focuses on equipping individuals with the knowledge, skills and resources to actively manage their health conditions through education, making informed decisions, adhering to treatment plans and engaging in healthy behaviours (Grady & Gough, 2014). These include one-to-one and group self-management education programmes delivered by occupational therapists in both community and hospital settings (refer to Chapter 24).

Furthermore, the growing burden on health and social care and advancements in technology and the digital age have significantly influenced the healthcare landscape. Digital health tools, such as mobile applications, wearable devices and telehealth platforms, have facilitated remote monitoring, self-assessment and virtual interactions between healthcare providers and individuals (Hamilton et al., 2023; Orlando et al., 2021; Prior & Wynn, 2023). These technological advancements have expanded access to healthcare services, improved communication and information sharing and empowered individuals to take an active role in their own care through education interventions delivered via digital platforms (Prior & Wynn, 2023).

In this context, education interventions in occupational therapy play a crucial role in the current healthcare landscape by empowering people, promoting health, self-management, enhancing functional independence, supporting transitions, addressing occupational injustice and adapting to technological advances. By incorporating education intervention into their practice, occupational therapists can equip individuals and collectives with the knowledge, skills and resources to actively participate in their own care, make informed decisions and promote their wellbeing through a collaborative relationship-focused practice (refer to Chapter 12). This is important to foster active occupational participation, encourage shared learning and knowledge exchange and support ongoing evaluation and adaptation.

In this chapter, models and theories relevant to education interventions will be described, an evidence-informed framework for education intervention presented and the integration of considerations related to equity, cultural sensitivity and social justice explored.

EDUCATION INTERVENTIONS IN OCCUPATIONAL THERAPY

While the role of education is relatively clear when it refers to training and practice, there are inconsistencies when education is used as an intervention (Goff et al., 2021). An example of the inconsistency is the use of materials that may not consider a range of factors such as a person's previous understanding of their condition, their social and financial backgrounds or previous levels of school and tertiary education. This may limit accessibility for groups of people who are unable to engage with the education provided (Heng et al., 2020). Education, when considered and delivered appropriately, can lead to a reduction in inequities in health literacy, disparities within social determinants and accessibility and show improvement in self-efficacy, therapeutic relationship and shared decision making (Krist et al., 2017). These benefits have a positive impact on health outcomes, quality of life and cost-effectiveness of services (Vahdat et al., 2014).

In practice, occupational therapists provide education interventions as 'a planned learning experience using a combination of methods such as teaching, counselling and behaviour modification techniques that influence [individual's] knowledge and health behaviour' (Bartlett, 1985, p. 323). These perspectives play a significant role in promoting the overall health and wellbeing of individuals and collectives and their ability to meaningfully engage in occupations.

Education interventions, in this context, refer to purposeful and structured strategies employed by occupational therapists to facilitate the acquisition of knowledge, skills and behaviours. These interventions aim to facilitate knowledge transfer and equip them with the necessary tools required for behaviour change to support self-management of their health condition(s) or injury.

For example, occupational therapists may employ ergonomic approaches in rheumatology (e.g. altered movement patterns and use of proper joint and body mechanics, restructuring activities, work simplification and altering the environment), which aim to reduce pain and fatigue during daily activities, work and leisure (Hammond et al., 2020) to facilitate symptom management. This consists of teaching ergonomic approaches as an education intervention, which must be tailored for individual needs, and the delivery of the intervention must be timed appropriately, that is, to those with less than 6 months' disease duration, minimal hand pain or activity problems, otherwise it may not be beneficial (Freeman et al., 2002). In this context, education intervention would be most beneficial as and when individuals are experiencing pain, particularly in the hands, and fatigue, which is not being adequately controlled by medication (Hammond et al., 2020). If they have little or no pain and fatigue, with few or no activity limitations, they are unlikely to perceive the need to change, and education may be of little value (Hammond et al., 2020). Therefore the emphasis would be on behaviour change and prevention. This can be done by supporting individuals and collectives using a shared decision-making process to make informed decisions, enabling these individuals and collectives to actively participate in their own care to achieve meaningful health and social outcomes (Krist et al., 2017). By providing individuals and collectives with information, guidance and resources, occupational therapists can support them in developing knowledge and skills to enhance their self-management.

THEORIES, MODELS AND FRAMEWORKS TO GUIDE EDUCATION

The use of education interventions should be guided by theories, models and frameworks to provide a foundation for practice, enabling occupational therapists to understand people's needs and design meaningful and effective interventions. These can assist occupational therapists gain insights into a range of factors that need to be considered and tailor education interventions accordingly. Additionally, theories and models support evidence-based practice, ensuring interventions align with established principles of learning and human functioning. They facilitate collaboration and communication among occupational therapists, the people receiving occupational therapy services and healthcare professionals, fostering shared understanding and effective teamwork. Continuously engaging with theories and models promotes professional development, enabling occupational therapists to refine their approaches, adapt to emerging evidence and enhance intervention quality. Overall, theories, models and frameworks provide occupational therapists with a theoretical foundation, optimising their ability to deliver effective and person-centred educational programmes.

Adult Learning Theory (Andragogy)

The idea that adults learn differently from younger people has been well documented. Adult learning is referred to as andragogy, building on the Greek routes of the word 'andra' [translates as the word adult], which makes andragogy the art and science of teaching adults (Knowles, 1980, p. 43). The central premise of adult learning theory/andragogy is that adult learners are self-directed, autonomous individuals who possess unique life experiences and prior knowledge (Knowles, 1980; Knowles et al., 2011; Mews, 2020). This theory highlights that the learning process of adults differs from children, and it is important to incorporate the experiences and knowledge of adult learners into the learning process to make it more relevant and meaningful for them. The theory suggests that adults are motivated to learn when they see the immediate application of knowledge to real-life situations. It emphasises learner-centred approaches, allowing adults to actively participate in setting their learning goals, designing educational activities and evaluating their progress (Knowles at al., 2011). Andragogy relies on adult learning being a product of a continuous process of development and learning that is based on six principles (Machynska & Boiko, 2020). These principles are based on an understanding that education and

learning experiences for those in the adult stage of life are shaped by personal experience, individual roles, self-expectations and ability to apply information to their own personal contexts (Machynska & Boiko, 2020). The six principles of adult learning are:

- Adults need to know why they need to learn something before beginning to learn it.
- Adults need to be actively involved in learning, rather than passive recipients of information, with the goal of empowering learners and encouraging them to become self-directed and responsible for their learning.
- Adults have a problem-centred orientation to learning.
- Adults enter the learning process with prior experience, and it is important that learners' life experiences are acknowledged and utilised throughout the learning process.
- Adults' readiness to learn will affect the outcomes of their learning.
- Adults are most motivated to learn when they see the content as relevant.

While andragogy highlights the significance of learner autonomy and relevance, critics of this learning theory argue that not all adults fit into the self-directed, experience-based model and andragogy lacks a well-evidenced explanatory framework (Rachal, 2002; St. Clair & Käpplinger, 2021). The concept of andragogy may lose its impact when social justice or cultural considerations are overlooked, particularly when compared to more contemporary adult education theories (Grace, 2001; Sandlin, 2005). The absence of a focus on these critical issues can render andragogy less effective or less relevant in addressing the diverse needs of adult learners in the contemporary educational landscape (St. Clair & Käpplinger, 2021).

Health Belief Model

The Health Belief Model (HBM) posits that the likelihood of engaging in a particular health behaviour depends on how an individual perceives the severity of the disease, their susceptibility to it and the perceived advantages and obstacles associated with that behaviour (Rosenstock, 1974).

This includes 'cues to action' which are triggers or stimuli that prompt individuals to take action towards a particular health behaviour (Janz & Becker, 1984; Meilier et al., 1997). These cues can be internal, such as experiencing symptoms or feeling a sense of urgency, or external, like receiving advice from a healthcare provider or seeing a health-related advertisement. Cues to action play a crucial role in motivating individuals to change their behaviour or take preventive measures in response to perceived health threats. They act as catalysts that initiate the decision-making process and drive individuals towards adopting healthier behaviours (Meilier et al., 1997).

The incorporation of self-efficacy into the evolving HBM has significantly enriched the comprehension of health behaviour dynamics (Lev, 1997). This represents an individual's belief in their competence to successfully execute a specific health-related behaviour (Bandura, 1986; Lev, 1997). Within the framework of the HBM, self-efficacy plays a pivotal role in determining whether a person engages in a recommended health action. This addition has strengthened the HBM by recognising that even when individuals perceive the severity and susceptibility of a health threat and acknowledge the benefits of taking action, they may remain inactive if they lack confidence in their ability to do so (Bandura, 1986; Lev, 1997). Self-efficacy addresses the psychological dimension of behaviour change, assessing an individual's confidence and belief in their capacity to overcome potential obstacles and achieve successful behaviour outcomes. Furthermore, self-efficacy is highly personalised, recognising that people possess varying levels of confidence for different behaviours (Bandura, 1986; Lev, 1997).

Occupational therapists can utilise self-efficacy assessments to tailor education interventions, providing targeted support and strategies to bolster an individual's confidence and increase the likelihood of behaviour modification. Importantly, self-efficacy is not a static trait but can evolve over time based on experiences, making it essential for interventions to remain adaptable to these fluctuations in self-confidence. In essence, self-efficacy's integration enhances the HBM's capacity to elucidate and foresee behaviour changes, rendering it an invaluable component of health promotion and education interventions.

Theories of Reasoned Action and Planned Behaviour

The Theory of Reasoned Action (TRA) and its extension, the Theory of Planned Behaviour (TPB) (Anzen & Fishbein, 1980; Fishbein & Anzen, 1975) are psychological models used to understand and predict human behaviour, including health-related actions. TRA posits that an individual's intention to perform a specific behaviour is the best predictor of whether they will actually engage in that behaviour. TPB extends TRA by introducing the concept of perceived behavioural control (Fishbein & Ajzen, 2010). It suggests that individuals are more likely to follow through with their intentions if they believe they have the necessary control and resources to perform the behaviour. This intention is influenced by two main factors: the individual's attitude towards the behaviour and subjective norms (Montaño & Kasprzyk, 2008). Attitude reflects an individual's personal evaluation of the behaviour, considering aspects like perceived benefits and drawbacks. Subjective norms involve the perceived social pressure or expectations from others regarding the behaviour (Montaño & Kasprzyk, 2015).

Similar to the HBM, the TRA and the TPB are also rooted in the value-expectancy theory. While they may not emphasise the concept of threat as prominently as the HBM does, their components partially mirror the considerations of perceived susceptibility, severity and the weighing of benefits and barriers that are integral to the HBM. The emphasis of these models on modifying knowledge levels rather than addressing other influential factors in behaviour change may be regarded as a critique.

Transtheoretical Model (Stages of Change Model)

The Transtheoretical Model (TTM), also known as the Stages of Change Model, is a framework that explains how individuals move through stages when making behavioural changes. It consists of six stages: Precontemplation (lack of awareness), Contemplation (awareness but no action), Preparation (intent to change), Action (active modification of behaviour), Maintenance (sustaining change) and Termination (complete integration of the new behaviour) (Prochaska & Norcross, 2002; Prochaska & Velicer, 1997). Central to the TTM is the idea that individuals progress through these stages at their own pace, and interventions should be tailored to their readiness for change. It also recognises that relapses are possible and part of the change process (Prochaska & Norcross, 2002). Originally applied to addiction recovery, the TTM has been adapted to various fields, including education and healthcare, to guide interventions aimed at promoting positive behavioural changes. Table 22.1 expands on this model with education interventions to offer potential strategies occupational therapists can employ to facilitate required behaviour change.

The Behaviour Change Wheel

The Behaviour Change Wheel is a comprehensive framework designed to guide the development and implementation of behaviour change interventions. At its core is the COM-B model – Capability, Opportunity and Motivation, three essential components that influence behaviour (Michie et al., 2011) which is widely used in health education interventions to support behaviour change.

■ Capability: This refers to an individual's psychological and physical capacity to engage in a particular behaviour. It encompasses both the person's knowledge and skills.
■ Opportunity: This pertains to the external factors and environmental conditions that facilitate or hinder a behaviour. It includes aspects like social influences, physical surroundings and time constraints.
■ Motivation: Motivation relates to the mental processes that drive behaviour. It involves an individual's desires, needs and intrinsic or extrinsic rewards associated with the behaviour.

TABLE 22.1		
The Transtheoretical Model (Stages of Change Model)		
Name of Stage	Characteristics	Education Interventions
Precontemplation	The person has no intention of changing their behaviour in the foreseeable future.	Raise awareness of the health issue and its consequences. Provide general information about the health condition, its risks and potential impact on daily life. Share success stories and testimonials to make the issue more relatable.
Contemplation	The person is ambivalent about change. Considering changing behaviour in the next 6 months.	Discuss the pros and cons of change. Provide information about different approaches to behaviour change. Help them identify their specific reasons for contemplating change and any perceived barriers to making this change.
Preparation	Change is planned within the coming month.	Assist in setting realistic goals and creating a plan. Help them identify specific, achievable goals (e.g. using SMART goals). Provide information on strategies for change. Offer resources and support for developing an action plan.
Action	The person has made the behaviour change within the last 6 months.	Support active efforts to change behaviour. Offer practical tools and techniques for implementing the action plan. Provide ongoing education about the benefits of the new behaviour and reinforcement of positive progress.
Maintenance	The health behaviour has been sustained for at least 6 months.	Help them sustain the new behaviour. Continue to offer support and encouragement. Discuss strategies for overcoming barriers and setbacks. Reinforce the long-term benefits of maintaining the behaviour change.
Termination (is included in some versions of the TTM)	In this stage, the new behaviour is seen as being fully established. There is no desire to return to prior negative behaviours.	Celebrate and reinforce the achieved behaviour change. Acknowledge their success in making a lasting change. Discuss strategies for preventing relapse and maintaining the behaviour in the long term.

Adapted from Prochaska, J. O., & Norcross, J. C. (2002). Stages of Change. In J. C. Norcross (Ed.), *Psychotherapy relationships that work: Therapist contributions and responsiveness to patients* (pp. 303–313). Oxford University Press.

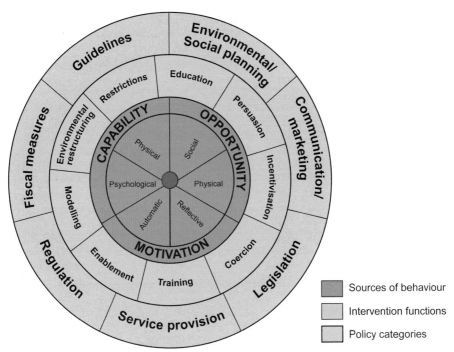

Fig. 22.1 ■ The Behaviour Change Wheel. From Michie, S., van Stralen, M. M., & West, R. (2011). The behaviour change wheel: A new method for characterising and designing behaviour change interventions. *Implementation Science, 6,* 42, with acknowledgement of Biomed Central. https://implementationscience.biomedcentral.com/articles/10.1186/1748-5908-6-42.

The Behaviour Change Wheel also incorporates the 'COM-B' components into the intervention functions (how to change behaviour) and policy categories (how to support behaviour change at the population level) (Michie et al., 2011) (Fig. 22.1).

Collaborative Relationship-Focused Practice and Shared Decision Making

Shared decision making is a collaborative process wherein the individuals or collectives and healthcare experts consider the advantages and disadvantages of each management option while also taking into account the individual's or collective's values and preferences (Hoffman et al., 2014). This supports the two-way exchange and deliberation of benefits or risks perceived in proposed interventions. This is a core element of collaborative relationship-focused practice that considers preference and choice through informed, respectful and integrated means. Collaborative relationship-focused practice (refer to Chapter 12) serves as a foundation to

enable shared decision-making process when considering the use of education intervention and strategies in occupational therapy (Elwyn et al., 2015; Restall & Egan, 2021). Stiggelbout et al. (2015) suggest that there are four steps to facilitating shared decision making (Fig. 22.2).

As indicated in the last step of the shared decision-making process, at this stage, people may feel unable to decide or prefer to defer the decision to a healthcare professional due to experiencing increased pressure or uncertainty around making a decision. This preference to defer the decision to the healthcare professional must be implemented carefully so that it does not default to the situation of the healthcare professional making all the decisions for the individual or collective (Elwyn, 2015). It is important to recognise that the impact of social deprivation on people's health has been extensively documented in the literature and should be considered by the occupational therapist to support the shared decision-making process. Social deprivation

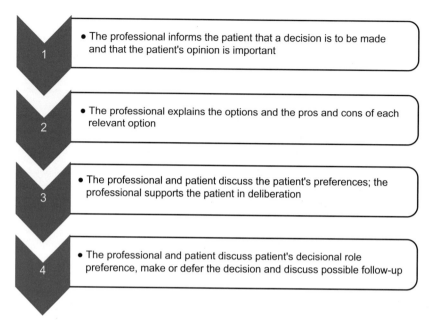

1. • The professional informs the patient that a decision is to be made and that the patient's opinion is important

2. • The professional explains the options and the pros and cons of each relevant option

3. • The professional and patient discuss the patient's preferences; the professional supports the patient in deliberation

4. • The professional and patient discuss patient's decisional role preference, make or defer the decision and discuss possible follow-up

Fig. 22.2 ■ Process of shared decision making. From Stiggelbout, A. M., Pieterse, A. H., & De Haes, J. C. J. M. (2015). Shared decision making: Concepts, evidence, and practice. *Patient Education and Counseling, 98*(10), 1172–1179. https://doi.org/10.1016/j.pec.2015.06.022.

encompasses more than just socioeconomic status and extends to factors like education level, social standing and access to resources available to the general population (Stephens et al., 2021). Therefore, when it comes to education, communication, cultural and health literacy factors play a significant role in building trust and fostering collaborative engagement (Groot et al., 2020; Jull et al., 2015).

In summary, by integrating shared decision making and collaborative relationship-focused practice, occupational therapists can optimise the educational experience and support people in achieving their goals and enhancing their overall quality of life.

APPLICATIONS OF THEORIES, MODELS AND FRAMEWORKS IN PRACTICE

This section aims to integrate the explored theories, models and framework to demonstrate how occupational therapists can effectively implement evidence-based practices when tailoring education intervention

within a collaborative relationship-focused practice, using three practice stories (Boxes 22.1 and 22.2) to put these into context.

Each practice story demonstrates that the focus on the person is paramount in delivering education interventions as it positively impacts health experiences, outcomes and the therapeutic relationship. Personalised interventions lead to increased confidence and improved attitudes towards illness, injury or impairment (Ricci et al., 2022). The practice stories illustrate how these concepts can be harmoniously combined to create a cohesive and impactful approach.

Practice Story: Antonia

In Antonia's story, applying andragogy and the behaviour change model within a collaborative relationship-focused practice supports tailoring education interventions. These principles, intertwined with micro and macro environmental considerations, help guide interventions by assessing Antonia's readiness for change and motivations. Employing a collaborative relationship-focused

BOX 22.1
ANTONIA

Antonia (she/her) is a 24-year-old woman of African-Caribbean heritage, who recently experienced a stroke following delivery of her baby. She experienced changes in her ability to communicate expressively and struggled with moving her left arm and leg in a coordinated manner. Through acute rehabilitation, Antonia made a significant recovery but continue to experience pain and reduced strength down the left side of her body, leading to increased frustration, anxiety and low mood. Prior to her stroke, she was able bodied and lived with her partner in a three-bedroom house, working full-time as a solicitor.

Using a collaborative relationship-focused approach, the occupational therapist had a conversation with Antonia about the different cultural, societal and wider contexts surrounding her daily life, environment and relationships to gain a fuller understanding of Antonio's personal experiences, values and circumstances. This included examining meaningful occupations, for example, roles, values, spirituality, occupations and sexual health and wellbeing as a young mother and a partner, living with a health condition. These conversations created an opportunity for Antonia to clarify her expectations from engaging in the service and how intervention priorities could be informed collaboratively to support her wellbeing.

The occupational therapist's use of this collaborative process was further informed by the Canadian Occupational Therapy Inter-relational Practice Process (COTIPP) Framework (see Chapter 12) to support understanding of the context in which Antonia experienced her limitations. This enabled the occupational therapist to consider and critically reflect on what was working and what was not working for Antonia, seeking to understand the layers of structural factors that influenced Antonia's health, wellbeing and occupational participation.

It was revealed that the focus of the acute rehabilitation Antonia received to date was around physical exercises and activities of daily living, but other important considerations were not addressed. This included recognising Antonia's sexual and reproductive rights, supporting her to be able to make her own decisions about her body and receive accurate information about these issues. She had concerns about engaging in intimacy and sexual relationship with her partner due to residual effects of stroke and as a young woman who recently delivered a baby. Her sexual self-esteem and identity were also negatively affected due to her changing body image and capabilities, loss of her able body and her job role. Antonia remarked that sexual activity had previously been a very important and regular part of her life with her partner and was worried that their relationship has changed forever.

The occupational therapist conducted a comprehensive assessment to gain a holistic understanding of Antonia's physical, cognitive and emotional abilities and limitations. Using a collaborative relationship-focused approach, the occupational therapist was able to initiate open discussions with Antonia about her concerns regarding intimacy and sexual relationships. By providing a safe space to discuss these topics, the occupational therapist was able to engage Antonia in tailored education around the impact of stroke on sexuality and its expression, the impact of childbirth, compensation strategies to explore alternative or adapted methods of experiencing and giving sensual and sexual pleasure, introducing positioning aids and negotiating practical support if needed from other agencies. The occupational therapist also provided an information booklet on 'Sex and intimate relationships after stroke' from the Stroke Association and signposted her to other sources of information, for example, https://www.sexwise.org.uk/ to find more about sexual and reproductive help and sexual wellbeing. This was to allow Antonia to consider this information in her own time and decide when would be the right time to resume sexual activities in the manner in which she would feel comfortable doing so. Exploring potential strategies helped Antonia to address her concerns and set meaningful and personalised goals, with a view to revisit and evaluate these at the follow-up appointment with the occupational therapist (refer to Chapter 25).

approach, her occupational therapist facilitates open, safe discussions on these sensitive subjects, respecting Antonia's preferences and values as per andragogy. The behaviour change model acknowledges Antonia's evolving journey through change stages, where Antonia's cultural, societal and personal concerns remain at the forefront. Open communication and recognising power dynamics ensure equitable, collaborative interactions, fostering a conducive learning environment (Haywood et al., 2019; Tabibian et al., 2017).

Practice Story Mel and Sam

For Mel and Sam, occupational therapists must consider their unique life experiences and backgrounds

---

BOX 22.2
MEL AND SAM

MEL

Mel (she/her) was diagnosed with chronic fatigue syndrome in the last 10 years. She is a white, middle-aged, heteronormative woman from a Eurocentric background. She lives with her partner in a Western country that has a publicly funded health and social welfare system and has access to private healthcare. She holds an honours degree and works in an office as a team manager.

Mel largely sees herself as independent and often plans her own holidays away. Mel often goes out to see her friends for a meal and frequents different music venues and gigs.

When asked to evaluate how she perceives her life, Mel reported that she can do the things that she wants to; however, she feels that people can be ignorant of her needs sometimes and they can treat her differently. She reports having fast access to healthcare but finds that she is having to spend more money on equipment or requires more planning when going to different places when thinking about accessibility. She also reports that while she feels respected and treated inclusively at work, she feels less so when working with people external to the team or out in public.

SAM

Sam (she/her/they) is a Black, trans woman, who is able bodied and lives in a Western country that has a publicly funded health and social welfare system. Sam holds an honours degree and works in an office as part of a team.

Sam has been on the waiting list for an assessment for ADHD for over a year and concerned about accessing timely diagnosis and support for her needs. Sam is very close with her family and is very engaged within her community. She spends most of her time at community events, parties and celebrations.

When asked to evaluate how Sam perceives her life, she highlights that she enjoys spending time with her community; however, she notes that some people are not accepting of her transition and still use her deadname* in the office. She notes that she often fidgets when she is having to sit down for a long time in places such as the office and restaurants and conscious about the looks she gets. She also gets random questions such as what her family thinks about her, which makes her feel uncomfortable. Outside of her community, Sam feels that she can go to places and do different things but feels isolated at times as she can often be in an environment where she perceives threats in the form of discrimination and does not feel welcomed in places like the gym, the office and new environments.

---

*Deadname: To refer to someone (especially a transgender person) who has changed names by a previous name (https://en.wiktionary.org/wiki/deadname).

---

to identify motivations, beliefs and attitudes to tailor education interventions.

Mel, a middle-aged woman with chronic fatigue syndrome, values her independence in planning activities like holidays and social outings. The occupational therapist should prioritise her accessibility needs and address instances of ignorance or differential treatment. While considering her privileged healthcare access, interventions aim to enhance wellbeing, being mindful of potential expenses.

Sam, a Black trans woman awaiting an ADHD assessment, cherishes her family and community ties. Focusing on her community engagement, interventions strengthen existing connections and support networks. Amidst workplace and public discrimination, the occupational therapist creates an inclusive, safe space, addressing concerns about isolation and discrimination.

Understanding Mel and Sam's unique needs empowers them towards desired health outcomes, respecting their diverse identities. This culturally sensitive approach personalises interventions to individual challenges and strengths, enhancing overall wellbeing (Machynska & Boiko, 2020).

CONSIDERATIONS WHEN PLANNING AND IMPLEMENTING EDUCATION INTERVENTIONS

This section focuses on a number of considerations to take into account when planning and implementing education interventions, with an overview of the key steps and decisions that an occupational therapist should take to ensure these are implemented effectively.

Determination of Educational Needs and Objective Setting

To deliver effective, tailored education interventions, the informational needs of learners and their support networks must be determined (Britton & Rosenwax, 2015). Individuals facing changes in health and wellbeing heavily rely on access to informative resources regarding treatments, interventions, care and self-management options. A lack of access to relevant information can significantly exacerbate anxiety levels and raise concerns about effectively managing occupations and coping with activities of daily living in the long term (Sleight & Duker, 2016).

Addressing this challenge is complex due to the multifaceted nature of health and wellbeing (Alsem, 2017; Knier et al., 2014). Alsem (2017) emphasises that information sources vary, including professional advice, experiential knowledge drawn from lived experiences, insights from peers and online platforms and input from wider communities. Understanding the information presented is a fundamental necessity for individuals and collectives (Barney & Perkinson, 2015). Occupational therapists must ensure that the language, format and timing of the information provided are tailored to support learners in adequately processing and comprehending the information, empowering them to make well-informed decisions.

Occupational therapists might also consider employing formal methods to assess informational needs, such as knowledge tests, attitude scales or behaviour checklists. Utilising a formal assessment offers the advantage of establishing a baseline measurement, which can be readministered after implementing the education strategy to evaluate its effectiveness (Hoffman & Eames, 2017). For example, self-management education needs can be effectively evaluated using the Educational Needs Assessment Tool, which includes 39 items, with many of them being relevant to occupational therapy. This assessment tool aids in identifying educational priorities and informing the process of goal setting and shared decision making to support individuals in their self-management journey (Ndosi et al., 2011).

Determination of educational needs is an ongoing and dynamic process as these needs can change over time and are influenced by wider personal, health and environmental factors, including the level of readiness to make changes. As individuals progress through different phases of their health condition, their educational needs evolve, necessitating continuous assessment and tailored interventions.

Once the educational needs are determined, the next stage involves working collaboratively with individuals or collectives to set clear and purposeful objectives that address these needs. SMART goals help create well-defined and realistic targets that can be monitored and adjusted over time. SMART stands for:

- **S**pecific (goals are clear and tailored to an individual's identified needs),
- **M**easurable (goals can be quantified or observed to track progress),
- **A**chievable (goals are realistic and attainable within the individual's capabilities),
- **R**elevant (goals align with the individual's broader objectives and are meaningful) and
- **T**ime-bound (goals have a set timeframe for completion).

Selecting the Optimal Education Delivery Format

When considering education interventions, a diverse array of formats can be employed, either individually or in combination, to effectively engage learners. These formats encompass verbal, written, audio/visual, internet-based and group-based resources, each offering unique advantages tailored to specific learning needs and preferences. Regardless of the chosen format, it is important to consider how information is presented within each approach and application in practice (Demir et al., 2007; Mayberry, 2007).

Verbal

Verbal education is commonly employed in occupational therapy practice due to its convenience and ease of implementation. When verbal education is incorporated as part of an education intervention, the dynamic between the occupational therapist and the learners takes on the roles of a teacher and a student, respectively. In this scenario, the occupational therapist assumes the responsibility of imparting knowledge and information to the learner, acting as the teacher. However, it is important to recognise that this format can sometimes overwhelm learners.

It is important to address the power dynamics within this relationship to ensure occupational therapists aligned with the principles of collaborative relationship-focused practice to support shared decision making and implement strategies to support learners in digesting information effectively. Providing and sharing information at appropriate time points in the intervention, tailoring it to specific stages of recovery and regularly assessing engagement and comprehension are essential approaches (Danzl et al., 2016).

When delivering verbal education, it is essential for healthcare providers to take into consideration various personal factors, including age and cognitive ability. These factors can significantly influence a learner's ability to comprehend and retain the information provided. As people age, their cognitive functions may naturally decline, affecting their capacity to process complex information. Additionally, hearing difficulties can further hinder effective communication during verbal education sessions. Barriers to information retention may also include anxiety, depression, denial, memory deficits, pain, stress or unfamiliarity (Maloney et al., 2014; Moran, 2016; Sandi, 2013). To ensure the effectiveness of verbal education, occupational therapists should employ strategies to accommodate learners' needs. Using clear and straightforward language, providing visual aids or written materials and allowing ample time for questions and clarification can enhance the understanding and retention of information for learners with varying cognitive abilities and hearing impairments. By tailoring verbal education to learners' needs, therapists can create a more inclusive and supportive learning environment, ultimately empowering people to take an active role in managing their health.

Further strategies to ensure the quality of verbal education include the use of clear, lay language in all communications. Using nonmedical language helps learners better comprehend the information without being overwhelmed by technical jargon (Bryant et al., 2022). Also, tailoring the language to the specific needs and backgrounds of the audience enhances their ability to relate to and engage with the content. Additionally, the delivery of information should be paced appropriately, allowing the recipients to process and absorb the information at a comfortable rate. Importantly, using clear and straightforward language facilitates better understanding and reduces the risk of confusion or misinterpretation (Marcus, 2014).

Combined Verbal and Visual

Education interventions that are verbal in nature are often accompanied by visual materials as a form of reinforcement (Bryant et al., 2022; Danzl et al., 2015).

This is often used to convey necessary information that supports the comprehension of health-related information.

The integration of verbal and visual delivery can be particularly effective when working with learners who identify themselves as having low literacy skills or when written materials might overwhelm or undervalue their understanding. By incorporating visual elements such as photos, flipcharts and illustrations, the communication of information becomes more accessible and engaging, transcending potential barriers arising from language or cultural differences (Camden et al., 2014). Visual elements can make the presentation of complex information easier to comprehend and more attractive. They can also reinforce written or spoken health messages and be used as effective tools for communicating health information (CDC, 2022). This multimodal approach can enhance the learners' comprehension and retention of the material, making it a valuable tool for promoting knowledge uptake.

However, it is essential to consider learners' needs and preferences when utilising this format. Different learners possess varying capacities for absorbing knowledge and processing visual and audio information over time. While some may benefit from the combined approach, others might find it overwhelming or challenging to process information delivered in multiple formats. Occupational therapists should be attentive to the preferences and learning styles of the people they work with, offering flexibility and providing options to tailor education interventions to meet diverse needs.

Written

Written materials provide learners with tangible materials to refer, enabling them to refresh their memory as needed. This format serves as a valuable support system, enabling them to retain and recall essential information about their health and wellbeing. Occupational therapists may provide written materials either with or without accompanying instructions, tailoring their approach to the learner's specific needs.

When creating written materials, occupational therapists must carefully consider the language used to ensure accessibility across a wide range of literacy abilities. Additionally, incorporating visual images alongside the written information can significantly enhance comprehension, adherence and recall of the material (Wittink & Oosterhaven, 2018). The effective display of written information is equally important, as it directly impacts the motivation to read and the overall comprehension of the content.

Despite being one of the most used formats, concerns have been raised regarding the effectiveness of written materials in isolation (Nutbeam et al., 2017; Giguere et al., 2020). Therefore, to enhance the impact of written education, occupational therapists should adopt a multimodal approach to education intervention, by combining written information with other formats, such as verbal explanations, visual aids or interactive activities, to create a more comprehensive and engaging educational experience.

Recommendations for designing effective written health education materials are provided in Box 22.3. These guidelines serve as valuable tools for occupational therapists to design written materials that are engaging, informative and tailored to specific learning preferences and needs.

Audio-Visual

Audio-visual information, encompassing visual media, motion and sound, such as films, videos and television, offers a dynamic and innovative format for delivering education interventions (Fuady & Mutalib, 2018). This mode of educational delivery presents a powerful opportunity to engage and effectively reach a diverse audience (Nicolaou et al., 2019). The combination of visual and auditory elements enhances the communication of complex information and concepts, making it easier for learners to comprehend and retain knowledge. Audio-visual materials can cater to different learning styles and preferences, accommodating learners with varying literacy levels, cognitive abilities and language skills.

Incorporating audio and video into education interventions opens a world of creative possibilities. Narrations, anecdotes and musical backgrounds can be skilfully integrated to enhance the learning experience, making it more captivating and memorable (Nicolau et al., 2019). Furthermore, navigator aids and interactive elements provide learners with a sense of autonomy, allowing them to explore and engage with the content in a way that suits their preferences and learning styles. Games, simulations and virtual reality

experiences offer interactive and immersive learning opportunities, fostering active participation and deeper understanding (Mayer, 2019).

Audio-visual information in education interventions offers immediacy, accessibility and engagement, benefiting learners with language barriers or difficulty with written language (Nicolau et al., 2019). However, challenges lie in ensuring the content's comprehensiveness, relevance and inclusivity. By carefully planning and structuring the material, therapists can strike a balance between simplicity and effectiveness. Culturally sensitive and accessible content, such as closed captions and transcripts, promotes equitable learning. Tailoring information to learners' needs enhances engagement and application in daily life. Well-designed audio-visual resources empower learners to make informed decisions and promote positive change (Nicolau et al., 2019).

Online/Virtual Environments and eHealth

People commonly turn to the Internet and social media to seek information about their injury, illness or impairment (Zhao & Zhang, 2017). The rise of telemedicine and eHealth is bridging health informatics and medical technologies for personalised medicine, health education, prediction and prevention (Prior & Wynn, 2023). These advancements support clinical diagnosis, treatment, participatory health and research.

However, the advancement of virtual environments, telemedicine and eHealth technologies presents new challenges regarding equitable access and user safety. While these innovations offer promising benefits, not everyone may have equal access to these services due to issues like digital poverty, lack of technological literacy or limited internet connectivity in certain regions (Najm et al., 2019; Prior & Wynn, 2023). This digital divide could lead to disparities in healthcare access and education outcomes. Additionally, concerns about data privacy and security arise as these technologies store sensitive health information (Prior & Wynn, 2023). Ensuring that these technologies are accessible, user-friendly and secure for all individuals and collectives is essential for promoting equitable and safe healthcare delivery in the digital age.

Occupational therapists must be proactive in assessing people's ability to access, comprehend and evaluate online information, as assuming universal digital

BOX 22.3
RECOMMENDATIONS FOR DESIGNING EFFECTIVE WRITTEN HEALTH EDUCATION MATERIALS

- Involve all key stakeholders, including the person receiving occupational therapy services, in the development and testing of the written material.

CONTENT

- Clearly state the purpose of the material.
- Provide information that is behaviour focused (e.g. 'It is important that you do the exercises every day').
- Ensure that the content is accurate, up-to-date and evidence-based and that sources are appropriately referenced.
- Include the authors' names on the material and the publication date.

LANGUAGE

- Avoid judgemental or patronising language.
- Aim for a fifth- to sixth-grade reading level.
- Use short sentences, expressing only one idea per sentence.
- Use short words, preferably one to two syllables, where possible.
- Use common words wherever possible. Avoid the use of jargon or abbreviations.
- Include a glossary if jargon or unfamiliar words are necessary.
- Write in the active voice and in a conversational style.
- Write in the second person (e.g. 'you' rather than 'the client').
- Structure sentences so that the context or old information is presented before new information. (e.g. 'To lower your risk of stroke [context], you will need to make changes to what you eat' [new information]).

ORGANISATION

- Sequence the information so that the information that individuals most want to know is at the beginning.

- Use subheadings.
- Present the information using bulleted lists where possible.
- Group related information into lists, with no more than five points in each list, and label each list descriptively.
- Keep paragraphs short and express only one idea per paragraph.
- Summarise the main points, either at the end of sections or at the end of the material.

LAYOUT AND TYPOGRAPHY

- Use a minimum 12-point font size.
- Avoid the use of italics and all capitals.
- Only use bold type to emphasise key words or phrases.
- Ensure good contrast between the font colour (e.g. black) and the background (e.g. white).

ILLUSTRATIONS

- Only use illustrations if they will enhance the reader's understanding.
- Use simple line drawings that are likely to be familiar to the reader.
- Use an explanatory caption with each illustration.
- Refer to the illustration in the text.

LEARNING AND MOTIVATION

- Incorporate features that actively engage the reader (e.g. blank space to write questions down, short quiz, 'list three things that you should do').

From Hoffmann, T., & Worrall, L. (2004). Designing effective written health education materials: Considerations for health professionals. *Disability and Rehabilitation, 26*, 1166–1173, with permission from Taylor and Francis Journals. http://www.informaworld.com.

literacy can lead to inaccurate assumptions (Gordon & Hornbrook, 2018). Online resources offer various benefits, including readability, easy access to relevant information and the creation of virtual communities for emotional support. It empowers people to explore at their own pace and supports shared decision making for those with good health literacy and motivation.

Group-Based

Group-based educational interventions can provide unique benefits beyond individualised approaches,

leading to long-term cost-effectiveness and improved management of health conditions (Molsted et al., 2011). Group interventions foster a sense of belonging and security, empower group members to seek peer support and enhance understanding and application of health information (Poscia et al., 2018). Participating in behaviour-based coping strategies within group settings can significantly boost coping self-efficacy and overall wellbeing, potentially leading to improved mental health self-efficacy and wellbeing (Ngooi et al., 2022). Vicarious experiences in activity-based groups can positively influence self-efficacy and wellbeing, as members observe and learn from others' efforts and successes in managing mental illness (Kukla et al., 2017; Silverman, 2019).

However, occupational therapists should consider individual differences when implementing group-based interventions. Some individuals, such as those who are neurodiverse or introverted, may face challenges in group settings, hindering their full engagement and benefit from the intervention. Further challenges include differing needs and goals, confidentiality concerns, group dynamics, time constraints, limited individual attention, language barriers, cultural considerations, cognitive or communication challenges, unequal participation and dropouts. To address these challenges, occupational therapists must carefully assess individual suitability for group interventions, foster a supportive and inclusive atmosphere, provide alternative options when needed and continually evaluate the intervention's effectiveness and participants' feedback for necessary adjustments.

Deciding When to Provide the Information

Ensuring the effectiveness and application of education strategies hinges on providing information at the right time. However, there is no guidance as to the optimum time to provide information as this greatly varies across individuals and collectives, their circumstances and the needs and the type of information provided (Hoffmann & Eames, 2017). It is important to consider individual factors, such as anxiety levels, coping strategies and the availability of support, in line with where people are in their unique journey of understanding their illness, injury or impairment. Careful thought should be given to whether the education intervention or information offered is beneficial to the learner at that specific moment and aligns with their current circumstances. Adopting various approaches to reiterate and clarify information over time further reinforces its impact and enhances the overall educational experience.

Gauging the timing of interventions demands a high level of emotional intelligence from the occupational therapist to guide their interactions. Emotional intelligence refers to the ability of a person to perceive and manage their own emotions while effectively interpreting, supporting and influencing the emotions of

others (Gribble et al., 2019). By harnessing emotional intelligence, occupational therapists can effectively support learners and their support networks, creating a conducive environment for meaningful and impactful educational experiences (Andonian, 2017). Using a collaborative relationship-focused approach (Restall & Egan, 2021) can also assist in determining the timing of educational input, by encouraging a reflective, shared ownership around the 'when' and 'how' education is delivered. This approach can support individuals and collectives to learn at their own pace by providing relevant and nuanced health information. It can allow ample time between consultations to process the information provided. It also encourages the asking of questions of the occupational therapist to ensure information is contextualised to the unique experience of the health condition by the learner.

Enhancing Accessibility to Education: Considering Health Literacy, Digital Poverty and Universal Design Principles

Occupational therapists take various accessibility considerations into account when providing education to ensure that the information is accessible and beneficial for all. This requires a careful assessment of the impact of language and communication style, health literacy, digital poverty and universal design to meet learners' accessibility needs. This assessment helps to tailor the delivery format for the education interventions.

Health Literacy

Health literacy plays a vital role in tailoring effective health communication and education. Understanding the literacy levels and information-processing abilities of the target audience is essential when delivering health information through verbal and written materials. Understanding of health literacy relates to an individual's ability to procure, read, understand and make legible decisions based on information regarding health and wellbeing (Cusack, 2018). Health literacy is variable across populations, with those at the lower ends of the social determinants of health experiencing poorer outcomes (Al Sayah et al., 2013).

Occupational therapists are well placed in fostering a more health-literate society (Attard et al., 2021). This involves recognising the literacy and numeracy skills of individuals and honing communication and education abilities to aid their comprehension of information. It is equally important for occupational therapists to reflect on their own health literacy and refine their communication styles to establish an environment of openness and support for individual growth.

Digital Poverty

Digital poverty refers to the lack of interaction and access to the online world due to socio-economic, geographic or educational reasons (Ferris et al., 2022). Holmes and Burgess (2022) suggest that digital poverty may not solely result from financial limitations. Exclusion and poverty arise from a complex interplay of social factors and technological access. Those classified as digitally poor may encounter challenges accessing the online world, experience limited connectivity, lack awareness of its benefits and possess insufficient education in navigation (Allmann, 2022). Occupational therapists must thoroughly consider health literacy, digital poverty and overall accessibility when considering the format of their education interventions and materials. These considerations are essential in overcoming barriers to engagement and ensuring inclusivity, thus enabling learners to benefit fully from the interventions provided.

Universal Design Principles

Universal design principles should be considered by occupational therapists when developing education interventions and accompanying materials to ensure maximum accessibility for learners (Nelson, 2014; Nelson & Basham, 2014; Rogers-Shaw et al., 2017). Universal design principles, entail the creation of learning materials following three fundamental principles:

1. Identify potential barriers and biases and determine ways to prevent or mitigate them.
2. Allow learner choice, when and where possible, to increase interest and achievement.
3. Empower learners to become experts in their process for learning and, ultimately, allow learners to self-assess and improve their learning over time.

In the context of blended and online learning environments, universal design can be particularly advantageous due to the diverse array of options offered by technology-enhanced education (Educause, 2015).

According to Keiran and Anderson (2018), universal design principles serve as a culturally responsive tool that can effectively support learners with diverse needs and backgrounds, considering various levels of understanding and intersectionality. Additionally, Roski et al. (2021) found that the application of universal design principles has resulted in heightened satisfaction, improved experiences and enhanced accessibility.

EVALUATING THE OUTCOME OF EDUCATION INTERVENTIONS

Occupational therapists should evaluate the outcomes of their education interventions, to ascertain their effectiveness, assess if the intended goals have been achieved and ensure the desired impact on the learners. Correctly interpreting the outcomes of an evaluative process for education interventions is essential to uphold evidence-based practice. Additionally, occupational therapists must be reflexive during evaluation, acknowledging the influence of personal views and thought processes on education interventions (Rettke et al., 2018).

The evaluation of education interventions can be conducted using both formal and informal methods, each offering unique insights. Informal evaluation involves gathering feedback from learners to ascertain if they understood the information that the occupational therapist provided to them, if their informational needs have been met and if they have any unanswered questions (Hoffmann & Eames, 2017). This feedback can be obtained through open-ended discussions, surveys or questionnaires. By asking learners about their experiences, satisfaction levels and perceptions of the intervention, occupational therapists can gain valuable insights into its strengths, weaknesses and areas for improvement. Subjective reviews and reflections by occupational therapists themselves can also contribute to the informal evaluation process. Additionally, informal evaluation can include observations made during consultations and follow-up appointments. Occupational therapists may assess engagement levels, learners' reactions and any immediate changes in behaviour or knowledge resulting from the educational intervention applied.

Formal evaluation of education interventions involves the use of standardised and systematic methods to measure specific outcomes and assess the effectiveness of the intervention. To do this, occupational therapists can employ standardised assessments, which are carefully developed and validated tools designed to measure changes in various areas such as knowledge, skills, attitudes, behaviour, self-efficacy and symptom severity.

Using patient-reported outcome measures (PROMs) is one common approach to quantitatively evaluate the impact of the education strategy or intervention. PROMs involve collecting data directly from the recipients of the intervention, allowing occupational therapists to gather valuable insights into their experiences and the effectiveness of the education provided (Prior et al., 2018). The timing of the measure should align with the specific objectives and goals set for the intervention. Occupational therapists need to consider when the intended changes or improvements are expected to occur based on the content and duration of the education intervention.

In some cases, occupational therapists may choose to administer the outcome measure immediately after the completion of the education intervention. This immediate postintervention assessment allows for an assessment of short-term changes and immediate impact on knowledge, skills or attitudes. However, in other cases, the occupational therapist may decide to schedule the outcome measure later, after the learners have had the opportunity to apply the newly acquired knowledge or skills in their daily life. This delayed assessment enables the occupational therapist to evaluate the long-term impact of the education intervention.

The timing of the outcome measure may also be influenced by the nature of the condition being addressed and the expected trajectory of improvement or change. For example, if the education intervention is focused on improving pain management for a long-term condition, the occupational therapist might choose to administer the outcome measure at different intervals over several weeks or months to capture changes in symptom management, functional abilities and self-management.

CONCLUSION

Education interventions are common in occupational therapy practice, promoting occupational participation for learners dealing with injury, illness or impairment. Within a collaborative relationship-focused occupational therapy approach, education interventions should be thoughtfully designed by occupational therapists, placing a strong emphasis on understanding and attending to the relational aspects of both the self and the individuals and collectives they serve. This approach recognises the significance of building trust and rapport between the occupational therapist and the individuals and collectives.

By cultivating a compassionate and empathetic environment, occupational therapists can create a safe space for learning and growth. The design of education interventions should be tailored, considering the unique goals, preferences and needs of learners. Occupational therapists should actively involve learners in the decision-making process, promoting shared ownership and co-creation of the education plan. Moreover, occupational therapists should be attentive to the dynamics of power and privilege within the therapeutic relationship. By fostering an inclusive and equitable environment, they can empower the learners to actively participate in their own education and decision-making processes. Through this relational and collaborative approach to education, occupational therapists can facilitate meaningful and sustainable outcomes for people they serve.

REFERENCES

Ajzen, I. (1989). Attitude structure and behavior. In A. R. Pratkanis, S. J. Breckler, & A. G. Greenwald (Eds.), *Attitude structure and function* (pp. 241–274). Lawrence Erlbaum Associates, Inc.

Ajzen, I., & Fishbein, M. (1980). *Understanding attitudes and predicting social behavior*. Prentice-Hall.

Al Sayah, F., Majumdar, S. R., Williams, B., Robertson, S., & Johnson, J. A. (2013). Health literacy and health outcomes in diabetes: A systematic review. *Journal of General Internal Medicine, 28*(3), 444–452.

Allmann, K. (2022). UK Digital Poverty Evidence Review 2022. https://digitalpovertyalliance.org/wp-content/uploads/2022/06/UK-Digital-Poverty-Evidence-Review-2022-v1.0-compressed.pdf

Alsem, M. W., Ausems, F., Verhoef, M., Jongmans, M. J., Meily-Visser, J. M. A., & Ketelaar, M. (2017). Information seeking by parents of children with physical disabilities: An exploratory qualitative study. *Research in Developmental Disabilities, 60*, 125–134. https://doi.org/10.1016/j.ridd.2016.11.015.

Andonian, L. (2017). Emotional Intelligence: An opportunity for occupational therapy. *Occupational Therapy in Mental Health, 33*(4), 299–307. https://doi.org/10.1080/0164212x.2017.1328649.

Attard, E., Musallam, A., Vaas, K., Chaney, T., Fortuna, J. K., & Williams, B. (2021). Health literacy in occupational therapy research: A scoping review. *The Open Journal of Occupational Therapy, 9*(4), 1–18. https://doi.org/10.15453/2168-6408.1832.

Bandura, A. (1986). *Social foundations of thought and action: A social cognitive theory.* Prentice-Hall.

Barney, J., & Perkinson, M. A. (2015). *Occupational therapy with aging adults: Promoting quality of life through collaborative practice.* Elsevier.

Bartlett, E. E. (1985). Patient education: A planned learning experience. *In Patient Education and Counseling, 7*(3), 323.

Birkeland, S., Bismark, M., Barry, M. J., & Möller, S. (2022). Is greater patient involvement associated with higher satisfaction? Experimental evidence from a vignette survey. *BMJ Quality & Safety, 31*(2), 86–93. https://doi.org/10.1136/bmjqs-2020-012786.

Bonsaksen, T., Dolva, A. S., Horghagen, S., Sveen, U., Hagby, C., & Arntzen, C. (2020). Characteristics of community-based occupational therapy: Results of a Norwegian survey. *Scandinavian Journal of Occupational Therapy, 27*(1), 39–46. https://doi.org/10.1080/11038128.2019.1609085.

Britton, L., Rosenwax, L., & McNamara, B. (2015). Occupational therapy practice in acute physical hospital settings: Evidence from a scoping review. *Australian Occupational Therapy Journal, 62*(6), 370–377. https://doi.org/10.1111/1440-1630.12227.

Bryant, A. M., Gee, B. M., & Gitlow, L. (2022). Health literacy and occupational therapy: A Discussion on assessing and addressing limited health literacy. *The Open Journal of Occupational Therapy, 10*(4), 1–5. https://doi.org/10.15453/2168-6408.1996.

Camden, C., Shikako-Thomas, K., Nguyen, T., Graham, E., Thomas, A., Sprung, J., Morris, C., & Russell, D. J. (2014). Engaging stakeholders in rehabilitation research: A scoping review of strategies used in partnerships and evaluation of impacts. *Disability and Rehabilitation, 37*(15), 1390–1400. https://doi.org/10.3109/09638288.2014.963705.

Centers for Disease Control and Prevention (CDC). 2022. Health Literacy. https://www.cdc.gov/healthliteracy/learn/index.html

Cusack, L., Del Mar, C. B., Chalmers, I., Gibson, E., & Hoffmann, T. C. (2018). Education interventions to improve people's understanding of key concepts in assessing the effects of health interventions: A systematic review. *Systematic Reviews, 7*(1), 2–9. https://doi.org/10.1186/s13643-018-0719-4.

Danzl, M. M., Harrison, A., Hunter, E. G., Macario, E., & Thomas, L. (2016). Evaluation of a peer-led asthma self-management program and benefits of the program. *Journal of Asthma, 53*(6), 630–636. https://doi.org/10.1111/jrh.12124.

Danzl, M. M., Harrison, A., Hunter, E. G., Kuperstein, J., Sylvia, V., Maddy, K., & Campbell, S. (2015). A Lot of Things Passed Me by: Rural Stroke Survivors' and Caregivers' Experience of Receiving Education From Health Care Providers. *The Journal of Rural Health, 32*(1), 13–24. https://doi.org/10.1111/jrh.12124.

Demir, F., Ozsaker, E., & Ilce, A. O. (2007). The quality and suitability of written education materials for patients*. *Journal of Clinical Nursing, 17*(2), 259–265. https://doi.org/10.1111/j.1365-2702.2007.02044.x.

Dineen-Griffin, S., Garcia-Cardenas, V., Williams, K., & Benrimoj, S. I. (2019). Helping patients help themselves: A systematic review of self-management support strategies in primary health care practice. *PLoS One, 14*(8), e0220116. https://doi.org/10.1371/journal.pone.0220116.

Elwyn, G., Frosch, D. L., & Kobrin, S. (2015). Implementing shared decision making: Consider all the consequences. *Implementation Science, 11*(2), 7. https://doi.org/10.1186/s13012-016-0480-9.

Ferris, R., Clarke, M., Raftery, D., Liddy, M., & Sloan, S. (2022). Digital poverty in a country that is digitally powerful: Some insights into leadership of girls' schooling in India under Covid-19 restrictions. *Asia Pacific Journal of Education, 42*(supp1), 34–51. https://doi.org/10.1080/02188791.2022.2031871.

Fishbein, M., & Ajzen, I. (1975). *Belief, attitude, intention and behavior: An introduction to theory and research.* Addison-Wesley.

Fishbein, M., & Ajzen, I. (2010). *Predicting and changing behavior: The reasoned action approach.* Psychology Press.

Freeman, A., & Dolan, M. (2001). Revisiting Prochaska and DiClemente's stages of change theory: An expansion and specification to aid in treatment planning and outcome evaluation. *Cognitive and Behavioral Practice, 8*(3), 224–234.

Fuady, R., & Mutalib, A. A. (2018). Audio-visual media in learning. *Journal of K6 Education and Management, 1*(2), 1–6. https://doi.org/10.11594/jk6em.01.02.01.

Giguère, A., Zomahoun, H. T. V., Carmichael, P.-H., Uwizeye, C. B., Légaré, F., Grimshaw, J. M., Gagnon, M.-P., Auguste, D. U., & Massougbodji, J. (2020). Printed education materials: Effects on professional practice and healthcare outcomes. *Cochrane Database of Systematic Reviews*, Issue 8. Article No.: CD004398. https://doi.org/10.1002/14651858.CD004398.pub4.

Goff, A. J., De Oliveira Silva, D., Merolli, M., Bell, E. C., Crossley, K. M., & Barton, C. J. (2021). Patient education improves pain and function in people with knee osteoarthritis with better effects when combined with exercise therapy: A systematic review. *Journal of Physiotherapy, 67*(3), 177–189. https://doi.org/10.1016/j.jphys.2021.06.011.

Gordon, N. P., & Hornbrook, M. C. (2018). Older adults' readiness to engage with eHealth patient education and self-care resources: A cross-sectional survey. *BMC Health Services Research, 18*(18). https://doi.org/10.1186/s12913-018-2986-0.

Grace, A. P. (2001). Using queer cultural studies to transgress adult educational space. In V. Sheared & P. A. Sissel (Eds.), *Making space: Merging theory and practice in adult education* (pp. 257–270). Bergin & Garvey.

Grady, P. A., & Gough, L. L. (2014). Self-management: A comprehensive approach to management of chronic conditions. *American Journal of Public Health, 104*(8), e25–e31. https://doi.org/10.2105/AJPH.2014.302041.

Greene, S. M., Tuzzio, L., & Cherkin, D. (2012). A framework for making patient-centered care front and center. *The Permanente Journal, 16*(3), 49–53. https://doi.org/10.7812/TPP/12-025.

Gribble, N., Ladyshewsky, R. K., & Parsons, R. (2019). The impact of clinical placements on the emotional intelligence of occupational therapy, physiotherapy, speech pathology, and business students: A longitudinal study. *BMC Medical Education, 19*(1). https://doi.org/10.1186/s12909-019-1520-3.

Groot, G., Waldron, T., Barreno, L., Cochran, D., & Carr, T. (2020). Trust and world view in shared decision making with indigenous patients: A realist synthesis. *Journal of Evaluation in Clinical Practice, 26*(2), 503–514. https://doi.org/10.1111/jep.13307.

Hamilton, D. F., Akhtar, S., Griffiths, B., Prior, Y., & Jones, R. K. (2023). The use of technology to support lifestyle interventions in knee osteoarthritis: A scoping review. *Osteoarthritis and Cartilage Open, 5*(2), 100344. https://doi.org/10.1016/j.ocarto.2023.100344.

Hammond, A., Adams, J., & Prior, Y. (2020). Chapter 26: Occupational therapy. In D. Scott, J. Galloway, A. Cope, A. Pratt, & V. Strand (Eds.), *Oxford textbook of rheumatoid arthritis.* Oxford University Press.

Haywood, C., Martinez, G., Pyatak, E. A., & Carandang, K. (2019). Engaging patient stakeholders in planning, implementing, and disseminating occupational therapy research. *American Journal of Occupational Therapy, 73*(1), 7301090010p1. https://doi.org/10.5014/ajot.2019.731001.

Heng, H., Jazayeri, D., Shaw, L., Kiegaldie, D., Hill, A.-M., & Morris, M. E. (2020). Hospital falls prevention with patient education: A scoping review. *BMC Geriatrics, 20*(1), 9. https://doi.org/10.1186/s12877-020-01515-w.

Hoffman, T. & Eames, S. (2017) Education. In M. Curtin, M. Egan, & J. Adams. *Occupational therapy for people experiencing illness, injury or impairment. Promoting occupation and participation.* (7), (pp. 342–358). Elsevier.

Hoffmann, T. C., Montori, V. M., & Del Mar, C. (2014). The connection between evidence-based medicine and shared decision making. *The Journal of the American Medical Association, 312*(13), 1295–1296. https://doi.org/10.1001/jama.2014.10186.

Hoffmann, T., & Worrall, L. (2004). Designing effective written health education materials: Considerations for health professionals. *Disability and Rehabilitation, 26*(19), 1166–1173. https://doi.org/10.1080/09638280410001724816.

Holmes, H., & Burgess, G. (2022). Digital exclusion and poverty in the UK: How structural inequality shapes experiences of getting online. *Digital Geography and Society, 3*, 100041. https://doi.org/10.1016/j.diggeo.2022.100041.

Janz, N. K., & Becker, M. H. (1984). The health belief model: A decade later. *Health Education Quarterly, 11*(1), 1–47. https://doi.org/10.1177/109019818401100101.

Jones, N. L., Gilman, S. E., Cheng, T. L., Drury, S. S., Hill, C. V., & Geronimus, A. T. (2019). Life course approaches to the causes of health disparities. *American Journal of Public Health, 109*(S1), S48–S55. https://doi.org/10.2105/AJPH.2018.304738.

Jull, J., Giles, A., Lodge, M., Boyer, Y., & Stacey, D. (2015). Cultural adaptation of a shared decision-making tool with Aboriginal women: A qualitative study. *BMC Medical Informatics and Decision Making, 15*(1), 1–13. https://doi.org/10.1186/s12911-015-0129-7.

Kieran, L., & Anderson, C. (2018). Connecting universal design for learning with culturally responsive teaching. *Education and Urban Society, 51*(9), 1202–1216. https://doi.org/10.1177/0013124518785012.

Knier, S., Stichler, J. F., Ferber, L., & Catterall, K. (2014). Patients' perceptions of the quality of discharge teaching and readiness for discharge. *Rehabilitation Nursing, 40*(1), 30–39. https://doi.org/10.1002/rnj.164.

Knowles, M. S. (1980). *The modern practice of adult education: From pedagogy to andragogy.* Association Press.

Knowles, M. S., Holton, E. F., & Swanson, R. A. (2011). *The adult learner: The definitive classic in adult education and human resource development* (7th ed.). Elsevier: Butterworth-Heinemann.

Krist, A. H., Tong, S. T., Aycock, R. A., & Longo, D. R. (2017). Engaging patients in decision-making and behavior change to promote prevention. *Studies in Health Technology and Informatics, 240*, 284–302.

Kukla, M., Strasburger, A. M., Salyers, M. P., Rattray, N. A., & Lysaker, P. H. (2017). Subjective experiences of the benefits and key elements of a cognitive behavioral intervention focused on community work outcomes in persons with mental illness. *The Journal of Nervous and Mental Disease, 205*(1), 66–73. https://doi.org/10.1097/NMD.0000000000000601.

Kuruvilla, S., Sadana, R., Montesinos, E. V., Beard, J., Vasdeki, J. F., Araujo de Carvalho, I., Thomas, R. B., Drisse, M. B., Daelmans, B., Goodman, T., Koller, T., Officer, A., Vogel, J., Valentine, N., Wootton, E., Banerjee, A., Magar, V., Neira, M., Bele, J. M. O., … Bustreo, F. (2018). A life-course approach to health: Synergy with sustainable development goals. *Bulletin of the World Health Organization, 96*, 42–50.

Lev, E. L. (1997). Bandura's theory of self-efficacy: Applications to oncology. *Scholarly Inquiry for Nursing Practice, 11*(1), 21–43.

Machynska, N., & Boiko, H. (2020). Andragogy – The science of adult education: Theoretical aspects. *Journal of Innovation in Psychology, Education and Didactics, 24*(1), 25–34. https://jiped.ub.ro/wp-content/uploads/2020/03/JIPED_24_1_2020_2.pdf.

Maloney, E. A., Sattizahn, J. R., & Beilock, S. L. (2014). Anxiety and cognition. *Wiley Interdisciplinary Reviews: Cognitive Science, 5*, 403–411. https://doi.org/10.1002/wcs.1299.

Marcus, C. (2014). Strategies for improving the quality of verbal patient and family education: A review of the literature and creation of the EDUCATE model. *Health Psychology and Behavioral Medicine, 2*(1), 482–495. https://doi.org/10.1080/21642850.2014.900450.

Mayberry, J. F. (2007). The design and application of effective written instructional material: A review of published work. *Postgraduate Medical Journal, 83*(983), 596–598. https://doi.org/10.1136/pgmj.2006.053538.

Mayer, R. E. (2019). Computer games in education. *Annual Review of Psychology, 70*(1), 531–549. https://doi.org/10.1146/annurev-psych-010418-102744.

Meillier, L. K., Lund, A. B., & Kok, G. (1997). Cues to action in the process of changing lifestyle. *Patient Education and Counseling, 30*(1), 37–51. https://doi.org/10.1016/s0738-3991(96)00957-3.

Mews, J. (2020). Leading through Andragogy. *Campus Viewpoint, 95*(1), 65–68.

Michie, S., van Stralen, M. M., & West, R. (2011). The behaviour change wheel: A new method for characterising and designing behaviour change interventions. *Implementation Science, 6*(42). https://doi.org/10.1186/1748-5908-6-42.

Molsted, S., Tribler, J., Poulsen, P. B., & Snorgaard, O. (2011). The effects and costs of a group-based education programme for self-management of patients with Type 2 diabetes. A community-based study. *Health Education Research, 27*(5), 804–813. https://doi.org/10.1093/her/cyr053.

Montaño, D. E., & Kasprzyk, D. (2008). Theory of reasoned action, theory of planned behavior, and the integrated behavioral model. In K. Glanz, B. K. Rimer, & K. Viswanath (Eds.), *Health behavior and health education: Theory, research, and practice* (pp. 67–96). Jossey-Bass.

Montaño, D. E., & Kasprzyk, D. (2015). Theory of reasoned action, theory of planned behavior, and the integrated behavioral model. In K. Glanz, B. K. Rimer, & K. V. Viswanath (Eds.), *Health behavior: Theory, research, and practice* (pp. 95–124). Jossey-Bass/Wiley.

Moran, T. P. (2016). Anxiety and working memory capacity: A meta-analysis and narrative review. *Psychological Bulletin, 142*, 831–864. https://doi.org/10.1037/bul0000051.

Najm, A., Nikiphorou, E., Kostine, M., Richez, C., Pauling, J. D., Finckh, A., Ritschl, V., Prior, Y., Balazova, P., Stones, S. R., Szekanecz, Z., Iagnocco, A., Ramiro, S., Sivera, F., Dougados, M., Carmona, L., Burmeister, G., Gossec, L., & Berenbaum, F. (2019). EULAR Points to consider for the development, evaluation and implementation of mobile health applications aiding self-management in people living with rheumatic and musculoskeletal diseases. *RMD Open, 5*(2), e001014. https://doi:10.1136/rmdopen-2019-001014.

National Institute for Health and Care Excellence. (2022). Shared decision making. https://www.nice.org.uk/guidance/ng197

Ndosi, M., Tennant, A., Bergsten, U., Kukkurainen, M. L., Machado, P., de la Torre-Aboki, J., Vlieland, T. P., Zangi, H. A., & Hill, J. (2011). Cross-cultural validation of the educational needs assessment tool in RA in 7 European countries. *BMC Musculoskelet Disord, 12*, 110.

Nelson, L. L. (2014). *Design and deliver: Planning and teaching using universal design for learning.* Paul H. Brookes Publishing.

Nelson, L. L., & Basham, J. D. (2014). *A blueprint for UDL: Considering the design of implementation.* UDL-IRN. https://udl-irn.org.

Ngooi, B. X., Wong, S. R., Chen, J. D., & Yin Koh, V. S. (2022). Exploring the use of activity-based group therapy in increasing self-efficacy and subjective well-being in acute mental health. *Hong Kong Journal of Occupational Therapy, 35*(1), 52–61. https://doi.org/10.1177/15691861221075798.

NHS. (2019). The NHS long term plan. https://www.longtermplan.nhs.uk/

Nicolaou, C., Matsiola, M., & Kalliris, G. (2019). Technology-enhanced learning and teaching methodologies through audiovisual media. *Education Sciences, 9*(3), 196. https://doi.org/10.3390/educsci9030196.

Nutbeam, D., McGill, B., & Premkumar, P. (2017). Improving health literacy in community populations: A review of progress. *Health Promotion International, 33*(5), 901–911. https://doi.org/10.1093/heapro/dax015.

O'Mara-Eves, A., Brunton, G., Oliver, S., Kavanagh, J., Jamal, F., & Thomas, J. (2015). The effectiveness of community engagement in public health interventions for disadvantaged groups: A meta-analysis. *BMC Public Health, 15*(129).

Office for Health Improvement and Disparities (OHID). (2022). Community-centred practice: Applying all our health. Guidance. https://www.gov.uk/government/publications/community-centred-practice-applying-all-our-health/community-centred-practice-applying-all-our-health

Orlando, G., Prior, Y., Reeves, N. D., & Vileikyte, L. (2021). Patient and provider perspective of smart wearable technology in diabetic foot ulcer prevention: A systematic review. *Medicina, 57*(12), 1359. https://doi.org/10.3390/medicina57121359.

Parliamentary Under Secretary of State for Public Health and Primary Care. (2019). *Advancing our health: prevention in the 2020s - consultation document.* Presented to Parliament by Command of Her Majesty. https://www.gov.uk/government/consultations/advancing-our-health-prevention-in-the-2020s/advancing-our-health-prevention-in-the-2020s-consultation-document.

Poscia, A., Stojanovic, J., La Milia, D. I., Duplaga, M., Grysztar, M., Moscato, U., Onder, G., Collamati, A., Ricciardi, W., & Magnavita, N. (2018). Interventions targeting loneliness and social isolation among the older people: An updated systematic review. *Experimental Gerontology, 102*, 133–144. https://doi.org/10.1016/j.exger.2017.11.017.

Prior, Y., & Wynn, M. (2023). Digital Innovation in Healthcare. In C. Vasilica, E. Gillaspy, & N. Withnell (Eds.), *Digital skills for nursing studies and practice.* SAGE Publications. https://uk.sagepub.com/en-gb/eur/digital-skills-for-nursing-studies-and-practice/book280020#contents.

Prior, Y., Tennant, A., Tyson, S., Kjeken, I., & Hammond, A. (2018). Measure of activity performance of the hand (MAP-Hand) questionnaire: Linguistic validation, cultural adaptation and psychometric testing in people with rheumatoid arthritis in the UK. *BMC Musculoskeletal Disorders, 19*(1), 275. https://doi.org/10.1186/s12891-018-2177-5.

Prochaska, J. O., & Norcross, J. C. (2002). Stages of change. In J. C. Norcross (Ed.), *Psychotherapy relationships that work: Therapist contributions and responsiveness to patients* (pp. 303–313). Oxford University Press.

Prochaska, J. O., & Velicer, W. F. (1997). The transtheoretical model of health behavior change. *American Journal of Health Promotion, 12*(1), 38–48. https://doi.org/10.4278/0890-1171-12.1.38.

Rachal, J. R. (2002). Andragogy's detectives: A critique of the present and a proposal for the future. *Adult Education Quarterly, 52*(3), 210–227. https://doi.org/10.1177/0741713602052003004.

Restall, G. J., & Egan, M. Y. (2021). Collaborative relationship-focused occupational therapy: Evolving lexicon and practice. *Canadian Journal of Occupational Therapy, 88*(3), 000841742110228. https://doi.org/10.1177/00084174211022889.

Rettke, H., Pretto, M., Spichiger, E., Frei, I. A., & Spirig, R. (2018). Using reflexive thinking to establish rigor in qualitative research. *Nursing Research, 67*(6), 490–497. https://doi.org/10.1097/nnr.0000000000000307.

Ricci, L., Villegente, J., Loyal, D., Ayav, C., Kivits, J., & Rat, A. C. (2022). Tailored patient therapeutic educational interventions: A patient-centred communication model. *Health Expectations: An International Journal of Public Participation in Health Care and Health Policy, 25*(1), 276–289. https://doi.org/10.1111/hex.13377.

Rogers-Shaw, C., Carr-Chellman, D. J., & Choi, J. (2017). Universal design for learning: Guidelines for accessible online instruction. *Adult Learning, 29*(1), 20–31. https://doi.org/10.1177/1045159517735530.

Rosenstock, I. M. (1974). The health belief model and preventive health behavior. *Health Education Monographs, 2*(4), 354–386.

Roski, M., Walkowiak, M., & Nehring, A. (2021). Universal design for learning: The more, the better? *Education Sciences, 11*(4), 164. https://doi.org/10.3390/educsci11040164.

Sandi, C. (2013). Stress and cognition. *Wiley Interdisciplinary Reviews: Cognitive Science, 4*, 245–261. https://doi.org/10.1002/wcs.1222.

Sandlin, J. A. (2005). Andragogy and its discontents: An analysis of andragogy from three critical perspectives. *PAACE Journal of Lifelong Learning, 14*, 25–42.

Schiavone, F., & Ferretti, M. (2021). The futures of healthcare. *Futures, 134*, 102849. https://doi.org/10.1016/j.futures.2021.102849.

Silverman, M. J. (2019). Music therapy for coping self-efficacy in an acute mental health setting: A randomized pilot study. *Community Mental Health Journal, 55*(4), 615–623. https://doi.org/10.1007/s10597-018-0319-8.

Sleight, A. G., & Duker, L. I. S. (2016). Toward a broader role for occupational therapy in supportive oncology care. *American Journal of Occupational Therapy, 70*(4), 7004360030p1. https://doi.org/10.5014/ajot.2016.018101.

St. Clair, R., & Käpplinger, B. (2021). Alley or Autobahn? Assessing 50 years of the andragogical project. *Adult Education Quarterly, 71*(3), 272–289. https://doi.org/10.1177/07417136211027879.

Stephens, A. R., Potter, J. W., Tyser, A. R., et al. (2021). Evaluating the impact of social deprivation on Press Ganey® outpatient medical practice survey scores. *Health Qual Life Outcomes, 19*, 167. https://doi.org/10.1186/s12955-020-01639-y.

Stiggelbout, A. M., Pieterse, A. H., & De Haes, J. C. J. M. (2015). Shared decision making: Concepts, evidence, and practice. *Patient Education and Counseling, 98*(10), 1172–1179. https://doi.org/10.1016/j.pec.2015.06.022.

Tabibian, B. E., Kuhn, E. N., Davis, M. C., & Pritchard, P. R. (2017). Patient expectations and preferences in the spinal surgery clinic. *World Neurosurgery, 106*, 595–601. https://doi.org/10.1016/j.wneu.2017.07.018.

Tuntland, H., Aaslund, M. K., Espehaug, B., Førland, O., & Kjeken, I. (2015). Reablement in community-dwelling older adults: A randomized controlled trial. *BMC Geriatrics, 15*, 145. https://doi.org/10.1186/s12877-015-0142-9.

Vahdat, S., Hamzehgardeshi, L., Hessam, S., & Hamzehgardeshi, Z. (2014). Patient involvement in health care decision making: a review. *Iranian Red Crescent Medical Journal, 16*(1), e12454. https://doi.org/10.5812/ircmj.12454.

Waldman, S. A., & Terzic, A. (2019). Health care evolves from reactive to proactive. *Clinical Pharmacology & Therapeutics, 105*(1), 10–13. https://doi.org/10.1002/cpt.1295.

Wittink, H., & Oosterhaven, J. (2018). Patient education and health literacy. *Musculoskeletal Science and Practice, 38*, 120–127. https://doi.org/10.1016/j.msksp.2018.06.004.

Zhao, Y., & Zhang, J. (2017). Consumer health information seeking in social media: A literature review. *Health Information & Libraries Journal, 34*(4), 268–283. https://doi.org/10.1111/hir.12192.

REFLECTION

1. Describe the four steps discussed to support the shared decision-making process. Discuss the impact of social deprivation on the learner's capacity to engage in this process and the occupational therapists' role in facilitating engagement.

2. Explore the reasons why occupational therapists should take into account factors like health literacy, digital poverty and overall accessibility while shaping the format of their educational interventions and materials.

3. Reflect on the significance of occupational therapists actively participating in an evaluative process for their educational interventions.

23

HEALTH PROMOTION

ERIN E. EPLEY ■ JENICA LEE

Overview

Definitions, history and practical application of health promotion in the field of occupational therapy are presented in this chapter. The central role of the World Health Organization (WHO) in health promotion is explored, and then underlying theories and models of health promotion as well as practical application skills used within the field of occupational therapy are presented. Those skills are then applied to two practice stories to connect theories, models and practice skills and illustrate the application of these at the individual and collective levels. The first practice story addresses secondary and tertiary prevention for a person with chronic disease, while the second practice story addresses all levels of prevention in an underserved population experiencing health disparities.

KEY POINTS

- Health promotion is defined by the World Health Organization (WHO) as 'the process of enabling people to increase control over and improve their health' (WHO, 1986, p. 1).

- Health promotion supports well-being and quality of life for individuals and collectives and drives public policies designed to improve population health.

- While health promotion encompasses primary, secondary and tertiary levels of prevention, its primary focus is on the goals of wellness and improved quality of life.

- Early concepts of well-being from the field of occupational therapy included participation in occupation as a core construct of promoting health (Andersen & Reed, 2017).

- Using occupation-based theories in combination with public and behavioural health theories from other disciplines provides a comprehensive view to better support the development and implementation of evidence-based assessments and interventions in health-promotion practice.

INTRODUCTION

Health promotion is a concept central to public health and policy initiatives and an integral value of the allied health professions. In this chapter, a brief history of health promotion, definition of terms and examination of theories underpinning the movement will be presented. Then the role and work of occupational therapists in providing health promotion for individuals and collectives will be explored through practice stories.

DEFINITION AND TERMS

Health promotion supports well-being and quality of life for individuals and collectives and drives public policies designed to improve population health. The World Health Organization (WHO) defines health promotion as 'the process of enabling people to increase control over, and improve, their health' (WHO, 1986, p. 1). This definition, widely used globally, originates from the *Ottawa Charter*, a health promotion historical document discussed (WHO, 1986). Health promotion, at its core, centres on empowering individuals and collectives to take action toward their own health and well-being (Kumar & Preetha, 2012).

The term *wellness* is often used in discussions of health promotion, though the two are not synonymous. Schell and Gillen (2019) define *wellness* as the 'perception of and responsibility for psychological and physical well-being as these contribute to overall satisfaction with one's life situation' (p. 1215). While health promotion is the overarching process, *wellness* is one of the products of the health promotion movement.

Still another term that must be differentiated is the term *prevention*. While health promotion is a broad construct that includes improving health and empowering individuals and collectives to control their health through organisational and governmental policies and programs, *prevention* is one component of this broad umbrella. According to the *Geneva Charter for Well-Being*, an update to the seminal *Ottawa Charter*, the promotion of health includes health-centred governance, improved health literacy and a push for healthy cities, among other sweeping public health initiatives (WHO, 2021). Health promotion is a complex, multi-layered systems approach and does not simply target disease prevention. Instead, it is a multi-faceted, global initiative designed to benefit individual and population health and quality of life through political, social and environmental policies (WHO, 2021).

The term *quality of life* (QoL), the twin outcome to *wellness* in the health promotion movement, is defined by the WHO as 'an individual's perception of their position in life in the context of the culture and value systems in which they live and in relation to their goals, expectations, standards and concerns' (WHO-QOL Group, 1995, p. 1405) In fact, QoL is often listed as one of the outcomes of occupational therapy, thus again connecting health promotion to the profession (American Occupational Therapy Association (AOTA), 2020b; Pizzi & Richards, 2017). Pizzi and Richards (2017) note that because QoL differs widely among individuals and collectives, its notion must account for perspectives unique to each individual and collective receiving occupational therapy services.

A BRIEF HISTORY OF HEALTH PROMOTION

While the nexus of the health promotion movement is multifactorial and influenced by many disciplines, the WHO has long sought to promote health and well-being across world populations. The WHO held its First International Conference on Health Promotion in 1986, out of which was borne the *Ottawa Charter*, a seminal document in the history of the movement (WHO, 1986). The *Ottawa Charter* elucidated and defined key points and concepts of health promotion, and the movement has continued to gain momentum since the document was created.

Since the *Ottawa Charter* was generated, the WHO has held a number of global conferences on health promotion. The *Geneva Charter for Well-Being* was generated after the 10th Global Conference on Health Promotion held in 2021 (WHO, 2021). The *Geneva Charter for Well-Being* outlines five opportunities for improvement, including economies, public policies, health coverage, digital media impact and planetary concerns (WHO, 2021). In congruence with the definition of health promotion, the *Geneva Charter for Well-Being* ultimately emphasises a mission of empowering people to take control of their health (WHO, 2021). Yet another connection between health promotion and occupational therapy is the mention of the outcome 'meaningful participation' within the *Geneva Charter* (WHO, 2021, p. 2). The Canadian Association of Occupational Therapists (CAOT) has recently adopted the *Canadian Model of Occupational Participation* (CanMOP) (refer to Chapter 11), which aligns with the *Geneva Charter of Well-Being's* emphasis on meaningful participation (Restall & Egan, 2021). According to the CanMOP, occupational therapy's primary outcome is meaningful *occupational* participation, which dovetails seamlessly with the overarching goal of the health promotion movement (Restall & Egan, 2021).

Canada has been a leading nation in the health promotion movement since the publication of *A New Perspective on the Health of Canadians*, also known as the *Lalonde Report* (Tulchinsky, 2018). The *Lalonde Report* was written by Canada's Minister of National Health and Welfare at the time, Marc Lalonde, and highlighted the term health promotion, linking health and QoL to the social determinants of health such as environment, lifestyle and biology (Tulchinsky, 2018). Since then, Canada has demonstrated continued dedication to public health and health promotion, including acting as co-sponsor for the WHO's First International Conference on Health Promotion as noted in the *Ottawa Charter* (WHO, 1986). Health Promotion Canada (HPC), the nationwide organisation to promote population health across Canadian territories, follows the guidance and values of the *Ottawa Charter* (HPC, n.d.).

Another international organisation dedicated to global health promotion is the International Union for Health Promotion and Education (IUHPE), created in 1951 (IUHPE, n.d.). The IUHPE is an international, nongovernmental organisation closely involved with WHO endeavours (IUHPE, n.d.). The IUHPE serves as another information hub for health promotion theory and initiatives and public policy development.

Since the beginnings of health promotion and through the efforts of the WHO and the IUHPE, health promotion movements have burgeoned worldwide. Guided by the tenets of the WHO, nations across the globe have created public health initiatives aimed at population health.

GLOBAL PUBLIC HEALTH AND SOCIAL DETERMINANTS OF HEALTH

Incorporating the WHO definition of health, unchanged since first drafted in 1948, public health may be defined as 'a state of complete physical, mental and social well-being and not merely the absence of disease or infirmity' seen in populations (WHO, 1948, p. 1). Furthermore, Cabaj et al. (2019) note that public health concerns the 'health of populations, has a future orientation, and requires societal/collective action' (p. 341), consistent with the tenets of the *Ottawa* and *Geneva Charters*. Accordingly, the health promotion movement is designed to improve public health, and the two are inextricably connected.

Drawing on a social model of health, global public policies often seek to mitigate the health disparities caused by social determinants of health, such as lack of access to healthcare, employment and education. The WHO identifies social determinants of health as factors influencing health into which people are 'born, grow, work, live, and age, and the wider set of forces and systems shaping the conditions of daily life' (WHO, n.d.b). Due to factors outside of an individual or collective's control, disparities may emerge, impacting overall health and QoL.

Worldwide health promotion initiatives aimed at reducing these disparities are manifold and include the following national and continental examples: Canada's *Healthy Early Years* campaign aimed at improving the health of children birth to age six; the United States' *Healthy People 2030*, a multiobjective framework aimed at national population health; the European Union's *EU4Health Programme 2021–2027*, aimed at health promotion and disease prevention; the African union's *Agenda 2063*, a comprehensive framework dedicated to continental improvement including but not limited to population health; and Australia's *Indigenous Australians' Health Programme* aimed at mitigating the unique racial disparities seen on that continent. The foregoing list, a mere handful of the public health initiatives seen globally, represents differing foci on the health of large populations, smaller groups and inherently, individual health.

HEALTH PROMOTION AND OCCUPATIONAL THERAPY

Through the profession's history and core values, occupational therapy has presciently addressed health-promoting measures since its inception with roots in the curative nature of occupations (Andersen & Reed, 2017). Early concepts of well-being included

TABLE 23.1			
Three Approaches to Prevention			
Level:	Primary	Secondary	Tertiary
Definition:	Prevention of disease, injury and/or impairment in healthy individuals and collectives	Screening for detection of subclinical disease, injury and/or impairment in at-risk individuals and collectives	Management of a diagnosed disease, injury and/or impairment to prevent and/or slow progression and reduce further impairment
Example:	Population: Public health campaigns aimed at prenatal health	Group: Screenings for depression and anxiety in groups experiencing occupational deprivation due to social determinants of health	Individual: Education in medication management and self-management strategies for an individual with diabetes or cardiovascular disease

participation in occupation as a core construct of promoting overall health and QoL, as seen in the early work of Swiss-born psychiatrist Adolf Meyer (1866–1950), who encouraged individuals in asylums to engage in occupations in order to improve their mental health (Andersen & Reed, 2017). American social worker and early pioneer of occupational therapy Eleanor Clark Slagle's (1871–1942) early interest in the curative value of occupations also points to the value the profession has long placed upon the importance of participation in occupation as a key to well-being (Andersen & Reed, 2017).

The World Federation of Occupational Therapy (WFOT) embraced the definition of health promotion put forth by the WHO, stating, 'Occupational therapy is a client-centred health profession concerned with promoting health and well-being through occupation' ((WFOT, 2013, p. 4). The very definition of the field includes the promotion of health. In fact, a majority of nations use this definition of occupational therapy within their member organisations (WFOT, 2013).

The American Occupational Therapy Association (AOTA) utilises the definition of health promotion from the *Ottawa Charter* in their position statement on occupational therapy in the Promotion of Health and Well-Being (AOTA, 2020a). The statement includes a focus on improved health and well-being and is further developed into a set of occupation-based strategies for occupational therapists to promote health for individuals and collectives. Strategies are occupation-based and include primary, secondary and tertiary prevention measures (Table 23.1),

including education on occupation-focused health-promoting topics such as leisure and meal preparation, health management and increasing participation in meaningful occupations (AOTA, 2020a). Ruth Brunyate Wiemer, an American visionary within the field of occupational therapy, advocated in the 1970s for occupational therapy to play a role in all three categories of preventive health (Reitz, 2010). While occupation has long been used in a curative and rehabilitative manner at the secondary and tertiary levels, Wiemer advocated for an occupational therapy role within the primary category of prevention (Reitz, 2010).

According to AOTA, the role of occupational therapy in health promotion is to serve individuals and collectives at risk for occupational participation restrictions with the goal of increasing participation in context (AOTA, 2020a). AOTA embodies the belief that occupational participation is inherently health promoting and labels health promotion and prevention as intervention approaches, with wellness and QoL as outcomes, consistent with WHO values (AOTA, 2020a). Reitz and Graham clarify the role of the profession, stating that 'occupational therapy directed health promotion is the client-centred use of occupations, adaptations to context or alteration of context to maximise [sic] pursuit of health and QOL' (Reitz & Graham, 2019, p. 675).

Canadian Model of Occupational Participation

Building on the WHO focus on supportive mechanisms for health and well-being, the CanMOP emphasises 'collaborative relationship-focused practice' over client-centred practice (Restall & Egan, 2021, p. 222). This shifted focus away from client-at-centre to collaboration and shared power increases congruence with the WHO health promotion initiatives and integration of the concepts of social determinants of health, which inherently explain health and wellness as the result of multiple factors (Restall & Egan, 2021). The CanMOP, a model to guide occupational therapy practice, argues that 'relational elements, along with a focus on valued occupations, are required in collaborative therapy relationships to work in partnership with individuals, families, groups, communities, and populations to promote occupational participation, justice, and equity' (Restall & Egan, 2021, p. 222).

The CanMOP supports a comprehensive and inclusive look at the complex interaction between multiple contextual levels, history, relationships and meaningful occupations with participation at the centre (Restall & Egan, 2021). Using the CanMOP allows an occupational therapist to gain valuable insight into the many factors impacting participation in occupation and, thus, overall wellness and QoL.

UNDERLYING THEORIES OF HEALTH PROMOTION

Using occupation-based theories and public health theories from other disciplines provides a comprehensive view to better support developing and implementing evidence-based assessments and interventions in health-promotion practice. Theories and frameworks also enhance communication and understanding between interdisciplinary teams. A selection of well-researched and prominent health behaviour theories and models that are mainly derived from the social and behavioural sciences are reviewed in this section. These health behaviour theories focus on behaviour change and prevention and can be applied to individuals and collectives (National Cancer Institute (NCI), 2005; Reitz, 2010). In addition, exercising a multi-model approach by systematically applying complementary knowledge from occupational therapy perspectives and health behaviour theories helps direct best practice decisions related to evaluation, interventions and outcomes in health promotion.

Health Belief Model

One of the first theories of health behaviour, the Health Belief Model (HBM), was developed in the 1950s by a group of U.S. Public Health Service social psychologists to explain the failure of people to adopt disease prevention strategies or screening tests for the early detection of disease (NCI, 2005). The HBM focuses on the individuals' perceptions of the health problems, benefits of action and barriers to action and other factors influencing a person's decision to act. There are six constructs of the HBM and the definitions of each construct and its application are described in Table 23.2. (NCI, 2005; Rosenstock, 1974).

The HBM model posits that a person will take action or engage in behaviour change if they believe that they are susceptible to the condition (perceived susceptibility), believe that the condition has serious consequences (perceived severity), believe that taking action would reduce their susceptibility to the condition or its severity (perceived benefits), believe that the benefits outweigh costs of taking action (perceived barriers) are exposed to factors that prompt action and feel confident in their ability to successfully perform an action (self-efficacy) (Champion & Skinner, 2008; NCI, 2005).

HBM remains one of the most widely used frameworks for health behaviour change (Champion & Skinner, 2008) and has been applied to a broad range of populations and health behaviours. For example, the HBM has been used to establish educational programs for individuals and collectives to prevent different diseases and their complications, including heart failure (Baghianimoghadam et al., 2013), type-2 diabetes (Shabibi et al., 2017), medication adherence with tuberculosis and HIV/AIDS (Munro et al., 2007), screening with breast and colorectal cancer (Champion & Skinner, 2008), physical activity for fall prevention with older adults (Punlomso et al., 2020) and most recently to understand COVID-19 prevention behaviour (Limbu et al., 2022; Zewdie et al., 2022).

While empirical evidence supports the HBM as moderately effective in predicting health-related behaviours (Abraham & Sheeran, 2015), the model also has limitations. For example, the HBM does not consider that habitual behaviours (e.g. smoking and wearing a seatbelt) may become independent of conscious

TABLE 23.2

Health Belief Model Constructs and Definitions

Concept	Definition
Perceived susceptibility	Individual's beliefs of their risks of acquiring an illness or disease.
	Example: People with hypertension may not follow a prescribed treatment because they are not experiencing any symptoms.
Perceived severity	Individual's beliefs about the seriousness of a condition and its consequences.
	Example: They must understand that hypertension can lead to strokes and heart attacks.
Perceived benefits	Individual's beliefs about the effectiveness of various actions available to reduce or cure the threat of illness or disease.
	Example: Taking prescribed medications or following a weight-loss program will reduce the risks.
Perceived barriers	Individual's beliefs of the obstacles to performing a recommended action (e.g. cost, time, discrimination, SES, attitudes, culture).
	Example: Taking prescribed medications will not have side effects.
Cues to action	Factors that activate 'readiness to change'. Cues can be internal (e.g. chest pains, wheezing, etc.) or external (e.g. advice from others, illness of a family member, newspaper article, etc.).
	Example: A recent family member who had a stroke or the use of reminder strategies may motivate them to adhere to the prescribed treatment.
Self-efficacy	Individuals' level of confidence in their ability to act.
	Example: Setting short-term goals and action plans to build confidence to better adhere to weight loss plans or medications management.

Adapted from National Cancer Institute (NCI). (2005). Theory at a Glance: A guide for health promotion practice. U.S. Department of Health and Human Services National Institutes of Health.

health-related decision-making processes. The HBM also does not consider behaviours performed for non-health-related reasons, such as social acceptability. Additionally, it does not account for economic or environmental factors that may prohibit or promote the recommended action (Abraham & Sheeran, 2015; Champion & Skinner, 2008). Despite these limitations, the health belief model framework has good potential to assist in designing and developing health promotion or disease prevention programs and can be combined with other theories or models (NCI, 2005; Reitz, 2010).

Transtheoretical Model

Developed in the late 1970s by Prochaska and DiClemente, The Transtheoretical Model (TTM), also called the Stages of Change Model, explains the stages people experience as they engage in behaviour change to maximise health and well-being (Reitz, 2010). The model emphasises that behaviour change occurs dynamically through a cyclical process and that individuals move through six stages of change: pre-contemplation, contemplation, preparation, action, maintenance and termination (Table 23.3). Termination was not part of the original model, and because this stage is difficult to achieve, it is not frequently included in the stages of

change. The TTM recognises that behaviour change is not a discrete event and takes time to evolve. Thus, an individual may enter the change process at any stage, relapse to an earlier stage and begin the process again. For each stage of change, different intervention strategies are most effective at progressing the person to the next stage of change and, subsequently, through the model to maintenance, the ideal stage of behaviour. (NCI, 2005; Prochaska et al., 2015; Reitz, 2010).

The TTM also includes the following factors that impact an individual's stage progression: processes of change, decisional balance and self-efficacy ((Prochaska et al., 2015). Ten processes of change have been identified, with some deemed more relevant to a specific stage of change than others (Prochaska et al., 2015; Table 23.4). An empirical study by Prochaska and colleagues (1992), suggests that in early stages, individuals apply cognitive, affective and evaluative processes to progress through the stages. In later stages, individuals rely more on commitments, conditioning, contingencies, environmental controls and support for moving towards maintenance or termination.

Decisional balance considers the advantages and disadvantages of changing behaviours and validly predicts progression through the different stages of change.

TABLE 23.3

The Transtheoretical Model Stages of Change, Definitions and Strategies

Stage	Definition	Potential Change Strategies
Precontemplation	Unaware of the need to change and thus has no intention to start the healthy behaviour within the next 6 months.	■ Increase awareness of the need for change
Contemplation	Can identify and acknowledge a problem. They try to understand the problem and are motivated to engage in behaviour change to fix the problem in the next 6 months.	■ Resolve ambivalence ■ Assist to choose change ■ Encourage making specific plans
Preparation	Intends to take action within the next thirty days and has taken some behavioural steps in this direction (e.g. acquiring needed resources or making public statements about intention to change).	■ Assist with developing and implementing concrete action plans ■ Help set goals
Action	Has changed behaviour for less than 6 months. This stage requires time, energy and commitment.	■ Provide feedback ■ Assist with problem-solving, social support and reinforcement
Maintenance	Has changed behaviour for more than 6 months.	■ Assist with coping, providing reminders, finding alternatives and avoiding slips/relapses (as applicable)
Termination	Behaviour change is so well integrated that there is minimal chance of relapse. However, since this is rarely reached and people tend to stay in the maintenance stage, this stage is often not considered in health promotion programs.	

Adapted from National Cancer Institute (NCI). (2005). Theory at a Glance: A guide for health promotion practice. U.S. Department of Health and Human Services National Institutes of Health.

TABLE 23.4

Transtheoretical Model: Processes of Change Descriptions

Processes of Change	Definition
Consciousness raising	Increase awareness of healthy behaviour (i.e., feedback)
Dramatic relief	Emotional arousal about health behaviour, whether positive or negative arousal
Self-re-evaluation	A person realising that the behaviour change is an important part of their identity
Environmental re-evaluation	A person realising the negative or positive impact of the unhealthy behaviour on their social and/ or physical environment
Self-liberation	Making a firm commitment to change
Helping relationships	Seeking and using social support for healthy behaviour change
Counterconditioning	Substitution of healthier alternative behaviour change and decreasing the rewards of the unhealthy behaviour
Reinforcement management	Increasing the rewards for positive behaviour change and decreasing the rewards for the unhealthy behaviour
Stimulus control	Incorporating reminders and cues to support healthy behaviour and removing reminders or cues that encourage unhealthy behaviour
Social liberation	Environmental opportunities that exist to show society is supportive of the healthy behaviour

Individuals tend to adopt new behaviour when the benefits outweigh the negatives. The further an individual progresses through the stages the more significant the advantages of change are valued over the disadvantages (Grimley et al., 1993; Prochaska et al., 2015). Drawing from Bandura's self-efficacy theory (1982), self-efficacy is also integrated as an essential construct in the TTM. Self-efficacy refers to the level of confidence a person has in achieving and maintaining a positive change despite the temptation to relapse. Confidence typically increases linearly across the stages of change (Liu et al., 2018; Prochaska et al., 2015).

The TTM has been extensively applied to smoking cessation and other addictive behaviours, including alcohol abuse and illicit drug use (Felicissimo et al., 2014; Rios et al., 2019). In addition, the TTM has been used to guide interventions to address other problematic behaviours, including stress management, medication compliance, exercise participation, weight control and chronic pain management (Bridle et al., 2005; Hashemzadeh et al., 2019; Prochaska et al., 2015). While some studies point out some weaknesses of TTM effectiveness in various healthcare contexts, such as quitting smoking, diet intervention in diabetic patients and the call for additional basic and applied research to validate its use (Champion & Skinner, 2008; Hashemzadeh et al., 2019; Prochaska et al., 2015); the TTM can be clinically useful for practitioners to help identify what stage of change someone may be in and then intentionally respond accordingly to promote positive behaviour change and promote health.

Social Cognitive Theory

In contrast to the HBM and TTM, which are applied at an individual level, the Social Cognitive Theory (SCT) focuses on the interpersonal level (NCI, 2005). According to the NCI, at the interpersonal level, health behaviour theories posit that individuals exist within and are influenced by a social environment. The social environment includes family members, co-workers, friends, health professionals and others, and their opinions and attitudes can influence the individual's thoughts and behaviours and thereby impact health (NCI, 2005).

The SCT was first known as Social Learning Theory (SLT) as its learning principles were first operationalised by Albert Bandura (1977). It was renamed Social Cognitive Theory in 1986 after developing and integrating concepts from cognitive psychology (Bandura & National Institute of Mental Health, 1986). The SCT emphasises social influences and external and internal social reinforcement on behaviour. The SCT posits that human behaviour is the product of the dynamic interplay of the person, environment and behaviour. SCT aims to explain how individuals regulate their behaviour through control and reinforcement to achieve goal-directed behaviour that can be maintained over time. The SCT also stresses the 'human capacity for collective action' (McAlister et al., 2008, p. 170). This fosters individuals to work together in organisations and social systems to achieve changes that benefit the entire group. The SCT has six primary constructs; its definitions and potential strategies are summarised in Table 23.5. The most important construct of the theory is self-efficacy, which is considered a major motivator of action and mediator and a fundamental requirement for behaviour change. 'Self-efficacy' refers to an individual's confidence in their capability to take a specific action or to overcome barriers to engaging in a specific behaviour (Bandura, 2004).

The SCT provides a comprehensive and well-supported conceptual framework for understanding factors that influence human behaviour and processes through which learning occurs, offering insight into a wide variety of health-related issues. There is evidence to support that the SCT is an adequate and practical theoretical framework to guide the design, implementation and evaluation of health intervention programs for some chronic health conditions, including obesity, type II diabetes, cancer, heart conditions, arthritis and asthma (Sebastian et al., 2021; Stacey et al., 2015; Tougas et al., 2015).

As healthcare providers, occupational therapists need to understand how people learn about their health conditions and how their perceptions and attitudes impact their motivation to make therapeutic changes. Therefore, when working on health promotion and wellness goals, occupational therapists can draw from occupation-based theories and behavioural health theories to understand what motivates the individual, family, group, community and population to stop their poor habits, adopt better lifestyle routines or learn more effective self-management strategies (Reitz, 2010).

APPLYING PROFESSIONAL REASONING

When practitioners begin planning health promotion interventions or health behaviour change, they need to draw from theory to guide their decisions and ensure that appropriate design, measures and procedures are chosen for the health problem, organisation, population or intervention. Different theoretical

TABLE 23.5		
Social Cognitive Theory		
Construct	Definition	Potential Change Strategies
Reciprocal determinism	The dynamic interaction of the person, behaviour and the environment in which the behaviour is performed.	■ Consider multiple ways to promote behaviour change, including adapting to the environment or influencing personal attitudes.
Behavioural capability	Person's ability to perform a given behaviour through knowledge and skills.	■ Promote mastery learning through skills training.
Expectations	Anticipated consequences of a person's behaviour.	■ Model positive outcomes of healthy behaviour.
Self-efficacy	Confidence in their ability to successfully perform a behaviour.	■ Approach behaviour change in small steps (i.e. setting incremental goals). ■ Use formal contracts with specified goals and rewards. ■ Provide feedback from self-monitoring and record keeping.
Observational Learning (Modelling)	Process whereby people learn the behaviour through witnessing and observing others.	■ Offer credible role models.
Reinforcements	Internal or external responses to a person's behaviour that impact the likelihood of continuing or discontinuing the behaviour.	■ Promote self-initiated rewards and incentives.

Adapted from National Cancer Institute (NCI). (2005). Theory at a Glance: A guide for health promotion practice. U.S. Department of Health and Human Services National Institutes of Health.

frameworks are called upon depending on the unit of practice and the type of health behaviour or issue. Practitioners may find that using multiple theories to address a problem is often needed and produces a more substantial impact, especially when developing comprehensive health promotion programs. The ability to apply theories of health behaviour is one of the most critical skills needed in designing health promotion programs. The PRECEDE-PROCEED planning model can facilitate the application of theory as it provides a step-by-step guide on integrating multiple theories and addressing health problems (Gielen et al., 2015; NCI, 2005). An overview of the model is presented in the next section.

PRECEDE-PROCEED Model

The PRECEDE-PROCEED model (PPM) was first developed in the 1970s by Green and colleagues (1980), and it aims to provide a structure for applying theories and concepts systematically for planning and evaluating health behaviour change programs. The first part of the framework, PRECEDE, provides a structure for planning targeted and focused public health programs. The acronym stands for

Predisposing, Reinforcing and Enabling Constructs in Educational/Environmental Diagnosis and Evaluation (Gielen et al., 2015). The second part of the framework, PROCEED, provides the structure for implementing and evaluating the public health program. Its acronym stands for Policy, Regulatory, Organisational Constructions in Educational and Environmental Development (Gielen et al., 2015). The model strongly emphasises the importance of active participation from the intended audience while defining their problems, establishing their goals and developing solutions (Gielen et al., 2015). Audience involvement is important to best capture their issues and ideas about resolving them and build community ownership of the interventions (Gielen et al., 2015; Green & Kreuter, 2005).

The PPM consists of a total of eight phases. PRECEDE has four assessment and planning phases to guide the audience in selecting what problem to address, examining its underlying causes and planning an intervention. PROCEED, on the other hand, includes four implementation and evaluation phases. Each planning step and touch points for applying health behaviour theories are summarised

TABLE 23.6
PRECEDE-PROCEED Model Phases

	Phase/Planning Step	Function
PRECEDE phases	Phase 1: Social assessment and situational analysis	Assess the social problems and needs of a given population and identify goals. Planners can use multiple data collection activities including, but not limited to interviews with key stakeholders, focus groups with community members, observations and surveys.
	Phase 2: Epidemiological assessment	Assess the health determinants (e.g. genetics, behaviour and environment) impact on the identified problem(s) and set priorities and goals. Planners can conduct secondary data analysis using existing data sources (e.g. vital statistics, state and national health surveys, etc.). The SCT can be useful to apply at this stage because of the interaction between individuals and their environment.
	Phase 3: Educational and ecological assessment	Analyse behavioural and environmental determinants (determined in Phase 2) that predispose, reinforce and enable the behaviours and lifestyles that are identified. – **Predisposing factors** provide motivation or rationale for the behaviour (i.e. knowledge, attitudes, beliefs, attitudes). Individual-level theories (e.g. HBM and TTM) are most appropriate for addressing these factors. – **Reinforcing factors** give the reward or incentive to promote the repetition of a behaviour. Interpersonal-level theories (e.g. SCT) are most appropriate for reinforcing factors. – **Enabling factors** promote motivation, including personal skills, assets and community resources. Therefore, community-level theories (e.g. Diffusion of Innovation) are most appropriate for enabling factors.
	Phase 4: Administrative/policy assessment	Identify resources, organisational barriers and facilitators and policies needed for program implementation. This will inform mapping of the program's components or interventions with the priority determinants previously identified. Again, community-level theories would be appropriate in this phase.
PROCEED phases	Phase 5: Implementation	Setting up and carrying out the planned intervention.
	Phase 6: Process Evaluation	Determines the extent to which the program was implemented according to protocol. Includes evaluations of community reaction to the program as well as staff performance.
	Phase 7: Impact Evaluation	Assesses the impact of the program on the designated target behaviours. This includes examining factors from Phase 3 (i.e. predisposing, enabling and reinforcing factors).
	Phase 8. Outcomes Evaluation	Determines the effect of the program on health and QoL indicators.

in Table 23.6 (Gielen et al., 2015; NCI, 2005; Reitz, 2010).

The PPM is a widely used planning model and has been successfully applied across a range of health promotion programs, including symptom or disease management (e.g. menopause, diabetes, hypertension and asthma), health behaviour promotion (e.g. diet, physical activity and sleep), psychological health (e.g. suicide and stress), improvement in QoL and health screenings (e.g. dental, cancer and cystic fibrosis) (Kim et al., 2022; Saulle et al., 2020). In addition, there is strong evidence to support the PPM to enhance the

TABLE 23.7
Occupational Therapy Preventative Interventions in a Hypothetical LGBTQ+ Clinic

Primary	Secondary	Tertiary
Movement groups to encourage maintenance of a healthy weight and prevention of cardiovascular disease (Lavie et al., 2019)	Motivational interviewing to encourage behaviour-change aimed at reducing substance use (Brown et al., 2015)	Relaxation methods such as movement and breathwork for individuals experiencing anxiety disorders (Jerath et al., 2015)

BOX 23.1
DIABETES

Diabetes mellitus type two (TD2) is a significant public health problem worldwide, and it continues to increase in incidence and prevalence as one of the leading causes of human suffering and deaths (Liu et al., 2020). It was estimated that the prevalence of diabetes in adults aged 18–99 years was 8.4% in 2017 and is expected to increase to 9.9% by 2045 (Cho et al., 2018). The worldwide increase in TD2 has primarily been driven by global ageing, economic growth, rapid urbanisation and nutritional transitions in different income-level countries (Liu et al., 2020). In diabetes, as with many chronic diseases, much of the potential to maintain health and prevent secondary complications stems from a person's ability to consistently carry out self-management activities according to the prescribed diabetes management regimen (e.g. dietary recommendations, self-monitoring and medication adherence). However, these activities are often experienced as burdensome and ongoing adherence is a challenge (Pyatak et al., 2018; Shen & Shen, 2019).

As a result of the importance of habits and routines in managing TD2, occupational therapy is increasingly being incorporated into intervention models for preventing and managing chronic disease (O'Toole et al., 2013; Pyatak et al., 2018). In a recent scoping review on habits and health promotion, Epley et al. (2021) report that habits, as one of the human performance patterns outlined in American Occupational Therapy Association's practice framework (American Occupational Therapy Association, 2020a), are of particular relevance to occupational therapy in chronic disease prevention, self-management of disease and health promotion. Interprofessional care is also considered best practice for those with TD2, and occupational therapists can play a vital role on an interprofessional team in diabetes education and self-management for both diagnosed individuals and those at risk of acquiring the disease (Feldhacker and Doll, 2020).

The expertise of occupational therapists lies in activity analysis: analysing an occupation to determine the demands, which may include space, time, material, physical, cognitive and social components. Once an occupation is deconstructed, practitioners can then observe a person performing the occupation and understand the specific barriers to participation. Using CanMOP, an occupational therapy practitioner considers occupational participation as central and uses the concepts of collaborative relationship-focused practice to consider what is meaningful and valuable to an individual (Restall & Egan, 2021). For example, consider a person who has difficulty taking insulin consistently due to a fear of injections; an occupational therapy practitioner might address this by offering relaxation strategies and addressing hypersensitivity to pain (Pyatak et al., 2018). The occupational therapist might also consider adapting the health management occupation by using an injection port, icing the site prior to injection and suggesting a change of environment to facilitate calm and relaxation during injection (Pyatak et al., 2018).

Feldhacker and Doll (2020) recommend further ways an occupational therapist can support a person with T2D, including providing health education and self-management techniques in consideration of a person's individual goals and social supports, encouraging self-efficacy in educating family and friends about the condition and providing strategies to promote emotional well-being and reduce anxiety. Applying the Health Belief Model and Social Cognitive Theory, occupational therapists might address a person's beliefs about the severity of the disease and therefore increase knowledge, self-efficacy and problem-solving skills in their ability to manage their T2D (Champion & Skinner et al., 2008; McAlister et al., 2008).

---

evaluation of health problems, health behaviours and desired changes (Gielen et al., 2015).

Two practice stories are presented in Boxes 23.1 and 23.2 that illustrate the application of health promotion by occupational therapists.

CONCLUSION

Health promotion is a global movement, informed and driven by the World Health Organization, aimed at supporting well-being and QoL of individuals and collectives. The field of occupational therapy has

long understood the importance of participation in meaningful occupation as critical to achieving a state of health and well-being (Hammell, 2020). Using primary, secondary and tertiary levels of prevention, occupational therapists can play a vital role in health promotion. Drawing from a combination of occupation-based models, health behaviour theories and frameworks and evidence-based interventions, occupational therapists are poised to contribute to the use of participation in meaningful occupation to promote health and wellness for individuals and collectives.

BOX 23.2
UNDERSERVED POPULATION

Health promotion serves as an invaluable framework for improving the health and well-being of underserved groups. Individuals identifying with the LGBTQ+ community (those identifying as lesbian, gay, bisexual, transgender, queer or those questioning their gender) are often marginalised and subject to unique barriers to healthcare (WHO, n.d.a). In the United States, the National Institute on Minority Health and Health Disparities (NIMHD) has identified the LGBTQ+ community as a health disparity population (NIMHD, 2016).

Research indicates that this group is subject to inequalities of care and less favourable outcomes in six main areas: sexually transmitted infections (STIs), violence, substance abuse, mental health conditions, eating disorders and heart disease (Medina-Martinez et al., 2021). These health inequities, in conjunction with other injustices felt by the LGBTQ+ population can lead to a decreased sense of well-being, one of the target outcomes of a health promotion approach (Semlyen et al., 2016).

In a community clinic for LGBTQ+ where an interprofessional team works in concert to address the health disparities unique to this population; each profession offers a unique lens. To begin, the multidisciplinary healthcare team uses the PRECEDE-PROCEED framework to guide the assessment approach to identify and prioritise the needs of this group, leading to the development and delivery of tailored interventions designed to address prevention from primary, secondary and tertiary levels, based upon the needs identified. Honing the mental health needs of the LGBTQ+ community, the PRECEDE phases 1–4 guide the healthcare team to utilise the most effective strategies to identify the socio-environmental and behavioural factors that impact the mental health of this vulnerable population. LGBTQ+ people experience high stress levels and stigma related to managing their sexual orientation. Thus, understanding their life experiences (e.g. experiences of prejudice, fear of rejection from family members and friends, internalised homophobia, etc.) is essential to inform the development of relevant interventions (Gielen et al., 2015; Kalra et al., 2012). In addition, assessing the clinic's resources and the community's surrounding support provides a comprehensive assessment and further contributes to impactful, evidence-based interventions (Gielen et al., 2015).

In the community clinic, doctors and nurses provide early detection and medical management of STIs, cancer and heart disease and refer individuals to a social worker or psychiatrist, who respectively screen and diagnose mental illness in this at-risk population. Occupational therapists serve a unique role on the interdisciplinary team, addressing the common health conditions experienced by the LGBTQ+ community from an occupational participation standpoint. Guided by the CanMOP, therapists holistically examine the many contributing factors to the disparities experienced by the LGBTQ+ community, considering factors at the micro, macro and meso levels that may expand or limit occupational participation (Egan & Restall, 2022). The CanMOP supports a focus on occupational participation in meaningful contexts, ensuring that valued occupations occur in their physical and social contexts, making CanMOP an ideal model for a community clinic setting (Egan & Restall, 2022). Importantly, CanMOP encourages occupational therapists to take the unique perspective of each individual and collective to ensure that their wishes and needs are met in the therapeutic process (Egan & Restall, 2022).

Occupational therapists also evaluate and address the habits, routines and roles of the people attending the clinic and promote health at all levels of prevention – primary, secondary and tertiary (Table 23.7). Practitioners assess meaningful occupations using assessments to tap into motivation and then promote participation in these occupations through leisure and social groups. In addition, occupational therapists target risk behaviours and mental health symptoms through such techniques as motivational interviewing, cognitive behavioural approach and relaxation techniques (e.g., guided meditation and abdominal breathing) (Brown & Stoffel, 2019). Health management and medication management for individuals with mental illness is yet another area where occupational therapists intervene with this underserved population.

From a physical rehabilitation model perspective, occupational therapists address heart disease and cancer through the occupation of health management strategies via education and promotion of safe sex, healthy eating and physical activity. In addition, occupational therapists promote social participation and physical well-being to the LGBTQ+ community, thus reducing health disparity and promoting public health within this marginalised group. Using models, theories and frameworks, occupational therapists play an integral part in the multidisciplinary team serving LGBTQ+ in the community clinic.

REFERENCES

Abraham, C., & Sheeran, P. (2015). The health belief model. In M. Conner & P. Norman (Eds.), *Predicting health behavior* (2nd ed., pp. 28–80). Open University Press.

American Occupational Therapy Association. (2020a). Occupational therapy in the promotion of health and well-being. *American Journal of Occupational Therapy, 74*(3), 7403420010p1–7403420010p14. https://doi.org/10.5014/ajot.2020.743003.

American Occupational Therapy Association. (2020b). Occupational therapy practice framework: Domain and process (4th ed.). *American Journal of Occupational Therapy, 74*(Suppl. 2), 7412410010p1–7412410010p87. https://doi.org/10.5014/ajot.2020.74S2001.

Andersen, L. T., & Reed, K. (2017). *The history of occupational therapy: The first century.* SLACK.

Baghianimoghadam, M. H., Shogafard, G., Sanati, H. R., Baghianimoghadam, B., Mazloomy, S. S., & Askarshahi, M. (2013). Application of the health belief model in promotion of self-care in heart failure patients. *Acta Medica Iranica, 51*(1), 52–58.

Bandura, A. (1977). *Social learning theory.* Prentice-Hall.

Bandura, A. (1982). Self-efficacy mechanism in human agency. *American Psychologist, 37*(2), 122–147. https://doi.org/10.1037/0003-066X.37.2.122.

Bandura, A. (2004). Health promotion by social cognitive means. *Health Education Behavior, 31*, 143–164.

Bandura, A., & National Institute of Mental Health. (1986). *Social foundations of thought and action: A social cognitive theory.* Prentice-Hall.

Bridle, C., Riemsma, R. P., Pattenden, J., Sowden, A. J., Mather, L., Watt, I. S., & Walker, A. (2005). Systematic review of the effectiveness of health behavior interventions based on the transtheoretical model. *Psychology & Health, 20*(3), 283–301. https://doi.org/10.1080/08870440512331333997.

Brown, C., & Stoffel, V. C. (2019). Appendix C: Index of interventions. In C. Brown & V. Stoffel C. (Eds.), *Occupational therapy in mental health: A vision for participation* (2nd ed., pp. 946–951). F. A. Davis.

Brown, R. A., Abrantes, A. M., Minami, H., Prince, M. A., Bloom, E. L., Apodaca, T. R., Strong, D. R., Picotte, D. M., Monti, P. M., MacPherson, L., Matsko, S. V., & Hunt, J. I. (2015). Motivational interviewing to reduce substance use in adolescents with psychiatric comorbidity. *Journal of Substance Abuse Treatment, 59*, 20–29. https://doi.org/10.1016/j.jsat.2015.06.016.

Cabaj, J. L., Musto, R., & Ghali, W. A. (2019). Public health: Who, what, and why? *Canadian Journal of Public Health, 110*, 340–343. https://doi.org/10.17269/s41997-019-00207-2.

Champion, V. L., & Skinner, C. S. (2008). The health belief model. In K. Glanz, B. K. Rimer, & K. Viswanath (Eds.), *Health behaviour and health education: Theory, research, and practice* (pp. 45–65). Jossey-Bass.

Cho, N. H., Shaw, J. E., Karuranga, S., Huang, Y., da Rocha Fernandes, J. D., Ohlrogge, A. W., & Malanda, B. (2018). IDF Diabetes Atlas: Global estimates of diabetes prevalence for 2017 and projections for 2045. *Diabetes Research and Clinical Practice, 138*, 271–281. https://doi.org/10.1016/j.diabres.2018.02.023.

Egan, M., & Restall, G. (2022). The Canadian model of occupational participation. In M. Egan & G. Restall (Eds.), *Promoting occupational participation: Collaborative relationship-focused occupational therapy* (pp. 73–95). Canadian Association of Occupational Therapists.

Epley, E., Wolske, J., Lee, J., Mirza, M., & Fisher, G. (2021). Habits and health promotion in occupational therapy: A scoping review. *Annals of International Occupational Therapy, 4*(4), 269–277. https://doi.org/10.3928/24761222-20210921-04.

Feldhacker, D. R., & Doll, J. D. (2020). An interprofessional approach to diabetes management in primary care for older adults. *SIS Quarterly Practice Connections, 5*(1), 23–26.

Felicíssimo, F. B., de Barros, V. V., Pereira, S. M., Rocha, N. Q., & Lourenço, L. M. (2014). A systematic review of the transtheoretical model of behaviour change and alcohol use. *Psychologica, 57*(1), 9–24.

Gielen, A. C., McDonald, E. M., Gary, T. L., & Bone, L. R. (2015). Using the PRECEDE-PROCEED model to apply health behavior theories. In K. Glanz, B. K. Rimer, & K. Viswanath (Eds.), *Health behavior and health education: Theory, research, and practice* (pp. 407–433). Jossey-Bass.

Green, L., & Kreuter, M. (2005). *Health program planning: An educational and ecological approach* (4th ed.). McGraw Hill.

Green, L. W., Kreuter, M. W., Deeds, S. G., & Partridge, K. B. (1980). *Health education planning: A diagnostic approach* (4th ed.). Mayfield.

Grimley, D. M., Riley, G. E., Bellis, J. M., & Prochaska, J. O. (1993). Assessing the stages of change and decision-making for contraceptive use for the prevention of pregnancy, sexually transmitted diseases, and acquired immunodeficiency syndrome. *Health Education Quarterly, 20*(4), 455–470. http://www.jstor.org/stable/45049493.

Hammell, K. W. (2020). Action on the social determinants of health: Advancing occupational equity and occupational rights. *Cadernos Brasileiros de Terapia Ocupacional, 28*(1), 378–400. https://doi.org/10.4322/2526-8910.ctoARF2052.

Hashemzadeh, M., Rahimi, A., Zare-Farashbandi, F., Alavi-Naeini, A. M., & Daei, A. (2019). Transtheoretical model of health behavioural change: A systematic review. *Iranian Journal of Nursing and Midwifery Research, 24*(2), 83–90. https://doi.org/10.4103/ijnmr.IJNMR_94_17.

Health Promotion Canada. (n.d.). *Our history.* Retrieved March 31, 2023, from https://www.healthpromotioncanada.ca/about-us/our-history/.

International Union for Health Promotion and Education. (n.d.). *The IUHPE at a glance: History.* Retrieved March 31, 2023, from https://www.iuhpe.org/index.php/en/iuhpe-at-a-glance.

Jerath, R., Crawford, M. W., Barnes, V. A., & Harden, K. (2015). Self-regulation of breathing as a primary treatment for anxiety. *Applied Psychophysiology and Biofeedback, 40*(2), 107–115. https://doi.org/10.1007/s10484-015-9279-8.

Kalra, G., Christodoulou, G., Jenkins, R., Tsipas, V., Christodoulou, N., Lecic-Tosevski, D., Mezzich, J., Bhugra, D., & European Psychiatry Association. (2012). Mental health promotion: Guidance and strategies. *European Psychiatry: The Journal of the Association of European Psychiatrists, 27*(2), 81–86. https://doi.org/10.1016/j.eurpsy.2011.10.001.

Kim, J., Jang, J., Kim, B., & Lee, K. H. (2022). Effect of the PRECEDE-PROCEED model on health programs: A systematic review and meta-analysis. *Systematic Reviews, 11*(1), 213. https://doi.org/10.1186/s13643-022-02092-2.

Kumar, S., & Preetha, G. (2012). Health promotion: An effective tool for global health. *Indian Journal of Community Medicine: Official Publication of Indian Association of Preventive & Social Medicine, 37*(1), 5–12. https://doi.org/10.4103/0970-0218.94009.

Lavie, C. J., Ozemek, C., Carbone, S., Katzmarzyk, P. T., & Blair, S. N. (2019). Sedentary behaviour, exercise, and cardiovascular health. *Circulation Research, 124*(5), 799–815. https://doi.org/10.1161/CIRCRESAHA.118.312669.

Limbu, Y. B., Gautam, R. K., & Pham, L. (2022). The health belief model applied to COVID-19 vaccine hesitancy: A systematic review. *Vaccines, 10*(6), 973. https://doi.org/10.3390/vaccines10060973.

Liu, J., Ren, Z. H., Qiang, H., Wu, J., Shen, M., Zhang, L., & Lyu, J. (2020). Trends in the incidence of diabetes mellitus: Results from the Global Burden of Disease Study 2017 and implications for diabetes mellitus prevention. *BMC Public Health, 20*(1), 1415. https://doi.org/10.1186/s12889-020-09502-x.

Liu, K. T., Kueh, Y. C., Arifin, W. N., Kim, Y., & Kuan, G. (2018). Application of transtheoretical model on behavioural changes, and amount of physical activity among university's students. *Frontiers in Psychology, 9*, 2402. https://doi.org/10.3389/fpsyg.2018.02402.

McAlister, A. L., Perry, C. L., & Parcel, G. S. (2008). How individuals, environments, and health behaviors interact: Social cognitive theory. In K. Glanz, B. K. Rimer, & K. Viswanath (Eds.), *Health behavior and health education: Theory, research, and practice* (pp. 169–188). Jossey-Bass.

Medina-Martínez, J., Saus-Ortega, C., Sánchez-Lorente, M. M., Sosa-Palanca, E. M., García-Martínez, P., & Mármol-López, M. I. (2021). Health inequities in LGBT people and nursing interventions to reduce them: A systematic review. *International Journal of Environmental Research and Public Health, 18*(22), 11801. https://doi.org/10.3390/ijerph182211801.

Munro, S., Lewin, S., Swart, T., & Volmink, J. (2007). A review of health behaviour theories: How useful are these for developing interventions to promote long-term medication adherence for TB and HIV/AIDS? *BMC Public Health, 7*, 104. https://doi.org/10.1186/1471-2458-7-104.

National Cancer Institute (NCI). (2005). *Theory at a glance: A guide for health promotion practice* (2nd ed.). National Institutes of Health. Retrieved March 28, 2023, from https://cancercontrol.cancer.gov/sites/default/files/2020-06/theory.pdf.

National Institute on Minority Health and Health Disparities. (2016). *Director's message: Sexual and gender minorities formally designated as a health disparity population for research purposes.* Retrieved March 31, 2023, from https://www.nimhd.nih.gov/about/directors-corner/messages/message_10-06-16.html.

O'Toole, L., Connolly, D., & Smith, S. (2013). Impact of an occupation-based self-management programme on chronic disease management. *Australian Occupational Therapy Journal, 60*(1), 30–38. https://doi.org/10.1111/1440-1630.12008.

Pizzi, M. A., & Richards, L. G. (2017). Promoting health, well-being, and quality of life in occupational therapy: A commitment to a paradigm shift for the next 100 years. *American Journal of Occupational Therapy, 71*(4), 7104170010p1–7104170010p5. https://doi.org/10.5014/ajot.2017.028456.

Prochaska, J. O., DiClemente, C. C., & Norcross, J. C. (1992). In search of how people change. Applications to addictive behaviours. *The American Psychologist, 47*(9), 1102–1114. https://doi.org/10.1037/0003-066x.47.9.1102.

Prochaska, J. O., Redding, C. A., & Evers, K. E. (2015). The transtheoretical model and stages of change. In K. Glanz, B. K. Rimer, & K. V. Viswanath (Eds.), *Health behaviour: Theory, research, and practice* (pp. 125–148). Jossey-Bass/Wiley.

Punlomso, S., Srimuang, P., & Tudpor, K. (2020). Fall prevention by Otago exercise program based on health belief model in community-dwelling older persons. *Indian Journal of Physiotherapy & Occupational Therapy Print, 14*(1), 245–252. https://doi.org/10.37506/ijpot.v14i1.3478.

Pyatak, E. A., Carandang, K., Vigen, C. L. P., Blanchard, J., Diaz, J., Concha-Chavez, A., Sequeira, P. A., Wood, J. R., Whittemore, R., Spruijt-Metz, D., & Peters, A. L. (2018). Occupational therapy intervention improves glycemic control and quality of life among young adults with diabetes: The Resilient, Empowered, Active Living with Diabetes (REAL Diabetes) randomised controlled trial. *Diabetes Care, 41*(4), 696–704. https://doi.org/10.2337/dc17-1634.

Reitz, S. M. (2010). Historical and philosophical perspectives of occupational therapy's role in health promotion. In M. E. Scaffa, S. M. Reitz, & M. A. Pizzi (Eds.), *Occupational therapy in the promotion of health and wellness* (pp. 1–15). F. A. Davis.

Reitz, S. M., & Graham, K. (2019). Health promotion theories. In B. A. B. Schell & G. Gillen (Eds.), *Willard and Spackman's occupational therapy* (13th ed., pp. 675–692). Wolters Kluwer.

Restall, G. J., & Egan, M. Y. (2021). Collaborative relationship-focused occupational therapy: Evolving lexicon and practice. *Canadian Journal of Occupational Therapy, 88*(3), 220–230. https://doi.org/10.1177/00084174211022889.

Rios, L. E., Herval, Á. M., Ferreira, R. C., & Freire, M. D. C. M. (2019). Prevalences of stages of change for smoking cessation in adolescents and associated factors: Systematic review and meta-analysis. *The Journal of Adolescent Health: Official Publication of the Society for Adolescent Medicine, 64*(2), 149–157. https://doi.org/10.1016/j.jadohealth.2018.09.005.

Rosenstock, I. M. (1974). The health belief model and preventive health behaviour. *Health Education Monographs, 2*(4), 354–386.

Saulle, R., Sinopoli, A., De Paula Baer, A., Mannocci, A., Marino, M., De Belvis, A. G., Federici, A., & La Torre, G. (2020). The PRECEDE-PROCEED model as a tool in public health screening: A systematic review. *La Clinica Terapeutica, 171*(2), e167–e177. https://doi.org/10.7417/CT.2020.2208.

Schell, B. A. B., & Gillen, G. (2019). Glossary. In B. A. B. Schell & G. Gillen (Eds.), *Willard and Spackman's occupational therapy* (13th ed., pp. 1191–1215). Wolters Kluwer.

Sebastian, A. T., Rajkumar, E., Tejaswini, P., Lakshmi, R., & Romate, J. (2021). Applying social cognitive theory to predict physical activity and dietary behavior among patients with type-2 diabetes. *Health Psychology Research, 9*(1), 24510. https://doi.org/10.52965/001c.24510.

Semlyen, J., King, M., Varney, J., & Hagger-Johnson, G. (2016). Sexual orientation and symptoms of common mental disorder or low well-being: Combined meta-analysis of 12 UK population health surveys. *BMC Psychiatry, 16*, 67. https://doi.org/10.1186/s12888-016-0767-z.

Shabibi, P., Zavareh, M. S. A., Sayehmiri, K., Qorbani, M., Safari, O., Rastegarimehr, B., & Mansourian, M. (2017). Effect of educational intervention based on the health belief model on promoting self-care behaviours of type-2 diabetes patients. *Electronic Physician, 9*(12), 5960–5968. https://doi.org/10.19082/5960.

Shen, X., & Shen, X. (2019). The role of occupational therapy in secondary prevention of diabetes. *International Journal of Endocrinology, 2019*, 3424727. https://doi.org/10.1155/2019/3424727.

Stacey, F. G., James, E. L., Chapman, K., Courneya, K. S., & Lubans, D. R. (2015). A systematic review and meta-analysis of social cognitive theory-based physical activity and/or nutrition behaviour change interventions for cancer survivors. *Journal of Cancer Survivorship: Research and Practice, 9*(2), 305–338. https://doi.org/10.1007/s11764-014-0413-z.

The WHOQOL Group. (1995). Position paper from the World Health Organization. *Social Science & Medicine, 41*(10), 1403–1409. https://doi.org/10.1016/0277-9536(95)00112-k.

Tougas, M. E., Hayden, J. A., McGrath, P. J., Huguet, A., & Rozario, S. (2015). A systematic review exploring the social cognitive theory of self-regulation as a framework for chronic health condition interventions. *PLoS One, 10*(8), e0134977. https://doi.org/10.1371/journal.pone.0134977.

Tulchinsky, T. H. (2018). Marc Lalonde, the health field concept and health promotion. In T. H. Tulchinsky (Ed.), *Case studies in public health* (pp. 523–541). Academic Press. https://doi.org/10.1016/B978-0-12-804571-8.00028-7.

World Federation of Occupational Therapists. (2013). *Definitions of occupational therapy from member organisations.* https://www.wfot.org/resources/definitions-of-occupational-therapy-from-member-organisations

World Health Organization. (1948). *Constitution of the World Health Organization.* Retrieved March 21, 2023, from https://apps.who.int/gb/bd/PDF/bd47/EN/constitution-en.pdf?ua=1.

World Health Organization. (1986). *Ottawa charter for health promotion: First international conference on health promotion.* Retrieved March 31, 2023, from https://www.healthpromotion.org.au/images/ottawa_charter_hp.pdf.

World Health Organization. (2021). *The Geneva charter for well-being.* Retrieved March 31, 2023, from https://www.who.int/publications/m/item/the-geneva-charter-for-well-being.

World Health Organization. (n.d.a). *Improving the health and well-being of LGBTQI+ people.* Retrieved March 31, 2023, from https://www.who.int/activities/improving-the-health-and-well-being-of-lgbtqi-people.

World Health Organization. (n.d.b). *Social determinants of health.* Retrieved March 31, 2023, from https://www.who.int/health-topics/social-determinants-of-health#tab=tab_1.

Zewdie, A., Mose, A., Sahle, T., Bedewi, J., Gashu, M., Kebede, N., & Yimer, A. (2022). The health belief model's ability to predict COVID-19 preventive behavior: A systematic review. *SAGE Open Medicine, 10*, 20503121221113668. https://doi.org/10.1177/20503121221113668.

REFLECTION

1. Why is occupational therapy considered to be inherently health promoting?

2. Explain the role that health education has in relation to health promotion. Suggest how health education can be used to support the implementation of effective health promotion strategies.

3. Explain the link between collaborative relationship-focused practice and health promotion.

4. Taking into account that the focus of occupational therapy is occupational participation, create an argument for why occupational therapists should be more involved in planning, creating, developing, implementing and evaluating health promotion strategies.

24

LIFESTYLE AND SELF-MANAGEMENT

MIRANDA MICHELLE M. THEW ■ SUZANNE HENSHALL

CHAPTER OUTLINE

Overview

How occupational therapists support people within community settings to self-manage chronic conditions to enable them to participate in daily and desired occupations is the focus of this chapter. The chapter offers an exploration of strategies that empower people to shape their current and future health by interventions that focus on their assets/strengths and capabilities. The evidence-based for self-management of long-term conditions is synthesised followed by a discussion of how collaborative self-management approaches provide co-efficiency in promoting health to prevent secondary conditions. Strategies built on the assets, values and lifestyles of individuals that increase the opportunities for people with chronic conditions to participate in a range of occupations are presented. Three practice stories are included to illustrate a range of occupation-centred lifestyle management interventions and strategies to demonstrate how occupational therapists can strengthen personal assets, occupational choices, participation and fulfilment in people's lives.

KEY POINTS

Working with people to develop self-management strategies to manage living with chronic and persistent diseases and conditions is consistent with promoting occupational participation.

■ Empowering people by supporting and promoting self-management strategies can facilitate better health outcomes and well-being even with often debilitating lifelong chronic diseases and conditions.

■ Using collaborative relationship-focused strategies that build on personal assets and personally derived quality occupations can motivate and reduce reliance on formal health and social care sectors.

■ Occupation-focused lifestyle management incorporated within daily routine can increase occupational participation and future-proof quality of life.

INTRODUCTION

Improvements in health care have increased the life expectancy of people (Grady & Gough, 2014); however, this has meant that many people are living their lives alongside symptoms from a variety of long-term conditions such as pain from osteoarthritis, breathlessness from chronic obstructive pulmonary disease (COPD) or fatigue from multiple sclerosis (MS), long-COVID or cancer (Gardetto, 2011; Kyu et al., 2018). These symptoms can lead to significant and prolonged occupational disruption and deprivation and impact a person's occupational participation. This impact on occupational participation is a public health issue of growing importance, which presents opportunities for the growth of occupational therapy roles and scope of practice within primary care settings (Grady & Gough, 2014; Lewis et al., 2022).

The burden of long-term disease rises with age, with an increasing number of people globally living with multiple chronic symptoms and experiencing resultant years of life being affected by decreasing quality of life due to illness, injury and/or impairment (Li et al., 2020; Lim et al., 2017). This leads to pressures on healthcare providers and consequently, the treatment and prevention of chronic diseases are now a major focus of health care (Li et al., 2020). Despite the increased attention on approaches to prevent disease and promote health and quality of life, even in countries that have subsidised or free health care (such as the National Health Service in the United Kingdom or the Unified Health Care System in Brazil), rates of mortality have either levelled out or are increasing, particularly postpandemic (WHO, 2023). Inequalities in access to healthcare provision remain a significant worldwide issue, with resultant disparities in both mortality and morbidity rates from often preventable and lifestyle-modifiable risk factors despite targeted health campaigns (Marmot, 2020; Negm et al., 2019). These key 'lifestyle' risk factors such as smoking, prolonged sedentary activities, alcohol abuse and poor dietary habits can adversely affect health and well-being and often are a response to social injustices such as poverty, social isolation, unemployment and lack of community resources (Ng et al., 2020).

Occupational Therapists as Facilitators for Self-Management in People Living With Chronic Conditions

A variety of strategies can be used under the umbrella of self-management, and these can vary widely in form, duration and intensity (Koller et al., 2012). However, typical generic interventions have included increasing daily exercise, cognitive symptom management techniques, nutrition, fatigue and sleep management, engagement with community resources and self-administration of medications (Lorig & Holman, 2003). These interventions are generally facilitated by education (advice), motivational activities, social networking, goal setting and self-monitoring of progress to initiate and sustain occupational participation of the person (Lim et al., 2017; Restall & Egan, 2021; Restall et al., 2022). Barriers to self-management can include cognition, computer literacy, finances, cultural expectations of health service provision and age (Hammell, 2022a).

Occupational therapists have the skills to support and address both physical and emotional needs through occupational participation. They are equipped to identify environmental, social and intrinsic barriers that can affect full participation in valued occupations and meaningful relationships in different micro, meso and macro contexts (Curtin & Robinson, 2019; Egan & Restall, 2022; Scaffa & Reitz 2020; Whiteford et al., 2020).

Occupational identity, potential and justice can be realised when people feel they have the agency to participate in valued occupations of choice (Egan & Restall, 2022; Hammell, 2020). However, prolonged episodes of illness can impede the natural flow of life and routine, whether that is facing typical symptoms of chronic disease such as fatigue, pain, breathlessness or weakened muscular strength. Additionally, occupational disruption can occur due to time off from work or suspension of a leisure occupation because of symptom relapse or deterioration of the condition, leading to possible occupational deprivation.

One of the factors behind the lack of progress towards healthier lifestyles to prevent disease and improve quality of life, particularly within marginalised populations, is arguably the lack of 'buy in' from people to take control of their health compared to reliance on health professionals to provide a remedy for the symptoms following acute episodes (Baum & Fisher, 2014). This is particularly relevant where people's self-beliefs about their health risks (such as sedentary lifestyle) may not align with the health professional's view (Thillainadesan et al., 2020). Hence, there is a shift in health care towards self-management, a term widely used to describe the day-to-day management of symptoms by an individual living with a chronic condition (usually at home or out of a healthcare setting) (Lorig & Holman, 2003). Self-management offers a strategy for empowering and supporting individuals with chronic conditions to identify their occupational choices and find opportunities to increase their occupational participation rather than merely follow prescribed health professional's advice (Restall & Egan, 2021; Grady & Gough, 2014; Pyatak et al., 2017; Restall & Egan, 2023).

Health professionals, including occupational therapists, are expected to be holistic and encourage people's autonomy by considering their health expectations, capabilities and life circumstances (Estall et al., 2023; Hyett et al., 2016). Yet enabling people to be independent and empowered to self-manage chronic conditions is yet to be fully established (Lewis et al., 2022). Possibly reflecting the historical Western paradigm of health care that has been predominantly paternalistic and disempowering (Hammell, 2020). This may be due to the approaches used to improve and promote health historically being based on a biomedical model, focusing on identifying needs and deficits that require professional resources and interventions. These approaches have not been effective and have led to increased pressures on healthcare services (Morgan & Ziglio, 2007).

Therefore it is important that the focus is on the empowerment and motivation of the person requiring occupational therapy. The person needs to learn how to self-monitor their symptoms and the impact of occupational participation and apply self-management strategies if they are able. If not, it is important to empower their family and carers to assist in this process (e.g. dementia and neuro-cognitive impairment) (Richardson et al., 2014).

Occupational identity, potential and justice can be realised when people feel they have the agency to participate in valued occupations of choice (Egan & Restall, 2022; Hammell, 2020). These need to be considered within the assessment and interventions provided. Accordingly, health professionals, including occupational therapists, are expected to be holistic and encourage people's autonomy by considering their health expectations, capabilities and life circumstances, all of which fall under the remit of SM (Estall et al., 2023; Hyett et al., 2016).

BUILDING ON A PERSON'S ASSETS AND SOCIAL CAPITAL IN SELF-MANAGEMENT STRATEGIES

Healthcare professionals, including occupational therapists, should work collaboratively with the person with chronic health condition to design and implement self-care/management strategies that consider all variables, including a person's assets and social capital (Yildirim, 2021). Building on a person's assets or strengths is key to enabling each person to regain the authorship of their future health story (Pyatak et al., 2022). The unique strengths that an individual has together with relevant social capital can empower them to achieve improvements in the quality and control of their lives (Van-Bortel et al., 2019; Zhang et al., 2012).

Assets

Cassetti et al. (2020, p. 19) proposed three different assets that can be mobilised within self-management interventions:

A. **Connecting assets:** for example, linking people with community leisure or support groups.
B. **Raising awareness on available assets:** for example, mobilising the use of community green space using information on allotments or walks in the park.
C. **Enabling assets to thrive**: essentially exploring opportunities for the person to become an asset within their communities – such as becoming 'patients as expert' or peer group leaders.

Enabling assets shifts the power of the therapeutic relationship from a paternalistic and ableist approach of 'the therapist knows best' to a 'person as partner' approach (Hammell, 2022a; Elwyn et al., 2012). This centres the person firmly within their own care pathway where they are considered a legitimate expert and changes the way in which services are delivered so that they are steered by the person (Elwyn et al., 2012).

Exploring occupations of choice (however limited these may be) and focusing on doing more of what is personally meaningful, achievable and pleasurable, rather than prioritising improving independence in areas of deficit (e.g. in personal care), can promote a 'positive' mindset. This is arguably more holistic and motivating for people to effect change within their lives (Ehsan et al., 2019; Restall & Egan 2021; Hammell, 2020). This focus on personal strengths has been found to slow down deterioration in conditions such as frailty in older adults (Collins et al., 2020; Thillainadesan et al., 2020).

Social Capital

Enhancing some assets can be realised through increasing or incorporating individual social capital within self-management techniques (Moore & Kawachi, 2017). Social capital is the amount of time and energy invested and embedded in a social network or community rich in support, trust, advice or information and comfort and can provide resources that help people achieve health goals (Lin, 2019). Social capital can be found in a variety of settings, including informal and formal social and support relationships within the family, friendship groups, workplace/work colleagues, local neighbourhoods, community groups, religious groups and peer support groups (Moore & Kawachi, 2017). Ehsan et al. (2019) conducted a meta-review of systematic and literature reviews that explored the influence of social capital on health outcomes and concluded that there is good evidence that social capital is associated with better health outcomes. Furthermore, it has been found that community-based groups can increase social capital and empowerment in hard-to-reach groups for example, young men (Robinson et al., 2018) or previously cared for young adults (Moore & Thew, 2023). Utilising an individual's social networks can also ensure that techniques are followed or encouraged (e.g. grading occupations to manage fatigue) or that co-occupations are pursued, rather than waiting for symptoms to be relieved before participating in meaningful occupation. This also empowers people to believe that it is possible to take action to improve their own health and well-being (Cassetti et al., 2020; Hammell, 2022b).

OCCUPATION FOCUSED SELF-MANAGEMENT LIFESTYLE STRATEGIES

Occupation-centred lifestyle management (or modification) is commonly used when implementing self-management strategies. The management combines collaborative goal setting, increased participation in active, meaningful and social occupations, health promotion advice and techniques to promote occupational choice and autonomy in daily life (Davies, 2011; Mountain et al., 2017; Pyatak et al., 2017; Pyatak et al., 2022; Shomer & Roll, 2022). Occupation-centred lifestyle management sits comfortably within an occupational therapist's repertoire of skills when working with individuals to 'develop a shared understanding of how a [person's] occupational history and imagined future influences participation in current daily activities' (Pyatak et al., 2022, p. 2). It includes linking and promoting self-management of health-relevant behaviours such as restful sleep, establishing routines, following a healthy diet, pacing and grading daily occupations to mediate against a variety of preventable diseases. They also need to apply them continuously and within a collaborative and dynamic process encompassing the capability to self-monitor the effects of participation in occupations to retain or attain a meaningful quality of life (Richardson et al., 2014).

Lifestyle Redesign (Clark et al., 2012) is a well-established occupation-centred lifestyle management approach, with particularly promising outcomes with older adults in maintaining wellness. Lifestyle Redesign involves the development of health-promoting performance patterns through the application of core techniques such as occupational self-analysis, narrative reasoning, collaborative problem-solving and autonomy-enhancing communication (Clark et al., 2012; Pyatak et al., 2022). Occupational therapists have the skills to support and address both physical and emotional needs through occupational participation. They are equipped to identify environmental, social and intrinsic barriers that can affect full participation in valued occupations and meaningful relationships in different micro, meso and macro contexts (Curtin et al., 2019; Egan & Restall, 2022; Scaffa & Reitz, 2020; Whiteford et al., 2020).

When working with people in a way that enables them to be in control of their lives, it is important that the strategies used are culturally relevant, person-focused and addressing inequitable factors that shape, constrain and dictate the occupations in which people choose to participate (Hammell, 2020). Ultimately, occupational therapists' endeavours should be focused on sustaining the person to feel that once some direction and support have been provided, their journey towards managing their condition or promoting their health should be sustained once the occupational therapist has ceased their support (Cruz et al., 2023; Pyatak et al., 2017). An occupational model, such as the Canadian Model of Occupational Participation (CanMOP) (Egan & Restall, 2022) (refer to Chapter 11), can be used to guide the assessment and intervention process to establish a person's values and connections regarding what they do each day.

The following sections present several occupation-focused self-management strategies. These strategies are illustrated in the three practice stories (Boxes 24.1–24.3).

BOX 24.1
THE LIVE WELL GROUP

Frailty in older adults is a global area of concern and increased referrals and repeated admissions are causing a considerable strain on services (Lambrinou et al., 2019). Health-promoting self-management strategies and interventions that support older at-risk adults to maintain and retake control over their occupational participation in daily life can increase subjective quality of life as well as improving health outcomes and reducing hospital admissions (Hauser et al., 2022) (refer also to Chapter 48).

This practice story illustrates strategies to enhance the occupational participation of older people at risk of decline into frailty. The focus is on motivating people to engage in personally authentic and culturally relevant leisure occupations, which can decline significantly due to physical and environmental barriers associated with age (Hauser et al., 2022).

The Living Well Group was a community-based group established by an occupational therapist working in a primary care setting, in collaboration with primary care providers. The Group ran as a 'rolling programme' into which primary care health professionals and individuals themselves could refer. Key information about the group is provided in Table 24.1.

A typical session plan for the Living Well Group is provided in Table 24.2.

BOX 24.2
TYPE 2 DIABETES PEER SUPPORT GROUP

Diabetes mellitus is the ninth major cause of death globally, with approximately 1 in 11 adults worldwide diagnosed and of whom 90% have type 2 diabetes mellitus. Typically, people with diabetes have at least one complication, with cardiovascular complications contributing to both morbidity (e.g. lower-limb amputations) or mortality (Zhang et al., 2018). Healthy lifestyles (such as no smoking, regular physical activity, low consumption of alcohol, keeping to a healthy body weight and maintaining a healthy diet) can positively impact both total life expectancy and incidence of chronic diseases such as type 2 Diabetes (Li et al., 2020).

An outline example of the session content of a peer-support group for people who had type 2 diabetes, which was set up by occupational therapy students on a role emerging placement within a GP practice, is presented in Table 24.3. The focus of the session was to maintain self-management of the condition initially taught by a local diabetes charity. By the use of a mixture of advice and guidance sheets (to take home), practical tasks (e.g. setting stealthy exercise goals into the occupational lifestyle diaries), sharing diaries and experience in carrying out the strategies at home or listening to ideas to improve sleep or fatigue, the group participants were empowered and motivated to manage their condition (Pyatak et al., 2022). Some were able to reduce their risk of diabetes, even to reverse the condition and achieve 'remission'.

One of the practice stories relates to an individual and two refer to community-based peer support groups. These practice stories are included to illustrate a range of self-management strategies and techniques that occupational therapists have successfully applied to empower individuals to take part in occupations that they need

---

BOX 24.3
TOMMY

Tommy lived with his partner, Sam. He had retired from being a full-time postman a few years ago. Recently, after walking the family dog, he experienced a stroke. The stroke has caused Tommy to have visual and cognitive problems. He is at risk of a further stroke due to his lifestyle which involves a sedentary routine, an imbalanced diet, late nights watching television and regularly consuming alcohol.

Examples of self-management strategies use with Tommy can be found in Table 24.4.

BOX 24.4
EXAMPLE OF A BANK DAILY LIFESTYLE DIARY

Week Commencing:

Hours of Day	Monday	Tuesday	Wednesday	Thursday	Friday	Saturday	Sunday
7–8 am							
8–9 am							
9–10 am							
10–11 am							
11 am–12 pm							
12–1 pm							
1–2 pm							
2–3 pm							
3–4 pm							
4–5 pm							
5–6 pm							
6–7 pm							
7–8 pm							
8–9 pm							
9–10 pm							
10–11 pm							

Note:
Complete with how you occupy your time, rate fatigue levels on a scale of 0 (no fatigue) to 10 (worst fatigue).

Use colours to highlight your emotions attached to what you do each hour, to help highlight areas that trigger pain/fatigue/low mood. For example, Pink = pleasure, Yellow = happy/ relaxed, Red = stress/anger/frustration, Blue = low mood. Leave blank for unmemorable/bored. Or use own colour scale.

Notice the patterns in your mood and in your fatigue levels in relation to how you occupy your time.

and want to do. The practice stories illustrate that the role of the occupational therapist is to collaboratively support and advocate for the person in order that they may be able to shape and orchestrate their own valued choice of everyday occupations (Egan & Restall, 2022; Kim et al., 2022; Hammell, 2020).

Occupational Lifestyle Diaries

Assessing occupational lifestyle needs requires assessment and evaluation of the person's capabilities, occupational disruption and their daily routine and the contexts in which they live their life. An occupational lifestyle diary can be used to document and understand how the person feels and reacts to their occupational participation and allows the establishment of incremental goals so that occupational participation and progress can be monitored and compared and motivation sustained.

An occupational Lifestyle Diary (Box 24.4 and Fig. 24.1) helps the person, the family/carer and occupational therapist understand how people are occupying their time, how this makes them feel and how they want to shape their occupations in the day. This occupational self-analysis involves

Date- From-To	FRIDAY Occupation	Feeling	SATURDAY Occupation Feeling		SUNDAY		Key-
8-10 am	Called bank-£ and Worked	:{	Snoozed-texting-lie in	☺	Shower-big breakfast	*	;)) = Pleasure (pink)
10-12 noon	Phone calls- office work	:{	Breakfast Tidied	:{	Got ready tidied	:{	
12-2 pm	Lunch at desk- meeting	☺	Lie on sofa -TV	☹	Family Sunday lunch-out	;))	☹ =Low (blue)
2-4 pm	Meetings/ office work	:{	Food- sandwich- TV- fell asleep-Tired	☹	Family Sunday lunch-out	;))	
4-6 pm	Home/bus/ tea	*	Grand-daughter- made tea	;))	Tidied	*	:{ Stressed/ Frustrated (red)
6-8 pm	Get ready to go out-walk to pub	☺	TV/played i-Pad	☺	Chatted to neighbour	☹	
8-10 pm	Meet G and B at pub-!	;))	TV-fell asleep-sofa	☺	TV- fell asleep on sofa	☹	☺ Relaxed (yellow) *other emotion
Night-time	Bed at 11.30-	;))	Bed at 12am.	*	Bed at 12am.	:{	

Fig. 24.1 ■ Completed occupational lifestyle diary.

recording how they choose to occupy every hour and how the occupations impact emotions or symptoms empower people to identify their own goals (Restall & Egan, 2021). By collaborative analysis of the self-completed diary and by analysing the pattern of symptoms and/or emotions in response to daily occupational participation, can identify the need for changes or grading and pacing of occupations. Recording the amount of time spent in an occupation can also indicate any imbalance or over exertion which may exacerbate pain or inexertion which may lead to muscle deconditioning. Ultimately, such diaries allow for goal setting, self-monitoring and feedback, which encompasses the main strategies of self-management of conditions (Morton et al., 2017).

Establishing Meaning in Daily Occupations

Using colours to code the diary entries (Fig. 24.1) can allow a person to visually identify:

- The occupations gave them pleasure (highlighted in pink),
- The occupations that caused 'stress/anxiety' (highlighted in red),
- When they were feeling relaxed (yellow),

- Where there were episodes of pain or fatigue or sadness/low mood (highlighted in blue) and
- When they felt no emotion (no colour).

Colour coding can be used to highlight other emotions or experiences of symptoms, such as feeling 'purposeful', bored or frustrated. The choice of colours and what to identify can be a decision of the person completing the diary.

Colour coding the diary can contribute to a discussion of prioritising occupations and obtaining a satisfactory balance of occupations. For example, the discussion may focus on how to integrate occupations that provide more pleasure and are more purposeful and relaxing in daily life. Having tangible occupations noted per hour also may identify barriers or enablers of occupation. Diaries and colour coding options are unique to the individual and place the person at the centre of the intervention (Restall et al., 2022); it also enables the person to identify the pattern and routines of occupations and where there may be loss or absence of desired occupations.

Goal Setting: Grading and Pacing of Occupations to Manage Symptoms

Through mutually reviewing and discussing the diaries both the occupational therapist and the person completing it become more aware of the individual's daily patterns, time use, values, drivers and motivations embedded in the daily range and choice of occupations. These factors become the shared assets which can be harnessed to progress therapy. Through the mutually agreeing and setting of Specific, Measured, Achievable, Realistic and Timed (SMART) goals (Doran, 1981), which increase or change the balance of the occupations, the person is able to work towards achieving their desired lifestyle.

Evidence suggests that when a person aligns their lifestyle towards their values and choices, this can contribute to greater health and well-being (WHO, 2023). Through using the diaries along with a person's values and motivations, the occupational therapist can introduce the concept of goal setting to move towards a more purposeful and meaningful lifestyle. The benefits of collaborative goal setting include increasing a person's occupational participation and facilitating a greater opportunity for collaboration between the person and the occupational therapist (Restall & Egan, 2023).

When setting goals with a person living with pain or fatigue, the initial step is to establish a baseline of activity that the person can manage without triggering or exacerbating an increase in symptoms. Through establishing this baseline, the person is initially encouraged to 'peg back' their activity levels to eliminate the 'crash and boom' of activity, reducing the risk of their being exhausted or experiencing increased pain following the activity (Thew & Pemberton, 2008). Through recognising the factors that lead to a crash of energy, a more stable baseline emerges. Once this is achieved, goals can be set incrementally either within the duration or the complexity of the occupational participation to increase engagement in a more sustained way. This can often be a highly frustrating process and therefore it is important the occupational therapist provides a comprehensive explanation and gains the support of other people in their lives.

The core skills of occupational therapists enable them to expertly support a person to grade and pace their current life as well as introduce new occupations, possibly in a different way. For example, sometime after Tommy (Box 24.3) completed his occupational therapy and was confident about implementing self-management strategies, he and his partner decided to move from their ground-floor flat to a small two-bedroom house. Tommy was able to draw on the self-management strategies he had learnt so that he did not overexert himself when packing household items into boxes. Over-exertion could have resulted in him having an increase in symptoms of fatigue and being unable to help for several days (crash and boom). However, Tommy was aware of how to grade and pace his occupational participation and could adopt the approach of sitting down to pack items, packing smaller boxes and taking regular breaks to ensure he was able to contribute to packing household items and not become fatigued. Although Tommy was not able to work quickly, he was able to assist his partner with preparing to move to their new house.

Occupation Focused Sleep Management Strategies

Exploring daily patterns of occupation can identify factors that could be inhibiting sleep at night, for example, when there are daytime naps or sleep, drinking caffeinated drinks or poor ergonomic positions while in prolonged sedentary occupations. Offering advice to promote greater levels of deep sleep, such as daily exercise earlier in the day, using relaxation or sleep apps to facilitate falling asleep, environmental adaptations (suitable mattress, blackout blinds, layering of bedding for temperature control) can be explored.

By explaining biorhythms and how the brain behaves in response to occupations, (e.g. the brain needs to 'switch off' from controlling bodily functions, like the gut digesting food or processing alcohol through the liver) can reinforce when to engage in daily occupations. Ultimately, exploring the unique daily occupational routine and habits of the individual can highlight a connection between the patterns of their daily life and its consequences on the quality of sleep and promotes a collaborative problem-solving strategy rather than following 'do' and 'do not' paternalistic lists (Hammell, 2022a).

Stealthy Exercise: Using Daily Occupations to Maintain Fitness, Flexibility and Physical Strength

A way to develop daily exercise to maintain fitness, flexibility and strength is to incorporate it within the daily routines of occupations that people spend time doing. This can allow a routine of gentle exercise which can be increased.

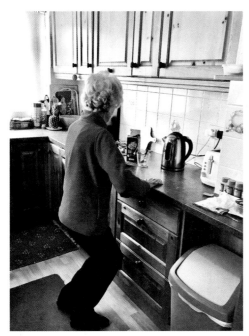

Fig. 24.2 ■ Each time a drink is made, carry out several leg squats.

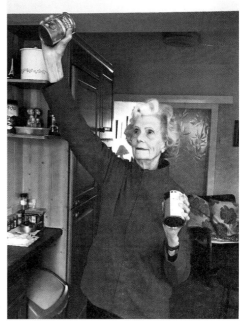

Fig. 24.3 ■ While in the kitchen, do some exercise.

Examples of 'exercise by stealth' include:

■ Doing squats each time someone makes a cup of tea (Fig. 24.2).
■ Going up and down three steps each time the person uses the stairs or going up the stairs quickly as opposed to very slowly.
■ Putting tea/coffee in a higher cupboard or using tins of food to do arm lifts (Fig. 24.3).
■ Putting the washing in a basket on the top of a washing machine and squatting while putting one item at a time into the washing machine.

Incorporating Supportive Social Networks

Social isolation is a common issue facing older adults and those who experience reduced mobility due to chronic disease (Negm et al., 2019). It is important to recognise a person's social assets (e.g. friends, family, neighbours and local groups), how regularly they are in contact (even via social media or telephone) and how they feel about each of their social connections. It can be important to identify who they share their occupations with and how this affects their mood or

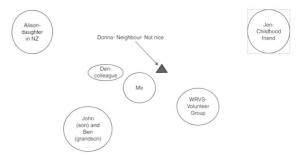

Fig. 24.4 ■ Social network.

motivation/volition. Co-occupations with people who lift mood or provide fun can enhance quality of daily life, and naturally, reduce feelings of loneliness and isolation. Providing a visual representation (Fig. 24.4) of a person's 'social assets' allows the person to make decisions about how they can increase their social capital.

This visual representation of someone's social network involves a person drawing themselves as a circle in the middle of a piece of paper and then using the rest

TABLE 24.1
Key Information About the Live Well Group

Aims of the group:

■ Provide a peer-support group that increases social contact and connects people with local community-based agencies.

■ Understand people's level of activity and enjoyment in living at home and learn about factors which affect this (barriers and enablers).

■ Maintain health, vitality and autonomy to live at home.

Inclusion criteria:

Older people are either self-identifying or referred with mild and moderate frailty including mobility problems, social isolation and decreased occupational participation.

Environment

The group was run in a community hall to promote a social model of care. Peer volunteers helped run the group, including organising refreshments. They encouraged social connections and promoted meet-ups outside of the group time (e.g. at pop-up café events and groups in the local area), paving the way for attendees to engage more in the local community.

Access to the group

The group was marketed to primary care staff – general practitioners, practice receptionists, primary care nurses, health support workers, pharmacy technicians and link workers for social prescribing groups. Flyers were placed in the waiting areas and promoted on the GP practice waiting room TV screens, so individuals could enquire at reception and book in (self-referral).

Session resources

Each session was built around the needs of the people attending and therefore was interactive. A range of topics could be covered in the group, including:

■ What do you do when you are well? (explore motivators, drivers and current occupations)

■ Frailty video

■ Ideas to keep actively participating in a range of occupations

■ Falls prevention strategies

■ Stealthy exercise

■ Eating a balanced diet

■ Social participation

■ Community groups

Representatives from local community services

Brief presentations were provided by a number of local services including:

■ Occupational therapy

■ Local disability living service equipment and mobility devices for a range of problems to enable occupational participation

■ Local community carers centre that provided carers' support groups and advice on financial support for caring roles

■ Live-at-home scheme/services

■ Social prescribing service

■ Volunteer scheme (voluntary work opportunities)

■ The local ambulance

---

of the space on the paper to draw circles that represent the other people in their life. The size of the circle represents how important that person is to them; the larger the circle the more important the person (the friend, daughter, neighbour, etc.) is. The position of a person/circle indicates the frequency of contact with that person, closer circles to the person's own drawn circle, represent frequency of contact; this can help identify who they could reach out to or with whom they can increase social contact.

TABLE 24.2
Typical Session Plan for the Living Well Group

Occupational goals for the group:

To empower and support the development of strategies to prevent deterioration of health

To enhance and increase occupational participation and socialisation

To recognise risks and barriers to occupational participation

To overcome occupational disruption (e.g. from falls or period of time in hospital)

To learn to self-monitor symptoms

Welcome:

Meet and greet by group facilitators and two service user volunteers. Ask all individuals to self-rate themselves on a Likert scale of 'how confident do they feel in managing their own health currently'

- Ground rules/confidentiality – explored and agreed
- Respect others' views and needs
- Opportunities to speak as little/as much as you want

Discussion and exploration:

What does living 'well' mean to you? Occupational focused questions provided to stimulate discussions:

- What do I do when I am well?
- What do I stop doing when I am well?
- What things affect my health?
- How are they doing in each occupational area?

Some guidelines for the group today:

- Ground rules/confidentiality – explored and agreed
- Respect others' views and needs
- Opportunities to speak as little/as much as you want

Personalised discussion:

Factors that can reduce our ability to live well (frailty): Summary of key points made on a video to prevent frailty in older age to reinforce. Followed by opportunity to personalise the information to themselves via discussion and reflection along with peer support – hearing other people's stories.

- Reduced mobility and falls
- Preventing acute illnesses (such as UTIs)
- Living with long-term conditions (Explain these can often be managed)
- Lack of support and social isolation
- Low mood/stress/anxiety/depression

'Focus of the day':

Key areas that group wants to discuss in more depth:

Education and group discussion on:

- Frailty video
- Keeping active
- Falls prevention
- Stealthy exercise
- Eating well with additional nutritional recommendations for older persons – calcium/vit D bone density
- Grading and pacing activities within daily occupations
- Social participation
- Community groups

With some practical demonstrations of stealthy exercises – attendees were encouraged to practice self-management strategies within the session. For example:

Reduced mobility and physical activity levels in general and falls prevention. For example, muscle re-conditioning (physical fitness) guidance and therefore – trying out simple stealthy exercises they can do in their home safely, for example, balanced leg squats while standing at the kitchen worktops (examples of such exercises given in a worksheet with plan to grade up if necessary to attain/maintain muscle strength).

Self-reflection:

An opportunity to personalise the education and information. Individuals were encouraged to self-rate themselves against the frailty criteria and identify areas they wished to address and/or gain more support with.

Each person left the group with a personalised plan.

Breaks agreed with the group:

Can involve trying out nutritional snacks and types of vitamins fortified drinks as well as tea/coffee.

Meet local community groups: (5 = minute explanation from each)

Representatives from community groups chatted with the group in the breaks to generate interest.

Group attendees were also able to have refreshments and a chance to mingle and meet others.

Summary and close:

Repeat outcome measure on whether individuals felt more confident and informed on what keeps them well.

TABLE 24.3	
Type 2 Diabetes Peer-Led Support Group	
Occupational goals	To explore strategies that promote occupational participation
	To discuss and share issues that prevent or act as barriers to occupation
	To identify weekly goals that can reintroduce meaningful occupation into daily life
	To teach and develop strategies that can manage fatigue, pain and stress
	To promote and encourage application of techniques at home by self-monitoring
Duration,	Two hours
location	Community Hall
frequency	Every 8 weeks
Who for?	People who have been newly diagnosed with type 2 diabetes
How accessed?	Self-referral/attendance – via GP recommendation, local diabetes charity, receptionist at well-being centre and social prescribing link workers.

Content (rotated every 9 months) provided by a variety of speakers organised by the leader of the peer-led group.
Understanding type 2 diabetes and medicines, risks (GP)
1. Eating a healthy diet and weight management (Diabetes Charity)
2. Stealthy exercise and occupational lifestyle diary (Occupational Therapist)
3. Getting a good night's sleep (Occupational Therapist)
4. Getting help from local support agencies/volunteer groups
5. Portable relaxation techniques to enable you to do more (Occupational Therapist)
6. Good foot health – watching out for problems (Chiropodist)
7. Managing fatigue to maximise occupational participation (Occupational Therapist)
8. Managing your blood sugars (Practice Nurse)
9. Ad hoc sessions from others in local services which the group was interested in

TABLE 24.4	
Examples of Self-management Strategies for Tommy	
Person	**Details of the Self-Management Occupation Focused Intervention**
Residual poststroke cognitive intrinsic barriers (identified in hospital) that reduced attentional capacity to attend to a task such as using the computer and/or impulsiveness that poses safety risks.	Used lifestyle diary to help Tommy and his partner highlight the areas that both wanted Tommy to work on. This identified areas that he was struggling with since his stroke.
Assets: Relatively fit as had continued walking over five kilometres a day postretirement (due to habit as a postman). Use this to get back to playing football with grandchildren and walking to local park and shop every day.	Occupation-focused interventions using educational strategies motivate Tommy to apply compensatory or coping strategies to promote occupational participation. For example:
Valued role: Family man – regularly sees his grown-up children and grandchildren.	■ Visual scanning – Tommy quickly learnt helpful visual scanning techniques which became a strong asset for him in enabling him to re-engage in home and community activities. Examples included following a prompt/reminder to scan his head completely from side to side in crossing roads and navigating unfamiliar environments so that he could walk to shops and cafes using these techniques.
	■ Attention – Education on cognition building the time and complexity provided to Tommy and his partner jointly. Self-management home exercise programme to build up attentional skills. Examples include sustaining attention on specific tasks within an occupation and grading/building this up. Introducing more complexities such as introducing distractions, switching and dividing attention between multiple elements within an occupation.
	■ Harnessed the support of his partner (asset) to follow the strategies and motivate Tommy in between planned sessions.
	■ Support and advice given to goal set, grade and pace his daily occupations to build up activity levels in a manageable way. This was underpinned by helpful fatigue management strategies (Thew & Pemberton, 2011). Able to self-manage and do this himself following this.

Continued

TABLE 24.4
Examples of Self-management Strategies for Tommy—cont'd

Person	Details of the Self-Management Occupation Focused Intervention
Environment/Social	Explored role changes following his stroke and the impact this was having on him and his partner. Explored how since his stroke he had been doing less in the house and his partner was doing considerably more.
Lives in a ground-floor flat, familiar area and local shops in a local urban area, including local park to walk his dog (prior to stroke).	Explored ways in which he could take back some independence and roles, through grading and pacing his activities.
Good relationship with partner, who was happy to support Tommy, but was feeling tired and demoralised.	This work improved their relationship further (asset) and reduced carer strain.
Change in social role – struggling in going to local working men's club Friday night.	**Occupational Self-management strategies:**
Occupations Tommy wants and still chooses to participate in	■ Returning to crosswords, computer work and taking responsibility for decision making (paying bills).
■ Still loved to walk every day and be active despite retiring prior to his stroke.	■ Occupational therapist used valued activities of puzzles, reading and recapping short articles.
■ Used to kick ball around park opposite flat with young grandson and go to football matches with son.	■ Graded therapy plan to increase tolerance, time and complexity of involvement of family to practice re-attending.
■ Enjoys attending the pub every Friday with his friends and ex-work colleagues.	■ Then further activities left with him to do and grade himself.
■ Enjoys reading/puzzles.	■ Supported him to complete activity planning/ establish helpful routines, scheduling, using calendars and whiteboards to help embed this into day-to-day life.
■ Has interests in local history and enjoys using laptop to browse web and source information on this.	■ Encouraged him to continue going to the pub with friends – able to do this. (social/leisure)
■ Enjoyed holidays.	
Resources used	At the end of the intervention:
	Self-management strategies summarised and documented into a personalised booklet/file and left with Tommy for his continued use and as a helpful memory aid to be able to be referred to.

CONCLUSIONS

Self-management strategies use a collaborative intervention approach which focuses on a person's abilities, their meaningful relationships, history and their environments rather than their deficits. They tend to involve self-monitoring and analysis of how they currently live their lives and consider ways and in what manner they choose to participate in occupations. These strategies are essential to empower people who are living with or potentially facing, long-term conditions or illnesses, to be able to choose their own life-path towards positive health outcomes and quality of life.

Occupational therapists with their focus on increasing occupational participation, apply, link and promote self-management of health-focused options for daily life – such as restful sleep, establishing routines, pacing and grading daily occupations and increasing social connection, which can mediate against a variety of chronic diseases and can retain or attain a meaningful quality of life. Finally, this chapter has illustrated the role of occupational therapists in primary care and shone a light on how this role could potentially empower individuals to manifest a greater sense of self-efficacy and empowerment over often life-limiting conditions and arguably address occupational injustices which can impinge on quality of life and occupational potential.

REFERENCES

Baum, F., & Fisher, M. (2014). Why behavioural health promotion endures despite its failure to reduce health inequities. *Sociology of Health and Illness, 36,* 213–225. http://doi.org/10.1111/1467-9566.12112.

Clark, F., Jackson, J., Carlson, M., Chou, C., Cherry, B., Jordan-Marsh, M., & Azen, S. (2012). Effectiveness of a lifestyle intervention in promoting the well-being of independently living older people: Results of the Well Elderly 2 randomised controlled trial. *Journal of Epidemiology and Community Health, 66,* 782–790. https://doi.org/10.1136/jech.2009.099754.

Cassetti, V., Powell, K., Barnes, A., et al. (2020). A systematic scoping review of asset-based approaches to promote health in communities: Development of a framework. *Global Health Promotion, 27*(3), 15–23.

Collins, T., Davys, D., Martin, D., Russell, R., & Kenney, C. (2020). Occupational therapy, loneliness and social isolation: A thematic review of the literature. *International Journal of Therapy and Rehabilitation, 27*(10), 1–23.

Cruz, D. D. C., Taff, S., & Davis, J. (2023). Occupational engagement: some assumptions to inform occupational therapy. *Cadernos Brasileiros de Terapia Ocupacional, 31*, e3385.

Curtin, S., Galvin, R., & Robinson, K. (2019). The relationship between cancer survivors' well-being and participation in work, activities of daily living and social engagement: Findings from the European Social Survey. *Scandinavian Journal of Occupational Therapy, 28*(7), 531–541. https://doi.org/10.1080/11038128.2019.1695932.

Curtin, M. (2017). Preface: 'The Right Attitude'. In M. Curtin, M. Egan, & Adams, J. (Eds.), *Occupational therapy for people experiencing illness, injury or impairment: Promoting occupation and participation* (7th ed., pp. ix–x). Elsevier.

Davies, N. (2011). Promoting healthy ageing: the importance of lifestyle. *Nursing Standard. 25*(19), 43–49.

De Coninck, L., Bekkering, G. E., Bouckaert, L., Declercq, A., Graff, M. J. L., & Aertgeerts, B. (2017). Home- and community-based occupational therapy improves functioning in frail older people: A systematic review. *Journal of the American Geriatrics Society, 65*(18), 63–69. https://doi.org/10.1111/jgs.14889.

Doran, G. T. (1981). There's a S.M.A.R.T. way to write management goals and objectives. *Management Review, 70*(11), 35–36.

Egan, M., & Restall, G. (2022). Canadian model of occupational participation: Collaborative relationship-focused occupational therapy. In M. Egan & G. Restall (Eds.), *Promoting occupational participation: Collaborative relationship-focused occupational therapy* (pp. 77). Canadian Association of Occupational Therapists.

Ehsan, A., Klaas, H. S., Bastianen, A., & Spini, D. (2019). Social capital and health: A systematic review of systematic reviews. *Population Health, 8*, 100425. https://doi.org/10.1016/j.ssmph.2019.100425.

Elwyn, G., Frosch, D., Thomson, R. et al. (2012), Shared Decision Making: A Model for Clinical Practice. *Journal of General Internal Medicine, 27*, 1361–1367 (2012). https://doi.org/10.1007/s11606-012-2077-6.

Gardetto, N. (2011). Self-management in heart failure: Where have we been and where should we go? *Journal of Multidisciplinary Healthcare, 4*, 39–51. https://doi.org/10.2147/JMDH.S8174.

Grady, P., & Gough, L. (2014). Self-management: A comprehensive approach to management of chronic conditions. *American Journal of Public Health, 104*(8), e25–e31. https://doi.org/10.2105/AJPH.2014.302041.

Hammell, K. W. (2020). Making choices from the choices we have: The contextual-embeddedness of occupational choice. *Canadian Journal of Occupational Therapy, 87*(5), 400–411. https://doi.org/10.1177/0008417420965741.

Hammell, K. W. (2022a). Securing occupational rights by addressing capabilities: A professional obligation. *Scandinavian Journal of Occupational Therapy, 29*(1), 1–12. https://doi.org/10.1080/11038128.2021.1895308.

Hammell, K. W. (2022b). A call to resist occupational therapy's promotion of ableism. *Scandinavian Journal of Occupational Therapy, 30*(6), 745–757. https://doi.org/10.1080/11038128.2022.2130821.

Hauser, D. R., Tripathi, N. S., Smith, M. N., Williams, C. L., Lefebvre, B. M., Ly, A., & Higgins, M. K. (2022). The impact of chronic conditions on leisure participation among community-dwelling older adults. *Physical & Occupational Therapy in Geriatrics, 40*(4), 419–443. https://doi.org/10.1080/02703181.2022.2056672.

Hyett, N., McKinstry, C. E., Kenny, A., & Dickson-Swift, V. (2016). Community-centred practice: Occupational therapists improving the health and wellbeing of populations. *Australian Occupational Therapy Journal, 63*(1), 5–8.

Kim, S., Xu, Y., Dore, K., Gewurtz, R., Larivière, N., & Letts, L. (2022). Fatigue self-management led by occupational therapists and/or physiotherapists for chronic conditions: A systematic review and meta-analysis. *Chronic Illness, 18*(3), 441–457. https://doi.org/10.1177/17423953211039783.

Koller, A., Miaskowski, C., De Geest, S., Opitz, O., & Spichiger, E. (2012). A systematic evaluation of content, structure, and efficacy of interventions to improve patients' self-management of cancer pain. *Journal of Pain and Symptom Management, 44*, 264–284.

Kyu, H. H., Abate, D., Abate, K. H., et al. (2018). Global, regional, and national disability-adjusted life-years (DALYs) for 359 diseases and injuries and healthy life expectancy (HALE) for 195 countries and territories, 1990–2017: A systematic analysis for the Global Burden of Disease Study 2017. *Lancet, 392*, 1859–1922.

Lambrinou, T., Hansen, J., & Beulens, W. (2019). Lifestyle factors, self-management and patient empowerment in diabetes care. *European Journal of Preventive Cardiology, 26*(2_suppl), 55–63. https://doi.org/10.1177/2047487319885455.

Lewis, S., Willis, K., Franklin, M., & Smith, L. (2022). Challenging times: Disconnects between patient and professional temporalities in chronic condition management. *Critical Public Health, 32*(4), 438–449. https://doi.org/10.1080/09581596.2022.2046705.

Li, Y., Schoufour, J., Wang, D., Dhana, K., Pan, A., Liu, X., et al. (2020). Healthy lifestyle and life expectancy free of cancer, cardiovascular disease, and type 2 diabetes: Prospective cohort study. *BMJ, 368*, l6669. https://doi.org/10.1136/bmj.l6669.

Li, X., Cao, X., Guo, M., Xie, M., & Liu, X. (2020). Trends and risk factors of mortality and disability adjusted life years for chronic respiratory diseases from 1990 to 2017: systematic analysis for the Global Burden of Disease Study 2017, 368. https://doi.org/10.1136/bmj.m237.

Lim, C. Y., Berry, A. B., & Hirsch, T. (2017). Understanding what is most important to individuals with multiple chronic conditions: A qualitative study of Patients' Perspectives. *Journal of General Internal Medicine, 32*(12), 1278–1284. https://doi.org/10.1007/s11606-017-4154-3.

Lin, N. (2019). Building a network theory of social capital. In N. Lin, K. Cook, & R. S. Burt. (Eds.), *Social capital: Theory and research* (pp. 3–29). New York.

Lorig, K. R., & Holman, H. (2003). Self-management education: History, definition, outcomes, and mechanisms. *Annals of Behavioral Medicine, 26*(1), 1–7. https://doi.org/10.1207/S15324796ABM2601_01.

Marmot M. (2020). Health Equity in England: the Marmot review 10 years on BMJ ; 368 :m693. https://www.10.1136/bmj.m693.

Morgan A, Ziglio E. (2007). Revitalising the evidence base for public health: an assets model. Promot Educ.; Suppl 2:17-22. PMID: 17685075. https://doi.org/10.1177/10253823070140020701x.

Moore, E. J., & Thew, M. (2023). Exploring the perspectives of 'young adults' (18–24) who have been in formal care and their experiences of attending a socially prescribed community allotment gardening group. *British Journal of Occupational Therapy, 86*(1), 26–32.

Moore, S., & Kawachi, I. (2017). Twenty years of social capital and health research: a glossary. *Journal of Epidemiological Community Health, 71*(5), 513–517.

Morton, K., Dennison, L., May, C., Murray, E., Little, P., McManus, R. J., & Yardley, L. (2017). Using digital interventions for self-management of chronic physical health conditions: a meta-ethnography review of published studies. *Patient Education and Counseling, 100*(4), 616–635.

Mountain, G., Windle, G., Hind, D., Walters, S., Keertharuth, A., Chatters, R., Sprange, K., Craig, C., Cook, S., Lee, E., Chater, T., Woods, R., Newbould, L., Powell, L., Shortland, K., & Roberts, J. (2017). A preventative lifestyle intervention for older adults (lifestyle matters): A randomised controlled trial. *Age and Ageing, 46*(4), 627–634. https://doi.org/10.1093/ageing/afx021.

Negm, A. M., Kennedy, C. C., Thabane, L., Veroniki, A. A., Adachi, J. D., Richardson, J., Cameron, I. D., Giangregorio, A., Petropoulou, M., Alsaad, S. M., Alzahrani, J., Maaz, M., Ahmed, M. M., Kim, E., Tehfe, H., Dima, R., Sabanayagam, K., Hewston, P., Alrob, H. A., & Papaioannou, A. (2019). Management of frailty: A systematic review and network meta-analysis of randomized controlled trials. *Journal of the American Medical Directors Association, 20*(10), 1190–1198.

Ng, R., Sutradhar, R., Zhan, Y., Wodchis, W., & Rosella, L. (2020). Smoking, drinking, diet and physical activity – Modifiable lifestyle risk factors and their associations with age to first chronic disease. *International Journal of Epidemiology, 49*(1), 113–130. https://doi.org/10.1093/ije/dyz078.

Pyatak, E. A., Carandang, K., Rice Collins, C., & Carlson, M. (2022). Optimizing occupations, habits, and routines for health and well-being with Lifestyle Redesign®: A synthesis and scoping review. *The American Journal of Occupational Therapy, 76*(5), 7605205050. https://doi.org/10.5014/ajot.2022.049269.

Pyatak, E. A., Carandang, K., Vigen, C. L. P., Blanchard, J., Diaz, J., Concha-Chavez, A., & Peters, A. L. (2017). Occupational therapy intervention improves glycemic control and quality of life among young adults with diabetes: The resilient, empowered, active living with diabetes (REAL Diabetes) randomized controlled trial. *Diabetes Care, 41*, 696–704. https://doi.org/10.2337/dc17-1634.

Restall, G. J., & Egan, M. (2021). Collaborative relationship-focused occupational therapy: Evolving lexicon and practice. *Canadian Journal of Occupational Therapy, 88*(3), 220–230. https://doi.org/10.1177/00084174211022889.

Restall, G., & Egan, M. (2023). *Canadian Occupational Therapy Inter-relational Practice Process (COTIPP)*. Webinar offered by the Canadian Association of Occupational Therapists. Retrieved February 08, 2023, from. https://caot.ca/uploaded/web/education/2022_2023/Webinars/Egan_Restall_2022.

Restall, G., Egan, M., Valavaara, K., Phenix, A., & Sack, C. (2022). Canadian occupational therapy inter-relational practice process.

In M. Egan, & G. Restall (Eds.), *Promoting occupational participation: Collaborative relationship-focused occupational therapy.* Canadian Association of Occupational Therapists.

Richardson, J., Loyola-Sanchez, A., Sinclair, S., Harris, J., Letts, L., MacIntyre, N. J., Wilkins, S., Burgos-Martinez, G., Wishart, L., McBay, C., & Martin Ginis, K. (2014). Self-management interventions for chronic disease: A systematic scoping review. *Clinical Rehabilitation, 28*(11), 1067–1077. https://doi.org/10.1177/0269215514532478.

Robinson, J., Bailey, E., Witt, K., Stefanac, N., Milner, A., Currier, D., & Hetrick, S. (2018). What works in youth suicide prevention? A systematic review and meta-analysis. *EClinicalMedicine, 4*, 52–91.

Scaffa, M., & Reitz, M. (2020). Occupational therapy in the community and population health practice. *Occupational Therapy in Mental Health, 36*(3), 303–305. https://doi.org/10.1080/0164212X.2020.1782306.

Shomer, L., & Roll, S. (2022). Lifestyle Redesign® intervention for psychological well-being and function in people with fibromyalgia: A retrospective cohort study. *The American Journal of Occupational Therapy, 76*(6), 7606205060. https://doi.org/10.5014/ajot.2022.049243.

Sprange, K., Mountain, G., Brazier, J., Cook, S., Craig, C., Hind, M., Walters, S., Windle, G., Woods, R., Keetharuth, A., Charter, T., Horner, K., et al. (2013). Lifestyle Matters for maintenance of health and wellbeing in people aged 65 years and over: Study protocol for a randomised controlled trial. *Trials, 14*, 302. https://doi.org/10.1186/1745-6215-14-302.

Thew, M. & Pemberton, S. (2008). Energy for life. In Thew, M & McKenna, J. (Eds.). Life-style Management in Health and Social Care. Oxford: Blackwell/Wiley Publishing.

Thillainadesan, J., Scott, I. A., & Le Couteur, D. G. (2020). Frailty, a multisystem ageing syndrome. *Age and Ageing, 49*(5), 758–763. https://doi.org/10.1093/ageing/afaa112.

Van Bortel, T., Wickramasinghe, N. D., Morgan, A., & Martin, S. (2019). Health assets in a global context: A systematic review of the literature. *BMJ Open, 9*(2), e023810. https://doi.org/10.1136/bmjopen-2018-023810.

Whiteford, G., Jones, K., Weekes, G., et al. (2020). Combatting occupational deprivation and advancing occupational justice in institutional settings: Using a practice-based enquiry approach for service transformation. *British Journal of Occupational Therapy, 83*(1), 52–61. https://doi.org/10.1177/0308022619865223.

World Health Organization, (WHO). (2023). *Global health estimates: Leading causes of death.* World Health Organization. Retrieved February 22, 2023, from. https://www.who.int/data/gho/data/themes/mortality-and-global-health-estimates/ghe-leading-causes-of-death.

Yildirim, D. (2021). Self-management of chronic diseases: A descriptive phenomenological study. *Social Work in Public Health, 36*(2), 300–310. https://doi.org/10.1080/19371918.2020.1859034.

Zhang, Y, Chapman, A., Plested, M, Jackson, D, Purroy, F. (2012). The Incidence, Prevalence, and Mortality of Stroke in France, Germany, Italy, Spain, the UK, and the US: A Literature Review, *Stroke Research and Treatment*, 1–11. https://doi.org/10.1155/2012/436125.

Zhang, A., Franklin, C., Currin-McCulloch, J., Park, S., & Kim, J. (2018). The effectiveness of strength-based, solution-focused brief therapy in medical settings: A systematic review and meta-analysis of randomized controlled trials. *Journal of Behavioral Medicine, 41*, 139–151. https://doi.org/10.1007/s10865-017-9888-1.

REFLECTION

1. What are assets or strengths-based approaches and how do they differ from a focus on deficits or the disability that the person has?

2. What strategies can promote a collaborative, occupation-centred approach to identify areas for goal setting and promote self-management of chronic symptoms?

3. Consider some strategies that people can employ to self-manage chronic fatigue or pain?

25

SEXUALITY

CHLOE BRYANT ■ CLAIRE LYNCH

CHAPTER OUTLINE

Overview

The information provided within this chapter aims to enable occupational therapists to begin confidently and safely supporting the sexuality of individuals. This chapter draws from established research and knowledge to provide foundational understandings on sexuality and intimacy relevant to the discipline of occupational therapy. Numerous sections are included to inform occupational therapists on various sexuality-related topics such as definitions and terminology, the individualised nature of sexuality, healthcare approaches, sexuality models and frameworks and the role of occupational therapy. The Canadian Occupational Inter-Relational Practice Process (COTIPP) is used to guide occupational therapists in their understanding of the importance of self-reflection, connecting with people and initiating the topic, promoting occupational participation in sexual and intimate activities, co-designing sexuality goals, utilising enablement skills and planning for transition. Information learnt is also applied to practice and interactive questions are provided throughout.

KEY POINTS

- Sexuality is the central aspect of being human, and occupational therapists have an important role in supporting the sexual well-being of people living with injury, illness or impairment.
- Supporting sexual well-being provides people with access to express their sexuality and recognises them as sexual beings.

337

■ Occupational therapists can support the sexual well-being of people at multiple levels including the individual, interpersonal, services and community and societal levels.

■ Occupational therapists play a crucial role in supporting the diverse and individualised nature of sexuality, encompassing physical, emotional and relational aspects and by addressing the *doing, being, becoming* and *belonging* of an individual's sexuality.

■ It is important that occupational therapists continually reflect on their own values and beliefs towards sexuality to be able to provide sensitive and high-quality support.

■ Occupational therapists are encouraged to initiate the conversation and to draw from their foundational occupational knowledge, skills and strategies when providing sexuality support.

UNDERSTANDING SEXUALITY

This chapter provides a foundational understanding of sexuality relevant to occupational therapy practice. It is intended that after reading this chapter, occupational therapists will be better prepared and more confident to support the sexuality of individuals and collectives. Sexuality is a fundamental dimension of each person's existence and a person's sexual health is part of their overall health. Living with an illness, injury or impairment has the potential to affect all aspects of a person's sexuality and therefore impact their overall health and quality of life. Understanding the nuance of a person's sexuality is therefore vital when working with people. Sexuality is a multifaceted aspect of human identity encompassing, sex, gender identities and roles, sexual orientation, eroticism, pleasure, intimacy and reproduction. Sexuality is experienced and expressed in thoughts, fantasies, desires, beliefs, attitudes, values, behaviours, practices, roles and relationships. While sexuality can include all of these dimensions, not all of them are always experienced or expressed. Sexuality is influenced by the interaction of biological, psychological, social, economic, political, cultural, legal, historical, religious and spiritual factors.

As the above definition indicates, a person's sexuality can be complex and highly varied for each person and requires in-depth consideration.

A person's sexuality consists of four key pillars: sexual well-being, sexual health, sexual justice and sexual pleasure (Mitchell et al., 2021). Sexual well-being

pertains to the holistic health of an individual's sexual life, encompassing physical, emotional and relational aspects. Sexual health emphasises the importance of safe, consensual and satisfying sexual experiences, irrespective of a person's physical or cognitive abilities. Sexual justice and rights advocate for equal access to sexual expression, education and healthcare, recognising that people experiencing illness, injury or impairment often face systemic barriers that impede their sexual autonomy. Sexual pleasure underscores the significance of fulfilling and enjoyable sexual experiences. Recognising and respecting the diverse ways in which individuals experiencing illness, injury or impairment feel and express their sexuality is pivotal in promoting a more inclusive and equitable society where everyone can fully participate in the human experience (Mitchell et al., 2021).

THE INDIVIDUALISED NATURE OF SEXUALITY

Sexuality is a central aspect of being human and includes numerous aspects of a person; hence no two individual's sexuality is the same. A person's sexual identity, sexual expression and sexual preferences are highly personal and multifaceted. It is therefore important that assumptions are not made. Critical discourse analysis research has discussed that within Australian, American and British healthcare environments, it appears that harmful heteronormative and ableist assumptions can influence how sexuality is supported (Bryant et al., 2024). Healthcare professionals appear to prioritise addressing sexuality with heterosexual people who are in established relationships and of reproductive age. It is also apparent that where sexual expression and behaviours are concerned, there is a misconception that people only engage in sexual intercourse (involving a penis and vagina). This has also been discussed in a recent article where the authors describe these same heteronormative approaches within occupational therapy (Morrison & Poblete-Almendras, 2023). Further, there appear to be ableist and ageist assumptions, where those of a certain age, or with an injury, illness or impairment, are often nonsexualised within society (Bryant et al., 2024; DeLamater, 2012; Morrison & Poblete-Almendras, 2023). These normative perspectives appear to impact on how sexuality is approached in health care, as there is often a focus on 'fixing' issues of sexual health and function rather than focusing on potential enjoyment and pleasure of sexual activities and intimacy (Bryant et al., 2024), regardless of age or ability. These harmful assumptions neglect to realise the breadth of ways that humans may express their sexuality along with the diverse sexual orientations and gender identities that exist within society, which all require equal consideration, support and respect.

Along with understanding that an individual's sexuality is unique to them and that it is important not to make assumptions, it is also essential to recognise that a person's sexuality may change across their life. Sexuality can evolve over time in response to developmental stages and life circumstances. For example, adolescence is often a period marked by pubescence, curiosity and self-discovery, where individuals may start to recognise their sexual preferences and identities. As people progress into adulthood, their sexuality can continue to evolve. Life circumstances such as relationships, trauma, personal growth and societal influences can all shape and reshape one's sexuality. For some people, entering intimate relationships can lead to the exploration of various aspects of a person's sexuality, deepening their understanding of what brings them pleasure and fulfilment (Portellos et al., 2023). Similarly, major life events like marriage, parenthood or career changes can impact the ways in which an individual perceives and engages with their sexuality. Furthermore, as individuals age, their sexuality often experiences shifts and adaptations (Fileborn et al., 2017). What was once a primary focus for someone in their younger years may take on different forms and meanings as the person enters middle and older age. For example, this could include a shift from a primarily physically oriented expression of sexuality to a more emotionally driven one, with a focus more on companionship rather than sexual activity (Portellos et al., 2023). However, for others, there may be an increase in sexual activity over time (DeLamater, 2012). Understanding and embracing these changes is a crucial aspect of an individual's overall well-being and self-acceptance as it allows them to navigate their evolving sexuality with openness, self-awareness and a deeper appreciation for the complexity of sexuality (Portellos et al., 2023). Although important to recognise that a

person's sexuality may continuously evolve, for others, many aspects of their sexuality, such as their sexual orientations and preferences, will remain constant across their lifetime. This too should be embraced by occupational therapists as part of understanding the individualised nature of sexuality.

Occupational therapists can play a pivotal role in providing support in all aspects throughout a person's life. To provide comprehensive and empathetic health care, the foundational step for occupational therapists is to recognise and respect the individualised nature of sexuality. A one-size-fits-all approach falls short in addressing the diverse and unique needs of individuals. By understanding and appreciating the multitude of factors that contribute to an individual's sexuality, occupational therapists can create a more inclusive and supportive environment (Lynch & Fortune, 2019; Lynch & Joosten, 2022; Rose & Hughes, 2018). An individual's personal factors both influence and are informed by their sexuality. In research, which has explored how health care supports sexuality with people living with spinal cord injury, in-depth consideration of an individual's personal factors was highlighted as critical for comprehensive care (Bryant et al., 2022a). Various personal factors are considered important such as an individual's cultural background, age at the time of the injury, gender, previous sexual experiences and relationship status. Some of these factors are presented in Table 25.1. Occupational therapists may wish to refer to different occupational models, such as the Canadian Model of Occupational Participation (CanMOP) (refer to Chapter 11) to consider different types of personal factors.

Application of Knowledge

In this 'application of knowledge' section, information learnt will be applied to Dr Kate Allatt's lived experience of receiving support after a stroke. Kate has generously provided information about herself, reviewed the information presented in this chapter for accuracy and has allowed her quotes to be used. Throughout this chapter, Kate's lived experience and how this impacted her sexuality will be explored. An introduction to Kate is in Box 25.1.

As indicated in Table 25.2, there was a lot of information missing that should have been discussed when Kate was an inpatient. If more questions were asked

TABLE 25.1
Examples of Personal Factors (Not an Exhaustive List) for Occupational Therapists to Consider as Part of a Person's Sexuality

Personal Factors	Potential Relevance to Sexuality
Age	The age of a person is highly important to consider as this can influence the various occupational roles or sexual health functions that a person may be experiencing. It is therefore important to consider the sexual well-being needs of people across the lifespan (Fileborn et al., 2017). Often healthcare professionals tend to focus on the sexual health needs of people within particular age ranges (McGrath et al., 2021). This may be due to a heteronormative assumption that sexual activity is reserved for people in heterosexual relationships (between a cisgender male and cisgender female) of a reproductive age. Healthcare professionals should aim to challenge harmful assumptions and normalise support for sexuality across all age groups. This can also include support for children and adolescents (WHO, 2023a). Often paediatric sexuality support is neglected; however, healthcare professionals can play an important role in supporting the sexual well-being of children and adolescents. For example, an occupational therapist may educate a child on the difference between public and private places to engage in self-pleasuring activities.
Gender	Along with gender being considered an aspect of sexuality, the World Health Organization (WHO) states that gender is a social construct that can change over time, whereas sex may refer to different biological and physiological characteristics (2023b). It is critical that occupational therapists are aware of potential normative assumptions that they (and society more broadly) may hold. Occupational therapists should aim to provide inclusive and empathetic support by creating a safe environment for individuals of all gender identities (Taylor, 2020). There is insufficient space within a textbook chapter to comprehensively address this topic, and occupational therapists are encouraged to seek out further learning opportunities. There are many resources and supports available to refer to for further in-depth understanding and knowledge on how to provide inclusive and safe practice when working with people who identify as lesbian, gay, bisexual, transgender, queer, intersex, asexual, plus (LGBTQIA+).
Sexual orientation	As indicated by the WHO (2006), a person's sexual orientation is also an aspect of their sexuality. There is no agreed definition of sexual orientation; however, it is thought to encompass a person's sexual behaviours, sexual identity, sexual attraction and sexual arousal, in relation to people of the same or opposite sex or both (Rokach & Patel, 2021). Occupational therapists should aim to create a safe space to support individuals of diverse sexual orientations and should challenge heteronormative assumptions (Taylor, 2020).
Health condition	A person's diagnosis and medical history can indicate potential impacts that may affect a person's sexual well-being. The medical treatments that a person receives may also further impact their sexual health, causing sexual dysfunction. There are many factors, not just biomedical, that can cause sexual dysfunction; however, there is a plethora of literature that can inform healthcare practitioners of the many ways different health conditions may impact sexuality. Health conditions that impact different body structures and functions may impact a person's sexual health in various ways; for example, urinary tract symptoms can cause dyspareunia (pain during sexual activity) or difficulties with orgasm (Rokach & Patel, 2021).
Relationship status	There are many different relationship status classifications, for example, people may identify as single, dating, married, defacto, widowed or in a relationship (among others). Additionally, many people may choose to be in monogamous, polyamorous, open, platonic or autoromantic relationships, among many other types. Although this personal factor can provide an initial piece of information, it is important that the occupational therapist does not make assumptions. Instead, they should seek further information where it is relevant to their occupational roles and participation. When doing so, they should use inclusive language, for example, 'partner'.
Decision-making capacity	Like other decisions in life, a person's capacity to consent to sexual and intimate activities may change over time. Decisions to participate in sexual and intimate occupations are often made in private and may change from one moment to the next (Srinivasan et al., 2019). Sexual consent cannot be predetermined and must be determined at the moment (Hillman, 2017). Understanding a person's decision-making capacity is a highly complex but important part of supporting an individual's sexuality. It is important that the occupational therapist works with the multidisciplinary team to obtain as much information as possible about the person's decision-making capacity and consider the laws and regulations relevant to their practice context.
Cultural background	The cultural background of the individuals can have a major influence on their attitudes and understandings of sexuality. Cultural systems can shape people's sexual perspectives and experiences and the ways in which they understand sexual behaviours (Aggleton et al., 2015). Different cultures may have varying perspectives on what is considered 'normal', for example, in some cultures, sexual activity with multiple partners outside of marriage may be frowned upon, whereas in other cultures, this may be considered acceptable. It is important that the occupational therapist considers this when working with individuals living with illness, injury or impairment in sexual and intimate occupations.

Kate (Figs. 25.1 and 25.2) is a passionate advocate for improving the health and well-being of people living with illness, injury or impairment. When asked to describe herself, Kate stated:

> In short, I am 53 years old and had a brainstem stroke with Locked-In Syndrome (LIS) at 39 caused by burnout and severe stress. LIS is where you can think, feel, see, hear but move absolutely nothing and not speak. Think buried alive and you will get a good idea.

Information about Kate's personal factors is presented in Table 25.2. Kate's personal information and story will be built upon throughout this chapter.

To find out more about Kate and her journey, go to www.kateallatt.com or https://x.com/kateallatt.

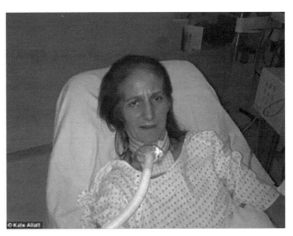

Fig. 25.1 ■ Kate in hospital.

while she was an inpatient, the healthcare team would have learnt more about personal factors related to her sexuality which were important to Kate. For example, Kate had not experienced any sexual dysfunction prior to her stroke and had never received medical or psychological counselling for sexuality. Additionally, Kate attended a Catholic school where she received limited sex education, which mostly consisted of basic information on menstruation. Therefore Kate may have benefited from more education on sexuality and sexual function along with information on how healthcare providers could support her sexual readjustment after her stroke. Further, no information was obtained about Kate's sexual function after her stroke as no discussions or investigations were had at the time. Therefore Kate felt unprepared to return to sexual and intimate activities after being discharged from inpatient rehabilitation.

Kate's reflection on her hospital experience is in Box 25.2.

SUPPORTING SEXUALITY WITHIN HEALTH CARE

Approaches towards sexuality and illness, injury or impairment in health care have previously been reflective of the attitudes towards disability broadly. Throughout history, many prominent and arguably harmful thinkers, such as Sigmund Freud, shaped how people viewed sexuality at the time. For example, Freud believed many typical sexual functions and sexual

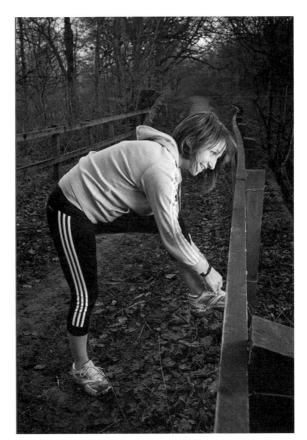

Fig. 25.2 ■ Kate out for a run.

expressions to be indicative of health disorders (Sayers, 2020). Thankfully, support for sexuality has evolved over time as attitudes towards sexuality have also progressed. Though it appears that healthcare support for

TABLE 25.2

Kate's Personal Factors that the Healthcare Team was Aware of While she was an Inpatient at the Hospital

Personal Factor	Information
Age	39
Gender	Cisgender female
Sexual orientation	Heterosexual
Health condition	Brainstem stroke impacting Kate's ability to complete activities of daily living and mobilise, with some impact on cognition. Kate had issues with bladder and bowel control and initially required a catheter for bladder management.
Relationship status	Married
Decision-making capacity	As Kate recovered from the coma and many of her cognitive symptoms resolved, Kate regained full decision-making capacity.
Cultural background	Kate grew up within a white, Catholic, British household in the United Kingdom. Following secondary schooling, Kate had received further education and had been working in marketing prior to the stroke.

sexuality continues to be dominated by a biomedical approach (refer to Chapter 8), which neglects to consider many other aspects of a person's sexuality and can result in ableist discourses (Bryant et al., 2022a; Bryant et al., 2024). A recent systematic review that investigated how sexuality is addressed for people living with

BOX 25.2
KATE'S REFLECTION

If anyone had given me advice on sexuality in hospital, I would have laughed. I was trying to walk, talk, eat, and control my bladder and bowel again, and to get home to hug my young kids! Sex or intimacy was the last thing on my mind. But if I had been told, I would have known there were issues I probably would not be able to control with my sexual function. I may not have felt the shame and guilt I have done. It would also have signposted for me to get help when I was ready [...] it would have prevented months of shame thinking there was something wrong with me.

chronic disease and impairment also found that despite societal progress, research spanning 40 decades shows there has not been increase in the amount of support provided (McGrath et al., 2021). As McGrath et al. (2021) highlight, failure to address sexuality in practice can result in poorer health outcomes for individuals living with an illness, injury or impairment. Therefore it is imperative that healthcare services and professionals, including occupational therapists, endeavour to improve the support provided for sexuality. The Socio-Health Framework of Sexuality and Disability (SHFSD) was recently developed in response to these identified gaps in practice (Bryant, 2023).

Socio-Health Framework of Sexuality and Disability

The Socio-Health Framework of Sexuality and Disability (SHFSD) (Fig. 25.3) was developed in response to several research studies that explored healthcare approaches to supporting the sexual well-being of people with spinal cord injuries. The interpersonal, services and community, and societal levels of the SHFSD represent the various levels that can impact the individual. These levels can influence the individual's sexual well-being and therefore require consideration. At each level, many factors can both facilitate or hinder the person from expressing their sexuality in meaningful and safe ways.

The individual level sits at the centre, demonstrating that the person with an illness, injury or impairment should be the focus of support as part of a person-centred approach. The interpersonal level refers to those people who the individual interacts with, such as healthcare professionals, intimate partners or family. For example, healthcare professionals may hinder the individuals from expressing their sexuality by avoiding the topic. This denies the person sexual access and fails to recognise the person as a sexual being (Bryant, 2023; Shuttleworth, 2006; Shuttleworth & Mona, 2021). The services and community level refers to the wider systems and supports which interpersonal dynamics exist within, such as public hospitals, community centres and meet-up groups. The societal level refers to the high-level systems and structures that can filter down to the individual level. This may include federal legislation, funding and economic structures and mass media, among many others. Importantly, all

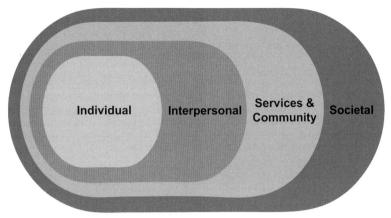

Fig. 25.3 ■ The Socio-Health Framework of Sexuality and Disability. (Reproduced with permission (Bryant, 2023), this figure depicts the Socio-Health Framework of Sexuality and Disability (SHFSD) and the associated four levels.)

four levels are interconnected and have the potential to impact sexual well-being. Occupational therapists may wish to provide support at each of these levels as they can draw from various skills and strategies to work with individuals and collectives, as is discussed further within '*Providing sexuality support*'. When working with people with injury, illness, or impairment, it is therefore encouraged that occupational therapists consider the SHFSD to determine at which level support is most needed.

Application of Knowledge

Drawing from Kate's life experiences, Table 25.3 is provided to help demonstrate how occupational therapists may apply information according to the SHFSD. This can be a helpful process for occupational therapists to undertake so that they are better able to understand what social and environmental issues they may wish to target as part of their therapy. An example is provided for each level relevant to Kate's experience while in hospital.

Kate's further reflection related to her hospital experience is in Box 25.3.

SEXUALITY WITHIN THE OCCUPATIONAL THERAPY PRACTICE PROCESS

The CanMOP was developed to conceptualise occupational participation (refer to Chapter 11). At the core of the CanMOP is occupational participation, that is having access to, initiating and sustaining valued occupations within meaningful relationships and contexts. Alongside the CanMOP is the process framework, the Canadian Occupational Therapy Inter-Relational Practice Process (COTIPP) which can be used to guide occupational therapist interactions (refer to Chapter 12). The COTIPP details numerous concepts to guide the practice process: connect, seek an understanding and define purpose, explore occupational participation, co-design priorities, goals, outcomes and plans, trial the plan, explore change and refine plans and plan for transition.

When providing support for sexuality for individuals, key concepts within both the CanMOP and the COTIPP can be applied. For the remainder of this chapter, the foundational understandings of sexuality, as described above, are 'put into practice' so that readers can better understand what sexuality support looks like within the practice process. The information presented is structured around concepts of the COTIPP.

CEMENTING THE ROLE OF OCCUPATIONAL THERAPY

In accordance with the International Classification of Functioning Disability and Health (ICF) model (refer to Chapter 8), healthcare professionals have the responsibility of guiding interventions aimed

TABLE 25.3		
Utilising the SHFSD to Understand Kate's Experience Within the Inpatient Rehabilitation Unit. Limited Example is Provided for Each Level		
SHFSD Level	**Information**	**Supporting Kate at this Level**
Individual	While receiving support at the inpatient rehabilitation unit, Kate was not ready to return to sexual activities. However, as no one had initiated the topic of sexuality, Kate was unaware of the potential impacts that her stroke may have had on her sexual well-being. Once learning this later, Kate wished someone had initiated the topic while in hospital.	By actively normalising sexuality, healthcare professionals may encourage individuals to begin thinking about sexuality earlier in their recovery journey. Kate may have therefore been more ready to address any sexuality issues/concerns earlier.
Interpersonal	The multidisciplinary team often had reduced capacity to explore goals outside of self-care or mobility goals. Therefore sexuality was not considered during Kate's rehabilitation. It is also likely that the team felt unprepared to address sexuality and appeared to handball these conversations to each other.	An occupational therapist could have better supported Kate's sexual well-being by seeking out learning opportunities and by taking responsibility for initiating the conversation.
Services and community	Kate was able to receive public healthcare support for her stroke within an inpatient rehabilitation setting under the National Health Service (NHS) in the United Kingdom. Within this service setting, there was also no education on sexuality for patients. Due to resource limitations, it appeared that the general approach was to make patients fit the service rather than providing a person-centred approach.	The occupational therapist could advocate for more resources and training to be provided at the service level. This may increase the likelihood that the multidisciplinary team would initiate the conversation and would increase the person-centred approach of this service.
Societal	Although public healthcare systems can increase citizen access to affordable healthcare, public funding may create a barrier to sexual expression for people living with an illness, injury or impairment. Conversative societal values and normative assumptions may reduce the likelihood that national leaders endorse and administer increased funding for services to support sexuality for people living with an illness, injury or impairment.	Occupational therapists could advocate for federal funding to increase resources and support for sexuality within services and the community. Occupational therapists may also actively challenge normative assumptions and conservative values which might impede on the sexual well-being of people living with an illness, injury or impairment.

BOX 25.3
KATE'S REFLECTION

I felt like an object in hospital (Fig. 25.4). There were exceptions like my physio and a nurse who made me feel human and got to know my humour and music. Both of which are very important to my sexuality and ability to cope. For example, my physio recorded a CD of all my favourite bands – The Smiths and Foo Fighters – because it was important for me to feel 'cool'. When I walked out of hospital my sexuality was very important to me which you could see from my outfit (leather jacket, blow-dried hair, gel nails) (Fig. 25.5) but also the fact I had videoed my historic walk. Me proving people wrong who had doubted me was important to my sexuality.

at enabling people living with an illness, injury or impairment to engage in desired activities and fostering their full participation in all aspects of life (WHO, 2001). In addition, the primary objective of occupational therapy is to empower individuals to reconstruct personally satisfying, resilient, and meaningful occupational lives. For many, sexuality plays a pivotal role in achieving such fulfilment. Previously there has been debate about the role of occupational therapists in supporting the sexuality of individuals. However, it is now recognised that occupational therapists are well positioned within the multidisciplinary team to provide essential support in addressing sexuality (Lynch & Fortune, 2019; O'Mullan et al., 2021). Lynch and Fortune (2019)

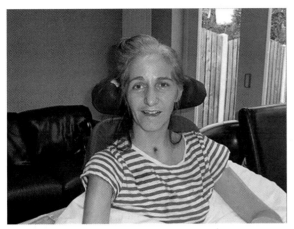

Fig. 25.4 ■ Kate is pictured in the hospital during her admission within the inpatient rehabilitation unit.

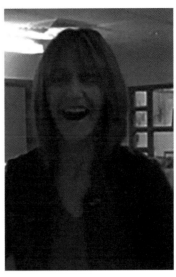

Fig. 25.5 ■ Kate is pictured on her last day, walking out of hospital in her leather jacket with blow-dried hair.

illustrated that on a social and occupational level, an individual's sexuality contributes to their identity, what they like to do (their occupational needs and desires), what they actually do (their level of participation in various occupations) and how they recognise/accept their sexuality. Exploring sexuality from this lens and providing access to sexuality support means that healthcare professionals, which includes occupational therapists, recognise the person as a sexual being with sexual rights. Further to this, they recognise the person as a whole being and are able to competently provide person-centred care.

Existing peer-reviewed research has largely focused on barriers to addressing sexuality, with many studies finding that occupational therapists can lack confidence, knowledge, skills and discomfort about addressing the topic (Hyland & Mc Grath, 2013; Lepage et al., 2021; Lynch & Joosten, 2022; McGrath & Lynch, 2014; Spaseska et al., 2022). Although numerous barriers interact and subsequently sexuality is often avoided or forgotten, research has indicated that additional education at a university, clinical and individual level can support occupational therapists to address sexuality more effectively (Auger et al., 2022; Low et al., 2022; Lynch & Joosten, 2022; McGrath et al., 2021). A call-to-action paper by Auger and colleagues (2022) highlighted that rather than focusing on barriers, literature should instead focus on ways in which occupational therapists can provide support. A seminal paper by

O'Mullan et al. (2021) focused on how occupational therapists can address sexuality effectively when there are clear personal and professional boundaries and can address sexuality within routine practice utilising core occupational therapy skills, such as communication, collaborative problem solving, pacing, positioning and adaptive equipment. This paper also argued that this can be done within a range of settings and that good support starts with commitment and motivation to address the topic. The remainder of this book chapter therefore will take this approach of focusing on ways to provide support for sexuality in practice rather than focusing on barriers.

Occupational Perspective of Sexuality: Doing, Being, Becoming and Belonging

As mentioned in the previous section, Lynch and Fortune (2019) devised a framework that intentionally integrates internationally recognised concepts from the occupational perspective of health – *doing, being, becoming* and *belonging* – to establish a connection between occupational-informed practice and sexuality. This framework, referred to as the Occupational Perspective of Sexuality, is represented in Fig. 25.6.

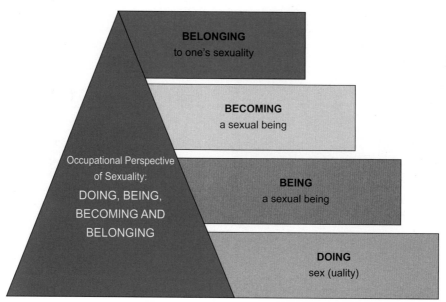

Fig. 25.6 ■ Occupational Perspective of Sexuality: Doing, being, becoming and belonging. (This figure is repurposed with permission by original authors (Lynch & Fortune, 2019).)

Within Fig. 25.6, the rectangular shapes symbolise the four occupation-related concepts: *doing* sex(uality), *being* a sexual being, *becoming* a sexual being and *belonging* to one's sexuality. The foundational position of 'doing' within the concepts indicates its relatively less complex nature, primarily addressing the physical aspect of doing sexual activity rather than the entirety of sexuality. The subsequent rectangle, being, illustrates the importance of a person's sexual identity and roles as a critical aspect of participation in life as a sexual being. Next, becoming, the importance of accompanying people on a journey to discover and grow and to eventually become who they want to be regarding their sexuality and sexual concerns. Finally, belonging, is acknowledging the hopes and aspirations that can lead a person to a sense of connectedness and belonging to their relationships/sexuality.

Each rectangle, concept, is inclusive of the previous one and hierarchically arranged to illustrate that a comprehensive understanding of sexuality involves an exploration of how individuals become the sexual beings they desire to be and how they engage and find their place within the various sexual aspects that represent their sexual identity. The triangle featured in the figure signifies the interconnection among all four categories, emphasising that occupational therapists who conceptualise sexuality through the lens of doing, being, becoming and belonging simultaneously address the biopsychosocial dimensions of an individual's sexuality. This visual representation underscores the importance of considering sexuality on multiple levels, guiding practice through a holistic and interconnected perspective rather than isolating specific aspects of the occupational experience.

Application of knowledge

Utilising the occupational perspective of sexuality, the dimensions of doing, being, becoming and belonging of Kate's sexuality are applied during the later stages of her rehabilitation, specifically when she transitioned back home and expressed the need to 'fend for myself'. At this juncture, Kate's focus shifted towards understanding and defining the evolving aspects of her sexuality. It is at this stage that the occupational therapist could have supported Kate with these aspects. To do this, the Occupational Perspective of Sexuality framework could have been used to explore Kate's experiences and perspectives. The information provided by Kate about her sexuality is mapped according to the four dimensions of doing, being, becoming and belonging as shown in Fig. 25.7.

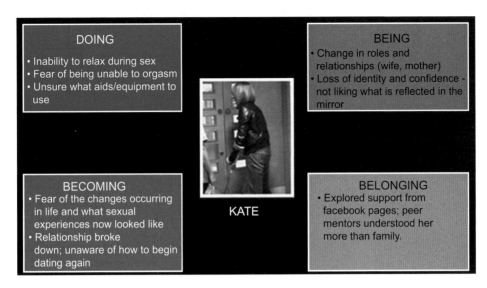

DOING
- Inability to relax during sex
- Fear of being unable to orgasm
- Unsure what aids/equipment to use

BEING
- Change in roles and relationships (wife, mother)
- Loss of identity and confidence - not liking what is reflected in the mirror

KATE

BECOMING
- Fear of the changes occurring in life and what sexual experiences now looked like
- Relationship broke down; unaware of how to begin dating again

BELONGING
- Explored support from facebook pages; peer mentors understood her more than family.

Fig. 25.7 ◼ Applying Kate's life experience according to the Occupational Perspective of Sexuality framework.

Doing: Kate's journey with sexuality post-stroke was challenging as previously effortless sexual activities now carried newfound complexities. Kate spoke about the inability to relax during intimate moments and the fear of being unable to orgasm. She also spoke about the provision of lots of information about assistive technology and equipment to assist with other aspects of her life but not her sex life. The occupational therapist could have facilitated and educated Kate about sexual techniques and positioning, energy conservation and the use of sexual assistive devices to engage in sexual activities both solely and within her relationships. The occupational therapist could have supported Kate in discussing with medical professionals about the impact of the stroke on her sexual functioning.

Being: Kate roles and relationships dramatically changed after her stroke. Prior to the stroke, she saw herself as an active mum and wife and a confident, independent woman. Upon returning home after her rehabilitation, she felt she had lost her identity and did not like what was reflected in the mirror. Kate explained how her roles as a mother and wife were impacted:

When I overheard my 8-year-old son tell his father in the garage that, 'Mum's back but not as she was', my heart was broken into a million pieces. I had tried so damned hard to prove everyone wrong – to

walk, eat again to return to my role as matriarch of our family. The wonderful family life I had created was changed forever and the only thing I ever wanted to be was a hands-on, loving, and reliable mother. My only purpose and sense of worth were annihilated in that one innocent statement from my 8-year-old, traumatised son. I was all alone trying to navigate motherhood doubly incontinent, physically weak, poor mobility, no self-worth and self-esteem with my own shame and trauma, emotional, psychological and relationship challenges. Sexually my body did not respond like it used to and sex became awkward, and I felt very unsexy and unconfident and unconnected.

As occupational therapists, working with individuals in relation to both their physical and mental health, support could have been provided to explore a journey of 'self-love' with Kate and allow her to be who she wanted to be from a sexual perspective. Kate talked about how 'bloody hard' it was to do this alone and having the guidance would have perhaps avoided many of the relationship difficulties she experienced along the way.

Becoming: Kate experienced many major shifts in her identity and purpose after returning home from hospital. Initially, Kate had to navigate many changes as a wife and mother which at times could be difficult, and after many years, Kate's marriage ended. Kate reflected

Identity was wrapped up in overachieving because of my childhood experiences. I over people-please as a mum, wife, friend, daughter, but my stroke made me incapable of being just average. I was in denial. But the guilt at the curve ball affecting my kids racked me with huge guilt. If someone professional had counselled and explained my stroke was not my fault and what I needed was my kids and ex-husband to do more to accommodate me, I would absolutely not have blamed and shamed myself, or felt so useless, worthless, unloved and redundant. Education on the ripple effects of stroke on everyone and signpost support would have been very helpful.

Having guidance, even a *'cheer squad'* to support and discuss what her life now looked like was something Kate echoed throughout her story. From an occupational perspective addressing *becoming* with an individual allows an opportunity to focus attention on the hopes, goals and aspirations related to the sexual being of a person.

Belonging: Kate longed for a feeling of being valued and respected in the context of her relationships. It was difficult to obtain this at home, but Kate obtained this sense of connectedness and belonging through the support of online support groups, from people who were experiencing similar challenges and concerns. Kate also began a registered charity organisation to help others in a similar situation as her to feel this *'sense of belonging'.*

Frankly, so many people in my support groups are so sad and lonely. Some talk about having never enjoyed intimacy for 15 years, others about how their partner cannot make the leap back to being a lover after being their partner's carer. But the worst comment that was post which truly horrified me was when one husband said to his wife after her stroke, 'It is like having sex with a dead body'. That is when I realised quite how many people are living in the community without experiencing any intimacy. That is utterly shocking. Disabled people, like able bodied people deserve to love and be loved. It is a basic human right.

BOX 25.4
KATE'S REFLECTION

For months after I returned home, I had problems with the physical side of our relationship [DOING]. Psychologically I had issues, I could not handle intimacy. For so long my body had been the public property of the doctors and nurses, who probed and prodded all my private nooks and crannies. Once I was home, I could say, 'Sod off, it is my body, I have had enough invasion' [BEING]. It took some time, but gradually Mark and I were able to rekindle our physical relationship with an emotional intensity that I never thought was possible [BECOMING and BELONGING] (Allatt, 2011).

Not all people who live with an illness, injury or impairment will be like Kate and be able to find their support network or indeed support others. Occupational therapists are well-positioned to lead an individual to find this sense of connectedness and belonging within their physical, social, community and cultural environment and to advocate for their sexual rights to be maintained.

Kate's reflection related to the concepts of doing, being, becoming and belonging is in Box 25.4.

Relevant Models to Support Practice

Occupational therapists are encouraged throughout their training and professional careers to refer to models and frameworks to support their practice. This is an important way for occupational therapists to ensure they are comprehensively and accurately providing meaningful and occupation-focused approaches. Although the SHFSD and the Occupational Perspective of Sexuality are two helpful frameworks, numerous models exist to support practice, such as the PLISSIT (Annon, 1976), Ex-PLISSIT (Taylor & Davis, 2007) and Recognition Model (Couldrick et al., 2010). It is encouraged that occupational therapists seek to understand the different models available and choose one that they are most comfortable using to support their practice in addressing sexuality.

The PLISSIT model is a well-established multidisciplinary model that is used commonly in practice. Initially introduced by Annon (1976) to aid healthcare professionals in addressing sexuality-related needs, the acronym PLISSIT signifies the four levels of intervention **P**ermission, **L**imited **I**nformation, **S**pecific

Suggestions and Intensive Therapy. The Ex-PLISSIT model serves as an extension of the PLISSIT model (Taylor & Davis, 2007). Unlike the linear PLISSIT model, within the Ex-PLISSIT model all interventions with individuals should begin with permission-giving; therefore the stages of Limited Information, Specific Suggestions and Intensive Therapy are underpinned by permission-giving (Taylor & Davis, 2007). Other features of the Ex-PLISSIT model include the requirement to review all interactions with the person and the incorporation of reflection as a means of increasing self-awareness by challenging assumptions. An occupational therapist can engage in all phases of the Ex-PLISSIT model. Some occupational therapists may predominantly specialise in sexual healthcare; however, for all occupational therapists, it is imperative for them to have a foundational understanding of sexuality to be able to provide limited information and specific suggestions. Occupational therapists must also then recognise when referrals to other services are necessary. For instance, psychosexual problems should be directed to psychosexual therapists and relationship issues should be referred to relationship counsellors, ensuring that individuals receive the specialised care they require (Taylor & Davis, 2007).

Similar to the PLISSIT and EX-PLISSIT models, the Recognition Model was published in 2010 to provide a team approach to supporting the sexual well-being of people with illness, injury or impairment (Couldrick et al., 2010). The authors noted several limitations of the PLISSIT model, most notably, a lack of a team approach. They therefore created the Recognition Model, drawing from the definitions of sexuality and sexual health as described by the WHO (2006) and developed in consultation with people with lived experience of injury, illness or impairment. The overall intention of the model was to enable therapists to work in a more sexually affirming way. The model involves five stages: recognition of the service user as a sexual being; provision of sensitive, permission-giving strategies; exploration of the sexual problem/concern; address issues that fit within the team's expertise and boundaries; and referral on when necessary. As Couldrick et al. (2010) indicated, it is expected that every occupational therapist should be working at the stage, 'recognition of the service use as a sexual being'. Occupational therapists may then draw on their own

existing skills and the skills within the team, in alignment with the outlined stages.

Reflect, Critically Reflect and Reason

Self-reflection allows occupational therapists to uncover personal biases, values and preconceptions that may inadvertently influence their interactions with people living with illness, injury or impairment (Dawson et al., 2022). By delving into their own beliefs and attitudes regarding sexuality, occupational therapists can cultivate a heightened awareness that fosters a more empathetic and unbiased therapeutic environment. There can be dominant discourses that exist within society that can impact on how healthcare professionals approach the topic of sexuality with people with injury, illness or impairment. By actively questioning and challenging their preconceived notions, occupational therapists can dismantle the barriers that biases pose in providing comprehensive care to individuals and collectives (Bryant et al., 2023). This reflective process not only promotes a more inclusive therapeutic environment but also reinforces the idea that critical reflection is not just a one-time task but an ongoing commitment (Taylor & Davis, 2007), allowing occupational therapists to adapt and grow continually. This also further ensures that their interventions remain responsive to the diverse needs of the individuals they work with.

Self-reflection can be done through formal means, such as attending professional development courses, special interest groups or supervision sessions. Informal methods can create a more fluid and dynamic exchange of ideas, for example, conversation with colleagues can allow occupational therapists to share experiences, learn from one another and collectively navigate the nuances of addressing sexuality (Spaseska et al., 2022).

The aim of this exploration is not to change an occupational therapist's personal values or attitudes. Rather, the aim for each occupational therapist is to recognise their own personal values and attitudes to become aware of these and identify if, and when, these values and attitudes may impact how they work.

Application of Knowledge

Before providing support to individuals on sexuality, it is crucial for an occupational therapist to understand their own personal values and attitudes. An occupational therapist should consider what approaches they could use to ensure thoughtful reflection on their own sexuality and its integration into their professional practice? Additionally, an occupational therapist should contemplate how their own sexuality aligns with the occupational perspective of sexuality – embracing the dimensions of doing, being, becoming and belonging. Occupational therapists should challenge themselves and spend some time reflecting and writing on their own values, beliefs and experiences related to sexuality. Further, they should reflect on how comfortable they would feel discussing sexuality topics with a healthcare provider and consider what might make these experiences more comforting for themselves if they were a person receiving healthcare services.

Promoting Occupational Participation in Sexual and Intimate Activities

There are many ways to explore and promote occupational participation in daily activities, and this is no different for sexual and intimate activities. The importance of co-design within therapy is particularly relevant in sexuality as this topic is so highly individualised and nuanced (refer to Chapter 19). Occupational therapists should promote participation in sexual and intimate activities across the continuum of care including in acute, inpatient, outpatient, transitional, community and private practice settings (Bryant et al., 2022a). Occupational therapists should also ensure that they are using a co-design approach to promote participation and decide on priorities with the person. This includes when exploring the person's occupational participation.

Use of Assessments, Observations and Questionnaires

To determine strengths and limitations of a person's occupational participation, an occupational therapist may draw upon standardised assessments, purpose-built questionnaires or use observations. Obtaining information on a person's sexuality, including their participation in sexual and intimate occupations, should be a routine part of practice. An occupational therapist could seamlessly integrate questions on sexuality during various other occupational therapy assessments, including functional capacity evaluations or even assessments related to the home environment or community access. For example, the occupational therapist may explore a person's community access to understand how they could independently use transport to attend romantic dates safely at night. By weaving questions about the individual's sexuality into typical assessments, observational or otherwise, occupational therapists can ensure that this crucial aspect of human experience is not overlooked.

Along with integrating questions and assessments into the usual occupational therapy schedule, the occupational therapist may also develop purpose-built questionnaires to ensure they are obtaining sufficient information. Within occupational therapy, and in health care more broadly, healthcare professionals commonly obtain sexual histories from individuals. However, the information asked when taking a sexual history can vary between occupational therapists (Brookmeyer et al., 2021). Often a sexual history will include information on the five Ps – partners, practices, protection from sexually transmitted infections (STIs), previous history of STIs and prevention of pregnancy. However, it has also been argued that the five Ps neglect many important aspects of sexuality (Brookmeyer et al., 2021). Pendleton & Schultz-Krohn (2011) discuss how occupational therapists may wish to undertake a sexual history questionnaire which could include the five Ps, along with questions on sexual behaviours, responses, sexual scripts, their medical history, psychological history and current relationships (where relevant). Therefore occupational therapists may seek to develop questionnaires to suit their practice.

There are limited validated standardised assessments that occupational therapists can use in the area of sexuality. Due to this lack of standardised assessments, the Occupational Performance Inventory of Sexuality and Intimacy (OPISI) (Walker et al., 2020) was created to screen, assess and measure performance related to sexuality. The OPISI includes a screening tool, in-depth self-assessment and a performance measure (Walker et al., 2020); however, it is still yet to be evaluated. There is also a component of the OPISI that can be used to assist with goal setting, which is another important component of promoting occupational participation.

Kate was unable to co-design her rehabilitation goals and it appeared that her rehabilitation team did not regard relationships and sexuality as important for the individuals who were in hospital.

> My OT gave me rehab based on what mattered to her as opposed to what mattered to me. There was no relationship advice.

Instead, Kate's goals were related to walking, balance, dressing, eating and bladder and bowel management. Kate would have liked to have also received other support. If Kate had been aware of the potential impact of a stroke on her sexuality, she might have been able to receive support for this and avoided some of the shame and guilt she experienced upon returning home.

> I wish someone would have informed me more about the effects of my stroke on my bladder and orgasm. I would have felt that they cared and thought about how my stroke had affected me on an emotional and sexual level. That they would have helped reduce some of my guilt and shame I later felt [...] I would not let my husband do my personal care. We avoided it. [I was worried] There was no way of coming back from that.

Co-Designing Sexual and Intimate Occupational Goals

Occupational therapists can enact co-design within their practice process by collaboratively creating goals with the person (refer to Chapter 19). Occupational therapists may wish to use sexuality specific goals sheets, as is provided in the OPISI (Walker et al., 2020), or they may wish to use other goal-setting tools such as the Canadian Occupational Performance Measure (Law, 1991) (refer to Chapter 16). It is important that goals are reviewed throughout the practice process. It is common for goals to change over time, and the occupational therapist should adapt with the person as required as part of a true co-design approach.

Application of Knowledge

Promoting occupational participation is a key component of occupational therapy; therefore understanding how to apply this in practice is vital. Kate had not received any support for sexuality; however, there were many occupational issues that Kate felt were relevant to her sexuality. Had an occupational therapist initiated

the topic of sexuality with her consent, this could have been explored when Kate was ready to do so. If the occupational therapist had conducted an informal or formal assessment, they likely would have learnt that as Kate required personal care support and had reduced ability to perform many occupations within her role as a wife and mother, there was increased tension in her marital relationship. This in turn resulted in fear and shame, decreased self-esteem and poor self-confidence impacting her sexuality. Kate had difficulty expressing her sexuality and returning to sexual and intimate occupations. If an occupational therapist had initiated the topic of sexuality and explored her occupational participation, numerous co-designed goals could have been developed with Kate. Several potential occupational goals may have included:

1. Prior to discharge, Kate will be able to independently paint her fingernails with bright colours to feel sexier and more connected to her sexual identity.
2. To improve her self-confidence and sense of belonging as a sexual being by receiving affirming sexuality support from her healthcare team and by engaging with peers within local or online communities.
3. To receive education and counselling to improve her self-esteem and symptoms of posttraumatic stress disorder (PTSD) with the aim of improving her self-confidence to return to sexual activities.
4. To receive education on managing changes to her sexual health and well-being so that Kate is better able to prepare for and engage in sexual and intimate activities.

Kate's reflection on the goals set for her in the hospital is in Box 25.5.

PROVIDING SEXUALITY SUPPORT

As highlighted in the previous section, occupational therapists can have toolbox of frameworks, models, assessments and strategies to address sexuality from an occupational perspective. This physical and metaphorical toolbox provides occupational therapists with the resources to support the individuals and collectives they work with; however, it should also have 'tools' to support, protect and guide the therapists themselves.

This section therefore explores therapeutic use of self, cultural humility and trauma-informed practice, initiating the conversation and use of enablement skills and strategies for sexuality.

Therapeutic Use of Self

Occupational therapists possess many tools within their metaphorical (or literal) toolbox that they can use when working with individuals, such as their therapeutic use of self. In the book, *The Intentional Relationship: Occupational Therapy and Use of Self*, Taylor (2020) describes how occupational therapists can utilise their own perspectives, insights, communication style and personality to support the therapeutic relationship. Although good therapeutic use of self is integral to all areas of practice within occupational therapy, this is particularly the case for sexuality. Sexuality is often a stigmatised topic and can be difficult for many individuals to discuss, further exemplifying why a well-considered, sensitive and individualised approach is warranted which draws on 'therapeutic use of self'. Taylor describes many ways that occupational therapists can use therapeutic use of self when providing support, such as utilising effective verbal and nonverbal communication. A couple of examples that Taylor discusses that are particularly relevant to the area of sexuality include being responsive to the individualised needs of the person, responding to suggestive verbal remarks and employing judicious use of touch.

As Taylor (2020) states, there are typical situations where people may attempt to push the boundaries of the therapeutic relationship, such as initiating physical touch with the occupational therapist or making suggestive comments/innuendos. Occupational therapists are encouraged to set professional boundaries and may wish to directly address verbal innuendos. Occupational therapists must also never accept attempts of sexualised or other inappropriate touch from individuals. Conversely, it is also vital that occupational therapists respect the person's boundaries. Touch can be a great way to demonstrate empathy; however, there can be negative consequences of touch, such as triggering trauma. Therefore Taylor (2020) suggests a judicious use of touch, where occupational therapists demonstrate good reasoning and judgement. This is essential considering that the global rate of sexual violence or assault is significant.

As part of an intentional relationship, Taylor also discusses the importance of providing culturally sensitive and safe support. As stated, '*developing cultural sensitivity is fundamental to effective use of self in occupational therapy*' (Taylor, 2020, p. 77). As discussed in the section immediately below, numerous sociocultural factors impact on how sexuality is viewed and approached between cultures within wider society.

Cultural Humility and Safety

Sexuality is an integral part of the human experience, deeply intertwined with socio-cultural norms. Therefore to understand how to provide sexuality support, occupational therapists are required to understand how to approach sexuality in a culturally safe manner. Culture is a concept that refers to patterns of human behaviour while cultural humility refers to an ongoing commitment to critically self-reflect and respectfully learn about others' cultural and structural backgrounds which is devoid of assumption (Curtis et al., 2019). Cultural safety is also grounded by self-reflection and recognises that sociological factors, such as historical, economic and social factors can create power differences within health care. In their book 'Cultural Safety in Trauma-Informed Practice from a First Nations Perspective', Tujague and Ryan (2023, p. 54) state 'You cannot be culturally safe unless you know your own culture, unless you know what it is about your culture that's different from the culture of the person or people you're working with'; further indicating the importance of reflection.

It is essential that occupational therapists review and reflect when supporting sexuality, and this also involves reflecting on their own culture. It is with critical self-reflection that occupational therapists can aim to dismantle existing power imbalances, particularly between the occupational therapist and the person and/or their family (Bryant et al., 2023; Morrison & Poblete-Almendras, 2023). This may help to ensure that harmful socio-cultural assumptions are not perpetuated within healthcare environments. There are numerous examples where socio-cultural factors can impose limitations on a person's sexual expression. For example, there has been limited research on people with injury, illness or impairment accessing sex work services and research on care workers supporting sexual expression. Bryant et al. (2023) discussed how there can be major differences in legislative and cultural approaches to facilitated sex and sex work, particularly between Western and non-Western cultures. Occupational therapists should better explore sociocultural issues in the context of sexuality and should include people with lived experienced as active participants in decision making, research and scholarship.

A major factor in providing culturally safe support for sexuality is to ensure that support is provided using a trauma lens. Tujague and Ryan (2023) argue that without a trauma-informed approach, it is difficult to practice in a culturally safe way.

Trauma-Informed Approach

It is important that occupational therapists understand and can draw from trauma-informed knowledge and skills when supporting people living with illness, injury or impairment. In relation to traumatic conditions, trauma may be defined as, 'exposure to an extremely threatening or horrific event or series of events'. However, trauma-informed care may be defined as a strengths-based approach to support a person's well-being, grounded in understanding and responsiveness to the impact of trauma on the person. There is emphasis on physical, psychological and emotional safety to support the person's sense of empowerment, and in turn, improve their health outcomes (Kimberg & Wheeler, 2019).

Understanding why occupational therapists should be able to utilise a trauma-informed approach, within the context of sexuality, is multifaceted. One way that an occupational therapist may utilise a trauma-informed approach may be when directly supporting a person's sexual well-being which has been impacted by their experience of trauma (whether of a sexual nature or not). Alternatively, an occupational therapist may work with a person on goals that are unrelated to sexuality though these goals may be impacted by their experience of sexual trauma (whether this has been disclosed or not). For example, previous research has highlighted that people who have experienced sexual trauma have increased negative impacts on their participation in employment occupations (Twinley, 2021).

Although not every person that the occupational therapist may work with may have experienced trauma, trauma-informed care is important for many individuals. There are also particular groups of people for which there may be an increased risk of experiencing trauma such as people who identify as LGBTQIA+ and those with intellectual disability (Sciolla, 2017; Tomsa et al., 2021). However, it is not always likely that the person the occupational therapist is working with will disclose an experience of trauma. It is therefore vital that occupational therapists do not make assumptions, as has been discussed throughout this chapter. Instead, occupational therapists should aim to be adequately educated in trauma-informed approaches to ensure they are able to provide competent and safe support for sexuality.

Initiating the Conversation

Along with utilising cultural humility and safety, therapeutic use of self and a trauma-informed approach, it is vital for occupational therapists to understand that it is their individual responsibility to initiate the conversation of sexuality when providing support. Research with people with lived experience of illness, injury or impairment has called for healthcare professionals to take responsibility for initiating the topic across all practice settings (Bryant et al., 2022a; Bryant et al., 2023; McGrath et al., 2021). Occupational therapists should first aim to develop and maintain rapport throughout the provision of sexuality support. Rapport will greatly increase the trust built with the person and therefore will improve their participation throughout the therapeutic process (Townsend & Polatajko, 2013). Occupational therapists and students have often noted that this can be daunting, and they are unsure when or how to address the topic, and further, what language to use in practice (Lynch & Joosten, 2022).

A lack of confidence has often been cited as to why occupational therapists are reluctant to initiate the topic (Spaseska et al., 2022). However, avoiding this topic fails to recognise the person as a sexual being with sexual rights. Occupational therapists are encouraged to initiate the conversation about sexuality by creating a safe and open space, reassuring individuals that discussions about sexuality are not only welcome but can be integral to their holistic well-being (Piantedosi et al., 2023). When initiating the conversation, the occupational therapist must also gain consent to discuss sexuality with the person, and importantly, must gain consent with the person on their own prior to discussing sexuality with any intimate partners (Bryant et al., 2022b).

It can be challenging to know what language to use when initiating or addressing the topic as people with lived experience of illness, injury or impairment can have very differing views of what sexuality means. For example, when asked to describe what sexual intimacy meant to them, one woman living with spinal cord injury described it as 'I really do not know for sure; when your body parts are really involved with each other?' While another described it as, 'Just having a normal life, a married life, and being able to smile' (Fritz et al., 2015, p. 3). Differences in understandings can create uncertainty for healthcare professionals on how to initiate the topic of sexuality and to know what language to use in practice confidently and safely. The umbrella definition of sexuality by the WHO (2006) therefore provides a helpful definition which can be used internationally to guide practice. Further, it is important that key concepts such as sexual well-being and sexual health are also understood. Though what is most important is for occupational therapists to recognise the person as a sexual being, to seek out their individualised understanding of sexuality and intimacy and to be guided by them, as discussed further below.

Although definitions can be helpful for guiding practice, people may be inclined to use terms that they feel more comfortable or familiar with. Therefore occupational therapists are encouraged to seek an individual's own understanding of sexuality and drawing from their 'therapeutic use of self' skills, they may wish to mirror the language the individual appears most comfortable using. The key lies in employing language that not only aligns with the occupational therapist's comfort level but also resonates with the person's preferences. It is crucial for occupational therapists to explore and understand the person's perspective on language, ensuring that the terms used are not only accurate but also culturally and personally meaningful. This mutual exploration fosters a sense of collaboration and trust, allowing the occupational therapist and the person receiving occupational therapy services to embark on a shared journey towards addressing and integrating sexuality.

Further, it is essential that practising and preregistered occupational therapists are also provided with opportunity to practice initiating the conversation (Lynch & Joosten, 2022). Occupational therapists have found with more experience that they become more comfortable when initiating the conversation (O'Mullan et al., 2021).

Enabling occupational therapists to practice and modify their language over time, whether during tertiary education or continual professional development opportunities, can help them become more comfortable with addressing the topic. This progressive and evolving process illustrates that there is not one singular, prescriptive approach to addressing sexuality, and the discovery for the occupational therapist is to find the approach that suits them and the individuals and collectives they work with.

Application of Knowledge

Given below are three examples of how the occupational therapist may initiate the conversation. However, it is vital that each occupational therapist practices what feels more natural and comfortable to them. The three examples are therefore only provided as a guide.

Examples of how to initiate the conversation of sexuality:

- I find some people also want to talk with me about their relationships or have questions about sex. I am happy to discuss these if you do have any concerns (Couldrick et al., 2010).
- I know we are suggesting it is necessary to move out of your double bed, but I wonder what that means to you both and to your relationship? (Couldrick et al., 2010).
- Many people with this condition have concerns about sexuality. Is there anything you would like to talk about or ask? (Taylor & Davis, 2007).

Kate's reflection on what she would have liked the healthcare team to ask is in Box 25.6

BOX 25.6
KATE'S REFLECTION

When I was in hospital, I wish that someone in the healthcare team had have just said to me, 'Perhaps this is the last thing on your mind and I totally get that, but I would like you to know that you may feel very differently, have physical struggles and your body may respond to intimacy and sex unlike before your stroke. So, I think it is important to explain to you that that is entirely normal for most people, but it can make people feel sad, anxious, even guilty and worried which is not right at all. It is not your fault [...] There is so much help, resources and support out there. I just want you to know this for when this is something you feel ready to explore'.

Enablement Skills and Strategies

The enablement skills and strategies, proposed by Townsend et al. (2007) and also depicted in the 7th edition of this textbook, are a set of skills that occupational therapists can utilise (Curtin, 2017). These skills and strategies can be applied across all areas of practice, including when supporting sexuality. There are seven strategies and ten enablement skills that the occupational therapist may wish to draw upon depending on the co-designed goal when working with individuals. The six strategies include remediation, compensation, education, community development, transformation and redistributive justice. The enablement skills include adapt, advocate, coach, collaborate, consult, coordinate, design/build, educate, engage and specialise.

Although all strategies and skills can be implemented into practice effectively, *education* is often a key enablement strategy used when supporting sexuality (refer to Chapter 22). Education may be targeted towards individuals or collectives. The occupational therapist may *engage* with the individual or collective and *educate* and *coach* them on sexuality-related topics, such as (though not limited to) the potential impact of illness, injury or impairment on sexuality, returning to intimacy or safe sex practices. The occupational therapist may wish to educate using various means such as face-to-face, virtually (e.g. email) or through resource provision. It is important that occupational therapists do not rely on written hand-outs and simply provide written information without opportunity for discussion (Bryant et al., 2022b). When providing education, occupational

	TABLE 25.4	
	Example of Enablement Skills Relevant to Kate	
Skill	**Goal (Brief)**	**Examples**
Adapt	To feel sexier and more connected to her sexual identity	This skill could have been employed by the occupational therapist who may have worked with Kate to see if there are different types of nail polishes that were easier to apply, such as quick-drying polishes.
Advocate	Education and counselling for self-esteem	The occupational therapist may have needed to advocate on behalf of Kate to her primary care physician for a referral to a psychologist for ongoing support for her reduced self-esteem and posttraumatic stress disorder (PTSD).
Coach	Engaging with peers within local or online communities	The occupational therapist could have established a partnership with Kate to explore what types of communities Kate would have wanted to participate in. The occupational therapist could have guided Kate while Kate remained responsible for her own decisions.
Collaborate	Receiving sexuality support from healthcare team	The occupational therapist could have collaborated with the multidisciplinary team to ensure the entire team was collectively working towards Kate's goals.
Consult	Engaging in sexual and intimate activities	The occupational therapist might have consulted with an equipment supplier to identify if there were any sexual assistive devices that could been prescribed for Kate.
Coordinate	Engaging with peers within local or online communities	The occupational therapist could have run group sessions on returning to sexual activity after a stroke. The occupational therapist may have coordinated with peer-support workers to also attend these sessions.
Design/build	Engaging in sexual and intimate activities	This skill could have been required by the occupational therapist if they were to have prescribed sexual assistive devices to support Kate's participation in sexual intercourse.
Educate	Engaging in sexual and intimate activities	The occupational therapist could have implemented this skill when working with both Kate and her husband to transfer knowledge on participating in sexual activities after a stroke.
Engage	Engaging with peers within local or online communities	As Kate was experiencing symptoms of PTSD, the occupational therapist could have used this skill to help motivate Kate to seek out more opportunities to engage with peers.
Specialise	Education and counselling for self-esteem	Drawing from experience within mental health, the occupational therapist could have provided specialist skills in counselling for self-esteem and for managing symptoms of PTSD if they have had received extra training and experience in this type of support.

therapists should monitor verbal and nonverbal communication to monitor the person's comfort and understanding (Taylor, 2020). Further information and examples of how the enablement skills can be applied to area of sexuality can be found in Table 25.4.

Application of Knowledge

To apply the information learnt about enablement skills, examples relevant to Kate's goals are presented in Table 25.4. The examples provided within this table are not exhaustive and are used to help demonstrate potential ways that the occupational therapist could enact different enablement skills within their practice process.

Refine Plans and Plan for Transition

It is important that occupational therapists continuously reflect on their practice, check in with individuals as part of a co-design approach, refine the plan and plan for transition. Occupational therapists are encouraged to evaluate what worked or did not work well and should seek feedback throughout. The practice process may conclude when the person has achieved their co-design goals related to sexuality, wishes to cease therapy or requires more specialised sexuality support from an alternative healthcare professional. Although important to refer onto other services, it is cautioned that occupational therapists do not refer on too early. As this chapter has highlighted occupational therapists possess the foundational knowledge and skills to be able to support individuals and collectives in achieving

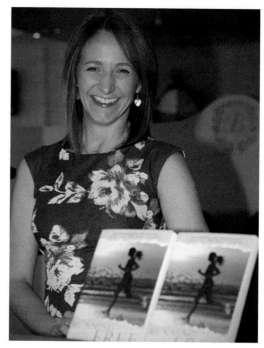

Fig. 25.8 ■ Kate at a book signing for her book 'Running Free: Breaking Out Of Locked In Syndrome'.

their sexual goals. Occupational therapists have an opportunity to play a pivotal role in being creators of change in this emerging area of practice.

Kate's reflection and advice for healthcare professionals are in Box 25.7.

CONCLUSION

Sexuality is an evolving area of practice, and increased research and implementation of knowledge into practice is required. This chapter has provided an overview of foundational understandings of sexuality for occupational therapists new to the discipline or to this area of practice. Occupational therapists are encouraged to reflect on their own attitudes and assumptions towards sexuality and consider ways in which they can further support the sexuality factor. The invitation to reflect on personal attitudes and assumptions towards sexuality is the initial step required for growth and enhanced support in this area. Beyond reflection, occupational therapists hold a distinct opportunity to become creators of change, actively shaping and advancing this

---

BOX 25.7
KATE'S REFLECTION

In Kate's book, *Running Free: Breaking Out of Locked-In Syndrome* (Fig. 25.8), Kate talks about how her stroke impacted her relationships. Overall, Kate describes her experience receiving support for sexuality as *'non-existent'*. As Kate did not receive support, she had to learn to return to intimacy on her own. She found her own strategies – *'They were about pleasuring my partner'*. However, had a healthcare professional supported her sexuality earlier, Kate feels she would, *'Have enjoyed sex as much as my partner'*. Kate believes that it is important for all healthcare professionals to address sexuality within their practices as, *'To love and be loved is a basic human right for everyone'*.

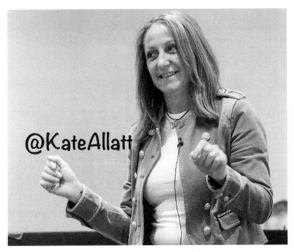

Fig. 25.9 ■ Dr Kate Allatt.

emerging area of practice. By embracing continuous learning opportunities, fostering open communication, assessing and evaluating the various aspects of sexuality, and championing inclusivity, occupational therapists can be a leading professional when creating change and ensuring the sexuality of *ALL* individuals and collectives with illness, injury or impairment is addressed.

Acknowledgement

The authors of this chapter want to acknowledge the invaluuable input from Dr Kate Allatt (Fig. 25.9) who generously provided her time story and images enhance this book chapter. Kate is an internationally renowned speaker, sexuality and health consultant, published author, researcher, disability advocate and peer mentor (Allatt, 2023). Kate's contribution to this chapter has been invaluable and her vulnerability and generosity are greatly appreciated. It is hoped that readers of this chapter will be able to learn from Kate's experiences and reflections and use the knowledge gained to improve their practice when supporting individuals with disabilities in their own practice.

Bryant and Lynch also acknowledge the traditional custodians of the lands on which this work was conducted – in Meanjin, the Yuggera and Turrbal people and the Wurundjeri Woi-wurrung and Bunurong Boon Wurrung people of the Easten Kulin Nation.

REFERENCES

Aggleton, P., Parker, R. G., & Thomas, F. (2015). *Culture, health and sexuality: An introduction*. Routledge.

Allatt, K. (2011). *Running free: Breaking out from locked-in syndrome*. Accent Press Ltd.

Allatt, K. (2023). *Bio*. www.kateallatt.com.

Annon, J. S. (1976). The PLISSIT model: A proposed conceptual scheme for the behavioral treatment of sexual problems. *Journal of Sex Education and Therapy, 2*(1), 1–15. https://doi.org/10.1080/01614576.1976.11074483.

Auger, L.-P., Masse, J., & Higgins, J. (2022). Sexuality in occupational therapy: A call to action. *The British Journal of Occupational Therapy, 85*(9), 627–628. https://doi.org/10.1177/03082226221107769.

Brookmeyer, K. A., Coor, A., Kachur, R. E., Beltran, O., Reno, H. E., & Dittus, P. J. (2021). Sexual history taking in clinical settings: A narrative review. *Sexually Transmitted Diseases, 48*(6), 393–402. https://doi.org/10.1097/olq.0000000000001319.

Bryant, C. (2023). *Enhancing sexual wellbeing after spinal cord injury: A multimethodological investigation using exploratory, critical, and partnered approaches to improve sexuality support*. [The University of Queensland, School of Health and Rehabilitation Sciences]. https://doi.org/10.14264/a7ef273.

Bryant, C., Aplin, T., & Setchell, J. (2022b). Sexuality support after spinal cord injury: What is provided in Australian practice settings? Sexuality support after spinal cord injury. *Sexuality and Disability, 40*(3), 409–423. https://doi.org/10.1007/s11195-022-09756-w.

Bryant, C., Gustafsson, L., Aplin, T., & Setchell, J. (2022a). Supporting sexuality after spinal cord injury: A scoping review of non-medical approaches. *Disability and Rehabilitation, 44*(19), 5669–5682. https://doi.org/10.1080/09638288.2021.1937339.

Bryant, C., Aplin, T., Piantedosi, D. K., & Setchell, J. (2024). It's Not, Can You Do This? It's … How Do You Feel About Doing This? A Critical Discourse Analysis of Sexuality Support After Spinal Cord Injury. *Sexuality and Disability, 42*(2), 259–275. https://doi.org/10.1007/s11195-024-09837-y.

Couldrick, L., Sadlo, G., & Cross, V. (2010). Proposing a new sexual health model of practice for disability teams: The recognition model. *International Journal of Therapy and Rehabilitation, 17*(6), 290–299. https://doi.org/10.12968/ijtr.2010.17.6.48152.

Curtin, M. (2017). Overview of enabling skills and strategies. In M. Curtin, M. Egan, & J. Adams (Eds.). *Occupational therapy for people experiencing illness, injury or impairment: Promotion occupation and participation*. (8th Ed.). Edinburgh: Elsevier. pp. 322–333.

Curtis, E., Jones, R., Tipene-Leach, D., Walker, C., Loring, B., Paine, S.-J., & Reid, P. (2019). Why cultural safety rather than cultural competency is required to achieve health equity: A literature review and recommended definition. *International Journal for Equity in Health, 18*(1), 174. https://doi.org/10.1186/s12939-019-1082-3.

Dawson, J., Laccos-Barrett, K., Hammond, C., & Rumbold, A. (2022). Reflexive practice as an approach to improve healthcare delivery for indigenous peoples: A systematic critical synthesis and exploration of the cultural safety education literature. *International Journal of Environmental Research and Public Health, 19*(11), 6691. https://doi.org/10.3390/ijerph19116691.

DeLamater, J. (2012). Sexual expression in later life: A review and synthesis. *The Journal of Sex Research, 49*(2–3), 125–141. http://www.jstor.org/stable/23249140.

Fileborn, B., Lyons, A., Hinchliff, S., Brown, G., Heywood, W., & Minichiello, V. (2017). Learning about sex in later life: Sources of education and older Australian adults. *Sex Education, 17*(2), 165–179. https://doi.org/10.1080/14681811.2016.1273829.

Fritz, H. A., Dillaway, H., & Lysack, C. L. (2015). 'Don't think paralysis takes away your womanhood': Sexual intimacy after spinal cord injury. *The American Journal of Occupational Therapy, 69*(2). 6902260030p1–10. https://doi.org/10.5014/ajot.2015.015040.

Hillman, J. (2017). Sexual consent capacity: Ethical issues and challenges in long-term care. *Clinical Gerontology, 40*(1), 43–50. https://doi.org/10.1080/07317115.2016.1185488.

Hyland, A., & Mc Grath, M. (2013). Sexuality and occupational therapy in Ireland – A case of ambivalence? *Disability and Rehabilitation, 35*(1), 73–80. https://doi.org/10.3109/09638288.2012.688920.

Kimberg, L., & Wheeler, M. (2019). Trauma and trauma-informed care. In M. R. Gerber (Ed.), *Trauma-informed healthcare approaches: A guide for primary care* (pp. 25–56). Springer International Publishing. https://doi.org/10.1007/978-3-030-04342-1_2.

Law, M. (1991). *Canadian occupational performance measure.* CAOT Publications ACE.

Lepage, C., Auger, L.-P., & Rochette, A. (2021). Sexuality in the context of physical rehabilitation as perceived by occupational therapists. *Disability and Rehabilitation, 43*(19), 2739–2749. https://doi.org/10.1080/09638288.2020.1715494.

Low, M. A., Power, E., & McGrath, M. (2022). Sexuality after stroke: Exploring knowledge, attitudes, comfort and behaviours of rehabilitation professionals. *Annals of Physical and Rehabilitation Medicine, 65*(2), 101547. https://doi.org/10.1016/j.rehab.2021.101547.

Lynch, C., & Fortune, T. (2019). Applying an occupational lens to thinking about and addressing sexuality. *Sexuality and Disability, 37*(2), 145–159. https://doi.org/10.1007/s11195-019-09566-7.

Lynch, C., & Joosten, A. V. (2022). Addressing sexuality: The comfort and preparedness of occupational therapy students. *Journal of Occupational Therapy Education, 6*(1), 1–16. https://doi.org/10.26681/jote.2022.060107.

McGrath, M., & Lynch, E. (2014). Occupational therapists' perspectives on addressing sexual concerns of older adults in the context of rehabilitation. *Disabil Rehabil, 36*(8), 651–657. https://doi.org/10.3109/09638288.2013.805823.

McGrath, M., Low, M. A., Power, E., McCluskey, A., & Lever, S. (2021). Addressing sexuality among people living with chronic disease and disability: A systematic mixed methods review of knowledge, attitudes, and practices of health care professionals. *Arch Physical Medicine and Rehabilitation, 102*(5), 999–1010. https://doi.org/10.1016/j.apmr.2020.09.379.

Mitchell, K. R., Lewis, R., O'Sullivan, L. F., & Fortenberry, J. D. (2021). What is sexual wellbeing and why does it matter for public health? *The Lancet. Public health, 6*(8), e608–e613. https://doi.org/10.1016/S2468-2667(21)00099-2.

Morrison, R., & Poblete-Almendras, M. J. (2023). Discourses on sexuality and occupations: Reflections for occupational therapy and occupational science. *Sexes, 4*(3), 392–401. https://doi.org/10.3390/sexes4030025.

O'Mullan, C., O'Reilly, M., & Meredith, P. (2021). Bringing sexuality out of the closet: What can we learn from occupational therapists who successfully address the area of sexuality in everyday practice? *Australian Occupational Therapy Journal, 68*(3), 272–281. https://doi.org/10.1111/1440-1630.12723.

Pendleton, H. M., & Schultz-Krohn, W. (2011). *Pedretti's occupational therapy.* Elsevier.

Piantedosi, D. K., Reed, K., & O'Shea, A. (2023). Supporting occupational therapists to initiate conversations about sexuality with people with intellectual disability: Co-design by deliberative dialogue. *Australian Occupational Therapy Journal, 70*(5), 581–598. https://doi.org/10.1111/1440-1630.12888.

Portellos, A., Lynch, C., & Joosten, A. (2023). Sexuality and ageing: A mixed methods explorative study of older adult's experiences, attitudes, and support needs. *The British Journal of Occupational Therapy, 86*(7), 515–526. https://doi.org/10.1177/03080226231164277.

Rokach, A., & Patel, K. (2021). *Human sexuality* (1st ed.). Elsevier Science & Technology. https://doi.org/10.1016/C2018-0-04449-7.

Rose, N., & Hughes, C. (2018). Addressing sex in occupational therapy: A coconstructed autoethnography. *The American Journal of Occupational Therapy, 72*(3). 7203205070p7203205071–7203205070p7203205076. https://doi.org/10.5014/ajot.2018.026005.

Sayers, J. (2020). *Sigmund FREUD: The basics.* Routledge.

Sciolla, A. F. (2017). An overview of trauma-informed care. In K. L. Eckstrand & J. Potter (Eds.), *Trauma, resilience, and health promotion in LGBT patients: What every healthcare provider should know* (pp. 165–181). Springer International Publishing. https://doi.org/10.1007/978-3-319-54509-7_14.

Shuttleworth, R. (2006). Sexual access. In G. L. Albrecht (Ed.), *Encyclopedia of disability,* (Vol. 4, pp. 1443–1445).

Shuttleworth, R., & Mona, L. (2021). *The Routledge handbook of disability and sexuality.* Routledge.

Spaseska, C., Lynch, C., Joosten, A., & Josefsson, K. A. (2022). Experience of recently graduated occupational therapists in addressing sexuality with their clients. *Sexuality and Disability, 40*(4), 769–783. https://doi.org/10.1007/s11195-022-09762-y.

Srinivasan, S., Glover, J., Tampi, R. R., Tampi, D. J., & Sewell, D. D. (2019). Sexuality and the older adult. *Current Psychiatry Reports, 21*(10), 97–99. https://doi.org/10.1007/s11920-019-1090-4.

Taylor, B., & Davis, S. (2007). The extended PLISSIT model for addressing the sexual wellbeing of individuals with an acquired disability or chronic illness. *Sexuality and Disability, 25*(3), 135–139. https://doi.org/10.1007/s11195-007-9044-x.

Taylor, R. e. R. (2020). *The intentional relationship: Occupational therapy and use of self* (2nd ed.). F.A. Davis Company.

Tomsa, R., Gutu, S., Cojocaru, D., Gutiérrez-Bermejo, B., Flores, N., & Jenaro, C. (2021). Prevalence of sexual abuse in adults with intellectual disability: Systematic review and meta-analysis. *International Journal of Environmental Research and Public Health, 18*(4), 1–17. https://doi.org/10.3390/ijerph18041980.

Townsend, E., Beagan, B., Kumas-Tan, Z., Versnel, J., Iwama, M., Landry, J., Stewart, D. & Brown, J. (2007). Enabling: Occupational therapy's core compeencey. In E. Townsend & H. Polatajko (Eds.). *Enabling Occupation II: Advancing an Occupational Therapy Vision for Health, Well-Being and Justice Through Occupation* (pp. 87–135). Ottawa: CAOT Publications ACE.

Townsend, E. A., & Polatajko, H. J. (2013). *Enabling occupation II: Advancing an occupational therapy vision for health, well-being, and justice through occupation* (2nd ed.). Canadian Association of Occupational Therapists.

Tujague, N., & Ryan, K. (2023). Towards Cultural Safety: Cultural Safety in Trauma-Informed Practice from an indigenous perspective. In N. Tujague, K. Ryan (Eds.), *Cultural Safety in Trauma Informed Practice from a First Nations Perspective.* Springer International Publishing. https://doi.org/10.1007/978-3-031-13138-7_3.

Twinley, R. (2021). *Illuminating the dark side of occupation: International perspectives from occupational therapy and occupational science.* Routledge.

Walker, B. A., Otte, K., LeMond, K., Hess, P., Kaizer, K., Faulkner, T., & Christy, D. (2020). Development of the occupational performance inventory of sexuality and intimacy (OPISI): Phase one. *The Open Journal of Occupational Therapy, 8*(2), 1–18. https://doi.org/10.15453/2168-6408.1694.

WHO. (2001). International classification of functioning, disability and health (ICF). Geneva: World Health Organization.

WHO. (2023a). *Adolescent sexual and reproductive health.* Retrieved October 9, 2023, from https://www.who.int/news-room/questions-and-answers/item/adolescent-sexual-and-reproductive-health.

WHO. (2023b). *Gender and health.* Retrieved October 9, 2023, from https://www.who.int/health-topics/gender.

REFLECTION

1. This chapter has explored the multifaceted aspects of sexuality. How does this influence, challenge or expand your previous understanding of sexuality?

2. How can the Socio-Health Framework of Sexuality and Disability (SHFSD) enhance your ability to address the interconnected levels of individual, interpersonal, services and community and societal factors that contribute to a person's sexuality?

3. In considering the Occupational Perspective of Sexuality as a framework for occupational therapy practice, how might you integrate the concepts of doing, being, becoming and belonging to shape your understanding of a person's sexuality?

4. How can the Canadian Occupational Therapy Inter-Relational Practice Process (COTIPP) support and guide your practice when addressing sexuality?

26 WORK PARTICIPATION

YELIZ PRIOR ■ TRACEY PARNELL

Overview

In this chapter, work as an important human occupation is explored, with a particular focus on paid work or employment. The benefits and challenges of participating in employment are explored in relation to health and well-being, and unemployment and underemployment as complex public health concerns that may contribute to reinforcing health inequities are discussed. The impact of illness, injury and impairment on participating in employment is provided, and the importance of a proactive approach to assessment and intervention is presented as a strategy to minimise work disability. The role of occupational therapists in collaborating with people to facilitate participation in work is also addressed, including discussion regarding assessment and intervention approaches that may be used.

KEY POINTS

■ Work is an important human occupation; participating in work-related occupations is a significant health outcome due to its impact on health and well-being.

■ Work is influenced by the context in which it occurs, and understandings of work are simultaneously influenced by a range of contextual factors, including societal and cultural factors.

■ Participation in paid work or employment can have both positive and negative impacts on health and well-being. Unemployment and underemployment are complex public health concerns that may contribute to reinforcing health inequities.

■ Proactive intervention is recommended to prevent or minimise absenteeism and presenteeism due to illness, injury or impairment that may lead to work disability. The impact of work disability extends beyond individuals to affect broader society.

■ Occupational therapists are well placed to collaborate with people to promote participation in work occupations due to their inherent understanding of occupation as a biopsychosocial construct.

AN INTRODUCTION TO UNDERSTANDING WORK AS AN OCCUPATION

Work defines us in myriad ways. Except for family, nothing is so central to our place in society, how others perceive us, and how we see ourselves [...] Work is also universal: only the most privileged are exempt from its demands, and only the most helpless and unlucky are denied the dignity and pride conferred by even the humblest job.

(Protzman, 2006, dust jacket)

Work is an integral part of contemporary life and is acknowledged as an important human occupation. Work is central to individual identity, provides a route to social inclusion and economic security, and being employed is generally associated with good health and well-being. Conversely, various physical and psychosocial aspects of work can pose risks to health and well-being. There is a strong association between worklessness and poor physical and mental health, including higher morbidity and mortality (Waddell & Burton, 2006). In this chapter, work as a human occupation is explored with a particular focus on paid work or employment and occupational therapists' role in supporting people to remain at or return-to-work, so they can lead healthier and fulfilled lives.

To many people, work is an activity that requires physical and mental effort, resulting in the production of and services of value to other people (Cook & Lukersmith, 2010). Work contributes to the maintenance of life and helps individuals to meet basic life needs; work also contributes to self-esteem, identity, social connectedness, sense of achievement and status (Harpaz & Fu, 2002; Sinnicks & Reeves, 2023). The World Health Organization (1986) recognised work as one of the determinants of health due to the impacts it can have on well-being. In reporting to the International Labour Organization (ILO), Somavia (2001, p. 5), described work as 'an expression of our unique talents, a way of contributing to the common good, an avenue for engaging deeply and meaningfully with a community'.

Work is not an easily defined concept. In his philosophical essay addressing the uniqueness of work for humans, Overell (2008, p. 12) stated that 'defining that grim little word is a notoriously difficult matter'. Occupational therapy has a long history of promoting the importance of work participation (see Harvey-Krefting, 1985; Jones, 1993; Toulmin, 1995; Jones 1998). From an occupational perspective (Njelesani et al., 2014), work is a significant occupation throughout the course of life that includes both paid and unpaid productive occupations (World Federation of Occupational Therapists, 2018) and contributes 'to the social and economic fabric of […] communities' (Law et al., 1997, p. 34). In considering the meaning of work to asylum seekers, Lintner and Elsen (2018, p. 76) found that work was not 'merely a rational and economic activity but a human occupation' that contributed to well-being, identity and connectedness. There is enormous variation in how people perceive work and what it means to them (Sinnicks & Reeves, 2023). For example, employment, voluntary work, caring for family and studying may all be considered to be work. However, within Western societies, the term 'work' is often synonymous with employment (Noon & Morrell, 2017). Some definitions consider work only to include employment; that is, work done for fiscal reward (Cambridge University Press, n.d.). Christiansen and Townsend (2004) noted that many publications and writings about work in the wider community are about employment.

Definitions of work that predominantly focus on employment have been criticised, and it has been suggested that 'defining work as paid employment is a modern prejudice' (Overell, 2008, p. 12). Indeed, narrow conceptions of work as synonymous with employment may well be a legacy of the increased focus on labour during the 19th and 20th centuries (Pocock, 2006). Grint (1991) proposed that in many modern Western societies, the importance placed on paid employment may have resulted in unpaid forms of work being deemed less important; other authors (see Jones, 1998) have argued for a redefinition of work to include unpaid work, which is often done at home. Unpaid work occupations may include occupations such as parenting, housework and volunteer duties (O'Halloran & Innes, 2005). Other definitions of work overtly acknowledge that employment is only one aspect of work. For example, Kielhofner et al. (1999) included both paid and unpaid productive occupations in their definition of work. More recently, Asaba et al. (2021, p. 83) defined work 'as an occupation encompassing a broad range of day-to-day activities, and as something situated in a socio-political landscape of conditions that afford more or fewer possibilities for participation.'

Like all occupations, work is influenced by the context within which it occurs; context is a multi-dimensional construct that includes micro, meso and macro elements (Egan & Restall, 2022). Understandings of work and the nature of work that people participate in are influenced by a range of contextual factors, including societal and cultural factors (Brown et al., 2001; Overall, 2008). Primeau (1996) suggested that attempts to define work as a separate entity from non-work are a convention of modern Western culture and fail to consider the impact of culture or experience on understandings of work. Other researchers have also found that opinions about work are influenced by a person's social and cultural origins and that these ideas are particularly developed and shaped during adolescence (Kirkpatrick Johnson & Mortimer, 2011). Similarly, in a naturalistic study with young children, Chapparo and Hooper (2002) found that the children's definitions of work were dependent on contextual factors such as age, culture, experience and issues of choice and agency. In addition to finding that, people make distinctions between work and non-work occupations, Chapparo and Hooper found that definitions of work vary between individuals and that this changes throughout the course of life. They also found that at a very young age, children had already begun to construct ideas about what work is, and what it is not, and contrasted work to other occupations such as self-care, play and rest.

The remainder of this chapter will focus particularly on paid work. Paid work is a significant aspect of the lives of many people due to financial reasons, societal expectations and acceptance, and mastery of competence. Supporting individuals to regain or enhance their ability to work is an important goal in occupational therapy, promoting personal fulfilment, financial independence, social integration, skill development, routine and positive health outcomes. By addressing work-related challenges, occupational therapists support individuals to achieve a meaningful and satisfying life. The focus on paid work does not intend to demean the value and importance of other forms of work or privilege paid work over other forms of work; however, a broader exploration of all aspects of work is not possible within the restrictions placed on chapter length.

EMPLOYMENT

The factors that drive people to seek out and maintain employment vary, and the nature of the employment

people engage in may also be motivated by different reasons. Work motivation has been extensively researched and is a topic of significant importance to organisational and societal success and to understanding the well-being of people in relation to work (Kanfer et al., 2017). Numerous extrinsic motivators have been shown to influence individuals' engagement in the labour force. For example, it is an expectation of most Western societies that people of working age will participate in employment (van Krieken et al., 2010). For some individuals, this societal expectation may be the most significant motivator to participate in employment. Other authors have suggested that financial recompense is a significant factor motivating people to participate in employment (O'Halloran & Innes, 2005). Whereas others (e.g. Jones, 1998; Schwartz, 2015) have proposed that people are motivated to work by factors other than fiscal gain, such as feeling accepted within society and the establishment of competence.

Many of the positive consequences of participating in employment are also positive intrinsic motivators that enhance a person's desire to work. Intrinsic factors that motivate people to participate in employment include: creating and maintaining identity (Jakobsen, 2001; Pocock, 2003; Stone, 2003; Unruh, 2004), having a sense of purpose and structure for each day (Jakobsen, 2001; Schwartz, 2015), experiencing a sense of accomplishment and competence (Jones, 1998; Pocock, 2003; Schwartz, 2015), community involvement (Jones, 1998; Pocock, 2006), achievement of status within society (Harpaz & Fu, 2002), and pleasure, gratification and independence (Pocock, 2003; Schwartz, 2015). For some people, employment can be a way of managing symptoms such as pain and anxiety (Jakobsen, 2001).

Extrinsic factors may operate to limit individual agency and set parameters about the nature of a person's participation in employment. For example, in Australia, there are programmes mandating when a person is required to engage and re-engage with the workforce, such as mutual obligation programmes and government policies that require parents to return to work when their youngest child reaches 6 years of age (Workforce Australia, 2023). Masterman-Smith and Pocock (2008) found that many individuals who are forced into employment under these conditions are often left financially worse off and with a poor quality of life.

Benefits of Employment

There are many positive outcomes associated with participating in employment. Pocock (2006) highlighted the central role that paid work or employment plays in the lives of people of working age in Western society and argued that for many people, the course of life is often structured around decisions related to employment and careers. Christiansen and Townsend (2004, p. 164) proposed that 'having a job provides individuals with a sense of identity and contributes to the common good'. Previous research has demonstrated the significant impact that participation in employment can have on a person's sense of identity (Pocock, 2006; Somavia, 2001; Unruh, 2004). Somavia (2001, p. 5) reflected that paid work is an 'activity through which individuals affirm their own identity, both to themselves and to those around them'. In the 2003 Australian Survey of Social Attitudes, 55% of respondents listed their employment as being one of the top three ways they describe themselves (Pocock, 2006). The relationship between a person's identity and their employment may also be dependent on the nature of the employment they participate in. In considering the link between paid work and identity, Selenko et al. (2017) found that job insecurity negatively impacts social identity, in turn impacting well-being. In addition to contributing to a person's identity, the worker role has also been found to contribute to self-esteem, health, well-being and quality of life (Cook & Lukersmith, 2010; Stone, 2003). It is likely that not all people's participation in employment will have a positive impact on their sense of identity. Indeed, some authors (e.g. Beck, 2002; de Botton, 2009) have challenged the centrality of paid work to the modern sense of self.

Paid work or employment provides opportunities for people to develop social contacts, develop routines and structure for daily life, define non-work time more clearly, and to contribute to their community through the sharing of knowledge, skills and capacities (Christiansen & Townsend, 2004). Paid work can also provide opportunities to contribute to the needs of others and foster a sense of belonging within a community (Baker & Jacobs, 2003; Brown et al., 2001). Harpaz and Fu (2002) found that people's status within society is linked to their worker roles and, more specifically, to their professions, their roles within an organisation, and the employment activities they perform. Pocock's (2006)

analysis of work and its impact on people from the perspectives of children and young people reinforced the findings of other researchers that the positive outcomes of participating in employment include the enhancement of self-esteem, engagement in social interactions, creation of a sense of belonging, the use of skills and experience and financial reward.

The distribution of the benefits linked to employment is, in some instances, inequitable and impacted by a range of social factors. For example, in the United States, paid work affords employees the benefit of access to private health insurance. Those people without employment and who cannot afford private health insurance or who do not qualify for government-funded health insurance are left without affordable access to health services; in 2021, this accounted for around 10% of the US population (Keisler-Starkey & Bunch, 2021). Similarly, Kiepek et al. (2022, p. 268) described the 'citizenship rights' present in the Global North and afforded to those citizens who are considered to contribute to society in a useful manner, for example, through employment. It is evident that participation in employment can provide privilege to those who have the capacity to participate in it.

The Dark Side of Employment

Although there is strong research evidence indicating that work is beneficial, what the evidence suggests is that 'good work' is good for a person; that is, a job that pays fairly and offers lasting security, ensures good working conditions, enables a life balance, and provides training and opportunities to progress (Waddell & Burton, 2006). Harmful aspects of employment have been identified and are particularly evident in some industries. These factors may impact the health and safety of individuals and impact their motivation to participate in employment. Workplace injuries, illnesses and deaths continue to be a major concern in many countries, despite significant improvements in workplace health (Schofield, 2009). The nature and quality of employment can influence whether an individual's employment contributes to their well-being or results in ill health (Faragher et al., 2005). There is evidence that working in some types of employment may be worse for individual well-being than the experience of unemployment (Butterworth et al., 2011); indeed, 'being unsatisfactorily employed is detrimental to psychological health and is psychologically as bad as being unemployed' (Dollard & Winefield, 2002, p. 4).

Masterman-Smith and Pocock (2008) highlighted the detrimental impact of being employed in low-paid positions on workers, their families and communities. The results of their study found that engaging in low-paid work increased an individual's vulnerability to poor health and decreased overall well-being. Masterman-Smith and Pocock also found that low-paid, working-class jobs are often exploitative, have higher rates of bullying and other psycho-social hazards, and regularly leave workers feeling demoralised and disconnected. Similarly, Zuzanek (2010) outlined that jobs demanding long working hours can have detrimental effects on individuals, including physical exhaustion, family tension and negative emotional and well-being outcomes. Kiepek et al. (2022) suggested that work that includes indentured labour or excessive hours may not contribute to personal meaning or may negatively impact health and quality of life and are examples of occupational injustice.

The Changing Nature of Employment

Employment has changed over time, and it will continue to evolve as technology continues to advance. The first industrial revolution saw the advent of urbanised, factory-based employment, with the coal-fired steam engine and other machinery setting a faster pace for labour; the hours were often long, remuneration low, and the conditions detrimental to health and well-being. Fast forward to the 2020s to what is being termed Industry 4.0 or the Fourth Industrial Revolution, and it is likely further changes to employment will be seen. As with the first industrial revolution, this new revolution brings both advantages and disadvantages for individuals and collectives. Industry 4.0 may mean employees are less likely to be exposed to harmful employment settings due to technology that can detect and mitigate these risks. However, new risks or an increase in existing risks may become apparent, for example, an increase in shift work and the associated health risks such as cancer, increased work insecurity, and an increase in on-demand employment or the gig economy (Min et al., 2019; Pratap et al., 2021). The benefits of new workplace technologies are not necessarily experienced equitably, for example, the introduction of some technological advancements creates demand

for more highly skilled workers while simultaneously decreasing the demand for workers with lower education and skills (European Parliament, 2018). Changes to the nature of employment require that occupational therapists be attuned to new employment possibilities and to the risks associated with these possibilities.

The global COVID-19 pandemic significantly impacted the way employment is structured. At the height of the pandemic, to slow the spread of the virus, many employees were forced to work from home. This change required rapid adaptation to virtual forms of communication to continue participating in employment duties and changes to the home environment to accommodate work-related equipment for one or more people. In contrast, people classified as essential workers, such as many healthcare workers, were required to attend their place of employment potentially placing them at risk of acquiring the virus. Post-pandemic employment has seen a shift in the use and acceptance of flexible work arrangements. In their study of 1400 workers, Ruppanner et al. (2023) found that pre-pandemic ways of participating in employment were not suitable for all employees, particularly those with competing demands (e.g. those with caring responsibilities and people with chronic illness). They also found that flexible work arrangements adopted during the pandemic resulted in some employees experiencing increased motivation for job duties and increased productivity; in addition, many study participants reported they would consider leaving a current position to seek out another that offered more flexible employment conditions. Ruppanner et al. (2023) concluded that creating new ways of working, including access to flexible work arrangements, is essential to ensure the workforce is resilient to future challenges and that a focus on a culture of inclusivity and improving labour market outcomes for vulnerable groups is paramount to ongoing workforce developments.

Unemployment/Underemployment

Not all people are afforded the privilege of being employed or are employed in a position that is meaningful and contributes to a sense of purpose and well-being. Both unemployment and underemployment are complex public health concerns, impacted by a range of contextual factors, and have the potential to contribute to reinforcing health inequities (Pratap et al., 2021).

Unemployment has been defined as 'those who do not have a job but are available for work' (Pratap et al., 2021, p. 8), it is synonymous with a lack of paid employment (O'Halloran et al., 2018). Research has highlighted the connection between unemployment and poor health outcomes, such as reduced physical health, increased mortality and increased risk of mental health problems, such as depression and anxiety (Kasl et al., 2007), as well as the negative impact of unemployment on the sense of identity and belonging (Crooks et al., 2009; Jakobsen, 2009; Stone, 2003). In contrast, underemployment generally refers to work that is inferior relative to a particular standard, such as level of experience, education, skill or hours desired to work (Feldman, 1996; Maynard et al., 2006). Underemployed individuals participate in jobs that are lower than their expectations and goals (Manjeet et al., 2020). Allan et al. (2020, p. 111) reported that people who are underemployed, and therefore unable to 'fully employ their skills and abilities may be at particular risk for poorer well-being.'

Understanding Work Disability

The International Classification of Functioning (ICF) (World Health Organization, 2001) defines disability as a complex interaction between a person (with a health condition) and that person's contextual factors (environmental and personal), thus proposing a biopsychosocial approach to disability. This approach is also aligned with the occupational therapy approach, in which participation in productive occupations (that is, work) requires a person (that is, worker) to interact with complex physical, psychosocial, personal and environmental demands. Thus a mismatch between a person's abilities and the person's job demands results in work instability (Gilworth et al., 2003). If work instability is not resolved in a timely manner, it can lead to work disability, which is broadly defined as ceasing to work before retirement age due to ill health.

Work disability is a complex construct, just like the definition of what constitutes 'work' and 'disability' in and of themselves. The impact of work disability is vast, transcending the individual and shaping the wider society due to its socio-economic and cultural consequences. Researchers have attempted to quantify this concept and introduced an array of new terminology specifically used to describe such phenomena to measure the impact of work disability and identify a range of health and social targets to inform interventions. Perhaps the most common and familiar notion in work disability is the quantification of the working hours/days lost due to illness, injury or impairment, when an employee is absent at work during a normally scheduled work period (that is off sick); this is often referred to as absenteeism in the literature. Absenteeism is relatively easier to identify compared to presenteeism, which is when people are at work (or working from home) but are unable to be productive, due to illness, injury or impairment. Frequent and unresolved presenteeism can also lead to absenteeism, and prolonged absenteeism can lead to work disability. It is understood that once people are work disabled, they are unlikely to return to work. Thus it is important to intervene early, when work instability is identified, to provide support to help people remain in employment.

Definitions of common terminology used in the field of work rehabilitation are presented in Table 26.1.

TABLE 26.1	
Definition of Key Terms Related to Work	
Key Terms	**Definition Used in This Chapter**
Work	Productive occupations performed within an employment setting.
Worker	A person who participates in paid or unpaid productive occupation.
Work instability	A mismatch between the duties and the abilities of an individual.
Work disability	Ceasing to participate in work before retirement age because of illness, injury or impairment.
Absenteeism	A state that occurs when an employee is absent from work during a normally scheduled work period.
Presenteeism	A loss of workplace productivity resulting from an employee's illness, injury or impairment or personal issues.
Work rehabilitation	A process to overcome the barriers an individual faces when accessing, remaining or returning to work after injury, illness or impairment.
Job retention intervention	Interventions to help people with health problems overcome the barriers to staying at work.
Return-to-work intervention	Interventions to help people return to work after an injury, illness or impairment.
Ergonomics	The study of people's efficiency in their working environment.

OCCUPATIONAL THERAPY AND WORK REHABILITATION

Work is integral to the ethos of occupational therapy, as the profession was founded upon principles related to the benefits of work and supporting people with health conditions to gain or return to paid employment (Royal College of Occupational Therapists [RCOT], 2021). Work rehabilitation is defined as 'a process to overcome the barriers an individual faces when accessing, remaining or returning to work following injury, illness or impairment' (Department for Work and Pensions, 2004, p. 12). Although work rehabilitation can be a stand-alone process in health and social care, in occupational therapy it should be a part of the individualised complex intervention provided to people with health problems and rehabilitation needs, tailored to suit the changing needs of the person as therapy progresses, with prevention of work loss or return-to-work (if desired and achievable) as the primary objective.

The work rehabilitation process in occupational therapy takes place when individuals identify problems at work or need help to support their return to work. Work rehabilitation can influence many factors relating to work instability and work disability, including but not limited to:

■ Job-related factors: environmental barriers; lack of specialised equipment; physically demanding jobs; inflexible working hours; problems with transportation; long-term sick leave; and lack of employer/team support and issues relating to equity, diversity and inclusion at the workplace, which can systematically impact people with protective characteristics.

■ Psychological factors: job strain, depression, lack of family/social support; poor work self-efficacy; lack of knowledge and/or advocacy skills to request and obtain help; and unwillingness to disclose condition and limited use of self-management strategies.

■ Condition-specific factors: symptoms such as pain, fatigue and activity limitation relating to a specific health condition interfering with daily activities and work, side effects of medication and a mismatch between the individual's capacity and the job demands.

Occupational therapists should work collaboratively with people, using a shared decision-making process to address the above factors when resolving work-related problems. The process undertaken to assess, plan and deliver work rehabilitation interventions will differ from one setting to another, depending on the availability of service provision, knowledge and experience of the team and cultural practices within that setting. It is important to note that, work rehabilitation is an essential part of occupational therapy practice and is not an isolated intervention. A comprehensive discussion of all approaches to work rehabilitation, including specialised services, standardised/non-standardised assessments and interventions to meet individuals' different health and social care needs, is not possible in this chapter. The focus in this chapter is on the approach to work rehabilitation, as part of a collaborative relationship-focused approach to occupational therapy (Egan & Restall, 2022).

Occupational Therapy's Role in Supporting Employment Participation

Occupational therapists are well placed to support people to participate in employment due to their inherent understanding of occupation as a biopsychosocial construct and have historically used therapeutic work activities in rehabilitation (Hammond et al., 2022; Prior et al., 2017; Prior & Hammond, 2014; Preston & Prior, 2013). As the only healthcare profession to train across physical and mental health, focusing on occupation (RCOT, 2021) and supporting people to maintain and optimise their participation in work is an important goal for occupational therapists.

Work rehabilitation interventions are delivered by occupational therapists when people report difficulties with participating in work due to physical, psychological, or social dysfunction, which might result from illness, injury or impairment (Prior et al., 2014). In spite of the occupational therapy profession's long history of providing work rehabilitation to individuals with work-related injuries (Cook & Lukersmith, 2010), the role of occupational therapists for people with health-related work problems to stay at work, or return to work after a period of ill-health or unemployment is highly variable, and not perceived as an intervention priority in many health and social care settings (Prior et al., 2014). However, socio-political changes across the globe to tackle health inequalities in populations, coupled with the socio-economic and health burden caused by work disability, have led to increased demand for health and social services to consider the consequences of health and injury on work participation. This provides an excellent opportunity for occupational therapists, whose profession has traditional values embedded in using occupation as a therapeutic medium, to drive and lead the delivery of work rehabilitation services across the globe.

Traditionally, these services have been embedded within existing health and social care services to support people with health conditions and disabilities to better manage themselves in the workplace. Nowadays, occupational therapists are deploying their expertise in new ways, for example, in primary care and tertiary services (occupational health), as well as developing new paths to vocational support, for example, in community mental health teams and working independently as work/career/personal development coaches, and vocational rehabilitation experts, providing occupation-focused interventions to help people experiencing difficulties at work or getting into paid employment.

Occupational therapists have a role working with individuals experiencing unemployment and underemployment to support them in finding work that is meaningful, that supports them in achieving their life goals, and that provides a 'just right' challenge by facilitating the use of their experience, knowledge and skills, which contributes to a positive sense of purpose, meaning and identity. Individualising the issue of unemployment has been challenged (O'Halloran, 2022) and instead, the creation of interventions and processes that do not start from the assumption that unemployed people do not want to work but rather aim to understand and address the barriers to employment, is advocated for. In addressing unemployment and underemployment, occupational therapists are encouraged to consider broad contextual issues, to look beyond neoliberal perspectives that individualise these issues, and to consider how to facilitate change at systemic or macro levels (Farias & Laliberte Rudman, 2019; Kirsh, 2015). These perspectives highlight the complexity of work participation from individual, societal and broader health and socioeconomic perspectives.

Work Assessment and Intervention Approaches in Occupational Therapy

Assessment of a person's work situation should start during the initial interview. This can be done by first establishing the person's work status and then by asking a question such as, 'Are you having any problems at work?' This question can be supported by further questions about the nature of the work (e.g. manual/professional/self-employed) and the identification of any areas for concern, for example, motivation to work, personal and contextual factors, past, current and anticipated difficulties and the role of environmental barriers and facilitators on work participation. It is preferable to support people to remain at work, as the research suggests that once people are out of work, they are much less likely to return to employment (Ravinskaya et al., 2023). People may be reticent to mention work problems in a health setting unless they are prompted to do so (Prior et al., 2017). Therefore occupational therapists should aim to identify work problems even when these are not highlighted in the initial interview and goal-setting stage.

Occupational therapy assessment of a person's work strengths and challenges would typically consist of applying ergonomic principles (i.e. the study of a person's efficiency in that person's work environment) with an emphasis on a biopsychosocial approach to examine:

- *The physical, neurodevelopmental and psychological consequences* of a person's health status on their activities at work (e.g. the impact of the person's illness, injury and/or impairment on their physical functioning; the impact of the person's mood, motivation and beliefs on undertaking certain tasks at work), and work participation (e.g. reduced productivity at work, increased absenteeism and work instability).
- *Contextual factors (personal and environmental factors)* affecting a person's work performance (e.g. personal factors such as being able to afford childcare, environmental barriers such as difficulties in using public transport or driving to access work, and/or mobility issues preventing the person from moving in and around the workplace).

Following the assessment of work participation, which can be conducted using standardised (e.g. disease-specific Patient Reported Outcome Measures and semi-structured interviews) or non-standardised assessments (e.g. as part of the initial interview), an occupational therapist would work collaboratively with key stakeholders to devise a work rehabilitation programme. In this context, work rehabilitation is devised under two main umbrellas, either with an aim to support individuals to remain in work, that is, a 'job retention vocational rehabilitation' (JRVR), or to help the person to regain employment either in the same or a new position, that is, a 'return-to-work job rehabilitation' (RTWJR). These are explored in more detail in the next section.

Once the type of intervention programme is identified, the occupational therapy work rehabilitation programme is devised as a complex and targeted intervention. This may involve:

1. physical (e.g. hand exercises to improve range of movement and strength; fatigue management through energy conservation and graded activity),
2. psychological (e.g. working on self-efficacy using counselling skills to increase the person's belief in their own capabilities),
3. environmental interventions (e.g. providing advice on ergonomic equipment),
4. advice on current work legislation, statutory and third-sector employment, support and advisory services and
5. the employee's rights to facilitate increased confidence in their ability to work.

Legislation, policies and services vary from one setting to another. Despite these variations, it is important to understand that the aim of workplace legislation, policies and services is to facilitate work participation of people experiencing illness, injury or impairment that impacts their ability to participate in work. It is therefore important that occupational therapists have knowledge and understanding of contemporary local and national policies and services to ensure they can support the people they are collaborating with to remain in or return to work.

Engagement with Stakeholders to Facilitate Work Participation

As work participation is deemed to be an important health outcome due to its impact on health and well-being, professional bodies in the United Kingdom have signed up to the Consensus Statement on Health and Work (https://www.councilforworkandhealth.org.uk/wp-content/uploads/2019/05/Health-and-Work-Consensus-Statement.pdf) which outlines four principles for health and care professionals, as a statement of action. These principles are:

1. Understand the health benefits of good work and the long-term effects of avoidable health-related worklessness.
2. Have the skill to incorporate discussions about working in the context of a health outcome with patients in their care, as appropriate to the health or disability of that individual.
3. Feel supported to understand and interact with the wider health and work system, employers, occupational health services and other bodies that have a role in assisting individuals who are not working for health-related reasons.
4. Recognise their own role in supporting healthy and safe working environments, looking after their own health and well-being and those of their colleagues.

2019 Healthcare Professionals' Consensus
Statement for Action
Statement for Health and Work

Occupational therapists' role in increasing work participation transcends the need to liaise with employers to negotiate work accommodations, and it is recommended that for the achievement of sustainable employment outcomes, the process should include facilitation of broad stakeholder engagement in the job retention or return-to-work process. Promotion of engagement across multidisciplinary teams (e.g. physiotherapists, psychologists, general practitioners and consultants) in health and social care, occupational health services, governmental departments, other bodies (e.g. employee benefit schemes), as well as family and carers, is also advised to ensure people receive timely and appropriate support. Occupational therapists can also provide tailored education and advice for family, carers and employers to support people with difficulties at work and/or planning to return to work within the environmental and cultural contexts they live and work in. Effective stakeholder liaison is also necessary to enable onward referral and collaboration, where additional specialist input is required.

Occupational therapists may be working with people who have complex health needs and multiple comorbidities. They may be responsible for coordinating their care across different healthcare providers and settings and ensuring they have access to the services and resources they need to achieve their goals. Occupational therapists have a role to play in the advocacy space, advocating for and working with individuals to secure safe, meaningful and sustainable employment, and working with collectives to advocate for their rights at work. This advocacy work supports aspects of Goal 8 of the 2030 Agenda for Sustainable Development (International Labour Organization, 2016), specifically the right to participate in full and productive employment and decent work.

Another example of occupational therapists working with stakeholders to support work participation is the introduction of 'fit notes' to certify the ability to work, as opposed to 'sick notes' which were traditionally issued for why people are 'not fit to work'. Fit notes are issued to people to provide evidence of the advice they have been given by a healthcare professional about their fitness for work. These notes record details of the functional effects of an individual's condition so the person and their employer can consider ways to facilitate their return to work (Department of Work and Pensions, 2013). More than 10 million fit notes are signed every year across the UK, mostly for sickness absence from work or welfare benefits. Previously, only doctors, through a fit note, could legally certify whether someone needed assistance returning or was unable to return to work; due to new legislation introduced by the UK government in July 2022, occupational therapists are also able to legally certify fit notes. This legislation covers all occupational therapists, at the point of registration with the Health and Care Professions Council (HCPC), therefore recognising occupational therapists as experts at providing work and health advice. The focus on what people can do, rather than what they cannot is an area of growing international interest and importance, as demonstrated by the introduction of a certificate of capacity in Australia in 2015, building on the fit note (Brijnath et al., 2015). This is a positive step in supporting people to retain or return to employment, however, the effectiveness of this initiative will be determined by the level of stakeholder engagement (e.g. effective liaison between the person, occupational therapist, employer

and occupational health) to facilitate work participation in the coming years.

Job Retention Interventions

Job retention interventions are aimed at people who are at work but experiencing problems affecting their productivity (e.g. work instability and presenteeism), which may have resulted in short-term sick leave (i.e. absenteeism), which is usually less than three months in duration. Job retention intervention provision varies between countries. In the UK, National Health Service (NHS), work-related support in many occupational therapy departments is sporadic. Where this exists, it is usually provided only to a few people who were originally referred for other reasons. Brief work advice lasts on average 45 minutes, without a structured work assessment, and includes signposting to work services, providing information booklets and self-management education related to work (Hammond et al., 2020).

Effective job retention assessment requires a thorough job analysis to establish the impact of a person's health on their ability to perform their work role as well as the impact of their work demands on their health and well-being. Informally, this could consist of a discussion about the person's physical work environment, role within the team and their workplace, daily tasks and responsibilities, working hours, transportation, relationships with colleagues, culture at the workplace, main stressors and knowledge of workplace policies to outline the support available for people when work performance is affected by illness, injury or impairment. It is also important to assess the impact of work life on a person's home life and relationships.

Throughout this process, therapists can utilise standardised assessments/outcome measures to facilitate the delivery and evaluation of job retention interventions. There are several standardised work assessments that can be used to identify job-specific limitations, concerns, and help inform the development of goal setting (Table 26.2). These include assessments widely used in occupational therapy practice, such as the Canadian Occupational Performance Measure (COPM) (Law et al., 2005) (refer to Chapter 16).

There are also disease-specific work assessments, which are developed and tested for use in specific populations for clinical and research purposes. For example, the UK Work Experience Survey-Rheumatic Conditions

TABLE 26.2
Examples of Standardised Work Assessments

Name of Work Assessment Scale	Description
Ergonomic Assessment Tool for Arthritis (EATA) (Backman et al., 2008)	The EATA was developed to be used as an assessment for people with arthritis. It is individualised to each person through five screening questions: Does your work involve (1) Prolonged sitting? (2) Prolonged standing, kneeling, walking or stair climbing? (3) Gripping or grasping objects or hand tools? (4) Frequent lifting or carrying? (5) Pushing or pulling items?
Rheumatoid Arthritis Work Instability Scale (RA-WIS) (Gilworth et al., 2003)	The disease-specific RA-WIS includes 23 yes/no scale questions that measure any mismatch between people's functional abilities and the demands of their jobs. Originally developed to measure work instability in people with RA, it has subsequently been validated for other musculoskeletal disorders.
Workplace Activities Limitations Scale (WALS) (Tang et al., 2011)	This 12-item questionnaire aims to measure the amount/level of difficulty in performing work tasks, with additional items for each question regarding whether the participant received help from others at work with the task or has any adaptation.
Work Environment Impact Scale (Moore-Corner et al., 1998)	A semistructured interview and rating scale focusing on people with physical or psychosocial conditions and their work problems. There are 17 items to examine the social and physical environment, supports, changing demands, objects used and daily job functions.
Work Experience Survey – Rheumatic Conditions (WES-RC) (Allaire & Keysor, 2009)	This is a structured interview for identifying barriers and formulating solutions for people with rheumatic conditions. The WES-RC can be administered through either face-to-face or telephone interviews.
Work Limitations Questionnaire (WLQ) (Lerner et al., 2001)	This 25-item questionnaire, with four subscales, measures physical work demands, time work demands, mental-interpersonal work demands and output work demands.

(WES-RC) (Hammond et al., 2013) is a structured work interview that supports an assessment of the person's job, roles and responsibilities in relation to their condition, disease severity and activity limitations, and allows a detailed assessment of work barriers. This is followed by the occupational therapist and the person collaboratively prioritising work problems, and agreeing to an action plan, which then supports a tailored, individualised programme, including self-management at work, job accommodations, employment rights information and other strategies as relevant (Hammond et al., 2020; Hammond et al., 2022). This process may include a work site visit if identified as relevant to a person's needs and there is an agreement by both the individual and their employer to conduct this. According to the individual's needs, the therapist or the person may need to liaise with the UK government-funded services, for example, Access to Work and Disability Employment Advisors (https://www.gov.uk/access-to-work), and any occupational health support available in their workplace to support access to work accommodations.

In addition to structured interviews, there are a number of work-specific reported outcomes available to provide direct reports from individuals with work problems to help identify targets for interventions. An example of this is the Work Activity Limitations Scale (WALS), which measures the amount of difficulty with work activities (work ability) (Beaton et al., 2016; Gignac et al., 2007; Hammond et al., 2023; Tang et al., 2014; Verstappen et al., 2019). The British English WALS consist of 12 items, measured on a scale of 0–3 for difficulty in performing work activities (0 = no difficulty; 3 = unable to do), which includes: eight physical activity items; three about managing work; and concentration at work. Psychometric testing of the British English WALS demonstrated good validity and reliability in employed people with rheumatic and musculoskeletal conditions, that is, rheumatoid arthritis, axial spondyloarthritis, osteoarthritis and fibromyalgia in the UK (Hammond et al., 2023).

The effectiveness of job retention interventions for employed people is limited. A systematic review of randomised controlled trials identified two trials with positive results and one with no effects (Hoving et al., 2014). A small UK trial of occupational therapy and job retention vocational rehabilitation showed a reduction in work instability and improvement in self-reported ability to manage at work, at 6 months (Macedo et al., 2009). A brief job retention intervention in the United States led to reduced job losses for 4 years (Allaire et al., 2003). A randomised control trial (RCT) of a multidisciplinary job retention programme in the Netherlands identified no changes in work outcomes, though, four out of 10 participants were already on long-term sick leave (De Buck et al., 2005). Other RCTs in the United States identified positive outcomes at two-year follow-ups. An occupational therapy-led workplace ergonomic intervention resulted in significant improvement in self-reported work impairment but not pain, job satisfaction, physical function, or mood (Baldwin et al., 2012). Another brief job retention intervention provided by occupational therapists and physiotherapists led to reduced job loss but no reduction in presenteeism (Keysor et al., 2016; Keysor et al., 2018). A recent job retention vocational rehabilitation RCT was conducted in the UK (Hammond et al., 2020; Hammond et al., 2023) to determine the clinical and cost-effectiveness of vocational rehabilitation and written self-help (intervention) or written self-help advice only (control) with 240 participants with inflammatory arthritis, including RA, psoriatic arthritis (PsA) and undifferentiated inflammatory arthritis (UIA). The results of this RCT are not yet available at the time this textbook was published.

Return-to-Work Interventions

Restoring the ability to work is a key element in the rehabilitation of working-age adults in occupational therapy. Return-to-work interventions are aimed at people who are either already on long-term sick leave (less than 3 months) and/or unable to work due to ill health (i.e. work disabled). Defining return-to-work interventions is complex, as this process can include those who have been away from work due to long-term sickness, as well as those who have been unemployed for various reasons, including long-term health conditions (e.g. stroke), illness (e.g. long-term COVID) or injury (e.g. an amputation). The approach to the return-to-work process may vary depending on whether the injury, illness or impairment was sustained at work or away from the work setting and will be informed by relevant legislation and/or procedures.

If the person is currently not working, it is essential to understand whether this is by choice (i.e. they could have taken time out to study, care for dependents, relocate, etc.). Similarly, if the person is retired, it is imperative to establish whether retirement was a choice or due to illness, injury or impairment to identify if return-to-work may be an appropriate goal. An international multi-stakeholder Delphi study to develop a core outcome set for work participation asked participants which outcomes should always be measured in intervention studies for improving work participation for people with a health problem (Ravinskaya et al., 2023). Due to the lack of consensus regarding the definition of 'returning to employment', new terminology has been proposed as 'duration of absence from work due to a health problem over a period of time'. They have also added another outcome, 'having lost employment', to this stage, as an indicator of workers who do not return to work at all after a period of health-related absence (Ravinskaya et al., 2023).

The process in which the work assessment is conducted, and the interventions are planned and delivered in occupational therapy-led return-to-work interventions closely mirror the process followed in job retention interventions. The role of occupational therapists in this process may involve supporting people during their transition back into the worker role after an injury or accident or recovering from a long-term illness. This includes working with people to collaboratively develop individualised rehabilitation goals aimed at re-building specific work skills, and the confidence needed to facilitate a return to work. The approaches to support return-to-work may include: job demand analysis, worksite visits, ergonomic assessment, use of assistive technologies, assessing function in relation to job demands, graduated return-to-work planning, return-to-work monitoring, vocational assessment and identification of work accommodations. Occupational therapists can also advocate for return-to-work options with the employer and provide on- and off-site coaching to facilitate job skills.

It is important that occupational therapists are skilled and confident in exploring realistic expectations, as return-to-work interventions can involve working with highly vulnerable people, and therefore careful management of expectations during this collaborative process is essential. For example, there is a growing number of people returning to work following cancer treatment while managing ongoing symptoms of cancer and side effects of treatment; many of these people are also living with multiple co-morbidities (Fowler et al., 2020). In line with the increased number of people living longer with cancer, the term 'cancer survivor' was coined to describe any person diagnosed with cancer, irrespective of the stage of treatment (Hewitt & Ganz, 2006). Thus regardless of the setting they work in, occupational therapists are likely to encounter cancer survivors, including supporting them in the return-to-work process, if appropriate. A qualitative study conducted in Australia explored the perceptions of occupational therapists about the facilitators and barriers for return-to-work for someone with cancer. This study found, 'that the person with cancer, employers, family members, co-workers and society underestimate the impact of ongoing cancer symptoms on return to work' (Hatton et al., 2021, p. 1). The study findings suggested that cancer survivors experienced symptoms such as ongoing fatigue and cognitive difficulties and had to deal with fear of relapse, while concerns regarding disclosure and how this would impact co-workers' perceptions of them also affected return-to-work (Hatton et al., 2021). In another study exploring the meaning of work for females with a breast cancer diagnosis, it was found that work remained an important priority as a way of maintaining a sense of self and control, but that the women desired an increased focus on life balance (MacLennan et al., 2022). It is therefore important that careful consideration be given to the individual person's goals, needs, diagnosis and symptoms in determining suitable work duties and hours, and the support required to facilitate a sustainable employment outcome.

Similar to job retention interventions, the evidence to support return-to-work interventions in occupational therapy is limited. A scoping review to identify best practice guidelines for occupational therapy to support people with trauma and stress-related mental health conditions suggested that return-to-work interventions in these populations are limited, and the interventions described were more often person-focused versus environment- and occupation-focused, and many were carried out by multidisciplinary teams (Edgelow et al., 2020). Another study investigated an

early, specialist vocational rehabilitation approach to facilitate the return-to-work after traumatic brain injury through a multi-centre feasibility, parallel-group RCT (Radford et al., 2018). Early specialist traumatic brain injury vocational rehabilitation was delivered by occupational therapists in the community using a case coordination model. The study concluded that it is feasible to assess the cost-effectiveness of vocational rehabilitation in this population, and return-to-work was most strongly related to social participation and work self-efficacy. The challenges identified for the definitive trial included employing experienced occupational therapists (Radford et al., 2018). Radford et al. are conducting ongoing research to increase the evidence base for occupational therapy-led return-to-work interventions in neurorehabilitation; they are conducting a multicentre randomised controlled trial to determine whether an early stroke specialist vocational rehabilitation service plus usual care is a clinically and cost-effective therapy to facilitate return-to-work after stroke, compared with usual care alone (Radford et al., 2022). The intervention is intended for delivery in the community and includes the following: (1) assessing stroke impact on the person and their job, (2) educating individuals, employers and families about stroke impact on work and strategies to lessen impact (e.g. memory aids and fatigue management), (3) work preparation, including opportunities to practice work skills and (4) liaison with employers to plan and monitor a phased return-to-work (Radford et al., 2022). There is a process evaluation embedded within this trial to inform future complex interventions. This will include fidelity data, which is necessary to interpret intervention outcomes, but despite extensive literature supporting its importance, fidelity is commonly underreported in studies of complex rehabilitation interventions. This RCT is an example of a complex intervention that involves interfaces between multiple stakeholders, is highly targeted, and requires behavioural change by the person, their family, and the employer to support a return-to-work (Radford et al., 2022).

Despite improvements in some aspects of employment, it is not uncommon for people to sustain injuries when undertaking employment duties. These injuries vary greatly and include acute, short-term injuries that resolve quickly through to long-term injuries that result in chronic illness or permanent disability, and in some instances, death. The return-to-work process following a work-related injury or illness is determined by legislation relevant to the industry and geographical context where the injury occurred (see for e.g. https://www.safeworkaustralia.gov.au/workers-compensation/national-return-work-strategy). In developed countries, such as Australia, legislation is in place to protect and support injured employees, and facilitate a timely, safe, positive and sustainable return to employment (Safe Work Australia, 2019). As with non–employment-related injuries and illness, the return-to-work process following an employment-related injury or illness aims to help employees return to meaningful duties or to remain in employment while recovering, and is impacted by individual, organisational and system-level factors (Safe Work Australia, 2019). For a successful and sustainable return to employment to occur, stakeholders at all levels must work together collaboratively.

Occupational therapists may be involved in various aspects of facilitating a successful return to employment for an individual injured at work. A previous review of the literature found that occupational therapy interventions positively contribute to return-to-work programs (Désiron et al., 2011). In considering the return-to-work process, the occupational therapist is likely to be involved in a range of assessments and return-to-employment strategies to facilitate the process, as outlined in previous sections of this chapter. These assessments and strategies include worksite assessment and modification, including a focus on ergonomic factors (Innes, 2008), functional capacity evaluation (De Baets et al., 2018), goal setting, graduated return-to-work planning and implementation, and communication and negotiation with key stakeholders to facilitate the return-to-work process and address barriers to success (Robart & Boyle, 2021). The specific approach to the return-to-work will vary depending on the injury or illness and the nature of work duties. The occupational therapist will use a range of skills, including task analysis and professional reasoning, to ensure an appropriate match between an individual's current capacity and the work demands, and to appropriately grade the return-to-work process.

Occupational therapists may also be involved in working with employers to develop and deliver education and injury prevention programs that aim to change workplace behaviours, ultimately reducing the risk of work disability. In a study exploring preventative behaviours at work, Lecours (2020) found that, in addition to increasing workplace safety, the establishment of work-preventative behaviours can contribute to positive physical, social and mental health outcomes. With their understanding of the link between positive work experiences, health and well-being, knowledge of approaches to enhance the interaction between the person, environment and occupation and strategies to facilitate safe work contexts, occupational therapists are well-placed to provide valuable contributions to educational and preventative programs to promotion participation in work.

CONCLUSION

Work, in its broadest sense, is defined as 'an activity involving mental or physical effort done in order to achieve a result' (British Psychological Society [BPS], 2018). However, the concept of work can hold different meanings, ranging from paid employment to volunteering to being a person's purpose in life. Regardless of which meaning is used, work provides a structure to people's lives, helping them identify with a perceived role in society, and a path to social inclusion, whether it is paid or unpaid.

The focus of this chapter is on employment, as being able to participate in employment is an important occupation, inherent to the health, well-being and livelihood of individuals. Widespread participation in employment is the motivating force for economies and provides structure and meaning to individual people and the communities in which they live. There is clear evidence that good work improves the health and well-being of people and protects against social exclusion. Conversely, unemployment impacts negatively on health and well-being and is associated with an increased risk of mortality and morbidity, including limiting long-term illness, cardiovascular disease, poor mental health, suicide and health-harming behaviours (Black, 2008). Similarly, underemployment and employment in positions that are unsafe and/or unsatisfying can be detrimental to health and well-being. Thus the impact of an unhealthy workforce on the economy and society is wide ranging and may include lost productivity, reduction in income tax receipts, and growing costs associated with increased health care and informal caregiving.

Occupational therapy has a long history of supporting work participation. Enabling people with illness, injury or impairment to obtain, return to, or retain work and be productive within the workplace sits well within the occupational therapy's philosophical stance; occupational therapists have the professional capabilities to work with people to meet goals to develop, recover, improve and maintain skills needed for daily living and working (Allchin et al., 2016; Prior et al., 2017). Occupational therapists' involvement in work rehabilitation includes job retention and return-to-work interventions, and the evidence base to support the effectiveness of these interventions has scope for further development.

REFERENCES

Allan, B. A., Rolniak, J. R., & Bouchard, L. (2020). Underemployment and well-being: Exploring the dark side of meaningful work. *Journal of Career Development, 47*(1), 111–125. https://journals.sagepub.com/doi/pdf/10.1177/0894845318819861.

Allaire, S., & Keysor, J. (2009). Development of a structured interview tool to help patients identify and solve rheumatic condition related work barriers. *Arthritis Care & Research, 61*(7), 988–995. https://doi.org/10.1002/art.24610.

Allaire, S. H., Li, W., & LaValley, M. P. (2003). Reduction of job loss in persons with rheumatic diseases receiving vocational rehabilitation: A randomized controlled trial. *Arthritis & Rheumatology, 48*(11), 3212–3218. https://doi.org/10.1002/art.11256.

Allchin, B., Sanders, B., & Bourke, C. (2016). Letter to the Editor. Occupational therapists are well placed to develop, support and embed carer programmes. *Australian Occupational Therapy Journal, 63*(6), 438. https://doi.org/10.1111/1440-1630.12341.

Asaba, E., Aldrich, R. M., Gabrielsson, H., Ekstam, L., & Farias, L. (2021). Challenging conceptualisations of work: Revisiting contemporary experiences of return-to-work and unemployment. *Journal of Occupational Science, 28*(1), 81–94. https://doi.org/10.1080/14427591.2020.1820896.

Backman, C. L., Village, J., & Lacaille, D. (2008). The Ergonomic Assessment Tool for Arthritis: development and pilot testing. *Arthritis & Rheumatology, 59*(10), 1495–1503. https://doi.org/10.1002/art.24116.

Baker, N., & Jacobs, K. (2003). The nature of working in the United States: An occupational therapy perspective. *Work, 20*(1), 53–61. https://content.iospress.com/articles/work/wor00274.

Baldwin, D., Johnstone, B., Ge, B, Hewett, J., Smith, M., & Sharp, G. (2012). Randomized prospective study of a work place ergonomic intervention for individuals with rheumatoid arthritis and osteoarthritis. *Arthritis Care & Research, 64*(10), 1527–1535. https://doi.org/10.1002/acr.21699.

Beaton, D. E., Dyer, S., Boonen, A., Verstappen, S. M. M., Escorpizo, R., Lacaille, D. V., Bosworth, A., Gignac, M. A. M., Leong, A., Purcaru, O., Leggett, S., Hofstetter, C., Peterson, I. F., Tang, K., Fautrel, B., Bombardier, C., & Tugwell, P. S. (2016). OMERACT filter evidence supporting the measurement of at-work productivity loss as an outcome measure in rheumatology research. *The Journal of Rheumatology, 43*(1), 214–222. https://doi.org/10.3899/jrheum.141077.

Beck, U. (2002). *The brave new world of work*. Polity Press.

Black, C. (2008). Working for a healthier tomorrow: Dame Carol Black's review of the health of Britain's working age population. Department for Work and Pensions. https://assets.publishing.service.gov.uk/media/5a7c55bee5274a1b0042313c/hwwb-working-for-a-healthier-tomorrow.pdf.

Brijnath, B., Singh, N., & Mazza, D. (2015). Stakeholder perspectives on the new sickness certificate in Victoria: Results from a mixed-methods qualitative study. *Australian Health Review, 40*(1), 27–32. https://doi.org/10.1071/AH14136.

British Psychological Society. (2018). Good practice in the workplace. In *Guidelines for psychologists working with refugees and asylum seekers in the UK: Extended version*. https://doi.org/10.53841/bpsrep.2018.inf300b.

Brown, A., Kitchell, M., O'Neil, T., Lockliear, J., Vosler, A., Kubeck, D., & Dale, L. (2001). Identifying meaning and perceived level of satisfaction in the context of work. *Work, 16*(3), 219–226. https://content.iospress.com/articles/work/wor00154.

Butterworth, P., Leach, L. S., Strazdins, L., Olesen, S. C., Rodgers, B., & Broom, D. H. (2011). The psychosocial quality of work determines whether employment has benefits for mental health: Results from a longitudinal national household panel survey. *Occupational and Environmental Medicine, 68*, 806–812. http://dx.doi.org/10.1136/oem.2010.059030.

Cambridge University Press. (n.d.). Work. In Cambridge dictionary. Retrieved June 12, 2023, from https://dictionary.cambridge.org/dictionary/english/work.

Chapparo, C. J., & Hooper, E. (2002). When is it work? Perceptions of six-year-old children. *Work, 19*(3), 291–302. https://content.iospress.com/articles/work/wor00264.

Christiansen, C., & Townsend, E. (2004). The occupational nature of communities. In C. Christiansen & E. Townsend (Eds.), *Introduction to occupation: The art and science of living* (pp. 141–172). Prentice Hall.

Cook, C., & Lukersmith, S. (2010). Work rehabilitation. In M. Curtin, M. Molineux, & J. Supyk-Mellson (Eds.), *Occupational therapy and physical dysfunction: Enabling occupation* (6th ed., pp. 391–408). Elsevier.

Crooks, V., Sharon, D., & Owen, M. (2009). Multiple sclerosis and academic work: Socio-spatial strategies adopted to maintain employment. *Journal of Occupational Science, 16*(1), 25–31. https://doi.org/10.1080/14427591.2009.9686638.

De Baets, S., Calders, P., Schalley, N., Vermeulen, K., Vertriest, S., Van Peteghem, L., Coussens, M., Malfait, F., Vanderstraeten, G., Van Hove, G., & Van de Velde, D. (2018). Updating the evidence on Functional Capacity Evaluation methods: A systematic review. *Journal of Occupational Rehabilitation, 28*, 418–428. https://doi.org/10.1007/s10926-017-9734-x.

de Botton, A. (2009). *The pleasures and sorrows of work*. Penguin Group (Australia).

De Buck, P. D. M., le Cessie, S., van den Hout, W. B., Peeters, A. J., Ronday, H. K., Westedt, M., Breedveld, F. C., & Vliet Vlieland,

T. P. M. (2005). Randomised comparison of a multi-disciplinary job retention vocational rehabilitation programme with usual outpatient care in patients with chronic arthritis at risk of job loss. *Arthritis Care Res, 53*(5), 682–690. https://doi.org/10.1002/art.21452.

Department for Work and Pensions. (2004). *Building capacity for work: A UK framework for vocational rehabilitation.* London: Department for Work and Pensions.

Department of Work and Pensions. (2013). *Guidance for doctors, nurses, occupational therapists, pharmacists, physiotherapists, employers, and patients using fit notes* (statements of fitness for work). https://www.gov.uk/government/collections/fit-note.

Désiron, H. A., de Rijk, A., Van Hoof, E., & Donceel, P. (2011). Occupational therapy and return-to-work: a systematic literature review. *BMC Public Health, 11*(615). https://doi.org/10.1186/1471-2458-11-615.

Dollard, M. F., & Winefield, A. H. (2002). Mental health: overemployment, underemployment, unemployment and healthy jobs. *Australian e-Journal for the Advancement of Mental Health, 1*(3). https://psycnet.apa.org/record/2012-18262-004.

Edgelow, M., Harrison, L., Miceli, M., & Cramm, H. (2020). Occupational therapy return-to-work interventions for persons with trauma and stress-related mental health conditions: A scoping review. *Work, 65*(4), 821–836. https://content.iospress.com/articles/work/wor203134.

Egan, M., & Restall, G. (2022). *Promoting occupational participation: Collaborative relationship-focused occupational therapy.* Canadian Association of Occupational Therapists.

European Parliament. (2018). *The impact of new technologies on the labour market and the social economy.* https://www.europarl.europa.eu/RegData/etudes/STUD/2018/614539/EPRS_STU(2018)614539_EN.pdf.

Farias, L., & Laliberte Rudman, D. (2019). Practice analysis: Critical reflexivity on discourses constraining socially transformative occupational therapy practices. *British Journal of Occupational Therapy, 82*(11), 693–697. https://doi.org/10.1177/0308022619862111.

Faragher, E. B., Cass, M., & Cooper, C. L. (2005). The relationship between job satisfaction and health: A meta-analysis. *Occupational & Environmental Medicine, 62*, 105–112. https://oem.bmj.com/content/oemed/62/2/105.full.pdf.

Feldman, D. C. (1996). The nature, antecedents and consequences of underemployment. *Journal of Management, 22*(3), 385–407. https://doi.org/10.1016/S0149-2063(96)90030-6.

Fowler, H., Belot, A., Ellis, L., Maringe, C., Luque-Fernandez, M. A., Njeru Njagi, E., Navani, N., Sarfati, D., & Rachet, B. (2020). Comorbidity prevalence among cancer patients: a population-based cohort study of four cancers. *BMC Cancer, 20*(2). https://doi.org/10.1186/s12885-019-6472-9.

Gignac, M. A. M., Sutton, D., & Badley, E. M. (2007). Arthritis symptoms, the work environment, and the future: measuring perceived job strain among employed persons with arthritis. *Arthritis Care & Research, 57*(5), 738–747. https://doi.org/10.1002/art.22788.

Gilworth, G., Chamberlain, A., Harvey, A., Woodhouse, A., Smith, J., Smith, G., et al. (2003). Development of a work instability scale for rheumatoid arthritis. *Arthritis & Rheumatology, 49*, 349–354.

Grint, K. (1991). *The sociology of work.* Polity Press.

Hammond, A., Woodbridge, S., O'Brien, R., & Grant, M. (2013). *The UK Work Experience Survey for persons with rheumatic conditions (UK WES-RC).* University of Salford. http://usir.salford.ac.uk/29319.

Hammond, A., Sutton, C., Cotterill, S., Woodbridge, S., O'Brien, R., Radford, K., Forshaw, D., Verstappen, S., Jones, C., Marsden, A., Eden, M., Prior, Y., Culley, J., Holland, P., Walker-Bone, K., Hough, Y., O'Neill, T. W., Ching, A., & Parker, J. (2020). The effect on work presenteeism of job retention vocational rehabilitation compared to a written self-help work advice pack for employed people with inflammatory arthritis: protocol for a multi-centre randomised controlled trial (the WORKWELL trial). *BMC Musculoskeletal Disorders, 21*(607). https://doi.org/10.1186/s12891-020-03619-1.

Hammond, A., Radford, K. A., Ching, A., Prior, Y., O'Brien, R., Woodbridge, S., Culley, J., Parker, J., & Holland, P. (2022). The Workwell trial: protocol for the process evaluation of a randomised controlled trial of job retention vocational rehabilitation for employed people with inflammatory arthritis. *Trials, 23*(937). https://doi.org/10.1186/s13063-022-06871-z.

Hammond, A., Tennant, A., Ching, A., Parker, J., Prior, Y., Gignac, M. A. M., Verstappen, S. M. M., & O'Brien, R. (2023). Psychometric testing of the British English Workplace Activity Limitations Scale in four rheumatic and musculoskeletal conditions. *Rheumatology Advances in Practice, 7*(1). https://doi.org/10.1093/rap/rkad028.

Harpaz, I., & Fu, X. (2002). The structure and meaning of work: A relative stability amongst change. *Human Relations, 55*(6), 639–667.

Harvey-Krefting, L. (1985). The concept of work in occupational therapy: A historical review. *American Journal of Occupational Therapy, 39*(5), 301–307. https://doi.org/10.5014/ajot.39.5.301.

Hatton, R., Wallis, A., Chew, A., Stanley, M., & Smith, A. (2021). Return to work and cancer: Perspectives of occupational therapists. *Australian Occupational Therapy Journal, 68*(4), 298–307. https://doi.org/10.1111/1440-1630.12727.

Hewitt, M., & Ganz, P. A. (Eds.). (2006). From cancer patient to cancer survivor: lost in transition: an American Society of Clinical Oncology and Institute of Medicine Symposium. National Academies Press.

Hoving, J. L., Lacaille, D., Urquhart, D. M., Hannu, T. J., Sluiter, J. K., & Frings-Dresen, M. H. W. (2014). Non-pharmacological interventions for preventing job loss in workers with inflammatory arthritis. *Cochrane Database Systematic Reviews, 11*(CD010208). https://doi.org/10.1002/14651858.CD010208.pub2.

International Labour Organization. (2016). The 2030 Agenda for Sustainable Development. https://www.ilo.org/.

Innes, E. (2008). Ergonomics and work assessments. In K. Jacobs (Ed.), *Ergonomics for therapists* (3rd ed., pp. 48–72). Mosby Elsevier.

Jakobsen, K. (2001). Employment and the reconstruction of self. A model of space for maintenance of identity by occupation. *Scandinavian Journal of Occupational Therapy, 8*(1), 40–48. https://doi.org/10.1080/11038120120825.

Jakobsen, K. (2009). The right to work: Experiences of employees with rheumatism. *Journal of Occupational Science, 16*(2), 120–127. https://doi.org/10.1080/14427591.2009.9686651.

Jones, B. (1993). Sleepers, wake! Ten years on. *Journal of Occupational Science: Australia, 1*(1), 11–16. https://doi.org/10.1080/14427591.1993.9686374.

Jones, B. (1998). Redefining work: Setting directions for the future. *Journal of Occupational Science, 5*(3), 127–132. https://doi.org/10.1080/14427591.1998.9686440.

Kanfer, R., Frese, M., & Johnson, R. E. (2017). Motivation related to work: A century of progress. *Journal of Applied Psychology, 102*(3), 338–355. https://doi.org/10.1037/apl0000133.

Kasl, S. V., & Jones, B. A. (2007). Unemployment and health. In S. Ayers, A. Baum, C. McManus, S. Newman, K. Wallston, J. Weinman, & R. West (Eds.), *Cambridge Handbook of Psychology, Health and Medicine* (pp. 232–238). Cambridge University Press.

Keisler-Starkey, K., & Bunch, L. N. (2021). U.S. Census Bureau, current population reports. In *Health Insurance Coverage in the United States: 2021*. U.S. Government Publishing Office. https://www.census.gov/content/dam/Census/library/publications/2022/demo/p60-278.pdf.

Keysor, J. J., AlHeresh, R., Vaughan, M., LaValley, M. P., & Allaire, S. (2016). The work-it study for people with arthritis: study protocol and baseline sample characteristics. *Work, 54*(2), 473–480. https://content.iospress.com/articles/work/wor2331.

Keysor, J. J., LaValley, M. P., Brown, C., Felson, D. T., AlHeresh, R., Vaughan, M., Yood, R., Reed, J. I., & Allaire, S. J. (2018). Efficacy of a work disability prevention program for people with rheumatic and musculoskeletal conditions: A single-blind, parallel arm randomised controlled trial. *Arthritis Care & Research, 70*(7), 1022–1029. https://onlinelibrary.wiley.com/doi/full/10.1002/acr.23423.

Kiepek, N., Durocher, E., Hark, R., McKinnon, A., & Phelan, S. (2022). Justice, equity, and rights through occupation. In M. Egan, & G. Restall (Eds.), *Promoting occupational participation: Collaborative relationship-focused occupational therapy* (pp. 261–284). Canadian Association of Occupational Therapists.

Kielhofner, G., Braveman, B., Baron, K., Fisher, G., Hammel, J., & Littleton, M. (1999). The model of human occupation: Understanding the worker who is injured or disabled. *Work, 12*(1), 37–45. https://content.iospress.com/articles/work/wor00002.

Kirkpatrick Johnson, M., & Mortimer, J. T. (2011). Origins and outcomes of judgments about work. *Social Forces, 89*(4), 1239–1260. https://doi.org/10.1093/sf/89.4.1239.

Kirsh, B. H. (2015). Transforming values into action: Advocacy as a professional imperative. *Canadian Journal of Occupational Therapy, 82*(4), 212–223. https://journals.sagepub.com/doi/pdf/10.1177/0008417415601395.

Law, M., Baptiste, S., Carswell, A., McColl, M. A., Polatajko, H., & Pollock, N. (2005). Canadian Occupational Performance Measure (COPM) [Database record]. APA PsycTests.

Law, M., Polatajko, H., Baptiste, S., & Townsend, E. (1997). Core concepts of occupational therapy. In E. Townsend (Ed.), *Enabling occupation: An occupational therapy perspective* (pp. 29–56). Canadian Association of Occupational Therapists.

Lecours, A. (2020). Using an occupational perspective to understand behaviours fostering the prevention of work-related health problems: A proposed conceptual model. *Journal of Occupational Science, 27*(2), 222–235. https://doi.org/10.1080/14427591.2019.1600575.

Lerner, D., Amick, B. C., Rogers, W. H., Malspeis, S., Bungay, K., & Cynn, D. (2001). The Work Limitations Questionnaire. *Medical Care, 39*(1), 72–85. http://www.jstor.org/stable/3767701.

Lintner, C., & Elsen, S. (2018). Getting out of the seclusion trap? Work as meaningful occupation for the subjective well-being of asylum seekers in South Tyrol, Italy. *Journal of Occupational Science, 25*(1), 76–86. https://doi.org/10.1080/14427591.2017.1373256.

Macedo, A., Oakley, S. P., Panayi, G. S., & Kirkham, B. W. (2009). Functional and work outcomes improve in patients with rheumatoid arthritis who receive targeted, comprehensive occupational therapy. *Arthritis Care & Research, 61*(11), 1522–1530. https://doi.org/10.1002/art.24563.

MacLennan, S., Cox, T., Murdoch, S., & Eatough, V. (2022). An interpretative phenomenological analysis of the meaning of work to women living with breast cancer. *Chronic Illness, 18*(3), 503–516. https://journals.sagepub.com/doi/10.1177/1742395320987883.

Manjeet, K., Pratibha, G., & Mini, G. (2020). Individual, interpersonal and economic challenges of underemployment in the wake of COVID-19. *Work, 67*(1), 21–28. https://content.iospress.com/articles/work/wor203249.

Masterman-Smith, H., & Pocock, B. (2008). *Living low paid: The dark side of prosperous Australia*. Allen & Unwin.

Maynard, D. C., Joseph, T. A., & Maynard, A. M. (2006). Underemployment, job attitudes, and turnover intentions. *Journal of Organizational Behavior, 27*(4), 509–536. https://doi.org/10.1002/job.389.

Min, J., Kim, Y., Lee, S., Jang, T., Kim, I., & Song, J. (2019). The Fourth Industrial Revolution and its impact on occupational health and safety, worker's compensation and labor conditions. *Safety and Health at Work, 10*(4), 400–408. https://doi.org/10.1016/j.shaw.2019.09.005.

Moore-Corner, R. A., Kielhofner, G., & Olson, L. (1998). Work Environment Impact Scale (WEIS) Version 2.0. The University of Illinois at Chicago. https://moho-irm.uic.edu/productDetails.aspx?aid=12.

Njelesani, J., Tang, A., Jonsson, H., & Polatajko, H. (2014). Articulating an occupational perspective. *Journal of Occupational Science, 21*(2), 226–235. https://doi.org/10.1080/14427591.2012.717500.

Noon, M., & Morrell, K. (2017). *The realities of work: Experiencing work and employment in contemporary society*. Bloomsbury Publishing.

O'Halloran, D. (2022). *The Power to Persuade: Sofia's Story*. https://www.powertopersuade.org.au/blog/sofias-story/1/12/2022.

O'Halloran, D., & Innes, E. (2005). Understanding work in society. In G. Whiteford & V. Wright-St Clair (Eds.), *Occupation and practice in context* (pp. 299–316). Elsevier.

O'Halloran, D., Farnworth, L., Innes, E., & Thomacos, N. (2018). An occupational perspective on three solutions to unemployment. *Journal of Occupational Science, 25*(3), 297–308. https://doi.org/10.1080/14427591.2018.1474128.

Overell, S. (2008). *Work and the human claim to uniqueness: A contribution to the philosophy of work*. http://www.theworkfoundation.com/assets/docs/publications/210_uniqueness%20(2).pdf.

Pocock, B. (2003). *The work/life collision*. The Federation Press.

Pocock, B. (2006). *The labour market ate my babies: Work, children and a sustainable future*. The Federation Press.

Pratap, P., Dickson, A., Love, M., Zanoni, J., Donato, C., Flynn, M. A., & Schulte, P. A. (2021). Public health impacts of underemployment and unemployment in the United States: Exploring perceptions, gaps and opportunities. *International Journal of Environmental Research and Public Health, 18*(19), 10021. https://doi.org/10.3390/ijerph181910021.

Preston, A., & Prior, Y. (2013). A systematic review of work interventions for people with Rheumatoid Arthritis. *British Journal of Occupational Therapy, 76*(Suppl 1), 125–126.

Primeau, L. A. (1996). Work versus nonwork: The case of household work. In R. Zemke, & F. Clark (Eds.), *Occupational science: The evolving discipline* (pp. 57–69). F.A. Davis Company.

Prior, Y., Amanna, A. E., Bodell, S. J., & Hammond, A. (2017). A qualitative evaluation of occupational therapy-led work rehabilitation for people with inflammatory arthritis: participants' views. *British Journal of Occupational Therapy, 80,* 39–48.

Prior, Y., Bodell, S., Amanna, A., & Hammond, A. (2014). Rheumatoid arthritis patients' view of a vocational rehabilitation intervention provided by rheumatology occupational therapists. *Rheumatology (Oxford), 53*(Suppl 2), 125.

Protzman, F. (2006). *Work: The world in photographs.* National Geographic Society.

Radford, K., Sutton, C., Sach, T., Holmes, J., Watkins, C., Forshaw, D., Jones, T., Hoffman, K., O'Connor, R., Tyerman, R., Merchán-Baeza, J. A., Morris, R., McManus, E., Drummond, A., Walker, M., Duley, L., Shakespeare, D., Hammond, A., & Phillips, J. (2018). Early, specialist vocational rehabilitation to facilitate return-to-work after traumatic brain injury: The FRESH feasibility RCT. *Health Technol Assess, 22*(33), 1–156. https://doi.org/10.3310/hta22330.

Radford, K. A., McKevitt, C., Clarke, S, Powers, K., Phillips, J., Craven, K., Watkins, C., Farrin, A., Holmes, J., Cripps, R., McLellan, V., Sach, T., Brindle, R., Holloway, I., Hartley, S., Bowen, A., O'Connor, R. J., Stevens, J., Walker, M., Murray, J., Shone, A., & Clarke, D. (2022). Return-to-work After stroKE (RETAKE) Trial: protocol for a mixed-methods process evaluation using normalisation process theory. *BMJ Open, 12,* e053111. https://bmjopen.bmj.com/content/12/3/e053111.

Ravinskaya, M., Verbeek, J. H., Langendam, M., Madan, I., Verstappen, S. M. M., Kunz, R., Hulshof, C. T. J., & Hoving, J. L. (2023). Which outcomes should always be measured in intervention studies for improving work participation for people with a health problem? An international multistakeholder Delphi study to develop a core outcome set for Work participation (COS for Work). *BMJ Open, 13*(2), e069174. https://bmjopen.bmj.com/content/13/2/e069174.abstract.

Royal College of Occupational Therapists. (2021). *Good work for good health. The difference occupational therapy makes.* https://www.rcot.co.uk/

Robart, R., & Boyle, P. (2021). Supporting workers with lower back injuries to return-to-work: A meta-ethnography. *British Journal of Occupational Therapy, 84*(2), 79–91. https://journals-sagepub-com.ezproxy.csu.edu.au/doi/pdf/10.1177/0308022620930609.

Ruppanner, L., Churchill, B., Bissell, D., Ghin, P., Hydelund, C., Ainsworth, S., Blackhman, A., Borland, J., Cheong, M., Evans, M., Frermann, L., King, T., & Vetere, F. (2023). *2023 state of the future of work.* Work Futures Hallmark Research Initiative, The University of Melbourne. https://www.work-futures.org/publications.

Safe Work Australia. (2019). *National Return-to-Work Strategy 2020-2030.* https://www.safeworkaustralia.gov.au/doc/national-return-work-strategy-2020-2030.

Schofield, T. (2009). Workplace health. In J. Germov (Ed.), *Second opinion: An introduction to health sociology* (4th ed., pp. 112–130). Oxford University Press.

Schwartz, B. (2015). *Why we work.* Simon & Schuster Inc.

Selenko, E., Mäkikangas, A., & Stride, C. B. (2017). Does job insecurity threaten who you are? Introducing a social identity perspective to explain well-being and performance consequences of job insecurity. *Journal of Organizational Behavior, 38*(6), 856–875. https://doi.org/10.1002/job.2172.

Sinnicks, M., & Reeves, C. (2023). Work. In M. N. S. Sellars & S. Kirste (Eds.), *The Springer Encyclopedia of the Philosophy of Law and Social Philosophy.* Dordrecht: Springer. https://doi.org/10.1007/978-94-007-6730-0_1090-1.

Somavia, J. (2001). *Reducing the decent work deficit: A global challenge.* Report of the Director-General of the ILO International Labour Conference, 89th Session, Geneva.

Stone, S. D. (2003). Workers without work: Injured workers and well-being. *Journal of Occupational Science, 10*(1), 7–13. https://doi.org/10.1080/14427591.2003.9686505.

Tang, K., Beaton, D. E., Boonen, A., Gignac, M. A., Bombardier. C. (2011). Measures of work disability and productivity: Rheumatoid Arthritis Specific Work Productivity Survey (WPS-RA), Workplace Activity Limitations Scale (WALS), Work Instability Scale for Rheumatoid Arthritis (RA-WIS), Work Limitations Questionnaire (WLQ), and Work Productivity and Activity Impairment Questionnaire (WPAI). *Arthritis Care & Research (Hoboken), 63*(Suppl 11), S337–49. https://doi.org/10.1002/acr.20633.

Tang, K., Boonen, A., Verstappen, S. M. M., Escorpizo, R., Luime, J. L., Lacaille, D., Fautrel, B., Bosworth, A., Cifaldi, M., Gignac, M. A. M., Hofstetter, C., Leong, A., Montie, P, Petersson, I. F., Purcaru, O., Bombardier, C., Tugwell, P. S., & Beaton, D. E. (2014). Worker productivity outcome measures: OMERACT filter evidence and agenda for future research. *The Journal of Rheumatology, 41*(1), 165–176. https://doi.org/10.3899/jrheum.130815.

Toulmin, S. (1995). Occupation, employment, and human welfare. *Journal of Occupational Science: Australia, 2*(2), 48–58. https://doi.org/10.1080/14427591.1995.9686395.

Unruh, A. M. (2004). Reflections on: "So… what do you do?" Occupation and the construction of identity. *Canadian Journal of Occupational Therapy, 71*(5), 290–295.

van Krieken, R., Habibis, D., Smith, P., Hutchins, B., Haralambos, M., & Holborn, M. (2010). *Sociology: Themes and Perspectives* (3rd ed.). Pearson Longman.

Verstappen, S. M. M., Lacaille, D., Boonen, A., Escorpizo, R., Hofstetter, C., Bosworth, A., Leong, A., Legget, S., Gignac, M. A. M., Wllman, J. K., Ter Wee, M. M., Berghea, F., Agaliotis, M., Tugwell, P. S., & Beaton, D. E. (2019). Considerations for evaluating and recommending worker productivity outcome measures: an update from the OMERACT worker productivity group. *The Journal of Rheumatology, 46*(10), 1401–1405. https://doi.org/10.3899/jrheum.181201.

Waddell, G., & Burton, A. K. (2006). *Is work good for your health and well-being?* TSO (The Stationery Office). www.tsoshop.co.uk.

Workforce Australia. (2023). *Obligations.* https://www.workforceaustralia.gov.au/individuals/obligations.

World Federation of Occupational Therapists (WFOT), Freeman, A., Shaw, L., Turcotte, S., de Montenegro, A., Alzamora, C., Galzer Wertheimer, L., & Garcia, A. (2018). *Decent work project report.* WFOT. https://www.researchgate.net/

publication/327321313_Decent_work_project_report_ May_2018_World_Federation_of_Occupational_Therapists_ wwwwfotorg.

World Health Organization. (1986). *Ottawa Charter for Health Promotion*. World Health Organization. https://www.who.int/ publications/i/item/WH-1987.

World Health Organization. (2001). International Classification of Functioning, Disability and Health (ICF). Geneva: World Health Organization.

Zuzanek, J. (2010). Work, occupation, and leisure. In C. Christiansen & E. Townsend (Eds.), *Introduction to occupation: The art and science of living* (2nd ed., pp. 281–302). Pearson.

REFLECTION

1. Describe what is meant by unemployment and underemployment. Discuss the connection between unemployment and poor health outcomes, in relation to underemployment and its health and social consequences.

2. Why is it essential for occupational therapists to have knowledge and understanding of local and national policies and services related to work participation?

3. How can standardised assessments and outcome measures be beneficial in the delivery and evaluation of job retention interventions?

OCCUPATIONAL PERFORMANCE COACHING

FI GRAHAM ■ CHI-WEN CHIEN ■ MELISSA NOTT ■ DOROTHY KESSLER ■ CHARMAINE BERNIE

CHAPTER OUTLINE

Overview

Coaching as a family of interprofessional interventions that support people to achieve improved occupational participation in the life situations they value is described in this chapter. Coaching methods are explained as goal-directed, autonomy-supportive conversations grounded in compassion and shared visions of peoples' preferred futures. The relationship between coaching and other enabling tools that an occupational therapist might draw on is explored. One form of coaching designed by and for occupational therapists, occupational performance coaching (OPC), is described in detail. The OPC methods are illustrated through a practice story. An OPC session audio recording and an abbreviated transcript of the session maps use of specific OPC methods within the session.

KEY POINTS

■ Coaching is a distinct approach to engaging with people in a collaborative, creative process to identify and make real, desired future ways of being in the world. Distinct from counselling and educating, coaching explores peoples' most valued life roles and activities in life contexts and guides reflection and decision-making on more effective ways to achieve goals.

■ Key elements of coaching are an individual's experience of agency over the direction of coaching conversations and a compassionate, non-judgemental relationship between the coach and the person being coached.

■ Occupational performance coaching (OPC) is one coaching approach which aligns closely with the Canadian Model of Occupational Participation (CanMOP) (Egan & Restall, 2022) and with occupational therapists' belief in the capability and right to self-determination of people (Hammell, 2020).

■ Distinguishing features of OPC, in relation to other forms of coaching, are the occupational participation focus of goals and the use of collaborative performance analysis to guide the coachee's reflection and decision-making.

DEFINING COACHING

The International Coaching Federation defines coaching as 'partnering with people in a thought-provoking and creative process that inspires them to maximize their personal and professional potential' (International Coaching Federation, 2023). Coaching is a relationship-focused process that centres on people's goals (not the practitioner's goals), fosters self-learning and is grounded in self-awareness, personal values, strengths recognition, possibilities, choice and self-responsibility. Coaching can be used with individuals and collectives (including teams, networks and community groups).

At its core, coaching is a 'talking-based' intervention that draws much of its effect from the relationship between the coach and the person being coached (referred to in this chapter as the 'coachee'). The coach intentionally cultivates a therapeutic space within which a coachee can explore their strengths, challenges and aspirations. Critical to this is the avoidance of judgment, including professional opinion, appraisal or advice-giving. The quality of the relationship between the coach and the coachee is critical to successful outcomes (Stober & Grant, 2006).

With application in many different fields, specific coaching approaches inevitably emphasise different key elements. To distil the key features, Ives (2008) identified several common elements of coaching, including:

- Active process designed to facilitate development or change (whether cognitive, emotional or behavioural).
- Conversation-based with emphasis on the skills of listening and questioning through which the coach aims to develop a person's abilities to assume autonomy and make changes in their life.
- Highly collaborative and egalitarian (power-equal) relationships.
- Solution construction rather than problem analysis.
- Accesses and builds upon the person's knowledge, skills, experience and resources.

Coaching requires practitioners to adopt a coaching mindset that is open, curious and collaborative. It facilitates a person's insights and promotes individual autonomy to transform learning and insight into action (International Coaching Federation, 2023).

For occupational therapists coaching is an opportunity to sit in the passenger seat, alongside the coachee, rather than in the driver seat. The mantra to 'practice not knowing' the answer to people's dilemmas is often used as a mental guide by coaches. Thus coaching brings a sense of uncertainty for some experienced occupational therapists, as their expertise as coaches shifts from what they know about people to how they work with them.

Coaching approaches implemented by occupational therapists have distinctive elements: an iterative process of goal setting, analysis, planning, action and evaluation, varying levels of performance analysis and outcomes of improved occupational participation (Kessler & Graham, 2015). Unique to the way occupational therapists embody coaching is the emphasis placed on consideration of an individual's life context in the process and outcome of coaching. Context is included in the setting of goals, analysis of occupational participation and any other contexts that might influence the implementation of strategies. Occupational therapists adopt a specific and unique understanding of 'activity in context' in which the physical, sensory, social and cultural elements of individuals' environments are considered.

Before taking a deeper dive into coaching methods, a comparison with other therapeutic skills used by occupational therapists is provided (Townsend et al., 2007).

Counselling: The goal of counselling-based therapy is to raise awareness of potentially negative thoughts, feelings or behaviours and to help individuals to modify these feelings and thoughts. In contrast, the goal of coaching is to raise awareness of a situation, to stimulate ideas, insights and actions consistent with the individual's main life values and interests and ultimately to plan and carry out actions that lead to progressing their goals.

Educating: When using a traditional educational approach, the occupational therapist is located as the 'expert', which emphasises the knowledge and expertise of the therapist. Educational approaches traditionally take on the form of advice-giving or instruction rather than information exchange between the coach and coachee. Advice-giving carries an unspoken expectation that the recipient of care will see information as useful and will comply with it. In coaching, the coachee's authority to decline or suggest alternative information or ideas is encouraged, thus supporting the development of their self-agency and autonomy.

Mentoring: Mentoring approaches share several common traits with coaching. They are goal-oriented processes that are part of a supportive relationship, and often involve methods similar to coaching such as creating a plan, using strategies and providing support (Doyle et al., 2019). Mentors typically have greater experience and expertise than the mentee, and the sharing of knowledge is predominantly from mentor to mentee. This is distinct from coaching, which is characterised by the reciprocal sharing of information, ideas and collaborative problem solving (Parsloe & Wray, 2000).

COACHING INTERVENTIONS: SIMILARITIES AND DIFFERENCES

Many different coaching approaches are used by occupational therapists. An in-depth scan of the literature revealed that occupational performance coaching (OPC) is the most widely tested intervention, either being used by itself or in conjunction with other approaches such as CO-OP (Araujo et al., 2021), contextual intervention (Azari et al., 2020), four-quadrant model of facilitated learning (Ghaffari et al., 2022) and parental occupational executive training (Frisch et al., 2020). Other named interventions include occupation-based coaching (Little et al., 2018; Wallisch et al., 2019) and coaching-in-context (Cadematori et al., 2021; Mulcahey et al., 2022).

Among these interventions, there are common elements that align with the definition of coaching in occupational therapy. For example, most are individual-led and include goal setting and a process for problem solving (i.e. planning, acting and evaluating) that is solution-focused. However, the degree to which the relationship with the occupational therapist-coach is emphasised varies and is often not described. The role that education plays in coaching approaches also varies, as does the degree to which coaching is led by the occupational therapist as opposed to being led by the coachee.

THEORIES, CONTEXTS, MECHANISMS AND OUTCOMES IN COACHING MODELS

The theories, mechanisms, contexts and outcomes that many coaching approaches share are summarised in this section, with an expanded explanation of

---

BOX 27.1
INTRODUCING MARIA AND TUI

Tui is a 10-year-old boy who lives with his adoptive parents and two siblings. Prior to adoption as an infant, Tui was exposed to alcohol, drug use and violence. Tui's adoptive family has been stable, nurturing and his parents, Maria and Dave are deeply committed and involved in Tui's health and education. Tui is physically mature for his age. His mother is concerned about his frequent and increasingly violent emotional outbursts, which have resulted in Tui being excluded from school several times and are becoming difficult to manage at home. Tui regularly leaves bruises on Maria as she attempts to restrain him during his outbursts. A psychiatrist and paediatrician diagnosed Tui with attention deficit hyperactive disorder, developmental coordination disorder and high verbal IQ but poor visuospatial skills. One occupational therapy consultation was undertaken in which Tui's motor, visual and sensory systems were assessed, and a home programme of sensory-motor activities was provided. After trying the home programme, Maria saw no change in his motor skills, sensory sensitivity or outbursts. Maria sought occupational therapy a second time from an alternative service to address his learning and behavioural difficulties. Tui's mother has just bought tickets to go on a world trip with the whole family in 9 months and is worried about how Tui will handle it. The occupational therapist, Fiona, decided to use occupational performance coaching (OPC) with Maria. She began by asking Maria what was most important to her for herself and Tui.

OPC. OPC is one of the most researched coaching approaches in occupational therapy and the approach used in the practice story of Maria and Tui (Box 27.1). A more detailed comparison of these approaches related to coaching is also provided by Graham (2021).

Theoretical Underpinning of Coaching

The theoretical underpinning of coaching interventions is important for coherent linkage between an intervention's key ingredients, and their intended responses and outcomes for people. Theory also enables a systematic approach to research and development of interventions (Moore et al., 2015).

Self-Determination Theory

Self-determination theory (SDT) (Ryan & Deci, 2017) posits that a person's motivation toward an action, such as taking up dance lessons, is influenced by how well their three psychological needs for autonomy, relatedness and competence are met. From an SDT perspective, the intrinsic motivation to act is high when a person feels autonomous over this decision to act (e.g. they enjoy dancing and see it as valuable), connected with others in their decision to join a dance class (e.g. they decide to join a dance class because they like the people at dance class) and competent to carry out the task (e.g. to join and take part in dance lessons).

During coaching conversations, exploration of autonomy, relatedness and competence can clarify uncertainty about what is most important to the coachee (i.e. identifying the goal) and resolve ambiguity about taking action to achieve the goal. In adopting a SDT lens, motivation is viewed as fluid and influenced, moment-by-moment, through the coaching conversation. When using OPC, the occupational therapist remains attuned to the need for autonomy, motivation and competence of the coachee.

Self-Regulation Theory

Self-regulation theories applied to coaching explain occupational therapists' use of cognitive scaffolding methods during coaching (e.g. goal clarification, preparing for change, implementing change and self-reflection) to help people to regulate their emotional responses. Emotional regulation is a key skill in maintaining calm, focus and clarity of thought, necessary for making choices and changing behaviour related to coaching goals (Zimmerman & Moylan, 2009). The self-regulation methods within coaching, particularly guiding individuals to explore and plan the steps of implementing their ideas, enhance each person's ability to navigate the anxiety that often occurs as they implement change in their lives.

Adult Learning Theory

Adult learning theory is also linked to several coaching approaches including OPC, lifestyle health coaching (Gordon et al., 2017), integrative health coaching (Caldwell et al., 2020; Smith et al., 2013) and contextual intervention (Dunn et al., 2012). Adult learning theory emphasises the role of the individual as a proactive learner, capable of addressing their own learning needs. The role of the coach is to create the conditions for this self-directed learning within the coaching conversation.

Systems Theories

Systems theories recognise and address the multiple interacting systems that influence the ability of an individual (or group) to create change (Brock, 2008; McMorris & Hale, 2006). Systems include those internal to the person, such as the musculoskeletal system, sensory and cognitive systems (Darrah & Bartlett, 1995; World Health Organization, 2001), through to the macro levels of the social and physical environments (Bandura, 1986; Bronfenbrenner & Morris, 2007). The influences of micro, meso and macro contexts on occupational participation are also acknowledged in the Canadian model of occupational participation (CanMOP).

Systems theories also posit that change in any one part of a system is likely to impact change in other parts of that system. Aligned with systems theory, coaching is open to change occurring through any system or set of systems. For example, a child may be impaired in their social and communication functions, but effective solutions to achieve participation in mealtimes with the family may be to place a fun game on the table during meals (a visual and motivational strategy), to remind the child what will happen after dinner. Non-coaching approaches that an occupational therapist may use, might focus on only one part of the system, such as one body impairment (e.g. muscle tone), or one type of strategy that targets the impairment (e.g. a sensory strategy). From a systems perspective, these are examples of just one small part of all systems influencing progress towards an occupational participation goal.

Models of Occupation

Occupational therapy models also reflect systems theories of thinking and are responsible for the close attention to a person's contexts in most occupational therapy approaches (Dunn et al., 1994; Graham, 2020). Models of occupation that are described as underpinning coaching include: Model of human occupation (MOHO) in the LifeSteps health promotion programme (Austin-McCain, 2015), value and meanings in occupation model (Persson et al., 2001) in the redesigning daily occupations (ReDO) programme (Erlandsson, 2013), and the person, environment, occupation (PEO) model (Law et al., 1996) in OPC. OPC is also consistent with the more contemporary CanMOP (refer to Chapter 11), particularly given the integration of relationships in our understanding of how occupational participation is achieved (Egan & Restall, 2022a).

A literature scan of coaching interventions used in occupational therapy (Graham et al., in press), identified that few coaching interventions have well-described theoretical bases. Instead, coaching principles are referred to or intervention components are described but without details of their theoretical base.

CONTEXTS OF APPLICATION OF COACHING IN OCCUPATIONAL THERAPY

A scoping review on the use of coaching in occupational therapy published in 2015 (Kessler & Graham, 2015) identified 11 articles. Since that time, the use of coaching has increased across the world, suggesting cross-cultural relevance. Coaching is most frequently implemented with parents of children who have a variety of participation challenges and health conditions including autism spectrum disorder, cerebral palsy, intellectual disability, attention deficit hyperactivity disorder and developmental coordination disorder. Coaching in occupational therapy has also been explored with people living with neurological conditions such as stroke (Fusari et al., 2020; Kessler et al., 2017; Nott et al., 2021), spinal cord injury (Cadematori et al., 2021), Huntington's disease (Quinn et al., 2016), multiple sclerosis (Askari et al., 2022), other chronic conditions (Alcorn & Broome, 2014; Austin-McCain, 2015; Brandt et al., 2018) (Austin-McCain, 2015; Brandt, 2018), workplace support (Erlandsson, 2013; Sundar & Brucker, 2021) and students in postsecondary education (Harrington et al., 2021; Egan et al., 2023).

Occupational therapists are primarily using coaching in community settings but have also applied coaching in acute care and inpatient rehabilitation settings. While coaching was initially used for in-person interactions, recent years have seen the growth of coaching via tele-heath (Jamali et al., 2022; Kessler et al., 2021; Kronberg et al., 2021; Little et al., 2018; Shin et al., 2022; Smith et al., 2023; Wallisch et al., 2019), and the exploration of coaching via human-computer interaction, such as apps (Fusari et al., 2020; Setoguchi et al., 2020). Coaching is also often described as a component of other occupational therapy interventions such

as cognitive orientation to daily occupational performance (CO-OP) (refer to Chapter 28) (Araujo et al., 2021) and parental occupational executive training (POET) (Azari et al., 2019).

The wide-ranging contexts in which occupational therapists use coaching approaches are evidence of the congruence of the principles of coaching with relationship-focused occupational therapy values. Although reports of coaching in occupational therapy are positive, the strength of this evidence varied greatly with few randomised controlled trials currently reported. The relationship between the contexts coaching is applied in and the specific coaching methods used warrant further research to clarify what works best, for who, and in what context.

EFFECTIVENESS OF COACHING USED IN OCCUPATIONAL THERAPY

Common outcomes within research on the effectiveness of coaching in occupational therapy include occupational performance and satisfaction using the Canadian occupational performance measure (Law et al., 1990), goal attainment, self-efficacy and impairments (e.g. executive function and motor outcomes).

The strongest evidence for coaching is to improve educational, motor and language outcomes in specific populations (Novak, 2014). Moderate evidence exists for coaching that integrates the use of collaborative goal setting, modelling and guided participation to improve play and leisure outcomes (Laverdure & Beisbier, 2021) while moderate to low evidence exists for coaching to improve occupational participation and functional mobility (Laverdure & Beisbier, 2021; Novak, 2014). There is limited evidence for coaching in combination with sensory systems-focused interventions to improve child behaviour, parent knowledge and self-efficacy (Allen et al., 2021).

Broadly, research evidence supports the use of coaching by occupational therapists with parents and teachers. However, the definition of coaching within these interventions varies and very few studies report evaluation or monitoring of intervention fidelity (i.e. what was specifically delivered by occupational therapists and how well). Therefore it is currently unclear which coaching techniques are critical to achieving outcomes. It is anticipated that occupational participation will become a primary outcome of studies evaluating the effectiveness of coaching (American Occupational Therapy Association, 2020).

OCCUPATIONAL PERFORMANCE COACHING

OPC is a specific coaching intervention used in a wide range of rehabilitation contexts, by several health professions. Like other coaching approaches, OPC is a conversation in which individuals and collectives are guided to identify their most highly valued goal, reflect on what works best for them to progress towards achieving that goal, evaluate their progress and apply their success to wider areas of their life. OPC is a goal-oriented approach that uses relational methods, envisioning and collaborative performance analysis (CPA) to guide people towards insight and change. Individual's reflection, decision-making and action lead to improved participation in personally valued life situations, that is, occupational participation. The processes of OPC contrast starkly with teaching or advising methods often used by occupational therapists and with interventions targeting bodily impairments (e.g. muscle tone and integration of sensory systems).

Occupational therapists using OPC apply three domains of enabling action:

(1) Consciously <u>Connect</u> with individuals;
(2) Guide individuals through a conversation <u>Structure</u> from envisaging to action; and

(3) Encourage individuals to <u>Share</u> what they already know about progressing toward their envisaged future (goal) (see Fig. 27.1).

Occupational therapist enactment of these domains is described below and illustrated with extracts of OPC with the practice story of Maria and Tui (Boxes 27.1–27.5). The OPC fidelity measure (Graham, 2020) details the specific occupational therapist behaviours that should be observed during OPC delivery.

OPC has considerable alignment with the CanMOP (Egan & Restall, 2022), and the key characteristics of collaborative relationship-focused occupational therapy (Restall et al. 2022). Both the foundational processes and the six action domains of the occupational therapy inter-relational practice process framework (COTIPP) (refer to Chapter 12), also demonstrate synergy with the three domains that underpin OPC; connect, structure and share (Graham, 2020, Restall et al. 2022). Connection and the building and sustaining of relationships are identified as essential principles in both the therapeutic and coaching processes described in OPC and the COTIPP. Also described in both processes, occupational therapists are encouraged to have self-awareness of their own emotional states, attitudes and behaviours, and processes that support relationship building, which can shift the balance of power or affect the exploration of possibilities if not appropriately positioned (Restall et al. 2022). OPC encourages the exploration of ways in which coachees can act, evaluate and generalise plans under consideration.

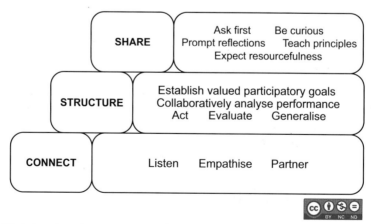

Fig. 27.1 ■ Three enabling domains of occupational performance coaching. (Reprinted with permission from Graham, F. (2020). *Occupational performance coaching resources*. https://www.otago.ac.nz/opc. This work is licensed under a Creative Commons Attribution-NonCommercial-NoDerivatives 4.0 International License. University of Otago.)

BOX 27.2

POSSIBLE QUESTIONS THE OCCUPATIONAL THERAPIST MIGHT ASK TO ELEVATE MARIA'S SENSE OF CHOICE AND CONTROL

What is most important to you today?
  Through all the things you've raised today, what is your top priority?
    What feels most useful to tackle first?
    Where is the best place to start?

BOX 27.3

OCCUPATIONAL THERAPIST BEING AWARE OF THEIR INTERNAL RESPONSES

In the case of Tui and Maria,
    What did you notice in yourself as you read of Maria being bruised by Tui? Did you notice a peak in your own arousal level (emotionality)? Did you feel frightened of meeting Tui, judgement towards him or a distancing from him? Were you reminded of a situation you or a loved one have experienced?
    Any of these responses are understandable, and they will affect the way an occupational therapist interacts with Maria. When an occupational therapist is aware of their internal responses, they can choose how they respond outwardly and focus on meeting the coachee's psychological needs.

These are mirrored in COTIPP's description of the trial and refinement of plans, as well as reflections around outcomes that can assist transition, by being generalised to real-world contexts. Critically, collaboratively developed or co-designed goals that help a coachee envision their purpose and participation-related priorities are specified and aligned features of both OPC and the COTIPP.

Connect, Structure, Share

The Connect Domain

The connect domain underpins all other coaching strategies within OPC; hence its position as a foundation domain in Fig. 27.1. The development of trusting, respectful relationships with individuals, underpinned by compassion, goes beyond the usual expectations of professional communication. Using OPC, the occupational therapist communicates in ways that intentionally fosters a relationship of partnership. The occupational therapist uses words and processes that add weight to individuals' choices and control over the direction and focus of therapy (Box 27.2).

In inviting the coachee to lead the direction of sessions, the occupational therapist positions themselves as the *listener* and guide, and the coachee as the expert. The occupational therapist also cultivates an expectation from the coachee that they are active *partners* in achieving their goals, and not passive recipients of the occupational therapist's advice and direction. As the coachee responds to the coach's questions, the coach remains conscious of their own internal emotional response. An authentic empathic response conveys recognition of the coachee's emotional experience and compassion toward them, rather than judgement. These relational methods require high levels of self-awareness by the therapist and a willingness to acknowledge and rest in their own emotional discomfort at times (Box 27.3).

The Structure Domain

The Structure domain of OPC offers a framework to guide the coachee's problem solving, from goal identification to the generalisation of successful strategies. Here, the distinctive feature of OPC is the absence of an occupational therapist's interference in shaping the coachee's goals, other than asking clarifying questions about the goal. Once the coachee has described an occupational participation goal that is highly meaningful to them, questioning shifts to guide the coachee to envision how the goal could be achieved, then how these ideas could be enacted, and then to evaluate how successful the strategies have been.

Valued Participatory Goals

OPC conversations open with the question: *What is most important to you?* An in-depth explanation of the occupational therapist's role, profession or expertise is not provided. In OPC the occupational therapist does not ask 'what is your goal' because this question seldom provides the level of guidance a coachee needs to articulate their most valued occupational participation goal. This type of goal setting is a complex and usually a very therapeutic process in and of itself. Goal setting is a key therapeutic element of coaching.

BOX 27.4
EXAMPLES OF GOAL STATEMENTS FOR MARIA

Component	Longer term goal	Immediate goal
Who[a]	Tui and the whole family	Tui
Will do what activity[b]	Will experience new things	Will get off technology
In what life context[c]	In the world trip	After school
To what extent[d]	Having a good time together	Calmly, 4/5 weekdays
By when[e]	In 9 months (date of planned trip)	In 1 month

[a]**Who** might refer to an individual, a dependent being cared for, a caregiver, a family or a community group.

[b]**Will do what activity** refers to a meaningful (to the recipient of coaching) unit of 'doing' of daily life. This could be attending a dance class, playing at a local park, brushing teeth, or getting to work on time. The meaning and scope of the activity are determined by the individual. The occupational therapist does not interfere with the scope of the activity, for example, because they feel it is too ambitious, not ambitious enough or it is unfamiliar. Achievability of goals is not a criterion for OPC goals. Often, powerful individual motivation is activated through highly ambitious goals. ***If a person shoots for the stars, they may find they land on the moon. How amazing to have reached the moon!***

[c]**In what life context** specifies where this desired future goal will occur. Specifying the context reminds the occupational therapist and coachee that the success of the coaching will be in daily life, not in any other measurement of things related to the goal activity. Specifying the context also starts the envisioning process, as it is easier to imagine things being better when a specific place/setting has been imagined.

[d]**To what extent** deepens attention to what it is about the doing of the activity in the life context that will be different when the person has progressed towards the goal. This goal element often clarifies what is most meaningful about the goal. For example, for one individual, the extent may be about attending a class more regularly, while for others it might be about being independent in a wider range of activities during the class.

[e]**By when** is a brief conversation once a goal is established about when (what date) the coachee thinks they can reasonably achieve this goal. Establishing a timeframe for goal achievement, usually within 1 to 3 months, and rarely longer than 6 months, provides transparency to expectations of both the occupational therapist and the coachee. Focusing attention intensively for a defined period also supports behaviour change and the implementation of planned actions. Be open to goals changing as the coachee's life priorities change or as they share their more private concerns.

Valued, participatory goal identification ensures that meaning and purpose are articulated and developed from the coachee's perspective, one of the fundamental considerations described in CanMOP (Egan & Restall, 2022). The meaningfulness of goals, reflecting what the coachee states are most important, is central to OPC goal statements. Goal statements specify who, will do what activity, in what life context, to what extent, and by when – thereby reflecting occupational participation (Box 27.4 and Table 27.1). Additional specificity of the extent of participation and timeframe to achievement are then clarified.

The practice story in Box 27.4 illustrates how the coach, Fiona, clarifies Maria's goal using the OPC process. As Maria's primary goal is for a travel event in 9 months, Fiona guides Maria to identify an occupation within her current routine that reflects her concerns about the longer-term goal. Listen to the audio clip (https://youtu.be/IyG4W839sc4) to observe how Fiona coached Maria to arrive at these goal statements. Notice how many cycles of question, reflection and silence Fiona prompts before Maria clearly articulates her core occupational participation goal for her son: that he ends his daily gaming time at home promptly and calmly.

Collaborative Performance Analysis

CPA describes the occupational therapist's 'roadmap' in guiding a person from an initial problem-focus to a solutions-oriented exploration of alternative ways of approaching goals and creating change (Fig. 27.2). Detailed explanations of CPA and other OPC methods are provided elsewhere (Graham & Ziviani, 2021b). Central to CPA is an orientation to engaging in the analytical process in partnership (i.e. collaboratively) with the coachee. Questions are asked to further the coachee's analysis, rather than to further the occupational therapist's analysis. This is a critical distinction

	Mindset quality	Occupational therapist thought	Occupational therapist words/action	Maria's response	Maria's action
TABLE 27.1					
An OPC Mindset in Contrast to an Expert Mindset Applied to Maria and Tui					
OPC Mindset	Compassion	They're juggling a lot and trying so hard	I can see how determined you are about this, despite what you're juggling.	(feels acknowledged) Jeez, thought you were going to tell me off for not doing the sensory diet! Thanks!	Reflects on how useful the sensory diet was, decides to drop most of it and let Tui decide if he finds any of it useful.
	Curiosity	I wonder where she finds the strength to carry on	What do you do in the week that fills your tank, to keep you so able to cope with this?	(laughs) Knowing when my next smoke break is! My doctor keeps trying to make me quit, but having a puff is my only me time, I love it.	Plans out 'me time' each morning for the day ahead– away from Tui, in the fresh air.
Therapist as expert	Occupational therapist knows the best	Still not doing the sensory diet. Therapy is pointless with Maria and Tui until they are committed.	The sensory diet really is important to Tui's nervous system. How about I make a tick chart so you can remember to use it?	I'm such a bad carer. I'm not doing enough.	Maria watches as the occupational therapist entertains Tui with the sensory diet. Maria and Tui do not attend the next scheduled session.

from an occupational therapist-as-expert approach, in which the occupational therapist would ask questions to gather data for their own analysis of situations and to prescribe or advise on solutions (Table 27.1).

CPA comprises three key phases: envision, explore and engage. Conversations start with Envision and move to Explore once a clear vision of the goal is established. The annotated transcript of Fiona and Maria's coaching session https://hdl.handle.net/10523/41402 illustrates how the dialogue moves through the CPA phases during the session.

ENVISION. In guiding a coachee to envision desired future aspirations, the occupational therapist invites the coachee to describe goal achievement in sufficient detail so that they can both 'see' it occurs. Envisioning enables exploration of what a future alternative to the current situation might look and feel like. At the same time, the process of describing the imagined, ideal future raises a broad range of possibilities for doing things. A possibilities orientation is also a distinct concept in CanMOP's essential considerations (Egan & Restall, 2022). Envisioning an imagined ideal future can be difficult for people when they feel despondent or stuck. It is common for the coachee to express grief or frustration at confronting the contrast between how things currently are and how they want them to be. The relational elements of OPC – empathy, non-judgement, compassion – guide the occupational therapist's response. Inviting the coachee to describe how they want things to be may involve repeating this question in several different ways, and possibly over several sessions. Envisioning is critical to the coachee shifting their behaviour and choices toward achieving their goals. If a person cannot imagine change occurring, change is unlikely to occur. Strengthening the coachee's experience of trust, empathy and compassion may be helpful.

EXPLORE. Like task analysis and dynamic performance analysis (refer to Chapters 17 and 18), the occupational therapist attends to the coachee's perspective

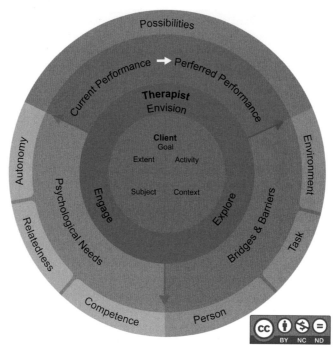

Fig. 27.2 ■ Collaborative performance analysis. (Reprinted with permission from Graham, F. (2020). *Occupational performance coaching resources*. https://www.otago.ac.nz/opc. This work is licensed under a Creative Commons Attribution-NonCommercial-NoDerivatives 4.0 International License. University of Otago.)

of what happens, in their context as they attempt a specific goal task. CPA in OPC is oriented to how the coachee wants things to be (rather than current performance) and thus relies heavily on the coachee's ability to visualise a desired future approach to a situation. Although the occupational therapist's knowledge of grading of tasks simply influences their questioning, it is the coachee's analysis of performance that leads this process, not the occupational therapist.

The Explore element requires the occupational therapist to engage with the coachee-as-expert, by following their lead, and asking questions that expand on their reflection and insight. At the same time, the occupational therapist maintains an awareness of their professional knowledge (i.e. knowledge of the OPC methods, health and disability and common solutions to occupational challenges) without privileging this over the coachee's opinion or ideas. OPC's success is entirely dependent on the coachee implementing strategies in the lived environment, usually at times when the occupational therapist is not present (e.g. during the morning or bedtime

routine). In addition, people are vastly more likely to implement a strategy that they have discovered; hence, coachee self-discovery is an important mechanism for change in OPC. The process of discovering a successful strategy also builds a person's sense of competence and autonomy, thus their capacity to self-manage situations in the future. Capacity building is a key long-term outcome of OPC.

ENGAGE. Throughout the OPC session, the occupational therapist attends to the engaging elements of CPA. Engage is aligned with addressing the three basic psychological needs highlighted in self-determination theory; it guides the occupational therapist to pay attention to what influences the coachee's level of engagement throughout the coaching conversation and their motivation for goal-related change. The coachee's motivation and engagement can fluctuate moment-by-moment and are influenced by their evolving relationship with the therapist, how difficult it is to discuss the topic matters and how they feel about their ability to achieve their goal.

ACT. Each OPC session concludes with the coachee identifying actions they plan to do over the coming days and weeks that they believe will enable them to progress towards their goals. The act phase includes a collaborative discussion of both the development of ideas for action and the exploration of factors that support the coachee's implementation of the plan. The occupational therapist asks questions to elicit action statements once the coachee has engaged in deep reflection on the goal situation.

EVALUATE. Evaluate occurs after an action has been attempted or implemented in the coachee's daily routine or specific context. This step generally occurs when the occupational therapist is not present, but this might occur within a session if it is appropriate for a strategy to be practised in this context. Evaluation is always based on the coachee's opinion, as it is their view of the success of a plan that will determine if they continue to use it.

Evaluate is approached with an open mind and has two key components that occur in the following order:

1. Evaluating goal progress; and
2. Evaluating the success of any strategies used.

Evaluation of progress occurs first. The initial goal statements (alongside the Canadian Occupational Performance Measure (COPM) or the Goal Attainment Scale (GAS) rating) are useful tools to explore progress. At this point in OPC, it is critical that the OPC goal statement formula was applied in the initial session, otherwise progress on goals is unclear and the discussion can quickly become lost. In the case of Maria and Tui, to explore goal progress, the occupational therapist may ask 'How many times did Tui get off technology calmly over the past week?' The occupational therapist does not seek further proof that Maria's report is accurate. Instead, they then interview Maria further about the circumstances of Tui getting off calmly, or more calmly than he has previously, thus transitioning directly into another, deeper round of CPA.

When evaluating the use of a strategy, it is important that strategy use is considered separately from goal progress because it is not uncommon that progress towards the goal occurs when the coachee perceives that the plan was not implemented, or that they used a different strategy to the one discussed. Diverging from the plan is a sign of independent problem solving, competence and

> **BOX 27.5**
> ## GENERALISABLE PRINCIPLE FOR MARIA
>
> Maria might arrive at a strategy of letting Tui know how long he has on technology before he starts, making sure he is aware of his finish time before he begins. The generalisable principle here is 'provide structure'/'no surprises'. Framed as this generalisable principle, Maria spontaneously identified that giving Tui a written timetable for the weekend helped Tui to be willing to try new things because he was less anxious about the unpredictability of his weekends.

initiative, all important for self-management of occupational participation issues. The coachee is guided to explore and reflect on what they observed, and what could explain what they observed. Usually, the coachee will have at least observed the goal situation more keenly and report more detailed observations, forming the basis of a renewed CPA. When individuals have not attended to the goal at all, the occupational therapist guides an exploration of the importance of the goal (being open to the possibility that this goal may no longer be the priority) and an exploration of the barriers to focusing on the goal if it is still a priority.

Generalise

The 'generalise' step is applied whenever the coachee reports that their chosen strategy was successful. To encourage generalisation, the occupational therapist asks questions that help the coachee identify the underlying principle of this successful strategy, where else it could be useful, and how it would need to be modified to suit the context of a different situation (Box 27.5).

Often a successful strategy addresses a recurrent underlying need or difficulty that is experienced by the coachee, thus it can have widespread applicability. Sometimes a coachee will spontaneously apply a successful strategy in multiple situations (Mezirow, 2012). However, increasing a coachee's awareness of how or why their strategy can be generalised to many situations can contribute to an amplified sense of competence and a self-management mindset.

Common generalisable strategies arising from OPC include planning ahead, allowing time; taking one step at a time; getting ready (mentally or physically); keeping it calm (or taking a breath) (Graham et al., 2016).

Generalise questions could include:

- Who else might benefit from knowing about your strategy?
- What is important for [teacher aid, paid carer, partner] to know if they are to use this strategy effectively?
- What other tasks do you do where this idea of 'one thing at a time' might be helpful?

The Share Domain

The share domain (Fig. 27.1) of OPC guides the occupational therapist in supporting the coachee to share their knowledge and ideas for moving toward achieving their goals. When using OPC, occupational therapists only share their knowledge with the coachee as a last resort and always invite the coachee to reject or critique any suggestions (Graham & Ziviani, 2021b, p. 85). The occupational therapist uses a range of techniques to elevate the coachee's awareness of the relevance of knowledge that they already hold, rather than what the occupational therapist knows.

In OPC, an 80:20 rule is applied to sharing information. 80% of the dialogue should be the coachee sharing their knowledge and ideas or the occupational therapist prompting them to share more. 20% (or less) of the dialogue should be the occupational therapist sharing specialist knowledge.

There are two good reasons for coaching the person to lead information sharing. First, when goals reflect occupational participation in everyday life situations, a coachee usually already knows of the kinds of actions they could take that can be sustainably applied in life contexts. It is not a lack of knowledge that has limited their ability to apply that knowledge. It is often, a lack of awareness of the usefulness of that knowledge to the goal they are aspiring to achieve. Sometimes, however, specialist knowledge is the key to goal progress and there is a place for this in OPC, but only used sparingly. Second, people are much more likely to implement change when the action is their idea. Furthermore, when goals reflect meaningful change in life situations, only the coachee can make the change happen. Attention to strategies that support the enactment of the plan arrived at during OPC is critical to a

coachee's progress. Strategies to encourage a coachee to share knowledge in OPC relate to the occupational therapists' mindset, and their communication strategies. Example questions that could be used during OPC, in relation to each of the OPC components are presented in Fig. 27.3.

Mindset

Several coaching interventions stress the importance of occupational therapists adopting a particular mindset for intervention techniques to have the intended effect (Caperton et al., 2018; King et al., 2006). Compassion, curiosity and an expectation of resourcefulness (or capability for growth) are signature elements of the OPC mindset. During OPC, an open mind to the possibilities of how a coachee might take action towards their goals, is needed. Holding a curious mindset also helps the occupational therapist to follow the coachee's lead and avoid attachment to their own analysis or opinion. Occupational therapists' development of mindful attention to their own internal dialogue during coaching is a core element of learning OPC. Maintaining the OPC mindset requires the occupational therapist to quieten tendencies for judgement and analysis. How an OPC mindset supports the discovery of strategies by the coachee rather than the occupational therapist is illustrated in Table 27.1.

Coaching Communication

Communication strategies within OPC that enable the coachee to identify solutions start from the envisioning phase. Often solutions can emerge simply by imagining that the goal is achieved. Asking first (before, if at all, telling), prompting reflection and teaching the principles (rather than advising on details) are useful, with examples provided in Fig. 27.3.

SELF-ASSESSMENT AND REFLECTION ON OPC SKILLS

To determine if OPC is being delivered as intended, the OPC fidelity measure (Graham, 2020) guides self- or peer-assessment of the quality of the most critical OPC behaviours (Graham & Ziviani, 2021a). The OPC Casenote Audit Tool guides and evaluates the occupational therapist's implementation of OPC through written communication. Both evaluation tools are freely available at

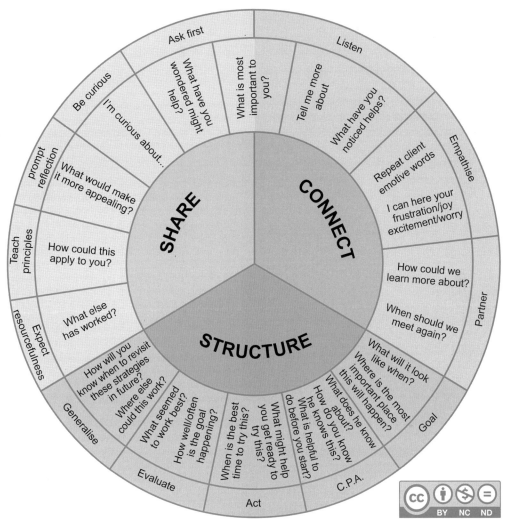

Fig. 27.3 ■ Occupation performance coaching question wheel provides examples of questions that could be used in for each OPC domain. (Reprinted with permission from Graham, F. (2023). *Occupational performance coaching resources*. https://www.otago.ac.nz/opc. This work is licensed under a Creative Commons Attribution-NonCommercial-NoDerivatives 4.0 International License. University of Otago.)

https://www.otago.ac.nz/opc/resources. An example of the Casenote Audit Tool and OPC-FM applied to the first session of Maria and Tui (Boxes 27.1–27.5) is available at/in the https://hdl.handle.net/10523/41402.

CONCLUSION

The context of coaching approaches in rehabilitation has been described in this chapter, with a particular focus on OPC. OPC is a form of coaching designed specifically for rehabilitation contexts, grounded in occupation theory and values.

Like other coaching approaches, OPC is a conversation in which individuals and collectives are guided to identify their most highly valued goal, reflect on what works best for them to progress towards achieving that goal, evaluate their progress and apply their success to wider areas of their life. Distinctively, OPC targets goals of improved occupational participation, from the perspective of individuals and aligns with concepts within the Canadian model of occupational participation as a lens for guiding individual reflection and insight. In applying OPC, the expertise of an occupational therapist is their skillful communication with individuals to optimise each coachee's engagement in their rehabilitation and sense of autonomy in their lives, coupled with knowledge of health conditions, activity grading and health and social systems.

OPC is supported by a rapidly growing evidence base. However, many questions about its use remain unanswered including who OPC is appropriate for (e.g. minimal research has been conducted with Indigenous populations), which elements of OPC are most critical for goal progress, and how much and what form of training in OPC leads to high fidelity implementation by most occupational therapists. Future research on OPC is likely to refine how OPC is applied, with whom, and how to ensure occupational therapist adherence to its intended principles.

REFERENCES

Alcorn, K., & Broome, K. (2014). Occupational performance coaching for chronic health conditions: A review of the literature. *New Zealand Journal of Occupational Therapy, 61*(2), 49–56.

Allen, S., Knott, F. J., Branson, A., & Lane, S. J. (2021). Coaching parents of children with sensory integration difficulties: A scoping review. *Occupational Therapy International*, 2021.

American Occupational Therapy Association. (2020). Occupational therapy practice framework: Domain and process – Fourth Edition. *American Journal of Occupational Therapy*, 74 (Suppl. 2): 7412410010p1–7412410010p84.

Araujo, C. R. S., Cardoso, A. A., Polatajko, H. J., & de Castro Magalhães, L. (2021). Efficacy of the cognitive orientation to daily occupational performance (CO-OP) approach with and without parental coaching on activity and participation for children with developmental coordination disorder: A randomized clinical trial. *Research in Developmental Disabilities, 110*, 103862.

Askari, S., Kessler, D., Smyth, P., & Finlayson, M. (2022). Evaluating occupational performance coaching to support fatigue management for people with multiple sclerosis: A feasibility study. *Clinical Rehabilitation 36*(9), 1244–1256.

Austin-McCain, M. (2015). LifeSteps: An evidence-based health promotion program for underserved populations–A community service learning approach. *The Open Journal of Occupational Therapy, 3*(2), 8.

Azari, Z., Hosseini, S., Rassafiani, M., Samadi, S., & Dunn, W. (2020). A Contextual Intervention Adapted for Autism Spectrum Disorders: A Pilot Study With Single-Subject Design. Archives of Rehabilitation, 21(1), 120-137. https://doi.org/10.32598/RJ.21.1.2932.1.

Azari, Z. P., Hosseini, S. A., Rassafiani, M., Samadi, S. A., Hoseinzadeh, S., & Winnie, D. (2019). Contextual intervention adapted for autism spectrum disorder: An RCT of a parenting program with parents of children diagnosed with autism spectrum disorder (ASD). *Iranian Journal of Child Neurology, 13*(4), 19.

Bandura, A. (1986). *Social foundations of thought and action*. Prentice-Hall.

Brandt, C. J., Søgaard, G. I., Clemensen, J., Søndergaard, J., & Nielsen, J. B. (2018). Determinants of successful eHealth coaching for consumer lifestyle changes: Qualitative interview study among health care professionals. *Journal of medical Internet Research, 20*(7), e237.

Brock, V. G. (2008). *Grounded theory of the roots and emergence of coaching*. International University of Professional Studies.

Bronfenbrenner, U., & Morris, P. A. (2007). The bioecological model of human development. In W. Damon & R. M. Lerner (Eds.), Handbook of child psychology, Vol. 1: Theoretical models of human development (6th ed., pp. 793–828). New York: Wiley.

Cadematori, C., Alpajora, B., Sivori, T., Betz, S., Gerhardt, N., Dunn, W., & Mulcahey, M. (2021). Preliminary examination of coaching in context with clients with spinal cord injury. *Spinal Cord Series and Cases, 7*(1), 27.

Caldwell, K. L., Vicidomini, D., Wells, R., & Wolever, R. Q. (2020). Engaging patients in their health care: Lessons from a qualitative study on the processes health coaches use to support an active learning paradigm. *Global Advances in Health and Medicine, 9*, 2164956120904662.

Caperton, D. D., Atkins, D. C., & Imel, Z. E. (2018). Rating motivational interviewing fidelity from thin slices. *Psychology of Addictive Behaviors, 32*(4), 434–441.

Darrah, J., & Bartlett, D. (1995). Dynamic systems theory and management of children with cerebral palsy: Unresolved issues. *Infants and Young Children, 8*(1), 52–59.

Doyle, N. W., Gafni Lachter, L., & Jacobs, K. (2019). Scoping review of mentoring research in the occupational therapy literature, 2002–2018. *Australian Occupational Therapy Journal, 66*(5), 541–551.

Dunn, W., Brown, C., & McGuigan, A. (1994). The ecology of human performance: A framework for considering the effect of context. *The American Journal of Occupational Therapy, 48*(7), 595–607.

Dunn, W., Cox, J., Foster, L., Mische-Lawson, L., & Tanquary, J. (2012). Impact of a contextual intervention on child participation and parent competence among children with autism spectrum disorders: A pretest-posttest repeated-measures design. *American Journal of Occupational Therapy, 66*(5), 520–528.

Egan, M. & Restall, G. (2022). The Canadian model of occupational participation. In M. Egan & G. Restall (Eds.). Promoting occupational participation: Collaborative relationship-focused occupational therapy (pp. 73–95). Canadian Association of Occupational Therapists.

Egan, M. Y., Toal-Sullivan, D., Kessler, D., Kristjansson, E., & Del Bel, M. J. (2023). Student-led occupational performance coaching in a university setting. *British Journal of Occupational Therapy, 86*(6), 413–422.

Egan, M., & Restall, G. (2022a). The canadian model of occupational participation. In M. Egan, & G. Restall (Eds.), *Promoting occupational participation: Collaborative relationship-focused occupational therapy.* CAOT Publications ACE.

Erlandsson, L.-K. (2013). The redesigning daily occupations (ReDO)-program: Supporting women with stress-related disorders to return to work – Knowledge base, structure, and content. *Occupational Therapy in Mental Health, 29*(1), 85–101.

Frisch, C., Rosenblum, S., & Tirosh, E. (2020). Parental occupational executive training: Feasibility and parental perceptions. *OTJR: Occupation, Participation and Health, 40*(3), 203–210.

Fusari, G., Gibbs, E., Hoskin, L., Dickens, D., Leis, M., Taylor, E., Jones, F., & Darzi, A. (2020). Protocol for a feasibility study of OnTrack: A digital system for upper limb rehabilitation after stroke. *BMJ Open, 10*(3), e034936.

Ghaffari, A., Azad, A., Zarei, M. A., Rassafiani, M., & Sharif Nia, H. (2022). Effect of occupation performance coaching with four-quadrant model of facilitated learning on children with specific learning disorder. *Occupational Therapy International, 6*(14), 1–13.

Gordon, N. F., Salmon, R. D., Wright, B. S., Faircloth, G. C., Reid, K. S., & Gordon, T. L. (2017). Clinical effectiveness of lifestyle health coaching: Case study of an evidence-based program. *American Journal of Lifestyle Medicine, 11*(2), 153–166.

Graham, F., Rodger, S., Ziviani, J., & Jones, V. (2016). Strategies identified as effective by mothers during occupational performance coaching. *Physical & Occupational Therapy in Pediatrics, 36*(3), 247–259.

Graham, F., & Ziviani, J. (2021a). Chapter 4, fidelity processes. In F. Graham, A. Kennedy-Behr, & J. Ziviani (Eds.), *Occupational performance coaching: A manual for practitioners and researchers* (pp. 92–109). Routledge.

Graham, F., & Ziviani, J. (2021b). Chapter 3, implementation procedures. In F. Graham, A. Kennedy-Behr, & J. Ziviani (Eds.), *Occupational performance coaching: A manual for practitioners and researchers* (pp. 40–91). Routledge.

Graham, F. (2020). Coaching in telehealth delivery of occupational therapy. *Occupational Therapy Telehealth Summit.*

Graham, F., & Ziviani, J. (2021). Theoretical and conceptual foundations. In F. Graham, A. Kennedy-Behr, & J. Ziviani (Eds.), *Occupational Performance Coaching: A manual for practitioners and researchers* (pp. 8–39). Routledge.

Graham, F., Kessler, D., Nott, M., Bernie, C., Kanagasabai, P. & Barthow, C. (in press). *A scoping review of coaching in occupational therapy: mapping methods, populations and outcomes.* Australian Occupational Therapy Journal.

Hammell, K. W. (2020). *Engagement in living: Critical perspectives on occupation, rights, and wellbeing.* Canadian Association of Occupational Therapists.

Harrington, E. E., Santos, G. O., & Potvin, M.-C. (2021). Postsecondary education students with disabilities' perceptions of occupational therapy-led coaching. *The Open Journal of Occupational Therapy, 9*(2), 1–13.

International Coaching Federation. (2023). *The international coaching federation.* Experience Coaching.

Ives, Y. (2008). What is' coaching'? An exploration of conflicting paradigms. *International Journal of Evidence Based Coaching & Mentoring, 6*(2), 100–113.

Jamali, A. R., Alizadeh Zarei, M., Sanjari, M. A., AkbarFahimi, M., & Saneii, S. H (2022). Randomized controlled trial of occupation performance coaching for families of children with autism spectrum disorder by means of telerehabilitation. *British Journal of Occupational Therapy, 85*(5), 308–315.

Kessler, D., Anderson, N. D., & Dawson, D. R. (2021). Occupational performance coaching for stroke survivors delivered via telerehabilitation using a single-case experimental design. *British Journal of Occupational Therapy, 84*(8), 488–496.

Kessler, D., Egan, M., Dubouloz, C. J., McEwen, S., & Graham, F. P. (2017). Occupational performance coaching for stroke survivors: A pilot randomized controlled trial. *American Journal of Occupational Therapy, 71*(3). 7103190020p1–7103190020p7. https://doi.org/10.5014/ajot.2017.024216.

Kessler, D., & Graham, F. (2015). The use of coaching in occupational therapy: An integrative review. *Australian Occupational Therapy Journal, 62*(3), 160–176.

King, G. A., Tucker, M. A., Baldwin, P. J., & Laporta, J. A. (2006). Bringing the life needs model to life: Implementing a service delivery model for pediatric rehabilitation. *Physical & Occupational Therapy in Pediatrics, 26*(1–2), 43–70.

Kronberg, J., Tierney, E., Wallisch, A., & Little, L. M. (2021). Early intervention service delivery via telehealth during COVID-19: A research-practice partnership. *International Journal of Telerehabilitation, 13*(1) e6363.

Laverdure, P., & Beisbier, S. (2021). Occupation-and activity-based interventions to improve performance of activities of daily living, play, and leisure for children and youth ages 5 to 21: A systematic review. *The American Journal of Occupational Therapy, 75*(1) 7501205050p7501205051–7501205050p7501205024.

Law, M., Baptiste, S., McColl, M., Opzoomer, A., Polatajko, H., & Pollock, N. (1990). The Canadian occupational performance measure: An outcome measure for occupational therapy. *Canadian Journal of Occupational Therapy, 57*(2), 82–87.

Law, M., Cooper, B., Strong, B., Stewart, D., Rigby, P., & Letts, L. (1996). The person-environment occupation model: A transactive approach to occupational performance. *Canadian Journal of Occupational Therapy, 63*(1), 9–23.

Little, L. M., Pope, E., Wallisch, A., & Dunn, W. (2018). Occupation-based coaching by means of telehealth for families of young children with autism spectrum disorder. *American Journal of Occupational Therapy, 72*(2), 1–7.

McMorris, T., & Hale, T. (2006). *Coaching science: Theory into practice.* John Wiley & Sons.

Mezirow, J. (2012). Learning to think like an adult: Core concepts of transformation theory. In E. W. Taylor, & P. Cranton (Eds.), *Handbook of transformative learning: Theory, research and practice* (pp. 73–95). Wiley.

Moore, G. F., Audrey, S., Barker, M., Bond, L., Bonell, C., Hardeman, W., Moore, L., O'Cathain, A., Tinati, T., Wight, D., & Baird, J. (2015). Process evaluation of complex interventions: Medical research council guidance. *British Medical Journal, 350*, h1258.

Mulcahey, M., Gerhardt, N., Alpajora, B., Thielen, C. C., & Dunn, W. (2022). Coaching-in-context with informal maternal care partners of children with spinal cord injury. *Topics in Spinal Cord Injury Rehabilitation, 28*(1), 99–113.

Nott, M., Wiseman, L., Seymour, T., Pike, S., Cuming, T., & Wall, G. (2021). Stroke self-management and the role of self-efficacy. *Disability and Rehabilitation, 43*(10), 1410–1419.

Novak, I. (2014). Evidence to practice commentary new evidence in coaching interventions. *Physical & Occupational Therapy in Pediatrics, 34*(2), 132–137.

Parsloe, E., & Wray, M. (2000). *Coaching and mentorship: Practical methods to improve learning.* Kogan.

Persson, D., Erlandsson, L. K., Eklund, M., & Iwarsson, S. (2001). Value dimensions, meaning, and complexity in human occupation – A tentative structure for analysis. *Scandinavian Journal of Occupational Therapy, 8*(1), 7–18.

Quinn, L., Trubey, R., Gobat, N., Dawes, H., Edwards, R. T., Jones, C., Townson, J., Drew, C., Kelson, M., & Poile, V. (2016). Development and delivery of a physical activity intervention for people with Huntington disease: Facilitating translation to clinical practice. *Journal of Neurologic Physical Therapy, 40*(2), 71.

Restall, G., Egan, M., Valavaara, K., Phenix, A., & Sack, C. (2022). Canadian occupational therapy inter-relational practice process. In M. Egan, & G. Restall (Eds.), *Promoting occupational participation: Collaborative relationship-focused occupational therapy.* Canadian Association of Occupational Therapists.

Ryan, R. M., & Deci, E. L. (2017). *Self-determination theory: Basic psychological needs in motivation, development, and wellness.* Guilford Press.

Setoguchi, M., Motruk, S., Frank, V., & Kessler, D. (2020). A review of mobile applications to enhance coaching in occupational therapy. *British Journal of Occupational Therapy, 83*(9), 549–560.

Shin, J., Jewell, V. D., Abbott, A. A., Russell, M., Carlson, K., & Gordon, M. (2022). Fidelity protocol development for a telehealth type 1 diabetes occupation-based coaching intervention. *Canadian Journal of Occupational Therapy, 89*(2), 159–169.

Smith, L. L., Lake, N. H., Simmons, L. A., Perlman, A., Wroth, S., & Wolever, R. Q. (2013). Integrative health coach training: A model for shifting the paradigm toward patient-centricity and meeting new national prevention goals. *Global Advances in Health and Medicine, 2*(3), 66–74.

Smith, S. L., Aytur, S. A., & Humphreys, B. P. (2023). Effects of telehealth parent coaching in supporting family participation, cohesion, and adaptability. *OTJR: Occupational Therapy Journal of Research, 43*(1), 24–34.

Stober, D., & Grant, A. (2006). *Evidence based coaching handbook.* John Wiley & Sons.

Sundar, V., & Brucker, D. (2021). 'Today I felt like my work meant something': A pilot study on job crafting, a coaching-based intervention for people with work limitations and disabilities. *Work, 69*(2), 423–438.

Townsend, E., Beagan, B., Kumas-Tan, Z., Versnel, J., Iwama, M., Landry, J., Stewart, D., & Brown, J. (2007). Enabling: Occupational therapy's core competencies. In E. Townsend, & H. Polatajko (Eds.), *Enabling occupation ii: Advancing and occupational therapy vision for health, well-being and justice through occupation* (pp. 87–133). CAOT.

Wallisch, A., Little, L., Pope, E., & Dunn, W. (2019). Parent perspectives of an occupational therapy telehealth intervention. *International Journal of Telerehabilitation, 11*(1), 15.

World Health Organization. (2001). *International classification of functioning, disability and health: ICF.* World Health Organization.

Zimmerman, B. J., & Moylan, A. R. (2009). *Self-regulation: Where metacognition and motivation intersect.* In *Handbook of metacognition in education* (pp. 311–328). Routledge.

REFLECTION

For the first three questions, you can refer to the practice story of Maria.

1. List three questions an OPC coach could use to elicit Maria's goal.

2. Describe two communications strategies within OPC that may enable Maria to identify solutions themselves.

3. How is Maria's autonomy supported in OPC and why?

4. Describe the key differences between educational approaches and coaching.

28

COGNITIVE ORIENTATION TO DAILY OCCUPATIONAL PERFORMANCE (CO-OP) APPROACH*

HELENE J. POLATAJKO

CHAPTER OUTLINE

Overview

The cognitive orientation to daily occupational performance (CO-OP) approach is a performance-based, problem-solving intervention that uses a global problem-solving strategy at its core. Rather than focusing on impairments or problems related to performance components, CO-OP is a capabilities approach that helps individuals develop cognitive strategies to solve occupational performance problems. This chapter describes how cognitive strategies can improve occupational performance and participation by providing an overview of cognitive strategy use, a description of the CO-OP approach and

illustrations of cognitive strategy use with practice stories. Finally, the chapter provides a summary of evidence that supports cognitive strategy use with adults who have experienced cerebrovascular or traumatic brain injury, as well as lessons learned from several studies.

KEY POINTS

CO-OP approach is:

- an occupation-based intervention that directly works on improving occupational performance;
- embedded in a learning paradigm and is focused on performance, NOT impairments in performance components;
- a task-oriented approach that enables occupational performance through a process of dynamic performance analysis and guided discovery;

*Updated from Polatajko, H. J., McEwen, S. E., Dawson, D. R., & Skidmore, E. R. (2017). Cognitive orientation to daily occupational performance. In M. Curtin, J. Adams, & M. Egan (Eds.), *Occupational therapy for people experiencing illness, injury or impairment* (Chapter 42, 7th ed.). Elsevier.

- an approach that uses cognitive strategies to change performance;

- an evidence-based approach;

- an approach that was first introduced for use with children with motor-based performance problems; and

- now used with a number of populations, including adults who have experienced a cerebrovascular accident or traumatic brain injury.

- Numerous peer-reviewed publications investigating the CO-OP Approach with adults who have experienced a cerebrovascular accident or traumatic brain injury suggest that this approach improves performance on trained and untrained self-selected goals and may also positively influence occupational participation in these populations.

INTRODUCTION

Cognitive orientation to daily occupational performance (CO-OP) is a client-centred, performance-based, problem-solving approach that uses global and domain-specific strategies to solve performance problems. Drawing on knowledge from cognitive science and human movement science, the CO-OP approach guides people in the discovery of strategies that are specific to their individual occupational performance needs. Rather than focusing on impairment and performance components such as balance, bilateral coordination or visual perception, CO-OP stimulates individuals to develop cognitive strategies to solve occupational performance problems. Emerging evidence demonstrates that this approach leads to better occupational performance, and consequently participation.

Traditionally, occupational performance, or more particularly, occupational performance issues have been ascribed to underlying impairments and the approaches to intervention have focused on remediating these underlying impairments. Although such impairment-focused interventions may have led to impairment reduction, research shows that this does not necessarily result in changes in meaningful occupations. Indeed, it is now generally recognised that task-oriented approaches are superior to impairment-reduction approaches in improving occupational performance (Chua et al., 2007; French et al., 2008; Hubbard et al., 2009).

Unfortunatley, improvement in performance in therapy does not generally transfer to other tasks or occupations, or generalise to other contexts. For example, improvement in dressing seen in therapy does not necessarily translate into improvements in the home, or in other related tasks. A growing body of evidence suggests that these limitations can be overcome by adding global cognitive strategy training to a task-specific approach (Dawson et al., 2009; Dawson et al., 2013; Geusgens et al., 2007; Liu et al., 2004; McEwen et al., 2010; McEwen et al., 2015; Skidmore et al., 2015). Much of this evidence is drawn from the CO-OP approach.

There is mounting evidence that the CO-OP approach not only supports performance during therapy but also, more importantly, enables people to generalise what is learned in therapy to their own environments and transfer this learning to other occupations. In other words, gains made through the CO-OP approach not only improve performance but also participation. Interestingly, emerging literature suggests that CO-OP can also reduce impairments and build capacity. The purpose of this chapter is to draw on the findings from research investigating the CO-OP approach and to describe how cognitive strategies can improve occupational performance and participation. The chapter begins with an overview of cognitive strategy use, followed by a description of the CO-OP approach. Next, the use of the CO-OP approach with adults with neurological impairments is presented and illustrated with two practice stories (Boxes 28.1 and 28.2). Finally, the evidence to support its use with adults who have experienced a cerebrovascular accident (CVA) or traumatic brain injury (TBI) and lessons learned conclude the chapter. But first, a word about CO-OP and participation.

CO-OP and Participation

The CO-OP approach, as the name indicates, is focused on occupational performance. However, this book is focused on occupational participation. Hence a brief detour to discuss the fit of CO-OP in a book on occupational participation is warranted.

The International Classification of Functioning, Disability and Health (ICF) (World Health Organization, 2001) ICF depicts *participation* as the desired outcome of rehabilitation, relating it, in part, to *body*

BOX 28.1
ADDRESSING OCCUPATIONAL PERFORMANCE ISSUES AFTER CVA – MS FINE

Ms Fine was a 56-year-old teacher, living with her husband, who experienced a right middle cerebral artery cerebrovascular accident (CVA). This resulted in moderate hemiparesis of her left arm and leg, sensory loss throughout her left side, and issues with initiation, planning and spatial perceptual judgement. Ms Fine spent 1 week in an acute care hospital and was then transferred to an inpatient rehabilitation programme. Her occupational therapist, Genevieve, conducted an extensive assessment that began with a goal-setting interview.

During this interview, Ms Fine discussed her valued occupations with Genevieve and reflected on the occupations she most wanted to work on during her rehabilitation. She decided that her priority occupational performance issues were difficulty getting around with the wheelchair (including transfers), reading books and eating 'properly'. Together Ms Fine and Genevieve identified the following four goals – Ms Fine would be able to:

1. Transfer from the bed to the wheelchair and back again;
2. Propel the wheelchair from her bed to the door of her bathroom;
3. Hold a book with two hands; and
4. Cut and eat food 'properly' (which she defined as neatly and with a knife and fork).

As a starting point for intervention Genevieve conducted an analysis of Ms Fine's pre-intervention performance of her identified goals. She asked Ms Fine to demonstrate transferring to the bed from the wheelchair, propelling her wheelchair, holding and reading a book and cutting food and eating. During these demonstrations, Genevieve ensured Ms Fine was safe but did not provide any verbal or physical assistance to help her complete the tasks. Genevieve used the performance quality rating scale (PQRS) to evaluate initial performance in these tasks. Ms Fine scored a 2/10 on wheelchair transfer, 4/10 on wheelchair propulsion, 5/10 on holding and reading a book and 2/10 on using both hands to cut and eat food.

While observing Ms Fine perform these activities, Genevieve carried out a dynamic performance analysis (refer to Chapter 18). She noticed that while Ms Fine had motor limitations, this was not the only problem limiting her ability to perform the tasks. Ms Fine also did not seem to know all the steps in the activities or mixed up the sequence of the steps. For example, while attempting to perform a transfer from bed to a wheelchair, she started to try to get up before ensuring the wheelchair was located beside the bed and before having moved herself forward into a position to best facilitate standing up. As a result, her performance of the task broke down into several steps.

After the baseline assessment, Genevieve taught Ms Fine the global cognitive strategy GOAL-PLAN-DO-CHECK. Ms Fine's specific GOAL was to be able to transfer from her bed to her wheelchair and back again, safely and without physical assistance. Over the next two sessions, Genevieve guided her to discover a PLAN. Through multiple small experiments carrying out potential plans (PLAN, DO and CHECK), Ms Fine solved multiple problems related to a good angle for the wheelchair to be positioned beside the bed and the best height of the bed to facilitate standing up and discovered that standing up was easier if her heels were a little behind her knees. Learning through discovery took more time than it would have taken for Genevieve to simply tell Ms Fine what to do. However, this would not have optimally engaged Ms Fine in the problem-solving process. That is, it would not have drawn on her cognitive skills, and it may not have resulted in domain-specific strategies that worked particularly well for her.

In this specific situation, Genevieve found that the GOAL-PLAN-DO-CHECK process took longer than it generally does when she works with people who have had a CVA. This was because initially Ms Fine seemed to have difficulty responding to open-ended questions. For example, when Genevieve said, 'Where do you think the wheelchair should be positioned to make the transfer easier?' Ms Fine did not respond. Eventually Ms Fine replied that she did not know.

To avoid frustrating Ms Fine, Genevieve switched to a closed form of questioning. While still encouraging her to think through the problem, Genevieve provided Ms Fine with options to try to solve the problems presented in each step of the task. For example, at the step of positioning the wheelchair Genevieve asked, 'Do you think it would be easier to transfer if the wheelchair was directly in front of you, or angled at the side of the bed?' 'Should we put it on the left or the right?' 'Once you are standing up, will it be easier to turn to the left or the right?' By the end of the third session, Ms Fine was problem solving more, responding to open-ended questions and engaging in discussions with Genevieve about possible strategies. Through this process, Ms Fine discovered a strategy that helped her to remember the sequence of steps 'chair, feet, up', and her PQRS score for transferring became a 7/10.

As she was now feeling very confident in her abilities, she added a new goal of propelling her wheelchair to the dining room to eat her meals. She and Genevieve worked on this together and accomplished the goal in a single session. After 3 weeks in the inpatient rehabilitation unit, Ms Fine had accomplished her goals with PQRS scores of 10/10, except for eating with a knife and fork, for which she scored a 6/10. She had added additional goals during her stay, including a tub transfer, a car transfer, dressing and walking to the toilet independently with her four-point cane.

Genevieve encouraged Ms Fine to apply the process to new challenges she would meet at home. Once she was home, these activities included unloading the dishwasher, folding laundry and taking her dog out on a leash. She was able to confidently apply the global cognitive strategy GOAL-PLAN-DO-CHECK to learn these activities to her satisfaction.

BOX 28.2

ADDRESSING OCCUPATIONAL PERFORMANCE ISSUES
AFTER TRAUMATIC BRAIN INJURY – MS ROLE

Ms Role sustained a severe traumatic brain injury (TBI) in a motor vehicle crash at age 28, emerged from a coma after 9 days and then spent about 2 months in an inpatient rehabilitation unit. On discharge home, she received community-based therapy (occupational therapy, physiotherapy, speech therapy) for 9 months. More than 20 years later, at age 50, she enrolled in a research study on the CO-OP approach. She had never been competitively employed since her TBI but did participate in several hours of community volunteer work each month.

Due to the length of time since her injury, details about her immediate postinjury impairments were not available. Her research pre-test, administered by a trained research assistant, included a test that allowed her premorbid IQ to be estimated to have been in the superior range. During this assessment she complained of mood difficulties, pain (headaches) and fatigue, noting that the latter interfered with her day-to-day activities more than half the time. In addition, she complained of significant difficulties with organisation, memory and distraction.

Further assessments (Table 28.3), also carried out for research purposes, suggested that Ms Role was mild to moderately depressed and moderately anxious. In terms of executive functioning, she scored in the impaired range on a standardised measure (the Behaviour Rating Inventory of Executive Function – Adult Version (Roth et al., 2005)). At the pre-test, she also indicated on the Mayo-Portland Adaptability Inventory Participation Index (www.tbims.org/combi/) that her ability to participate in leisure and social activities was substantially limited.

A research occupational therapist administered the Canadian Occupational Performance Measure (Law et al., 2014) (refer to Chapter 16), during which Ms Role identified five areas of difficulties. From these difficulties, related goals that she wanted to address during her therapy were identified. As per the research protocol (Dawson et al., 2013), she was able to select one of these to address during therapy: the other four were randomised such that two were addressed in therapy and two remained untrained (Table 28.4).

The occupational therapist, Mary, identified baseline performance on the three trained goals through conversation, as observation was not possible. Once Mary felt she had a good understanding of the situation she began the process of guiding Ms Role to develop plans that would facilitate her goal attainment.

Mary found the first several sessions with Ms Role particularly difficult, as Ms Role would move from topic to topic in conversation very quickly. Mary shared this observation with Ms Role, stating, 'I'm getting quite confused during our sessions – I lose track of what is happening. Is that something you are experiencing?' Ms Role immediately confirmed that she was also having this experience and so a plan was generated that when either of them started to feel confused they would stop the session and ask themselves what goal they were working on. This plan worked well and was used throughout the intervention.

As per the research protocol, Mary provided Ms Role with goal sheets in a binder. These sheets included columns for plans, the desired outcome for the plan, whether the plan was executed and whether the plan worked. For example, in working on the goal of organising her finances using a commercial software program, Ms Role made a plan to watch the instructional video so that she could learn how to synchronise her bank account with the program. Part of her plan included the domain-specific strategy of paying attention to her fatigue level and stopping to rest as needed throughout the activity.

Ms Role watched the video but was not able to synchronise her bank account with the program. In analysing her performance with Mary, she realised that she had not set enough time aside to fully understand the video and then do the synchronisation. Her next plan was to take more time. She did this but was still not able to accomplish the synchronisation. She then made a plan to call the helpline. She used the domain-specific strategy of writing relevant information (e.g., account number) on Post-It notes and putting these on the computer screen. In this way, she was ultimately able to accomplish her goal.

As shown in Tables 28.3 and 28.4, Ms Role received considerable benefit from the CO-OP Approach intervention. Her performance and satisfaction with performance improved substantially on all of her goals (trained and untrained) and her gains were maintained 3 months after the intervention was finished. These findings suggest that Ms Role had learned strategy use and was transferring it to new situations. This is considered far transfer, that is, transfer of learning to a context and task that is different from where the original learning occurred (Barnett & Ceci, 2002).

---

function & structure and, in part to *activity*. The former refers to what are often called performance components in occupational therapy, and are not a focus of CO-OP. As used in the ICF, the term activity refers

to the execution of a task or action, akin to the term performance in occupational therapy and, more specifically, in CO-OP. Participation, in the ICF, refers to involvement in a life situation of people in the actual context in which they live, the intended outcome of CO-OP.

While the name of the CO-OP approach identifies it as being focused on performance, it is important to note that the performances actually addressed in the intervention are determined by the individual receiving the intervention in response to the question: What do you need to, want to, or are expected to do that you can't do to your own satisfaction[1]. In other words, using the language of the ICF (WHO, 2001), the problems CO-OP addresses are problems in participation. Nonetheless, the focus of the intervention is on performance, whether it is delivered in the context of the clinic or the individual's real-world environment. The underlying premise being that participation is dependent on performance – that performance issues contribute to participation problems and performance competencies support participation.

In CO-OP, the skills that are the focus of the intervention (the skills that the individual receiving the intervention chooses to address) are those that they identify as issues in their day-to-day living. In other words, performance issues that affect their ability to participate in life, fully. In many instances, the CO-OP intervention is conducted in the real-world context of the individual's goal. Where it is not, the intervention is designed to support the generalisation and transfer of skills addressed in the therapy context to the real-world environment. Being an intervention that targets the performance issues that individuals identify as affecting their day-to-day participation, CO-OP is, by implication, an intervention that supports occupational participation. Thus from here forward, in this chapter, when discussing participation the focus is on performance and participation.

COGNITIVE STRATEGY USE: AN OVERVIEW

Cognitive strategies are conscious, goal-directed plans of action (Toglia et al., 2012). Effective goal-directed

behaviour tends to rely on higher-level cognitive functions (Luria, 1966). For the purposes of CO-OP, Polatajko and Mandich (2004) identified two types of cognitive strategies: global and domain specific.

Global Cognitive Strategies

Global cognitive strategies, also referred to as executive or metacognitive strategies, are evaluative or regulatory in nature and include processes to make decisions about which actions to take or which domain-specific strategies to use if a goal has not been reached. Global cognitive strategies make use of executive cognitive functions, those 'integrative cognitive processes that determine goal-directed and purposeful behaviour and are superordinate in the orderly execution of daily life functions […] includ[ing]: the ability to formulate goals; to initiate behaviour; to anticipate the consequences of actions; to plan and organise behaviour according to spatial, temporal, topical or logical sequences; and to monitor and adapt behaviour to fit a particular task or context' (Cicerone et al., 2000, p. 1605). These abilities are largely mediated by the systems and networks involving the frontal lobes. Executive functions are used as a term to cover a broad range of mental processes; these can be placed into four functional categories (Aharon-Peretz, 2017):

1. Executive functions involved in the control of more automatic functions, such as planning, monitoring, inhibiting and switching.
2. Behavioural self-regulatory functions involved in controlling emotional and behavioural responses in order to produce a more adaptive response.
3. Activation or energising functions that allow people to persist in working towards a goal.
4. Metacognitive processes that further link the first three functions.

Metacognition refers to a person thinking about how they think in the context of being self-aware and being able to evaluate these thoughts. For example, when planning a complex activity such as a summer vacation not only does a person think about what needs to be done (choose dates, choose a destination, etc.) but also about organising and sequencing plans to attain the goal (e.g. need to know if accommodation is available on specific dates before booking air

---

[1]The CO-OP protocol calls for the use of the Canadian Occupational Performance Measure (COPM) (Law et al., 2019) to initiate the goal-setting process, i.e. the individual is asked to identify performance problems in their everyday life [refer to Chapter 16].

TABLE 28.1
Examples of Global Strategies Used in a Variety of Strategy Training Approaches

Authors	Global Strategy
Bash and Camp (1986) Adopted by Meichenbaum (1991); by Polatajko et al. (2001)	GPDC: <u>G</u>oal; <u>P</u>lan; <u>D</u>o; <u>C</u>heck
Lawson and Rice (1989)	WSTC: <u>W</u>hat should I be doing?; <u>S</u>elect a strategy; <u>T</u>ry the strategy; <u>C</u>heck the strategy
van Heugten et al. (1998)	Initiation; Execution; Controlling
Ylvisaker et al. (1998)	Goal; Plan; Predict; Do; Review
von Cramon et al. (1991)	Problem-Solving Therapy (PST): Orient to problem; Define problem; Generate alternatives; Make a decision; Do it; Verify the solution
Levine et al. (2000)	Stop; Define; List; Learn; Do; Check
Levine et al. (2011)	Stop; Be in the present; State; Split; Check

travel), forming intentions about when things need to be done (e.g. awareness of the date by which balance must be paid in full and making a plan to execute payment before that date), making decisions about potential behaviour changes if a specific outcome cannot be achieved (e.g. travel partner is not responding to emails about potential destinations, therefore make a decision to try communication by telephone) and making conscious changes to plans (e.g. preferred destination is not available during current vacation dates, so make arrangements to switch vacation dates or look at other destinations). Clearly, metacognition is necessary for problem solving and goal attainment.

Research into metacognitive strategy training became prevalent in the 1970s, particularly in education and psychology. Donald Meichenbaum (1977, 1991), a prominent psychologist considered a founder of cognitive behavioural modification therapy, adopted the rubric *goal, plan, do and check,* introduced by Bash and Camp (1986), as part of his approach to using a problem-solving strategy to support behavioural change. This paved the way for occupational therapists and researchers to begin to use this and similar rubrics

as a 'cognitive scaffold' to address executive difficulties among people with neurological problems. Table 28.1 shows a sample of various problem-solving rubrics used in different global problem-solving approaches.

Domain-Specific Strategies

In contrast to global strategies, domain-specific strategies are generated to solve specific problems that occur while working through a particular occupational performance problem (Mandich et al., 2001). Toglia et al. (2012) refer to domain-specific strategies as 'mind tools' and developed a classification system that places them in three broad groupings: modality-specific strategies (sensory cues or prompts provided by the person themselves), mental or self-verbalisation strategies and task modification strategies (modifying or adapting the task or environment). As described by Mandich et al. (2001), CO-OP uses both a global strategy and domain-specific strategies.

THE CO-OP APPROACH

The CO-OP approach is 'a client-centred, performance-based, problem-solving, approach that enables skill acquisition through a process of strategy use and guided discovery' (Polatajko & Mandich, 2004, p. 2). The approach is designed to achieve four goals: skill acquisition, cognitive strategy use, skill and strategy generalisation and skill and strategy transfer.

It comprises seven key features: client-centred[*2], occupation-based goal setting; dynamic performance analysis; cognitive strategy use; guided discovery; enabling principles; significant other involvement; and intervention format. In this section, an overview of the CO-OP approach's development is provided, followed by a detailed description of the seven key features.

Development of the CO-OP Approach

The CO-OP approach was developed in response to an identified need for a new approach for helping children diagnosed with developmental coordination disorder (DCD) meet occupational performance goals. Previously, the majority of intervention approaches were impairment focused, derived from a neurodevelopmental perspective on motor performance. Polatajko

---

[2]Although the term *person-centred* is the preferred term for this book, the term *client-centred* is used in this chapter when referring to a key feature of the CO-OP approach.

et al. (2001) decided to adopt a learning paradigm – to consider skilled motor performance as the outcome of skill learning rather than neuromotor development. An intervention was created that was modelled after Meichenbaum's cognitive behaviour modification approach where, as mentioned earlier, children were taught to use verbal self-guidance for problem solving with a *global* cognitive strategy, GOAL-PLAN-DO-CHECK, to learn new skills.

Meichenbaum's approach was adapted to fit within an occupation-based, client-centred framework and augmented by principles taken from motor learning. The approach focused on the acquisition of client-chosen occupational goals through a collaborative process of using the GOAL-PLAN-DO-CHECK global strategy to solve performance problems. The role of the occupational therapist was to guide the child to test out potential strategies to improve performance, evaluate the results and ultimately acquire the desired skill.

Original investigations of the approach, then called verbal self-guidance (VSG), indicated that the approach did indeed support motor skill acquisition through a process of cognitive strategy use, therapist verbal guidance and verbal self-guidance (Polatajko et al., 2001). The approach was called VSG to emphasise the importance of verbal guidance to the approach; however, careful analysis of videotapes of VSG intervention sessions revealed that cognitive strategy use was essential to the approach. Hence, the name was changed from cognitive orientation to daily occupational performance (CO-OP).

From the videotaped analysis, it also became clear that during the sessions the children used not only the global cognitive strategy GOAL-PLAN-DO-CHECK but also a number of domain-specific strategies (Mandich et al., 2001). These domain-specific strategies, derived from a process of dynamic performance analysis (refer to Chapter 18) and guided discovery, were found to be specific to the child and the task. In addition, as skill performance improved, specific strategies were used less and less and then not at all once the skill was well established. In contrast, children learned and continued to use the global strategy over time within the same task and across different tasks.

Subsequent studies have continued to provide evidence of the effectiveness of cognitive strategies, identified through a client-centred problem-solving approach, in supporting skill acquisition. Studies now reveal that the CO-OP approach is not only effective with children with DCD but can also be used with adult populations, including individuals with neurological impairments that result from CVA or TBI (Scammels et al., 2016).

The CO-OP Approach: The Seven Key Features

As originally described by Polatajko et al. (2001), CO-OP approach comprises seven key features: client-chosen, occupation-based goals, dynamic performance analysis, cognitive strategy use, guided discovery, enabling principles, parent or significant other involvement and intervention format. In 2011 an international invitational meeting of CO-OP approach scholars was held to consider, among other things, the essential elements of the approach. In particular, the scholars examined the relevance of the original seven key features. Based on current evidence and the collective experience with administering and teaching others to administer the approach, they determined that the seven key features should be maintained but their relevance should be further specified. Accordingly, the original seven key features were specified as either essential or structural elements. Essential elements are key features that must be present for the intervention to be considered CO-OP approach. Structural elements are key features that are preferred or suggested elements but may be altered to meet the specific needs of the person or practice setting. An overview of the refined key features, now divided into essential and structural elements, is presented in Table 28.2.

In the CO-OP approach, through these key features, the cognitive, affective and physical components of performance are addressed simultaneously, as are the occupational and environmental contributions to performance. *Goals* must be identified through collaboration with the individual and must address identified occupation-based needs. The Canadian Occupational Performance Measure (COPM) (Law et al., 2014) is used to support the identification of priority occupational performance issues to be addressed using CO-OP (refer to Chapter 16).

After the identification of these issues, *dynamic performance analysis (DPA)* is used to investigate current performance. DPA is an active, iterative process

TABLE 28.2
The CO-OP Approach Seven Key Features: The Essential and Structural Elements

Seven Key Features Essential Elements	Critical Attributes
Occupation-focused goals	Collaborative, client-centred, occupation-based
Dynamic performance analysis (DPA)	Active, iterative process, evoked initially by occupational therapist; becomes a collaborative process with both therapist and person; in many cases, the person eventually conducts DPA spontaneously and independently
Cognitive strategy use	Global (metacognitive) or domain specific
Guided discovery	Optimises client's role in learning
Enabling principles	Promotes learning, generalisation, transfer
Structural Elements	**Variable Attributes**
Parent or significant other involvement	May be critical for children; may or may not be necessary for adults, depending on the person
Intervention format	May vary in session sequence, format, length, frequency, duration or materials needed

TABLE 28.3
Pre-test, Post-test and Follow-up Scores for Ms Role

Executive Function Measure	Pre-test Score	Post-test Score	Follow-up Score
Depression: PHQ-9 (lower better)	9	4	10
Anxiety: GAD-7 (lower better)	12	8	14
DKEFS Letter Fluency (higher better) (scaled score)	9	12	11
DKEFS Tower Test – first move time (scaled score)	9	14	14
BRIEF-A (t-score) (lower better)	77	68	77
MPAI Participation Index (lower better)	16	10	14

BRIEF-A, Behaviour Rating Inventory of Executive Function – Adult Version; *DKEFS,* Delis-Kaplan Executive Function System; *GAD-7,* Generalised Anxiety Disorder 7-item Questionnaire; *MPAI,* Mayo-Portland Adaptability Inventory; *PHQ-9,* Patient Health Questionnaire.

TABLE 28.4
COPM Scores

COPM–performance	Pre-test Score	Post-test Score	Follow-up Score
To get funding to pay for online course	4	9	10
To stick to budget while grocery shopping	1	10	7
To organise finances using a specific software program	1	6	8
To plan menus and cook meals (**untrained**)	6	8	10
To organise day in order to manage fatigue (**untrained**)	1	8	8
COPM–satisfaction	Pre-test Score	Post-test Score	Follow-up Score
To get funding to pay for online course	1	9	10
To stick to budget while grocery shopping	1	10	9
To organise finances using a specific software program	1	6	5
To plan menus and cook meals (**untrained**)	5	6	10
To organise day in order to manage fatigue (**untrained**)	1	6	8

through which therapists and those receiving therapy services examine person, occupation and environmental aspects to identify performance breakdowns (Polatajko et al., 2000). DPA typically occurs while observing performance (refer to Chapter 18).

Cognition is explicitly brought into play in the CO-OP approach through the key feature of *cognitive strategy use*. The CO-OP approach global strategy, GOAL-PLAN-DO-CHECK, provides the cognitive scaffold for performance and applies to all goals. It is a metacognitive strategy as it provides a mechanism for a person to think about his or her thinking. It also provides a structure for self-monitoring with CHECK, a built-in evaluation of performance.

The complementary domain-specific strategies support task-specific performance. Domain-specific strategies are sometimes but not always transferable across tasks. For example, developing a domain-specific strategy of using a timer for cooking may be transferable to using a timer for remembering to move the washing to the dryer or leave in time to make an appointment. On the other hand, a domain-specific strategy of using a specialised cutting board for one-handed cutting during meal preparation is specific to this task and is therefore less likely to be useful with another goal.

Guided discovery is the method of instruction in the CO-OP approach. It supports self-discovery by the person, as they are guided to 'discover' solutions to performance problems with guidance from the occupational therapist. The person's self-discovery ensures that cognition is used; the occupational therapist's guidance ensures the person does not become overly frustrated with repeated unsuccessful performance attempts using the same ineffective strategy.

Supporting the guided discovery process are the *enabling principles*. This key feature comprises a group of instructional and feedback methods designed to optimise learning, generalisation and transfer of skills.

Two of the key features, *significant other involvement* and *intervention format,* are considered structural rather than essential elements; that is, they are considered important to the CO-OP Approach but are modifiable based on the needs of the person, practice setting and other factors. *Significant other involvement* is recommended so that important people in the person's life are aware of the approach, know the global cognitive strategy, GOAL-PLAN-DO-CHECK, and can enable generalisation and transfer of achievements in therapy to the person's real-world environment. Although the setting and number of sessions can vary based on the person's needs, the *intervention format* should include a preintervention assessment phase, an intervention phase with homework, and a postintervention assessment phase.

In terms of pre- and post-intervention, typically subjective and objective measures are used. The COPM (Law et al., 2014) is used to measure the person's own judgement of their pre- and post-intervention performance and satisfaction with the performance of the targeted tasks (refer to Chapter 16). The performance quality rating scale (PQRS) (Gimeno et al., 2021; Martini et al., 2015; Polatajko & Mandich, 2004) is a reliable and responsive tool to be used by the occupational therapist to evaluate the pre- and post-intervention performance of client-selected goals objectively.

The PQRS is a 10-point scale, designed for use in the CO-OP approach, to rate the performance quality of the targeted tasks, with 1 indicating that the activity is not done at all and 10 indicating that the activity is done very well.

THE CO-OP APPROACH AND ADULTS WITH NEUROLOGICAL IMPAIRMENTS

As mentioned earlier, the CO-OP approach was originally designed for use with children with DCD as an alternative to traditional neurodevelopmental approaches that lacked evidence of efficacy. Around the same time, researchers working with other populations, including adults with neurological impairments, were also seeking to replace impairment-focused neurodevelopmental techniques. Evidence emerged to support the use of task-specific training (e.g. French et al., 2008). However, over time it became apparent that although these approaches were associated with improvements in the activities trained, they were not followed by long-term change in the performance of the trained tasks, and transfer to other activities did not occur.

Although task-specific training clearly had promise, additional intervention components were needed to optimise outcomes. Early testing of CO-OP, which combines cognitive strategy use with task-specific training, demonstrated that it can help adults with neurological injury improve their performance in client-chosen tasks (Dawson et al., 2009; Henshaw et al., 2011; McEwen et al., 2009). In addition, this approach appeared to promote longer-term change in performance. Importantly, once people had learned the method, they seemed to be able to apply it to improve their performance in other tasks (McEwen et al., 2009, 2010, 2015; Skidmore et al., 2014, 2015). The use of the CO-OP approach to improve the occupational performance of two people who have experienced neurological impairment as a result of CVA or head injury is illustrated in Boxes 28.1 and 28.2.

Evidence for the CO-OP Approach with Individuals with Neurological Injuries

Taken together, the evidence to date suggests that for individuals who have experienced CVA or TBI, the

CO-OP approach can be expected to improve performance on trained self-selected goals and have transfer effects for improved performance on untrained self-selected goals. The CO-OP approach may also yield improvements in selected impairments and behaviours, as well as positively influence occupational participation. At present, there are several additional clinical trials examining the use of the CO-OP approach, or some derivation, for improving outcomes after acute stroke (Linkewich et al., 2020; McEwen et al., 2015; Song et al., 2019), chronic stroke (Henshaw et al., 2011; McEwen et al., 2009, 2010; Polatajko et al., 2012), youth with dystonia (Gimeno et al., 2019, 2021), adults with cerebral palsy or spina bifida (Öhrvall et al., 2020) and traumatic brain injury (Dawson et al., 2009; Ng et al., 2011).

Impact on Occupational Performance Goals

The primary expected outcome of the CO-OP approach is improvement in occupational performance. Evidence from several studies with people who have experienced CVA or TBI provides support for this expected outcome. Evidence from 12 single-case experimental design participants (Dawson et al., 2009; McEwen et al., 2009, 2010; Ng et al., 2013), three single-case studies (Henshaw et al., 2011; Skidmore et al., 2011) and five pilot randomised controlled trials (Dawson et al., 2013; McEwen et al., 2015; Polatajko et al., 2012; Poulin et al., 2017; Skidmore et al., 2015) suggests that the CO-OP approach leads to improvement in performance in self-selected goals.

Furthermore, CO-OP intervention has been associated with larger improvements in the objectively rated PQRS scores compared with usual care occupational therapy, with one study demonstrating a medium effect of between-group differences immediately after treatment and a large effect on between-group differences three months later (McEwen et al., 2015). These data provide convincing evidence that CO-OP intervention is associated with improved performance in self-selected goals.

Perhaps more important is the evidence that addresses some of the transfer effects of the CO-OP approach. These transfer effects have been demonstrated in performance improvements on untrained goals, as measured by the self- and significant other-reported

COPM and the observer-rated PQRS (Dawson et al., 2009, 2013; McEwen et al., 2010, 2015; Ng et al., 2013; Poulin et al., 2017). Of note, transfer effects have also been noted in measures of impairments and behaviours that were not the direct target of CO-OP approach intervention. For example, two separate pilot randomised controlled trials demonstrated significantly greater improvements in measures of executive functions compared with an attention control condition in acute CVA (Skidmore et al., 2015) and compared with usual care in subacute CVA (Wolf et al., 2016). Additional evidence suggests that CO-OP intervention has an effect on self-efficacy (McEwen et al., 2015; Poulin et al., 2017) and sustained goal-directed behaviour (i.e. low levels of apathy symptoms) (Skidmore et al., 2014).

Impact on Participation

Perhaps the best measure of the overall impact of a CVA and TBI rehabilitation intervention is the effect of the intervention on participation. Evidence from pilot randomised controlled trials suggests that CO-OP intervention is associated with a moderate effect on participation, as measured by the Stroke Impact Scale and the Community Participation Index, compared with usual care (McEwen et al., 2015) and with improvements in the Mayo Portland Adaptability Inventory Participation Index (Dawson et al., 2013).

Impact on Impairment

Evidence suggests that metacognitive strategy training, based heavily on the CO-OP approach, is feasible to administer during acute inpatient rehabilitation (Skidmore et al., 2011, 2014) and is associated with significantly greater reductions in disability (measured with the Functional Independence Measure) and improvement in executive cognitive functions (measured with selected indices of the Delis Kaplan Executive Functioning System) among adults with cognitive impairments after acute CVA (Skidmore et al., 2015). A separate research group found similar results for people in the subacute phase after a CVA (Wolf et al., 2016). Further, Wolf and colleagues reported a moderate effect of CO-OP compared with contemporary therapy on arm and hand capacity using the Action Research Arm Test. These changes came after an average of 12, 45-minute intervention sessions, about nine hours of treatment.

LESSONS LEARNED FROM THE CO-OP APPROACH USED WITH PEOPLE WHO HAVE HAD A CEREBROVASCULAR ACCIDENT OR TRAUMATIC BRAIN INJURY

From the experience of using the CO-OP approach with individuals after CVA or TBI a number of important lessons were learned regarding whether a person might benefit from the CO-OP approach, session structure and strategy specifics.

Who Will Benefit from the CO-OP Approach?

To benefit from the use of CO-OP, the person must have occupational performance goals and sufficient language abilities to participate in the GOAL-PLAN-DO-CHECK process, which includes engaging in problem-solving discussions with the occupational therapist.

In terms of physical or cognitive capacity, nature of the injury or length of time since the injury, boundaries are still being tested. The CO-OP approach or a very similar strategy training approach has been used successfully with people as early as three days after a neurological event and as long as decades later. CO-OP approach has been used with people with very limited motor recovery, including people with Chedoke-McMaster Stroke Assessment Impairment Inventory (Miller et al., 2008) scores as low as 2/7 for arm, hand and foot (indicating spasticity present but no voluntary movement) and 3/7 for leg (indicating marked spasticity present and voluntary movement only within synergistic patterns). It has been used with people with moderate cognitive impairment, scoring as low as 21 on the Montreal Cognitive Assessment (Nasreddine et al., 2005), and with people with moderate to severe executive function impairments after TBI (Dawson et al., 2009).

Although these scores describe the minimum levels of physical and cognitive function of previous CO-OP approach participants, the minimum physical and cognitive capabilities required to benefit from the CO-OP approach have not yet been established. However, it is likely that insight into, or awareness of, deficits is not necessarily a prerequisite since the focus in CO-OP is on applying a problem-solving strategy to identify occupational performance breakdown, and effective strategies to solve the problems. Thus if a person has occupational goals and wishes to try a cognitive strategy-based approach, then implementing CO-OP approach may be a possibility.

Facilitating Goal Setting

In the original CO-OP approach format with children, a daily activity log and the COPM were used to facilitate goal setting. With adults with neurological injuries, it is recommended that, if time permits, they complete the daily activity log over a week, to provide a fuller idea of the activities in which they are engaged. Other methods to help with the identification of valued occupations before administering the COPM that might be considered include the Activity Card Sort (Baum & Edwards, 2008) and the elucidation module of Personal Projects Analysis (Egan et al., 2016; Little, 2011).

Evaluating Performance Before and After Intervention

Many people living with the effects of neurological injury, particularly those who have lived with the effects of the injury for longer periods, have complex participation goals, such as planning a wedding or obtaining a job interview. For these goals, it may not be possible to administer the PQRS as part of the baseline assessment, as the related activities stretch out over time and over environments. In these cases, the person's self-report of performance and satisfaction with performance using the COPM is relied upon for preintervention and postintervention evaluation. If an additional perspective on the person's performance is desired or required, it is sometimes possible to also ask a significant other to rate the person's performance using, for example, the COPM.

Significant Other Involvement

The involvement of significant others in the CO-OP approach is a structural key feature. It is recommended that they attend the first few sessions so that they have an understanding of GOAL-PLAN-DO-CHECK and the process within which it is used. This involvement is believed to be an important facilitator of generalisation and transfer. However, with adults, it may be difficult for family members to attend sessions and should not be considered as a prerequisite for the person's participation in the CO-OP approach.

Intervention Format

The CO-OP approach key feature *intervention format* is considered a structural feature rather than an essential element. All iterations of the CO-OP approach should include a pre-intervention assessment phase, an intervention phase, which includes teaching the global cognitive strategy in the first session and using it in subsequent sessions, and homework, and a post-intervention assessment phase. The specific details of each of these phases can vary depending on the characteristics of the population, the setting and the individual's needs. Some of the alterations from the classic intervention format described in 2004 (Polatajko & Mandich, 2004) include using scripts and presentations to teach the global cognitive strategy and maintaining flexibility regarding the number of intervention sessions.

Adults with neurological injuries are far from a homogeneous group in terms of the type or severity of their impairments. Those with more severe impairments may require more than the originally suggested 10 intervention sessions. Adults with subacute CVA have required, on average, about 12 sessions (McEwen et al., 2015). Adults with TBI with identified executive dysfunction have been trialled with both 20 and 15 sessions, with 15 sessions seeming to work for most. Some people with relatively minor impairments and relatively intact cognition may require only 5 or 6 sessions.

CONCLUSION

Since 2009, numerous peer-reviewed publications investigating the CO-OP approach with adults with CVA and TBI have suggested that the CO-OP approach improves performance on trained and untrained self-selected goals and may also positively influence participation in these populations. Using the CO-OP approach with adults with neurological injuries requires that occupational therapists focus on occupational performance rather than occupational performance components during assessment and treatment, that they embrace client-centred, occupation-based goals setting, and that they give up a degree of control to people receiving their services by using guided discovery as the instructional method and enabling people to self-discover their own strategies. Although implementing the CO-OP approach may at first present some challenges, occupational therapists can expect to be rewarded by long-term significant improvements in the occupational performance of people who are receiving their services.

REFERENCES

Aharon-Peretz, J. (2017). Traumatic brain injury. In B. L. Miller & J. L. Cummings (Eds.), *The human frontal lobes: Functions and disorders* (3rd ed., pp. 402–435). Guilford Publications.

Barnett, S. M., & Ceci, S. J. (2002). When and where do we apply what we learn? A taxonomy for far transfer. *Psychological Bulletin, 128*(4), 612–637.

Bash, M. A., & Camp, B. W. (1986). Training teachers in the think aloud classroom program. In G. Cartledge & J. F. Milburn (Eds.), *Teaching social skills to children: Innovative approaches* (2nd ed.). Pergamon Press.

Baum, C., & Edwards, D. F. (2008). *The activity card sort* (2nd ed.). American Association of Occupational Therapy.

Chua, K. S., Ng, Y. S., Yap, S. G., & Bok, C. W. (2007). A brief review of traumatic brain injury rehabilitation. *Annals of the Academy of Medicine, Singapore, 36*(1), 31–42.

Cicerone, K. D., Dahlberg, C., Kalmar, K., Langenbahn, D. M., Malec, J. F., Bergquist, T. F., … Morse, P. A. (2000). Evidence-based cognitive rehabilitation: Recommendations for clinical practice. *Archives of Physical Medicine and Rehabilitation, 81*(12), 1596–1615.

Dawson, D. R., Binns, M. A., Hunt, A., Lemsky, C., & Polatajko, H. J. (2013). Occupation-based strategy training for adults with traumatic brain injury: A pilot study. *Archives of Physical Medicine and Rehabilitation, 94*(10), 1959–1963.

Dawson, D. R., Gaya, A., Hunt, A., Levine, B., Lemsky, C., & Polatajko, H. J. (2009). Using the cognitive orientation to occupational performance (CO-OP) with adults with executive dysfunction following traumatic brain injury. *Canadian Journal of Occupational Therapy, 76*(2), 115–127.

Egan, M., Scott-Lowery, L., De Serres Larose, C., Gallant, L., & Jaillet, C. (2016). The use of personal projects analysis to enhance occupational therapy goal identification. *The Open Journal of Occupational Therapy, 4*(1), 4.

French, B., Leathley, M., Sutton, C., McAdam, J., Thomas, L., Forster, A., … Watkins, C. (2008). A systematic review of repetitive functional task practice with modelling of resource use, costs and effectiveness. *Health Technology Assessment, 12*(30). http://doi.org/10.3310/hta12300.

Geusgens, C. A., Winkens, I., van Heugten, C. M., Jolles, J., & van den Heuvel, W. J. (2007). Occurrence and measurement of transfer in cognitive rehabilitation: A critical review. *Journal of Rehabilitation Medicine, 39*(6), 425–439.

Gimeno, H., Brown, R. G., Lin, J.-P., Cornelius, V., & Polatajko, H. J. (2019). Cognitive approach to rehabilitation in children with hyperkinetic movement disorders post-DBS. *Neurology, 92*(11), e1212–e1224. https://doi.org/10.1212/WNL.0000000000007092.

Gimeno, H., Farber, J., Thornton, J., & Polatajko, H. (2021). The relative merits of an individualized versus a generic approach to rating functional performance in childhood dystonia. *Children, 8*(1), 7. https://doi.org/10.3390/children8010007.

Gimeno, H., Polatajko, H. J., Cornelius, V., Lin, J.-P., & Brown, R. G. (2021). Rehabilitation in childhood-onset hyperkinetic movement disorders including dystonia: Treatment change in outcomes across the ICF and feasibility of outcomes for full trial evaluation. *European Journal of Paediatric Neurology, 33*, 159–167. https://doi.org/10.1016/j.ejpn.2021.04.009.

Henshaw, E., Polatajko, H. J., McEwen, S. E., Ryan, J. D., & Baum, C. M. (2011). Cognitive approach to improving participation after stroke: Two case studies. *The American Journal of Occupational Therapy, 65*(1), 55–63.

Hubbard, I. J., Parsons, M. W., Neilson, C., & Carey, L. M. (2009). Task-specific training: Evidence for and translation to clinical practice. *Occupational Therapy International, 16*(3–4), 175–189.

Law, M., Babtiste, S., Carswell, A., McColl, M. A., Polatajko, H. J., & Pollock, N. (2014). *Canadian occupational performance measure* (5th ed.). CAOT Publications ACE.

Lawson, M. J., & Rice, D. N. (1989). Effects of training in use of executive strategies on a verbal memory problem resulting from closed head injury. *Journal of Clinical and Experimental Neuropsychology, 11*(6), 842–854.

Levine, B., Robertson, I. H., Clare, L., Carter, G., Hong, J., Wilson, B. A., … Stuss, D. T. (2000). Rehabilitation of executive functioning: An experimental-clinical validation of goal management training. *Journal of the International Neuropsychological Society, 6*(3), 299–312.

Levine, B., Schweizer, T. A., O'Connor, C., Turner, G., Gillingham, S., Stuss, D. T., … Robertson, I. H. (2011). Rehabilitation of executive functioning in patients with frontal lobe brain damage with goal management training. *Frontiers in Human Neuroscience, 5*(9), 1–9.

Linkewich, E., Avery, L., Rios, J., & McEwen, S. (2020). Minimally clinically important differences in functional independence after a knowledge translation intervention in stroke rehabilitation. *Archives of Physical Medicine and Rehabilitation, 101*, 587–591. https://doi.org/10.1016/jp.apmr.2019.10.185.

Little, B. R. (2011). *Personal Project Analysis* [Workbook]. http://www.brianrlittle.com/Topics/research/assessment-tools/.

Liu, K. P., Chan, C. C., Lee, T. M., & Hui-Chan, C. W. (2004). Mental imagery for promoting relearning for people after stroke: A randomized controlled trial. *Archives of Physical Medicine and Rehabilitation, 85*(9), 1403–1408.

Luria, A. R. (1966). *Higher cortical functions in man* (B. Haigh Trans.) Basic Books.

Mandich, A. D., Polatajko, H. J., Missiuna, C., & Miller, L. T. (2001). Cognitive strategies and motor performance in children with developmental coordination disorder. *Physical & Occupational Therapy in Pediatrics, 20*(2/3), 125–143.

Martini, R., Rios, J., Polatajko, H. J., Wolf, T., & McEwen, S. E. (2015). The performance quality rating scale (PQRS): Reliability, convergent validity, and internal responsiveness for two scoring systems. *Disability and Rehabilitation, 37*(3), 231–238.

McEwen, S., Polatajko, H. J., Baum, C., Rios, J., Cirone, D., Doherty, M., & Wolf, T. (2015). Combined cognitive-strategy and task-specific training improves transfer to untrained activities in sub-acute stroke: An exploratory randomized controlled trial. *Neurorehabilitation and Neural Repair, 29*(6), 526–536. http://nnr.sagepub.com/content/early/2014/11/14/1545968314558602.

McEwen, S. E., Polatajko, H. J., Huijbregts, M. P., & Ryan, J. D. (2009). Exploring a cognitive-based treatment approach to improve motor-based skill performance in chronic stroke: Results of three single case experiments. *Brain Injury, 23*(13-14), 1041–1053.

McEwen, S. E., Polatajko, H. J., Huijbregts, M. P., & Ryan, J. D. (2010). Inter-task transfer of meaningful, functional skills following a cognitive-based treatment: Results of three multiple baseline design experiments in adults with chronic stroke. *Neuropsychological Rehabilitation, 20*(4), 541–561.

Meichenbaum, D. (1977). *Cognitive-behavior modification: An integrative approach*. Plenum Press.

Meichenbaum, D. (1991). *Cognitive behavior modification*. Workshop presented at Child and Parent Research Institute Symposium.

Miller, P., Huijbregts, M., Gowland, C., Barreca, S., Torresin, W., Moreland, J., … Barclay-Goddard, R. (2008). *Chedoke-McMaster stroke assessment development, validation and administration manual*. McMaster University and Hamilton Health Sciences.

Nasreddine, Z. S., Phillips, N. A., Bedirian, V., Charbonneau, S., Whitehead, V., Collin, I., … Chertkow, H. (2005). The Montreal Cognitive Assessment, MoCA: A brief screening tool for mild cognitive impairment. *Journal of the American Geriatrics Society, 53*(4), 695–699.

Ng, E. M., Polatajko, H. J., Marziali, E., Hunt, A., & Dawson, D. (2013). Telerehabilitation for addressing executive dysfunction after traumatic brain injury. *Brain Injury, 27*(5), 548–564.

Öhrvall, A. M., Bergqvist, L., Hofgren, C., & Peny-Dahlstrand, M. (2020). "With CO-OP I'm the boss" – experiences of the cognitive orientation to daily occupational performance approach as reported by young adults with cerebral palsy or spina bifida. *Disability and Rehabilitation, 42*(25), 3645–3652. https://doi.org/10.1080/09638288.2019.1607911.

Polatajko, H. J., & Mandich, A. D. (2004). *Enabling occupation in children: The cognitive orientation to daily occupational performance (CO-OP) approach* (1st ed.). CAOT Publications ACE.

Polatajko, H. J., Mandich, A. D., & Martini, R. (2000). Dynamic performance analysis: A framework for understanding occupational performance. *The American Journal of Occupational Therapy: Official Publication of the American Occupational Therapy Association, 54*(1), 65–72.

Polatajko, H. J., Mandich, A. D., Missiuna, C., Miller, L. T., Macnab, J. J., & Malloy-Miller, T. (2001). Cognitive orientation to daily occupational performance (CO-OP): Part III – the protocol in brief. *Physical & Occupational Therapy in Pediatrics, 20*(2/3), 107–123.

Polatajko, H. J., McEwen, S. E., Ryan, J. D., & Baum, C. M. (2012). Pilot randomized controlled trial investigating cognitive strategy use to improve goal performance after stroke. *The American Journal of Occupational Therapy, 66*(1), 104–109.

Poulin, V., Korner-Bitensky, N., Bherer, L., Lussier, M., & Dawson, D. R. (2017). Comparison of two cognitive interventions for adults experiencing executive dysfunction post-stroke: A pilot study. *Disability and Rehabilitation, 39*(1), 1–13.

Roth, R. M., Isquith, P. K., & Gioia, G. A. (2005). *Behavioral rating inventory of executive function - adult version (BRIEF-A)*. Psychological Assessment Resources, Inc.

Scammell, E., Bates, S., †Houldin, A., & Polatajko, H. J. (2016). The Cognitive Orientation to Daily Occupational Performance: A Scoping Review. *Canadian Journal of Occupational Therapy, 83*(4), 216–225. http://doi.org/10.1177/0008417416651277.

Skidmore, E. R., Dawson, D. R., Butters, M. A., Grattan, E. S., Juengst, S. B., Whyte, E. M., … Becker, J. T. (2015). Strategy training shows promise for addressing disability in the first 6 months after stroke. *Neurorehabilitation and Neural Repair, 29*(7), 668–676.

Skidmore, E. R., Dawson, D. R., Whyte, E. M., Butters, M. A., Dew, M. A., Grattan, E. S., … Holm, M. B. (2014). Developing complex interventions: Lessons learned from a pilot study examining strategy training in acute stroke rehabilitation. *Clinical Rehabilitation, 28*(4), 378–387.

Skidmore, E. R., Holm, M. B., Whyte, E. M., Dew, M. A., Dawson, D. R., & Becker, J. T. (2011). The feasibility of meta-cognitive strategy training in acute inpatient stroke rehabilitation: Case report. *Neuropsychological Rehabilitation, 21*(2), 208–223.

Song, C.-S., Lee, O.-N., & Woo, H.-S. (2019). Cognitive strategy on upper extremity function for stroke: A randomized controlled trials. *Restorative Neurology and Neuroscience, 37*(2019), 61–70. doi: 10.3233/RNN-18053.

Toglia, J. P., Rodger, S. A., & Polatajko, H. J. (2012). Anatomy of cognitive strategies: A therapist's primer for enabling occupational performance. *Canadian Journal of Occupational Therapy, 79*(4), 225–236.

van Heugten, C. M., Dekker, J., Deelman, B. G., Stehmann-Saris, J. C., & Kinebanian, A. (1998). Outcome of strategy training in stroke patients with apraxia: A phase II study. *Clinical Rehabilitation, 12*(4), 294–303.

von Cramon, D. Y., Matthes-von Cramon, G., & Mai, N. (1991). Problem-solving deficits in brain-injured patients: A therapeutic approach. *Neuropsychological Rehabilitation, 1*(1), 45–64.

Wolf, T., Polatajko, H., Baum, C., Rios, J., Cirone, D., Doherty, M., & McEwen, S. (2016). Combined cognitive-strategy and task-specific training affects cognition and upper extremity function in sub-acute stroke: An exploratory randomized controlled trial. *American Journal of Occupational Therapy, 70*(2). 7002290010 p1-p10. http://doi.org/10.5014/ajot.2016.017293.

World Health Organization. (2001). International classification of impairments, disabilities, and health (ICF). World Health Organization.

Ylvisaker, M., Feeney, T., & Szekeres, F. (1998). Cognitive rehabilitation: Executive functions. In M. Ylvisaker (Ed.), *Traumatic brain injury rehabilitation: Children and adolescents* (2nd ed.). Butterworth-Heinemann.

REFLECTION

1. List the two type of cognitive strategies used in the CO-OP Approach and describe the importance of each to the CO-OP objectives.

2. Define metacognition and discuss why GOAL-PLAN-DO-CHECK is considered a metacognitive strategy.

3. Describe the CO-OP instructuional approach and distinguish it from direct instruction.

4. CO-OP Approach is described as occupation-based, not component-focused. What does this mean?

5. What is the evidence to support the use of the CO-OP Approach over a component-focused approach.

29

HOME MODIFICATION AND UNIVERSAL DESIGN

CATHERINE ELIZABETH BRIDGE ■ PHILLIPPA CARNEMOLLA

CHAPTER OUTLINE

Overview

Home modifications and universal design as relevant to occupational therapy practice are the focus of this chapter. Key concepts in home modifications and universal design are presented along with a justification for why home modification should be considered a critical occupational therapy practice area. Knowledge about home modification assessments and interventions that may be used by occupational therapists as a part of implementing a collaborative relationship-focused practice is also included in this chapter. The practice stories illustrate how to approach home modification for people who have an illness, injury or impairment. The research evidence base in terms of what is known about home modification efficacy as an intervention strategy is presented.

KEY POINTS

- There is a tension between built environment changes that benefit a person experiencing illness, injury or impairment and changes that benefit the majority of a population. This tension can be understood through knowledge of home modification and universal design approaches.

- Policy changes, such as the move towards self-directed funding, make it critical to understand how a person's home and the objects within can best enable autonomy, control and life quality.

- Home modifications can be effective in reducing falls, improving occupational participation, increasing social participation and reducing caregiving and disability-related expenses.

- Access standards and building codes, although useful for general guidance, cannot account for a person's need as they do not account for their occupational habits and preferences and generally assume standardised mobility device usage or full upper-limb range of motion.

- Self, and informal and formal, care are correlated to how enabling or disabling an environment is for occupational participation.

- Detailed knowledge of a person's everyday occupations, such as entering, passing through, listening, viewing, toileting, feeding and bathing, are critical to effective home modification.

INTRODUCTION

The evidence base for and the key concepts of home modification and universal design practice for occupational therapists are set out in this chapter. Rapid technological advances increase levels of specialisation, and this is no different with home modification, where the connected home of the future will be the next frontier presenting new possibilities and challenges. Collaborative relationship-focused practice facilitates outcomes that meet the needs of a range of people. However, this approach can be difficult to implement as health care and rehabilitation practices have become more technical and are increasingly driven by impersonal standards, protocols and guidelines. In the home space the person and their preferred occupations, rhythms and routines, and support system are central, and personal preferences are critical to good outcomes. There is an increasing body of evidence that home modification and changes in the structural design and fabric of the dwelling can reduce care burden, improve quality of life and afford greater autonomy and independence across the lifespan. Ensuring a safe, accessible, affordable and secure home base enables people with an illness, injury or impairment to build on their abilities while maintaining participation in valued occupations and dignity in a place of their choosing and with a degree of control over their daily activities and social participation.

KEY CONCEPTS IN UNIVERSAL DESIGN

Before discussing home modifications more directly, it is important to outline the key concepts involved in universal design (UD), which include equitable use, flexibility in use, simple and intuitive use, perceptible information, tolerance for error, low physical effort, and size and space for approach and use (Story, 2001). The potential for change to the physical environment to reduce the impact of illness, injury or impairment has been well documented (Woolf & Aron, 2013). Housing interventions that ameliorate dependence on home and community-based services are important because they help maintain independence and enable individuals to live in their own homes and communities (Gamble, 2015). Further, home design and population health and well-being outcomes are linked (Bridge et al., 2003; Thomson et al., 2013).

UD inspiration may arise by noticing users who either have difficulty with available assistive technology or who use products in unintended ways. One example of the successful implementation of UD principles is the story of how a simple vegetable peeler became an award-winning design icon. Farber created a more ergonomic and user-friendly peeler that would be easier for his wife and others with similar impairments to use: the peeler featured a large, soft, and easy-to-grip handle that was suitable for people with limited hand strength or mobility. Farber went on to create Oxo Utensils and the commercial success of Oxo as a company is due in part to its commitment to user-centred design, which stems from understanding a broad range of users' needs and its focus on making assistive products that are both functional and aesthetically pleasing (Pearson, 2011).

Focusing on a broad range of users has not been an overt nor well-documented process for the development of UD housing. Nevertheless, due to the advent of both population ageing and deinstitutionalisation, there are a number of UD housing design approaches specific to increasing the availability of more accessible and liveable housing. All UD housing approaches seek to make new housing more flexible and adaptable so as to better accommodate change over people's lifespans. These approaches include the UK's Lifetime homes (Robinson et al., 2020), Livable housing in Australia (Winkler et al., 2020), and visitable design initiatives in North America and Europe (Langdon, 2022). UD housing approaches try to ensure that the general layout and fabric of a home facilitate access while enabling basic modifications to be undertaken at minimal cost; for example, bathroom walls that are able to have grab rails installed if required.

A major benefit of UD implementation in initial building construction is that it potentially decreases the need for, and cost of, future home modifications, alterations or retrofits. Importantly, UD allows customisation of the home for a particular person or family depending on the illness, injury or impairment and occupational participation needs. This customisation can enable people to live in their homes as long as possible and facilitate ageing in place. Enabling people to age in place reduces pressure on health and aged care systems by reducing dependence on institutional care and is, therefore a preferred option for government policymakers and providers (Tinker, 1997; Wiles et al., 2012). On an individual level, the ability of a person to remain in their home while ageing or experiencing illness, injury or impairment helps support and maintain independence, autonomy and social connections (Wiles et al., 2012). At a community level, having older people and people who have an illness, injury or impairment remain active members of the community from their own homebase can better ensure that their civic contributions are maintained and that the greater community retains its diversity.

Many advocate that UD should be integrated into all aspects of design not just housing, from the physical and built environments to products, teaching and technology (Joines & Payne, 2017). The three principles that Joines and Payne (2017) set out for occupational therapists are (1) universal usability, (2) inclusion of people experiencing illness, injury or impairment, and (3) alignment with occupational therapy core values.

While UD principles are used to create products and environments that are accessible and usable for a wide range of people, it is a population-based approach. Hence, it is important to recognise that personal needs and preferences can vary greatly and accommodating them all can be difficult (Burgstahler, 2015). This difficulty can be illustrated using the example of curb cuts referred to by Joines and Payne as a UD exemplar (2017). Curb cuts were mandated for pedestrian design after World War II wheelchair veterans advocated for them to them to be able to cross roads independently (Williamson, 2019). However, the original curbs, without curb cuts, facilitated mobility for people with vision impairments. An unanticipated consequence of putting in curb cuts meant that people with vision impairments were placed at risk necessitating the rollout of tactile markings to indicate a curb cut (Matthews et al., 2015). This example highlights that

one approach cannot meet the needs of all people. This is particularly true for individuals with impairments, who may have unique physical, sensory, or cognitive needs that require specific adaptations or accommodations (Burgstahler, 2015).

Joines and Payne (2017) emphasised the importance of involving people with impairments in the design process, as their input can provide valuable insights into the needs and preferences of different user groups. While involving people with impairments in the design process is important, it is not sufficient to ensure a successful outcome. For example, some individuals with impairments may have limited experience with design processes, or may not be representative of the wider disability community, which can result in incomplete or biased feedback (Kujala, 2003). Instead, it is recommended that a participatory design approach be used, which involves working closely with end-users throughout the design process, and engaging them in ongoing dialogue and feedback (Lewis et al., 2008; Newell et al., 2000). Participatory design recognises that the needs and experiences of end-users are diverse and complex and that their input is valuable but can be difficult to implement as different approaches yield different outcomes throughout the design process; it is often cheaper and quicker to get user input after the product has been developed. Nevertheless involving end-users in co-creation rather than just as advisory or reference group participants, designers can gain insights into the lived experiences of different user groups, and use this knowledge to develop more effective and user-friendly products and environments (Lewis et al., 2008).

Joines and Payne (2017) argued that UD is a critical component of occupational therapy practice and can play a key role in promoting inclusion, participation, and health for all individuals. However, this sits somewhat contrary to the idea that occupational therapy values and practices are grounded in collaborative relationship-focused and occupation-centered approaches, which emphasise the importance of individualised care and tailored interventions that consider the unique needs, goals and contexts of each person (American Occupational Therapy Association [AOTA], 2020; Restall & Egan, 2022). This approach recognises that standardisation is not always appropriate or effective, as it may fail to address the unique

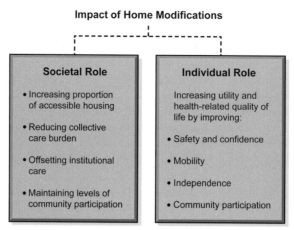

Fig. 29.1 ■ Dual role of home modifications.

needs and experiences of individual people (AOTA, 2021).

A systematic review concluded that limited rigorous evidence-based research exists to confirm that occupational therapy participation in UD projects in the built environment improves occupational participation despite anecdotal stories of some success (Young et al., 2019). However, increasing the practice of more universal or inclusive home design as part of the practice of home modifications has individual, collectives and societal and benefits, as illustrated in Fig. 29.1.

KEY CONCEPTS IN HOME MODIFICATION

Home modification is a complex process that requires an understanding of environmental factors, building codes, and the needs of the individual being served. The practice of home modification involves the assessment of a person's functional abilities, identifying environmental barriers, developing solutions to address these barriers, and evaluating the effectiveness of the interventions. For example, for anyone with impairments that make using the stairs uncomfortable or difficult, having the ease of access to a lift or home elevator can be life-changing. Thus knowledge about the prescription and pitfalls of home elevators, stair climbers and automated hoists is now also crucial for home modification practice, especially for occupational therapists working with older adults or people experiencing illness and injury impairments. These assistive

technologies can greatly enhance independence, safety, and quality of life for individuals with mobility limitations. However, they can also present significant risks if not prescribed and installed appropriately. Similarly, automated hoists or stair climbers that are not appropriately installed or operated can result in falls, injuries, or damage to the device or surrounding environment. Therefore occupational therapists and other professionals involved in home modification should have a thorough understanding of the prescription and installation guidelines for any assistive devices or technologies being recommended so as to ensure their safe and effective use by people (Pappalettera et al., 2023). Proper installation and use of assistive devices in the home can greatly enhance independence and safety for individuals and enable them to age in place.

IMPORTANCE OF COLLABORATIVE RELATIONSHIP-FOCUSED PRACTICE IN HOME MODIFICATIONS

Collaborative relationship-focused and self-funding approaches to disability and ageing service provision call for transparency and consistency of principles with practice as well as individual, service sector and community knowledge and capacity building. This service paradigm can lead to individualised and occupationally appropriate intervention, and a collaborative approach to purchasing and management approach.

Many individuals and families are presented with options that do not support occupational lifestyles of choice but instead demand that they stay indefinitely in the family home or move into more institutional environments. Importantly, living outside institutions and within communities and neighbourhoods does not mean people who have an illness, injury or impairment are truly 'at home'. This is because the autonomy, safety and emotional comfort afforded by being able to accomplish valued occupations may not be available.

SMART HOME ASSISTIVE TECHNOLOGIES

Smart homes can be defined as the use of computing technologies to offer user control of home appliances and devices through an interface or voice-activated virtual assistant. The ambient intelligence systems built into these devices may monitor the home to provide customisations and optimisations that can be tailored to user's preferences and behaviours (Alam et al., 2012). The whole smart home ecosystem and its relationship to smart devices that have the ability to control aspects is illustrated in Fig. 29.2.

Smart home assistive technologies are increasingly supporting ageing in place and disability housing. These technologies have the potential to improve the quality of life, reduce reliance on care and reduce the cost of care for those with occupational participation limitations associated with ageing or the onset of illness, injury or impairment (Bridge et al., 2021). Additionally, as discussed by Bridge et al. (2021) these technologies may indirectly support a range of ongoing benefits potentially including extended independent living, smart home energy efficiency, safety and security, physical and mental activity, and healthcare monitoring.

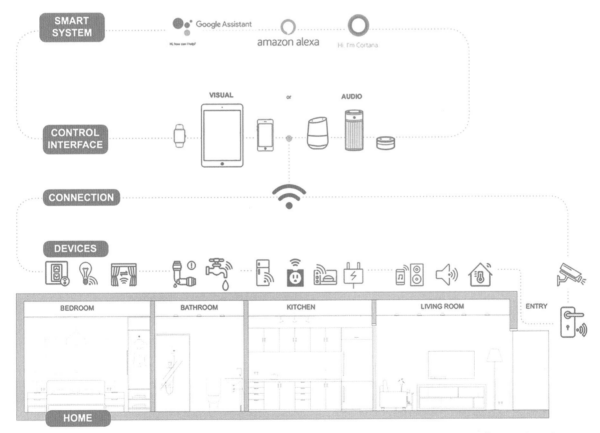

Fig. 29.2 ■ Smart home ecosystem diagram. (From Bridge, C., Zmudzki, F., Huang, T., Owen, C., & Faulkner, D. (2021). *Impacts of new and emerging assistive technologies for ageing and disabled housing*. AHURI Final Report No. 372. Australian Housing and Urban Research Institute Limited, Melbourne. https://www.ahuri.edu.au/research/final-reports/372, doi: 10.18408/ahuri7122501.)

There are key challenges to the widespread adoption of smart home assistive technologies, including issues related to affordability, accessibility and usability. Importantly addressing concerns around privacy and security to ensure the safety and well-being of users of these technologies is critical to efficiency and long-term impact on users. Nevertheless, the majority of end-users report overall high satisfaction with their smart home assistive technology (Bridge et al., 2021).

SELF-DETERMINATION AS EXEMPLIFIED THROUGH PRACTICE STORIES

Internationally significant shifts in policy are underway towards a more individualised planning and support approach for home modification intervention that better promote self-determination. This approach is increasingly part of a self-directed funding approach where management of public (government) monies (funds) are given to individuals in contrast with the former block funding model where funds were provided to services and the individual applied to the service for completion of housing modification interventions (Lynch & Findlay, 2007).

Technological advances, including simpler and easier-to-use hand tools and kits that are widely available via hardware retailers, such as a handheld shower kit, have facilitated a 'do-it-yourself' (DIY) building and renovation culture that is actively promoted via the media, through lifestyle shows and publications. The available technology and the ways in which materials can be put together in an aesthetically pleasing manner are features of the DIY phenomenon, whose origins and determinants are not well known (Bogdon, 1996). This phenomenon is occurring not only in mainstream renovation but also in home modification for people who have an illness, injury or impairment. For instance, the British television programme Grand Designs' featured the house that Jon built (Grand Designs, 2014). Jon had both legs amputated above the knee and his right arm amputated at his elbow as a consequence of active duty in Afghanistan. Having learnt on the job with mentoring and support during his own home build, Jon is now running a project management consultancy specialising in building projects. Jon's story and many other DIY stories exemplify the importance of a shift in focus towards aspirations, goals and individual choices, not just apparent need. High home ownership and the move to self-managed funding in combination with the increased popularity and growth of self-help media mean this approach is likely to continue to grow in coming years, especially as it is easy to obtain information, with the Internet and YouTube providing a growing plethora of 'how to' guidance (Bleasdale et al., 2014).

The four practice stories presented in this chapter represent a diversity of issues covering a number of variables that have been identified as being of relevance to effective home modification practice (Boxes 29.1–29.4). The practice stories explore how aspirations, goals and individual experiences

---

BOX 29.1

THE HOME I DESIGNED AND BUILT MYSELF – CHRIS'S STORY

In 2000 Chris (Fig. 29.3) moved from the United Kingdom to Australia to take up an information technology (IT) management position. After an accident that resulted in a complete T6 paraplegia, he met his wife, an occupational therapist, changed careers and now works in an access consultancy business in partnership with his wife.

Funded by accident compensation, Chris was able to design and purpose-build a house to accommodate his impairment and the needs of his family of four children. The house was five minutes from the consultancy business where he worked.

Chris and his wife had no family members living close by for support, so they used order and routine to keep life running smoothly. Their children assisted Chris in reaching things when the floor became too cluttered with their toys. Chris designed items like an accessible pool filter, workbench and rubbish disposal system that allowed him to be independent and have the opportunity to do as many domestic tasks as possible.

As Chris worked in IT he was familiar with computer-aided design software. He expanded his ability to use this software to design his new house, and became what he described as super 'teched up'.

Chris was incredibly well-informed through both his personal and work interests in the design of the home. He used universal and adaptable design principles when designing his house. His product choices were a result of rigorous research, mostly online but also through conversations with friends, visiting retailers, advice from builders and trade workers and some creative adaption of 'not for that purpose' products. Grab rails were the only do-it-yourself modification Chris did not incorporate, regarding them as not necessary for his needs.

To listen to Chris' home modification story, go to https://www.youtube.com/watch?v=GqdDZc_kH4M.

BOX 29.2
IMPLEMENTING A SMART HOME ECOSYSTEM – RICHARD'S STORY

Richard, an older man, was married when his smart technology journey started. His wife was diagnosed with a neurodegenerative illness and started wandering during both the day and night and was having trouble walking. Richard's son started looking for devices that could track his mum and alert the family if she wandered off or fell over. Richard and his wife both purchased a waterproof smartwatch (Fig. 29.4) that offered fall detection with an emergency services alert and enabled Richard and his son to track and locate Richard's wife should she wander off.

Richard, like his tech-savvy son, was amenable to acquiring other smart home devices because he liked technology and because he preferred using voice control due to the progressive vision loss he was experiencing increasing difficulty reading and writing. With his son's assistance, Richard decided to supplement the watch and existing iPad, with other smart home devices such as temperature sensors, automatic curtains, air conditioning and lighting systems.

The devices were located throughout their home. Richard's son lived in the apartment directly below and helped resolve issues as needed. For instance, setting up the fall detection notifications and then ensuring the ambulance services had the necessary information to gain access into the security building and into Richard's apartment as both were electronic code-based locks. This technology enabled Richard now living alone with severe vision loss after his wife died, to age in place and to access the ambulance automatically if an emergency occurred even if his son was at work or travelling. Their smart home devices provided both peace of mind for Richard and his son, and effectively addressed most of the limitations of vision loss and cognitive failure plus provided peace of mind regarding the risk of falling and not being found. This story illustrates that home modification can start with small changes that can build to investment in more technology if they meet occupational performance preferences.

To read Richard's full story and others like him experiencing smart home technology go to https://www.ahuri.edu.au/research/final-reports/372.

BOX 29.3
AGEING AT HOME IN THE COUNTRY – PAUL'S STORY

Two years ago Paul and his wife, Robyn, 'sold up' their 100-acre 'retirement project' property and moved into a nearby country town because the property maintenance was becoming too much for them. Paul had a fall two years prior to their move and was consequently diagnosed with epilepsy, and had a back operation that left him with double incontinence and in constant pain. Robyn was driving Paul the 200-km return trip to the nearest hospital at least weekly for his medical needs. More recently, Paul had a hip replacement that temporarily left him immobile.

Paul and Robyn's daughter was about to move to the United States of America with their 'one and only' grandson so that her American husband could fulfil his family obligations. Paul's son-in-law was an engineer and had installed many of Paul's do-it-yourself home modifications.

Robyn had a mobile phone, but did not like to use it. They had a computer at home, which Paul used to write grant applications for the Lions Club they belonged to and Robyn used it to find quilting patterns.

Paul felt the hospital staff were not very helpful in considering his housing needs and preferences and gave no advice about assistive technology and home modification. As a result, he felt he and his family had to 'wing it'. Consequently, Paul relied on word of mouth from their friends in regard to receiving community services such as the building service used for constructing access ramps. Paul used the Internet to find a walker tall enough and also talked with retail assistants at their nearest hardware outlet to find a suitable handheld shower and grab rails (Fig. 29.5).

To listen to Paul's home modification story, go to https://www.youtube.com/watch?v=liiyitT3cJc.

---

shape home modification strategies and personal engagement. The stories include differences in how people who have an illness, injury or impairment may differ in terms of their context, knowledge, skill, motivation, self-efficacy and competence, and in such factors as the following:

- Age and life stage
- Profession/education level
- Impact of illness, injury or impairment on occupational participation
- Recency of illness, injury or impairment
- Urban or rural location
- Financial means
- Access to retail stores
- Help with installing products
- Uptake of smart technology
- Engagement with internet technology

The key characteristics of the people in the practice stories in relation to five relatively simple home modification interventions are presented in Table 29.1. More detail can be obtained by reading each practice story and watching the associated short videos.

BOX 29.4
SERIAL RENOVATION EXPERIENCE – TONI'S STORY

After a few years in her apartment, Toni felt the bathroom and laundry were too small, so she engaged a builder to remodel the space according to her vision. Toni referred to herself as a 'serial renovator' and loved keeping up with the latest products by looking online and in retail stores. Toni sourced most of her components through a local bathroom retailer (Fig. 29.6).

Toni worked part time as a disability consultant despite her sometimes very debilitating autoimmune disease. The disease affected all her joints and her mobility. When her condition was severe she required a wheelchair and when her condition was less severe she could do most things around the house independently.

Toni lived alone with her two cats in a two-bedroom apartment in a modern block. Downstairs was a trendy café where she often caught up with friends. Toni had a strong friend network and had built relationships with her neighbours through mutual assistance arrangements such as child minding, looking after keys and sharing in potluck dinners. Toni paid a cleaner to come once a week to clean her apartment.

Toni's daughter lived locally and Toni regularly looked after her two grandchildren. Toni and her daughter's family also socialised at least twice a week. Toni was quite technically savvy; she had a smartphone and a new iMac for work and personal use.

To listen to Toni's home modification story, go to https://www.youtube.com/watch?v=TWIhSD-79Qo.

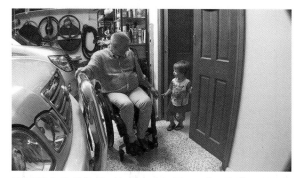

Fig. 29.3 ■ Chris in his garage. (Photo by Shelley O'Neil, www.jumpthefence.com)

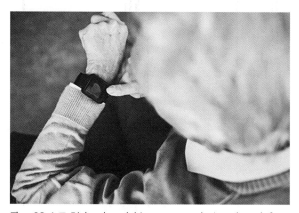

Fig. 29.4 ■ Richard and his smartwatch (purchased from istock). (Photo by Shelley O'Neil, www.jumpthefence.com)

HOME MODIFICATION IN OCCUPATIONAL THERAPY PRACTICE

Where a person is at risk of losing the ability to live independently or safely in the home, home modification can be undertaken to improve the accessibility and enabling characteristics of that home. Thus where structural changes are made specifically to improve independence and safety, decisions about housing changes are made based on the existing structure and design of the dwelling, and the health and well-being of the person or collective living there. This approach is an expression of the interplay among location, structure, person and modification.

The term *home modification* is a composite of two words: *home* and *modification*. Housing studies indicate that the concept of home has a plethora

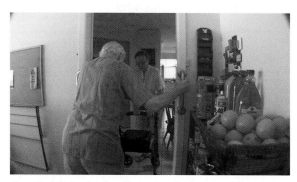

Fig. 29.5 ■ Paul using his grab rail to move down a step. (Photo by Shelley O'Neil, www.jumpthefence.com)

of characteristics, some of which are not mutually exclusive (Booth, 1982; Fallis, 2014; Harvey, 2010). For instance, a home can be thought of as a commodity having the following key features, which make it, like a person, unique:

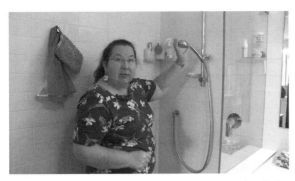

Fig. 29.6 ■ Toni and her handheld shower. (Photo by Shelley O'Neil, www.jumpthefence.com)

- Heterogeneous in type, quality, space, age, upkeep
- Spatially fixed (services such as water, power and waste cannot be easily moved)
- A commodity that people cannot do without
- Durable (lifespan of housing can be 200 years)
- Changes ownership infrequently
- Land is permanent and improvements have a long life expectancy

- Changeable: the ability to be retro-fitted, modified and updated
- Various uses (e.g. shelter, privacy and status) that are not mutually exclusive

Historically the term *home modification* has been closely associated with the notion of home renovation or remodelling but was thought of as less extensive and is more associated with disability (Bridge, 2009). The term *modification* implicitly de-emphasises fashion, aesthetic or stylistic concerns that are inherent in the notion of remodelling. More formally, in a programme or block funding sense, the term *home modification* typically refers to structural changes to a person's home to improve occupational participation, safety and/or accessibility.

Home modifications are not assistive technology, and they are not the act of moving a rug across a room. Home modifications do not include general repairs to the home or improvements designed for lifestyle, fashion or aesthetics alone. Home modification is often associated with other assistive technology interventions such as grab rails or bars, the dynamics

						TABLE 29.1
						Overview of Home Modifications for Chris, Paul, Richard and Toni
Name and Brief Background	Handheld Shower	Grab Rail	Hand Rail	Level Access Shower	Ramps	Smart Home Assistive Technology
Chris ■ Middle aged ■ Access consultant ■ Married with four kids ■ Urban location	✓		✓	✓	✓	
Richard ■ Older person ■ Carer and widower ■ Retired ■ Father		✓	✓			✓
Paul ■ Older person ■ Husband ■ Grandparent ■ Retired pharmacist ■ Rural location	✓	✓	✓		✓	
Toni ■ Middle aged ■ Small business owner ■ Grandparent ■ Divorced	✓	✓		✓		

of which have been described as 'complex' in a number of research studies (Johansson et al., 2007; Lord et al., 2006).

Home modification work typically involves working with builders and designers who may sit outside the health and social care services. Although legislation varies from country to country and region to region, there are typically a number of requirements, which apply everywhere (Bridge, 2009). For example, a grab rail/bar is a piece of assistive technology. Its correct placement and installation are not unlike assistive technology that sits with health and therapeutic goods legislation and regulation. The installation of a grab rail is governed by building codes and requires, in addition, an understanding of the who, what, where and why specifications associated with the domain of building and construction.

It is important to consult relevant environmental legislation and regulations before making any home modification recommendation (Bridge, 2009), especially as zoning laws and development legislation may directly affect home modification options. Knowledge of accessibility guidelines, local and national building codes and other relevant legislation (i.e. negligence, product liability and trespass) is helpful. Building codes stipulate the minimum necessary standards to achieve health, safety, amenity and sustainability of the building; accessibility codes provide guidance on aspects of physical accessibility relevant to some if not all home modifications.

The human experience of housing is highly personal and each person's physical health and level of ability is unique, which directly affects what occupations they can participate in within the home. As inclusive housing design standards or policies for home modification do not exist and because UD is about populations or the majority, even when housing is fully based on UD, modifications are typically still required to meet the needs of an individual. In many countries where UD guidelines do exist, they have exceptions, are voluntary and differ significantly resulting in limited availability of UD housing (Heller et al., 2022). Consequently, current UD housing options are haphazard at best and the majority of people who have an illness, injury or impairment are often able to manage with very minor changes to their home in response to a functional crisis.

EVIDENCE OF HOME MODIFICATIONS' EFFECTIVENESS

There is an increasing quantity of available research evidence since the 1990s that demonstrates an encouraging trend towards the positive impacts of home modifications on caregiving, safety, health, well-being and social participation. A systematic review (Carnemolla & Bridge, 2015) commissioned by Home Modifications Australia (MOD.A), the peak organisation for home modification services within Australia, enabled a first-of-its-kind, bird's-eye overview or mud map of what is currently globally known about the effectiveness of home modifications as a practice area. Within the 77 studies included in the review, it was noted that a large number of terms were used to refer to either home modifications or a multifactorial intervention that included home modifications. These terms ranged from the very specific (i.e. *bath grab bar*) to the very general (i.e. *environmental adaptation*).

Seven key themes have been identified within home modification publications. These themes provide an understanding of what home modifications might achieve for individuals. For instance, fall reduction research and activities of daily living (ADLs) or function-related effects are strongly supported by high-quality studies, whereas the impact of home modifications on physical health and well-being, caregiving, economic effectiveness, the ageing process and social participation are not well understood. The seven themes are illustrated in Fig. 29.7.

Theme 1: Fall Prevention

The strongest evidence for home modification effectiveness has been associated with falls (Carnemolla & Bridge, 2015). Several systematic reviews found positive evidence that a home modification intervention can reduce the likelihood of a fall or fall-related injury occurring (Chang et al., 2004; Clemson et al., 2008; Tse, 2005; Turner et al., 2011). Despite some contradictory evidence on the effect of home modifications on falls prevention (Wahl et al., 2009), five systematic reviews found home modifications effective in reducing the likelihood of a fall or injury occurring as a part of a *multifactorial intervention* (i.e. home modification in combination with assistive technology and exercise) (Chang et al., 2004; Clemson et al., 2008; Tse, 2005;

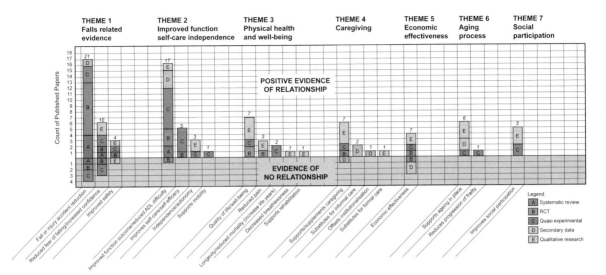

Fig. 29.7 ■ Results of a systematic review of home modification impacts. (From Carnemolla, P., & Bridge, C. (2015). *Systematic review; evidence on home modifications.* Home Modifications Information Clearinghouse.)

Turner et al., 2011). Overall it was found that home modifications may have a positive effect by:

■ Improving confidence and reducing fear of falling (Chase et al., 2012)
■ Reducing injuries in older people living at home (i.e. those persons with osteoporotic changes and/or the loss of skeletal muscle mass and strength as a result of ageing) (Plautz et al., 1995).

Theme 2: Self-Care and Independence

The impact of home modifications on autonomy and the ability to carry out valued self-care activities without assistance and subsequently eliminating, changing or reducing caregiving has been a focus of research. Two systematic reviews (Chase et al., 2012; Wahl et al., 2009) and several randomised controlled trials (Gitlin et al., 2001; Mann et al., 1999; Szanton et al., 2014; Wilson et al., 2009) found that home modifications led to an improvement in a person's function and/or a reduction in occupational participation difficulty. Additionally, others found improvements in the following:

■ Feelings of self-efficacy (Gitlin et al., 1999, 2006; Ostensjo et al., 2005; Petersson et al., 2012)
■ Mobility (Berg et al., 2002; Ostensjo et al., 2005); and
■ Cognitive function (Guo et al., 2014)

For people who have cognitive impairment, their homes act as a vessel of memories and a cue to action and can contribute to keeping people at home longer via sensitive modifications (Van Hoof et al., 2010).

Theme 3: Physical Health and Well-being

Physical health and well-being are explored in 'quality of life' and life satisfaction research. Research has demonstrated improvements in the following areas after completion of home modifications:

■ Health, comfort and happiness by the person with an illness, injury or impairment. (Ahmad et al., 2013; Lin et al., 2007).
■ Breathing as a result of reducing moulds, pollens and pollutants, accommodating respirators and reducing steam build-up.
■ Reduction in pain as a result of less strain on joints and muscles.

Theme 4: Caregiving

Caregiver impact can be best understood in terms of who provides the care. Three types of caring have been identified (Aronson & Neysmlth, 1997; Australian Bureau of Statistics, 2012):

■ Care delivered by paid staff or trained volunteers (i.e. formal care)

- Care delivered by unpaid carers, usually family members (i.e. informal care)
- Self-care, or the capacity of a person to undertake tasks associated with showering or bathing, dressing, eating, toileting and bladder or bowel control

Home modification has the potential to make caregiving easier, safer and more time efficient by ensuring adequate circulation space and by the installation of mechanical lifters and other devices (Agree et al., 2005; Anderson & Wiener, 2013; Newman et al., 1990). Increased ease of care provision is particularly important in the context of funding formal care and taking time out of paid work to provide informal care. Caregiver stress is exacerbated by workforce shortages which is the result of the demand for care exceeding its supply (Carnemolla & Bridge, 2011; Gray & Heinsch, 2009). Davy et al. (2014) found that home design and modification considerations needed to consider the perspectives and views of carers and other members of the household, as well as those of the person with an illness, injury or impairment, particularly in regard to how the proposed modification of the home could do the following:

- Assist carers in specific care activities
- Provide a private space to retreat to
- Facilitate activities of other household members

Carnemolla (2015) used a quasi-experimental mixed-methods research design to examine how 157 participants changed their care patterns after a home modification intervention. Results from quality-of-life scores and informal and formal care hours were compared before and after home modifications, and the key finding was that home modification directly substituted for care. Informal care was the most sensitive, with reductions in care as high as:

- 63% for bathing and showering;
- 47% for toileting; and
- 41.1% for moving about the house.

The greatest reduction in formal care occurred in moving about the house, followed by bathing and showering. These results clearly indicate that care is sensitive to home modifications, with a 47% overall reduction in the care provided. As shown in Fig. 29.8,

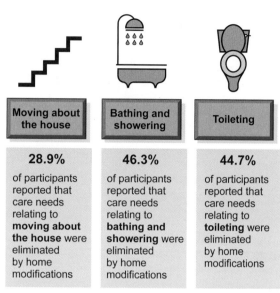

Where is care likely to be substituted by home modifications?

Moving about the house	Bathing and showering	Toileting
28.9%	**46.3%**	**44.7%**
of participants reported that care needs relating to **moving about the house** were eliminated by home modifications	of participants reported that care needs relating to **bathing and showering** were eliminated by home modifications	of participants reported that care needs relating to **toileting** were eliminated by home modifications

Fig. 29.8 ■ How home modifications substitute for care in the home. (Adapted from Carnemolla, P. (2015). *Measuring non-shelter effects of housing design: A mixed-methods exploration of home modifications, care-giving and health-related quality of life.* Unpublished PhD thesis.)

home modifications may not only support caregiving but substitute for it, and this suggests a strong relationship between home modification and improved health-related quality of life.

Theme 5: Economic Effectiveness

Home modification is typically a large one-off cost compared with ongoing smaller costs such as providing a formal caregiver to assist someone with bathing. This large one-off cost has been shown to be effective as an economic strategy for reducing overall cost, but is dependent on a number of factors, and perspectives vary regarding who is financially responsible and the payment period. Nevertheless, home modifications as a multifactorial intervention are generally viewed as cost-effective (Heywood & Turner, 2007; Jutkowitz et al., 2012; Lansley et al., 2004; Mann et al., 1999).

Theme 6: Ageing Process

There is a lack of strong experimental data that has focused on the impact of home modification on the ageing process. However, home modifications have been linked to the following:

- Slower progression of frailty (Hwang et al., 2011; Mitoku, 2014; Safran-Norton, 2010)
- Enhanced meaning of home for some people (Tanner et al., 2008), but not others (Ahn & Hegde, 2011)

Given the mixed findings about the emotive impact of home modifications, it can be conjectured that non-aesthetic or stigmatising interventions such as ramps could have a negative effect, whereas an intervention that improves value and home pride may have the opposite effect.

Theme 7: Social Participation

Studies on social participation, although scarce, suggest that home modifications may have a positive effect on social participation in the form of reduced effort, greater visit-ability and increased perceptions of competence and control (Heywood et al., 2001; Ostensjo et al., 2005; Randström et al., 2012; Vik et al., 2007). The fact that international policy and World Health Organization (WHO) guidelines promote 'active ageing' and greater social participation (Cannuscio et al., 2003) is important as modifying the home environment appears to be one means of improving a person's ability to leave the home, entertain at home and contribute to a sense of purpose for themselves and others.

HOME ASSESSMENT AND FOLLOW-UP

Occupational therapists receive training in home modification as part of their undergraduate training and during practice placements. However, this training is not comprehensive nor always in context. For example, the assessment of a domestic environment in the hospital context for a person who has a spinal cord injury is very different to that carried out for a person with dementia living in public housing.

Occupational therapists undertaking home assessments should consider the physical features and subfeatures, characteristics and subcharacteristics

(relevant to the people receiving occupational therapy services) as outlined in Table 29.2. The items in Table 29.2 are indicative only but demonstrate the level of analysis the therapist should consider before making a recommendation. Careful examination and analysis of the person and the person's abilities and environment guided by a collaborative relationship-focused approach, is crucial before making recommendations about the modification of a person's home.

Basic task and activity analysis is the key to quality assessment of restrictions to occupational participation (refer to Chapters 17 and 18). However, as stated in Millikan (2012), the competent therapist needs to look more widely than just task analysis and observations when proposing home modification intervention. For example, in addition to a person's level of ability to clean his or her body, it is critical to reflect on the following:

- Physical attributes and design of the room
- Body cleansing tools available
- Alternative body cleansing techniques, assistive products and technologies

Looking at each aspect of the task, including the environmental and tool-based requirements, the therapist may be able to collaborate with the person to identify additional issues, modifications, equipment or a change in the process that could be trialled. Looking at each aspect of the task enables the therapist to collect the evidence required to support the recommendations for an environmental modification.

Fishpool and Bridge (2012) stated that most home modification interventions include post-assessment follow-up with people. Some form of post-modification follow-up is needed to gather information about the impact of the modification on the person, as modifications can be complex. Failure to follow-up can risk missing important feedback necessary both for optimal outcomes and one's own personal learning (Sanford & Butterfield, 2005).

A variety of checklists, attention direction frameworks, surveys and observation techniques can be used to guide the assessment and follow-up process, measure the completion of recommendations (Cumming et al., 1999) and review changes to the person's occupational participation. However, as Barras (2005) noted,

TABLE 29.2				
Features and Subfeatures, Characteristics and Subcharacteristics Relevant to Assessment for Home Modification				
Feature	Subfeature	Characteristics	Subcharacteristics	Impact on Function
Access	■ Street frontage (or equivalent) ■ Driveway ■ Front access ■ Back access ■ Side access ■ Internal access	■ Gutter/kerbing ■ Stairs/steps ■ Ramp ■ Driveway ■ Lift/elevator ■ Lighting	■ Material (concrete, wood, tiles, etc.) ■ Slope/gradient ■ Ownership	■ Mobility
Bath	■ Main or en suite ■ Indoor or outdoor ■ Large/small ■ Upstairs/downstairs	■ Shower ■ Bath ■ Hand shower ■ Sliding glass door ■ Shower enclosure ■ Flooring ■ Taps, faucet (single or double) ■ Storage ■ Drainage	■ Materials (tiled, linoleum, timber, concrete sheet, concrete slab) ■ Tap type, faucet type, tap control	■ Transfers ■ Mobility ■ Personal care
Toilet	■ Main or en suite ■ Indoor or outdoor ■ Size ■ Location	■ Style ■ Seat height ■ Seat position ■ Cistern location ■ Grab rails/assistive technology ■ Bidet	■ Materials ■ Floor covering ■ Flush control mechanism ■ Toilet paper ■ Storage	■ Transfers ■ Personal care
Hallway	■ Size ■ Length ■ Purpose	■ Lighting ■ Access/egress	■ Floor surface/covering ■ Direction/prompts ■ Control of lighting	■ Mobility
Bedroom	■ Location and access to room ■ Main/secondary/spare ■ Use/size ■ Upstairs/downstairs	■ Access/egress ■ Furniture ■ Users – shared, sole occupant, activity	■ Windows/window dressings and control thereof ■ Thermoregulation (passive) and temperature management tools and control thereof ■ Power sources and control thereof ■ Lighting and control of lighting	■ Transfer ■ Mobility ■ Personal care ■ Domestic tasks

Kitchen	■ Location
	■ Size
	■ Set out (galley, square, rectangle, open plan)
		■ Access/egress
		■ Users
		■ Use of room (eating or preparation only)
			■ Appliances: type of and location of:
			  - fridge/freezer/kettle, etc.
			  - stove type and controls
			  - oven type and controls
			  - microwave type and controls
			  - direction of the door opening
			■ Source of drinking water
				■ Transfer
				■ Mobility
				■ Eating/drinking
				■ Domestic tasks

Continued on following page

		TABLE 29.2		
		Features and Subfeatures, Characteristics and Subcharacteristics Relevant to Assessment for Home Modification— *(Continued)*		
Feature	**Subfeature**	**Characteristics**	**Subcharacteristics**	**Impact on Function**

Lounge	▪ Location
	▪ Size
	▪ Position/aspect
		▪ Access/egress
		▪ Seating
		▪ Furniture position and use
			▪ Thermoregulation (passive), and temperature management tools and control
			▪ Windows/window dressings
			▪ Power sources
			▪ Lighting
			▪ Appliances:
			  – television
			  – DVD/video player/stereo/remote control
			  – fans/air conditioners
			▪ Seating – type and control (if relevant)
				▪ Transfer
				▪ Mobility
				▪ Eating/drinking
				▪ Domestic tasks

Garden	▪ Location ▪ Size ▪ Position/aspect	▪ Access/egress ▪ Yard furniture position and use ▪ Seating ▪ Yard equipment (clothesline) ▪ Verandah/pergola ▪ Roofed area ▪ Pool ▪ Garden tap ▪ Fencing	▪ Materials (tiled, paving, timber, concrete sheet, concrete slab) ▪ Tap type, faucet type, tap control ▪ Paths	▪ Transfer ▪ Mobility ▪ Eating/drinking ▪ Domestic tasks ▪ Home maintenance ▪ Yard care ▪ Pet care ▪ Security

From Millikan, L. (2012). *Environmental assessment & modification for Australian occupational therapists.* Home Modification Information Clearinghouse, University of New South Wales. www.homemods.info.

no consistent and standardised assessment tool currently exists. Home modification follow-up, as distinct from the initial assessment, requires additional specific attention to the following:

▪ Installation (i.e. asking if the modification has been correctly installed to specification by the agreed installer)
▪ Usage (i.e. to ascertain if the person is using the modification and if there are any questions about how to use the modification)
▪ Functionality (i.e. to determine that this modification has solved the functional issue satisfactorily)
▪ Safety (i.e. questioning regarding any risks or unintended consequences associated with the modification)

It is important to be aware that, although home modification service funders typically place the highest priority on functional outcomes, failure to factor in personal preferences and aesthetics can lead people to reject the modifications (Bridge et al., 2007; Clemson et al., 1999). Homes fulfil many needs for the occupants: they provide a place of self-expression, a vessel of memories, and a place of refuge from the outside world, in addition to affording a place to transact self-care and other care tasks. The introduction of home modifications may impact the meaning of the home environment. For instance, Ainsworth et al. (2022) found that 'people's prior experience of home, the circumstance of and time to plan modifications, the perceived value of the modifications, and the home modification process and funding influenced perceptions of outcomes' (p. 1, 2022).

BARRIERS TO HOME MODIFICATION INTERVENTION

There are a number of factors external to the person that present barriers to home modification intervention. Bridge et al. (2007) suggested the seven barriers illustrated in Fig. 29.9. The seven barriers fall into two main categories: practical and psychological. Practical barriers include financial problems, lack of knowledge, aesthetics/desirability and tenure. Practical barriers can be significant; however, the psychological barriers to home modifications, which include concerns about stigma, lack of social support and perception of need, may be more problematic and are often underexplored by therapists.

Bridge et al. (2007) also outlined research that found people with modification needs may often have a low socioeconomic status, high unemployment rates and may be women who tend to live alone and not own their dwellings. Significantly, many people with illness, injury or impairment are unaware of relevant existing services and funding that can be used for home modifications. General knowledge and acceptance of the formal service system are viewed as better predictors of home modification service usage than the demographics of functional capacity (Naik & Gill, 2005). Indeed, reliable information regarding what works, how much it will cost and the implications can be difficult to locate as most governments and services have not systematically gathered or invested in these data and may erroneously believe that less information available to the general public may help cap modification services and associated government funding. Tenure is another significant issue impacting home modification. It has been demonstrated that if a person lacks a secure home base, or has to get building approval from others such as relatives, landlords or a body corporate, this can result in significant differences in home modification rates even after controlling for age (ERMA et al., 2007).

The stigma of being viewed by others as less capable and the need a person has to protect his or her self-image in the onset of traumatic change and loss of

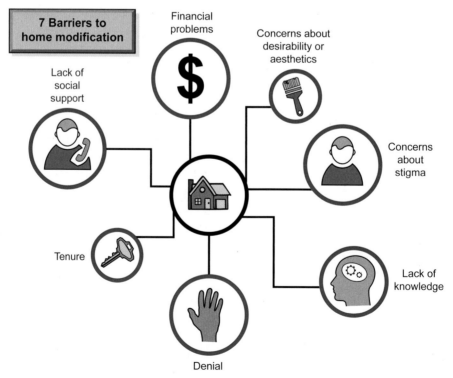

Fig. 29.9 ■ Barriers to home modification interventions.

functional capacity often leads people to implement psychological strategies to help them cope with the anxiety associated with functional losses. These strategies preserve individuals' sense of self-worth during adjustment to the physical, functional and environmental limitations being experienced even though they may appear to be irrational from the perspective of outsiders (Katz et al., 2002). It is important to be aware that the psychological strategies may involve either a gradual psychological adaptation process (Calabro, 1990), brief defensive mechanisms such as denial and repression (Katz et al., 2002), or a mixture of the two strategies (Calabro, 1990). It is therefore important in home modification practice to be aware that denial can involve a belief system that considers the functional impairment to be temporary, views the residential situation as safe and comfortable, and/or perceives the financial implications of home modifications as being too great. Further, any decision-making entails predicting the future, and oftentimes people imagine how the outcomes of their choices will make them feel (emotional consequences), so it is not uncommon to avoid what they fear (Douglas & Jones, 2007). However, when the level of dysfunction tips from intermittent or moderate to severe, denial is typically replaced by action (Gitlin, 1995). Giving people time to adjust and reflect is important to helping to achieve optimal home modification outcomes.

CONCLUSION

An overview of the importance of home modification has been presented in this chapter. With regards to home modifications, a better understanding of who, what, where and why is critical for occupational therapists in presenting information to the people they serve and for the people themselves in choosing to either accept or reject modifications to their homes that may improve occupational participation and quality of life.

Home modification interventions are complex and are shaped by a variety of factors. Importantly, there is strong evidence that home modifications can reduce the likelihood of falls and injury, reduce fear of falling and improve confidence of those at risk of falls. Additionally, improvements in confidence and reduction of fear are also related to the well-being effects of improving a person's living space by modifying it.

REFERENCES

Agree, E., Freedman, V., Cornman, J., Wolf, D., & Marcotte, J. E. (2005). Reconsidering substitution in long-term care: When does assistive technology take the place of personal care? *The Journals of Gerontology Series B: Psychological Sciences and Social Sciences, 60*(5), S272–S280.

Ahmad, J., Shakil-ur-Rehman, S., & Sibtain, F. (2013). Effectiveness of home modification on quality of life on wheelchair user paraplegic population. *Rawal Medical Journal, 38*(3), 263–265.

Ahn, M., & Hegde, A. (2011). Perceived aspects of home environment and home modifications by older people living in rural areas. *Journal of Housing for the Elderly, 25*(1), 18–30.

Ainsworth, E., Aplin, T., de Jonge, D., & Bennett, S. (2022). Understanding home modification outcomes from the perspective of older people and people with a disability: informing home modification evaluation. *Disability and Rehabilitation, 45*(24), 4101–4110.

Alam, M. R., Reaz, M. B. I., & Ali, M. A. M. (2012). A review of smart homes—Past, present, and future. *IEEE Transactions on Systems, Man, and Cybernetics, Part C (Applications and Reviews), 42*(6), 1190–1203.

American Occupational Therapy Association. (2020). Occupational therapy practice framework: Domain and process (4th ed.). *American Journal of Occupational Therapy, 74*(Suppl. 2), 7412410010. https://doi.org/10.5014/ajot.2020.74S2001.

American Occupational Therapy Association. (2021). Standards of practice for occupational therapy. *American Journal of Occupational Therapy, 75*(Suppl. 3), 7513410050. https://doi.org/10.5014/ajot.2021.75S3004.

Anderson, W., & Wiener, J. (2013). The impact of assistive technologies on formal and informal home care. *The Gerontologist, 55*(3), 422–433.

Aronson, J., & Neysmlth, S. (1997). The retreat of the state and long-term care provision: Implications for frail elderly people, unpaid family carers and paid home care workers. *Studies in Political Economy, 53*, 37–66.

Australian Bureau of Statistics. (2012). *Disability, aging and carers.* Australia: Summary of Findings, 2012. (4430.0). Australian Bureau of Statistics. http://www.abs.gov.au/AUSSTATS/abs@.nsf/Lookup/4430.0Explanatory%20Notes5002012?OpenDocument.

Barras, S. (2005). A systematic and critical review of the literature: The effectiveness of Occupational Therapy Home Assessment on a range of outcome measures. *Australian Occupational Therapy Journal, 52*(4), 326–336.

Berg, K., Hines, M., & Allen, S. (2002). Wheelchair users at home: Few home modifications and many injurious falls. *American Journal of Public Health, 92*(1), 48.

Bleasdale, M., McNamara, N., Zmudzki, F., & Bridge, C. (2014). *Positioning paper: DIY home modifications: Point-of-sale support for people with disability and their carers.* Home Modification Information Clearinghouse, UNSW Australia. Retrieved from www.homemods.info.

Bogdon, A. S. (1996). Homeowner renovation and repair: The decision to hire someone else to do the project. *Journal of Housing Economics, 5*(4), 323–350.

Booth, P. (1982). Housing as a product: Design guidance and resident satisfaction in the private sector. *Built Environment, 8*(1), 20–24.

Bridge, C. (2009). Home modification: Occupation as the basis for an effective practice. In M. Curtin, M. Molineaux, & J. Supyk (Eds.), *Occupational therapy and physical dysfunction: Enabling occupation* (6th ed., pp. 409–430). Churchill Livingstone Elsevier.

Bridge, C., Flatau, P., Whelan, S., Wood, G., & Yates, J. (2003). *Housing assistance and non-shelter outcomes: Australian Housing and Urban Research Institute*. AHURI. www.ahuri.edu.au/attachments/80188_final_housingassist.pdf.

Bridge, P., Gohar, N., & Chaudhary, K. (2007). *Evidence based research: Identifying barriers to home modifications*. Home Modification Information Clearinghouse, UNSW Australia. www.homemods.info.

Bridge, C., Zmudzki, F., Huang, T., Owen, C., & Faulkner, D. (2021). *Impacts of new and emerging assistive technologies for ageing and disabled housing*. AHURI Final Report No. 372. Melbourne: Australian Housing and Urban Research Institute Limited. doi:10.18408/ahuri7122501. https://www.ahuri.edu.au/research/final-reports/372.

Burgstahler, S. E. (2015). In S. E. Burgstahler (Ed.), *Universal design in higher education: From principles to practice* (2nd ed.). Harvard Education Press.

Calabro, L. (1990). Adjustment to disability: A cognitive-behavioral analysis and clinical management. *Journal of Rational-Emotive and Cognitive-Behavior Therapy, 8*(2), 17–22.

Cannuscio, C., Block, J., & Kawachi, I. (2003). Social capital and successful aging: The role of senior housing. *Annals of Internal Medicine, 139*(5 Part 2), 395–399.

Carnemolla, P. (2015). *Measuring non-shelter effects of housing design: A mixed-methods exploration of home modifications, caregiving and health-related quality of life*. Unpublished PhD thesis.

Carnemolla, P., & Bridge, C. (2011). *Home modifications and their impact on waged care substitution*. Home Modifications Information Clearinghouse.

Carnemolla, P., & Bridge, C. (2015). *Systematic review; evidence on home modifications*. Home Modifications Information Clearinghouse.

Chang, J., Morton, S., Rubenstein, L., Mojica, W. A., Maglione, M., Suttorp, M. J., Roth, E. A., & Shekelle, P. G. (2004). Interventions for the prevention of falls in older adults: Systematic review and meta-analysis of randomised clinical trials. *BMJ, 328*(7441), 680.

Chase, C., Mann, K., Wasek, S., & Arbesman, M. (2012). Systematic review of the effect of home modification and fall prevention programs on falls and the performance of community-dwelling older adults. *American Journal of Occupational Therapy, 66*(3), 284–291.

Clemson, L., Cusick, A., & Fozzard, C. (1999). Managing risk and exerting control: Determining follow through with falls prevention. *Disability and Rehabilitation, 21*, 531–541.

Clemson, L., Mackenzie, L., Ballinger, C., Close, J., & Cumming, R. (2008). Environmental interventions to prevent falls in community-dwelling older people a meta-analysis of randomized trials. *Journal of Aging and Health, 20*(8), 954–971.

Cumming, R. G., Thomas, M., Szonyi, G., Salkeld, G., O'Neill, E., Westbury, C., & Frampton, G. (1999). Home visits by an occupational therapist for assessment and modification of environmental hazards: A randomized trial of falls prevention. *Journal of the American Geriatrics Society, 47*(12), 1397–1402.

Davy, L., Adams, T., & Bridge, C. (2014). *Caring for the carer: Home design and modification for carers of young people with disability*. Home Modification Information Clearinghouse, University of New South Wales Australia. www.homemods.info.

Douglas, K., & Jones, D. (2007). How to make better choices. *New Scientist, 194*(2602), 35–43.

Environmental Resources Management Australia (ERMA), Phibbs, P., & Bridge, C. (2007). *Research into the nature of the need for home modification products and services in Queensland (final report)*. Queensland Department of Housing and Public Works.

Fallis, G. (2014). *Housing economics*. Butterworth-Heinemann.

Fishpool, J., & Bridge, C. (2012). *Follow-up efficacy post environmental modifications; a guide for clinical practice*. Home Modification Information Clearinghouse, University of New South Wales. www.homemods.info.

Gamble, P. (2015). *Building in Inclusive Design: A modern housing perspective*. Housing Learning & Improvement Network.

Gitlin, L. N. (1995). Why older people accept or reject assistive technology. *Generations, XIX*(1), 1–9.

Gitlin, L., Corcoran, M., Winter, L., Boyce, A., & Hauck, W. (2001). A randomized, controlled trial of a home environmental intervention: Effect on efficacy and upset in caregivers and on daily function of persons with dementia. *The Gerontologist, 41*(1), 4.

Gitlin, L., Hauck, W., Winter, L., Dennis, M., & Schulz, R. (2006). Effect of an in-home occupational and physical therapy intervention on reducing mortality in functionally vulnerable older people: Preliminary findings. *Journal of the American Geriatrics Society, 54*(6), 950–955.

Gitlin, L., Miller, K., & Boyce, A. (1999). Bathroom modifications for frail elderly renters: Outcomes of a community-based program. *Technology and Disability, 10*(3), 141–149.

Grand Designs. (2014). *The Crooked Chocolate Box Cottage: Revisited. Series 13, Ep 4*. British Broadcasting Commission. http://docuwiki.net/index.php?title=Grand_designs:_series_14#The_Crooked_Chocolate_Box_Cottage_Revisited.

Gray, M., & Heinsch, M. (2009). Aging in Australia and the increased need for care. *Aging International, 34*(3), 102–118.

Guo, J., Tsai, Y., Liao, J., Tu, H., & Huang, C. (2014). Interventions to reduce the number of falls among older adults with/without cognitive impairment: An exploratory meta-analysis. *International Journal of Geriatric Psychiatry, 29*(7), 661–669.

Harvey, D. (2010). *Social justice and the city* (Vol. 1). University of Georgia Press.

Heller, C., Ekstam, L., Haak, M., Schmidt, S. M., & Slaug, B. (2022). Exploring housing policies in five Swedish municipalities: alternatives and priorities. *BMC Public Health, 22*(1), 1–15.

Heywood, F., Oldman, J., & Means, R. (2001). *Housing and home in later life*. McGraw Hill Education.

Heywood, F., & Turner, L. (2007). *Better outcomes, lower costs. Implications for health and social care budgets of investment in housing adaptations, improvements and equipment: Review of the evidence*. Office for Disability Issues/Department of Work and Pensions.

Hwang, E., Cummings, L., Sixsmith, A., & Sixsmith, J. (2011). Impacts of home modifications on aging-in-place. *Journal of Housing for the Elderly, 25*(3), 246–257.

Joines, S., & Payne, A. (2017). *Universal design.* In *Occupational therapy for people experiencing illness, injury or impairment: Promoting occupation and participation* (7th ed.). Elsevier.

Johansson, K., Lilja, M., Petersson, I., & Borell, L. (2007). Performance of activities of daily living in a sample of applicants for home modification services. *Scandinavian Journal of Occupational Therapy, 14*(1), 44–53.

Jutkowitz, E., Gitlin, L., Pizzi, L., Lee, E., & Dennis, M. (2012). Cost effectiveness of a home based intervention that helps functionally vulnerable older adults age in place at home. *Journal of Aging Research, 2012*, 680265.

Katz, N., Fleming, J., Keren, N., Lightbody, S., & Hartman-Maeir, A. (2002). Unawareness and/or denial of disability: Implications for occupational therapy intervention. *Canadian Journal of Occupational Therapy, 69*(5), 281–292.

Kujala, S. (2003). User involvement: a review of the benefits and challenges. *Behaviour & Information Technology, 22*(1), 1–16.

Langdon, N. (2022). *Evaluating the dwelling satisfaction of households with disabled members in Ontario, Canada.* Doctoral dissertation.

Lansley, P., McCreadie, C., & Tinker, A. (2004). Can adapting the homes of older people and providing assistive technology pay its way? *Age and Aging, 33*(6), 571–576.

Lewis, A., Parsons, S., Robertson, C., Feiler, A., Tarleton, B., Watson, D., Byers, R., Davies, J., Fergusson, A., & Marvin, C. (2008). Participation in research: Reference, or advisory, groups involving disabled people: reflections from three contrasting research projects. *British Journal of Special Education, 35*, 78–84. https://doi.org/10.1111/j.1467-8578.2008.00376.x.

Lin, M., Wolf, S., Hwang, H., Gong, S., & Chen, C. (2007). A randomized, controlled trial of fall prevention programs and quality of life in older fallers. *Journal of the American Geriatrics Society, 55*(4), 499–506.

Lord, S., Menz, H., & Sherrington, C. (2006). Home environment risk factors for falls in older people and the efficacy of home modifications. *Age and Aging, 35*(2), ii55–ii59.

Lynch, K., & Findlay, I. (2007). *A new vision for Saskatchewan: Changing lives and systems through individualized funding for people with intellectual disabilities* [a research report]. Community-University Institute for Social Research and Centre for the Study of Co-operatives.

Mann, W., Ottenbacher, K., Fraas, L., Tomita, M., & Granger, C. (1999). Effectiveness of assistive technology and environmental interventions in maintaining independence and reducing home care costs for the frail elderly: A randomized controlled trial. *Archives of Family Medicine, 8*, 210–217.

Matthews, B., Hibberd, D., & Speakman, K. (2015). The impact of street accessibility on travel and independence for disabled people. In: *14th International Conference on Mobility and Transport for Elderly and Disabled Persons (TRANSED)*, 28–31 Jul 2015, Lisbon, Portugal. (Unpublished).

Millikan, L. (2012). *Environmental assessment & modification for Australian occupational therapists.* Home Modification Information Clearinghouse, University of New South Wales. www.homemods.info.

Mitoku, K. (2014). Home modification and prevention of frailty progression in older adults: a Japanese prospective cohort study. *Journal of Gerontological Nursing, 40*(8), 40–47.

Naik, A. D., & Gill, T. M. (2005). Underutilisation of environmental adaptations for bathing in community-living older people. *Journal of the American Geriatric Society, 53*, 1497–1503.

Newell, A., & Gregor, P. (2000). User sensitive inclusive design: In search of a new paradigm. *Proceedings of the Conference on Universal Usability*, 39–44. https://doi.org/10.1145/355460.355470.

Newman, S., Struyk, R., Wright, P., & Rice, M. (1990). Overwhelming odds: Care-giving and the risk of institutionalization. *Journal of Gerontology, 45*(5), S173–S183.

Ostensjo, S., Carlberg, E., & Vollestad, N. (2005). The use and impact of assistive devices and other environmental modifications on everyday activities and care in young children with cerebral palsy. *Disability & Rehabilitation, 27*(14), 849–861.

Pappalettera, A., Bottiglione, F., Mantriota, G., & Reina, G. (2023). Watch the next step: A Comprehensive survey of stair-climbing vehicles. *Robotics, 12*(3), 74. https://doi.org/10.3390/robotics12030074.

Pearson, R. (2011). Design thinking: A new take on ADDIE. *Canadian Learning Journal, 15*(2), 24.

Petersson, I., Lilja, M., & Borell, L. (2012). To feel safe in everyday life at home a study of older adults after home modifications. *Ageing and Society, 32*(5), 791–811.

Plautz, B., Beck, D., Selmar, C., & Radetsky, M. (1995). Modifying the environment: A community-based injury- reduction program for elderly residents. *American Journal of Preventive Medicine, 12*(4 Suppl), 33–38.

Randstrom, K., Asplund, K., & Svedlund, M. (2012). Impact of environmental factors in home rehabilitation: A qualitative study from the perspective of older persons using the International Classification of Functioning, Disability and Health to describe facilitators and barriers. *Disability and Rehabilitation, 34*(9), 779–787.

Restall, G., & Egan, M. (2022). Collaborative relationship-focused occupational therapy. In M. Egan & G. Restall (Eds.), *Promoting occupational participation: Collaborative relationship-focused occupational therapy* (pp. 97–117). Canadian Association of Occupational Therapists.

Robinson, D., Green, S., & Wilson, I. (2020). Housing options for older people in a reimagined housing system: A case study from England. *International Journal of Housing Policy, 20*(3), 344–366.

Safran-Norton, C. (2010). Physical home environment as a determinant of aging in place for different types of elderly households. *Journal of Housing for the Elderly, 24*(2), 208–231.

Sanford, J., & Butterfield, T. (2005). Using remote assessment to provide home modification services to underserved elders. *Gerontologist, 45*(3), 389–398.

Story, M. F. (2001). Principles of universal design. In *Universal design handbook, 2E.* McGraw-Hill.

Szanton, S. L., Wolff, J., Leff, B., Thorpe, R. J., Tanner, E. K., Boyd, C., Xue, Q., Guralnik, J., Bishai, D., & Gitlin, L. N. (2014). CAPABLE trial: A randomized controlled trial of nurse, occupational therapist and handyman to reduce disability among older adults:

Rationale and design. *Contemporary Clinical Trials, 38*(1), 102–112.

Tanner, B., Tilse, C., & De Jonge, D. (2008). Restoring and sustaining home: The impact of home modifications on the meaning of home for older people. *Journal of Housing for the Elderly, 22*(3), 195–215.

Thomson, H., Thomas, S., Sellstrom, E., & Petticrew, M. (2013). Housing improvements for health and associated socio-economic outcomes. *Cochrane Database of Systematic Reviews, 2*, CD008657.

Tinker, A. (1997). Housing for elderly people. *Reviews in Clinical Gerontology, 7*(2), 171–176.

Tse, T. (2005). The environment and falls prevention: Do environmental modifications make a difference? *Australian Occupational Therapy Journal, 52*(4), 271–281.

Turner, S., Arthur, G., Lyons, R., Weightman, A. L., Mann, M. K., Jones, S. J., John, A., & Lannon, S. (2011). Modification of the home environment for the reduction of injuries. *Cochrane Database of Systematic Reviews, 2*, CD003600.

Van Hoof, J., Kort, H., van Waarde, H., & Blom, M. (2010). Environmental interventions and the design of homes for older adults with dementia: an overview. *American Journal of Alzheimer's Disease and Other Dementias, 25*(3), 202–232.

Vik, K., Nygard, L., & Lilja, M. (2007). Perceived environmental influence on participation among older adults after home-based rehabilitation. *Physical & Occupational Therapy in Geriatrics, 25*(4), 1–20.

Wahl, H., Fange, A., Oswald, F., Gitlin, L., & Iwarsson, S. (2009). The home environment and disability-related outcomes in aging individuals: What is the empirical evidence? *The Gerontologist, 49*(3), 355–367.

Wiles, J. L., Leibing, A., Guberman, N., Reeve, J., & Allen, R. (2012). The meaning of 'ageing in place' to older people. *The Gerontologist, 52*(3), 357–366.

Williamson, B. (2019). Accessible America. In *Accessible America.* New York University Press.

Wilson, D., Mitchell, J., Kemp, B., Adkins, R., & Mann, W. (2009). Effects of assistive technology on functional decline in people aging with a disability. *Assistive Technology, 21*(4), 208–217.

Winkler, D., Martel, A., Chen, Y., & Greaves, T. (2020). *Preliminary findings: Audit of accessible features in new-build house plans.* https://assets.summerfoundation.org.au/pdf_offload/2020/08/Preliminary_findings__new_housing_audit_31Aug2020-final.pdf.

Woolf, S. H., & Aron, L. (2013). Physical and social environmental factors. In *U.S. health in international perspective: Shorter lives, poorer health.* National Academies Press (US). https://www.ncbi.nlm.nih.gov/books/NBK154491/.

Young, D., Wagenfeld, A., & Rocker, H. V. V. (2019). Universal design and the built environment: Occupational therapy and interprofessional design teams—A scoping review. *Annals of International Occupational Therapy, 2*(4), 186–194.

REFLECTION

1. What is the difference between accessibility and universal design?

2. List three ways to help Chris learn about what modifications might be available and might work best for him within his home.

3. How important is it that the modification made by individuals to their own homes are safe, and how might this be assessed?

4. How does home modification practice differ from universal design practice?

30

EMBRACING A CRITICAL COMMUNITY DEVELOPMENT ORIENTATION AND STRATEGY IN OCCUPATIONAL THERAPY PRACTICE

LIESL PETERS ■ SITHEMBELENKOSINI BEAUTY NGCOBO ■ ROSHAN GALVAAN

Overview

Dominant discourses that frame occupational therapy practice can limit the contributions occupational therapists make to the well-being of individuals and collectives. It is argued that occupational therapists should work towards developing practices that more adequately engage with the issues of injustice and inequality that shape people's health. There is therefore a need to challenge and resist the discourses that keep practice framed in limited ways. Different frames of reference to guide occupational therapy practice are, however, required to create the openings through which occupational therapists might consider their practice imperatives differently. This chapter introduces community development as a form of critical occupational therapy practice that prompts occupational therapists to engage more directly with the conditions that shape people's lives and determine their experiences of health and well-being. The principles, strategies and competencies of the occupation-based community development framework are described to demonstrate how these enable an approach for occupational therapy practice that can more adequately engage with the situational aspects of exclusion for people experiencing illness, injury and impairment. Using two practice stories the value of applying frameworks like occupation-based community development to interrupt injustices and offer new ways of thinking and doing for occupational therapists is demonstrated.

KEY POINTS

■ Community development is a form of critical occupational therapy that enables occupational therapists to engage with the conditions shaping people's lives.

■ Dominant discourses can limit the practice of occupational therapists, particularly in biomedical settings. Evaluating, resisting and challenging these discourses can support the development of occupational therapy approaches that more adequately engage with issues of justice and exclusion that shape health and well-being.

■ Different practice frameworks can be drawn on to guide the implementation of a community development approach in occupational therapy practice. Elements of these frameworks may be helpful in shaping practice when working with people who experience illness, injury and impairment. The orientation and priorities of these frameworks guide the occupational therapist to focus on issues that ordinarily fall outside of conditional and diagnostic reasoning.

■ Principles and strategies drawn from the occupation-based community development framework are described and explained to demonstrate how they might shape practice when working in physical health.

■ The application of the principles and strategies of the occupation-based community development framework within settings where occupational therapists work with people with illness, injury and impairment assists occupational therapists in building a mutual understanding that can guide practice in more pertinent ways, addressing the multiple factors that contribute to health and well-being.

INTRODUCTION

Occupational therapists have been called upon to contribute as change agents to promote the participation of individuals and collectives. To contribute strategically to positive social change, occupational therapists need to be supported by theoretical frameworks that advance collaborative and relationship-focused approaches to practice (Restall & Egan, 2022) and practice with communities (Galvaan & Peters, 2013; Lopes & Malfitano, 2021). Central to these approaches is an appreciation of the situated nature of occupation (refer to Chapter 6) which recognises the influence of contextual factors, such as socio-political and economic factors on community participation. However, occupational therapists working in and with communities have mostly relied on clinical approaches, often practising from a rehabilitation or public health paradigm. Community development involves working with community members, through partnerships, to address priorities by drawing in collective local strengths and resources. Within occupational therapy, community development practice has adopted critical theoretical perspectives that shift practice towards addressing constraining discourses.

In this chapter, the orientation and priorities of community development practice in relation to occupational therapy are described. While community development is a distinct domain of practice in occupational therapy, the occupation-based community development framework is drawn on to suggest how community development principles, strategies and competencies could be applied within settings that do not ordinarily lend themselves to these forms of practice. Two practice stories illustrating the application of the occupation-based community development framework are referred to throughout the chapter.

COMMUNITY DEVELOPMENT PRACTICE AS CRITICAL OCCUPATIONAL THERAPY

Farias and Laliberte Rudman (2019) identified three dominant discourses that shape and perpetuate our practice limitations as occupational therapists. These discourses are the 'individualisation of social issues' where individuals are held responsible as workers and consumers of health services, rather than acknowledging the socio-political barriers limiting participation in occupations. Second, is an over-reliance on a 'biomedical lens and healthism' as a goal of occupational therapy practice, emphasising health as located within the physical body with individual behaviour as the cause of and solution to health concerns. Lastly, 'the growth of managerialism and maintaining our professional status' as occupational therapists (Farias & Laliberte Rudman, 2019, pp. 694-696) has continued to pressure occupational therapists, through neoliberal approaches to health management, to comply with guidelines and protocols that control costs by simplifying complex transactional understandings of participation to matters of individual performance. Together, these discourses implicitly govern occupational therapy practice and constrain the subjectivity of occupational therapists. They direct attention towards particular issues, shaping how, where and why occupational therapists might engage with people in attempting to contribute positively to their experience of health and well-being.

In Box 30.1 Part A, Ngcobo (the second author), recounts her encounter with dominant discourses

BOX 30.1
QUESTIONING AND CHALLENGING DOMINANT DISCOURSES IN OCCUPATIONAL THERAPY PRACTICE (NCGOBO)

PART A: CONSTRAINED BY DOMINANT DISCOURSES

I worked at a rural district hospital in South Africa with an in-patient capacity of 219 people. I worked in a small rehabilitation team that included two occupational therapists, one physiotherapist, two dietitians, one audiologist and one speech and language pathologist. Half of the team, including myself, were completing our compulsory community service[a] graduate placements. The team delivered outreach services to eight community-level clinics and served about 90,000[b] people from the surrounding areas. My designated primary role was to provide in- and out-patient occupational therapy services at the hospital and the clinics. This included home-based care to community members who came to the hospital seeking assistance for a range of medical conditions. Most people experienced acute and chronic physical conditions and sought relief for their conditions through our services.

Often, people's stories about their physical pains did not make sense clinically. The more I asked about the pain, the more people told me about the other difficulties in their lives. The pain of losing a loved one, loneliness and being ostracised by the community. The pain of no longer being able to work and provide for their families. The pain of not receiving the services and assistance they needed to live healthier lives. These individuals were often sent to occupational therapy because they were suspected of malingering since they frequently returned even though they were treated appropriately for their physical conditions. The rehabilitation team was required to take on the unenviable task of figuring out if their pain was real.

Was it 'real' enough to qualify them for a social welfare (SASSA[c]) grant?

Was it 'fake' enough for us to discharge them from our services because they could be wasting resources for people with more real, physical pain?

---

[a]In South Africa, graduates of the health professions are required to complete a compulsory year of service in a designated institution. They are allocated to institutions by the National Department of Health.

[b]http://www.mseleni.co.za/mselenihospital/facts.htm

[c]SASSA stands for the South African Social Security Agency. SASSA administers social grants of a variety of types, collectively referred to in everyday language as SASSA grants. Examples of types of grants include the disability grant, the child-care grant, the older persons grant etcetera [South African Social Security Agency. (2023). *SASSA Grants – Social Grants in SA*. Retrieved July 7, 2023, from https://www.sassagrants.co.za/]. At present, in South Africa, there is no basic income grant.

People returned repeatedly, but often were not seen as a high priority. There was pressure to figure out what was wrong with them quickly, to solve whatever the physical cause of the problem was, and discharge or refer them accordingly. The explicit and inferred messages the team received was that we had other individuals to attend to, whose presentations were seen as being more important given their more obvious biomedical needs. There was constant pressure to prove our 'worth' as a rehabilitation team by showing, through patient statistics, how many individuals we had seen and 'helped'. Patient statistics were one of the main measures of value and impact within the healthcare system. The more individuals we saw, the more the 'powers that be' would recognise the team's value and allocate additional financial and human resources towards our rehabilitation services. This created a tension for team members as we started to recognise that something was not working in the services we were offering. I constantly wondered whether the biomedical lens was really adequate for the issues we were noticing. Our services were not oriented to attend to the pain associated with the deep flaws and failures in our country's socio-economic and health system.

As team members, we spoke to our line manager about our observations and they acknowledged what we were saying, but they indicated that we would still need to 'do our jobs'. We had the sense that they were worried that if we took on the task of attempting to contribute to the broader issues we were noticing, team members would not have time to see the in-patients in the hospital. Consequently, we would not be able to record and show the work we were doing via the necessary statistics and monitoring systems. The lack of capacity (being understaffed) contributed to my line manager's response, but I also think that some of the shifts I was suggesting in terms of my role as an occupational therapist did not fall into what management saw as my 'scope' of practice.

PART B: BACK TO THE (SHARED) DRAWING BOARD

While listening to the stories about the things that caused individuals' pain, the team realised that there was a common thread. These individuals all mostly lacked social support and so the physiotherapist and I invited them to join pain management groups that we were jointly facilitating at the clinics we serviced. The decentralisation of our services was important so as not to add to the social burden (for example finding transport money) of those who wanted to attend these groups. These groups developed into both 'movement' and 'talk' groups. We made time to facilitate movement and stretching, sometimes providing heat and

Continued on following page

BOX 30.1

QUESTIONING AND CHALLENGING DOMINANT DISCOURSES IN OCCUPATIONAL THERAPY PRACTICE (NCGOBO)—*(Continued)*

cold therapies for those who needed them. We then shifted from the role of being the 'expert' practitioner who directs the session, to one where we facilitated the opportunity for the group to discuss what felt important for them – even if we (collectively as the group) could not solve these problems immediately. This was difficult because, although we wanted to position ourselves as part of the collective, the group members would often look to us or call on us for solutions. This included pushing us to advocate for their needs.

We attempted to navigate our stance as both insiders and outsiders in a fluid way, answering questions and giving advice if this felt right, but also prompting the community members to share their perspectives as a way of building a collective interpretation of what the solutions might be. Where relevant, we assisted with taking things up in terms of advocacy, choosing to view the community members' prompts for us to do so as an important expression of their own agency and an indication of the relationship that we had built with them. They felt capable, at times, of asking for what they needed from us and were not just waiting to be told what to do. However, we simultaneously challenged the hegemonic discourses that hindered them from advocating for themselves, both within the group space and in their personal lives. We did this through a process of facilitation over time. We asked critical questions, telling stories as a way of problem-posing and offering alternative perspectives. This led to renewed understandings of what the issues at hand were and led to a process where members were able to plan, take actions and then reflect on these during subsequent time together in the pain management groups. For instance, often the group would agree on a homework task, like choosing to do exercises at home or talking to family members about issues that concern them.

Recognising that the causes of the group members' issues were largely social in nature, the physiotherapist and I were not satisfied with working only with them. Collectively, the rehabilitation team decided to trial multiple initiatives for building the necessary understanding to unearth potential leverage points for creating change. We started a forum with health practitioners from other hospitals as part of a community trust initiative. This allowed the team to understand how health issues were experienced in the community and how people were interacting with health systems. We started learning about the community governance systems and leaning into what 'onomakhaya' (community health workers) were saying about what was needed outside of the hospital services. The dietitian shared their experience of working with community agricultural societies

so we could learn how to assist with community gardens. The team also began to attend community meetings that were usually run by nursing staff. Joining them meant that the team had an opportunity to position ourselves as 'community-facing'. Throughout these experiences, team members talked about what we were seeing and started working things out collectively with community members (both in and outside of the hospital).

Team members learnt a great deal about the time and investment that the process of building a mutual understanding takes. Most of the rehabilitation team were only there for our community service year and the approach started to gain ground towards the end of that year. This meant that we personally were not able to realise the systemic change in terms of what the hospital allowed. However, I changed and my colleagues changed. Critically, those we served began to interact differently with the rehabilitation team's services. Community members stopped waiting for us to initiate actions and they started to initiate small actions themselves – like taking ownership of the group spaces.

PART C: SHIFTING THE NEEDLE – SEEING CRITICAL COMMUNITY DEVELOPMENT AS AN ESSENTIAL PART OF THE OT ROLE IN PHYSICAL HEALTH PRACTICE SETTINGS

What I struggled with the most is that all the 'steps' I listed in Box 30.1 Part B were not being recognised as legitimate occupational therapy work within the hospital system. It was seen as an 'extracurricular' activity. Perhaps this is a point of contestation for occupational therapists: to advocate for a different kind of practice that embraces the wholeness of peoples' lives. When I think about my manager, I do not judge her as being against change. For the most part, I recognised that she was stuck in the same mechanics of the system that we were stuck in. I recognise also that there were missed opportunities in the rehabilitation team's interactions with her. We became stuck in seeing her as a manager who would not budge. The complexity of hierarchies is that we often cannot communicate with each other as partners who have shared experiences and shared grievances. As a junior occupational therapist, I was so aware of that status (being junior) and was obsessed with not appearing as unknowing and unskilled. eventually, it was easier to just sidestep her in our thought processes and our enactment. I thought that I could not afford to be vulnerable and invite my senior into my uncertainty.

I wonder what might have happened had I been more open to do so?

in her occupational therapy practice that lead her to question her reasoning.

Critical occupational therapy has been suggested as a form of occupational therapy practice where the conditions that shape peoples' participation and performance are engaged with more seriously (Hammell & Iwama, 2012) (refer to Chapter 2). Critical occupational therapy should aim to contest oppressive hegemonies as a way of contributing to well-being, equity and justice. As such, attempting to contribute by drawing on a critical occupational therapy practice allows attention to be directed differently, to address the underlying causes of peoples' ill-health. Community development practice has been offered as a form of critical occupational therapy, enabling occupational therapists to turn their attention to the multiple facets – outside of impairment – that construct peoples' experience of health and well-being. However, engaging community development practice in this way requires that occupational therapists draw on theories and approaches that make it possible to engage with the social determinants of health more effectively. It therefore makes sense that these theories and approaches are located within a critical approach to community development that aligns with and prompts a politically progressive stance. When community development is critical in nature it 'is community-led, develops a collective analysis about the drivers that create and perpetuate poverty, exclusion and disadvantage, and then organises and structures its processes beyond the local level to effect social change' (Lathouras, 2016, p. 32). Such an orientation to community development is essential if occupational therapists intend to contribute to inclusion and justice within communities.

ORIENTATION AND PRIORITIES OF A COMMUNITY DEVELOPMENT-FOCUSED OCCUPATIONAL THERAPY PRACTICE

In community development practice, the concept of a 'community' does not only refer to a group of people confined to a particular geographical location. Rather, a community is understood as a collective with common interests or a historical association. This means that different communities may present concurrently within different places and institutions. Consequently, which communities are worked with as part of community development practice is related to the evident needs that arise in relation to the situations that different communities experience. In any case, it is the community that sets the priorities within community development practice and occupational therapists are positioned as facilitators and resource persons, rather than experts when working with each community (Leclair et al., 2019). This is in contrast to practices that occur in healthcare settings where occupational therapists are often positioned as experts (Robertson et al., 2015). Community development approaches within occupational therapy have attempted to apply a different orientation to practice where the agenda is usually defined through a co-created process where multiple factors are considered, including the community's future plans. The community development process is open-ended, as it is shaped by events and factors affecting the community. This differs from community-based approaches, which focus on project outcomes and professional timelines.

Occupational therapists have drawn on interdisciplinary knowledge, including occupational science, to inform frameworks for community development practice. These include the occupation-based community development framework (Galvaan & Peters, 2017a), the community-centred practice framework (Hyett et al., 2019) and the community practice process derived from the Canadian Practice Process Framework (Leclair et al., 2019). Each framework describes how occupational therapists could work in participatory and collaborative ways *with* communities to address a community's priorities. According to these frameworks, occupational therapists partner with communities or community representatives to facilitate processes where they identify their priorities and strategies to promote community members' participation and the realisation of social inclusion, aiming to enhance local resources and self-sustainable solutions (refer to Chapter 14). In such a practice orientation, the creation of opportunities to work collaboratively with communities in ways that account for social, economic and political driving forces of participation in occupations is prioritised. This approach aligns with the occupational therapy values of promoting occupational justice and creating a more inclusive society (Bailliard et al., 2020).

Drawing on Ife's (2002) work community development in occupational therapy that intends to be critical should use and generate theories and practices that focus on:

- Challenging the marginalisation of communities while contributing to developing their capabilities, enhancing the power communities have over their opportunities and choices.
- Developing partnerships with communities and honouring their right to both define their needs and have them met.
- Eradicating injustices through political actions that draw on processes of education, social planning and policy development and implementation.

Ngcobo's story (Box 30.1 Parts A and B) illuminates a situation where occupational therapy practice paid little attention to the influence of social and occupational injustices in people's lives and institutional practices sustained this way of operating, making it difficult to break with the dominant discourses limiting occupational therapy practice. However, through drawing on theories in occupational therapy, occupational science and community development, occupational therapists can identify ways to contribute to addressing the impact of exclusion and injustices that shape people's health. Different ways to collectively understand and work with these issues in partnership with communities are required to guide practice. The next section begins by broadly outlining some of the key features of occupational therapy in community development that can assist occupational therapists working in the domain of physical health. Thereafter, those features that guide the ways in which partnerships and understanding might be built are presented. As signalled earlier, there are various frameworks for guiding occupational therapy practices within community development. For the purposes of this chapter, the occupation-based community development framework in a country context of elevated levels of inequality and ongoing injustices is presented.

OCCUPATION-BASED COMMUNITY DEVELOPMENT AS CRITICAL COMMUNITY DEVELOPMENT IN OCCUPATIONAL THERAPY: KEY FEATURES

The occupation-based community development framework was developed through practice-based evidence to guide reasoning in community development practice. Occupation-based community development (ObCD) has been defined as 'a value-based form of occupational therapy practice with communities where doing is both the means and ends of actions that are aimed at bringing about changes in human connection and occupational engagement. ObCD involves long-term discursive processes where discourses and practices in and of everyday life are challenged' (Galvaan & Peters, 2013, p. 1). The outcomes are centred around realising liberated occupational engagement through resisting and challenging entrenched mindsets, unequal power relationships and structural inequalities (Galvaan & Peters, 2013).

The ObCD framework comprises four iterative phases: initiation, design, implementation and monitoring and reflection and evaluation. An overview of each phase is presented in Table 30.1. A fuller description of the phases is documented in online resources and other texts (Galvaan & Peters, 2013; Galvaan & Peters, 2017a, b).

When applying ObCD in practice the four phases are generally applied in a non-linear fashion. However, when initiating new partnerships with communities the process always begins with the initiation phase. The focus from identifying a person's needs within their environment to identifying a community's needs and the resources available aligns with the Initiation phase. As can be inferred from Table 30.1, a need refers to a gap between the current reality and what all involved believe it should be. Assessing these needs in community development practice occurs through collaborating and negotiating with community role players and stakeholders. It involves partnering with these role players and stakeholders to decide the focus of change, based on how the situation is understood. Different people within a collective may view the situation, needs and resources available differently. This may be influenced by multiple needs, competing

	TABLE 30.1
	Phases of the ObCD Framework
Initiation	This phase focuses on building authentic relationships with communities and on facilitating the development of a mutual and contextually situated understanding of the community's needs and priorities. This involves developing a picture of the different occupations in which groups within the community participate and how sociohistorical, economic, cultural and physical factors shape this participation. Developing this perspective of participation in occupations occurs through dialogue and participation with the community, analysing the gaps and potential for participation in alternative occupations together. Informed by a critical theoretical perspective, this analysis also includes identifying what the dominant and alternate ideologies are that inform prevailing discourses.
	The process of building collaborative relationships and a common understanding of community priorities in the initiation phase of the ObCD framework elucidates a reasoning process that explores how people may experience contexts as marginalising and who the target group might be. In the context of ObCD a target group is defined as a group who experiences marginalisation and whose occupational engagement is the focus of the process of developing mutual understanding. Members of the target group are part of the collaborative process of developing mutual understanding, but the identification of issues or situations that contribute to their needs might mean that other role players and stakeholders are worked with while attempting to resolve these issues and contribute towards change.
	The goal of the initiation phase is to generate a mutual understanding of the issues/situation at hand rather than imposing a singular truth. Each party's understanding shapes and grows through engaging together. This assists with identifying the complexities of the challenges to participation that people must navigate. Taking this perspective on community needs into account requires that a practitioner identify what the needs – beyond those that are clinical – are. This requires delving into the socio-economic and political influences on participation.
Design	Building an understanding of the need is an ongoing process, but once the community feels that they have developed an adequate understanding to begin addressing facets of this need the process of design unfolds through collaboratively formulating the strategies that will contribute to meeting these needs. Simultaneously, the necessary resources to support the proposed design are identified.
	The process of design involves the selection and application of both occupational science and occupational therapy theories that support and further the analysis and co-conceptualisation of the needs. The selected theories should also have the potential to guide the development of strategies to address the needs identified. Given the focus on marginalised groups and inequality, the occupational science constructs utilised must illuminate the social, historical, economic and political influences on occupational engagement. The politics of human occupation construct cluster (Ramugondo, 2015) is helpful for this.
Implementation	Implementing the proposed actions follows Design by drawing on methods that are suitable, given how the needs associated with participation in the occupation have been understood. Consistently reflecting on and modifying implementation accordingly is central to the successful application of the ObCD framework.
Monitoring, reflection and evaluation	Monitoring, reflection and evaluation involve developing indicators and approaches through which the community will monitor and evaluate how needs have been met. Ongoing reflection and concordant adjustments remain central. The development of indicators happens early in the process so that monitoring occurs against agreed-upon 'manifestations' of the proposed outcomes of the ObCD process.

priorities, opposing views on addressing the needs, different values, beliefs and languages. The initiation process is therefore a negotiated and evolving process that requires the use of certain principles, strategies and competencies that relate specifically to building this mutual understanding.

Following Ngcobo's realisation that a different approach to practice would be needed to effectively meet people's needs (Box 30.1 Part A), they acknowledged that a critical community development approach could enhance their practice in a physical health setting. In Box 30.1 Part B, Ngcobo illuminates the application of principles, strategies and competencies that contributed to developing a mutual understanding and to the inevitable redirection of the practice approach used by the rehabilitation team. The relevant

TABLE 30.2

Principles and strategies for building a mutual understanding.

Aim	Principles	Key strategies	Examples of helpful methods/practices/theories to enact strategies
Collaboration	The occupational therapist develops insights and learns with those concerned about the occupational participation of those who experience marginalisation as a consequence of injustice and inequity. The process is participatory and co-operative. The occupational therapist works with people involved in the situation to come to an understanding and is not the bearer of answers and/or solutions.	Explores occupational participation with community members. Formulates an understanding of who the 'target group' is and how their occupational participation is shaped.	Participatory and naturalistic observation Occupational storytelling Productive inquiry (Jandernoa & Gillespie, 2007) Photovoice (Breny & McMorrow, 2020; Galvaan, 2008)
Facilitation	The occupational therapist is part of *facilitating* the process of coming to understand differently. There is an expectation that the occupational therapist's understanding will be influenced by this process. The occupational therapist explores with those involved in the situation what the different facets of it are, as well as how the situation is viewed and understood by different individuals and collectives.	Consults with community role players and stakeholders, building relationships to support the emergence of a shared understanding. Suspends own assumptions about the issues identified and is willing to be changed by the process. Poses critical questions that are capable of opening opportunities to explore alternative/new understanding and are not only about information for the occupational therapist. Analyses issues from the perspective of the systems involved in shaping everyday life. Employs strategies from development practice for facilitating processes.	Productive conversations (Senge, 2006) Problem-posing (Hope & Timmel, 1984) Action-learning (Taylor et al., 2005) System's thinking (Senge, 2006) Process-based facilitation (Olive-PPT Publications, 2007)
Identity work	The occupational therapist acts as both an objective and subjective insider.	Navigates and negotiates own identity in a relational way. Analyses how intersectionality dynamics play out and influence relationships in practice, shaping how mutual understanding emerges to prioritise particular groups and needs.	Intersectionality theory (Yuval-Davis, 2006) Critical questions that inform reasoning in the Initiation phase (Galvaan & Peters, 2013)

aims, principles and strategies drawn on from ObCD in Ngcobo's story are presented in Table 30.2 and the core competencies that are necessary to enact these are listed in Table 30.3.

The competencies occupational therapists should acquire to understand a community's needs are drawn from organisational learning and development theories (Taylor, 2000). These competencies are often taken for granted, expecting that they are automatic for practitioners. However, the development and implementation of the ObCD framework can show that the use of these competencies in practice requires considerable skill and should be given more attention in occupational therapy education and practice.

Since contributions towards a community's health and well-being are constructed in response to issues

TABLE 30.3
Core Competencies for Building Mutual Understanding (Taylor, 2000)

1. **The ability to question:** Embracing an openness to asking a series of questions when the problem is not well defined is key to development practice. Learning to construct incisive questions that enable observation, exploration and understanding of diverse perspectives, values and beliefs about a situation allows new ways of understanding what could be changed to emerge. Open-ended questions and follow-up questions inquiring into the situation aim to elicit more knowledge about the situation. These kinds of questions are 'reservoirs' for unlocking dialogue that can allow individuals and collectives to work together as they develop new ways of understanding that can support desired change. Surfacing incisive questions thrives with deep listening and observing.

2. **The ability to actively listen and observe:** Listening and observation are skills that are often employed by occupational therapists to extract diagnostic information. Emphasis is on listening and observing to see and understand afresh through deeply focusing on who is speaking, what is being said and how it is said. This active listening can inspire people to see and hear in ways that unlock unconscious bias that may exist. The thinking environment (Kline, 1999) and organisational learning theories (Senge, 2006) can support the development of this skill.

3. **The ability to bring meaning:** Bringing meaning is a process that can be orchestrated through different means but can also evolve organically. Storytelling and picture-building are tools very often used to initiate the opportunity to bring and build on meaning. It is important here to note that the occupational therapist is not an 'outsider' to the processes being facilitated, and the intent is not to colonise understanding and promote certain agendas. The idea is to offer a tentative meaning through drawing on the careful listening, questioning and observing being done 'with'. This then acts as an invitation to refute, further construct and shape the understanding being developed through these processes. The occupation-based community development framework recognises that this process can be facilitated in different ways. The ideas that Freire offers in his work on problem-posing (Hope & Timmel, 1984) are especially illuminating. Using constructed codes to bring meaning and initiate necessary dialogue can effectively shape the opportunity to bring meaning through this collectively oriented process (Hope & Timmel, 1984).

identified, designated approaches cannot be applied prescriptively (Galvaan, 2021). To ensure that the process is worked with fluidly, action-learning is a central tool used throughout the application of the phases of ObCD. Action-learning enables the co-reflection and co-analysis of actions and reactions as they emerge in reality. It provides the occupational therapist with a rigorous and accessible approach to engaging with emergent processes. The use of action-learning as it is embedded within ObCD is illustrated in Box 30.2.

The two practice stories in this chapter demonstrate the value that a community development practice 'lens' could contribute to already beneficial occupational therapy services. However, embracing such an approach to practice will take a concerted effort from occupational therapists to re-imagine their role and advocate for institutional changes that allow such a role to be enacted. This is not necessarily an easy task. This is illustrated in Box 30.1 Part C in which Ngcobo voices the frustration and tension of advocating for critical community development to be a complimentary aspect of the occupational therapy services offered in hospital-based settings.

CONCLUSION: AN INVITATION

When people who experience illness, injury and impairment choose to utilise occupational therapy services they are not just bringing their bodies, they are bringing their *whole lives*. This should make occupational therapists sit up and take more critical note of whether the services being offered truly address the needs that are part of this 'whole'. When occupational therapists deal with the intricacies, complexities and contradictions that are part of people's lives – particularly those whose lives are deeply impacted by issues of inequity and injustice – there are seldom quick fixes. However, working with and through the discomfort of not necessarily having fast and easy solutions to address the underlying causes of illness, injury and impairment should push occupational therapists to be more collaborative in order to innovate towards change.

This chapter has presented the opportunity that exists for occupational therapists working within services that address illness, injury and impairment to draw on a critical community development practice as

BOX 30.2

BONGIWE AND LIEZL'S STORY – ACTION-LEARNING SUPPORTS THE FACILITATION OF A SHARED UNDERSTANDING

Bongiwe and Liezl's story illustrates how action-learning might be applied as part of facilitating the development of shared understanding within an under-resourced community with an organisation focused on the needs of people with disabilities. In 2016 Bongiwe and Liezl were final-year occupational therapy students at the University of Cape Town. They were placed at an organisation known as the Cape Town Association for the Physically Disabed (CTAPD) to complete a practical learning placement.

At the time of their placement, CTAPD supported a group of disabled people in one of Cape Town's largest and oldest townships. The leader of this group was interested in having CTAPD invest their services to support the group in developing income generation and alternative participation opportunities. As part of this investment, the organisation requested that Bongiwe and Liezl contribute to the support that the group needed. Later this group developed into their own registered organisation, but at the time that Bongiwe and Liezl assisted them, they met each day in a local pastor's garage.

When the students first met with the group they were interested in positioning themselves as fellow 'learners' who would join with the group to collectively understand their needs and goals. Since the group was sure that they wanted to focus on income generation, the process of facilitating the development of a mutual understanding involved uncovering the various barriers that were preventing them from meeting this need. Bongiwe and Liezl recognised that action-learning (Taylor et al., 2005) would support both the process of further exploring this need through sharing their previous actions in attempting to address it, and in being able to reflect on and learn from new actions that they may plan to take in response. Action-learning involves four consolidated phases that are applied in an integrated way (Taylor et al., 2005):

1. Action: taking action/sharing previous actions taken;
2. Reflection: focusing intentionally on the actions that have occurred in order to interrogate how and why these actions emerged as they did;
3. Learning: drawing out key points of learning by focusing on the insights generated through reflection; and
4. Planning: determining which action(s) should be taken in response to this learning as a way of moving forward towards positive change.

The group's initial sharing of previous stories revealed that a key factor influencing their opportunity to participate in work was their limited transport options. In South Africa, many people who are not able to afford cars take public transport. One of the most common forms of public transport in South Africa is minibus taxis. Minibus taxis are often filled to capacity in order to ensure that their operators accrue enough profit. This means that people in wheelchairs and those using other mobility devices are frequently ignored when they attempt to hail a minibus taxi because their devices take up too much room. When they are picked up, they are required to pay an additional fee for their device. This makes the cost of seeking employment substantial and was leaving the members of the group with limited choices in being able to address this situation. As a result of the collaborative unpacking of these stories through action-learning the group recognised that, while they were the target group of any change they wanted to bring about, there were other stakeholders who would need to be involved in addressing this situation. Chief among these stakeholders were the taxi drivers. Through the facilitated process of the reflection and learning phases of action-learning, the members of the group recognised that they would need to partner with taxi owners and drivers if they wanted to change the situation in relation to this particular issue.

The group resolved to take action to have conversations with the taxi drivers at their local taxi rank as a way of beginning to self-advocate and develop a partnership with them. Group members planned for how they would do this and, with the support of Bongiwe and Liezl, they took these actions interdependently. While this was daunting and did not immediately resolve the situation, upon reflection the group realised that while the taxi drivers seemed to be reluctant to immediately agree, they were open to talking further. The group's actions had opened a pathway to further understanding. This led to the recognition that building a mutual understanding had to continue with taxi drivers and extend beyond the immediate target group.

Bongiwe and Liezl's story illustrates that the development of mutual understanding is a process that emerges over time and requires both action and facilitation. It is not passive, instead requiring the active involvement of multiple stakeholders. This is because as shared understanding is shaped it supports how mindsets might be differentially shaped. This can contribute to shifting the dominant hegemonies that constrain disabled peoples' lives and prevent their social inclusion in society. Working in this way to address the social determinants of health had the potential to positively change members of the group's lives.

a way of beginning to collaborate with collectives so that addressing the social determinants of health and well-being, through focusing on the causes of exclusion and injustice, becomes a more realistic probability. Through the use of Ngcobo, Bongiwe and Liezl's practice stories, the principles, strategies and competencies of occupation-based community development have been explained and demonstrated.

The World Federation of Occupational Therapist's position statement on community-centred practice (2019) encourages occupational therapists to establish community-level practice roles. Leaning into this invitation, relying more actively on a critical community development practice approach and being willing to change has the potential to lead occupational therapists towards a more responsive occupational therapy practice.

Acknowledgements

We acknowlege our final year occupational therapy students from 2016, Bongiwe Gumede and Liezl Putuma, who generously applied themselves during their practice learning block and whose practice story - shared in this text - provided an opportunity for deeper learning about how action-learning might be used in partership with communities.

REFERENCES

Bailliard, A. L., Dallman, A. R., Carroll, A., Lee, B. D., & Szendrey, S. (2020). Doing Occupational Justice: A Central Dimension of Everyday Occupational Therapy Practice. *Canadian Journal of Occupational Therapy, 87*(2), 144–152. https://doi.org/10.1177/0008417419899930.

Breny, J. M., & McMorrow, S. L. (2020). *Photovoice for social justice: Visual representation in action.* SAGE Publications Incorporated.

Farias, L., & Laliberte Rudman, D. (2019). Practice analysis: Critical reflexivity on discourses constraining socially transformative occupational therapy practices. *British Journal of Occupational Therapy, 82*(11), 693–697. https://doi.org/10.1177/0308022619862111.

Galvaan, R. (2008). Getting the Picture: The process of participation. In N. de Lange, C. Mitchell, & J. Stuart (Eds.), *Putting People in the Picture: Visual methodologies for social change.* Sense Publishers BV.

Galvaan, R. (2021). Generative disruption through occupational science: Enacting possibilities for deep human connection. *Journal of Occupational Science, 28*(1), 6–18. https://doi.org/10.1080/14427591.2020.1818276.

Galvaan, R., & Peters, L. (2013). *Open Education Resource: A strategy for occupation-based community development.* http://hdl.handle.net/11427/6651

Galvaan, R., & Peters, L. (2017a). Occupation-based Community Development: A critical approach to occupational therapy. In S. Dsouza, R. Galvaan, & E. Ramugondo (Eds.), *Concepts in Occupational therapy: Understanding Southern Perspectives.* Manupal University Press.

Galvaan, R., & Peters, L. (2017b). Occupation-based community development: Confronting the Politics of Occupation. In N. Pollard, & D. Sakeleriou (Eds.), *Occupational Therapies without Borders: Integrating justice with practice* (2nd ed.). Elsevier Limited.

Hammell, K. R. W., & Iwama, M. K. (2012). Well-being and occupational rights: An imperative for critical occupational therapy [Article]. *Scandinavian Journal of Occupational Therapy, 19*(5), 385–394. https://doi.org/10.3109/11038128.2011.611821.

Hope, A., & Timmel, S. (1984). *Training for Transformation: a handbook for community workers.* Mambo Press.

Hyett, N., Kenny, A., & Dickson-Swift, V. (2019). Re-imagining occupational therapy clients as communities: Presenting the community-centred practice framework. *Scandinavian Journal of Occupational Therapy, 26*(4), 246–260. https://doi.org/10.1080/11038128.2017.1423374.

Ife, J. (2002). *Community Development: Community-based alternatives in an age of globalisation* (2nd ed.). Pearson Education Australia.

Jandernoa, B., & Gillespie, B. (2007). *Leadership for Collective Learning and Action. Course 1.*

Kline, N. (1999). *Time to Think: Listening to ignite the human mind.* Cassell Illustrated.

Lathouras, A. (2016). A Critical Approach To Citizen-Led Social Work: Putting the political back into community development practice. *Social Alternatives, 35*(4), 32–36.

Leclair, L., Lauckner, H., & Yamamoto, C. (2019). An occupational therapy community development practice process. *Canadian Journal of Occupational Therapy, 86*(5), 345–356. https://doi.org/10.1177/0008417419832457.

Lopes, R. E., & Malfitano, A. P. S. (Eds.). (2021). *Social Occupational Therapy: Theoretical and Practical Designs.* Elsevier, Inc.

Olive-PPT Publications. (2007). *Part 1: Introducing Facilitation. Ideas, definitions and descriptions of key concepts.* In *Facilitating Development Processes.* Olive-PPT Publications.

Ramugondo, E. (2015). Occupational Consciousness. *Journal of Occupational Science, 22*(4), 1–14.

Restall, G., & Egan, M. (2022). Key characteristics of relationship-focused practice. In M. Egan, & G. Restall (Eds.), *Promoting occupational participation: Collaborative relationship-focused occupational therapy* (pp. 101). Canadian Association of Occupational Therapists.

Robertson, D., Warrender, F., & Barnard, S. (2015). The critical occupational therapy practitioner: How to define expertise? *Australian occupational therapy journal, 62*(1), 68–71. https://doi.org/10.1111/1440-1630.12157.

Senge, P. (2006). *The Fifth Discipline. The art and practice of the learning organisation.* Random House Business Books.

Taylor, J. (2000). *Organisations and Development. Towards Building a Practice*. Community Development Resource Association.

Taylor, J., Marais, D., & Kaplan, A. (2005). *Action Learning. A Developmental Approach to Change*. Community Development Resource Association. Retrieved 05/12 from. http://www.cdra.org.za/index.php?option=com_content&view=article&id=59:action-learning-a-developmental-approach-to-change.

World Federation of Occupational Therapists. (2019). Position Statement. Occupational Therapy and Community-Centred Practice.

Yuval-Davis, N. (2006). Intersectionality and Feminist Politics. *European Journal of Women's Studies, 13*(3), 193–209.

REFLECTION

1. Dominant discourses and resource limitations have been shown to limit the way occupational therapy can be practised. Do you have any experiences where the dominant discourses framing your occupational therapy practice and resource limitations did not allow you to address the needs of the people you were working with?

2. Briefly explain the priorities of a community-development focused occupational therapy practice.

3. Describe the key aims, principles and strategies that could be drawn on from the 'Initiation' phase of occupation-based community development to support practice with people who experience illness, injury and impairment.

4. Explain the key competencies occupational therapists should develop in order to support their skill in contributing to building a mutual understanding?

5. Critical community development is positioned to enable occupational therapists to engage with the conditions shaping peoples' lives more adequately. What opportunities exist within your practice setting to use the principles and strategies presented in this chapter in order to engage with the conditions that shape the lives of the people you work with?

Section 4

SKILLS AND STRATEGIES TO SUPPORT THE PROMOTION OF OCCUPATIONAL PARTICIPATION

ASSISTIVE TECHNOLOGY

NATASHA A. LAYTON

CHAPTER OUTLINE

Overview

The role of assistive technology (AT) in enabling occupational participation is the focus of this chapter. Using the Canadian Occupational Therapy Inter-relation Practice Process (COTIPP) the role of the occupational therapist in AT provision is reviewed. The societal and practice contexts in which occupational therapists recommend AT are discussed, as well as the challenges of balancing pragmatic concerns with collaborative relationship-focused outcomes. The dynamic pace of technology innovation and design movements, such as the universal and inclusive design movements, are altering perspectives of technology and the idea of mainstream or specialised assistive products. Good practice principles from the perspective of AT users and AT literature are presented in this chapter, providing a contemporary frame

of reference as a way forward to realise the potential of AT to meet people's occupational participation goals. These principles are described and illustrated in three practice stories of people who use AT.

KEY POINTS

- Assistive technology (AT) and accessible environments form a 'technology chain' used by all humans on the spectrum of human variation.

- AT can enable occupational participation when tailored to the person, environment and occupation.

- Effective matching of person, environment and AT to enable occupational participation often requires skilled service provision.

- Professional reasoning and person-empowerment are critical to AT provision.

- International good practice principles for AT provision exist and can be linked to the Canadian Occupational Therapy Inter-relation Practice Process.

- The availability, selection and uptake of AT are influenced by socio-political factors.

- Systemic/political practice of occupational therapy may be indicated where there are societal barriers to realising good practice.

INTRODUCTION

Occupational therapists engage with consumers to promote occupational participation. Assistive technology (AT) is a key strategy to facilitating this. Occupational therapists also understand that occupational participation is an outcome of the transaction among the person, environment and occupation (Law et al., 1996).

This chapter provides an overview of the role of the occupational therapist in prescribing AT to promote occupational participation. A range of theoretical approaches to design, outcomes measurement and coproduction are provided. Three practice stories are included to illustrate the implementation of AT strategies and interventions.

DEFINING ASSISTIVE TECHNOLOGY

A range of terms have been used to describe technology that mediates the effects of impairment or minimises barriers within the environment, for example, rehabilitation technology, everyday technologies, adapted technologies, healthcare technologies, or medical devices. In this chapter, the term AT or assistive product has been used. That is because AT is the *umbrella term* for assistive products and the services, often provided by occupational therapists, to fit the assistive product to the person, their occupations and their environments. The ICF describe AT as enabling individuals to 'perform tasks they would otherwise be unable to do or increases the ease and safety with which tasks can be performed' (WHO, 2001, p. 10). The international standard, ISO 9999, provides a classification and terminology of assistive products, 'especially produced or generally available, for persons to optimize functioning and reduce disability' (ISO, 2022, p. 7).

These definitions offer a critical departure from previous approaches and are in line with current approaches to inclusive design, as the definitions include commonly available products when these provide assistance to people living with impairment to participate and engage in occupations (ISO, 2022). How AT is defined is important as the definition can affect whether a particular technology will be funded. If having an impairment is seen to require *special* products this can lead to policies where mainstream items such as a digital tablet (e.g. iPad) are not eligible for funding, even if this could replace a more costly communication device.

Currently, the international taxonomy enables any assistive product to be theoretically classified. The International Organization for Standardization (ISO) 9999 classification system offers over 650 product categories across 11 classes, which are listed in Table 31.1. The non-consecutive numbering of the classes allows space for future categories to be added. Within each class, three levels of classification are offered: for example, class 12 denotes assistive products for personal mobility, with 18 subclasses including walking products, cars, cycles, wheelchairs and transferring and turning products, with additional divisions for powered wheelchairs, foot-driven wheelchairs and so on.

Within most of these broad classes, a range of complexity is evident. Some assistive products (e.g. an angled comb) may be categorised as *straightforward, noncomplex* or *low tech* (Cook & Polgar, 2015). Some assistive products have inherent technological complexity yet are relatively straightforward in terms of a therapy recommendation (e.g. noise-cancelling headphones). Other simple assistive products become complex in terms of their application and utility: a palmar pocket and pointer to maximise hand function for someone who has paralysis of upper limb muscles following a cervical spinal cord injury may be adapted for a range of small products (spoon, toothbrush) and even digital items. In this last example, generally available or *mainstream* technologies deliver significant outcomes if planned with a full spectrum of occupational participation goals in mind. Occupational therapists bring skills in professional reasoning to envision the potential of AT to support a person's occupational participation goals, grounded in an understanding of the interaction of AT and environmental factors. The next section considers the relationship between products and services or therapeutic supports.

TABLE 31.1

International Organization for Standardization (ISO) Classification

Class	Description	Example products	Within the scope of practice of (some examples)
04	Assistive products for measuring, stimulating or training physiological and psychological functions	■ Respiratory supports ■ Medication management systems ■ Memory training	■ Dietitians ■ Occupational therapists ■ Prosthetists/orthotists ■ Physiotherapists ■ Speech pathologists ■ Nurses ■ Educators
06	Orthoses and prostheses	■ Hand splints (orthotics) ■ In-shoe orthotics ■ Lower limb prosthesis	■ Occupational therapists ■ Prosthetists/orthotists ■ Physiotherapists ■ Podiatrists ■ Pedorthists
09	Assistive products for self-care activities and participation in self-care	■ Adapted clothing ■ Shower stool ■ Continence products	■ Occupational therapists ■ Nurses
12	Assistive products for activities and participation relating to personal mobility and transportation	■ Wheelchairs ■ Vehicle adaptations ■ Transfer supports ■ Mobile hoists	■ Occupational therapists ■ Physiotherapists ■ Exercise physiologists
15	Assistive products for domestic activities and participation in domestic life	■ Adapted cutting board ■ Wheeled laundry basket ■ Long-handled gardening equipment	■ Occupational therapists ■ Dietitians
18	Furnishings, fixtures and other assistive products for supporting activities in the indoor and outdoor human-made environments	■ Rise/recline lounge chair ■ Adjustable bed ■ Fold down grabrails ■ Portable ramps	■ Occupational therapists
22	Assistive products for communication and information management	■ Hearing loops; electronic communication devices; adapted computer mouse	■ Occupational therapists ■ Speech pathologists ■ Audiologists
24	Assistive products for controlling, carrying, moving and handling objects and devices	■ Environmental control units for operating devices from a distance ■ Assistive products for extended reach ■ Forearm support for computer use ■ Non-slip products	■ Occupational therapists ■ Physiotherapists
27	Assistive products for controlling, adapting or measuring elements of physical environments	■ Air filters ■ products for reducing vibration ■ Lighting management products ■ Noise-cancelling headphones	■ Occupational therapists ■ Physiotherapists ■ Dietitians ■ Audiologists
28	Assistive products for work activities and participation in employment	■ Workstations ■ Lifting platforms ■ Adapted tools ■ Alarms and monitors	■ Occupational therapists ■ Physiotherapists ■ Exercise physiologists ■ Rehabilitation counsellors/ergonomists
30	Assistive products for recreation and leisure	■ Adapted saddles ■ Sports wheelchairs ■ One-handed playing card holders	■ Occupational therapists ■ Physiotherapists ■ Exercise physiologists

ISO, International Organization for Standardization.

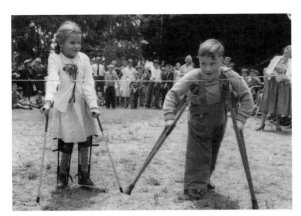

Fig. 31.1 ■ Children using callipers and crutches at the Yooralla Sports Day in Victoria, Australia, 1958. (Courtesy Rosslyn Pickhaver and Polio Australia.)

HUMANS AND TECHNOLOGY

From the time early human beings fashioned tools, technology has been a critical enabler of occupation participation. Technology use is ubiquitous and in many ways a seamless element of identity. Possessing the newest smartphone, for example, can be experienced as a marker of status. The same is rarely said for AT (Hocking, 1999; Barbareschi et al., 2021). Assistive technology developments over the 19th and 20th centuries were characteristically medically focused and institutionalised in intent and appearance (Albrecht, Seelman, & Bury, 2001; Liu, 2018). In line with the medical model lens, products focused on managing basic activities such as self-care and mobility. The resulting independent living market, although certainly providing necessary AT, dominated perceptions of what people living with impairment can and should aspire to and use, and in some ways has contributed to the othering, or problematic identity, of disability.

An example of identity related to assistive products is that of hiking poles versus a walking stick: both provide a point of support for walking, but one presents an image of outdoor recreation, whereas the other is more likely to be associated with age or infirmity. Historical images of assistive products (variously termed equipment, invalid aids, or appliances) include leather and buckle callipers (Fig. 31.1), medical implements and specially adapted homes. Current and future developments include robotics, exoskeletal products, augmented and virtual reality applications and smart home technology. Effectively, then, AT represents a strategy that can either enable or disable a person's occupational participation.

The reluctance of people to use compensatory and/or AT (Hansson, 2007) may speak to the fact that assistive products have been seen as markers of illness and loss, identity and stigma (Cook & Polgar, 2015; Hocking, 1999). Assistive products have typically been designed, manufactured and marketed by niche suppliers for the disabled other (Hobbs et al., 2009; Renda et al., 2016), and the resulting lack of consultation and consideration regarding the views, attitudes and tastes of individuals correlates with AT nonuse and abandonment (Scherer & Federici, 2015; Cruz et al., 2016; World Health Organisation, 2022).

A range of ethical issues has emerged in the wake of new inventions. Nonhuman designs such as prosthetic cheetah legs are no longer replacing or augmenting human functioning; they in fact provide superhuman capabilities (Fig. 31.2). A range of technologies such as robots to replace personal care from other humans (e.g. to perform the functions of a mobile hoist), or robotic pets to simulate nurturing, introduce the risk that technology will replace human contact. Critical writings from the disability perspective warn that the needs and autonomy of people living with impairment may become subordinated to the technologies in use. The rapid diversification of enabling technologies holds significant implications for AT users and for occupational therapists who recommend AT.

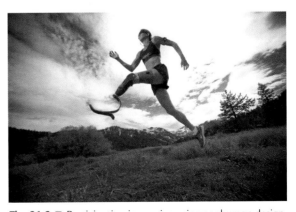

Fig. 31.2 ■ Participation in running using nonhuman design. (From Chabner (2012).)

The 2022 WHO/ UNICEF Global Report on Assistive Technology (2022) sets out a case for the value of assistive products and services and proposes that AT is provided as a human right, within universal health care. AT enables people to realised their human rights (Smith et al., 2022) and delivers on the United Nations' Sustainable Development Goals (Tebbutt et al., 2016). In many countries and jurisdictions, AT funding is limited to assistive products to support body functions and structures or for the purpose of safety or independence. This becomes problematic because it perpetuates the medical model view of disability and may prevent recognition of the potential of AT to support inclusion through diverse participation (Ripat & Woodgate, 2012). AT users are challenging this situation, asking if people living with disability have a 'right to the frivolous' (Barbareschi & Shakespeare, 2021).

THE CAPABILITY APPROACH

One contemporary theory that addresses human needs in a human rights paradigm is the capability approach (Nussbaum, 2011; Sen, 1999; Layton & Borg, 2023). The capability approach identifies what is needed for people, given their capabilities and the limitations of their environments, to achieve outcomes. The capability approach is congruent with occupational therapy practice. It relocates problems or deficits away from the individual, allowing for the social model of disability's notion of disablement by the environment, and embraces the political practice of occupational therapy (Pollard et al., 2008) and can be explained from the perspective of person, environment and occupation.

Person

To engage in occupation and to reach goals and aspirations, individuals call upon their capabilities. Human capabilities consist of abilities (capacities) and personal factors. Abilities include body structures and functions as well as personality and resilience. Personal factors include such things as demographics, circles of support and socioeconomic situation. The full set of capabilities for each person depends on three interrelated elements: innate skills and capacity to function; agency or freedom to choose to engage in valued occupations; and whether the environment enables or inhibits the person to flourish (e.g. whether the person is affected

by, for example, poverty or discrimination) (Whalley Hammell, 2015).

The term 'disability' has been used to describe impairment and/or the presence of barriers to promoting occupational participation. Usually, this is applied to people living with the effects of congenital or acquired impairment. Many people with an impairment note that the term *disability* is stigmatising and represents a focus on a person's limitations rather than strengths. A more holistic view is that impairments are part of universal human variation (Bickenbach et al., 1999; Patston, 2007). In other words, having strengths and challenges is a feature of being human, and, taking a lifespan view, will be experienced by all humans at some stage in their lives. In this view, mediating the capability gap is an ongoing, relational and human interaction and exchange. An example would be the personal support that a frail older person may receive from a neighbour. Many supports have profound impacts and are seen as entirely common such as glasses and hearing aids used to augment body functions and fill sensory capability gaps.

Environment

Disability scholars have observed that the experience of disability has a lot to do with barriers within the environment and low expectations from the nondisabled world. This social model of disability (Shakespeare, 2008) approach argues that the environment plays a key role in disablement, and as a result, issues of person/environment fit should not be perceived as problems within an individual.

As well as using capabilities to engage in tasks and to reach desired outcomes, people use a range of accommodations and supports. Examples include a continuous path of travel making it possible to move from home to work or using an elevator to arrive at the 20th floor of a building for a meeting. Some people require more accommodations and support than others, to mediate or fill the 'gap' between aspiration and capability. The concept of a capability gap (Nussbaum, 2011) is powerful in that it opens space for the idea of occupational fit.

Occupation

Occupational participation is influenced by the congruence – or lack of it – between a person's capabilities and occupational goals, that is, the occupations that a person wishes to engage and participate in and what the person must master to achieve this outcome. Professor Stephen Hawking, a world-renowned Cambridge-based physicist, participated in an active educational and economic life. His particular capability gap was significant, as his only reliable motor response was a blink of an eye gaze. This capability gap was mediated with a sophisticated AT solution including a specialised seating system, head-controlled wheelchair and eye-gaze-operated communication system. The occupational participation goal of an economic and educational life, given the accommodations in place, was achieved. In contrast, the capability gap of a person with vision impairment in the urban city of Bangalore, India, who wishes to learn a trade may require several relatively straightforward accommodations, including tactile indicators, education and resources in Braille and a reliable path of travel. Although this person may be able to move around their home through tactile sensing, they may be unable to rely on environmental supports outside their front door. There may be no tactile indicators present on the unmade roads and no safe access to transport or Braille supports at the trade college. Further, poverty, gender and their position in the caste system may represent additional barriers to the goal of a trade qualification and employment. This could lead to the capability gap remaining, the person's potential unrealised, and the occupational participation goals of education and work unmet.

ASSISTIVE, UNIVERSAL, INCLUSIVE DESIGN AND THE TECHNOLOGY CHAIN

As technology is all about augmenting human capabilities, it is difficult to think of any technology that is not assistive. However, there are many examples of products that require effort or adaptation on the part of the human user, such as complex mobile phone interfaces, poor colour contrast and tiny symbols on television remote controls and can openers that require two hands to operate. Design has typically focused on the archetypal user, usually understood to be an adult male. As a consequence, many products such as seating, workbench height and reach range are designed using anthropometric measurements that do not match the user requirements of the population as a whole (Imrie & Hall, 2001).

The first wave of user-focused design came to be known as the universal design movement. Universal design focuses on accommodating the needs of the majority of users through the application of universal design principles (equitable use, flexibility in use, simple and intuitive use, perceptible information, tolerance for error, low physical effort and size and space for approach and use) (Steinfeld & Danford, 2006). The majority of users is usually taken to mean a majority percentage of the population bell curve, up to the 80th or 90th decile. This is depicted in Fig. 31.3A and B. The

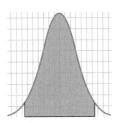

a) Frequency distribution Bell curve

Locating the human population as norms or outliers

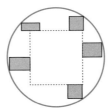

b) Specialist disability design

Does not address the population as a whole

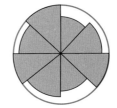

c) Designed for diversity

Design for diversity removes disable/able bias

Fig. 31.3 ■ Contrasting conceptualisations of the human population in ergonomics, universal design and inclusive design (Acknowledgement of these inclusive design concepts is made to Dong, H. (2007). Shifting paradigms in universal design. In C. Stephanidis (Ed.), *Universal access in human computer interaction: Coping with diversity* (pp. 66–74). Springer-Verlag and Wijk, M. (2001). The Dutch struggle for accessibility awareness. In W. F. Preiser & E. Ostroff (Eds.), *Universal design handbook* (pp. 1–28). McGraw-Hill.)

universal design approach therefore endeavours to meet the needs of 80% to 90% of users but is unlikely to cater for the needs of the outliers or last deciles on the curve.

Universal design tenets have shifted towards an inclusive view of the population (Steinfeld, 2010) and address the needs of most but not all. Inclusive design uses a 'deep understanding of diversity' (Dong, 2007, p. 70) to move beyond norms and outliers. From an inclusive design perspective, the traditional bell curve population is now characterised as a circular entirety with a series of segments that capture the ergonomic diversity of the population (Dong, 2007) (Fig. 31.3C). An inclusive design perspective can be illustrated by a common kitchen aid such as a potato peeler: a small moulded pistol-grip potato peeler suits both adolescent hand size and older people with weakened grip caused by arthritic conditions; a heavier cylindrical-grip potato peeler suits adults with large hands but poor dexterity as well as people with athetoid upper limb and hand movements. These examples illustrate that differently tailored designs can meet the diverse needs of the whole population, where a single design might only meet the needs of a proportion, albeit a large proportion, of that population. The special aspects of the designs are marketed in a way that does not distinguish disability but rather distinguishes particular design features. Such inclusivity has the potential for a paradigm shift from 'designing special aids and equipment for disabled people (an AT approach), to designing mainstream products for as many people as possible (a universal design approach)' (Dong, 2007, p. 67; Holloway & Barbareschi, 2022).

As design becomes democratised the role of AT users should also extend into the design and testing of AT products, a strategy that will address a long history of exclusion from research, design and development. Exciting developments are occurring between product and user experience designers, occupational therapists and AT users (Renda et al., 2016). Such inclusion strategies have the potential to ameliorate, in part, the abandonment and nonuse of assistive products and to normalise and universalise disability technologies (Scherer, 2020; Desmond et al., 2018)

Assistive products are always used in an environmental context, and the substantial relationship between AT and environmental interventions has been conceptualised as a technology chain. For example, the provision of products such as a bath seat will not be required if the shower over a bath is replaced with a step-less shower recess and a built-in propping ledge; in other words, the barriers or facilitators of environments create or remove the need for a specific AT or aspect of personal support.

ASSISTIVE TECHNOLOGY IN THE CONTEXT OF OTHER INTERVENTIONS

Occupational therapists have a range of skills and strategies available to them to promote occupational participation. A useful tool to understand the provision of assistive products in relation to other interventions, and to outcomes, is the IMPACT 2 Model developed by Roger Smith and colleagues (Smith, 2002, 2017) (Fig. 31.4). The model demonstrates that outcomes can be described by considering the following six stages: (1) pre-intervention, (2) context, (3) baseline, (4) intervention approaches, (5) outcome covariates and (6) outcomes. A left-to-right bold arrow indicates the direction.

Pre-intervention strategies to improve functional performance, universal design and health promotion, can be seen in the lower left-hand corner as part of the person–task–environment context. The Context stage is represented as the person using AT to perform a task within an environment. Intervention approaches consist of six methods available to improve functional performance. These are: (1) reduce the impairment, (2) compensate for the impairment, (3) use AT devices and services, (4) redesign the activity, (5) redesign the environment and (6) use personal assistance. Occupational therapists will often use one or more strategies in collaboration with the people with whom they work. To illustrate this strategies for a person living with arthritis in relation to gardening are presented in Table 31.2.

Measuring function before an intervention is a crucial step to be able to establish if performance, quality of life and participation, change for the person. It is also important to identify any covariates or variables that are happening at the same time and that may impact the person's outcomes. Measuring outcomes after the intervention involves reevaluation of the individual's performance, quality of life and participation. This will determine how effective the intervention is (Smith, 2002; Federici & Scherer, 2017).

THE IMPACT² MODEL

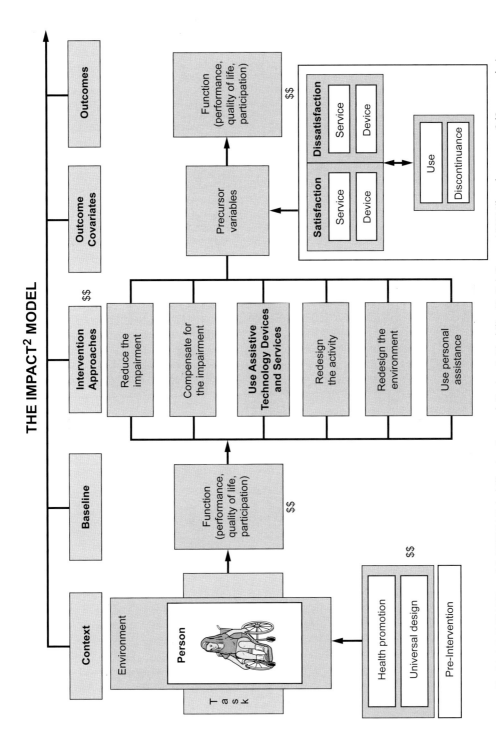

Fig 31.4 ■ IMPACT model. (©2004 Rehabilitation Research Design & Disability (R₂D₂) Center, UW-Milwaukee, www.r2d2.uwm.edu.)

TABLE 31.2

Strategies for a Person Living with Arthritis in Relation to Gardening

Intervention example: Participating in gardening with arthritis

Reducing the impairment
Medical or surgical procedures, for example, hand splinting to align and support joints

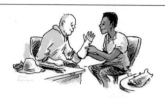

Compensating for the impairment
Use joint protection techniques; indoor garden only; have artificial plants

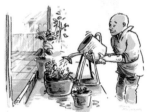

Redesigning the activity
Work simplification techniques, and work rest routines

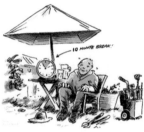

Using assistive products
For example, garden kneeler, long-handled tools; power grip on tools; robo-mower

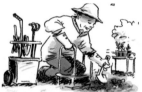

Redesigning the environment
No-dig garden design; raised garden beds, install an automatic watering system

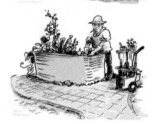

Using personal assistance
Paid gardener; exchange garden produce for in-kind garden help

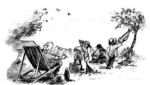

ASSISTIVE PRODUCTS, AND THE SERVICES OR SUPPORTS THAT FIT PRODUCTS TO PERSON, OCCUPATION AND ENVIRONMENT

A substantial evidence base demonstrates that assistive products are most effective when provided alongside key services and supports (Scherer & Federici, 2015; WHO/UNICEF, 2022). Imagine a non-ambulant person obtaining a wheelchair for the first time, planning to move around the home and community but with no prior knowledge or skills. They are likely to experience difficulty, when using the wheelchair, in reaching bench tops, manoeuvring through doorways and transporting the wheelchair in a car. Tailored supports are essential to ensure that assistive products meet the needs of the users, for example, wheelchair skills training (Dalhousie University, n.d.; International Society of Wheelchair Professionals, n.d.).

A range of terms have been used to identify the interrelated nature of support and product (Cook & Polgar, 2015). In Australia, the term wraparound support is used to articulate the 'human' ingredients of an AT bundle for funding purposes (Layton et al., 2024b) and is gaining traction in AT policy redesign.

The Occupational Therapist and Wraparound Supports

A range of stakeholders provide wraparound support. Work is underway globally to explore AT capabilities given global workforce shortages, as well as the consumer empowerment agenda (WHO/UNICEF, 2022; Layton et al., 2021). When delivering wraparound support, it is useful to consider the relationship with the person who will use the AT, what they may want from their service delivery, and good practice steps in providing wraparound support.

Firstly, at the foundation of any intervention is the therapeutic alliance between occupational therapists and the people with whom they work (Kayes & McPherson, 2012). Secondly, a valuable set of indicators of the effective use of soft technologies has emerged from research on the motivations and incentives of a range of AT stakeholders in Australia (De Jonge et al., 2017). An overview of what users want from AT services is in Box 31.1. Thirdly, a consensus set of good practice steps for AT provision draws on a range of

BOX 31.1
WHAT AT USERS WANT FROM AT SERVICES

- Determination of the best combination of products, personal support and environmental design.
- Access to sufficient funding for good quality and long-lasting products.
- Funding to meet AT needs in every area of life.
- Holistic assessment of needs, so that each product works well and does not interfere with other supports.
- Consideration of AT needs across the lifespan and as needs change.
- Support throughout the process of getting AT, including trial, training and maintenance.
- Access to resources when needed.
- Active involvement in decision making.
- Consideration of personal preferences and identity so that AT is chosen to suit lifestyle and participation.

international studies (de Witte et al., 2018; Layton et al., 2024a). The broad steps applicable to assessing and matching the AT to the person, occupation and environment are presented in Fig. 31.5. Implementing the good practice steps requires knowledge of assistive products as well as skills in wraparound supports, alongside professional reasoning regarding the individual goals and environment, and a capability-building approach that recognises the individual's own skills and knowledge as an AT user.

Pragmatic Constraints on Good Practice

Occupational therapists may find themselves working in situations where it is difficult to follow good practice steps because of the design of AT policy and therefore of AT service delivery. Pragmatic reasoning is the term used in the professional reasoning literature to describe practical considerations within the practice context of the occupational therapist, which may influence decision making (Unsworth, 2004). Occupational therapists may therefore need to engage in a range of systemic advocacy activities identifying shortfalls in policy or service provision guidelines, against benchmarks such as practice guidelines (where available) or good practice steps. Common scenarios and potential pragmatic actions to address these can be found in Table 31.3.

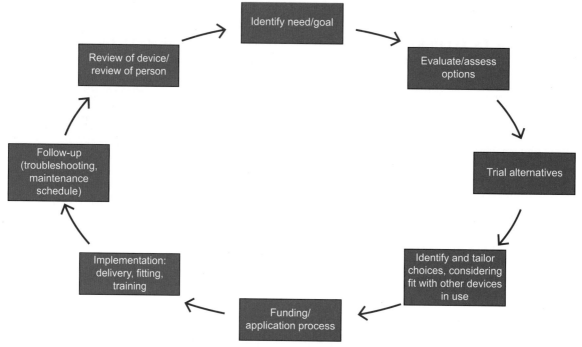

Fig. 31.5 ■ Good practice steps for assistive technology provision.

TABLE 31.3
Examples of Pragmatic Constraints and Possible Actions

Pragmatic constraint	Possible actions
The AT funding scheme generally funds assistive products but does not fund wrap-around supports.	Occupational therapists may need to articulate to managers and to policymakers that, to follow evidence-based practice principles, good practice steps should be adhered to. Informing and partnering with service users and service user advocates to argue for rights to support under the CRPD (United Nations, 2006) is changing policy in many countries.
The AT funding scheme provides a limited subsidy for a limited range of assistive products.	Occupational therapists who present a limited range of options to the consumer, in line with funding constraints, are operating pragmatically but not ethically. A more empowering approach would be to collaboratively discuss the full range of options and support the service user in making a decision taking into account factors such as funding constraints. This may include seeking alternate funds, making a representation as a self-advocate for consideration, or providing data on the unmet need to funders and policymakers to develop improved policy.

PRACTICE STORIES: OCCUPATIONAL THERAPY PRACTICE IN AT PROVISION AND THE IMPACT OF CONTEXT

To illustrate occupational therapy practice in AT provision, the practice stories of three people who use AT, Heather, Ricky and Peter, are included in this chapter (Boxes 31.2–31.4). These individuals are introduced using ICF language, and examples of AT interventions are described using the Canadian Occupational Therapy Inter-relation Practice Process (refer to Chapter 12). The impact of societal and practice contexts for each practice story and the frames of reference used are presented below.

BOX 31.2
RICKY

Ricky is a young blogger and web designer, and has a chronic illness. Ricky is a self-advocate who also works towards improving systems for others.

Body structures and functions: Ricky has several severe metabolic/systemic disorders that became incapacitating during her university years. Orthostatic intolerance and hyper-mobile joints mean Ricky spends most of her time in bed in a supine position and makes some short trips in her reclined power wheelchair. Ricky experiences severe fatigue, sensory sensitivity (vision and hearing) and fluctuating cognitive issues, such as word finding and concentration difficulties. Her hand dexterity is unaffected but her fluctuating systemic functioning means she fatigues quickly and experiences overuse symptoms when typing on her computer keyboard or hand sewing for moderate periods.

Occupational participation: Ricky actively seeks opportunities, within her limited physical capacity and occupationally deprived environment, to engage with the world. Ricky fosters cats in need of socialising and enjoys growing and tending many climbing plants. She builds meaning through her online contacts and takes every opportunity to read, learn and engage with the world via small engagements and projects (e.g. craft projects and organising feed for the birds outside her window). Before her illness, Ricky studied computer science. Ricky retains strong interests in artificial intelligence research, languages and assistive technology (AT). She actively engages in online dialogue and system advocacy regarding disability and human rights issues.

Environments: After a period of homelessness, Ricky was placed on the ground floor of an inner city Ministry of Housing flat, 45 minutes from her family and far from the semirural, outer suburban area in which she grew up. Her physical environment comprises an electrically adjustable bed in the living room, with a view of the hallway and living room window. The flat is wheelchair accessible but circulation spaces are too narrow for the bed to be moved into any other rooms. A wall between the living room and the kitchen prevents Ricky from viewing the kitchen or participating in kitchen-related activities, including supervising her support workers. Ricky runs her part-time web design business from her bed and is an active member of virtual communities using a combination of mainstream technologies, such as an Apple Mac computer, iPhone and large high-definition computer screen, and assistive technologies, such as a computer monitor stand attached to the hospital bed and foam postural supports for positioning (Fig. 31.6)

Occupational participation goals: Ricky wishes to maintain and extend her participation in virtual communities. She wants to spend less time and energy negotiating and navigating through different funding bodies and services and to participate in more formal education. She wishes to have some choice over where she lives and to be in closer proximity to family and friends to increase the ease with which they can visit.

The application of the Canadian Occupational Therapy Inter-relation Practice Process (COTIPP) with Ricky to improve information and communication technology performance can be found in Table 31.4

THE IMPACT OF SOCIETAL CONTEXT

Ricky, Heather and Peter live in urban or regional areas of Australia. The social contract that exists between individuals and the state differs according to country (e.g. the limited health safety net in the United States for those people who are uninsured compared with the national health scheme in the United Kingdom). The social contract also changes over time, with Australia and many countries moving from charitable approaches to social justice and human rights approaches, as enshrined in the Convention on the Rights of Persons with Disabilities (United Nations, 2006). The convention can be viewed as a tool for social justice and social change. Just as disabled persons'

organisations write 'shadow reports' to inform the UN as to how countries that are signatories to the convention are delivering on their commitment, occupational therapists and the people receiving their services may choose to document the achievement of occupational participation goals, or failure to achieve these goals, using the convention as a blueprint. Occupational therapists and the people receiving their services can use many of the Articles that specifically relate to access to AT and accessible environments to demonstrate whether outcomes are realised or unrealised, as part of the argument for resourcing.

For example, in relation to the three practice stories:

■ Ricky is dependent on government social security (pensions), rental accommodation (housing),

---

BOX 31.3
HEATHER

Heather is independent, artistic and a lover of cats. Living alone without hearing or sight, Heather is an active self-advocate in the deafblind community.

Body structures and functions: Heather is a female in her 50s who has Ushers syndrome, a genetic disorder affecting her hearing and sight. She has lived with complete deafness all her life and lost her sight in her 20s. Heather explains, 'Being Deafblind is very difficult and isolating and I am always determined to make my life the best as I can'.

Occupational participation: Heather's ability to participate in most occupations is facilitated through computer-based communication or tactile communication with another person. She works hard to structure her days and her weeks. Heather requires support workers or *communication guides* to be skilled in tactile communication techniques. Heather elects to use some of her limited personal support hours to enable her to swim and she feels 'fantastic after that'. She also uses her support worker hours for more basic needs; she provides the example of using her support worker to 'cancel swimming, to make contact calls [and to read] snail mail if it doesn't come through email'.

Environment: Heather receives approximately 25 hours per week of specialised support and 5 hours per week of council home care and lives independently in the company of her cat, in a house purchased with support through a housing association. Heather's combination of mainstream and adaptive technology, as well as extensive soft technology (training across environments), enables her to meet a range of life goals (mapped across education, community, civic and social areas). Simple labelling procedures at home such as Hi Mark (a tube of quick-hardening raised putty) on the microwave and washing machine and Dymo Braille tape or magnets on food ingredients, enable Heather to manage her domestic life. As the world around them is tangible only through touch and smell, vibrating alerts (e.g. clock, doorbell, smoke alarm and vibrating pager with four different alerts for phone) and tactile input via human or via computer, are the ways in which Heather can receive and impart communication. Emerging technologies such as the use of an iPhone with a Braille app connected to a refreshable Braille device enable Heather to, for example, use Facebook to connect with others. The known environments are easily managed by Heather, who is familiar with her dwelling, able to walk around the block with a white cane and perform transactions at known shops, and able to take the train to the city independently. Crossroads and unfamiliar terrain, especially if uneven and with poor tactile signage, present barriers. AT such as the Mini-Guide (a vibrating alert that detects objects in the vicinity) helps Heather to identify barriers such as traffic but does not help her to negotiate these barriers.

Occupational participation goals: Heather values 'regularity and personal activity' in her life and longs to be more active, stating 'I don't need any help for showers or things like that [...] I have my shower, eat my breakfast, open the computer to see if I've received any emails [....,] go outside and check the weather. All through the day [...] sometimes I'm quite bored, I put the computer on and I'm backwards and forwards checking for emails, I play with the cat, I do many laps of the block with my white cane'.

The application of the Canadian Occupational Therapy Inter-relation Practice Process with Heather's use of AT to enhance leisure and creativity options can be found in Table 31.5.

---

health care (medicines and monitoring) and disability supports (personal care, AT, environmental modifications). The difficulties she experiences coordinating all these supports can be examined in relation to Article 25 (Health), Article 26 (Habilitation & rehabilitation) and Article 28 (Adequate standard of living and social protection).

■ Limited access to information and communication technology means Heather cannot participate in further education, get around her neighbourhood or engage in community activities. Heather's rights to do so are called up in the following articles: Article 19 (Living independently and being included in the community),

Article 21 (Freedom of expression and opinion, and access to information), and Article 24 (Education).

■ Peter finds he is unable to access Parliament House through the main entrance as there are steps and the rear ramped entrance is closed because of renovations. This situation is addressed in Article 9 (Accessibility), Article 20 (Personal mobility) and Article 29 (Participation in political and public life).

In these examples, Ricky, Heather and Peter and their occupational therapists identify that policy systems 'lag behind' policy rhetoric and that available programmes have not yet realised the human right to

BOX 31.4
PETER

Peter is a retired bookseller, parent and highly dedicated volunteer who has lived with the effects of polio since he was four years old.

Body structures and functions: Peter is 65 years of age. He is a tall man who is approaching 100 kg in weight. He recently retired from work because of the effects of postpolio syndrome. Peter states that his capacity is limited by shortness of breath, difficulty exhaling, fatigue, loss of muscle strength in arms and legs and previous back and left shoulder injuries. He can walk around his home and garden with bilateral knee-ankle-foot orthoses and a single-point stick. However, if he walks for more than 5 minutes he is severely affected by fatigue, twitching or fasciculation and cognitive difficulties.

Occupational participation: Peter is a writer. He is currently researching postpolio syndrome and its management from a consumer perspective. He is active in systemic advocacy through consumer groups. For six months Peter attended counselling to come to terms with his life changes; currently, Peter describes a high level of reward from his community visits to people in nursing homes, and running the local polio network. He has applied for a disability support pension and self-funded his scooter last year.

Environment: Peter lives in an unrenovated brick single-storey dwelling in need of some maintenance, with his wife and young adult children. Only minimal modifications have been performed on Peter's home. Peter stated, 'When I knew this was happening I put the bricks out the back [forming level access around the house to the back entrance], and a single handrail adjacent to shower-overbath, but no alteration to the single step at front patio'. Peter is not in a position to purchase many of the major items of assistive technology that would minimise his capability gap, including improved respiratory equipment and an extensive home renovation. Peter currently uses AT such as a pickup stick around the house and a continuous positive airway pressure machine overnight.

Occupational participation goals: Peter is planning to demolish his home and build two smaller units on the block, both accessible, one for resale and one as the family home. He has found that the powered scooter does not provide the flexibility to traverse indoor areas and cannot be transported easily in a vehicle. As Peter's walking speed, endurance and balance change, he wishes to find a better way to mobilise and replace his walking.

The application of the COTIPP with Peter can be found in Table 31.6.

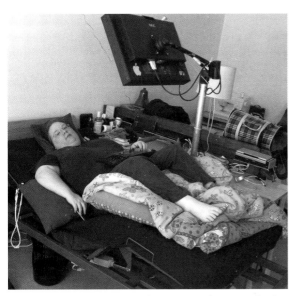

Fig. 31.6 ■ Ricky with her information and communication technology set up around her bed.

fulfilment capability gaps and therefore to equal outcomes. Thus the idea of systemic advocacy to influence societal and practice context is of relevance to occupational therapists (Pollard et al., 2008).

THE IMPACT OF PRACTICE CONTEXT

A good starting point is for occupational therapists to consider the practice context in which they are working. Practice contexts will vary in terms of resourcing and a range of other pragmatic constraints. For example, private and insurance-based facilities have caps on bed days and limit potential postdischarge follow-up, and specific-purpose clinics may not be set up to enable occupational therapists to follow through on aspects of a person's life that are not related to the clinic's purpose. A range of other implicit or hidden motivations and incentives can affect practice and professional reasoning. These may include departmental 'rewards' for statistics, prompt discharges and coming in on budget. In other words, the lens of occupational therapists will be influenced by the practice context in which they work (refer to Chapter 5).

TABLE 31.4

Application of the Canadian Occupational Therapy Inter-relation Practice Process with Ricky

Action domain of the Canadian Occupational Therapy Inter-relation Practice Process	Application of the COTIPP to address Ricky's assistive technology requirements
Connect	Ricky was referred to an independent nonprofit assistive technology consultancy service.
	In addition to completing the standard information form required by the service, Ricky provided a comprehensive written summary of her AT system and vision for what was needed. This demonstrated her depth of knowledge of technology and spoke from the outset of her right to seek equality and respect from the relationship between her and the consultant occupational therapist.
	The occupational therapist conducted the initial session on-site at Ricky's unit, as Ricky's sitting tolerance, fatigue and postural hypotension meant travelling to the service was not possible. The basic structure of the session was discussed with Ricky, who was invited to direct the session schedule, for example, the timing of breaks.
Seek understanding and define the purpose	Having the session at Ricky's home allowed the occupational therapist to observe the context of Ricky's home-based technology-related occupations. Initial active listening and validation by the occupational therapist led to a shared awareness and appreciation of Ricky's unique requirements as an expert user of AT, and her desire to collaborate on equal terms was established. As evidence of emerging trust, Ricky disclosed instances of prior discrimination by health professionals, attributing these to the lack of a formal diagnosis of her condition. She also shared her frustration at the lack of technical knowledge of some health professionals and her experiences of inequality arising out of hospital-based services.
Explore occupational participation	Information in the referral was reviewed together and feedback was sought as to its perceived currency and accuracy. Ricky demonstrated her AT use to the occupational therapist.
	Initial consideration was given to the possibility of integrating system components (i.e. integrated AT where one device can encompass multiple purposes to enhance efficiency of access ('reward for effort' equation) and potentially reduce costs of the system over the longer term.
	New AT options that the occupational therapist brought to the session were explored and trialled briefly. Key features of the AT options were highlighted in language appropriate to Ricky's level of experience and expertise and level of alertness at the time. Task analysis encompassed Ricky's physical, sensory and cognitive interactions with the equipment in the proposed environment of use (Ricky's bedroom/living area), and Ricky's observations as she explored each AT option were sought and noted.
	The occupational therapist talked through his observations of relevant environmental influencers and constraints and sought confirmation of these with Ricky. The availability of support to assist with the setup of the system, as well as potential requirements for maintenance and troubleshooting (technical support), were identified as key considerations.
Co-design priorities, goals, outcomes and plans	Based on the assessment outcomes, Ricky and the occupational therapist determined the following objectives and priorities of Ricky's proposed system requirements:
	■ Maintain and develop online relationships with friends, colleagues and health and other professionals via efficient and effective computer access (keyboard and mouse option that permits Ricky to work comfortably for the required duration).
	■ Independently set and edit alarms, voice reminders and calendar entries on computer and phone as these can assist in compensating for intermittent difficulties with recall and information retention.
	■ Take notes during phone conversations.
	■ Use the phone in speakerphone mode (possibility of portable voice amplification system).
	■ Access to entertainment (stored locally on disc & drive; online via streaming services).
	■ Establish home automation control of lights, TV, stereo and DVD. An action plan was developed that focused on trialling AT systems to meet the objectives and priorities. One option included trialling alternative ergonomic keyboards. The occupational therapist discussed funding options for the AT along with the time frame involved in arranging the trial of the options. Ricky and the occupational therapist also determined an evaluation criteria for the equipment trial that took into account the variability in Ricky's symptoms. It was decided that AT options would need to be on loan for at least 1 month for Ricky to be able to decide if they were suitable. It was also decided that as the various components were to be used as part of a system, the trial equipment was to be used concurrently rather than sequentially, even though at times it might have been preferred to trial AT options individually. The occupational therapist investigated funding options for the AT options (e.g. an Apple trackpad and X-Keys software and the ergonomic keyboard) assuming a successful trial is attained. The occupational therapist also further explored and evaluated both mainstream and purpose-built smart device–based reminder and calendaring apps and shared his findings with Ricky.

TABLE 31.4	
Application of the Canadian Occupational Therapy Inter-relation Practice Process with Ricky— (Continued)	
Action domain of the Canadian Occupational Therapy Inter-relation Practice Process	**Application of the COTIPP to address Ricky's assistive technology requirements**
Trial the plan, explore change and refine the plan	The occupational therapist facilitated the trial of an ergonomic keyboard, programmable number pad and portable voice amplifier by liaising with known specialist equipment suppliers, while respecting Ricky's rights to privacy and confidentiality and only disclosing the minimum required information to allow the trials to proceed.
	Once the equipment arrived, training was provided for Ricky and regular visiting support staff of her choice in the operational features of the system, including setup and positioning of trial items. The use of photographs and written instructions were employed to supplement verbal instructions. Ricky and the staff were encouraged to call or email the occupational therapist with concerns or queries should they arise during the trial period.
	Ricky was encouraged to maintain a log of her comfort levels and duration of use when interacting with the equipment during the trial phase. Ricky used her smartphone to take notes and record observations.
	A one-month trial of options was completed and a follow-up call was made to evaluate progress.
	Ricky reported that she found the split keyboard heavy when she was fatigued and that moving it in and out of the position of use (over her abdomen) caused pain in her left thumb. She provided a digital image via email of the thumb position when she relocated the keyboard and it was visibly hyperextended at the CMC joint. An alternative fully split tethered keyboard was suggested as this was lighter and could also allow her to type with her arms fully supported by her sides in bed. A trial of this was proposed to Ricky and she agreed to continue the exploration process.
	Ricky reported that she found setting up the voice amplifier cumbersome. She had independently located a simple and inexpensive phone mount online that positioned her phone close enough so the speaker on the phone could be used. An update to the operating system of the phone allowed her to use full hands-free mode for voice dialling of her contacts, which further reduced the effort involved in operating her phone.
	A programmable number pad was effective in allowing her to activate frequently required functions with prestored shortcuts, and Ricky reported she had already added to those initially programmed, demonstrating her competence and ownership of this component of her computer access system.
Plan for transition	During a subsequent planned follow-up call, Ricky reported that the second keyboard trial was successful.
	Funding for the system components was obtained from a philanthropic grant. The components were purchased and provided under a long-term loan scheme. Several months later Ricky reported that an operating system update on her Apple computer caused an issue with the keyboard. ComTEC Technical Support Officer contacted the manufacturer and a firmware update was issued and installed to fix the issue.
	Ricky and the occupational therapist agreed that this phase of the process was complete.

This practice story was provided by Ricky Buchanan and David Harraway, an occupational therapist with ComTEC Yooralla.

In the past, the rehabilitation approach, underpinned by a normative agenda, with its focus on achieving independence and remediating impairment, was an approach of choice when assessing for and providing AT. However, this approach has been severely critiqued by individuals living with impairment as it locates the problem with the individual (Swain et al., 2004), privileges professional priorities (Rist et al., 2008) and lacks appreciation of the diverse engagements with diversity (Shakespeare, 2008). The use of collaborative relationship-focused practice strategies ensure that the aspirations and capabilities of the person are foregrounded, even when working in settings with acute, rehabilitative or other foci. Hence, occupational therapists need to seek out approaches of specific relevance to the worldview of the person requiring the AT.

Selecting Frames of Reference

When occupational therapists choose one or more theories, models or approaches, they are constructing a frame of reference or lens through which to view and work with the consumer. For Ricky, Heather and Peter, the following frames of reference were considered:

TABLE 31.5	
Application of the Canadian Occupational Therapy Inter-Relation Practice Process with Heather	
Action domain of the Canadian Occupational Therapy Inter-relation Practice Process	**Application of the COTIPP to address Heather's leisure objectives**
Connect Seek understanding and define the purpose	Heather identified herself as a creative person and wished to enrich and fill her time. Heather essentially lived in a state of occupational deprivation because of her profound sensory losses. The primary absence of visual and auditory inputs was compounded by the secondary loss of incidental communication and environmental feedback. These losses resulted in significant occupational participation restrictions. A key strategy for Heather was her involvement in the deafblind self-advocacy movement. As well as teaching the community about deafblindness, this group met regularly for leisure activities. It was in this context that Heather sought to engage in art and craft.
Explore occupational participation	Heather had successfully constructed and given characters and backstories to a range of hand puppets for use in video storytelling. Heather wished to extend her repertoire and described her passions for animals and her childhood love of drawing and creating. Heather's objective was to reengage with drawing as a meaningful recreation. Heather described how she used to draw despite her vision loss, using her fingers to track her drawing progress, but being unable to see the final result. To achieve this objective, activity analysis and task adaptation were undertaken so that the occupation of drawing could occur in a way that used Heather's capabilities despite her sensory losses.
Co-design priorities, goals, outcomes and plans	As Heather and her colleagues within the deafblind advocacy group met regularly, enjoyed socialising and had similar needs and objectives, several sessions were planned for the group in a sunny courtyard with tables and seating, as well as a wet area. Clay tablets with a range of stylus tools were introduced. Carving into the tablets was demonstrated with hand-over-hand techniques, and participants were encouraged to experiment with the material and the effect of the different stylus tools (Fig. 31.7). They were also encouraged to share their results through tactile contact with each other's work.
Trial the plan, explore change and refine the plan	Mastery was gained over several sessions. Heather created two key pieces: one was a profile of a dog, and another, was the interlinking images of hands. Heather explained the strong visual image she had of the dog which she had drawn, and her delight in being able to feel the outline she had created in the clay. The interlinking hands were a strong symbol of tactile communication and connectivity; other group members used similar image metaphors, such as fences and linked chains. In addition to producing artworks, the occupational engagement enjoyed by Heather and the group was significantly enriched as a shared experience and provided opportunities for deep and important connections to themes that mattered to these individuals.

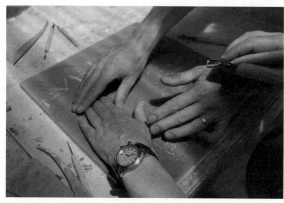

Fig. 31.7 ■ Heather learning to draw in clay. (Image courtesy Self-Advocacy Resource Unit.)

■ Ricky describes many negative experiences with medical or rehabilitation approaches. In Ricky's experience, professionals value recovery and 'trying harder', and this is problematic when the trajectory of chronic illness does not fit with the linear progression that is often the focus of many rehabilitation services. She also noted a tension between independence (as valued by health professionals) and her own version of independence, which she referred to as, 'My bossing, and someone else's hands'. Ricky based her service decisions on whether she was supported in her decisions around independence versus energy conservation in self-care activities. A frame of

TABLE 31.6

Application of the Canadian Occupational Therapy Inter-relation Practice Process with Peter

Action domains of the Canadian Occupational Therapy Inter-relation Practice Process	Application of the COTIPP to address Peter's assistive technology requirements
Connect Seek understanding and define the purpose	As a retiree living with the late effects of polio, Peter was planning for a likely change from ambulation with bilateral callipers to powered mobility. Peter researched his options online, with the local Independent Living Centre and with several AT suppliers. Through these actions, Peter became informed as to what options were on the market, and he was able to identify that a powered wheelchair rather than a scooter or any other type of wheeled mobility device would meet his needs. Peter was aware that he was the 'expert in his own condition', but identified a need for professional input regarding fitting an AT device to his current and future physical capacities and his lifestyle as well as impartial advice as to AT device performance in his environments of use – in other words, he was seeking advice on ensuring a fit between the powered wheelchair and the person–environment–occupation.
Explore occupational participation	Peter elected to collaborate with an occupational therapist specialising in polio, who was familiar with the progressive nature of his impairment as well as its contraindications. The occupational therapist met with Peter at his home, and evaluated his home environment, using person-centred planning principles to elicit Peter's occupational goals. Peter wanted to be able to move around his home and neighbourhood and continue his community visits to residents in a nursing home. He wanted the powered wheelchair to be able to manage gutters, tram tracks and some grassy terrain and to have a range of at least 10 km. As Peter was currently writing a book and intended to visit a range of libraries and archives, he also required the powered wheelchair to be taken on public transport. Finally, Peter intended to be able to transport the AT device in the boot of his car when he travelled.
	The occupational therapist's lens was influenced by their knowledge of the difficulty of obtaining funding and the need for the recommended device to meet Peter's needs for 3–5 years. The occupational therapist was also mindful of the progressive nature of postpolio syndrome and hence of the need to ensure the wheelchair would still be suitable for Peter in 3–5 years (e.g. it was possible that Peter would require postural trunk supports, and the occupational therapist felt that it was important that these supports could be added to the wheelchair in the future if required).
	Peter's perspective was somewhat different. He still drove a car and had been using a powered scooter; thus he envisaged a wheelchair that was flexible enough to be pushed, dismantled, travel over unknown terrain and be used on public transport.
Co-design priorities, goals, outcomes and plans	In light of Peter's extensive community mobility goals (travelling to archives and libraries where access is unsure, and using public transport as well as driving), Peter and the occupational therapist explored the compromise between seating integrity and the option to dismantle the wheelchair. This resulted in the selection of a folding powerchair that was able to be transported in vehicles.

Continued on following page

TABLE 31.6	
Application of the Canadian Occupational Therapy Inter-relation Practice Process with Peter—(Continued)	
Action domains of the Canadian Occupational Therapy Inter-relation Practice Process	**Application of the COTIPP to address Peter's assistive technology requirements**
Trial the plan, explore change and refine the plan	The occupational therapist discussed the options Peter had previously found during his research and did some additional research to establish which of the available powered wheelchairs that had suitable features would be eligible for funding. The number of wheelchairs trialled, and the schedule of trials, was influenced by Peter's fatigue (one per week, in the mornings) and the availability of the occupational therapist. Appointments were made with AT suppliers who provided powerchairs for trials. Each device was set up and Peter was trained in its use. Peter and the occupational therapist evaluated the performance of the powered wheelchairs on a similar 'circuit' for comparison. Peter then trialled each chair for a few days.
	After the trial periods, the preferred options were discussed by telephone, and the occupational therapist put in a funding application. A wait list of 18 months was experienced. Once Peter reached the top of the list, a further occupational therapy home assessment was conducted to ensure the features of the powered wheelchair remained suitable and reviewed the newer models that have become available. The powered wheelchair was then purchased and delivered.
	Peter was delighted to take delivery of the powerchair. Over the next 3 weeks, Peter identified that the castors provided were too small to cope with train track crossings. Peter discussed this with the occupational therapist over the phone, and they decided to try a larger set, mindful that this would affect the size of the turning circle. Peter funded this alteration himself, as it was quicker than waiting for the funding body to consider and approve this change.
	To tailor the situation still further, Peter wanted to explore alternatives to dismantling the power wheelchair to lift into the boot, which, although feasible, was physically tiring and time consuming. Although Peter was still physically able to dismantle and lift the wheelchair components into the boot of his car, the 18-month wait had seen deterioration in his physical capacity and endurance. Peter reviewed alternative vehicle apertures and found that a second-hand station wagon enabled him to merely fold the backrest, tilt the front wheels off the ground and push the chair in (Fig. 31.8)
Plan for transition	Peter was satisfied that he had a device that met his self-identified occupational performance outcome.
	The occupational therapist anticipated that the folding powerchair offered less stability and suspension than a rigid-framed wheelchair and noted that a rigid wheelchair with folding accessories, along with an appropriate vehicle, may have been a better selection. The occupational therapist reflected that at the time of the assessment, Peter was not prepared to alter his goals and change the car that he was driving, particularly as vehicle choices such as vans were not 'family friendly'. The occupational therapist felt that Peter had been supported in his choice and that this choice was made after a thorough assessment and trial.
	After Peter had received the powered wheelchair, the occupational therapist did recommend a drop-in postural seat and backrest that would provide Peter with better support than the standard seat and backrest that came with the wheelchair, and Peter accepted this recommendation.

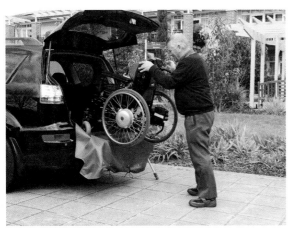

Fig. 31.8 ■ Peter putting his lightweight powerchair in the car.

reference comprising approaches which support individual autonomy and self-efficacy, such as chronic disease self-management and self-direction, are more likely to meet Ricky's needs.

■ Heather greatly values her independence and control, yet a feature of deafblindness is the lack of experiential knowledge of what is possible without direction from practitioners and others. Useful theoretical constructs for Heather then include occupational justice theory, to guide and inform a rights-based plan for occupational enrichment, as well as adult learner approaches to build iterative knowledge capital for Heather to make informed choices and decisions.

■ The experience of Peter and others who have had polio is embedded in the medical model. However, the postpolio community have been cautious regarding the rehabilitation approaches as they consider these approaches to be inappropriate for people with postpolio syndrome. Peter explains his experience and his preferred approach: 'My experience of the late effects of polio (LEoP) is that physical deterioration is from overuse, not a sedentary lifestyle. For many polio patients, a programme of healthy movement may have far greater and longer benefits than load bearing or repetitive movement. This has been my experience. My use of bracing, sticks, powered wheels and respiratory support has lessened the load on weakened muscles, reduced pain and enabled me to become more active. I believe more permanent benefits are likely to be a result of healthy weight management, supported movement, use of AT, an accessible environment and avoiding fatigue from overuse'. Useful theoretical lenses for working with Peter include life course approaches and the collaborative application of daily living skills, including self-help–based work simplification, energy conservation, occupational balance and relaxation strategies.

Note: A suitable framework to use to guide the collaborative relationship approach with Ricky, Heather and Peter is described in Chapter 10.

CONCLUSION

The assessment and prescription of assistive technologies are a key interventions used by occupational therapists to enable occupational participation. Occupational therapists are uniquely placed to implement AT strategies because of their professional reasoning capabilities and their understanding of the person–environment–occupation fit. The challenges for occupational therapists working with AT include keeping up with the rapid diversification of assistive products and design paradigms and managing the sociopolitical factors that influence AT supply and practice. Occupational therapists working in the field of AT, as in many other fields of practice, are encouraged to enact systemic advocacy roles in achieving the best possible outcomes with and for people with impairment. Strategies to do this include adhering to best practice principles for occupational therapy practice and AT service delivery, using key frameworks such as the WHO ICF and the UN Convention on the Rights of Persons with Disabilities to articulate and document practice, and contributing to the evidence base for AT as an intervention.

REFERENCES

Albrecht, G., Seelman, K., & Bury, M. (Eds.). (2001). *Handbook of disability studies*. SAGE.

Barbareschi, G., Carew, M. T., Johnson, E. A., Kopi, N., & Holloway, C. (2021). "When they see a wheelchair, they've not even seen me"—Factors shaping the experience of disability stigma and discrimination in Kenya. *International Journal of Environmental Research and Public Health, 18*(8). https://doi.org/10.3390/ijerph18084272.

Barbareschi, G., & Shakespeare, T. (2021). A right to the frivolous? Renegotiating a well-being agenda for AT research. *Assistive Technology, 33*(5), 237. https://doi.org/10.1080/10400435.2021.1984112.

Bickenbach, J., Chatterji, S., Bradley, E., & Ustun, T. (1999). Models of disablement, universalism and the international classification of impairments, disabilities and handicaps. *Social Science and Medicine, 48*, 1173–1187.

Chabner, D.-E. (2012). *Medical terminology: A short course* (6th ed.). Saunders Elsevier.

Cook, A., & Polgar, J. (2015). *Assistive technologie* (4th ed.). Mosby.

Cruz, D. M., Emmel, M. G., Manzini, M. G., & Braga Mendes, P. V. (2016). Assistive technology accessibility and abandonment: Challenges for occupational therapists. *The Open Journal of Occupational Therapy, 4*(1). https://doi.org/10.15453/2168-6408.1166.

Dalhousie University. (n.d.). *Wheelchair skills program*. https://wheelchairskillsprogram.ca/en/

de Jonge, D., Hoyle, M., Layton, N., & Verdonck, M. (2017). The occupational therapist: Enabling activities and participation using assistive technology. In F. Scherer (Ed.), *Assistive Technology assessment handbook* (pp. 211–234). CRC Press.

de Witte, L., Steel, E., Gupta, S., Ramos, V. D., & Roentgen, U. (2018). Assistive technology provision: towards an international framework for assuring availability and accessibility of affordable high-quality assistive technology. *Disability and Rehabilitation: Assistive Technology, 13*(5), 467–472. https://doi.org/10.1080/17483107.2018.1470264.

Desmond, D., Layton, N., Bentley, J., Boot, F. H., Borg, J., Dhungana, B. M., Gallagher, P., Gitlow, L., Gowran, R. J., Groce, N., Mavrou, K., Mackeogh, T. McDonald, R., Pettersson, C, & Scherer, M. (2018). Assistive technology and people: A position paper from the first global research, innovation and education on assistive technology (GREAT) summit. *Disability and Rehabilitation: Assistive Technology, 13*(5), 437–444. https://doi.org/10.1080/17483107.2018.1471169.

Dong, H. (2007). Shifting paradigms in universal design. In C. Stephanidis (Ed.), *Universal access in human computer interaction: Coping with diversity* (pp. 66–74). Springer-Verlag.

Federici, S., & Scherer, M. (Eds.). (2017). *Assistive technology assessment handbook*. CRC Press.

Hansson, S. O. (2007). The ethics of enabling technology. *Cambridge Quarterly of Healthcare Ethics, 16*, 257–267.

Hobbs, D., Close, J., Downing, A., Reynolds, K., & Walker, L. (2009). Developing a national research and development centre in assistive technologies for independent living. *Australian Health Review, 33*(1), 152–160.

Holloway, C., & Barbareschi, G. (2022). *Disability Interactions: Creating Inclusive Innovations*. Morgan & Claypool (Springer Nature). https://doi.org/10.1007/978-3-031-03759-7.

Hocking, C. (1999). Function or feelings: Factors in abandonment of assistive devices. *Technology and Disability, 11*, 3–11.

Imrie, R., & Hall, P. (2001). *Inclusive design: Designing and developing accessible environments*. Spon Press.

International Organization for Standardization. (2022). *Assistive products for persons with disability — Classification and terminology*. International Organisation for Standardisation.

International Society of Wheelchair Professionals. (n.d.). Wheelchair Service Training Packages (WSTP). https://wheelchairnetwork.org/.

Kayes, N., & McPherson, K. (2012). Human technologies in rehabilitation: 'Who' and 'how' we are with our clients. *Disability & Rehabilitation, 34*(22), 1907–1911.

Law, M., Cooper, B., Stewart, D., Rigby, P., & Letts, L. (1996). The Person-Environment-Occupation Model: A transactive approach to occupational performance. *Canadian Journal of Occupational Therapy, 63*, 9–23.

Layton, N., & Borg, J. (2023). Assistive technology and the wellbeing of societies from a capabilities approach. *Societies, 13*(2). https://doi.org/10.3390/soc13020019.

Layton, N., & Brusco, N. (2022). *The Australian Assistive Technology Equity Studies: Improving access to assistive technology for people with disability who are not eligible for the NDIS*. https://assistivetechforall.org.au/our-work/.

Layton, N., Harper, K., Martinez, K., Berrick, N., & Naseri, C. (2021). Co-creating an assistive technology peer-support community: Learnings from AT Chat. *Disability and Rehabilitation: Assistive Technology*, 1–7. https://doi.org/10.1080/17483107.2021.1897694.

Layton, N., Spann, A., Khan, M., Contepomi, S., Hoogerwerf, E. J., Bell, D., & de Witte, L. (2024a). Guidelines for assistive technology service provision – A scoping review. Disability and Rehabilitation: Assistive Technology, 1–12. https://doi.org/10.1080/17483107.2024.2327515.

Layton, N., Brusco, N., Callaway, L., Henley, L., & Wang, R. H. (2024b). It is time for nationally equitable access to assistive technology and home modifications in Australia: An equity benchmarking study. *Australian Journal of Social Issues, 59*(1), 244–263. https://doi.org/10.1002/ajs4.290.

Liu, L. (2018). Occupational therapy in the Fourth Industrial Revolution. *Canadian Journal of Occupational Therapy, 85*(4), 272–283. https://doi.org/10.1177/0008417418815179.

Nussbaum, M. (2011). *Creating capabilities: The human development approach*. Harvard University Press.

Patston, P. (2007). Constructive functional diversity. A new paradigm beyond disability and impairment. *Disability & Rehabilitation, 29*(20-21), 1625–1633.

Pollard, N., Sakellariou, D., & Kronenberg, F. (Eds.), (2008). *A political practice of occupational therapy*. Churchill Livingstone Elsevier.

Renda, G., Jackson, S., Kuys, B., & Whitfield, T. W. A. (2016). The cutlery effect: do designed products for people with disabilities stigmatise them? *Disability and Rehabilitation: Assistive Technology, 11*(8), 661–667. https://doi.org/10.3109/17483107.2015.1042077.

Ripat, J. D., & Woodgate, R. L. (2012). The role of assistive technology in self-perceived participation. *International Journal of Rehabilitation Research, 35*(2), 170–177.

Rist, P., Freas, D., Maislin, G., & Stineman, M. (2008). Recovery from disablement: What functional abilities to rehabilitation professionals value the most? *Archives of Physical Medicine and Rehabilitation, 89*, 1600–1606.

Scherer, M. J. (2020). It is time for the biopsychosocialtech model. *Disability and Rehabilitation: Assistive Technology, 15*(4), 363–364. https://doi.org/10.1080/17483107.2020.1752319.

Scherer, M., & Federici, S. (2015). Why people use and don't use technologies: Introduction to the special issue on assistive technologies for cognition/cognitive support technologies. *Neuro Rehabilitation, 37*(3), 315–319.

Sen, A. (1999). *Development as freedom*. Oxford University Press.

Shakespeare, T. (2008). Disability: Suffering, social oppression, or complex predicament? In D. M. C. Rehmann-Sutter, & D. Mieth (Eds.), *The contingent nature of life: Bioethics and limits of human existence* (pp. 235–246). Springer.

Smith, E. M., Huff, S., Wescott, H., Daniel, R., Ebuenyi, I. D., O'Donnell, J., Maalim, M., Zhang, W., Khasnabis, C, & MacLachlan, M. (2022). Assistive technologies are central to the realization of the Convention on the Rights of Persons with Disabilities. *Disability and Rehabilitation: Assistive Technology*, 1–6. https://doi.org/10.1080/17483107.2022.2099987.

Smith, R. O. (2002). *IMPACT 2 MODEL*. http://www.r2d2.uwm.edu/archive/impact2model.html.

Smith, R. O. (2017). Technology and occupation: Past, present, and the next 100 years of theory and practice. *The American Journal of Occupational Therapy, 71*(6), 7106150010p7106150011-7106150010p7106150015. https://doi.org/10.5014/ajot.2017.716003.

Steinfeld, E. (2010). Advancing universal design. In J. L. Maisel (Ed.), *The state of the science in universal design: Emerging research and developments* (pp. 1–19). State University of New York at Buffalo, Bentham Sciences Publishers.

Steinfeld, E., & Danford, S. (2006). Universal design and the ICF. *Living in Our Environment: The Promise of ICF Conference in Vancouver, June 4-5, 2006*. http://www.icfconference.com/New%20Presentations/ICF%20Presentation%20Notes.pdf.

Swain, J., French, S., Barnes, C., & Thomas, C. (Eds.). (2004). *Disabling barriers – Enabling environments* (2nd ed.). SAGE Publications.

Tebbutt, E., Brodmann, R., Borg, J., MacLachlan, M., Khasnabis, C., & Horvath, R. (2016). Assistive products and the Sustainable Development Goals (SDGs). *Globalization and Health, 12*, 1–6.

United Nations. (2006). *Convention on the rights of persons with disabilities and optional protocol*. http://www.un.org/disabilities/convention/conventionfull.shtml.

Unsworth, C. (2004). Clinical reasoning: How do pragmatic reasoning, worldview and client-centredness fit? *British Journal of Occupational Therapy, 67*(1), 10–19.

Whalley Hammell, K. (2015). Quality of life, participation and occupational rights: A capabilities perspective. *Australian Occupational Therapy Journal, 62*, 78–85.

Wijk, M. (2001). The Dutch struggle for accessibility awareness. In W. F. Preiser, & E. Ostroff (Eds.), *Universal design handbook*. McGraw-Hill.

World Health Organization. (2001). *International classification of functioning, disability and health: ICF*. World Health Organization.

WHO & UNICEF. (2022). *Global report on assistive technology*. (Licence: CC BY-NC-SA 3.0 IGO). https://apps.who.int/iris/handle/10665/354357.

REFLECTION

1. What might be some human reactions to assistive technology, and how might occupational therapists manage these in their occupational therapy practice?

2. Describe the universal design features of an everyday technology that you use, and identify an assistive technology (AT) device where several versions could fulfil an 'inclusive design' brief.

3. Apply the AT best practice steps to teh process of assessing a frail elderly person who wishes to continue to shower safely but is finding it difficult to stand in the shower recess.

32

WALKING AND FALLS

ALISON CATHERINE PIGHILLS ■ LINDY MAXTED CLEMSON ■ SUSAN STARK

CHAPTER OUTLINE

Overview

Walking is a complex task which requires the coordination of both motor and sensory systems, mediated by higher-order cognitive processes. A person's ability to walk can be affected by disruption to these systems, as well as by environmental, psychological, psychosocial, economic and cultural barriers. Walking enables people to participate in meaningful occupations and supports healthy ageing by maintaining functional independence, thereby reducing loneliness and the likelihood of falls and fall-related injuries.

Falls in older people are prevalent, cause serious injury, are costly to health services and are primarily caused by interactions between intrinsic, behavioural and extrinsic risk factors. High intensity, comprehensive environmental fall-hazard reduction, when it is tailored toward the needs of older people at high risk of falls, focused on falls prevention and delivered by occupational therapists is a clinically effective intervention, reducing falls by 38%–39%.

KEY POINTS

- Impaired ability to walk limits a person's occupational participation and can lead to physical dependence, impaired mental and physical well-being and reduced quality of life.

- Occupational therapists working in an expanded scope of practice are likely to assess mobility and prescribe walking aids.

- Half of all people over 65 have walking impairments which often lead to falls.
- Environmental fall-hazard reduction is an evidence-based occupational therapy intervention, which reduces falls by 38%–39% when targeted toward people at high risk of falls.

INTRODUCTION

Humans adopted a bipedal stance between 3.5 and 7 million years ago. An upright posture likely evolved to increase energy efficiency and to hunt and carry provisions. The evolution of this stance is closely linked to functional task performance as it freed up the hands to engage in functional activity and develop in-hand manipulation, enhanced reach and access to places and objects (Retallack, 2022). However, reliance on two limbs, as opposed to four, to move within the environment left humans vulnerable to imbalance and immobility following illness, injury or impairment.

Walking requires the seamless integration of physiological and cognitive systems to enable efficient and effective movement in the environment. It relies on the coordination of both motor and sensory systems, mediated by higher-order neurological processes, such as executive function (van der Wardt et al., 2015). Disruption of the integrated functioning of these systems can lead to walking impairment and immobility. Walking impairment can be caused by both physiological and psychological factors, including congenital disorders, acute and chronic diseases, injuries, chronic fatigue, or pain and ageing.

Walking impairment can be categorised as acute (short term), progressive or chronic (long term) and can be temporary, situation specific or permanent. The degree of severity can range from mild impairment to complete dependence (Wee & Lysaght, 2009). The underlying cause and severity will likely determine the complexity of walking impairments, which are also influenced by comorbidities, psychological, social and environmental factors. If the underlying cause is multifaceted or the walking impairment complex, intervention requires a multifactorial and multidisciplinary approach (Robson, 2017).

Walking is a crucial component of successful task performance, which in turn is linked to occupational participation. Occupational participation refers to a person's ability to engage in life situations and is associated with quality of life and psychosocial well-being (Che Had et al., 2023). Occupational participation is the core concern for occupational therapists, therefore occupational therapists have a significant role in addressing walking dysfunction to enhance occupational participation (Egan & Restall, 2022).

THE GAIT CYCLE

Understanding the principles of normal walking is important when analysing the impact of physical illness, injury, or impairment. Walking is usually an automatic movement that requires no thought (Wensley & Slade, 2012). Impairments often result in a conscious effort to walk to accommodate deficits. Usually, the occupational therapist will be unaware of a person's usual pattern of movement, prior to their walking impairment, so it is important to understand the normal gait cycle to inform a more accurate assessment of how a person deviates from this.

The gait cycle is a cyclic pattern of movement and describes the sequence of events from foot strike to successive foot strike on the same side, with propulsion of the centre of gravity in the direction of motion (Fig. 32.1). It consists of two phases, the stance or contact phase and the swing or non-contact phase. The stance phase comprises the time that the foot is on the floor. It begins with foot strike and ends with toe off and is the most stable phase of the cycle, accounting for 62% of the duration, with contact duration decreasing at faster walking speeds (Kharb et al., 2011). The swing phase comprises the time the foot is off the floor. It begins with toe off and ends in a foot strike and accounts for 38% of the cycle duration (Romkes & Bracht-Schweizer, 2017). The stance phase is divided into initial double limb support, single limb stance and second double limb support and the swing phase into initial, mid and terminal swing. The body is least stable during the mid-swing of the swing phase, as the body weight is supported, and balance maintained, through one limb. Normal gait alternates between losing and regaining balance with the centre of mass being propelled forwards during mid-swing and balance regained as the swinging foot strikes the floor. The centre of mass moves about 5 cm laterally during

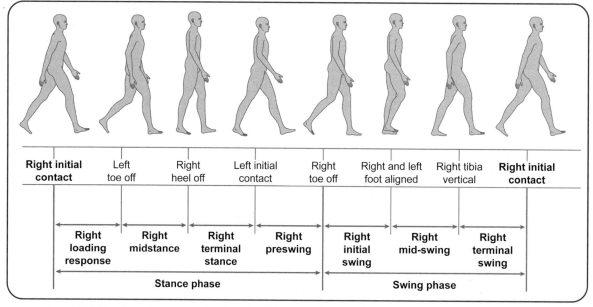

Fig. 32.1 ■ Overview of the gait cycle. (From Braddon, R. L. (2011). *Physical medicine and rehabilitation*. Saunders.)

the cycle. Cadence refers to the number of steps an individual takes in a minute and averages 114 steps in adults over 40 years of age (Chambers & Sutherland, 2002). Gait speed is the distance covered over time and is determined by cadence and stride length (Kharb et al., 2011). The mean gait speed in people aged 18–85 is 1.12 m/s and 0.96 m/s for people with a mean age of 84 (Bohannon & Wang, 2019). Poor balance, low cadence and slow gait speed are common signs of mobility impairment and predictors of falls in older adults (Urbanek et al., 2022).

The main tasks involved in walking are weight acceptance, single-leg support and limb advancement. The aim of weight acceptance is to stabilise the leg in preparation for taking the full body weight on one limb, absorb shock and allow forward motion of the body (Robson, 2017). Single-leg support involves moving and supporting the body weight through one limb while the centre of mass advances beyond the supporting foot, with the weight moving from the heel onto the ball of the foot. Limb advancement involves the foot clearing the ground and the limb swinging through the initial, mid and terminal swing phases (Urbanek et al., 2022).

Although walking primarily involves lower limb movement, the whole body is involved in walking.

During the gait cycle, the head and ears are aligned to the shoulders with no forward head posture. Forward head posture is common in older people and is associated with instability and impaired functional balance (Lin et al., 2022). The arms help to maintain and regain balance and the arm swing reduces the amount of energy expended. The speed of the arm swing increases in proportion to gait speed, and vice versa, and the arms move forward in synchrony with the opposite leg in a pendular action to maintain balance and momentum and to enable the opposite leg and pelvis to move forwards (Romkes & Bracht-Schweizer, 2017). The shoulder girdle and pelvis rotate in opposite directions and the upper body moves forward at varying speeds. The hips, knees and ankles flex and extend at varying times throughout the cycle.

The prerequisites of normal gait are stability of the weight-bearing foot throughout the stance phase, non-weight-bearing foot clearance in the swing phase, adequate positioning of the foot in the terminal swing phase, adequate step length and energy conservation (Chambers & Sutherland, 2002). However, given that the whole body is involved in gait, these prerequisites do not account for the dynamic interplay between the complex physiological and cognitive components of walking.

PHYSIOLOGICAL COMPONENTS OF WALKING

Walking involves the coordination of multiple body systems. From a physiological perspective, efficient walking involves a complex integration of muscle function, joint range of motion, skeletal stability, balance, cardio-pulmonary circulation, energy production and neuromuscular integration. The elements of the musculoskeletal system (muscles, bones and joints) work together to provide stability and generate movement (Martino et al., 2015). The circulatory system provides oxygen and nutrients to muscles during physical activity and the respiratory system supplies oxygen to generate energy and removes carbon dioxide as a waste product. Neuromuscular integration creates smooth and efficient movement and involves intricate coordination between the nervous system and muscles (Martino et al., 2015). Sensory information from receptors, such as proprioceptors (which detect body position and balance), is processed by the nervous system to generate motor commands, which activate the appropriate muscles. These motor commands, coordinated by neural pathways, trigger muscular contractions and relaxations to produce coordinated movement. Muscle activity is fine-tuned through feedback loops which enable adjustments in posture, balance and gait in response to changing environmental conditions. Neuromuscular integration is essential for generating power, maintaining stability and coordinating movements, to enable individuals to navigate their surroundings efficiently and safely (Menant et al., 2021).

COGNITIVE COMPONENTS OF WALKING

From a cognitive perspective, ambulant mobility relies on an integration of sensory input, perception, and higher-order cognitive processes, including topographical orientation, executive function, memory and attention. These higher-order cognitive processes are required to enable individuals to navigate their surroundings and avoid obstacles, plan and memorise routes and divide their attention. Sensory information, from the visual, auditory, vestibular and somatosensory systems, is processed to create a mental representation of the environment, which is used for motor planning and executing appropriate movements (Menant et al., 2021). Perception plays a role in the higher-order functions of motor planning and topographical orientation, as sensory information from the environment is processed to guide movement and spatial awareness. Topographical orientation enables a person to navigate in space by constructing cognitive maps. It includes the integration of spatial information such as direction, distance, location and orientation of objects or landmarks in the environment and involves perceptual processes such as spatial orientation and spatial memory, and the ability to interpret spatial information to navigate different surroundings (Iaria & Burles, 2016).

The higher-order executive function domain involves complex cognitive processes that are involved in goal-directed behaviours, such as reasoning, problem solving, decision-making, volition, motor planning, purposive action and action monitoring (Kearney et al., 2013). Motor planning involves the ability to plan and organise required movement sequences for task performance and selecting appropriate muscles, timing and sequencing movements, and coordinating different body parts to execute a motor task smoothly and efficiently. Both physical and cognitive impairments can have a negative impact on walking, and changes in gait often precede cognitive decline (Rosso et al., 2013). Indeed, executive function and motor function share neuroanatomy and are, thus closely related (Zhang et al., 2019).

BARRIERS TO WALKING

Walking can be limited by environmental, psychological, psychosocial, economic and cultural factors (Kalu et al., 2022).

Environmental Factors

A person's environmental context can either support or impede walking. For example, a person who uses a mobility aid in the home environment is likely to be more independent if the internal access is level and the home is modified and uncluttered. Equally, 'age-friendly' town planning and infrastructure can enhance outdoor walking, through the provision of well-designed and well-maintained footpaths, road

TABLE 32.1	
Dimensions of Potential Barriers to Walking Outdoors	
Dimension	**Example of Dimension**
Distance to cover	Long distances between available resting places
Temporal factors	Being able to cross a road in the allotted time, rushing for appointments
Ambient conditions	Light, temperature and weather conditions
Physical load	Carrying shopping, awkwardly shaped items, items which obscure visual field
Terrain characteristics	Uneven pavers, gravel, tree roots
Attentional demands	Noise levels, dual tasking
Postural transitions required by the environment	Reaching high shelves, bending
Density of people	Human traffic and objects in the immediate surroundings

From Shumway-Cook, A., Patla, A. E., Stewart, A., Ferrucci, L., Ciol, M. A., & Guralnik, J. M. (2002). Environmental demands associated with community mobility in older adults with and without mobility disabilities. *Physical Therapy, 82*(7), 670-681. https://doi.org/10.1093/ptj/82.7.670.

crossings and features to enhance accessibility, such as ramps and lifts. Ambient environmental conditions, such as extremes of hot or cold temperatures, excessively sunny, icy or wet weather and illumination levels affect an individual's safety when mobilising outdoors and their motivation to do so (Che Had et al., 2023). Eight dimensions of potential outdoor environmental barriers are listed in Table 32.1 (Shumway-Cook et al., 2002).

Psychological and Psychosocial Factors

Psychological factors that may influence an individual's willingness to walk include emotional well-being, motivation, self-efficacy, attitudes towards walking, perceptions of safety and habitual behaviour. A person's emotional well-being may affect their decision-making processes, perceptions of safety and motivation to walk. Motivation can be influenced by intrinsic factors, such as enjoyment of walking, or extrinsic factors, such as environmental concerns (Che Had et al., 2023; Kalu et al., 2022). Self-efficacy refers to an individual's level of confidence in their ability to successfully perform a task and influences the amount of effort and persistence an individual will employ in mastering it (Rogowska et al., 2020). Higher levels of self-efficacy enhance life satisfaction and can positively influence an individual's willingness to walk independently, such as feeling confident in navigating the environment or managing potential safety concerns. Thus self-efficacy is an important medium through which to enhance quality of life

(Kalu et al., 2022). Attitudes towards walking include an individual's values, beliefs and preferences. Positive attitudes, such as the perception of walking as enjoyable and environmentally responsible, can increase willingness to engage, whereas negative attitudes, such as perceiving walking as painful or physically challenging, are likely to have the reverse effect (Kalu et al., 2022). Concerns about safety while walking can include issues such as potential harassment or discrimination, the layout of the environment and fear of falling or heavy traffic. A perception that the environment is unsafe may restrict walking and is often linked to negative past experiences (World Health Organization, 2007). People for whom walking outdoors is established as a habitual behaviour may be more likely to engage in walking, leading to better health and well-being (van Soest et al., 2020).

Psychosocial factors shape a person's opportunities and motivation to walk and include social support and networks, living arrangements, home and work social environments, bereavement, loneliness, social status and level of social integration. These factors influence walking via thoughts, perceptions, beliefs, attitudes, emotions and subsequent behaviour. A person's belief and confidence in their ability to walk independently, their perception of their own physical ability and supportive social networks are likely to influence their motivation, willingness and opportunity to walk (Kalu et al., 2022). Fear of challenges and failure, a perception of being at risk of injury and limited opportunity will have a negative impact. Equally, perceptions of the safety, accessibility and aesthetics of the physical environment play a role in a person's motivation to walk.

Economic Factors

Economic factors that influence opportunities to walk outdoors include mobility options available, the cost of public or private transport and the availability of disability pensions (Che Had et al., 2023). People on a low income may not be able to afford to buy, maintain and run a private vehicle, thus rely on public transport or walking (van Soest et al., 2020). Equally, people who have a lower socioeconomic status may face barriers such as access to safe neighbourhoods, availability of well-maintained pedestrian-friendly infrastructure and may live long distances from urban centres due to housing costs (Che Had et al., 2023).

Cultural Factors

Cultural norms, values, attitudes and beliefs related to walking outdoors and using public transport vary widely and can impact a person's willingness to engage in, and perception of, walking as a viable mode of transportation (van Soest et al., 2020). In most cultures, walking in the community is accepted and positively encouraged for its health and environmental benefits; however, in other cultures travelling in private vehicles can be seen as a status symbol, or using other modes of transport is preferred and walking is seen as less socially acceptable. Gender-specific cultural norms, which require male family escorts for women, may restrict opportunity due to logistical arrangements. In some cultures, the streets are seen as 'male zones', particularly at certain times of the day, thus limiting access for women (Almahmood et al., 2017). These cultural attitudes will influence a person's willingness and autonomy to walk in the community; therefore it is important to be aware of cultural influences on walking outdoors, as understanding and considering these can inform interventions aimed at promoting walking in diverse cultural contexts.

WALKING AND OCCUPATIONAL PARTICIPATION

Walking enables people to move around and access their environment, and thus plays a pivotal role in participating in many occupations. Impaired walking can result in a loss of autonomy and increased dependence on others, which may negatively impact mental and physical well-being and quality of life (Smith et al., 2016).

The ability to walk enables people to access the wider community to participate in meaningful occupations, such as shopping, employment, accessing healthcare services, travelling and participating in social, recreational and cultural activities (Shumway-Cook et al., 2007). Independent walking enhances a person's ability to actively choose and participate in occupations that are personally meaningful and align with their values, interests and abilities. This participation contributes to motivation, a sense of purpose and personal achievement and promotes social connections, self-confidence, physical and mental well-being and quality of life (Wensley & Slade, 2012). Therefore maintaining or improving walking ability is an essential component of occupational participation both at home and in the wider community.

As a form of regular physical exercise, walking contributes to physical health by reducing the risk of sedentary lifestyle-related health issues. It helps to strengthen muscles, improve cardiovascular fitness, enhance bone density, maintain joint range of motion and balance and promote healthy weight management. Thus walking plays a vital role in reducing the risk of chronic conditions such as cardiovascular disease, pulmonary disease, obesity and diabetes. Walking also contributes to people feeling healthier and more socially connected. Walking supports healthy ageing by maintaining functional independence, reducing loneliness and the likelihood of falls and related injuries. Indeed, walking is the most common form of moderate physical exercise chosen by older adults, most likely because it is readily accessible, inexpensive and easy and safe for most people (Mizuta et al., 2023; Smith et al., 2016; Wensley & Slade, 2012). Maintaining the ability to walk through regular physical activity is essential for promoting optimal physical health, mental well-being and quality of life.

ASSESSING WALKING IMPAIRMENT

Occupational therapists understand people as occupational beings who spend most of their time engaged in 'doing' and derive meaning from what they do. Thus when a person's ability to walk is affected, the occupational therapist's role focuses on a person's occupational participation needs (Wensley & Slade, 2012). The focus of occupational therapy intervention is on the person's strengths and restoration of the areas of function challenged by their impaired walking ability. Occupational therapists assess the impact of a person's walking while participating in occupations within relevant environments, including analysing the activities and task components of the occupation (Christiansen et al., 2005). Occupational therapists assess the physical, cognitive and psychological aspects of the person engaging in occupations and identify barriers that impinge on participation.

Functional assessment of capabilities will identify how an individual's walking impairment is impacted by the environment and affects their occupational participation. The occupational therapist will identify existing adaptive strategies and determine ways in which the person may be able to participate in occupations. Environmental assessment will provide an understanding of the way in which the person currently walks within multiple environments; activity analysis will inform this assessment (refer to Chapters 17 and 18). Functional cognition is assessed, and formal validated cognitive assessments may also be indicated.

To assist with identifying the degree and impact of a walking impairment a range of performance-based mobility screening tools and tests can be used. A selection of these tools and tests is presented in Table 32.2 along with the likelihood of falls associated with poor test results.

Walking Aids

Occupational therapists and physiotherapists work closely together with people with walking impairments. Physiotherapists assess a person's ability to walk and prescribe walking aids if required; however, occupational therapists might also assess for and prescribe walking aids if working in an expanded scope of practice (Pighills et al., 2015). Walking aids (Fig. 32.2) may be prescribed for people with temporary or permanent injury, illness, or impairment to support walking. Walking aids fulfil two major functions: offload weight from a weak, painful, or injured limb; or support balance by increasing a person's supporting area; they can also increase confidence and autonomy (Resnik et al., 2009). Walking aids include walking sticks (single,

three and four point), crutches (axillary, elbow and gutter) and frames (no wheels, two and four wheeled, folding and gutter). Walking sticks are primarily used to compensate for impaired balance and provide mild weight offload, crutches are used for weight offload, and frames can be used to compensate for impaired balance, limb weakness and weight offload. Individual assessment and bespoke prescription are important to ensure the person is provided with the most suitable device, given their unique mobility impairments, environmental layout and cognitive capacity.

As people age, changes in posture and gait render them more susceptible to walking impairment. It is estimated that around 48% of people over 65 have impaired mobility, thus many require walking aids (Kalu et al., 2022). However, social pressures and stigma, due to the association with ageing and physical decline, often lead to older people rejecting walking aids, leaving them susceptible to falls. Providing people with choice and agency in selecting features (e.g. colour, finish, or amenities) may improve their acceptance of a walking aid (Resnik et al., 2009). Falls prevention in older people is an important, evidence-based area of occupational therapy practice.

FALLS IN COMMUNITY-DWELLING OLDER PEOPLE

One of the major risks of walking impairment is falls. Falls in older people are highly prevalent, cause serious injury and are costly to health services. A fall can be defined as "an unexpected event in which the participant comes to rest on the ground, floor, or lower level" (Lamb et al., 2005). Falls are sustained by approximately 35% of people aged 65–79 years and by 50% of people aged over 80 years (Moreland et al., 2020). These figures are likely underestimates, as studies which have prospectively monitored falls have reported fall rates of 64%–66% in people aged 70 and over (Cai et al., 2023; Pighills et al., 2011). Two-thirds of falls are occasional (defined as one fall in the preceding year) and one-third are recurrent (defined as two or more falls in the previous year) (Morris et al., 2004). Over 50% of people who have fallen will fall again within a year (Close et al., 1999). Falls are the leading cause of injury-related deaths (77%), injury-related hospitalisations (71%) and emergency department visits in people aged 75 years and

TABLE 32.2

Performance-Based Balance and Mobility Screening Tools and Tests

PERFORMANCE-BASED SCREENING TOOLS (IN DESCENDING ORDER OF PoTP[a])

	Description	Interpretation	Equipment Needed
Single Leg Stance (eyes open)	Unassisted stand on one leg. Time is measured from when the opposite foot leaves the ground to when the opposite foot touches the ground and/or when hands leave the hips.	Unable to maintain single-leg stance positions for >6.5 seconds indicates a **45% probability of falling.**	■ Stopwatch
Self-Selected Walking Speed (SSWS)	Measures gait speed over 4 metres walking at a normal pace (self-selected speed) through a 1-m acceleration zone, a central 4-m "testing" zone (timed with a stopwatch) and a 1-m deceleration zone.	Walking speeds of <1 m/s indicate a **39% probability of falling.**	Measured 6-metre distance with markers at the 1- and 5-metre points. ■ 4 markers ■ Stopwatch

PERFORMANCE-BASED TESTS (IN DESCENDING ORDER OF PoTP[a])

	Description	Interpretation	Equipment Needed
Berg Balance Scale	14 items scored on a scale of 0–4. 0 = unable to do the task 4 = able to do the task Maximum score = 56 Measures standing unsupported, sit-to-stand, transfers, single-leg stance, turning 360 degrees, etc.	Scoring <50 points indicates a **59% probability of falling.**	■ Stopwatch ■ Chair with armrests ■ Measuring tape ■ Object to pick up off the floor ■ Step stool
Timed Up and Go Test (TUG)	Time taken to rise from a chair, walk 3 metres at a normal pace with an assistive device (if used), turn, return to the chair and sit down.	A time of >11 seconds indicates a **47% probability of falling.**	■ Chair ■ Measured point of 3 metres ■ Stopwatch
5 Times Sit-to-Stand (STS)	Measures lower limb strength, speed and coordination. Time taken to complete five STS sequences as fast as possible from a chair.	A time of >12 seconds indicates a **41% probability of falling.**	■ Standard height chair (43 cm)

[a]PoTP Post-test probability of falls – values.

From Lusardi, M. M., Fritz, S., Middleton, A., Allison, L., Wingood, M., Phillips, E., Chui, K. K., et al. (2017). Determining risk of falls in community dwelling older adults: A systematic review and meta-analysis using posttest probability. *Journal of Geriatric Physical Therapy, 40*(1), 1–36.

over, with approximately one older person dying every three hours following a fall in Australia alone (Australian and New Zealand Falls Prevention Society, 2022; Australian Bureau of Statistics, 2018; Australian Institute of Health and Welfare, 2023). Men are more likely than women to sustain fatal falls (Yoshida, 2006). Only half of all older people admitted to hospital following a fall survive a year (Rubenstein, 2006). It is estimated that falls in older people account for 27% of hospital costs and cost the Australian health system $2.3 billion ($595 per capita of the entire population) in 2022 (Australian and New Zealand Falls Prevention Society, 2022).

Falls leave long-lasting adverse effects, such as physical injury, psychological trauma, functional decline and institutionalisation. Around 20%–30% of people who fall suffer injuries that reduce mobility and independence (World Health Organization, 2004). Approximately 20% of falls are serious and require

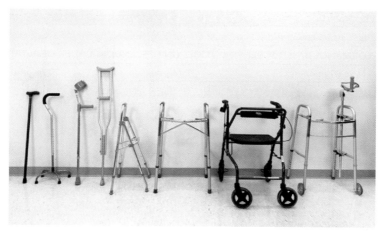

Fig. 32.2 ■ Mobility aids.

medical attention, with 5% leading to fractures, of which 1% are femoral breaks (Cockayne et al., 2021; Moreland et al., 2020). These statistics may be underestimates as many falls go unreported (Cumming, 2002).

Older people are more susceptible to falls and subsequent injury due to a higher prevalence of chronic disease and age-related physiological changes. Declining strength, coordination, flexibility and reflexes result in impaired postural control and balance. A stooped posture, arising from the weakening of the muscles that support spinal alignment and stiff joints can affect the smoothness and stability of gait, evoking compensations to maintain balance, such as spending more time in double support with both feet in contact with the floor (Lord et al., 2021). As a result, older adults may experience a slower and more cautious gait, a wider stance with shorter strides and a decreased arm swing and step height. This age-related decline impairs the ability to withstand environmental challenges to avoid falls (Che Had et al., 2023).

These factors predispose older people to falls and can make relatively mild falls dangerous. Recurrent falls commonly precipitate admission to institutional care, because they tend to be experienced by frail people in the older age range of 75 and over, who are more likely to sustain hip fractures due to slowed reflexes (Rubenstein, 2006). In contrast, those aged 65 to 74 are more likely to sustain wrist fractures following falls, due to faster reflexes initiating protective extension of the arm. In old age, the strategy for maintaining balance after a slip moves from a corrective 'hip'

movement, through a protective 'step' strategy, to a total loss of ability to correct balance in time to avoid a fall. Falls are a threat to older people because of the combination of high incidence, high susceptibility to injury, psychological trauma and functional decline, all of which are risk factors for future falls and often precipitate institutionalisation (Rubenstein, 2006). Falls have a high cost to both the individual and society in general.

There is a range of strategies delivered by interdisciplinary teams that are effective in reducing falls in older people. These strategies include exercise, medical review, medication review, psychological interventions, vision assessment and environmental fall-hazard reduction (Hopewell et al., 2018). Occupational therapists are the primary professionals who facilitate environmental fall-hazard reduction, which is effective in reducing the number of falls by around 38%–39% when targeted toward older people at high fall risk (Clemson et al., 2023; Pighills et al., 2011).

Fall Risk

Over 400 variables have been identified as potential risk factors for falls (CRD, 1996). Risk factors for recurrent falls are summarised in Table 32.3.

Older people with none of the risk factors for recurrent falls have a 10% probability of experiencing recurrent falls, increasing to 97% in older people with all nine factors present (Pluijm et al., 2006). Other studies have found that fall risk increases with the number of risk factors present, from 8% with no risk factors

TABLE 32.3
Risk Factors for Recurrent Falls in Older People

Risk Factors for Recurrent Falls

Two or more previous falls

Dizziness

Functional limitations

Weak grip

Low body weight

Fear of falling

Dogs/cats in the household

High educational level

Drinking 18+ units of alcohol per week

From Pluijm, S. M., Smit, J. H., Tromp, E., Stel, V., Deeg, D. J., Bouter, L., & Lips, P. (2006). A risk profile for identifying community dwelling elderly with a high risk of recurrent falling: Results of a 3-year prospective study. *Osteoporosis International, 2*, 1007–1015. https://doi.org/10.1007/s00198-005-0002-0.

to 78% with four or more (Tinetti et al., 1988). Risk factors are frequently categorised as intrinsic, behavioural or extrinsic (Pighills et al., 2019). Intrinsic risks (person-related) are those characteristics inherent to the individual. For example, impaired balance, gait, or walking problems (due to disease or motor disorders), poly-pharmacy, postural hypertension, visual, or cognitive impairment (Lusardi et al., 2017). Behavioural risks (activity-related) are an individual's self-imposed exposure to risk as a consequence of their behaviour, for example, hurrying, failing to concentrate or intentionally moving outside their base of support. Extrinsic risks (environment-related) are environmental features or characteristics that may pose a hazard to an older adult, given their unique composite of abilities and impairments (Pighills & Clemson, 2021).

The relationship between intrinsic, behavioural and extrinsic fall risk factors is complex. An older person may possess several risk factors from each category which interact with one another. It is estimated that 60% of falls have multiple causal factors (Karlsson et al., 2013). Extrinsic factors are identified as the primary cause of 30%–50% of falls in community-dwelling people aged 65 and over (Rubenstein, 2006), with behavioural factors attributed to 35% and intrinsic factors to 18% (Brace et al., 2003).

Rather than falls being attributable to a single cause, they can be viewed as additive combinations of risk factors, or interactions between increased individual susceptibility to hazards from the cumulative effect of age and disease, behaviour during task performance

and environmental variables. Falls are rarely depicted by older people as being the product of a single trigger, but rather the outcome of several causal factors. When given the option of ascribing falls to causal categories, older people often choose more than one category (Morris et al., 2004).

Intrinsic Risk Factors

Intrinsic risk factors can include fear of falling, advanced age, previous falls, muscle weakness, walking aid use, gait and balance problems, difficulty with everyday occupations, dizziness, urge incontinence, medical comorbidities, vision impairment, chronic diseases such as Parkinson's disease, depression, dementia and history of stroke (Lusardi et al., 2017).

Fear of Falling

Fear of falling is an important intrinsic risk factor that is strongly associated with falls. Following a fall, concern about sustaining further fall-related injuries can lead to psychological difficulties, such as fear and loss of self-confidence (Kalu et al., 2022). Fear of falling is defined as: 'A lasting concern about falling that leads to an individual avoiding activities that he/she remains capable of performing' (Tinetti & Powell, 1993, p. 36). Fear of falling contributes to activity avoidance (a behavioural risk factor) and subsequent impaired physical function (Makino et al., 2018). Fear of falling compromises the quality of life by diminishing an individual's sense of well-being, causes an older adult to self-limit mobility and functional activity, and is attributed to social withdrawal (Kalu et al., 2022). Around 40%–50% of older people limit their activity due to fear of falling and, as a consequence, it is thought to be a risk factor for falls due to reduced physical conditioning (Makino et al., 2018). Both falls and fear of falling are associated with age-related declines in functional ability, often leading to loss of independence and subsequent institutionalisation (Tinetti, 1986). The combination of these elements presents a cycle of fall-related physical decline which is represented in Fig. 32.3.

Self-efficacy relates to confidence and fear of falling relates to anxiety, often leading to activity avoidance. Through activity avoidance, fear of falling affects occupational participation, which in turn affects occupational behaviour and life satisfaction. Activity avoidance limits opportunities to use skills and maintain

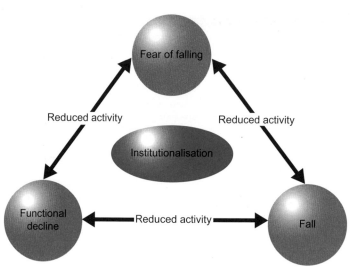

Fig. 32.3 ■ Cycle of fall-related physical decline.

a realistic sense of efficacy. Interventions positively addressing self-efficacy are likely to influence volition and improve occupational adaptation and ultimately participation (Peterson et al., 1999). However, increasing activity levels may increase risk and hence the incidence of falls; although, research has indicated that increasing activity levels usually assists people to mediate their risk, rather than increase exposure to it (Chou et al., 2005). Indeed, fear of falling is not always negative; it may also have a positive protective impact. It may be an appropriate response to a realistic threat preventing people from engaging in high-risk activities (Zijlstra et al., 2007). As fear of falling leads to people avoiding activities that they remain capable of doing, it is also significantly associated with decreased life satisfaction, depression, frailty and restrictions in mobility and social activity (Childs & Kneebone, 2002). Therefore decreasing the fear of falling is an important goal to improve psychological well-being. Enhancing self-efficacy through intervention is likely to reduce both fear of falling and subsequent falls.

Behavioural Risk

Behavioural risk factors can include behaviours such as rushing, not paying attention to the route ahead and poor ladder/climbing safety (Clemson, Cumming et al., 2003). Older people frequently engage in high-risk behaviour in their homes, with 66% reporting rushing, 80% hoarding clutter, 54% changing light bulbs, 43% engaging in do-it-yourself activities and many getting out of bed during the night or using stairs without switching on lights. Seventy-one percent of older adults leave objects on stairs and 29% report that they would not ask for help if an object was difficult to carry downstairs and would attempt to do it themselves (Brace et al., 2003; Hill et al., 2000). Clearly, opportunities exist to reduce fall risk in the home by addressing behavioural issues.

There are common patterns of behaviours that lead to falls. These include inattention to a walking route and environmental hazards, unfamiliarity with surroundings, walking quickly or hurrying, failing to compensate for visual impairment, lack of confidence and overexertion (Clemson, Manor et al., 2003). As environmental hazards are ubiquitous, and the environment is constantly changing, learning to manage environmental risk factors through behaviour is a more practical strategy than removing every potential hazard in the environment (Campbell et al., 2005).

Extrinsic Risk (Environment Related)

Environmental hazards are frequently identified by older people as causal in falls (Stevens et al., 2014). Environmental fall hazards are specific to individuals and their unique patterns of abilities and behaviours, thus many observational studies have not identified a direct association between the number of generic environmental hazards and falls. A longitudinal study, investigating the number of fall hazards in the home, identified a significant association between hazards and falls, with fall risk increasing by 19% for every additional hazard identified (Leclerc et al., 2010). Around 73%–88% of outdoor falls and 30%–50% of indoor falls in older people are ascribed to environmental hazards and up to 77% of all falls occur within the home and surrounding grounds (Li et al., 2006; Nyberg et al., 1996; Rubenstein, 2006; Tinetti et al., 1988). Women tend to fall indoors and men outdoors, in the presence of environmental hazards (Lee, 2021). Therefore the identification and remediation of potential environmental hazards have face validity. It is likely that an association between falls and environmental hazards is less clearly identified in causal studies because the role of environmental hazards is influenced by both intrinsic and behavioural risk factors (Pighills & Clemson, 2021). Therefore environmental fall-hazard reduction makes sense as a compensatory measure in the presence of other fall risk factors.

Research has identified that 80% of the homes of older people had one or more hazards and 39% had more than five. Bathrooms were identified as the most hazardous room, with 66% having at least one hazard. Thirty-percent of homes rated as very safe by older people had more than five hazards and 97% of people living in potentially hazardous environments rated their homes as safe (Carter et al., 1997). Indoor falls predominantly occur in the most frequently used rooms, listed in order of frequency of use; lounge/dining area, bedroom, kitchen and bathroom (Sattin et al., 1998). Most falls occur in the afternoon, which is a period when people are more active (Campbell et al., 1990). Falls during the night are more serious but less frequent and predominantly occur in the bathroom, or on poorly lit stairs, where harder surfaces that do not absorb the kinetic energy of falls increase the force of impact and potential for serious injury (Nyberg et al., 1996). Table 32.4 summarises hazards commonly identified as causal in falls.

Falls Risk Assessment

Falls are multifactorial and can be caused by an interaction of intrinsic, behavioural and extrinsic risk categories, comprising a multitude of risk factors. Therefore no single measure can accurately identify risk. Risk assessment measures include history questions, self-report measures, performance-based measures and a combination of these. To identify those older people, living in the community, who are more likely to fall, history questions, self-report measures and performance-based measurement tools with the highest probability of predicting falls should be used. The predictive ability of five history questions and two self-report measures are summarised in Table 32.5 and the predictive ability of

TABLE 32.4		
Common Environmental Causal FACTORS for Falls and Recommended Modifications		
Most Frequent Environmental Hazards Ascribed as Causal in Falls (Keglovits et al., 2020; Stevens et al., 2014; Walker-Peterson & Clemson, 2008)	Most Common Environmental Hazards Identified on Assessment (Clemson et al., 1997; McNulty et al., 2003; Peel et al., 2000)	Most Commonly Recommended Modifications (Tse, 2005)
Slippery surfaces	Mats	Removal of rugs
Obstacles/clutter	Floor surfaces	Contrast edge on steps
Poor illumination	Steps/stairs	Bathroom floors made slip-resistant
Throw rugs/carpets	Obstacles	Stair rails
Cords/wires	No grab rails in bathing areas	Rollator walking frames
Poorly placed light switches		Raised toilet seats
Items placed too low/too high		Lighting (improve indoors/install outdoors)
No grab bars		Repair indoor and outdoor floor surfaces
Toilet seats too low		Modify furniture
Uneven floor surfaces		Slip-resistant bathmats
Backless/unsupportive shoes		
Unsteady stairs		
Inadequate heating/cooling		
Step stools without railings		
Pets		

TABLE 32.5	
History Questions and Self-Report Measures with the Highest Probability of Predicting Falls (Lusardi et al., 2017)	
History Questions (in Descending Order of PoTP[a])	**Values for Post-test Probability of Falls**
Previous fall history	Yes, indicates a **44% probability of falling**
Use of psycho-active medications	Yes, indicates a **38% probability of falling**
Assistance required for activities of daily living	Yes, indicates a **38% probability of falling**
Fear of falling "are you concerned that you might fall?"	Yes, indicates a **38% probability of falling**
Use of an ambulatory assistive device indoors	Yes, indicates a **36% probability of falling**
Self-report Measures (in Descending Order of PoTP[a])	**Values for Post-test Probability of Falls**
Geriatric Depression Scale-15 (GDS-15)	Score of <6, indicates a **45% probability of falling**
Falls Efficacy Scale – International version (FES-I)	Score of ≥24, indicates a **42% probability of falling**

[a]PoTP Post-test probability of falls – values.

From Lusardi, M. M., Fritz, S., Middleton, A., Allison, L., Wingood, M., Phillips, E., Chui, K. K., et al. (2017). Determining risk of falls in community dwelling older adults: A systematic review and meta-analysis using posttest probability. *Journal of Geriatric Physical Therapy, 40*(1), 1–36.

two performance-based screening tools and three tests is summarised in Table 32.2 (Lusardi et al., 2017).

Falls-Hazard Assessment and Remediation

The theoretical approach underpinning environmental assessment posits that the person, environment and task being performed continually interact in ways that enhance or diminish a person's task performance (behaviour) and that environmental hazards are dynamic entities which occur through an interaction between these three elements (Law et al., 1996). Assessment and remediation of risk factors must take into account the relationships between intrinsic, behavioural and extrinsic fall risk factors (Pighills & Clemson, 2021). This is particularly relevant to extrinsic risk factor reduction. Early research studies focused on the removal of hazards in isolation of functional assessment (Day et al., 2002; Stevens et al., 2001). Using

a predetermined list of hazards without considering the personal capacity and context fails to recognise the dynamic nature of environmental hazards, which change constantly, depending on how the environment is being used. For example, a grandchild may leave a toy in a walkway, posing a tripping hazard which disappears when they leave. The toy (extrinsic risk) may present a threat to an older person who has a reduced step height (intrinsic risk) and fails to scan effectively for potential hazards (behavioural risk). It would be inappropriate to consider any one risk category in isolation from the others (Pighills & Clemson, 2021). The strength of occupational therapy falls-hazard assessment and remediation is that it considers the relationships between different risk categories. For example, circumstances of previous falls, the person's understanding of their fall risk, observation of mobility restrictions, the tasks they do, the usage of various areas of the home – and how they

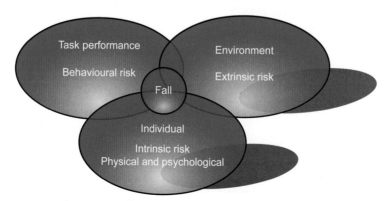

Fig. 32.4 ■ Relationship between the three risk categories.

all relate to fall risk. The relationship between the three risk categories is illustrated in Fig. 32.4.

The environment in relation to falls is defined as:

"The context within which the occupational performance of the person takes place. It influences behaviour and in turn is influenced by the behaviour of the person [...] The environment is considered to be more amenable to change than the person".

(Law et al., 1996, p. 17)

Since falls are a consequence of the relationship between physical competence, risk-taking behaviour and extrinsic risk, the extent to which environmental variables play a role in falls depends on intrinsic factors. More physical competence is required to cope in physically demanding environments and less competence in less demanding environments. Environmental factors are more commonly implicated in falls in vigorous, as opposed to frail, older people possibly because they are more mobile and spend more time outdoors facing challenging environmental conditions and having greater exposure to environmental risk (Northridge et al., 1995). Vigorous older people can tolerate more demanding environmental challenges, typically encountered outdoors, but may fall in the presence of extreme challenges, such as icy conditions. Frail people often stay indoors and live in modified environments or avoid hazards to avert environmentally initiated falls. Very frail older people are likely to fall regardless of their surroundings (Northridge et al., 1996). People who sustain extrinsic falls generally have fewer intrinsic risk factors, or a higher degree of physical competence (Nyberg et al., 1996). However, the linear categorisation of falls oversimplifies the phenomenon. For example, classic 'extrinsic' falls, such as trips, could have an intrinsic root cause, such as weakness, or a behavioural root cause, such as inattention. Indeed, it is conceivable that falls are predominantly caused by either intrinsic or behavioural factors and that all falls have a contributory environmental component (Pighills & Clemson, 2021).

The environment is only hazardous if people have several risk factors. Therefore environmental intervention needs to address all risk factors. In fact, intrinsic, behavioural and environmental factors could conceivably interplay during each phase of a fall, from its initiation

to its conclusion. Therefore it is likely that all falls are environmentally influenced, and within the context of the environment they could be categorised as predominantly intrinsic, behavioural or a combination of the two ("*combination falls*") (Pighills & Clemson, 2021).

Environmental Press

The demands that environments exert on individuals (extrinsic factors) relate directly to their level of functional ability or competence (intrinsic factors). This concept is known as '*environmental press*' and is a component of person/environment relations theory (Lawton et al., 1982). Behaviour is the product of a combination of individual and environmental variables. Although the individual and the environment produce behaviour, it is equally true that behaviour produces new person/environment situations, which lead to new behaviours. This relationship is reflected in Fig. 32.5.

When presented with environmental press, a person's behaviour is either adaptive or maladaptive. Low competence and high press, or low press and high competence may induce low moods and maladaptive behaviour, such as activity avoidance or risk taking, which could cause falls (Pighills et al., 2016). Adaptation level is the point at which a balance is struck between the level of an external stimulus and the degree of competence (Helson, 1964). For less competent people, small changes in the press produce greater changes in behaviour. Normal environmental variation often raises press to excessive levels and results in maladaptive behaviour with variations in behaviour being associated with environmental as opposed to intrinsic change (Fig. 32.6). This suggests that environmental change can influence behaviour (Lawton et al., 1982).

Active Engagement in Risk Identification and Solution Generation

In choosing environmental changes, individuals tend to design their environments appropriately with respect to their competence, highlighting the importance of active engagement of older people in risk identification and solution generation, recognising their agency and capacity to problem solve (Clemson, Mackenzie et al., 2008). Attempts to lower environmental press for older people, through the provision of support services, modifications, equipment, activity avoidance and institutionalisation, are often appropriate but can

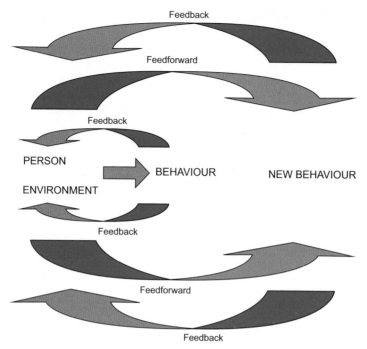

Fig. 32.5 ■ Relations between behaviour, the individual and the environment.

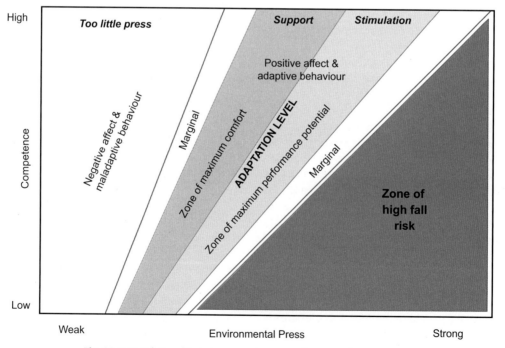

Fig. 32.6 ■ Relationship between environmental press and competence.

be overused and lead to low mood, maladaptive behaviour and decreased competence through environmental under-stimulation. There is a fine line separating protection from environmental stress and environmental deprivation. Conversely, a small relief in the environmental press or introduction of an appropriate level of support can bring behaviour back to an acceptable range for the person's level of competence (Lawton et al., 1982). This reinforces the importance of viewing human behaviour within its environmental context and environmental interventions that encompass assessment, rather than checklist-style hazard removal, provided by suitably qualified professionals with an understanding of the complexities of person/environment relations. This is the balance that occupational therapists are trained to strike, through activity/occupation analysis, requisite skills development and environmental modification to achieve optimal occupational participation and well-being.

ENVIRONMENTAL FALL-HAZARD ASSESSMENT

Given that environmental hazards are highly prevalent in the homes of community-dwelling older people, are associated with falls and are implicated in most falls, environmental intervention makes intuitive sense as a falls prevention strategy. Indeed, there is compelling evidence supporting the clinical effectiveness of high-intensity, comprehensive environmental fall-hazard reduction, when it is tailored toward the needs of older people at high risk of falls, focused on falls prevention and delivered by occupational therapists (Clemson et al., 2023). Occupational therapist-led environmental fall-hazard reduction has been shown to reduce falls by 19%–21% in all risk categories and around 38%–39% in high-risk groups, however, it has less effect when delivered by health care workers other than occupational therapists or to low-risk populations (Clemson et al., 2023; Pighills et al., 2011). During environmental fall-hazard reduction occupational "therapists assess the home environment and make recommendations for safety: provide advice and are actively involved in modifications; have an educating role in increasing awareness of falls and causes of falls; ensure self-monitoring of

some hazards; and ensure safe transfer techniques" (Clemson, 1997, p. 21).

An environmental fall-hazard intervention is different in its approach to a home assessment to assess independence in an area of functional difficulty, which primarily aims to improve task performance and access for people with physical limitations. Table 32.6 provides a comparison between a home visit to assess functional independence and an environmental fall-hazard assessment.

High-intensity environmental fall-hazard intervention comprises the following core components:

1. A comprehensive assessment of the older person considering personal, behavioural and environmental risks;
2. Using an assessment tool validated for a broad range of fall hazards;
3. Formal assessment of functional capacity within the context of the home environment;
4. Follow-up to support the implementation of recommendations; and
5. Active involvement of the older person in risk identification, problem solving and priority setting (Clemson, Bundy et al., 2008).

Environmental interventions consider the abilities of the person (intrinsic), their activity (behavioural) and their environment (extrinsic). Strategies to reduce hazards include the provision of assistive technology or equipment; material adaptations (e.g. clearing pathways, securing loose mats and providing slip-resistant strips on steps); behavioural and practical strategies to maintain or improve independence and safety (e.g. avoiding risky activities); structural modifications (e.g. installing a stair lift); and education about falls risks (Clemson et al., 2023). Environmental interventions for fall-hazard reduction are more complex than the simple removal or remediation of potential hazards, as intrinsic, behavioural and extrinsic risks are all contributing factors to falls (Pighills & Clemson, 2021). Assessment requires the interpretation and synthesis of information to inform clinical decision-making.

Low-intensity intervention comprises of a checklist-style environmental screen with limited or no functional observation or intervention (Clemson et al., 2008). Screening involves limited or no clinical reasoning and

TABLE 32.6

Occupational Therapy Home Assessments: Comparison Between a Home Assessment to Assess Independence and an Environmental Assessment for Fall-Hazard Reduction

Assessment Components	Home Assessment to Determine the Level of Independence and Modify the Environment for Occupational Participation and Access	Environmental Assessment and Fall-hazard Reduction for Falls Prevention
Target population	People of any age experiencing functional decline/difficulty at home	Older people (>65) at high risk of falls (history of 2+ falls in the previous year, injurious falls, functional decline, mobility/balance impairment, polypharmacy, vision impairment, comorbidities)
Focus	Secondary intervention to increase independence in an area of occupational participation difficulty	Primary prevention of falls. Look at falls hazards from a person-environment fit perspective using a person, environment, occupation approach. Considers the interaction between an individual's functional capacity (including behaviour) and the activities in which they engage, within the context of their home environment
Format	Specific assessment of an area of occupational participation difficulty, for example, assessing access to bathing/showering facilities. Not necessarily conducted within the person's own home, the assessment could take place within a similar environment, such as the bathroom in an occupational therapy department	Structured assessment of the older person carrying out occupations within their own home environment. Comprehensive evaluation process to identify hazards and set priorities, taking into consideration personal risk factors/markers (including behavioural risk), environmental hazards and the activities in which the person engages. Includes assessment of functional vision, balance, mobility and occupational participation.
Timeframe of visit	Approximately 1 hour	Approximately 1.5 hours
Clinician experience/training	No experience or training is required in addition to a graduate occupational therapy qualification	Completion of face-to-face or online training modules (https://fallspreventiononlineworkshops.com.au/) recommended to enhance knowledge of falls prevention and format of standardised assessment. No experience is required in addition to a graduate occupational therapy qualification
Approach/engagement	Prescriptive. The occupational therapist assumes the role of the 'expert', recommends solutions and prescribes intervention, modifications and/or equipment	Collaborative. Active involvement of the older person and/or their carer in problem identification, prioritisation and solution generation
Tools	Home-made checklists, environmental audits using service-specific non-validated home assessment forms, functional assessments and/or freehand case notes to record observations and actions	Standardised, valid and comprehensive assessment tool, for example, the Westmead Home Safety Assessment (WeHSA) which is a 72-item assessment grouped into 15 domains
Intervention intensity	Often incorporates 1–3/5 components of an intensive falls prevention intervention (Clemson, Mackenzie et al., 2008)	Incorporates 4–5/5 components of an intensive falls prevention intervention (Clemson, Mackenzie et al., 2008)
Recommendations	Further intervention and/or equipment, adaptations and/or modifications to the physical environment, written by the occupational therapist. A copy may or may not be given to the client	Action plan given to, and written in collaboration with, the client documenting what to do and why, including habits to change (risk-taking behaviours while engaged in activity); equipment to procure; modifications to the physical environment (including who will do these); other adaptations to implement; and future considerations

Continued on following page

	TABLE 32.6	
	Occupational Therapy Home Assessments: Comparison Between a Home Assessment to Assess Independence and an Environmental Assessment for Fall-Hazard Reduction (*Continued*)	
Assessment Components	**Home Assessment to Determine the Level of Independence and Modify the Environment for Occupational Participation and Access**	**Environmental Assessment and Fall-hazard Reduction for Falls Prevention**
Follow-up	Referral for equipment installation, modifications and adaptations. Telephone follow-up to check that recommendations have been carried out. Tailored instruction following installation, if required	Referral for equipment installation, modifications and adaptations. Telephone follow-up to check that recommendations have been carried out. Additional visit(s) to the person's home environment to re-assess function and re-prioritise risks and solutions once recommendations have been carried out

comprises a standardised process to collect and score information, using a template and has not been shown to be effective in reducing falls (Clemson & Pighills, 2021). Occupational therapists generally carry out environmental assessments, as opposed to environmental screens, thus occupational therapist-led environmental fall-hazard reduction always met the high-intensity intervention criteria in clinical trials. This reflects the natural alignment between occupational therapy theoretical frameworks and the aims of clinical environmental assessments, which require environment-person fit approaches to support change and may explain why occupational therapist-led environmental fall-hazard reduction is effective (Clemson et al., 2023).

Environmental and Behavioural Fall-Hazard Assessments and Screening Tools

There are 77 different assessments which screen or assess for environmental fall risk (Blanchet & Edwards, 2018). A review of 36 of these tools identified the environmental falls-hazard assessment, self-assessment, screen, outdoor assessment and falls behaviour assessment presented in Table 32.7, as possessing the best psychometric properties (Romli et al., 2018).

Conducting the Home Falls-Hazard Assessment

The Westmead Schema is a conceptual framework that can be used to structure the environmental falls-hazard assessment (Keglovits et al., 2020). It has been used to develop online learning modules, resources and tools on environmental interventions for falls prevention. The evidence-based online modules "Home and Community Safety" (https://fallspreventiononlineworkshops.com.au/) teach occupational therapists, and other allied health professionals, how to conduct a comprehensive home assessment, designed to reduce the risk of falls for community-dwelling older people. The Westmead Schema outlines foundations for clinical reasoning and comprises of three key areas (Clemson & Pighills, 2021):

1. 'Understanding the person': The environmental falls-hazard assessment begins with an initial discussion about the client's history of falling, the circumstances of previous falls, their beliefs and understanding of their fall risk, intrinsic risk factors, lifestyle, functional capacity, patterns of usage of areas in the home, risk-taking behaviour, strategies already adopted to reduce falls, environmental changes previously made, exercise, footwear and functional vision. This discussion may include a review of the Fall Behavioural Scale and administration of the Outdoor Falls Questionnaire (Chippendale et al., 2016; Clemson, Bundy et al., 2008).

2. 'Moving through the home environment and collaborative problem solving': The environmental falls-hazard assessment involves using a validated assessment tool, such as the Westmead

TABLE 32.7

Environmental and Behavioural Fall-Hazard Assessments and Screening Tools with the Best Psychometric Properties

Assessment/Screen	Details	Comments
Westmead Home Safety Assessment (Clemson, 1997; Clemson, Cusick et al., 1999; Clemson, Fitzgerald et al., 1999a, b; Keglovits et al., 2020)	Valid and reliable assessment tool. 72-item long form, 44-item short form. Assesses falls hazards inside and outside the home. Domains: internal/external traffic ways, general/indoors, living area, seating, bedroom, bathroom, kitchen, laundry, footwear, medication management.	Functional home falls-hazard assessment. Gold standard in home-fall hazard assessments. Used in the majority of the trials which have demonstrated clinical effectiveness of the intervention.
Home Safety Self-Assessment Tool (Horowitz et al., 2013; Tomita et al., 2014)	Validated, environmental self-assessment tool. 64-item.	Self-assessment for home falls-hazards.
HOME FAST (Mackenzie et al., 2000)	Validated environmental screening tool. 25-item. Consists of 18 environmental hazards and 7 mobility/transfer items.	Screening tool to identify for home falls-hazards. Not recommended for a tailored and comprehensive approach to fall prevention.
Outdoor Falls Questionnaire (Chippendale et al., 2016)	Validated tool. Assesses environmental factors and individual behaviours contributing to falls, perceived risks and strategies used for fall prevention in the community.	Identifies outdoor falls hazards.
Falls Behavioural Scale (FaB) (Clemson et al., 2003; Clemson et al., 2008)	Valid and reliable assessment tool. 30-item long form, 24-item short-form version which has been validated as an outcome measure. Identifies protective and high-risk behaviours which may cause indoor and outdoor falls.	Can be used as a self-assessment tool and discussed with the older person during a home falls-hazard assessment.

Home Safety Assessment, to functionally assess the older person in their home (Clemson, 1997). The occupational therapist and the client move through the house together and a functional evaluation is carried out. Items on the checklist are rated as either relevant (i.e. deemed to be a hazard), not relevant (i.e. not deemed to be a hazard), or not present.

3. 'Prioritising and Planning': The occupational therapist discusses any potential falls hazards (intrinsic, environmental and behavioural) identified during the assessment and collaboratively problem solves with the older person, recognising their right to make informed decisions about risk (Kessler et al., 2019). A list of recommendations is co-created. If possible, and in

consultation, identified hazards are addressed/ removed. If required, the occupational therapist makes referrals to other agencies for equipment or a handyman for minor modifications. The occupational therapist may also make recommendations for the private purchase of equipment, such as lightweight step ladders with handles and height-adjustable rotary washing lines. In such cases the occupational therapist will liaise with the older person or a family member regarding the purchase of such equipment. The occupational therapist makes a clinical judgement on whether a follow-up home visit is required. A co-created action plan is written and sent to the older person. Following the visit(s) the occupational therapist will contact the older person/carer to review follow-through with recommendations and provide further advice if necessary.

Community Mobility

Community mobility relates to "moving around in the community and using public or private transportation, such as driving, walking, bicycling, or accessing and riding in buses, taxi cabs, or other transportation systems" (Roley et al., 2008, p. 631) Environmental falls-hazard interventions generally focus on the immediate home surroundings, because bespoke changes cannot be made in the wider community and research into the effectiveness of falls prevention interventions in this context requires a population-level approach. However, some studies have seen a reduction in falls extend beyond the home, even though community safety was not a component of the environmental falls-hazard assessment (Campbell et al., 2005; Clemson et al., 2004; Cumming et al., 1999; Nikolaus & Bach, 2003). This outcome is likely due to older people generalising falls prevention strategies and adapting their behaviour to broader contexts (Clemson, Mackenzie, et al., 2008).

Given that most falls, attributable to extrinsic causes, occur in the community, improvements in the design and maintenance of community facilities are likely to be an effective population-level falls prevention strategy (Li et al., 2006). Universal design principles promote inclusion and participation and aim to create built environments that are accessible and safe for people, regardless of their age and ability (Gray et al., 2012). Implementation of universal design principles requires coordination at national, state and local levels to set and implement design, construction and maintenance standards. Examples of design improvements include even, cleared and maintained pavements, contrasting edges on curbs, stairs and changes of level, removal of tripping hazards, clear signage, adequate street lighting, timed traffic lights and provision of resting places and grab rails (Clemson & Pighills, 2021).

Falls Prevention Solutions

Potential hazards that may be identified during an environmental falls-hazard assessment, and possible solutions, are presented in Table 32.8. These potential hazards and possible solutions have been drawn from the literature and from the authors' experience of delivering the intervention in falls prevention trials. Many of the solutions have been suggested by trial participants themselves, as examples of strategies they have devised and implemented to reduce their risk of falling. Solutions should be co-created and tailored so they are relevant and acceptable to older people and target the behaviour for change.

Adherence to Recommendations

Adherence potentially dictates the outcome of environmental falls-hazard interventions (Ballinger & Clemson, 2006; Walker-Peterson & Clemson, 2008). Low levels of follow-through with recommendations are likely to reduce the potency of the intervention. Indeed, one study reported that those in the intervention group failing to implement any recommendations experienced the same fall rate as controls, but those who adhered to at least one recommendation experienced a 36% reduction (Nikolaus & Bach, 2003). In trials, home falls-hazard recommendations, provided by occupational therapists, have resulted in relatively high levels of adherence (between 53% and 90% full or partial adherence) (Campbell et al., 2005; Cumming et al., 1999; Nikolaus & Bach, 2003; Pighills et al., 2011). Factors Influencing the follow-through of recommendations include:

- Immediate follow-up to support the implementation of recommendations
- Collaborative problem solving and co-creating solutions (empowerment, ownership)
- Belief that the recommendation will reduce falls
- Perception of being at risk of falls
- Perceived ability to 'exert control' over the home environment
- Involvement of carers/relatives
- Degree of action required to implement the recommendation and
- Provision of equipment as opposed to modifications.

(Clemson, 1997; Clemson, Cusick et al., 1999; Clemson & Pighills, 2021; Cumming et al., 2001; Pighills et al., 2019)

Non-adherence has been attributed to older people not believing they are at risk of falling, concern about the stigma surrounding disability equipment, and the

TABLE 32.8
Environmental Falls Risk and Potential Solutions

Environmental Falls Risks	Potential Environmental and Behavioural Solutions
Hazardous flooring and mats	■ Use double-sided tape to secure mats or replace them with rubber-backed slip-resistant mats. ■ Avoid thick pile carpets that catch feet. ■ The colour of carpets should contrast with the walls to define the floor-wall boundary. ■ Avoid putting an overlay of protective carpeting of the same pattern on fitted carpets. ■ Use double-sided tape to secure mats or place a thin layer of foam underneath loose mats and rugs. ■ Mop up spills immediately; use a cleaner if there are oil or butter spills. ■ Clean up dust on smooth floor surfaces. ■ Replace patterned carpets with light-coloured plain ones, particularly on the stairs and particularly carpets with horizontal or vertical lines.
Steps and stairs	■ Replace poor-condition stair coverings. ■ Use adhesive strips/paint white strips on the edges of concrete steps. ■ Avoid leaving things on the stairs. ■ Stair rails should preferably be a round pole style with a diameter of 220 mm and extend 1 tread width beyond the last riser. ■ Only carry things that require one hand, leaving the other free to hold on; ask others to carry large objects. ■ Avoid carrying objects up/downstairs (restricts view of stair surface); use pockets/bags instead. ■ Avoid carrying large amounts of laundry downstairs, have a laundry basket next to the washing machine and bring dirty items down a few at a time or locate the washing machine and dryer upstairs where most laundry is generated. ■ Coming downstairs backwards, moving an item down a step at a time, poses the risk of misjudging the bottom of the stairs. ■ Have an additional vacuum upstairs. ■ Use a small handheld vacuum, a damp cloth or a dustpan and brush to clean stairs or ask others to do it. ■ Leave a walking aid at the top and bottom of the stairs. ■ Stair lifts should be able to be parked in a position that does not cause severe obstruction for other users. ■ Remove loose rugs from the top of stairs. ■ Avoid positioning smoke alarms over the stairs to allow for safe testing and battery changing.
Lighting	■ Install night lights beside the first and last steps and a light switch at the top and bottom of the stairs. ■ Switch on stair lights when descending at night (18% of older people do not do this). ■ Use a low-energy light bulb and leave it on all night. ■ Use a night light or a plug-in photosensitive light in a power point; these are soft enough not to 'awaken' you and automatically light up when dark, so you do not have to remember. ■ Use a 100-watt light bulb at the top and bottom of stairs. ■ Avoid sudden changes in light intensity, for example, going from a dimly lit room to bright lighting and vice versa (causes temporary blindness). ■ Use long-life bulbs (reduces the frequency with which they need changing but some have a delay in reaching full brightness which can be helpful in adjusting to changes in light intensity). ■ Avoid too low or too high wattage bulbs (check the safety of the lampshade and fittings with the light bulb – most lampshades and fittings are made for bulbs under 100 watts). ■ Avoid lampshades that reduce illumination (solid plastic design). ■ Turn on lights when getting up at night but allow time for eyes to accommodate to the change. ■ Use fluorescent lighting for traffic ways. ■ Get practical help to change light bulbs. ■ Make light switches more accessible, particularly traffic ways to reach them. ■ Make light switches more visible by contrasting colour with the walls. ■ Ensure that bedside lights have a secure base and an accessible switch or use a touch lamp or light on the bed headboard for easy access. ■ Use opaque light bulbs to reduce glare. ■ Use net curtains to counteract glare from sunlight. ■ Avoid changes in floor surfaces in areas prone to shifts in lighting (while eyes are adjusting, changes in surface might not be recognised in time to adjust gait). ■ Choose matt non-reflecting surfaces when re-decorating a room.

TABLE 32.8

Environmental Falls Risk and Potential Solutions (*Continued*)

Environmental Falls Risks	Potential Environmental and Behavioural Solutions
Pets	■ Keep pets confined overnight and during times of high activity to avoid tripping over them in poor light. ■ Give pets a fluorescent collar, jacket, or a bell so that they are noticed more easily. ■ Consider a pet training programme. ■ Position pet food bowls away from traffic ways to avoid tripping over pets while they eat.
Clothes	■ Dressing gowns and loose long pants can be a trip hazard on the stairs. ■ Wear well-fitting shoes that allow a good grip and a feeling of the floor surface. ■ Make sure your shoe soles are not slippery. ■ Wear a sari, trousers and long dresses slightly shorter. ■ Avoid baggy, ill-fitting clothes. ■ Apply a rubber solution to the heels of worn shoes/score the soles of leather shoes. ■ Avoid walking in stockinged feet. ■ Sleep in bed socks with a slip-resistant tread if nocturnal bathroom trips are necessary.
Bathroom	■ Consider a rail in the shower or toilet. ■ Use rubber-backed slip-resistant bathroom mats. ■ Increase accessibility of toiletries in bath/shower. ■ Place a light in the medicine cabinet. ■ Carpet bathroom floor to avoid slippery wet floors or use sheet rubber flooring. ■ Fit contrasting coloured toilet seats to the toilet to facilitate proper seating placement. ■ Contrast bathroom walls with the toilet pan to enable people to visualise the toilet.
Kitchen	■ Boil food in a chip basket to avoid lifting pans of boiling water to drain food. ■ Rearrange cupboards placing commonly used items on shelves that require the least reaching. ■ Re-hang fridge doors to avoid overreaching. ■ Avoid buying ovens with doors that drop down which are easy to trip over.
Public transport	■ Have money or ticket easily accessible and ready in advance. ■ Once off the bus, pause, gain balance and walk first in the direction the bus is travelling. ■ Be early to be first in the queue (it allows more time to sit down). ■ Travel at off-peak times to avoid the crowds. ■ Find out which bus routes have accessible buses. ■ Take a backpack to carry shopping. ■ Ask the driver not to set off until you are seated. ■ Take the first seat as close to the front as possible. ■ Keep a hand free to hold on. ■ Ask the driver to pull in as close to the pavement as possible. ■ Use the bus stop sign to help get from the road to the pavement.
Garden	■ Roughened concrete is a good slip-resistant surface. ■ Install external sensor lights. ■ Keep paths clear of moss. ■ Keep hose pipes on a reel.
Outdoors	■ Allow extra time to get to places, particularly when going somewhere new. ■ Have strategies for crossing roads safely. ■ Avoid windy conditions. ■ Slow down your pace. ■ Wear clothing that is easily seen. ■ Wear a rain hood rather than using an umbrella if you use a walking stick. ■ Avoid going out at peak times. ■ Plan outings carefully including toilet stops. ■ Wear woolly socks over the top of outdoor shoes in icy and slushy conditions; they stick to ice.

Continued on following page

	TABLE 32.8
	Environmental Falls Risk and Potential Solutions (*Continued*)

Environmental Falls Risks	Potential Environmental and Behavioural Solutions
Impaired vision to judge depth/ distance	■ Take extra care when getting new glasses prescriptions to adjust to changes, particularly on stairs and changes of level. ■ Avoid thick-framed glasses that may obscure the visual field. ■ Glasses without rims can make it difficult to distinguish where the glasses end and thus affect depth perception. ■ Bifocals (worn by 57% of older people) increase difficulty in judging depth and distance and can cause distortion; consider having two pairs of glasses instead of bifocals; discuss with an optician. ■ Varifocals (worn by 22% of older people) can cause blurred or double vision when walking around; discuss with the optician.
General risk mitigation strategies	■ Source a secure, lightweight step ladder with a wide base and a high handrail for climbing and reaching. ■ Avoid furniture with splayed legs. ■ Contrast furniture with floor and wall covers. ■ Ensure that furniture used for support while mobilising is stable. ■ Replace unstable chairs/tables. ■ Avoid pedestal-style tables which tip easily or position them away from traffic ways. ■ Select tabletops with a contrasting border to assist in identifying the boundary. ■ Use curtain pull cords to avoid overreaching. ■ Use fall detectors if living alone. ■ Use a door intercom upstairs to avoid rushing to answer the door. ■ Avoid rushing to answer the phone; find out the number you can call to find out who was your last caller. ■ Scan ahead when walking to observe hazards rather than watching feet. ■ Avoid taking alcohol and prescribed medication together if contra-indicated. ■ Rearrange your diary for two days after a change in medication to enable extra care to be taken. ■ Develop an awareness of potential hazards. ■ Have something at the entrance to put bags and shoes on that is above floor level. ■ Be aware that visitors often introduce new hazards to a home (handbag straps, toys, shoes at the entrance). ■ Avoid having throws or bedclothes that dangle onto the floor. ■ Move awkward or heavy things around on a trolley. ■ Use adhesive slip-resistant strips 50 mm apart on linoleum floors and surfaces used to support weight, for example, sink rim (colour should match the floor surface to prevent them being interpreted as ground elevations). ■ Walk heel to toe. ■ Hip protectors may be beneficial for older ladies with a slight build to cushion a fall. ■ Contrast the colour of the handrails with the walls to promote visibility. ■ Avoid chairs with seat edges that overhang the position of the legs which may tip during transfers. ■ Have a flu injection as illness renders people more prone to falling. ■ Talk to neighbours about having a routine to show you are ok such as opening a front blind when get up in the morning. ■ Use sensor lights at entrances.

From Clemson, L., & Pighills, A. (2021). Environmental interventions to prevent falls at home and in the community. In S. R. Lord, C. Shrerrington, & V. Naganathan (Eds.), *Falls in older people; risk factors, strategies for prevention and implications for practice* (3rd ed.). Cambridge University Press.

perception that the recommendation is unnecessary, with only 1% of people reporting non-adherence due to affordability (Cumming et al., 2001).

Environmental fall-hazard reduction has been incorporated into international guidelines (the recent world falls guidelines), is feasible to implement and cost-effective, with estimations indicating it takes 90 minutes to complete (Montero-Odasso et al., 2022; Pighills et al., 2011; Tynan et al., 2022). However, research suggests that it is not being implemented in

| | **TABLE 32.9** | |
| | **Summary of the Stepping On and LiFE Programmes** | |
Programme	Stepping On, Reducing Falls and Improving Confidence	Lifestyle-Integrated Functional Exercise Programme (LiFE) to Prevent Falls and Improve Function
Purpose	Community multi-component fall prevention programme for older people who have fallen once or twice in the past year.	Embedding balance and lower limb strength training into daily life activities and routines to reduce falls and improve function.
Sessions	Seven weekly sessions (1.5 hrs) and a follow-up booster at 3 months.	Home-based training over five sessions with follow-up. Adapted for group settings (7 sessions).
Content	Teaching balance and lower limb strengthening, community safety and safe mobility, footwear, home fall hazards and medication management.	What is balance and strength training; LiFE Balance and Strength activities; Upgrading; LiFE assessment tool; LiFE planners to set LiFE weekly goals.
Conceptual underpinning	Decision-making framework to prompt reflection and action. Practical strategies, problem solving and reflective motivation. Self-efficacy as a tool for change; guided homework.	Principles of balance and strength training. Habit reforming theory as a basis to support integration into daily habits and routines (Clemson & Munro, 2016).
Evidence	Randomised trial – fall reduction (Clemson et al., 2004). Numerous other studies support behaviour change, reduction of physical fall risks and reduction of fall-related health costs.	Randomised trial – reduced falls and increased functional capacity in daily life activities (Clemson et al., 2012). Other studies support implementation and a series led by M. Schwenk successfully adapted LiFE for group delivery (Kramer et al., 2020). Pilot studies support combining LiFE with home safety by occupational therapists.
Manual	Manual for facilitators (Clemson & Swann, 2019). Spanish version Pisando Fuerte (available: Wisconsin Institute Healthy Ageing (WiHA)).	Manuals for participants and trainer's tools (available Sydney University (SUP); Amazon.com). German and Chinese language versions (available: 2019 Springer; HKOT respectively) (Clemson et al., 2019). LiFE tools downloadable SUP.
Training	Australia (www.steppingon.com); North America (WiHA, www.wihealthyaging.org).	Online LiFE training for occupational therapists available 2024 (www.fallsprevention-onlineworkshops.com.au).

routine occupational therapy practice (Pighills et al., 2019). Implementation barriers include external contextual factors, conflicting organisational processes, limited clinician skills, lack of focus on prevention, perceived complexity of the intervention and consumer expectations (Clemson et al., 2014; Tynan et al., 2022). The occupational therapy profession needs to ensure that new graduates are skilled in environmental fall-hazard reduction, so they are confident and equipped to implement this evidence-based intervention in routine practice.

Other evidence-based occupational therapy interventions for falls prevention include a multi-component group-based fall prevention programme, Stepping On, which incorporates exercise, home and community safety and education and the LiFE programme, which embeds balance and strength exercises into daily activities and routines (Clemson et al., 2014; Clemson & Swann, 2019). Both programmes have been proven to be clinically effective in randomised controlled trials and are summarised in Table 32.9 (Clemson et al., 2004; Clemson et al., 2012; Jansen et al., 2021; Jansen et al., 2023).

CONCLUSION

Walking involves the complex integration of physiological and cognitive systems to produce smooth, efficient movement. Disruption of any element of these systems can cause walking impairment, which in turn has a profound effect on a person's occupational participation. A person's occupational participation can be further limited by environmental, societal, psychosocial, economic and cultural barriers. Impaired occupational participation can lead to dependence on others, limited access to services, financial hardship, a more sedentary lifestyle, activity avoidance, low self-efficacy, social isolation, loneliness, depression, poor physical and mental well-being, and, ultimately, poor quality of life. Occupational therapists facilitate occupational participation for people with walking impairments by enhancing capabilities, modifying activities and/or adapting environments to promote independence, health and well-being. Older adults are particularly susceptible to walking impairment due to physical decline from ageing and comorbidities. This combination often results in falls that can lead to a cycle of fall-related decline, institutionalisation and ultimately death. Occupational therapy intervention in falls prevention, underpinned by robust evidence, can reduce falls by 38%–39% (Clemson et al., 2023; Pighills et al., 2011).

REFERENCES

Almahmood, M., Scharnhorst, E., Carstensen, T. A., Jørgensen, G., & Schulze, O. (2017). Mapping the gendered city: Investigating the socio-cultural influence on the practice of walking and the meaning of walkscapes among young Saudi adults in Riyadh. *Journal of Urban Design, 22*(2), 229–248. https://doi.org/10.1080/13574809.2016.1273742.

Australian and New Zealand Falls Prevention Society. (2022). *Why investing in falls prevention across Australia can't wait*. https://fallsnetwork.neura.edu.au/invest-in-fall-prevention/#:~:text=Professor%20Kim%20Delbaere%2C%20NeuRA%20and,effective%20means%20to%20do%20this.

Australian Bureau of Statistics. (2018). *Australia's leading causes of death (2016 data)*. http://www.abs.gov.au/ausstats/abs@.nsf/Lookup/by%20Subject/3303.0~2016~Main%20Features~Australia's%20leading%20causes%20of%20death,%202016~3.

Australian Institute of Health and Welfare. (2023). *Falls in older Australians 2019–20: Hospitalisations and deaths among people aged 65 and over*. https://www.aihw.gov.au/reports/injury/falls-in-older-australians-2019-20-hospitalisation/contents/about.

Ballinger, C., & Clemson, L. (2006). Older people's views about community falls prevention: An Australian perspective. *British Journal of Occupational Therapy, 69*(6), 263–270.

Blanchet, R., & Edwards, N. (2018). A need to improve the assessment of environmental hazards for falls on stairs and in bathrooms: Results of a scoping review. *BMC Geriatrics, 18*(1), 272. https://doi.org/10.1186/s12877-018-0958-1.

Bohannon, R. W., & Wang, Y.-C. (2019). Four-meter gait speed: Normative values and reliability determined for adults participating in the NIH toolbox study. *Archives of Physical Medicine and Rehabilitation, 100*(3), 509–513. https://doi.org/10.1016/j.apmr.2018.06.031.

Brace, C. L., Haslam, R. A., Brooke-Wavell, K., & Howarth, P. A. (2003). *The contribution of behaviour to falls among older people in and around the home*. http://www.lboro.ac.uk/departments/hu/groups/hseu/publications/documents/home%20falls%20report%202003.pdf,

Cai, Y., Leveille, S. G., Andreeva, O., Shi, L., Chen, P., & You, T. (2023). Characterizing fall circumstances in community-dwelling older adults: A mixed methods approach. *The Journals of Gerontology: Series A, 78*(9), 1683–1691. https://doi.org/10.1093/gerona/glad130.

Campbell, A. J., Borrie, M. J., Spears, G. F., & Jackson, S. L. (1990). Circumstances and consequences of falls experienced by a community population 70 Years and over during a prospective study. *Age and Ageing, 19*(2), 136–141.

Campbell, A. J., Robertson, M. C., La Grow, S. J., Kerse, N. M., Sanderson, G. F., Jacobs, R. J., ... Hale, L. A. (2005). Randomised controlled trial of prevention of falls in people aged 75 with severe visual impairment: The VIP trial. *British Medical Journal, 331*(817), 1136–1143. https://doi.org/10.1136/bmj.38601.447731.55.

Carter, S. E., Campbell, E. M., Sanson-Fisher, R. W., Redman, S., & Gillespie, W. J. (1997). Environmental hazards in the homes of older people. *Age and Ageing, 26*(3), 195–202. http://ageing.oxfordjournals.org/content/26/3/195.full.pdf.

Chambers, H. G., & Sutherland, D. H. (2002). A practical guide to gait analysis. *Journal of the American Academy of Orthopaedic Surgeons, 10*(3), 222–231. https://journals.lww.com/jaaos/Fulltext/2002/05000/A_Practical_Guide_to_Gait_Analysis.9.aspx.

Che Had, N. H., Alavi, K., Md Akhir, N., Muhammad Nur, I. R., Shuhaimi, M. S. Z., & Foong, H. F. (2023). A scoping review of the factors associated with older adults' mobility barriers. *International Journal of Environmental Research and Public Health, 20*(5), 4243. https://www.mdpi.com/1660-4601/20/5/4243.

Childs, L., & Kneebone, I. I. (2002). Falls, fear of falling and psychological management. *British Journal of Therapy and Rehabilitation, 9*(6), 225–231.

Chippendale, T., Knight, R.-A., An, M. S. M., Cefalo, L., Lautman, T., Stoffel, C., ... Huang, D. (2016). Development and validity of the outdoor falls questionnaire (OFQ). *American Journal of Occupational Therapy, 70*(4), 1–7. https://doi.org/10.5014/ajot.2016.70S1-RP304D.

Chou, K., Yeung, F., & Wong, E. (2005). Fear of falling and depressive symptoms in Chinese elderly living in nursing homes: Falls efficacy and activity level as mediator or moderator? *Ageing and Mental Health, 9*(3), 255–261.

Christiansen, C. H., Baum, C. M., & Bass-Haugen, J. (2005). *Occupational therapy: Performance, participation and wellbeing* (3rd ed.). SLACK Incorporated.

Clemson, L. (1997). *Home fall hazards: A guide to identifying fall hazards in the homes of elderly people and an accompaniment to the assessment tool, the Westmead Home Safety Assessment (WeHSA)*. Co-ordinates Publications.

Clemson, L., Bundy, A. C., Cumming, R. G., Kay, L., & Luckett, T. (2008). Validating the Falls Behavioural (FaB) scale for older people: A Rasch analysis. *Disability and Rehabilitation, 30*(7), 498–506. https://www.tandfonline.com/doi/abs/10.1080/09638280701355546.

Clemson, L., Cumming, R. G., & Heard, R. (2003). The development of an assessment to evaluate behavioural factors associated with falling. *American Journal of Occupational Therapy, 57*(4), 380–388. http://ajot.aota.org/article.aspx?articleid=1869393.

Clemson, L., Cumming, R. G., Kendig, H., Swann, M., Heard, R., & Taylor, K. (2004). The effectiveness of a community-based program for reducing the incidence of falls in the elderly: A randomized trial. *Journal of the American Geriatrics Society, 52*(9), 1487–1494. http://www.swetswise.com/eAccess/viewAbstract.do?articleID=20971711&titleID=115510.

Clemson, L., Cusick, A., & Fozzard, C. (1999). Managing risk and exerting control: Determining follow through with falls prevention. *Disability and Rehabilitation, 21*(12), 531–541. https://doi.org/10.1080/096382899297189.

Clemson, L., Donaldson, A., Hill, K., & Day, L. (2014). Implementing person-environment approaches to prevent falls: A qualitative inquiry in applying the Westmead approach to occupational therapy home visits. *Australian Occupational Therapy Journal, 61*(5), 325–334. https://doi.org/10.1111/1440-1630.12132.

Clemson, L., Fiatarone Singh, M. A., Bundy, A., Cumming, R. G., Manollaras, K., O'Loughlin, P., & Black, D. (2012). Integration of balance and strength training into daily life activity to reduce rate of falls in older people (the LiFE study): Randomised parallel trial. *BMJ: British Medical Journal, 345*, e4547. https://doi.org/10.1136/bmj.e4547.

Clemson, L., Fitzgerald, M. H., & Heard, R. (1999a). Content validity of an assessment tool to identify home fall hazards: The Westmead Home Safety Assessment. *British Journal of Occupational Therapy, 62*(4), 171–179.

Clemson, L., Fitzgerald, M. H., Heard, R., & Cumming, R. G. (1999b). Inter-rater reliability of a home fall hazards assessment tool. *Occupational Therapy Journal of Research, 19*(2), 83–100.

Clemson, L., Mackenzie, L., Ballinger, C., Close, J., & Cumming, R. G. (2008). Environmental interventions to prevent falls in community-dwelling older people: A meta-analysis of randomized trials. *Journal of Ageing and Health, 20*(8), 954–971. https://doi.org/10.1177/0898264308324672.

Clemson, L., Manor, D., & Fitzgerald, M. H. (2003). Behavioural factors contributing to older adults falling in public places. *OTJR: Occupation, Participation and Health, 23*(3), 107–117. https://doi.org/10.1177/153944920302300304.

Clemson, L., & Munro, J. (2016). *Conceptual model of habit reforming to improve balance and prevent falls*. In *Encyclopaedia of geropsychology*. Springer.

Clemson, L., Munro, J., & Singh, M. F. (2014). *Lifestyle-integrated Functional Exercise (LiFE) program to prevent falls: Trainer's manual*. Sydney University Press.

Clemson, L., Munro, J., Singh, M. F., Schwenk, M., & Nerz, C. (2019). *Trainer-Manual-Aktiv und Sicher Durchs Leben Mit Dem LiFE Programm*. Springer.

Clemson, L., & Pighills, A. (2021). Environmental interventions to prevent falls at home and in the community. In S. R. Lord, C. Shrerrington, & V. Naganathan (Eds.), *Falls in older people; risk factors, strategies for prevention and implications for practice* (3rd ed.). Cambridge University Press.

Clemson, L., Roland, M., & Cumming, R. G. (1997). Types of hazards in the homes of elderly people. *Occupational Therapy Journal of Research, 17*(3), 200–213.

Clemson, L., Stark, S., Pighills, A. C., Fairhall, N. J., Lamb, S. E., Ali, J., & Sherrington, C. (2023). Environmental interventions for preventing falls in older people living in the community. *Cochrane Database of Systematic Reviews, 1465–1858*. https://doi.org/10.1002/14651858.CD013258.pub2.

Clemson, L., & Swann, M. (2019). *Stepping on building confidence and reducing falls a community based programme for older people* (3rd ed.). Sydney University Press.

Close, J., Ellis, M., Hooper, R., Glucksman, E., Jackson, S., & Swift, C. (1999). Prevention of falls in the elderly trial (PROFET): A randomised controlled trial. *The Lancet, 353*, 93–97.

Cockayne, S., Pighills, A., Fairhurst, C., Adamson, J., Crossland, S., & Drummond, A., ... (2021). Home hazard assessment and environmental modification to prevent falls in older people: The OTIS trial. *F1000Research, 10*(500). https://doi.org/10.12688/f1000research.52313.1.

CRD. (1996). Preventing falls and subsequent injury in older people2. Effective Health Care Number 4, ISSN 0965 0288).

Cumming, R. G. (2002). Intervention strategies and risk-factor modification for falls prevention. A review of recent intervention studies. *Clinics in Geriatric Medicine, 18*(2), 175–189. www.otseeker.com.

Cumming, R. G., Thomas, M., Szonyi, G., Frampton, G., Salkeld, G., & Clemson, L. (2001). Adherence to occupational therapist recommendations for home modifications for falls prevention. *American Journal of Occupational Therapy, 55*(6), 641–648. http://ajot.aota.org/article.aspx?articleid=1869052.

Cumming, R. G., Thomas, M., Szonyi, G., Salkeld, G., O'Neill, E., Westbury, C., & Frampton, G. (1999). Home visits by an occupational therapist for assessment and modification of environmental hazards: A randomised trial of falls prevention. *Journal of the American Geriatrics Society, 47*, 1397–1402.

Day, L., Fildes, B., Gordon, I., Fitzharris, M., Flamer, H., & Lord, S. (2002). Randomised factorial trial of falls prevention among older people living in their own homes. *British Medical Journal, 325*(7356), 128–131. https://www.ncbi.nlm.nih.gov/pmc/articles/PMC117228/pdf/128.pdf.

Egan, M., & Restall, G. (2022). *Promoting occupational participation: Collaborative relationship-focused occupational therapy; 10th Canadian occupational therapy guidelines; guidelines for occupational therapy in Canada*. Canadian Association of Occupational Therapists.

Gray, J. A., Zimmerman, J. L., & Rimmer, J. H. (2012). Built environment instruments for walkability, bikeability, and recreation:

Disability and universal design relevant? *Disability and Health Journal, 5*(2), 87–101. https://doi.org/10.1016/j.dhjo.2011.12.002.

Helson, H. (1964). *Adaptation level theory.* Harper and Row.

Hill, L. D., Haslam, R. A., Howarth, P. A., Brooke-Wavell, K., & Sloane, J. E. (2000). *Safety of older people on stairs: Behavioural factors.* Department of Trade and Industry.

Hopewell, S., Adedire, O., Copsey, B. J., Boniface, G. J., Sherrington, C., Clemson, L., … Lamb, S. E. (2018). Multifactorial and multiple component interventions for preventing falls in older people living in the community. *Cochrane Database of Systematic Reviews*(7).

Horowitz, B. P., Nochajski, S. M., & Schweitzer, J. A. (2013). Occupational therapy community practice and home assessments: Use of the Home Safety Self-Assessment Tool (HSSAT) to support aging in place. *Occupational Therapy in Health Care, 27*(3), 216–227. http://www.tandfonline.com/doi/abs/10.3109/07380577.2013.807450.

Iaria, G., & Burles, F. (2016). Developmental topographical disorientation. *Trends in cognitive sciences, 20*(10), 720–722.

Jansen, C.-P., Gottschalk, S., Nerz, C., Labudek, S., Kramer-Gmeiner, F., Klenk, J., … Schwenk, M. (2023). Comparison of falls and cost-effectiveness of the group versus individually delivered Lifestyle-integrated Functional Exercise (LiFE) program: Final results from the LiFE-is-LiFE non-inferiority trial. *Age and Ageing, 52*(1). https://doi.org/10.1093/ageing/afac331.

Jansen, C.-P., Nerz, C., Labudek, S., Gottschalk, S., Kramer-Gmeiner, F., Klenk, J., … Schwenk, M. (2021). Lifestyle-integrated functional exercise to prevent falls and promote physical activity: Results from the LiFE-is-LiFE randomized non-inferiority trial. *The International Journal of Behavioral Nutrition and Physical Activity, 18*(1), 115. https://doi.org/10.1186/s12966-021-01190-z.

Kalu, M. E., Bello-Haas, V. D., Griffin, M., Boamah, S., Harris, J., Zaide, M., … Tkachyk, C. (2022). Cognitive, psychological and social factors associated with older adults' mobility: A scoping review of self-report and performance-based measures. *Psychogeriatrics, 22*(4), 553–573. https://doi.org/10.1111/psyg.12848.

Karlsson, M. K., Vonschewelov, T., Karlsson, C., Cöster, M., & Rosengen, B. E. (2013). Prevention of falls in the elderly: A review. *Scandinavian Journal of Public Health, 41*(5), 442–454. https://doi.org/10.1177/1403494813483215.

Kearney, F. C., Harwood, R. H., Gladman, J. R., Lincoln, N., & Masud, T. (2013). The relationship between executive function and falls and gait abnormalities in older adults: A systematic review. *Dementia and Geriatric Cognitive Disorders, 36*(1-2), 20–35.

Keglovits, M., Clemson, L., Hu, Y.-L., Nguyen, A., Neff, A. J., Mandelbaum, C., … Stark, S. (2020). A scoping review of fall hazards in the homes of older adults and development of a framework for assessment and intervention. *Australian Occupational Therapy Journal, 67*, 470–478. https://doi.org/10.1111/1440-1630.12682.

Kessler, D., Walker, I., Sauvé-Schenk, K., & Egan, M. (2019). Goal setting dynamics that facilitate or impede a client-centered approach. *Scandinavian Journal of Occupational Therapy, 26*(5), 315–324. https://doi.org/10.1080/11038128.2018.1465119.

Kharb, A., Saini, V., Jain, Y., & Dhiman, S. (2011). A review of gait cycle and its parameters. *IJCEM International Journal of Computational Engineering & Management, 13*, 78–83.

Kramer, F., Labudek, S., Jansen, C.-P., Nerz, C., Fleig, L., Clemson, L., … Schwenk, M. (2020). Development of a conceptual framework for a group-based format of the Lifestyle-integrated Functional Exercise (gLiFE) programme and its initial feasibility testing. *Pilot and Feasibility Studies, 6*(1), 6. https://doi.org/10.1186/s40814-019-0539-x.

Lamb, S. E., Jorstad-Stein, E. C., Hauer, K., & Becker, C. (2005). Development of a common outcome data set for fall injury prevention trials: The Prevention of Falls Network Europe consensus. *Journal of the American Geriatrics Society, 53*(9), 1618–1622. https://doi.org/10.1111/j.1532-5415.2005.53455.x.

Law, M., Cooper, B., Strong, S., Stewart, D., Rigby, P., & Letts, L. (1996). The person-environment-occupation model: A transactive approach to occupational performance. *Canadian Journal of Occupational Therapy, 63*, 9–22.

Lawton, M. P., Windley, P. G., & Byers, T. D. (Eds.). (1982). *Ageing and the environment: Theoretical approaches.* Springer.

Leclerc, B. S., Bégin, C., Cadieux, E., Goulet, L., Allaire, J. F., Meloche, J., … Kergoat, M. J. (2010). Relationship between home hazards and falling among community-dwelling seniors using home-care services. *Revue D'epidemiologie Et De Sante Publique, 58*(1), 3–11. https://doi.org/10.1016/j.respe.2009.10.008.

Lee, S. (2021). Falls associated with indoor and outdoor environmental hazards among community-dwelling older adults between men and women. *BMC Geriatrics, 21*(1), 1–12. https://doi.org/10.1186/s12877-021-02499-x.

Li, W., Keegan, T. H. M., Sternfeld, B., Sidney, S., Quesenberry, C. P., Jr., & Kelsey, J. L. (2006). Outdoor falls among middle-aged and older adults: A neglected public health problem. *American Journal of Public Health, 96*(7), 1192–1200. https://doi.org/10.2105/AJPH.2005.083055.

Lin, G., Zhao, X., Wang, W., & Wilkinson, T. (2022). The relationship between forward head posture, postural control and gait: A systematic review. *Gait & Posture, 98*, 316–329. https://doi.org/10.1016/j.gaitpost.2022.10.008.

Lord, S. R., Shrerrington, C., & Naganathan, V. (Eds.). (2021). *Falls in older people; risk factors, strategies for prevention and implications for practice* (3rd ed.). Cambridge University Press.

Lusardi, M. M., Fritz, S., Middleton, A., Allison, L., Wingood, M., Phillips, E., … Chui, K. K. (2017). Determining risk of falls in community dwelling older adults: A systematic review and meta-analysis using posttest probability. *Journal of Geriatric Physical Therapy, 40*(1), 1.

Mackenzie, L., Byles, J., & Higginbotham, N. (2000). Designing the Home falls and Accidents Screening Tool (HOME FAST): Selecting the items. *British Journal of Occupational Therapy, 63*(6), 260–269.

Makino, K., Makizako, H., Doi, T., Tsutsumimoto, K., Hotta, R., Nakakubo, S., … Shimada, H. (2018). Impact of fear of falling and fall history on disability incidence among older adults: Prospective cohort study. *International Journal of Geriatric Psychiatry, 33*(4), 658–662. https://onlinelibrary.wiley.com/doi/10.1002/gps.4837.

Martino, G., Ivanenko, Y., d'Avella, A., Serrao, M., Ranavolo, A., Draicchio, F., … Lacquaniti, F. (2015). Neuromuscular adjustments of gait associated with unstable conditions. *Journal of Neurophysiology, 114*(5), 2867–2882. https://doi.org/10.1152/jn.00029.2015.

McNulty, M. C., Johnson, J., Poole, J. L., & Winkle, M. (2003). Using the transtheoretical model of change to implement home safety modifications with community dwelling older adults. *Physical and Occupational Therapy in Geriatrics, 21*(4), 53–66.

Menant, J., Hylton, B. M., & Chaplain, C. (2021). Gait characteristics and falls. In S. R. Lord, C. Sherrington, & V. Naganathan (Eds.), *Falls in older people; risk factors, strategies for prevention and implications for practice* (3rd ed.). Cambridge University Press.

Mizuta, S., Uchida, K., Sawa, R., Nakamura, J., Encho, H., Akisue, T., & Ono, R. (2023). Context of walking and loneliness among community-dwelling older adults: A cross-sectional study. *BMC Geriatrics, 23*(1), 326. https://doi.org/10.1186/s12877-023-04043-5.

Montero-Odasso, M., van der Velde, N., Martin, F. C., Petrovic, M., Tan, M. P., Ryg, J., ... Blain, H. (2022). World guidelines for falls prevention and management for older adults: A global initiative. *Age and Ageing, 51*(9), afac205.

Moreland, B., Kakara, R., & Henry, A. (2020). Trends in nonfatal falls and fall-related injuries among adults aged ≥65 years—United States, 2012–2018. *Morbidity and Mortality Weekly Report, 69*(27), 875. https://www.ncbi.nlm.nih.gov/pmc/articles/PMC7732363/pdf/mm6927a5.pdf.

Morris, M., Osborne, D., Hill, K., Kendig, H., Lundgren-Lindquist, B., Browning, C., & Reid, J. (2004). Predisposing factors for occasional and multiple falls in older Australians who live at home. *Australian Journal of Physiotherapy, 50*(3), 153–159. https://www.sciencedirect.com/science/article/pii/S0004951414601537?via%3Dihub.

Nikolaus, T., & Bach, M. (2003). Preventing falls in community dwelling frail older people using a home intervention team: Results from the randomised falls-HIT trial. *Journal of the American Geriatrics Society, 51*, 300–305. https://doi.org/10.1046/j.1532-5415.2003.51102.x.

Northridge, M., Nevitt, M., & Kelsey, J. (1996). Non-syncopal falls in the elderly in relation to home environments. *Osteoporosis International, 6*, 249–255.

Northridge, M., Nevitt, M., Kelsey, J., & Link, B. (1995). Home hazards and falls in the elderly: The role of health and functional status. *American Journal of Public Health, 85*, 509–515.

Nyberg, L., Gustafson, Y., Breggren, D., Brannstrom, B., & Bucht, G. (1996). Falls leading to femoral neck fractures in lucid older people. *Journal of the American Geriatrics Society, 44*, 156–160.

Peel, N., Steinberg, M., & Williams, G. (2000). Home safety assessment in the prevention of falls among older people. *Australian and New Zealand Journal of Public Health, 24*(5), 536–539.

Peterson, E., Howland, J., Keilhofner, G., Lachman, M. E., Assmann, S., Cote, J., & Jette, A. (1999). Falls self efficacy and occupational adaptation among elders. *Physical and Occupational Therapy in Geriatrics, 16*, 1–16.

Pighills, A., Ballinger, C., Pickering, R., & Chari, S. (2016). A critical review of the effectiveness of environmental assessment and modification in the prevention of falls amongst community dwelling older people. *British Journal of Occupational Therapy, 79*(3). https://doi.org/10.1177/0308022615600181.

Pighills, A., & Clemson, L. (2021). Environmental risk factors for falls. In S. R. Lord, C. Shrerrington, & V. Naganathan (Eds.), *Falls in older people; risk factors, strategies for prevention and implications for practice* (3rd ed.). Cambridge University Press.

Pighills, A., Drummond, A., Crossland, S., & Torgerson, D. J. (2019). What type of environmental assessment and modification prevents falls in community dwelling older people? *BMJ, 364*, l880. https://doi.org/10.1136/bmj.l880.

Pighills, A., Furness, L., Rawle, M., & Tynan, A. (2019). Occupational Therapist led environmental assessment and modification (EAM) to prevent falls: Current practice in an Australian rural health service district. *Australian Occupational Therapy Journal, 66*, 347–361. https://doi.org/10.1111/1440-1630.12560.

Pighills, A. C., Bradford, M., Bell, K., Flynn, L. J., Williams, G., Hornsby, D., ... Kaltner, M. (2015). Skill-sharing between allied health professionals in a community setting: A randomised controlled trial. *International Journal of Therapy and Rehabilitation, 22*(11), 524–534. https://www.magonlinelibrary.com/doi/pdf/10.12968/ijtr.2015.22.11.524.

Pighills, A. C., Torgerson, D. J., Sheldon, T. A., Drummond, A. E., & Bland, J. M. (2011). Environmental assessment and modification to prevent falls in older people. *Journal of the American Geriatrics Society, 59*(1), 26–33. https://doi.org/10.1111/j.1532-5415.2010.03221.x.

Pluijm, S. M., Smit, J. H., Tromp, E., Stel, V., Deeg, D. J., Bouter, L., & Lips, P. (2006). A risk profile for identifying community dwelling elderly with a high risk of recurrent falling: Results of a 3-year prospective study. *Osteoporosis International, 2*, 1007–1015. https://doi.org/10.1007/s00198-005-0002-0.

Resnik, L., Allen, S., Isenstadt, D., Wasserman, M., & Iezzoni, L. (2009). Perspectives on use of mobility aids in a diverse population of seniors: Implications for intervention. *Disability and Health Journal, 2*(2), 77–85. https://doi.org/10.1016/j.dhjo.2008.12.002.

Retallack, G. J. (2022). *Evolution of humans*. Salem Press.

Robson, K. M. (2017). Mobility. In M. Curtin, M. Egan, & J. Adams (Eds.), *Occupational therapy for people experienceing illness, injury or impairment: Promoting occupation and participation* (7th ed.). Elsevier.

Rogowska, A. M., Zmaczyńska-Witek, B., Mazurkiewicz, M., & Kardasz, Z. (2020). The mediating effect of self-efficacy on the relationship between health locus of control and life satisfaction: A moderator role of movement disability. *Disability and Health Journal, 13*(4). https://doi.org/10.1016/j.dhjo.2020.100923.

Roley, S. S., DeLany, J. V., Barrows, C. J., Brownrigg, S., Honaker, D., Sava, D. I., ... Lieberman, D. (2008) (2nd ed.)Occupational therapy practice framework: Domain & process62. American Occupational Therapy Association.

Romkes, J., & Bracht-Schweizer, K. (2017). The effects of walking speed on upper body kinematics during gait in healthy subjects. *Gait & Posture, 54*, 304–310. https://doi.org/10.1016/j.gaitpost.2017.03.025.

Romli, M. H., Mackenzie, L., Lovarini, M., Tan, M. P., & Clemson, L. (2018). The clinimetric properties of instruments measuring home hazards for older people at risk of falling: A systematic review. *Evaluation & the Health Professions, 41*(1), 82–128.

Rosso, A. L., Studenski, S. A., Chen, W. G., Aizenstein, H. J., Alexander, N. B., Bennett, D. A., ... Rosano, C. (2013). Aging, the central nervous system, and mobility. *The Journals of Gerontology: Series A, 68*(11), 1379–1386. https://doi.org/10.1093/gerona/glt089.

Rubenstein, L. Z. (2006). Falls in older people: Epidemiology, risk factors and strategies for prevention. *Age and Ageing, 35*(Supplement 2), ii37–ii41. https://doi.org/10.1093/ageing/afl084.

Sattin, R. W., Rodriguez, J. G., DeVito, C. A., & Wingo, P. (1998). Home environmental hazards and the risk of fall injury events among community dwelling older people. Study to Assess Falls Among the Elderly (SAFE) Group. *Journal of the American Geriatrics Society, 46*, 669–676.

Shumway-Cook, A., Guralnik, J. M., Phillips, C. L., Coppin, A. K., Ciol, M. A., Bandinelli, S., & Ferrucci, L. (2007). Age-associated declines in complex walking task performance: The walking in CHIANTI toolkit. *Journal of the American Geriatrics Society, 55*(1), 58–65. https://doi.org/10.1111/j.1532-5415.2006.00962.x.

Shumway-Cook, A., Patla, A. E., Stewart, A., Ferrucci, L., Ciol, M. A., & Guralnik, J. M. (2002). Environmental demands associated with community mobility in older adults with and without mobility disabilities. *Physical Therapy, 82*(7), 670–681. https://doi.org/10.1093/ptj/82.7.670.

Smith, A. R., Chen, C., Clarke, P., & Gallagher, N. A. (2016). Trajectories of outdoor mobility in vulnerable community-dwelling elderly: The role of individual and environmental factors. *Journal of Aging and Health, 28*(5), 796–811. https://doi.org/10.1177/0898264315611665.

Stevens, J. A., Mahoney, J. E., & Ehrenreich, H. (2014). Circumstances and outcomes of falls among high risk community-dwelling older adults. *Injury Epidemiology, 1*(1), 5. https://doi.org/10.1186/2197-1714-1-5.

Stevens, M., Holman, C., D'Arcy, J., Bennett, N., & de Klerk, N. (2001). Preventing falls in older people: Outcome evaluation of a randomised controlled trial. *Journal of the American Geriatrics Society, 49*, 1448–1455.

Tinetti, M. E. (1986). Performance-orientated assessment of mobility problems in elderly patients. *Journal of the American Geriatrics Society, 34*, 119–126.

Tinetti, M. E., & Powell, L. (1993). Fear of falling and low self efficacy: A cause for dependence in elderly persons. *Journal of Gerontology, 48*, 35–38.

Tinetti, M. E., Speechley, M., & Ginter, S. F. (1988). Risk factors for falls among elderly persons living in the community. *The New England Journal of Medicine, 319*(26), 1701–1707.

Tomita, M. R., Saharan, S., Rajendran, S., Nochajski, S. M., & Schweitzer, J. A. (2014). Psychometrics of the Home Safety Self-Assessment Tool (HSSAT) to prevent falls in community-dwelling older adults. *American Journal of Occupational Therapy, 68*(6), 711–718. http://ajot.aota.org/article.aspx?articleID=1934887.

Tse, T. (2005). The environment and falls prevention: Do environmental modifications make a difference? *Australian Occupational Therapy Journal, 52*(4), 271.

Tynan, A., Pighills, A., White, W., Eden, A., & Mickan, S. (2022). Implementing best practice occupational therapist-led environmental assessment and modification to prevent falls: A qualitative study of two regional and rural public health services in Australia.

Australian Occupational Therapy Journal, 70(2), 202–217. https://doi.org/10.1111/1440-1630.12849.

Urbanek, J. K., Roth, D. L., Karas, M., Wanigatunga, A. A., Mitchell, C. M., Juraschek, S. P., … Schrack, J. A. (2022). Free-living gait cadence measured by wearable accelerometer: A promising alternative to traditional measures of mobility for assessing fall risk. *The Journals of Gerontology: Series A, 78*(5), 802–810. https://doi.org/10.1093/gerona/glac013.

van der Wardt, V., Logan, P., Hood, V., Booth, V., Masud, T., & Harwood, R. (2015). The association of specific executive functions and falls risk in people with mild cognitive impairment and early-stage dementia. *Dementia and Geriatric Cognitive Disorders, 40*(3-4), 178–185.

van Soest, D., Tight, M. R., & Rogers, C. D. F. (2020). Exploring the distances people walk to access public transport. *Transport Reviews, 40*(2), 160–182. https://doi.org/10.1080/01441647.2019.1575491.

Walker-Peterson, E., & Clemson, L. (2008). Understanding the role of occupational therapy in fall prevention for community-dwelling older adults. *OT Practice, 13*(3), 1–8.

Wee, J., & Lysaght, R. (2009). Factors affecting measures of activities and participation in persons with mobility impairment. *Disability and Rehabilitation, 31*(20), 1633–1642. https://doi.org/10.1080/09638280902736346.

Wensley, R., & Slade, A. (2012). Walking as a meaningful leisure occupation: The implications for occupational therapy. *British Journal of Occupational Therapy, 75*(2), 85–92.

World Health Organization. (2004). *What are the main risk factors for falls amongst older people and what are the most effective interventions to prevent these falls? How should interventions to prevent falls be implemented?* http://www.euro.who.int/document/E82552.pdf.

World Health Organization. (2007). *Global age-friendly cities: A guide.* World Health Organization.

Yoshida, S. (2006). *Epidemiology of falls.* World Health Organization.

Zhang, W., Low, L.-F., Schwenk, M., Mills, N., Gwynn, Josephine D., & Clemson, L. (2019). Review of gait, cognition, and fall risks with implications for fall prevention in older adults with dementia. *Dementia and Geriatric Cognitive Disorders, 48*(1-2), 17–29. https://doi.org/10.1159/000504340.

Zijlstra, G. A. R., van Haastregt, J. C. M., van Rossum, E., van Eijk, J. T. M., Yardley, L., & Kempen, G. I. J. M. (2007). Interventions to reduce fear of falling in community-living older people: A systematic review. *Journal of the American Geriatrics Society, 55*(4), 603–615. http://www.blackwell-synergy.com/doi/abs/10.1111/j.1532-5415.2007.01148.x.

REFLECTION

1. List five behavioural risk factors for falls.

2. List five extrinsic (environmental) risk factors for falls.

3. What are the five core components of high-intensity environmental fall-hazard intervention?

4. Give five examples of universal design improvements which enhance safety when walking outdoors.

33

WHEELED MOBILITY AND SEATING SYSTEMS

W. BEN MORTENSON ▪ JAIMIE BORISOFF ▪
DANIELLE RAE ▪ FRANCINE MILLER ▪ MIKE PRESCOTT ▪
BONITA SAWATZKY ▪ WILLIAM C. MILLER

CHAPTER OUTLINE

Overview

Wheeled mobility and seating systems, which are prescribed using a collaborative relationship-focused approach that takes into consideration the person, their occupational participation priorities and the context in which they live, can have a powerful positive impact on the quality of life of people who require them. Using three practice stories, this chapter illustrates this process of wheeled mobility and seating system prescription following the World Health Organization's 8-stage process for wheeled mobility device provision. An overview of important considerations regarding how assessments should be conducted that solicit a user's occupational participation goals and determine their abilities and seating needs is provided. Training and follow-up are important parts of the process to ensure that users and their caregivers have the necessary skills to use wheeled mobility devices proficiently and safely. By fostering wheeled mobility occupational therapists can promote occupational participation in a way that upholds the rights of people with disabilities.

KEY POINTS

- Approximately 1% of the world's population uses wheeled mobility.

- Despite the potential benefits of wheeled mobility, many users experience negative outcomes, especially without a robust provision process.

- Wheeled mobility device prescribers need to follow a collaborative relationship-focused approach that takes into consideration the person and their caregivers, their occupational participation priorities and the context in which they live.

- There are many people who may be involved in the process (e.g. the user, the occupational therapist, family members, peers, caregivers, vendors). Wheeled mobility assessment should include documentation of users' physical abilities, postural needs and risk for skin breakdown.

- When it comes to wheeled mobility, equipment every choice represents a compromise (i.e. it has different pros and cons)

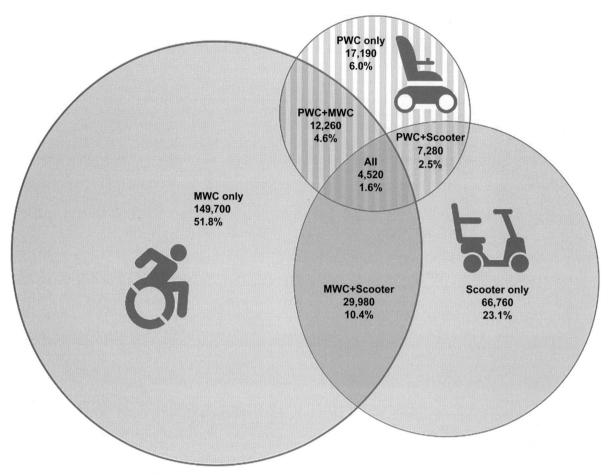

Fig. 33.1 ■ Wheelchair and scooter users by device type in Canada in 2012.

- Wheeled mobility training can help users be safer without sacrificing performance.
- Funding should not dictate the wheeled mobility options that are discussed with the people who need them.

INTRODUCTION TO WHEELED MOBILITY

The World Health Organization estimates that 1% of the world population needs a wheelchair for

[1]In this chapter the terms person/individual (and plural variations of these terms) refer to a person/collective receiving occupational therapy services, and the terms 'wheeled mobility user' or 'wheelchair user' or 'scooter user' and on occasion 'user' refer to a person/collective who needs a wheeled mobility device.

mobility; however, many people do not have access to these devices (2008). In 2012, it was estimated that there were 288,800 community-dwelling wheelchair and scooter users[1] aged 15 years and over in Canada, representing 1.0% of the Canadian population. Almost 20% of these individuals use multiple devices. However, this excludes children and those living in long-term care. Almost 20% use multiple devices (Fig. 33.1).

Wheeled mobility devices are provided to help people who have difficulty ambulating. Improving their mobility may facilitate social participation, by enabling users to go to school, work, take part in their communities and access health services (WHO, 2008). For example, participants in a qualitative study identified over 100 outcomes they wanted to achieve while using their wheeled mobility devices, which included occupation-related outcomes inside the home (e.g. personal care) and in the community (e.g. shopping), as well as corporeal outcomes (e.g. comfort and positioning). In this regard, a properly prescribed wheelchair (which takes into consideration the person's occupational participation goals, functional abilities and environmental factors) can create a positive feedback loop, which likely further facilitates their mobility and overall quality of life, including helping people escape poverty (i.e. spatial mobility improves social mobility) (de Madariaga & Neuman, 2020).

Common components of a manual wheelchair are illustrated in Fig. 33.2. Scooters with different wheel configurations are shown in Fig. 33.3A and B, and a rear-wheel drive power wheelchair in Fig. 33.3C. A tilt function on a wheelchair in which the entire seating system rotates in space is shown in Fig. 33.3D.

Wheelchair Physics

Wheelchairs are mechanical devices, which are strongly influenced by the laws of physics. The location of the centre of mass of a person in a manual wheelchair will greatly affect how the wheelchair performs. If the centre of mass moves outside the base of support, the wheelchair will tip over. The wheelie is a skill learned by many manual wheelchair users that changes their centre of mass in relation to their base of support and allows them to navigate obstacles such as curbs. To perform a wheelie (i.e. balancing only on the large rear drive wheels of the chair), wheelchair users move their centre of mass backwards so that it is directly over their rear axle (on the edge of the base of support). They do this by leaning backwards and popping their front casters off the ground (see the section below on the camber for information about how the wheel angle can impact stability). Rear-mounted anti-tippers are an option for manual wheelchairs that prevent wheelchairs from tipping backwards. While safer in static sitting,

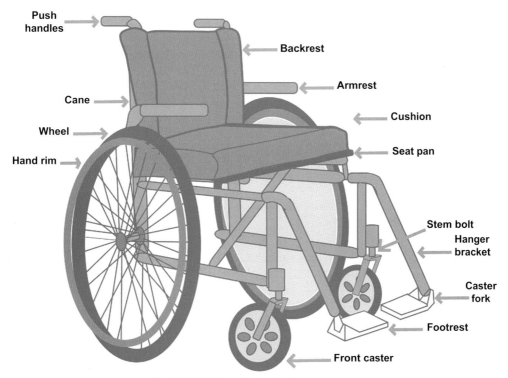

Fig. 33.2 ■ Manual wheelchair components.

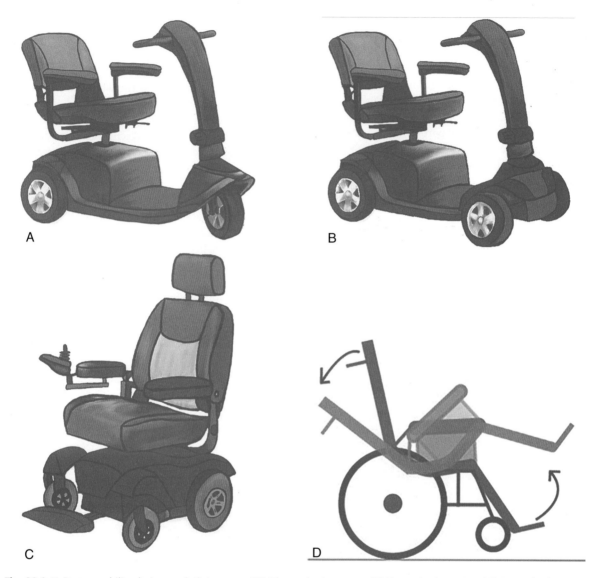

Fig. 33.3 ■ Power mobility devices and tilt-in-space. (A) Three-wheel scooter. (B) Four-wheel scooter. (C) Rear-wheel power-chair. (D) Tilt-in-space function on wheelchair.

anti-tippers will also make it impossible to perform an effective wheelie or to ascend most curbs. In this case, there may be a perceived compromise between safety and wheelchair performance; however, it should be noted this is a false dichotomy because wheelchair skill training could enable both safety and performance.

The centre of mass of a wheelchair shifts in relation to the base of support depending on the position of the rear axle of the wheelchair as illustrated in Fig. 33.4.

The further forward the centre of mass is in front of the rear axle, the more stable the chair will be front-to-back (i.e. tippiness). Unfortunately, this configuration will also make it more difficult to manage cross slopes (most sidewalks have a 2% cross slope for water drainage and curb cuts and driveways may have an 8% slope). The greater the distance the centre of mass is in front of the rear axle, the greater the cross-slope forces (torque) the wheelchair a user has to overcome. In

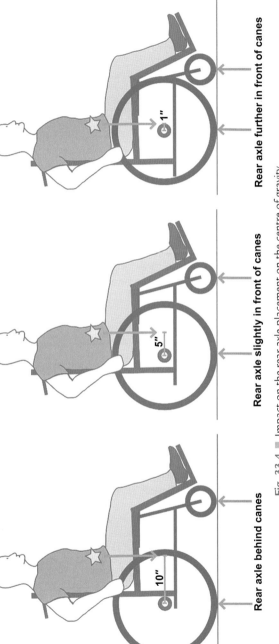

Fig. 33.4 ◾ Impact on the rear axle placement on the centre of gravity.

practice, this means that when going down a sidewalk with a manual wheelchair the user will need to push harder on the rim that is closest to the street so that the wheelchair will go straight rather than fall off the curb into the street. Power wheelchairs may be programmed to automatically adjust for these side slope forces.

To propel a manual wheelchair the user needs to contact the rim of the wheel usually with their hands. To have adequate contact with the rim it is recommended that the wheelchair user be able to touch the hub with their fingertips. This will enable them to contact the rim between 10 PM and 2 PM. Rear wheels frequently have some degree of camber (the top of the wheel is closer to the wheelchair user than the bottom of the wheel) (Fig. 33.5A and B). This makes it easier for the user to grasp the rim and decreases the forces exerted on the shoulder. A higher degree of camber increases the width of the wheelchair, which increases its lateral stability but poses problems trying to manoeuvre through narrow doorways. For example, wheelchairs used to play basketball have extreme camber to greatly increase their lateral stability.

A variety of strategies are available to improve mechanical efficiency with manual wheelchair propulsion. For example, wheelchairs with rigid frames are more mechanically efficient than folding chairs. The wheelchair's movable joints decrease the overall frame stiffness, which makes them less efficient to wheel. In another example, reducing rolling resistance will also improve efficiency. Rolling resistance is affected by the diameter and characteristics of the drive wheels and front casters, as well as by the weight distribution (percentage of weight on the drive wheels versus the front casters). Diameter, width, profile and hardness affect the rolling resistance of tyres (Sprigle et al., 2019). Larger drive wheels with the same width profile and hardness will have less rolling resistance than smaller wheels. In addition, when the centre of mass of the user and chair is closer to the rear axles (and this is combined with larger rear wheels), the weight is off-loaded from the front wheels and reduces the overall rolling resistance (see Fig. 33.4 for an explanation of the impact of the centre of gravity). This configuration also makes the chair more manoeuvrable. Although larger front casters would have lower rolling resistance, the effect is not very large if the front wheels are not heavily weighted (Zepeda et al., 2016; Chan et al., 2018). Therefore many wheelchair users elect to have smaller front casters because they reduce the footprint of the chair. In

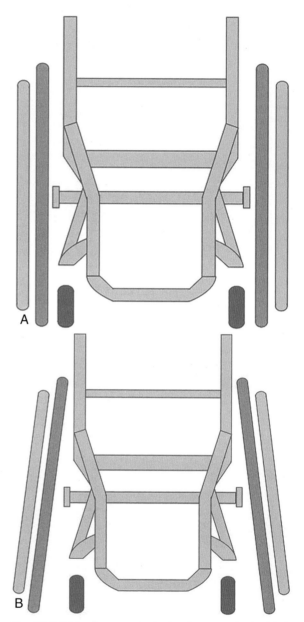

Fig. 33.5 ■ The frame and wheels of a manual wheelchair from the back. (A) Shows 0° camber. (B) Shows 7° camber.

addition, since front caster width, profile and hardness also affect rolling resistance, larger-diameter casters may not have lower resistance than smaller ones (Sprigle et al., 2019). Furthermore, high-performance rear wheels and casters likely have lower resistance because of these properties (Misch & Sprigle, 2021).

Potential Problems with Wheeled Mobility Devices

While wheelchairs may support occupational participation, potential issues associated with wheelchair use include overuse injuries and shoulder pain, falls, ineffective use due to limited training, problems with maintenance, pressure injuries, accessibility issues and problems with wayfinding.

Common concerns among wheelchair users are overuse injuries and shoulder pain. Although it is commonly assumed that manual wheelchair propulsion is a primary cause of these issues, a cross-sectional study of shoulder pain among people with spinal cord injury revealed pain was reported by 47% of power wheelchair users, 35% of manual wheelchair users, 50% of crutch or cane users and 33% of those who walked without devices (Jain et al., 2010). Thus pain and repetitive strain may also be caused, in part, by transfers or overhead reaching. These problems might also precipitate premature power mobility use.

Falls are also a major concern. A prospective study of wheelchair users with spinal cord injury found that over the course of one year, 64% of participants fell and 34% of them were injured (Forslund et al., 2017). The most common risk factors identified for falls include wheelchair-related factors (e.g. lack of maintenance), performance of transfers, poor sitting balance and environmental factors (e.g. uneven terrain) (Rice et al., 2015).

Despite the potential benefits of wheeled mobility skill training, relatively few users receive formal training, especially in more advanced skills required to move safely around a community (Best et al., 2015). An experimental study among a sample of community-dwelling wheelchair users found that 99% of wheelchairs required maintenance, and there was a significant decrease in accidents among those whose wheelchairs received a regularly scheduled maintenance check-up (Hansen et al., 2004).

Wheelchair users are at higher risk for developing pressure injuries (i.e. breakdown of the skin and underlying tissues, which are very difficult and expensive to treat), likely due to difficulties repositioning themselves as well as reduced or absent sensation (Sprigle et al., 2020).

Internationally, in many countries, laws exist to protect people with disabilities from discrimination in several areas of public life, such as transportation and physical barriers to accessibility. Despite the existence of the Americans with Disabilities Act since 1990, wheeled mobility accessibility appears to be a recalcitrant problem in the United States (Welage & Liu, 2011) and other jurisdictions (Carlsson et al., 2022). One issue related to a lack of universal accessibility is related to wayfinding (being able to plan trips between one location and another). Specifically, it is often challenging for wheeled mobility users to plan routes because accessibility information is either not available (e.g. usable and confusing) or not up-to-date. This challenge is compounded by the necessity of wheeled mobility users focusing much of their attention on the ground to avoid tipping hazards and other obstacles (Prescott et al., 2021).

WHEELED MOBILITY PROVISION PROCESS

The World Health Organization (2008) has identified a multi-stage process for manual wheelchair provision in less-resourced settings. These stages are also applicable to all wheeled mobility devices in more resourced settings. These stages are: (1) referral and appointment, (2) assessment, (3) prescription, (4) funding and ordering, (5) trialling, (6) product preparation, (7) fitting and adjusting, (8) user training and (9) maintenance, repairs and follow-up.

The remainder of this chapter is organised based on these eight stages; however, as occupational therapists, it is critical to understand that these stages must be implemented in a way that is congruent with the Canadian occupational therapy inter-relational practice process (COTIPP) (Egan & Restall, 2022). (NB: the *italics* text in the following paragraphs refer to different elements of COTIPP) (refer to Chapter 12).

Building and maintaining connection should be incorporated into all the WHO stages. *Seeking understanding and defining purpose and exploring occupational participation* are critical elements during Stage 2 (assessment). Since fostering occupational participation is at the heart of the relationship between the occupational therapist and the person, it is essential to foreground the valued occupations that the person wishes to perform before considering how they might achieve these occupations. Wheeled mobility may be one means to facilitate their occupational participation, but other approaches may be preferable. If the only tool an occupational therapist uses is a hammer, then every problem can look like a nail.

During the assessment stage, the person should be involved in *co-designing priorities, goals, outcomes and planning* (refer to Chapter 19) in recognition of the expertise they bring to the relationship and the need for ongoing collaboration to make the process successful. *Trialling plans, exploring changes and refining plans* occur during Stage 7 (fitting and adjusting), Stage 8 (user training) and Stage 9 (maintenance, repairs and follow-up). *Planning for transition* is an important element of follow-up to ensure the wheeled mobility device provided continues to meet users' needs over time.

To provide wheeled mobility devices successfully, occupational therapists must have a *nuanced understanding of context*. This includes understanding the physical and social environments where wheeled mobility is being considered as well as issues related to funding and accessibility. Throughout this process, occupational therapists must *critically reflect and reason* so that each person can achieve their occupational participation goals regardless of the means. Success also requires the use of justice, equity and rights-based lenses. For example, occupational therapists may need to work with people to appeal unjust funding decisions.

Practice Stories

To illustrate the application of the eight steps of the WHO framework and the collaborative relationship-focused occupational therapy (Egan & Restall, 2022) three practice stories will be drawn on. The practice stories are used to identify beneficial outcomes associated with appropriate wheeled mobility prescription, as well as to identify potential problems. An overview of the person who is the focus of each practice story is provided in Table 33.1.

TABLE 33.1
Practice Stories: Key Background Information

Name	Baljeet	Obama	Mel
Device trajectory	Initially provided with a manual wheelchair. Considering getting a new wheelchair.	Ambulating with difficulty. Considering powered mobility use.	Admitted to long term with a power wheelchair, but having safety concerns.
Age	28	55	75
Primary Diagnosis	Spinal cord injury	Multiple sclerosis	Parkinson's disease
Gender	Female	Male	Non-binary
Pronouns	She/her	He/him	They/them
Social support	Family	Wife and family	Pat, their long-term partner
Ethnic/racial origin	East Asian	Black	Caucasian
Narrative	Injured in a car accident at the age of 24. Sustained a C7 spinal cord injury. Experiencing overuse issues in shoulders	Has been reluctant to consider the possibility of wheeled mobility.	Admitted to long-term care because of problems managing in the community.
Wheelchair	Provided with a manual wheelchair when discharged from rehabilitation. Is wondering about getting a new wheelchair or powered add-on to be able to travel longer distances.	Has become more open to the idea of trialling a scooter because of advice from peers.	Currently using a power wheelchair with joystick control, but having increasingly frequent accidents.
Goals	Returning to medical residency. Socialising with friends and family. Returning to sports.	Continuing to work as a journalist. Parenting two young teenagers. Going on trails in local park.	Going to activities in the community centre. Going for "walks" with partner in the community. Making sure they eat at the dining room table with others.

Stage 1: Referral and Appointment

People who may require a wheeled mobility device and seating system will usually be referred to occupational therapists from a variety of different sources depending on the occupational therapist's practice setting. For example, some occupational therapists may have standing orders to see all people admitted to certain programmes or wards, while other people may be referred by other health care professionals or refer themselves. Those preliminary interactions represent the start of collaborative relationship-focused occupational therapy, and it is critical that they are handled professionally in a trauma-informed and culturally safe manner.

An intake form or interview may be helpful to ensure the referral is appropriate and determine who should take part in the initial assessment. Given that wheeled mobility is frequently a collaborative activity (e.g. family members or caregivers may help transport wheeled mobility devices or assist with pushing manual wheelchairs), it may be beneficial to ask permission from the person being assessed if family members and care partners can attend the initial assessment. Having family members or surrogate/substitute decision makers involved is necessary for those who are unable to provide their own consent (e.g. minors and adults who are unable to consent). Navigating the wheelchair provision system can be challenging, especially if a person has never used wheeled mobility previously.

Stage 2: Assessment

Obtaining Consent

Wheeled mobility assessment involves many components and areas. Consent should be obtained in an ongoing manner and in an assessment-specific fashion. This is especially important when administering assessments in which the person might be injured (e.g. assessing wheelchair skills like transfers or going down curbs). Obtaining consent is part of collaborative relationship-focused occupational therapy as a means of establishing and maintaining trust.

Identifying Occupational Participation Goals

The most important part of assessment is determining the occupations in which an individual wishes to participate. Once these occupational participation goals have been identified, or as part of the identification

process, the use of standardised person-specific outcome measures is recommended so that occupational participation achievement can be measured and documented. Change can then be documented by administering these measures after a wheeled mobility device has been delivered and used by the person. There are a variety of potential person-centred measures, including the Wheelchair Outcome Measure (Mortenson et al., 2007), which was developed specifically for wheelchair provision, and is freely available at https://millerresearch.osot.ubc.ca/tools/mobility-outcome-tools-2/the-wheelchair-outcome-measure-whom/.

The three most important occupational participation goals identified by Baljeet, Obama, and Mel are listed in Table 33.1.

Once these occupational participation outcomes have been identified and prioritised, the next step is to determine if they could be achieved either completely or in part by using wheeled mobility. One potential benefit of assistive technology is that, unlike the assistance of formal or family caregiving, it is generally always available (Agree & Freedman, 2000). It should be noted that some people may not have the capacity to use wheeled mobility independently in some or all situations or may elect to always use their wheeled mobility with the assistance of others.

In the case of Baljeet and Mel the question was not whether they would receive a wheelchair, but instead what type would be best for them? For Obama, he was reluctant to consider the use of wheeled mobility as he perceived scooters as disabling (i.e. a disability signifier.

(Jang et al., 2020)

Additional Biographical and Performance-Based Assessments

Additional assessments may be beneficial to inform decision-making about whether wheeled mobility is necessary or to assist with determining the type of wheeled mobility to be provided. Reviewing a person's medical history would help identify issues that may require further assessment. For example, people who have a spinal cord injury or advanced diabetes can have sensory impairments that may predispose them to pressure injuries. People who have had a stroke may experience spatial neglect that impacts safety. Several assessment tools that could be used when providing a wheel mobility device are referred to in the online Spinal Seating Modules offered by the Agency for Clinical Innovation (https://aci.health.nsw.gov.au/networks/spinal-cord-injury/spinal-seating/downloadable-resources (SSCIS, 2015)). These assessment tools include forms that document how to measure someone for a wheelchair and conduct a mechanical assessment test (MAT).

Mechanical Assessment Test

Most people who are provided with a wheeled mobility device should have a MAT. Space constraints in this chapter preclude an in-depth review of the MAT, but it should document positioning/posture in the person's current wheeled mobility device (if applicable) and include a supine and seated assessment that evaluates positioning and mobility of the pelvis, hips, spine, knees and ankles. During this assessment, it is important to determine if any deformities present are reducible (i.e. flexible) or nonreducible (i.e. fixed) and also to determine the person's sitting balance (e.g. can they sit unsupported (hands-free), sit with support of hands, or are unable to sit without external supports (i.e. a backrest/lateral support)), as well as their transfer ability. While seated, occupational therapists can use their hands to simulate the support needed to enable the person to either sit in a neutral posture or in as neutral a posture as possible. The assessment is ideally conducted on a firm plinth, but if no plinth is available, the assessment should be conducted on another surface (e.g. the person's bed) rather than not conducting the assessment at all, as valuable information can still be obtained.

> A MAT assessment for Baljeet revealed that she had hamstring and iliopsoas tightening (she was only able to extend her knees to 150 degrees in sitting). She also had mild scoliosis (convex left) in her thoracic region (reducible). She was able to sit without the support of her hands and had a low tone in her trunk and lower extremities. She indicated that her legs and trunk go into extensor spasm when she hits cracks on the sidewalk (Kawamura et al., 1989), which pulls her out of her seat and makes her slide forward.

> A MAT assessment for Obama did not reveal any nonreducible postural deformities, but he reported that fatigue causes his posture to become more stooped as the day progresses. No balance problems were noted in sitting, but he had fallen while walking in the community several times.

> Mel was unable to sit unsupported and had stiffness, rigidity and dystonia, all of which varied during the day. When sitting on a flat surface their head was forward, shoulders rounded (increased thoracic kyphosis; non-reducible), and they sat with their pelvis posteriorly tilted. When sitting they could only flex their hips to 80 degrees with a maximum thigh-to-trunk angle of 100°, and they had a fixed pelvic obliquity with a higher left side (non-reducible).

Assessing the Potential for Pressure Injury

Assessments like the Braden scale can be used to determine a person's risk for developing pressure injury (risk factors include lack of mobility, lack of sensation and moisture) (Braden, 2012). It can also be helpful to consider factors that can increase or mitigate the risk of developing pressure injuries that are not included in most published scales, such as caregiver support, equipment status and maintenance, diet and substance use. It is also important to determine a user's ability to and practice of regularly assess themselves for signs of skin breakdown. If there is any concern in this regard, with the person's consent and in a private space, the skin over bony prominences like the ischial tuberosities, sacrum and greater trochanters should be observed for any signs of breakdown.

Pressure mapping is a technology that measures interface pressure and can be a beneficial tool to assess the risk posed to the wheeled mobility user by surfaces including wheelchair cushions.

> In the past Baljeet had experienced a stage two pressure injury under her right ischial tuberosity. She has learnt to check her own skin with a mirror and now sits on a pressure-redistributing cushion.

> Mel has intact sensation and has no signs of pressure injuries. Mel has not had skin breakdown but is at high risk given their inability to weight shift and issues with continence.

Component-Based Assessments/Determining Capacity to Provide Consent

Some occupational therapists may also administer a variety of component-based assessments (e.g. vision, hearing, perceptual skills, neglect and memory). In a sample of 30 power mobility users, mostly living in the community, perceptual skills and cognition were strongly correlated with indoor driving skills (<.6) (Pellichero et al., 2021). Caution must be exercised as there are no component-based cut-off scores that can be used to predict whether someone would be safe or unsafe to use powered mobility. However, these component-based assessments may inform the overall assessment process.

It is also important to consider whether the person has the capacity to provide their consent to participate in the assessment process. The ability to provide consent is activity specific. For example, some people may be declared financially incompetent, but may still be considered competent to make health care decisions. For a person to provide informed consent, they need to be able to understand the risks and potential benefits of any proposed assessment or intervention. For example, when assessing power wheelchair skills, a person needs to understand there is a risk that they may be hurt, others may be injured, or property may be damaged, and they need to be able to accept this risk. An evaluation of a person's orientation to time and place will not determine whether they have the capacity to consent to wheeled mobility skills training.

Mel is experiencing mild cognitive impairment and has trouble understanding the risks associated with power mobility use. Pat is Mel's surrogate/substitute decision-maker for healthcare-related issues. Where possible Pat asks Mel for their preferences and involves Mel as much as possible in decision-making.

Wheeled Mobility Skills Assessment

If someone already has a wheelchair, it can be helpful to assess their wheelchair mobility skills. The Wheelchair Skills Training Programme (https://wheelchair-skillsprogram.ca/ (Kirby et al., 2022)) is freely available and contains evidenced-based resources to assess and train people to use manual wheelchairs, powered wheelchairs and motorised mobility scooters (with or without the assistance of caregivers).

Baljeet has good manual wheelchair mobility skills and can do most skills (e.g. independent transfers, wheelies, manoeuvre up and down small curbs) but does not go up or down high curbs or go down ramps while doing a wheelie.

Mel uses a power wheelchair but is having trouble stopping the chair reliably. Some facility staff would like Mel to stop using the power chair. However, this is a very serious decision to make because it would drastically reduce their independent mobility within their facility (Mortenson et al., 2005). The facility has a research-based practice guideline to make this decision: removal of power mobility only should be considered as a last resort once all other options are exhausted (modifications to the wheelchair, training, assessment for alternative underlying causes, and modification to the environment) (Mortenson et al., 2006).

After one accident, staff put Mel in another resident's manual chair. Using their arms, Mel could propel this wheelchair only short distances independently. Furthermore, they had poor sitting tolerance and became fatigued later in the day, which put them at risk for falls. This fatigue also occurred when Mel used their power chair, which did not have any dynamic seating features (tilt or recline). The manual chair did not accommodate Mel's postural support needs (limited hip flexion and obliquity) and the seat-to-back angle of the manual chair was 90 degrees. Mel has a thigh-to-trunk angle of 100° and could not tolerate sitting against the backrest at this angle, so slid forward to accommodate the hip flexion contracture. The closed seat-to-back angle also did not accommodate their thoracic kyphosis and pushed their trunk into more forward flexion, forcing Mel to gaze downwards. This shift in gaze affected Mel's swallowing, respiration, safety with wayfinding, and social interaction. Mel also required two people to assist with transfers. In addition, when Pat tried to push Mel outside in the manual wheelchair, they could negotiate curb cuts with effort, but were not able to go up and down curbs that did not have a curb cut.

It is critical to assess where the person intends to use wheeled mobility, for example, the person's home (including entrances) and the local community. It may also include places of employment, work, or other locations where desired occupational participation occurs. For example, some people may want a scooter only for outdoor community mobility. So, it might not be appropriate to assess the use of the scooter in their homes, although having a place to store and charge the device is critical.

Baljeet lives in a condo with automatic front doors and elevator access. She is unable to use her balcony independently because of there is a 4-inch (10 cm) lip.

Obama lives in a three-bedroom bungalow. To access the front entrance, he must climb three stairs to a landing, and then navigate either six stairs down to the basement or seven stairs up to the main floor. Alternatively, eight stairs lead up to a deck at the back of the house to access the main floor.

Mel lives in a long-term care facility and shares a room with one other resident. The entire facility is wheelchair accessible. Outside of the facility, some streets have curb cuts, but others do not, which limits the places Mel can go with Pat.

Some people may live in communities where there are no sidewalks and roads are gravel, which would affect the type of wheelchair provided.

Working as a Team

Occupational therapists involved in the seating and mobility assessment process should work within a team. The team includes the vendor that the person selects. The vendor should be knowledgeable about products so that, based on assessment and simulation, the occupational therapist can describe the parameters required such as functionality, materials, contour, size and other parameters and the vendor should be able to suggest products to trial that match these parameters. For complex seating, a seating technician, if available in the local context, is integral to helping design possible custom seating to meet goals. As the occupational therapist assesses for seating needs, other functional, health and medical issues may arise which are related to and impact on seating and mobility. It is important to recognise when referral to and collaboration with other team members is needed. Team members may include: assistive technology consultants for communication and environmental control input, orthotists, spasticity management clinics, physicians and specialists, physiotherapists, dysphagia consultants, wound nurses, respiratory therapists and others. It takes a village to best meet the many seating and mobility needs of a person and better outcomes are achieved with a team approach.

Stage 3: Prescription

Based on the findings of the assessments, and in consultation with the person and their family members, as well as with the input of vendors and in consideration of the intended environment of use, a potential wheeled mobility device is identified. Generally, these devices should be trialled before a final product is ordered. If a vendor is needed, the person should be free to choose the vendor they wish to work with. Most wheeled mobility devices will require the person's measurements to be documented. In addition, the device must accommodate their weight.

In Fig. 33.6, a simple flow diagram to provide a broad overview of the types of wheeled mobility devices that are commonly available is presented. Wheeled mobility is generally manual or powered; however, manual wheelchairs may be equipped with powered add-on devices to provide continuous ongoing assistance. Generally, the selection process involves weighing the pros and cons of each device. Some people may only be able to experience independent mobility using a power wheelchair, but these generally cannot be transported in un-adapted private vehicles. Many people prefer manual wheelchairs because of their transportability and flexibility (can be used with a powered add-on device).

A flow chart to illustrate different types of wheeled mobility seating that may be provided depending on a person's needs is provided in Fig. 33.7. There is a wide variety of seating options available, so it is important to perform a MAT assessment and work with a knowledgeable vendor to determine the most appropriate seating to trial.

Historically the mantra in rehabilitation was 'use it or lose it'. Unfortunately, this may have contributed

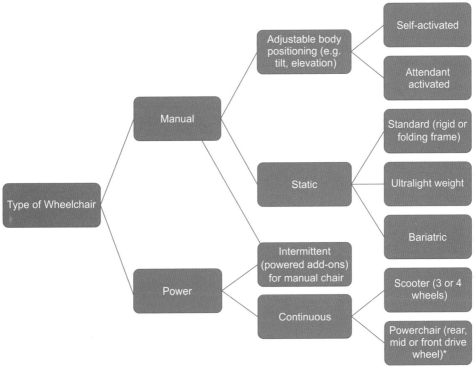

* Powerchairs may have a variety of powered body positioning options (e.g., tilt, recline, seat elevation, powered leg rests)

Fig. 33.6 ■ Types of wheeled mobility devices.

to devastating overuse injuries, which may further restrict a wheelchair user's upper extremity functioning (e.g. transfers, dressing and manual wheelchair use) (Kemp, 2005).

Baljit currently has an aluminium chair that weighs 25.5 lbs (11.6 kg). She is wondering about whether a new ultralight design would be better. On level ground, weight makes little impact on wheelchair performance and energy requirements. However, on hilly terrain weight makes a bigger difference in terms of energy required for propulsion on slopes and cross slopes. Weight is also an important consideration when transferring wheelchairs into vehicles. In terms of the type of tyre provided, research has shown that properly inflated pneumatic tyres have significantly lower rolling resistance than solid tyres, although there is a trade-off in terms of the potential for punctures and maintenance with pneumatic tyres (Sawatzky et al., 2004).

Baljeet is also wondering about the use of a power mobility add-on (Khalili et al., 2022,). As noted in Fig. 33.8, there are three types of add-ons that are generally available: powered wheels; powered front-end attachments (turns the manual wheelchair into a powered tricycle); and powered rear end attachments.

There are pros and cons with each wheeled mobility device, which reflect the adage that every choice is a compromise. The front-end attachments increase the base of support of the wheelchair and lift the front casters off the ground; the larger front wheel can help negotiate much larger obstacles than typical front casters. Some of them can go very quickly (18.5 miles/hour or 30 km/hour). One potential issue is where the device is stored when not in use. They also dramatically increase the turning radius, which may make it unusable in some indoor settings. In addition, the device would make it very difficult to perform a wheelie.

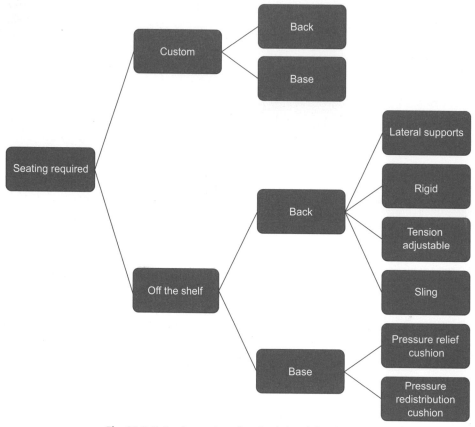

Fig. 33.7 ■ Seating options for wheeled mobility devices.

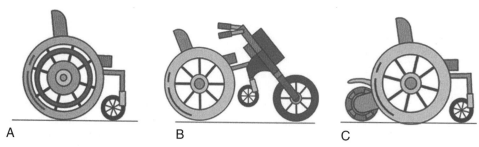

Fig. 33.8 ■ Power add-ons for wheelchairs. (A) Powered wheels. (B) Powered front-end attachments (turns the manual wheelchair into a powered tricycle). (C) Powered rear end attachments. (Image courtesy Dr. Mahsa Khalili).

Powered rear wheels (aka PAPAWs) have been around for the longest and are the best-researched powered add-on (Choukou et al., 2021). Powered wheels have been found to have a neutral impact on overall wheelchair skills scores, because they facilitate doing some skills (like going up ramps) but prevent them from doing wheelies (unless they are turned off) (Best et al., 2006). Rear-mounted attachments usually do not increase the turning radius of the chair. They operate at slower speeds than most front-end attachments. Some rear-end attachments permit users to do wheelies and significantly increase speed ascending longer ramps and slopes; however, some people have difficulty controlling them (Sawatzky et al., 2018). All these devices transform the manual wheelchair into a power chair, which requires users to relearn how they typically use their devices to avoid accidents (Sawatzky et al., 2018).

Baljeet is leaning towards using a rear-mounted attachment to avoid issues of device storage when indoors. Baljeet currently uses a pressure-redistributing air cushion, which she finds unstable. She would like to try a different cushion that offers more stability. This would be particularly important when a power-assist device that can start and stop quickly.

Obama has been resisting the idea of needing a powered mobility device for several years. He preferred to walk, despite increasing fatigue and falls. Recently he was chatting with a woman with multiple sclerosis who had obtained a scooter. She described how she had also resisted getting one, but that now that she had one it had completely changed her life by reducing the fatigue she feels at the end of the day. The importance of peers in decision making around wheeled mobility should not be overlooked (Mortenson et al., 2008). At this point, Obama would like to get a scooter since his home is not accessible and he wants to use it to facilitate his mobility in the community. Obama is interested in trialling a hybrid model scooter to reduce the turning radius but increase the base of support compared to the three-wheel scooter.

There are a variety of scooters to choose from. Some are very small to facilitate transportation. Others are larger to facilitate outdoor mobility. Scooters also vary in terms of the number and configuration of wheels (three-wheel, four-wheel and hybrid (front wheels are closer together than rear wheels)). Three-wheel scooters are more likely to flip if the user turns quickly because of their smaller base of support of the device (Fig. 33.9). Generally, scooters have very few seating options available.

For Mel, there are a variety of factors that need to be considered. Unfortunately, the lack of sufficient postural support in their current chair causes Mel to become fatigued later in the day. There are also safety concerns regarding Mel's use of their current device. To address hip flexion limitations, it would be beneficial to open up the seat to the back angle of their wheelchair. This could be accomplished by installing an angle adjustable backrest in their current chair that accommodates this non-reducible tightness or by increasing the back cane angle. To increase sitting tolerance, it might be helpful to provide the Mel with a wheelchair that tilts-in-space (Fig. 33.3D). Power wheelchairs can be equipped with power (self-controlled) tilt. There are also manual wheelchairs with tilt. Although most of these are attendant-controlled, power tilt is an option on some manual chairs. One of the big issues with power mobility for Mel is safety. However, you have recently learned from a vendor about an after-market system that helps prevent collisions. If this system worked, it would allow Mel to continue to mobilize independently at the facility where they live.

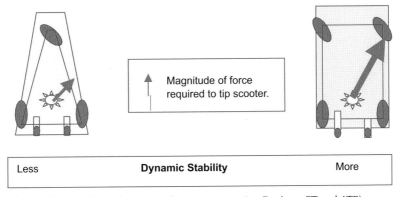

Dynamic Stability

Less   More

Magnitude of force required to tip scooter.

Fig. 33.9 ■ Stability of 3-wheel versus 4-wheel scooters. (Image courtesy Ian Denison, PT and ATP).

Stage 4: Funding and Ordering

Funding has a critical influence on the wheeled mobility device that a person can receive. Funders can include health maintenance organisations, workers, compensation boards, automobile insurances or government funding.

As Baljeet was injured in a car accident, she has relatively good funding for home modifications and equipment through her automobile insurance. That said, most funders will only provide a new wheelchair after a certain number of years and there may be restrictions on the types of devices they funded. It may be necessary to appeal decisions made by funders that appear unjust. However, it is critical to avoid letting funding constrain the types of devices discussed and considered by clients. In Canada and many other jurisdictions, if Baljeet had been injured in a non-work-related fall, she would have needed to rely on government programs to fund her equipment. In many jurisdictions, these programs fund devices based on medical needs, which may not be congruent with occupational participation. However, there are some jurisdictions that provide funding to support occupational participation more broadly. If Baljeet was ineligible for government assistance then it might have been necessary to approach charities to fund the equipment she needed, or pay out of pocket, perhaps with family assistance.

Obama has extended health benefits to cover the cost of a scooter if the proper procedures are followed. Health benefits funding will only provide one device every five years so it may be difficult to get a different device (e.g. a power wheelchair) if he has an exacerbation of his multiple sclerosis. However, it is already a huge step for him to consider using a scooter and he is unwilling to use a power wheelchair, which currently would not be needed for him to participate in his desired occupations. Difficulty predicting prognosis can make prescription challenging (Mortenson & Miller, 2008). If Obama did not have extended health benefits, he would need to pay privately for the device or investigate charitable options.

Mel does not have access to extended health benefits. They have had to pay privately for all their equipment. This has had a significant impact on their financial situation. The facility where they live only provides a basic manual wheelchair to residents. Residents or families are expected to pay for any additional devices. This situation is actually an improvement because historically, facilities in their health authority were not required to provide any wheelchairs. This demonstrates the potential for advocacy to make policy changes, which might eventually lead to the provision of other types of wheelchairs to residents. Knowing their financial situation, some occupational therapists might not identify more costly potential mobility options, but this approach is paternalistic (i.e. it tries to reduce the possibility of a person's disappointment based on the assumptions they could not problem-solve potential ways to obtain this equipment) and does not let Pat and Mel know about the full spectrum of options that are available. Although Mel has limited funding, Pat indicates they have been a well-respected member of their queer community for decades and believes it might be possible to raise funds through crowdsourcing for a wheelchair with these features if a trial indicates the device meets their needs.

In the United States, there are marked differences in the way that wheeled mobility devices are funded between programmes. For example, Medicare provides wheeled mobility devices for use only in the home, which may drastically limit and restrict users' community participation (Betz et al., 2022). In contrast, the Veteran's Health Administration and Medicaid provide coverage for wheeled mobility devices outside the home to support community engagement.

Stage 5: Trialling

Baljeet is able to trial a rigid carbon fibre wheelchair. Via some experimentation, she determined that having two inches (5 cm) of seat slope or dump was preferred (rear of seat lower than the front of seat). This is beneficial as it increases pelvic stability (e.g. gravity holds the pelvis back in the seat and improves balance by decreasing the angle between the between the thighs and the trunk) (Cooper et al., 2018). However, this means her seat is not level for transfers, which is something she needs to adapt to. She trials an off-loading cushion, which eliminates weight bearing on her ischial tuberosities to encourage skin health. She finds the cushion provides much more postural support but makes transfers more challenging since the surface is not as flat as her previous air-filled, pressure-redistributing cushion. She also trials a backrest with moderate trunk lateral support at the mid-thoracic region, which reduces her reducible scoliosis and subsequent lean. Lastly, Baljeet trials a recessed footplate that allows her to tuck her feet under her seat and a shorter seat depth, which accommodates her limited knee extension and reduces her tendency to slide out of her seat when she experiences spasms.

Obama tested the scooter around his home and in the community. He is able to park the scooter in his garage to charge it, so he does not need to bring it into his house. He is trained to use the scooter following the materials available on the Wheelchair Skills Training Program website. He reports that driving the scooter is fairly intuitive and similar to driving a car. He finds the scooter relatively easy to use on sidewalks but does encounter obstacles like business sandwich boards and bus stops that are hard to pass by. He finds the scooter a little challenging to use inside businesses that are wheelchair accessible because many aisles are cluttered with cardboard display items. He feels very self-conscious about using his scooter, especially indoors. He describes how he feels this may acerbate the racism he already experiences, as he will be hypervisible. Despite these concerns, at this point, he believes that the benefits of using a scooter would outweigh the potential drawbacks he might experience as he negotiates social environments using the device. His concerns about discrimination using a scooter are not unjustified (Labbé et al., 2020); and intersectional concerns have been raised about how the discrimination experienced by people with multiple marginalized identities is not purely additive (e.g. the racism experienced by people with disabilities may be different from the racism experienced by those without disabilities) (Fuentes et al., 2023). He wonders about whether a three-wheel scooter would be better for mobility in tight spaces, but given concerns about their tippiness he elects to proceed with the hybrid model.

Mel trials the new power wheelchair with anti-collision devices, a powered tilt function, and a more open back angle and backrest that accommodates their kyphosis. Opening the back angle is successful at accommodating Mel's hip flexion contractures and kyphosis. This makes their wheelchair much more comfortable and enabled Mel to be able to see where they are moving more clearly. Mel successfully trials a cushion with an accommodative pelvic obliquity buildup to level their pelvis and reduce trunk lean. Despite repeated attempts, Mel does not seem to be able to use the tilt function of the wheelchair independently. However, because it uses a similar joystick as their old power wheelchair Mel is able to drive the new chair. The anti-collision features prove invaluable for preventing Mel from hitting objects and people while travelling in the facility.

If the power mobility trial had been unsuccessful Mel would have then trialled a manual dynamic tilt in space wheelchair. Because many tilt-in-space wheelchairs are meant for the attendant population only, they might trial a chair with a low seat-to-floor height that allows for foot propulsion. When trialling their wheelchair, it is noted that during the mornings Mel can propel the wheelchair short distances with their feet. In the afternoons they are able to sit in the wheelchair for longer periods when it is tilted to counteract the forward pull of gravity on their thoracic kyphosis. With training, Pat can operate the tilt-in-space feature of the chair and is able to put the footplates on to take Mel outside the facility. One issue that Pat identifies is that the wheelchair is heavier than their older manual wheelchair, which makes it more difficult to negotiate slide slopes and curb cuts. The occupational therapist provides training to Pat about how to go down curb cuts backwards to make sure the descent from the curb is slow.

Either of these chairs would require fundraising. If funds were not available, Mel might be forced to use a facility chair that was completely unsuitable for their needs. The occupational therapist might need to look at other funding options as well (e.g. Parkinson's Society) to avoid this situation from creating occupational deprivation and drastically reduced quality of life for Mel.

Stage 6: Product Preparation

With some products like scooters, limited product preparation is required; however, many devices require assembly and set-up, often performed by the vendor. Some people may have postural asymmetry that cannot be accommodated by commercial solutions and custom seating may be needed with the help of a specialised seating clinic. It is also important to confirm that the wheeled mobility device and seating ordered are the same as those that were trialled, or that any substitutions do not adversely affect occupational participation goals (Barlow et al., 2009).

Stage 7: Fitting and Adjusting

Manual and power wheelchairs have several adjustable features. Wheelchairs and seating must be correctly fitted to the user. In the case of a wheelchair with commercial seating, the vendor will do the initial set-up of the seating, but it is imperative that the prescribing occupational therapist does a fitting with the user and the vendor to ensure that the wheelchair is set up to match the user's postural and functional needs. Depending on the equipment chosen, there may be many adjustable features that can be customised (e.g. backrest angle and height, armrest height, pelvic belt attachment point, footplate and headrest position, rear axle position) In the case of custom seating, the occupational therapist facilitates the fabrication and fitting process with a seating technician and the wheeled mobility user. In both situations, the wheeled mobility user and/or family/caregivers should participate in the process and be consulted about what they find the most comfortable and functional. Ultimately, the user is the expert in how their body works.

Stage 8: User Training

Most studies indicate low rates of training for wheeled mobility devices. Some preliminary training should be performed prior to deciding on the specific type of wheeled mobility that will be provided. Once the product has been delivered, additional training is required. It is especially important to provide training in the context where the device will be used to facilitate carry over. As mentioned previously, the Wheelchair Skills Training Programme is a free resource that provides information on manual and power wheelchair/scooter skills assessment and training for users

and their caregivers (Kirby et al., 2022). Users do not need to learn all possible wheelchair skills, instead, the wheeled mobility user may select the skills they wish to learn that are most applicable to their occupational participation goals. It is important to distinguish between wheeled mobility skills capacity (the ability of people to perform skills) versus their performance (which skills they perform on a day-to-day basis). Sometimes people have the capacity to perform some skills but do not because they lack the opportunity or need (e.g. being able to ascend a tall curb). Sometimes people may not use the skills they can do in practice because of a lack of confidence. The Wheelchair Skills Test Questionnaire includes items that assess capacity, performance and confidence, which may be useful in identifying areas to target for training.

Besides mobility skills, other skills may be beneficial for wheelchair users to learn, such as wheelchair maintenance, wayfinding and self-advocacy. An experimental study that evaluated the impact of offering users a scheduled wheelchair maintenance check-ups versus user-initiated contact found that 99% of chairs in the experimental group needed maintenance. Furthermore, the number of accidents remained unchanged in the control group (with no scheduled maintenance) whereas no accidents were reported in the experimental group (Hansen et al., 2004). It was noted that "most wheelchair users are unable to determine on their own when adjustments are needed." Tyre pressure has a profound effect on rolling resistance, so maintaining proper tyre pressure is a relatively easy way to reduce rolling resistance and improve chair performance (Sawatzky et al., 2004). Feasibility testing of a peer-led wheelchair maintenance training programme found that it resulted in significant improvements in wheelchair maintenance knowledge and confidence as well as significant decreases in wheelchair rolling resistance. Training materials from this programme are freely available at http://www.iwheel.ca/category/manual-wheelchair-maintenance/ (Eshraghi, 2016).

Wayfinding can be challenging for wheeled mobility users because services like Google Maps do not indicate the quality of sidewalks or the presence of curb cuts (Prescott et al., 2021). Research has shown that wheelchair users in novel environments plan routes that are significantly longer than the shortest possible distance and when they attempt to implement those plans they travel significantly further than the route they planned (Prescott, 2020). Presently there are no effective interventions that have been evaluated and shown to improve wayfinding; this is an area of consideration for occupational therapists working with wheeled mobility device users.

Furthermore, the ability to navigate the social environment is an important element of wheeled mobility success. Therefore the Wheelchair Confidence Measure includes four items about advocacy, five items about managing social situations, and three items about managing emotions (Rushton et al., 2011). Given that it is relatively easy for spaces that have been designed to be physically accessible to be made inaccessible via social practices (e.g. sandwich boards blocking sidewalks, accessible washrooms being used for storage and clutter blocking aisles) it may be helpful to work with wheeled mobility device users to develop skills to advocate for changes to improve accessibility. Depending on where wheeled mobility device users live, they may also be able to file formal complaints, especially where accessibility is legislated.

Stage 9: Maintenance, Repairs and Follow-Up

As noted previously wheeled mobility devices tend to be poorly maintained and this may contribute to accidents (Hansen et al., 2004). Given the cost of repairs, it would be ideal for funding programmes to cover the cost of ongoing maintenance and repair of wheeled mobility devices. Alternatively, it may be helpful for people who use wheeled mobility devices to learn to maintain them themselves, although this represents an example of off-shifting responsibility to people with disabilities, a common cost containment strategy. As most people use wheeled mobility devices for extended periods of time, ongoing follow-up is critical as insidious changes can result in serious secondary complications including pressure injuries, permanent deformities and chronic pain (Hogaboom et al., 2018).

CONCLUSION

Applying the 8-stage process for wheelchair provision outlined by the WHO can have significant benefits for individuals who use wheeled mobility devices. The process ensures that the individual receives a wheelchair tailored to their unique needs, environment and activities, thus improving their overall quality of life. Furthermore, occupational therapists can help individuals learn how to use and maintain their wheeled mobility devices properly, preventing injuries and promoting independence. Prioritising the 8-stage process and involving occupational therapists in the provision of new wheelchairs, can help to ensure that individuals who use wheeled mobility devices are provided with the best possible mobility solution to support their daily activities and improve their overall well-being.

REFERENCES

Agree, E. M., & Freedman, V. A. (2000). Incorporating assistive devices into community-based long-term care: An analysis of the potential for substitution and supplementation. *Journal of Aging and Health, 12*(3), 426–450. https://doi.org/10.1177/089826430001200307.

Barlow, I. G., Liu, L., & Sekulic, A. (2009). Wheelchair seating assessment and intervention: A comparison between telerehabilitation and face-to-face service. *International Journal of Telerehabilitation, 1*(1), 17–28. https://doi.org/10.5195/ijt.2009.868.

Best, K. L., Kirby, R. L., Smith, C., & Macleod, D. A. (2006). Comparison between performance with a pushrim-activated power-assisted wheelchair and a manual wheelchair on the Wheelchair Skills Test. *Disability and Rehabilitation, 28*(4), 213–220. https://doi.org/10.1080/09638280500158448.

Best, K. L., Routhier, F., & Miller, W. C. (2015). A description of manual wheelchair skills training: Current practices in Canadian rehabilitation centers. *Disability and Rehabilitation: Assistive Technology, 10*(5), 393–400.

Betz, M., Beauregard, T., Stojkov, A., Schein, R., & Digiovine, C. (2022). *Complex rehabilitation technology policy investigation*. Rehabilitation Engineering and Assistive Technology Society of North America. https://www.resna.org/sites/default/files/conference/2022/PublicPolicyandAdvocacy/103_Betz/103_Betz.pdf.

Braden, B. J. (2012). The Braden scale for predicting pressure sore risk: Reflections after 25 years. Advances in Skin & Wound Care, 25(2), 61.

Chan, F. H. N., Eshraghi, M., Alhazmi, M. A., & Sawatzky, B. J. (2018). The effect of caster types on global rolling resistance in manual wheelchairs on indoor and outdoor surfaces. *Assistive Technology, 30*(4), 176–182. https://doi.org/10.1080/10400435.2017.1307880.

Choukou, M. A., Best, K. L., Potvin-Gilbert, M., Routhier, F., Lettre, J., Gamache, S., Borisoff, J. F., & Gagnon, D. (2021). Scoping review of propelling aids for manual wheelchairs. *Assistive Technology, 33*(2), 72–86. https://doi.org/10.1080/10400435.2019.1595789.

Cooper, R. A., Cooper, R., & Susmarki, A. (2018). Wheelchair sports technology and biometrics. In J. A. De Luigi (Ed.), *Adaptive sports medicine: A clinical guide* (pp. 21–34). Springer Cham https://doi.org/10.1007/978-3-319-56568-2_2.

de Madariaga, I. S., & Neuman, M. (2020). *Engendering cities: Designing sustainable urban spaces for all.* Taylor and Francis. https://doi.org/10.4324/9781351200912.

Egan, M., & Restall, G. (Eds.). (2022). *Promoting occupational participation: Collaborative relationship-focused occupational therapy.* Canadian Association of Occupational Therapists.

Eshraghi, M. (2016). *Wheelchair maintenance training.* I-Wheel. http://www.iwheel.ca/category/manual-wheelchair-maintenance/.

Forslund, E. B., Jørgensen, V., Franzén, E., Opheim, A., Seiger, Å., Ståhle, A., Hultling, C., Stanghelle, J. K., Roaldsen, K. S., & Wahman, K. (2017). High incidence of falls and fall-related injuries in wheelchair users with spinal cord injury: A prospective study of risk indicators. *Journal of Rehabilitation Medicine, 49*(2), 144–151. https://doi.org/10.2340/16501977-2177.

Fuentes, K., Hsu, S., Patel, S., & Lindsay, S. (2023). More than just double discrimination: a scoping review of the experiences and impact of ableism and racism in employment. *Disability and Rehabilitation.* doi:10.1080/09638288.2023.2173315.

Carlsson, G., Slaug, B., Schmidt, S. M., Norin, L., Ronchi, E., & Gefenaite, G. (2022). A scoping review of public building accessibility. *Disability and Health Journal, 15*(2), 101227. doi.org/10.1016/j.dhjo.2021.101227.

Hansen, R., Tresse, S., & Gunnarsson, R. K. (2004). Fewer accidents and better maintenance with active wheelchair check-ups: a randomized controlled clinical trial. *Clinical Rehabilitation, 18*(6), 631–639. https://doi.org/10.1191/0269215504cr777oa.

Hogaboom, N. S., Worobey, L. A., Houlihan, B. V., Heinemann, A. W., & Boninger, M. L. (2018). Wheelchair breakdowns are associated with pain, pressure injuries, rehospitalization, and self-perceived health in full-time wheelchair users with spinal cord injury. *Archives of Physical Medicine and Rehabilitation, 99*(10), 1949–1956. https://doi.org/10.1016/j.apmr.2018.04.002.

Jain, N. B., Higgins, L. D., Katz, J. N., & Garshick, E. (2010). Association of shoulder pain with the use of mobility devices in persons with chronic spinal cord injury. *PM&R, 2*(10), 896–900. https://doi.org/10.1016/j.pmrj.2010.05.004.

Jang, S., Mortenson, W. B., Hurd, L., & Kirby, R. L. (2020). Caught in-between: Tensions experienced by community mobility scooter users. *Disability & Society, 35*(10), 1577–1595. https://doi.org/10.1080/09687599.2019.1696749.

Khalili, M., Jonathan, C., Hocking, N., Van Der Loos, M., Mortenson, B., & Borisoff, J. F. (2022). Perception of autonomy among people who use wheeled mobility assistive devices: Dependence on the type of wheeled assistive technology. *Assistive Technology, 34*(6), 725–733. https://doi.org/10.1080/10400435.2021.1934611.

Kawamura, J., Ise, M., & Tagami, M. (1989). The clinical features of spasms in patients with a cervical cord injury. *Paraplegia, 27*(3), 222–226. https://doi.org/10.1038/sc.1989.33.

Kemp, B. J. (2005). What the rehabilitation professional and the consumer need to know. *Physical Medicine and Rehabilitation Clinics of North America, 16*(1), I–vii. https://doi.org/10.1016/j.pmr.2004.06.009.

Kirby, R. L., Rushton, P. W., Smith, C., Routhier, F., Archambault, P. S., Axelson, P. W., Best, K. L., … Worobey, L. A. (2022). *Wheelchair Skills Program Manual Version 5.3.* Published electronically at *Dalhousie University.* Canada: Halifax, Nova Scotia. https://wheelchairskillsprogram.ca/en/skills-manual-forms/.

Labbé, D., Mortenson, W., Rushton, P., Demers, L., & Miller, W. (2020). Mobility and participation among ageing powered wheelchair users: Using a lifecourse approach. *Ageing & Society, 40*(3), 626–642. 10.1017/S0144686X18001228.

Misch, J., & Sprigle, S. (2021). Effects of wheels and tires on high-strength lightweight wheelchair propulsion cost using a robotic wheelchair tester. *Disability and rehabilitation. Assistive technology,* 1–11. Advance online publication. https://doi.org/10.1080/17483107.2021.2012274.

Mortenson, W. B., Miller, W. C., Boily, J., Steele, B., Odell, L., Crawford, E. M., & Desharnais, G. (2005). Perceptions of power mobility use and safety within residential facilities. *Canadian Journal of Occupational Therapy, 72*(3), 142–152. https://doi.org/10.1177/000841740507200302.

Mortenson, W. B., Miller, W. C., Boily, J., Steele, B., Crawford, E. M., & Desharnais, G. (2006). Overarching principles and salient findings for inclusion in guidelines for power mobility use within residential care facilities. *Journal of Rehabilitation Research and Development, 43*(2), 199–208. https://doi.org/10.1682/jrrd.2005.01.0031.

Mortenson, W. B., Miller, W. C., & Miller-Polgar, J. (2007). Measuring wheelchair intervention outcomes: Development of the wheelchair outcome measure. *Disability and Rehabilitation: Assistive Technology, 2*(5), 275–285. https://doi.org/10.1080/17483100701475863.

Mortenson, W. B., & Miller, W. C. (2008). The wheelchair procurement process: Perspectives of clients and prescribers. *Canadian Journal of Occupational Therapy, 75*(3), 167–175. https://doi.org/10.1177/000841740807500308.

Pellichero, A., Best, K., Leblond, J., Coignard, P., Sorita, É., & Routhier, F. (2021). Relationships between cognitive functioning and power wheelchair performance, confidence and life-space mobility among experienced power wheelchair users: an exploratory study. *Journal of Rehabilitation Medicine, 53*(9). https://doi.org/10.2340/16501977-2869.

Prescott, M. (2020). *Towards a conceptual framework of navigation for people who use wheeled mobility devices in the community.* University of British Columbia.

Prescott, M., Miller, W. C., Borisoff, J., Tan, P., Garside, N., Feick, R., & Mortenson, W. B. (2021). An exploration of the navigational behaviours of people who use wheeled mobility devices in unfamiliar pedestrian environments. *Journal of Transport & Health, 20*, 100975. https://doi.org/10.1016/j.jth.2020.100975.

Rice, L. A., Ousley, C., & Sosnoff, J. J. (2015). A systematic review of risk factors associated with accidental falls, outcome measures and interventions to manage fall risk in non-ambulatory adults. *Disability and Rehabilitation, 37*(19), 1697–1705. https://doi.org/10.3109/09638288.2014.976718.

Rushton, P. W., Miller, W. C., Lee Kirby, R., Eng, J. J., & Yip, J (2011). Development and content validation of the wheelchair use confidence scale: A mixed-methods study. *Disability and Rehabilitation: Assistive Technology, 6*(1), 57–66. https://doi.org/10.3109/17483107.2010.512970.

Sawatzky, B. J., Kim, W. O., & Denison, I. (2004). The ergonomics of different tyres and tyre pressure during wheelchair propulsion.

Ergonomics, 47(14), 1475–1483. https://doi.org/10.1080/0014013
0412331290862.

Sawatzky, B., Mortenson, W. B., & Wong, S. (2018). Learning to use a rear-mounted power assist for manual wheelchairs. *Disability and Rehabilitation: Assistive Technology, 13*(8), 772–776. https://doi.org/10.1080/17483107.2017.1375562.

Sprigle, S., McNair, D., & Sonenblum, S. (2020). Pressure ulcer risk factors in persons with mobility-related disabilities. *Advances in Skin & Wound Care, 33*(3), 146–154. https://doi.org/10.1097/01.ASW.0000653152.36482.7d.

Sprigle, S., Huang, M., & Misch, J. (2019). Measurement of rolling resistance and scrub torque of manual wheelchair drive wheels and casters. *Assistive echnology, 34*(1), 91–103. https://doi.org/10.1080/10400435.2019.1697907.

State Spinal Cord Injury Service [SSCIS]. (2015). *Spinal seating development project assessment form AF2.3: Basic MAT assessment.*

NSW Agency for Clinical Innovation. https://aci.health.nsw.gov.au/__data/assets/pdf_file/0004/312745/AF2.3_MAT_Assessment.pdf.

Welage, N., & Liu, K. P. (2011). Wheelchair accessibility of public buildings: a review of the literature. *Disability and Rehabilitation: Assistive Technology, 6*(1), 1–9. https://doi.org/10.3109/17483107.2010.522680.

World Health Organization [WHO]. (2008, May 13). *Guidelines on the provision of wheelchairs in less resourced settings.* https://www.who.int/publications/i/item/9789241547482

Zepeda, R., Chan, F., & Sawatzky, B. (2016). The effect of caster wheel diameter and mass distribution on drag forces in manual wheelchairs. *Journal of Rehabilitation Research and Development, 53*(6), 893–900. https://doi.org/10.1682/JRRD.2015.05.0074_.

REFLECTION

1. Why is it important not to let funding dictate the wheeled mobility options that are discussed with users?

2. What are some ways to improve the mechanical efficiency of manual wheelchairs?

3. What should the consent process look like when providing wheelchair assessment and training?

4. What aspects of the wheelchair provision process represent areas you want to learn more about?

5. How might you go about further developing those skills?

34

DRIVING AND TRANSPORTATION FOR COMMUNITY MOBILITY

LILIANA ALVAREZ ■ RUHEENA SANGRAR ■ APRIL VANDER VEEN

Overview

Driving and transportation are essential forms of occupational participation. An understanding of driving and transportation is necessary for occupational therapists to be effective partners in supporting not only the specific community mobility needs of people experiencing illness, injury or ipairment, but their meaningful overall occupational participation. As such, the necessary foundations for occupational therapists to connect, and collaboratively explore, design and advocate for people and collectives' needs for timely, safe, sustainable and accessible community mobility options are the focus of this chapter.

KEY POINTS

■ Community mobility is a human right and an enabler of participation in social, economic and cultural opportunities.

■ Occupational therapists must be equipped to partner with individuals and collectives to explore and support their community mobility needs.

■ When partnering with people who experience illness, injury or impairment, occupational therapists may address driving, public transportation or active transportation needs according to each person's values, priorities and contextual factors.

■ Occupational therapists have access to a varied and comprehensive toolbox to address community mobility needs including driving clinical screening, clinical, simulator and in-vehicle assessment and interventions, community mobility assessment and interventions.

■ Occupational therapists must critically examine the barriers to community mobility that discriminate, oppress and exclude equity-deserving groups and their community mobility needs.

■ Occupational therapists have an opportunity and responsibility to collaboratively explore and partner for transportation equity and justice.

INTRODUCTION

A person's participation in economic, social and cultural opportunities is largely dependent upon adequate access to community mobility (Coggin & Pieterse, 2015). Community mobility involves reaching meaningful places outside of a person's home, which fosters a sense of belonging and supports social participation by allowing people to engage in occupations that are necessary and of value to them (van Biljon et al., 2022). Not surprisingly, driving represents a primary means of community mobility across much of the Global North and South, where cities are largely car-centric in their infrastructure and planning (Pojani & Stead, 2018).

People experiencing illness, injury or impairment often face challenges pertaining to driving. Many individuals may require expensive vehicle modifications. For those who may not be able to drive or when access to a private vehicle is not affordable, practical, desired or possible, public transportation systems, private ride-sharing services or active transportation (e.g. walking or wheelchair rolling) may be an option. However, people experiencing illness, injury or impairment may face challenges with lack of adequate availability of such services, affordability and physical and social access barriers.

Occupational therapists must recognise the right of all people to community mobility (Classen, Alvarez et al., 2019) and support the complex community mobility needs of people and collectives. This chapter: (1) introduces driving and transportation and the corresponding occupational therapy scope of practice, (2) offers guiding principles and practical strategies across the continuum of community mobility practice and (3) challenges occupational therapists to critically examine the justice and equity issues that current driving and transportation systems perpetuate or overlook.

COMMUNITY MOBILITY CONCEPTS AND DEFINITIONS

Community mobility is deeply intertwined with social and cultural practices. For example, in many Western societies, obtaining a driver's licence is a rite of passage for teenagers and youth. Similarly, driving cessation marks a significant and often negative experience for older adults, whose occupational participation and social inclusion are severely restricted by the loss of

licensing privileges in car-centric communities. The centrality of community mobility as an area of practice for occupational therapists collaborating with people receiving their services cannot be overlooked. The following subsections provide an overview of key terminology related to community mobility practice and invite a transition to addressing community mobility as a right.

Fitness to Drive

Considering the importance of acknowledging the rights of people to community mobility, and based on a definition offered by Brouwer and Ponds (1994), the concept of fitness to drive is conceptualised as *having the ability and resources required to operate a motor vehicle, while abiding by the rules of the road and following normal and reasonable flow of traffic.*

Other definitions, such as that of the US Transportation Research Board's Taxonomy in Senior Mobility Circular (2016) or the UK Driver and Vehicle Licensing Agency (UK Driver and Vehicle Licensing Agency, 2021) emphasise the absence of functional or medical conditions as a central aspect of fitness to drive. This is consistent with reporting requirements in many jurisdictions, where certain healthcare professionals are required (mandatory) or allowed (discretionary) to report to the transportation authority any person who has or appears to have a medical condition or functional impairment that may make it dangerous to operate a motor vehicle (College of Occupational Therapists of Ontario, 2018). However, healthcare professionals and legal frameworks increasingly recognise that driver fitness should be based on an individual assessment. For example, in 1999 the Supreme Court of Canada ruled in favour of Terry Grismer, a person diagnosed with homonymous hemianopsia, loss of half of the peripheral field of view. The court determined that a functional assessment and not a diagnosis must be the standard by which fitness to drive is determined (Supreme Court of Canada, 1999).

Comprehensive Driving Evaluation

Comprehensive driving evaluation (CDE) refers to 'a complete evaluation of an individual's driving knowledge, skills, and abilities [...] that includes medical and driving history, clinical assessment of sensory-perceptual, cognitive, and/or psychomotor functional abilities [often through paper and pencil tests], an on-road assessment, an outcome summary and recommendations for an inclusive mobility plan, including transportation options' (Transportation Research Board, 2016, p. 9). CDEs are also referred to as 'functional assessments' by some transportation and medical authorities (Canadian Medical Association, 2017). Occupational therapists are recognised as professionals equipped to conduct CDEs in several regions including North America (Canadian Medical Association, 2017) and countries like South Africa, where they are recognised as uniquely positioned to make fitness-to-drive and driver rehabilitation recommendations (Classen, Groenewald et al., 2018).

Driving Cessation and Retirement

Driving cessation refers to the 'total discontinuation of operating a motor vehicle for productive, social, spiritual or any other purposes' (Chihuri et al., 2016, p. 333). Cessation is often recommended or required by a healthcare provider or licensing authority. With legislative changes and an ageing population, the tensions around addressing driving cessation, which can lead to significant physical and mental health decline among older adults (Edwards et al., 2009; Windsor et al., 2007), are increasingly prevalent in occupational therapists' caseloads.

Driving retirement refers to an individual deciding, often informed by healthcare providers and support networks, to reduce and/or eventually discontinue driving. The term driving retirement thus reflects the agency of the individual in preparing for and having time to consider this important transition (Jenkins & Holston, 2015). As such, driving retirement elevates this choice to the level of significant comparative choices such as end-of-life care, employment retirement and others.

Active Transportation

Active transportation refers to a person using their own body power to operate a device for movement such as bicycling, wheelchair rolling or scootering (Peruzzi et al., 2020). Active transportation, when adequately supported by the environment and infrastructure, can support people with their community mobility needs, and provide access to the health benefits of participation in physical activity (Buffart et al., 2009).

In addition to the above-mentioned forms of transportation, people increasingly rely on commercial non-public transportation such as taxis, Uber or Lyft,

as well as private transportation options aside from driving including rides by family or friends.

Transportation Poverty

The increased urbanisation of territories, population growth, systemic oppression of equity-deserving groups, and increased migration due to a variety of social (e.g. armed conflict) or geospatial (e.g. climate change) factors, are some of the determinants of growing transportation poverty. This term can be broadly defined as an *enforced lack of adequate* 'mobility options necessary for participation in society, resulting from an inaccessibility and/or unaffordability of transport' (Lowans et al., 2021, p. 2). Transportation poverty negatively affects health by limiting reliable access to healthcare services (Atuoye et al., 2015; Goswami et al., 2016), employment opportunities (Allen & Farber, 2019), education (Allen & Farber, 2018) and social participation (Boisjoly & Yengoh, 2017).

DRIVING AND COMMUNITY MOBILITY PRACTICE THROUGH THE CANADIAN MODEL OF OCCUPATIONAL PARTICIPATION LENS

Participation in community mobility influences occupational participation in other out-of-home occupations and can also be a meaningful occupation in and of itself. Through the Canadian Model of Occupational Participation (CanMOP) (refer to Chapter 11), Egan and Restall (2022) encourage occupational therapists to begin with two essential considerations: (1) Understand the meaning and purpose of participation in an occupation for an individual or collective, and (2) Collaborate with people and collectives to examine barriers to accessing, initiating and sustaining occupational participation at the level of microsystems, mesosystems and macrosystems.

1. *Understand the meaning and purpose of participation in an occupation for an individual or collective.*

Having pride in their identity as a driver or self-confidence to independently navigate public transit systems are examples of how individuals place value in these occupations. Occupational therapists can explore how transportation-related occupations might serve a need for a person's ability to access employment, food or health services (i.e. survival and safety);

the individual's view of driving as an occupation that makes them feel independent and productive (i.e. competence); the impact of paratransit services (i.e. publicly funded services that provide bookable rides without fixed routes or timetables) on the individual's community mobility (i.e. autonomy); or how participation in community mobility might depend on availability of a caregiver or attendant (i.e. relatedness).

Relationships and history can also influence the meaning and purpose of participating in occupations (Eagan & Restall, 2022). For example, driving can be valuable to a volunteer driver who delivers meals, or to a grandparent who takes a grandchild to after-school activities. Individual experiences (e.g. experiencing a car crash), as well as broader geographical and historical events (e.g. bus driver strikes), can also shape a person's perceived meaning of community mobility. Thus it is important to consider how driving and community mobility occupations support meaningful relationships across the lifespan, and to explore a person's history and personal meaning.

2. *Collaborate with people and collectives to examine barriers to accessing, initiating, and sustaining occupational participation at the level of microsystems, mesosystems, and macrosystems.*

At the level of the microsystem, an occupational therapist might evaluate a person's physical, affective, sensory and cognitive functions, as well as identify their financial and other personal resources such as their ability to plan a trip using a public bus, navigate to the bus stop, pay the fare and attend to announcements to get off at the correct destination. With the person, the occupational therapist can collaboratively identify challenges encountered, and assess financial barriers to afford the fare or the role of a caregiver or family member during the trip. At a mesosystem level, an occupational therapist working in a rural community might consider barriers people face when seeking to reinstate a suspended licence due to a medical event. If they need to undergo a comprehensive driving evaluation, the fact that such evaluations are only available in urban centres constitutes a barrier to participation. The occupational therapist might need to work with private practice organisations and community transportation systems to facilitate access to this return to driving service for their clients.

Occupational therapists need to consider how macrosystems might limit the occupational possibilities of collectives to engage in driving and/or transportation. People experiencing illness, injury or impairment are among the populations historically vulnerable to experiencing transportation poverty (Buliung et al., 2021; Currie & Delbosc, 2011). For example, Wolfe et al. (2020) found that in 2017 alone, 5.8 million persons in the United States delayed medical care because of a lack of transportation. Among them, people with a 'functional limitation' were more likely to report transportation as a barrier, when compared to others with similar sociodemographic and health characteristics. Moreover, transportation disadvantages have been linked to poor viral suppression among people living with human immunodeficiency virus (HIV) (Goswami et al., 2016), and limited use of assistive technology for people experiencing chronic conditions (Howard et al., 2022), just to list a few examples.

Occupational therapists can collaborate with collectives to understand how occupational participation in public transportation can be sustained by advocating for structural changes that promote community mobility. For example, The Minnesota Department of Health integrated *Inclusive Walk* audits for people with mobility impairments to promote their community mobility. *Inclusive Walk* audits are a public engagement activity where participants walk a predetermined route and identify barriers that impact their ability to walk safely and comfortably (Remillard et al., 2022). This initiative brought together people with mobility impairments and government officials to identify solutions to walkability issues and assess transportation improvements (Remillard et al., 2022). In 2020, the Spanish city of Barcelona installed electronic beacons in their bus fleet and in over 2500 bus stops. The beacons allow people with low vision waiting at a bus stop to receive live notifications about the next bus's destination, line and proximity to the stop. The user can message the driver to indicate they are a person with low vision and want to board the vehicle, among other features. This intervention was the result of years of collective advocacy and is part of a broader accessibility plan for the city's public transportation. Such initiatives illustrate the types of efforts that occupational therapists can partner to advocate for when working at the macrosystem level.

COMMUNITY MOBILITY PRACTICE WITH THE CANADIAN OCCUPATIONAL THERAPY INTER-RELATIONAL PRACTICE PROCESS FRAMEWORK

By employing the six action domains proposed by the Canadian Occupational Therapy Inter-Relational Practice Process (COTIPP) framework (refer to Chapter 12), occupational therapists can take a dynamic approach to understand, explore, co-design and refine community mobility transition strategies with individuals and collectives. The following sections and the practice story in Box 34.1 illustrate the professional reasoning and practical strategies that can be informed by each action domain in the framework.

Connect, Seek Understanding and Define Purpose

Mr Munro's Practice Story illustrates the importance of connecting with the person, which may include connecting and partnering with others in their network of support such as Mr Munro's wife and doctor. The fact that Mr Munro or his doctor are not concerned about his driving, but his wife is, can inform the professional reasoning of the occupational therapist in this early stage. For example, evidence has shown that the risk impression of caregivers who routinely drive with a person with Parkinson's disease are predictive of failing an on-road assessment, compared with the impressions of drivers themselves, or their physicians (Classen & Alvarez, 2016). However, it is important for the occupational therapist to consider the meaning that driving has for Mr Munro as

---

BOX 34.1
MR MUNRO

Mr Munro is a 76-year-old male, living in rural South-western Ontario. He lives with his wife of 53 years and is a retired teacher. He is involved in the Rotary Club and is an avid reader. He has two sons who live in other provinces. Mr Munro was diagnosed with Parkinson's disease ten years ago and is closely monitored by a movement disorders specialist. Mr Munro and his wife rely on his driving as his wife does not have a licence and public transportation options are limited where they live. He also enjoys driving and finds it a relaxing and mind-clearing activity. A few months ago, his wife noticed some changes in his driving, and she commented on this to his doctor. His doctor did not think Mr Munro had real issues with driving but made a referral to be supportive of Mrs Munro's concerns. Mr Munro himself is not too concerned but has agreed to see an occupational therapist to put his wife's mind at ease, plus he said that his wife, 'is always right', so 'better safe than sorry'.

SCREENING ASSESSMENT

Sadia, the occupational therapist, and Mr Munro agree upon an evidence-based screening plan, including tests listed in Table 34.3. Mr Munro's scores include: Trails B = 117s, intact contrast sensitivity, LFTN = 20 seconds, RPW = 6s, MMSE = 27 and his physician reported H&Y is 2. Mr Munro is surprised at how 'challenging' he found the Trails B. Collaboratively, Sadia, Mr Munro and his wife, agree that further assessment is warranted.

DRIVING SIMULATOR ASSESSMENT

To minimise the need for an out-of-pocket expense, Sadia recommends a driving simulator assessment to gain insights into driving performance and identify aspects in potential

need of intervention. Mr Munro is excited to try a simulator, and jokes that 'it makes him feel like his grandson with all his games on the computer'.

The simulator assessment identified that Mr Munro had some issues with visual scanning and vehicle positioning. This is consistent with evidence that shows visual scanning, signalling, vehicle positioning and under-speeding are predictive of failing an on-road assessment in people with Parkinson's disease.

Sadia and Mr Munro co-design a plan to address these driving errors. Consistent with the evidence, Mr Munro has developed insight into his skills and limitations on the road after this screening, and together they decide that reporting is not warranted at this time. Mr Munro's son is in town and doing most of the driving, and they agree that a comprehensive driving assessment will be conducted after the intervention plan is in place.

DRIVING REHABILITATION

Sadia and Mr Munro implemented their collaborative plan. The evidence-based plan includes:
- Education and on-road training with appropriate use of a Front Collision Warning System and Adaptive Cruise Control currently available in his vehicle;
- Remedial visual scanning training including road sign and landmark recognition with eye and head movements; and
- An extra mirror mounted in the car to compensate for limitations in head rotation movements.

Sadia conducts a CDE and Mr Munro passes, using the compensatory strategies he learned, and the improvements gained with specific skill training.

TABLE 34.1

Guiding Questions to Determine the Need for Driving Screening

Guiding Question	Considerations
Are there any clinical findings that would make driving screening redundant?	In the presence of known risks for driving, such as significant, apparent and persistent functional impairments impacting other daily activities and occupations, specific driving screening may be redundant. Such impairments warrant conversations with the person and may warrant notification of the local licensing authority. (Mr Munro has not experienced any apparent and significant changes in overall function, and as such, a specific driving screening may be appropriate.)
Is this the most appropriate time to screen the person?	Consider the person's current functional status and potential for improvement (Bédard & Dickerson, 2014). If the person is experiencing a transient/temporary functional change expected to improve, screening may be best deferred to allow time for functional recovery. Conversely, if the person's functional status is expected to remain stable, driver screening may be indicated. (This is the case with Mr Munro.)
What does the evidence say?	As evidence-based practitioners, occupational therapists must be knowledgeable of evolving best evidence for driver screening related to their area of practice. Existing best practice guidelines may inform their decision-making. Furthermore, the risk impressions of caregivers are predictive of driving outcomes when compared to neurologist or driver impressions (Classen & Alvarez, 2016). (For Mr Munro, a large body of evidence has documented the driving impairments that individuals with Parkinson's disease may experience.)
Are there more suitable time points for driver screening?	If there are concerns surrounding the person's medical status (i.e. blood sugar management, cardiac function) screening at follow-up with their family doctor might be most appropriate. Alternatively, in the event of a transient or temporary functional impairment, screening may be best completed later in the continuum of care (e.g. community vs. acute care).

driving is his family's only means of adequate transportation. As such, any findings from this process will shape his and his family's lives for years to come.

In this action point, occupational therapists must appraise the need for a comprehensive approach to community mobility along the journey. For example, the connection may happen in the acute care unit with a person who has experienced a stroke. In that setting, though not a driving-specific setting, people will be informed of the 30-day post-stroke mandatory driving cessation recommended by current guidelines (Frith et al., 2015). Thus occupational therapists should seek to identify and address alternative transportation options with the person and assist with seeking subsidised transportation where possible, and address the burden of in-person appointments (Vander Veen & Laliberte Rudman, 2022).

Explore Occupational Participation

Exploring participation in community mobility requires an understanding of the toolbox that occupational therapists have access to, and the factors that deem each tool most suitable in different contexts.

Driving Screening

The first approach to this exploration of driving is screening. Driving screening[1] is the administration of brief tests for the purposes of identifying whether a driver requires further detailed assessment to determine fitness to drive (Bédard & Dickerson, 2014). As such, screening is often conducted by an occupational therapist using paper and pencil tests in a community or health care setting. As with all occupational therapy assessments, a careful consideration of the person's presentation is required to understand when driver screening is appropriate. Guiding questions to inform professional reasoning to determine if it is appropriate to initiate driver screening are presented in Table 34.1 as they apply to Mr Munro (Box 34.1).

---

[1] The terms 'driver assessment', 'driver screening' and 'driver rehabilitation' are most used in the literature and field. However, these terms centre the action process around the person, instead of the specific occupation of driving. In line with collaborative relationship-focused occupational therapy, using actions verbs that address the occupation is less likely to reduce the individual to a set of skills deemed to be 'adequate' to access the regulated legal privilege of driving.

No single tool can inform decisions about fitness to drive (Bédard & Dickerson, 2014; Bennett et al., 2016). As such, occupational therapists will need to use professional reasoning to select appropriate evidence-based tools and other functional assessments to co-develop an appropriate screening plan with the person (Bédard & Dickerson, 2014). A series of assessment reflection questions developed by MacLachlan et al. (2019) applied to the context of driving are listed in Table 34.2.

Driving can be a contentious topic to broach with people, which underscores the need for a clear and transparent process. It is important for the occupational therapist to be aware of and communicate to the person the reporting requirements to the local licensing authority, their role in completing or contributing to such reports, and how a report would affect the person's driver's licence status. In some jurisdictions, reports received at the licensing authority can trigger a request for further documentation (from a family medical practitioner), licence suspension and/or requirement of a road test (as completed when initially attaining a licence) or comprehensive driving evaluation. People also need to be informed of potential fees for these requirements.

Examples of evidence-based driving screening tools, evidence-based populations studied and psychometrics of the tests are provided in Table 34.3. *A word of caution:* screening and assessment tools are only useful if they are supported by the best evidence when used to determine driving needs. Not all tools are appropriate for all people and the decision to use a tool must take into consideration the person's needs, context and condition. Periodic reviews of the evidence are required to maintain current with screening best practices.

The results of driving screening do not determine fitness to drive, they can only determine if a person is at risk and requires further assessment.

Driving Simulation Assessment

Driving simulators imitate real-world driving tasks, including the operation of a vehicle and its navigation (Classen et al., 2017). The driver's view when using a DriveSafety Driving Simulator is shown in Fig. 34.1. There is a wide variety of driving simulators currently available for clinical and research practice, including simulators with complete vehicle cabins and realistic controls, as well as motion platforms that can simulate cues from the vestibular, somatosensory and proprioceptive systems, also known as inertia cues (Classen & Evans, 2017).[2]

Clinical driving simulators are specially designed for use by healthcare professionals, to assist in the assessment and intervention of driving (Classen & Evans, 2017). These simulators can also be used to develop occupation-centred interventions that address underlying cognitive, sensory, perceptual or physical needs.

Compared to on-road assessments, driving simulator assessments are less expensive for the person, more easily controlled and standardised (which enables comparison across multiple sessions or individuals), reduce safety risks associated with on-road driving, provide objective data collection and reporting on driving performance and offer flexible customisation of scenarios to address driving skills in specific settings (e.g. inclement weather, highway driving, etc.) (Campos et al., 2017; Classen & Evans, 2017). Driving simulators alone cannot be used to determine a person's fitness to drive. Though valuable in a practice setting to assess and address the specific driving abilities of individuals, driving simulators cannot replace on-road assessments, given several limitations including a lack of common standards for their use, their susceptibility to triggering experiences of simulator sickness, specialised training requirements, access to funding and space limitations associated with their use, and the need for further evidence regarding their predictive and ecological validity (Caffò et al., 2020; Classen & Evans, 2017).

In the practice setting driving simulators can be used for assessments in a variety of ways. The multiple uses of driving simulators as proposed by Campos et al. (2017) are illustrated in Fig. 34.2. When conducting driving simulator assessments, occupational therapists are encouraged to develop assessment protocols that consider the evidence-based recommendations of Campos and colleagues (2017) contained in Table 34.4.

---

[2]The book 'Driving Simulation for Assessment, Intervention, and Training: A Guide for Occupational Therapy and Health Care Practitioners' (Classen, S., ed.) provides an extensive overview of the type of simulators and their features.

	TABLE 34.2	
	Screening and Assessment Action Points and Guiding Reflection Questions	
Screening action point	**Guiding questions**	**Considerations**
Reflect on assumptions	What assumptions does this assessment make?	The underlying assumption when broaching driver screening is that the person may be unfit to drive. Awareness of this assumption should inform how this sensitive conversation is approached. Understanding the person's values, the meaning of driving for them and the impact on their occupations is essential to this step.
	Whose agenda does this assessment align with?	Overwhelmingly, the decision to pursue driver screening is not the agenda of the person, but rather health professionals and family members. The occupational therapist must reflect upon the reason for the screening (and subsequent assessment). Is the source providing a reliable report? Do they have sufficient knowledge of the person's driving ability to convey a concern?
Determine if there are appropriate screening tools	Whose knowledge and values do the assessments align with?	Increasingly, recognising how different values and ways of knowing impact assessment is required to foster culturally safe assessment practices (Restall & Egan, 2022). Using tools that assume a certain level of education, for example, is problematic for inclusivity. To select appropriate driver screening tools, the occupational therapist needs to consider the demographics of the person (age, gender, language, culture, ethnic identity, etc.), as well as the diagnosis. Appropriate screening tools are validated with the same demographics and diagnostic category of the person to ensure helpful comparisons between norms/cut points and performance. If a specific tool is not validated for the same group membership, results should be considered with caution and transparently communicating this to the client is imperative.
Obtain informed consent for driver screening.	Can the person say no to this assessment, and what happens if they do?	A person may refuse driver screening for a myriad of reasons but avoiding the threat to licence status may be a common source of refusal. In this case, the occupational therapist can consider a more appropriate time to complete screening; and the risk to the person and public safety such that they have an ethical duty to send/recommend a report to the licensing authority if a person refuses screening. The potential impacts of the response to this question must be clearly discussed with the person.
Complete driver screening.	Does this assessment allow room for collaboration and partnership?	Completing a driving screening and assessment requires a partnership that leads to meaningful exploration. Understanding a person's occupational narrative is essential to such a partnership. Did they recently witness a loved one go through this process with a negative outcome? Do they have a history of test anxiety that was presented during the screening? Have they been in a motor vehicle collision?
	What can be done to reduce the power differential between the occupational therapist and the person?	The occupational therapist must consider how they can create conditions that are supportive of the person's agency including active listening, acknowledging and validating feelings and their physical positioning as an evaluator compared to the person.

TABLE 34.3

Examples of Evidence-Based Driving Screening Tools

Diagnostic group	Tools	Cut points/normative data	Psychometric properties and statistics
Stroke	Trails B	90 seconds (Devos et al., 2011)	PPV 68% NPV 84% (Devos et al., 2011)
	Motor-Free Visual Perceptual Test (MFVP)	30/36 (Korner-Bitensky et al., 2000; Mazer et al., 1998)	PPV 60.9% NPV 64.2% (Korner-Bitensky et al., 2000)
	Useful Field of View (UFoV)	Divided attention subtest >100 ms (George & Crotty, 2010)	Sensitivity 85.7% Specificity 69.4% predictive ability 77.5% (George & Crotty, 2010)
	Stroke Driver's Screening Assessment (SDSA)		Predicted pass/fail outcome in simulator-based driving evaluation with 87% accuracy (A. Akinwuntan et al., 2013)
	Compass (also within SDSA)	25	Sensitivity 85%, Specificity 54%, PPV 56%, NPPV: 84% for the outcome of the on-road test (Devos et al., 2021)
	Road Sign Recognition (also within SDSA)	8.5	Sensitivity 84%, Specificity 54%, PPV 56%, NPV 83% for the outcome of the on-road test (Devos et al., 2021)
Parkinson's disease	Trails B	108 seconds, with area under the curve = .86 (Alvarez & Classen, 2018)	Sensitivity = .89 Specificity = .74 PPV = .71 NPV = .91 (Alvarez & Classen, 2018)
	Contrast sensitivity	Impaired (Alvarez & Classen, 2018)	Sensitivity = .82 Specificity = .63 PPV = .61 NPV = .84 (Alvarez & Classen, 2018)
	Left Finger to Nose Test	A 1-unit speed decrease (1 s) for left FNT, the increase in odds of obtaining a pass was 47.3% over the fail group, and the increase in odds of obtaining a pass with recommendations was 55.9%. (Classen et al., 2015)	$B = -.749$ Exp. $(B) = .473$ $P = .024$ (Classen et al., 2015)
	Rapid Pace Walk	>6.22 seconds	AUC = .73
	Modified Hoehn and Yahr (H&Y), a measure of disease severity (AUC = .82)	≥ 2.5 (Crizzle et al., 2013)	AUC = .82 (Crizzle et al., 2013)
	Mini Mental Status Exam (MMSE)	<27 (Crizzle et al., 2013)	Internal consistency Cronbach's alpha = 0.78 Sensitivity = 0.83 Specificity = 0.99 (Kabátová et al., 2016)

Continued on following page

TABLE 34.3

Examples of Evidence-Based Driving Screening Tools *(Continued)*

Diagnostic group	Tools	Cut points/normative data	Psychometric properties and statistics
Multiple Sclerosis	Stroke Driver's Screening Assessment (SDSA)	Pass/Fail determined by predictive equation (available in manual).	Predicts 86% of pass versus fail outcomes on the behind-the-wheel test. Sensitivity, 88%, specificity 80%, PPV 67%, NPV 93%, (Akinwuntan et al., 2012)
	Useful Field of View (UFoV)	As per manual	When combined with the Stroop test (colour) SDSA, the UFOV (central visual processing speed, subtest 1) predicts 91% of pass versus fail outcomes on the behind-the-wheel test. Sensitivity 70%, Specificity 97%, PPV 88%, NPV 92% (Akinwuntan et al., 2013)
			Slower central visual processing speed on the UFOV (subtest 1) correlates with a higher number of gap acceptance errors ($\rho = 0.40$, p = .03) (Classen, Krasniuk, et al., 2018)
	Symbol Digit Modalities Test	As per manual	Specificity 98%, Sensitivity 25% for outcome on-road test (Schultheis et al., 2010)

Note: PPV = Positive predictive value (the probability of failing for drivers for whom the test has predicted will fail the on-road assessment); NPV = negative predictive value (the probability of passing for those drivers for whom the test has predicted will pass the on-road assessment).

Comprehensive Driving Evaluation

Referring a person for a CDE indicates a healthcare provider's or transportation authorities' concern and uncertainty about that person's fitness to drive (Kowalski et al., 2010). As such, a CDE aims to identify drivers who pose a significant risk to the safe operation of a vehicle. A CDE is most often an out-of-pocket expense that is rarely covered by public health care or extended health insurance (Stressel et al., 2014). Barriers to accessing a CDE include, but are not limited to, the financial cost, lack of accessible evaluation centres and medical care providers' understanding of the role and value of a CDE (Betz et al., 2014; Stav et al., 2011). Within these parameters, a CDE is only readily available to people who can afford them.

A CDE is conducted by occupational therapists with advanced training in driving assessment and rehabilitation alongside trained certified driving instructors. Training for occupational therapists seeking to pursue this area of expertise involves continuing professional development and supervised mentorship experience. Specific qualifications can be attained (e.g. Certified driving rehabilitation specialist [CDRS], driving rehabilitation professional [DRP], driver-trained occupational

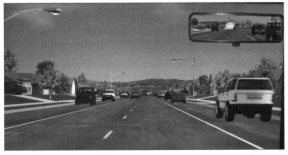

Fig. 34.1 ■ Driving simulation scene using a DriveSafety Inc. simulator (Utah, US). (From DriveSafety, Inc. (Utah, US)).

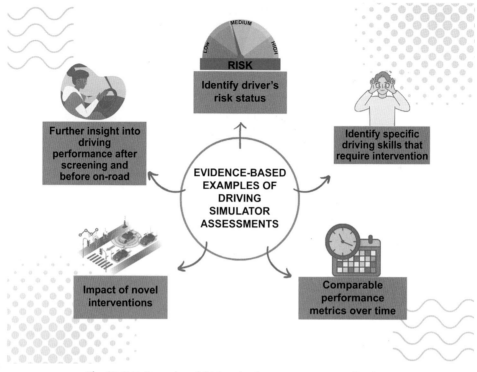

Fig. 34.2 ■ Examples of driving simulator assessment applications.

TABLE 34.4
Recommendations for the Design and Implementation of Driving Simulator Assessments
Recommendations for the design and implementation of driving simulator assessment protocols by Campos and colleagues (2017)
Maintain a consistent language
Establish fidelity, validity and reliability
Develop hypothesis-driven assessment protocols (targeted scenarios and metrics)
Customise scenarios to the driving behaviours of the population of interest
Use hypothesis-driven outcome measures

therapists [DTOT] or occupational therapy driving assessors [OTDA]). A CDE can last between 1 and 4 hours on a single day or span over multiple days (Dickerson, 2013).

Across transportation jurisdictions and countries, the protocol for a CDE can vary. However, there are two key components: An in-clinic medical assessment and an on-road driving performance evaluation.

In-Clinic Medical Assessment: The in-clinic medical assessment seeks to determine the effects of a person's medical condition, medication side effects and functional limitations on driving (Di Stefano & Macdonald, 2012). The in-clinic medical assessment includes medical and driving history, and valid and reliable assessments that are appropriate for the person's diagnosis and prognosis (Breidenbach & Hellrung, 2015; Dickerson, 2013). Examples include but are not limited to visual perceptual, cognitive skills and physical skills as well as seating considerations (Breidenbach & Hellrung, 2015; Dickerson, 2013). The result of the in-clinic medical assessment can lead to a referral to other services (e.g. wheelchair seating clinic, in-depth vision assessment), therapeutic rehabilitation to improve a person's candidacy for driving or an on-road assessment to further elucidate driving capacity (Breidenbach & Hellrung, 2015; Langereis et al., 2022; Vrkljan et al., 2015).

On-Road Driving Performance Evaluation: These road tests can vary in length from 30 minutes to over an hour (Kowalski et al., 2010), are conducted in a dual-brake vehicle, and the vehicle may need to be adapted to meet a person's accessibility needs (e.g. spinner knob on a steering wheel, extended rear-view mirrors, wheelchair adapted driver's seat). On-road driving performance evaluations might follow a standardised protocol and route (i.e. evaluators could use a psychometrically assessed test) or a non-standardised route that targets key driving tasks. Though susceptible to bias, on-road assessments are considered the gold standard in assessing driving performance (Berndt et al., 2015; Dickerson, 2013). While assessment criteria can vary across evaluators and protocols, on-road assessments will generally examine a person's performance of basic driving manoeuvres including pre-driving tasks (e.g. ingress/egress of the vehicle), basic manoeuvres (e.g. speed modulation, vehicle control during turns, navigating intersections), general environmental awareness and responsiveness (e.g. hazard perception) and a demonstration of recommended driving behaviours, such as blind-spot checks (Berndt et al., 2015; Breidenbach & Hellrung, 2015; Di Stefano & Macdonald, 2012). Instructions and components can increase in complexity as the evaluation unfolds (Justiss et al., 2006).

In-clinic medical assessment and on-road driving performance evaluation results are consolidated, and can generally lead to five possible outcomes (Kowalski et al., 2010; Langereis et al., 2022; Vrkljan et al., 2015). The person:

1. Demonstrates functional driving skills and capacity.
2. Demonstrates functional driving capacity, but requires some driving lessons to enhance their behind-the-wheel skills.
3. Is a novice driver who requires driver training to gain behind-the-wheel skills as well as adaptations or strategies to accommodate for their impairments.
4. Demonstrates deficits in behind-the-wheel skills and capacity that can be remediated or accommodated through rehabilitation and training.
5. Has significant deficits in functional driving skills and capacity whereby operating a vehicle is not recommended.

Depending on the transportation jurisdiction, the evaluator sends their assessment results directly to licensing regulators, particularly if they were the referral source. Such direct communication would be paramount where a person has undergone a CDE to reinstate a suspended driving licence, obtain a new driving licence, or evaluate capacity to continue driving. While the CDE determines driving capacity, it is often the prerogative of licensing regulators to decide licensing status.

Community Mobility Assessment

Community mobility assessment refers to the process of exploring a person's participation in places outside of their home by means different from driving a private vehicle. Examples of available tools include the Occupational Therapy Checklist of Community Mobility Skills (American Occupational Therapy Association, 2020), and the Life Space Assessment (Baker et al., 2003).

The Occupational Therapy Checklist of Community Mobility Skills uses 20 items representing functional areas to indicate whether the person can perform the task independently, with assistance, with difficulty, or unable to. The checklist provides a list of activity demands for public transportation such as buses or subways, transportation network services such as Uber or Lyft, and supplemental/assisted ride programmes such as door-to-door services. Using these activity demands, the checklist provides guidance regarding an appropriate type of transportation option. The checklist is available free of charge at https://www.aota.org/-/media/corporate/files/practice/aging/driving/community-mobility-skills-checklist.pdf.

The Life Space Assessment (Baker et al., 2003) is a self-report measure that evaluates the frequency of independent mobility in the past four weeks, across five life spaces (other rooms of the home, area outside the home such as deck or patio, place in the neighbourhood, places outside the neighbourhood but in the town, places outside town). Originally designed for older adults, the tool has demonstrated good psychometric properties for individuals with musculoskeletal, orthopaedic, neurological, balance, vestibular or general surgical needs who are engaged in community-based rehabilitation (Alshebber et al., 2020; McCrone et al., 2019). The validity and reliability of the LSA across different ethnic and cultural groups have also been established, including Latin-American males and females (Curcio et al., 2013; Snih et al., 2012), Chinese community-dwelling older adults (Ji et al., 2015) and community-dwelling Finnish older adults (Portegijs et al., 2014).

These tools approach community mobility from the perspective of what the person is 'able to do' and not what the infrastructure can or could offer. Non-standardised observations and explorations of available infrastructure are essential. For example, Stock and colleagues (2019) established the potential utility of a Smart Travel Concierge System (STCS) to support people with intellectual disabilities in planning and preparing for trips using fixed-route bus systems. Other approaches, such as that of Bezyak and colleagues (2017) have used quantitative and qualitative methods to explore the barriers to community mobility experienced by people with disabilities, in order to identify necessary infrastructure and system educational needs.

Co-design, Trial and Refine Priorities, Goals, Outcomes and Plans

Occupational therapists will use the information gathered in the exploration process, and collaboratively develop a plan with the person or collective. The following subsections describe various evidence-based approaches to driving interventions.

General Approaches to Driving Interventions

Dickerson et al. (2011) found a strong relationship between participant performance in a test of instrumental activities of daily living (IADL) and behind-the-wheel performance. The authors posit that IADL performance skills (such as scanning, sequencing and modifying actions in a dynamic environment), are also requisite skills for driving (Dickerson et al., 2011). As such, the occupational therapy process for addressing other IADLs may be applied to driving. In addition to occupational-based approaches, research has investigated skill-based interventions for driving. A recent systematic review and meta-analysis demonstrated that skill-specific training approaches (e.g. visual scanning, reaction time, etc.) and combining approaches (targeting multiple skills) improve driving performance and safety among older adults (Fausto et al., 2021). Moreover, Sangrar et al. (2019) highlights the importance of person-specific interventions informed by detailed, individualised assessments. Occupational

therapists with advanced training and expertise in driving rehabilitation (Dickerson et al., 2011) can employ specialised driving interventions including but not limited to graded driving practice, driving simulator-assisted practice or recommendations for adaptive devices (Langereis et al., 2022),

Technology Automation Approaches and Innovations

Currently, available vehicle automation technologies have the potential to enhance a person's driving capacity by enhancing comfort, improving vehicle safety, or automating the driving task itself and compensate for challenges with vehicle operation (Classen, Jeghers et al., 2019; Knoefel et al., 2019). As such, occupational therapists should understand what features people have in their vehicles when partnering with them to support their mobility needs, their understanding of how the features functions and how they use the technologies (or not) is critical to understanding driving as a highly personalised occupation as the vehicle fleet evolves.

SAE International (previously known as the Society of Automotive Engineers) provides a framework to describe six levels of vehicle automation that are helpful to occupational therapists when considering the impact of vehicle automation on the occupation of driving (SAE International, 2021):

■ Level 0 (No Driving Automation).
■ Level 1 (Driving Assistance).
■ Level 2 (Partial Driving Automation).
■ Level 3 (Conditional Driving Automation).
■ Level 4 (High Driving Automation).
■ Level 5 (Full Driving Automation).

Between Levels 0 and 2, the human driver is in control of the vehicle even if some technological systems provide driving support. For example, adaptive cruise control systems are characterised as Level 1 as they automatically adjust vehicle speed to assist the driver. Alternatively, a heads-up display can be categorised as Level 0 as it only provides the driver with information but does not take over any aspect of the driving task. Other examples include blind-spot detection, lane departure warning systems, or backup cameras. Some drivers perceive that accepting such technologies may lead to unconstrained trust and misuse of the systems

(Classen et al., 2020; Haghzare et al., 2023). However, further research is needed on the potential for occupational therapists to recommend these technologies as post-market adaptations or purchase of vehicles with these technologies as a form of compensating for limitations in driving ability (Liu, 2018). It is important for occupational therapists to understand how drivers learn to use these new technologies and integrate their use into everyday driving behaviours (Sangrar et al., 2018; Stinchcombe et al., 2017).

In Levels 3 to 5, the human driver is not primarily in control of the car. A Level 3 autonomous vehicle can request that the driver take full control when certain environmental conditions arise, whereas vehicles at Level 5 remain in control. Occupational therapists will likely encounter people who own and drive vehicles with such automations in the near future (Liu, 2018). Furthermore, self-driving or fully autonomous vehicles (i.e. Level 4 or 5) hold the promise of increasing community mobility for people who have never been able to operate a vehicle or those who have lost the capacity to do so (Dicianno et al., 2021). For example, Haghzare et al. (2023) found that people experiencing dementia may place higher levels of trust in fully versus partially automated vehicles. Emerging evidence suggests that these vehicles will greatly reduce traffic fatalities once widely adopted (Liu, 2018), but the actual impact of these transport options on out-of-home mobility has yet to be determined (Hutchinson et al., 2020).

At present, access to, affordability and availability of self-driving vehicles and autonomous public transit that enable community mobility are not ubiquitous (Hutchinson, 2020). In addition, further advancements in transportation system infrastructure are needed to make this mode of transportation a viable option that occupational therapists can draw upon to promote individuals' and collectives' occupational participation. This represents an opportunity for occupational therapists to advocate for solutions that are tailored to the needs of people experiencing illness, injury and impairment. Moreover, early exposure and education may enhance safe adoption and acceptance. For example, Classen and colleagues (2020) exposed older adults (N = 69) to an automated shuttle. Findings showed that exposure to the technology may positively impact participants' perceptions of trust and safety.

Finally, occupational therapists must be aware of emerging changes in the transportation landscape that are arriving much earlier than fully automated vehicles, including mobility apps such as Car2Go, Bus checker, Waze and Blindsq. Such apps can increase the social sustainability of transport, which may, in turn, increase the user's agency. For example, a review of mobility apps (Gebresselassie & Sanchez, 2018) found that such transportation tools address equity and inclusion issues by using universal design, including cost-conscious options, increasing language customisation, and by sceptically developing applications for people with impairments. Other increasingly common apps for ride-hailing, such as Uber and Lyft, represent opportunities but also potential exclusion barriers for people with impairments. For example, in a study exploring the experiences of people with impairments (N = 32) with ride-hailing apps, older adults and individuals with acquired impairments experienced difficulties with use, while younger individuals and those with more experience found them to be convenient, relatively more affordable than taxis, and reliable (Cochran, 2022).

Community Mobility Transition Strategies

Community mobility transitions are changes in how a person accesses their community that can be either permanent or temporary. This section will discuss transitions specific to driving retirement/cessation as well as temporary driving disruptions that impact community mobility.

Driving Retirement and Cessation Among Older Adults

Poor mental health, reduced quality of life, social isolation and financial stress are among the myriad outcomes of driving cessation among older adults (Schofield et al., 2023; Stinchcombe et al., 2021; Veerhuis et al., 2022). As such, it is not surprising that many older adults are inclined to delay discussions about driving transitions (Betz et al., 2013; Stinchcombe et al., 2021). Approaching this transition as a proactive process of retirement for whom individuals and collectives can plan and be supported in, may shift the approach to such conversations and support the person's community mobility needs and goals (Stinchcombe et al., 2021). Moreover, discussing community mobility planning prior to the onset of body changes that could impact driving provides the person with opportunities to make their own plans. A useful planning strategy may be to encourage the older driver to access alternate methods of transportation prior to changes in driving status to practice navigating without a car and identify preferred alternate methods (Veerhuis et al., 2022). This can allow the person and family to experiment with the transition without the pressures of imminent cessation. The presence of other life transitions also offers an opportunity to discuss driving retirement, such as vocational retirement or moving to a new home (Veerhuis et al., 2022). Supportive communities can also facilitate and normalise conversations about driving retirement (Schofield et al., 2023). Senior housing facilities, service clubs and church groups are among the settings suggested by older drivers to discuss driving with peers. For occupational therapists, this provides an opportunity to consider how driving could be addressed in group therapy sessions in both inpatient and community settings.

Driving Disruptions

Some unexpected medical conditions can signal unpredictable driving transitions, from temporary disruptions to permanent cessation. For example, following traumatic brain injury (TBI), individuals may not initially be able to drive but up to 60% eventually return to driving (Liddle et al., 2011). This temporary driving disruption is described as 'on hold' during which people report frustration, stress, depression and anger (Liddle et al., 2011). Clear communication about expectations for return to driving, including recovery indicators and assessments used to inform decisions, timeframes and practical support to access alternative transportation options can help to assuage the difficulties of being 'on hold' (Liddle et al., 2011).

Transportation Equity and Justice-focused Interventions

Occupational therapists have a responsibility to address the environmental and systems-level conditions that exclude and oppress equity between people with different abilities and access to services. In Khayelitsha and Nyanga in Cape Town, for example, disabled women who experienced transportation barriers partnered with the Department of Occupational Therapy at the University of Cape and the NGO South African Christian Leadership Assembly (SACLA) Health Project (Lorenzo, 2008). Based on the principles of emancipatory action research, their mobilisation resulted in effective advocacy for an accessible public transportation system (Lorenzo, 2008).

In another example, young people with disabilities, their parents, therapists and transportation stakeholders worked together to overcome challenges when accessing and navigating public transportation (Lindsay, 2020). Together, they formulated over 122 transportation solutions such as a user-friendly booking system for wheel trans (a door-to-door transportation service offered), transportation consultants for youth with complex needs, and disability awareness mandatory training for all transportation personnel. Other community-based approaches have integrated technology-leveraged solutions, such as Shaheen and colleagues' investigation of an electric vehicle (EV) car-sharing programme with 443 residents of the Rossmoor Senior Adult Community in Walnut Creek, California. Such insights provide opportunities for occupational therapists to partner in advocacy and collaborative practice to develop system-level changes.

CONCLUSION

Occupational therapists are optimally equipped to partner with individuals and collectives in exploring and supporting their community mobility needs. Occupational therapists must critically examine the implications of driving disruptions and transition and creatively address the assessment and rehabilitation needs of people who want and need to drive. This does not require a compromise of personal or public safety; it requires a holistic and critical understanding of community mobility as a right, and as existing in a continuum. Beyond driving, occupational therapists must also examine public and active transportation, and develop strategies for safe, accessible, equitable and timely access for all.

REFERENCES

Akinwuntan, A. E., Devos, H., Stepleman, L., Casillas, R., Rahn, R., Smith, S., & Williams, M. J. (2013). Predictors of driving in individuals with relapsing-remitting multiple sclerosis. *Multiple Sclerosis (Houndmills, Basingstoke, England)*, 19(3), 344–350. https://doi.org/10.1177/1352458512451944.

Akinwuntan, A. E., O'Connor, C., McGonegal, E., Turchi, K., Smith, S., Williams, M., & Wachtel, J (2012). Prediction of driving ability in people with relapsing-remitting multiple sclerosis using the stroke driver screening assessment. *International Journal of MS Care, 14*(2), 65–70. https://doi.org/10.7224/1537-2073-14.2.65.

Akinwuntan, A., Gantt, D., Gibson, G., Kimmons, K., Ross, V., Newman Rosen, P., & Wachtel, J. (2013). United States Version of the Stroke Driver Screening Assessment: A pilot study. *Topics in Stroke Rehabilitation, 20*(1), 87–92. https://doi.org/10.1310/tsr2001-87.

Allen, J., & Farber, S. (2018). How time-use and transportation barriers limit on-campus participation of university students. *Travel Behaviour and Society, 13*, 174–182. https://doi.org/10.1016/J.TBS.2018.08.003.

Allen, J., & Farber, S. (2019). Sizing up transport poverty: A national scale accounting of low-income households suffering from inaccessibility in Canada, and what to do about it. *Transport Policy, 74*, 214–223. https://doi.org/10.1016/J.TRANPOL.2018.11.018.

Alshebber, K. M., Dunlap, P. M., & Whitney, S. L. (2020). Reliability and concurrent validity of life space assessment in individuals with vestibular disorders. *Journal of Neurologic Physical Therapy, 44*(3), 214–219. https://doi.org/10.1097/NPT.0000000000000320.

Alvarez, L., & Classen, S. (2018). Driving with Parkinson's disease: Cut points for clinical predictors of on-road outcomes. *Canadian Journal of Occupational Therapy, 85*(3), 232–241. http://dx.doi.org/10.1177/0008417418755458.

American Occupational Therapy Assssociation. (2020). Occupational therapy checklist of community mobility skills. Bethesda, Maryland: AOTA Press. Retrieved from: https://www.aota.org/-/media/corporate/files/practice/aging/driving/community-mobility-skills-checklist.pdf.

Atuoye, K. N., Dixon, J., Rishworth, A., Galaa, S. Z., Boamah, S. A., & Luginaah, I. (2015). Can she make it? Transportation barriers to accessing maternal and child health care services in rural Ghana. *BMC Health Services Research, 15*(1), 1–10. https://doi.org/10.1186/S12913-015-1005-Y/FIGURES/2.

Baker, P. S., Bodner, E. V., & Allman, R. M. (2003). Measuring lifespace mobility in community-dwelling older adults. *Journal of the American Geriatrics Society, 51*(11), 1610–1614. https://doi.org/10.1046/J.1532-5415.2003.51512.X.

Bédard, M., & Dickerson, A. E. (2014). Consensus statements for screening and assessment tools. *Occupational Therapy in Health Care, 28*(2), 127–131. https://doi.org/10.3109/07380577.2014.903017.

Bennett, J. M., Chekaluk, E., & Batchelor, J. (2016). Cognitive tests and determining fitness to drive in dementia: A systematic review. *Journal of the American Geriatrics Society, 64*(9), 1904–1917. https://doi.org/10.1111/jgs.14180.

Berndt, A. H., May, E., & Darzins, P. (2015). On-road driving assessment and route design for drivers with dementia. *British Journal of Occupational Therapy, 78*(2), 121–130. https://doi.org/10.1177/0308022614562397.

Betz, M. E., Dickerson, A., Coolman, T., Schold Davis, E., Jones, J., & Schwartz, R. (2014). Driving rehabilitation programs for older drivers in the United States. *Occupational Therapy in Health Care, 28*(3), 306–317. https://doi.org/10.3109/07380577.2014.908336.

Betz, M. E., Jones, J., Petroff, E., & Schwartz, R. (2013). "I wish we could normalize driving health:" A qualitative study of clinician discussions with older drivers. *Journal of General Internal Medicine, 28*(12), 1573–1580. https://doi.org/10.1007/s11606-013-2498-x.

Bezyak, J. L., Sabella, S. A., & Gattis, R. H. (2017). Public transportation: An investigation of barriers for people with disabilities. *Journal of Disability Policy Studies, 28*(1), 52–60. https://doi.org/10.1177/1044207317702070.

Boisjoly, G., & Yengoh, G. T. (2017). Opening the door to social equity: local and participatory approaches to transportation planning in Montreal. *European Transport Research Review, 9*(3), 1–21. https://doi.org/10.1007/S12544-017-0258-4/TABLES/5.

Breidenbach, D. H., & Hellrung, J. (2015). *A Job Analysis Study of the Driver Rehabilitation Specialist.* www.goAMP.com.

Brouwer, W. H., & Ponds, R. W. (1994). Driving competence in older persons. *Disability and Rehabilitation, 16*(3), 149–161. http://www.ncbi.nlm.nih.gov/entrez/query.fcgi?cmd=Retrieve&db=PubMed&dopt=Citation&list_uids=7919398.

Buffart, L. M., Westendorp, T., Van Den Berg-Emons, R. J., Stam, H. J., & Roebroeck, M. E. (2009). Perceived barriers to and facilitators of physical activity in young adults with childhood-onset physical disabilities. *Journal of Rehabilitation Medicine, 41*(11). https://doi.org/10.2340/16501977-0420.

Buliung, R., Bilas, P., Ross, T., Marmureanu, C., & El-Geneidy, A. (2021). More than just a bus trip: School busing, disability and access to education in Toronto, Canada. *Transportation Research Part A: Policy and Practice, 148*, 496–505. https://doi.org/10.1016/J.TRA.2021.04.005.

Caffò, A. O., Tinella, L., Lopez, A., Spano, G., Massaro, Y., Lisi, A., Stasolla, F., Catanesi, R., Nardulli, F., Grattagliano, I., & Bosco, A. (2020). The drives for driving simulation: A scientometric analysis and a selective review of reviews on simulated driving research. *Frontiers in Psychology, 11.* https://doi.org/10.3389/fpsyg.2020.00917.

Campos, J. L., Bédard, M., Classen, S., Delparte, J. J., Hebert, D. A., Hyde, N., Law, G., Naglie, G., & Yung, S. (2017). The guiding framework for driver assessment using driving simulators. *Frontiers in Psychology, 8*(Aug). https://doi.org/10.3389/fpsyg.2017.01428.

Canadian Medical Association. (2017). *Determining medical fitness to operate motor vehicles: CMA driver's guide.* Joule Inc.

Chihuri, S., Mielenz, T. J., Dimaggio, C. J., Betz, M. E., Diguiseppi, C., Jones, V. C., & Li, G. (2016). Driving cessation and health outcomes in older adults. *Journal of the American Geriatrics Society, 64*(2), 332–341. https://doi.org/10.1111/jgs.13931.

Classen, S., & Alvarez, L. (2016). Caregivers' impressions predicting fitness to drive in persons with Parkinson's. *OTJR: Occupation, Participation and Health, 36*(1), 5–13. https://doi.org/10.1177/1539449215601117.

Classen, S., Alvarez, L., Bundy, A., Dickerson, A. E., Gelinas, I., Matsubara, A., Patomella, A.-H., Pfeiffer, B., Ross, P., Schold-Davis, E., & Swanepoel, L. (2019). *Position Statement: Occupational Therapy in Driving and Community Mobility.* https://www.wfot.org/resources/occupational-therapy-in-driving-and-community-mobility

Classen, S., Dickerson, A. E., & Rosenthal, T. J. (2017). Terminology and Taxonomy of Terms for Driving Simulation. In S. Classen (Ed.), *Driving simulation for assessment, intervention, and training: A guide for occuapional therapy and health care practitioners* (pp. 13–26). AOTA Press.

Classen, S., & Evans, D. F. (2017). Overview of simulators by type, characteristics, and attributes. In S. Classen (Ed.), *Driving simulation for assessment, intervention, and training: A guide for occuapional therapy and health care practitioners* (pp. 27–40). AOTA Press.

Classen, S., Groenewald, R., Kolling, J., Norval, H., Rule, C., & Swanepoel, L. (2018). Occupational Therapy Association of South Africa (OTASA) Position Statement. Enabling community mobility through driver evaluation and rehabilitation: The role of occupational therapists. *South African Journal of Occupational Therapy, 48*(3), 62–63. http://www.scielo.org.za/scielo.php?script=sci_arttext&pid=S2310-38332018000300010&nrm=iso.

Classen, S., Holmes, J., Alvarez, L., Loew, K., Mulvagh, A., Rienas, K., Victoria, W., & He, W (2015). Clinical assessments as predictors of primary on-road outcomes in Parkinson's disease. *OTJR: Occupation, Participation and Health, 35*(4), 213–220.

Classen, S., Jeghers, M., Morgan-Daniel, J., Winter, S., King, L., & Struckmeyer, L. (2019). Smart in-vehicle technologies and older drivers: A scoping review. *OTJR: Occupation, Participation and Health, 39*(2), 97–107. https://doi.org/10.1177/1539449219830376.

Classen, S., Krasniuk, S., Morrow, S. A., Alvarez, L., Monahan, M., Danter, T., & Rosehart, H. (2018). Visual correlates of fitness to drive in adults with multiple sclerosis. *OTJR Occupation, Participation and Health, 38*(1), 15–27. https://doi.org/10.1177/1539449217718841.

Classen, S., Mason, J., Wersal, J., Sisiopiku, V., & Rogers, J. (2020). Older drivers' experience with automated vehicle technology: Interim analysis of a demonstration study. *Frontiers in Sustainable Cities, 2,* 27. https://doi.org/10.3389/FRSC.2020.00027/BIBTEX.

Cochran, A. L. (2022). How and why do people with disabilities use app-based ridehailing? *Case Studies on Transport Policy, 10*(4), 2556–2562. https://doi.org/10.1016/J.CSTP.2022.11.015.

Coggin, T., & Pieterse, M. (2015). A right to transport? Moving towards a rights-based approach to mobility in the city. *South African Journal on Human Rights, 31*(2), 294–314. https://doi.org/10.1080/19962126.2015.11865248.

College of Occupational Therapists of Ontario. (2018). *Guide to discretionary reporting of fitness to drive in effect July 1, 2018.* https://www.coto.org/news/news-details/2019/06/13/guide-to-discretionary-reporting-of-fitness-to-drive-in-effect-july-1-2018.

Crizzle, A. M., Classen, S., Lanford, D. N., Malaty, I. A., Okun, M. S., Wang, Y., Wagle Shukla, A., Rodriguez, R. L., McFarland, R., & McFarland, N. R. (2013). Postural/gait and cognitive function as predictors of driving performance in Parkinson's disease. *Journal of Parkinson's Disease, 3*(2), 153–160. https://doi.org/10.3233/JPD-120152.

Curcio, C. L., Alvarado, B. E., Gomez, F., Guerra, R., Guralnik, J., & Zunzunegui, M. V. (2013). Life-Space Assessment scale to assess mobility: validation in Latin American older women and men.

Aging Clinical and Experimental Research, 25(5), 553–560. https://doi.org/10.1007/S40520-013-0121-Y.

Currie, G., & Delbosc, A. (2011). Transport disadvantage: A review. *New Perspectives and Methods in Transport and Social Exclusion Research,* 15–25. https://doi.org/10.1108/9781780522012-002.

Devos, H., Akinwuntan, A. E., Nieuwboer, A., Truijen, S., Tant, M., & De Weerdt, W. (2011). Screening for fitness to drive after stroke: A systematic review and meta-analysis. *Neurology, 76,* 747–756.

Devos, H., Hawley, C. A., Conn, A. M., Marshall, S. C., & Akinwuntan, A. E. (2021). Driving after stroke. In T. Platz (Ed.), *Clinical pathways in stroke rehabilitation* (pp. 243–260). Springer.

Di Stefano, M., & Macdonald, W. (2012). Design of occupational therapy on-road test routes and related validity issues. *Australian Occupational Therapy Journal, 59*(1), 37–46. https://doi.org/10.1111/j.1440-1630.2011.00990.x.

Dicianno, B. E., Sivakanthan, S., Sundaram, S. A., Satpute, S., Kulich, H., Powers, E., Deepak, N., Russell, R., Cooper, R., & Cooper, R. A. (2021). Systematic review: Automated vehicles and services for people with disabilities. *Neuroscience Letters, 761,* 136103. https://doi.org/10.1016/J.NEULET.2021.136103.

Dickerson, A. E. (2013). Driving assessment tools used by driver rehabilitation specialists: survey of use and implications for practice. *American Journal of Occupational Therapy, 67*(5), 564–573. https://doi.org/10.5014/ajot.2013.007823.

Dickerson, A. E., Reisletter, T., Schold Davis, E., & Monahan, M. (2011). Evaluating driving as a valued instrumental activity of daily living. *American Journal of Occupational Therapy, 65*(1), 64–75.

Edwards, J. D., Lunsman, M., Perkins, M., Rebok, G. W., & Roth, D. L. (2009). Driving cessation and health trajectories in older adults. *The Journals of Gerontology Series A: Biological Sciences and Medical Sciences, 64A*(12), 1290–1295. https://doi.org/10.1093/gerona/glp114.

Fausto, B. A., Adorno Maldonado, P. F., Ross, L. A., Lavallière, M., & Edwards, J. D. (2021). A systematic review and meta-analysis of older driver interventions. *Accident Analysis and Prevention, 149,* 105852. https://doi.org/10.1016/j.aap.2020.105852.

Frith, J., Hubbard, I. J., James, C. L., & Warren-Forward, H. (2015). Returning to driving after stroke: A systematic review of adherence to guidelines and legislation. *British Journal of Occupational Therapy*(6), 78. https://doi.org/10.1177/0308022614562795.

Gebresselassie, M., & Sanchez, T. W. (2018). Smart" tools for socially sustainable transport: A review of mobility apps. *Urban Science, 2*(2), 45. https://doi.org/10.3390/URBANSCI2020045.

George, S., & Crotty, M. (2010). Establishing criterion validity of the Useful Field of View assessment and Stroke Drivers' Screening Assessment: Comparison to the result of on-road assessment. *American Journal of Occupational Therapy, 64,* 114–122.

Goswami, N. D., Schmitz, M. M., Sanchez, T., Dasgupta, S., Sullivan, P., Cooper, H., Rane, D., Kelly, J., Del Rio, C., & Waller, L. A. (2016). Understanding local spatial variation along the care continuum: The potential impact of transportation vulnerability on HIV linkage to care and viral suppression in high-poverty areas, Atlanta, Georgia. *Journal of Acquired Immune Deficiency Syndromes, 72*(1), 65. https://doi.org/10.1097/QAI.0000000000000914.

Haghzare, S., Stasiulis, E., Delfi, G., Mohamud, H., Rapoport, M. J., Naglie, G., Mihailidis, A., & Campos, J. L. (2023). Automated vehicles for people with dementia: A "tremendous potential" that "has ways to go" – Reports of a qualitative study. *The Gerontologist, 63*(1), 140–154. https://doi.org/10.1093/GERONT/GNAC115.

Howard, J., Fisher, Z., Kemp, A. H., Lindsay, S., Tasker, L. H., & Tree, J. J. (2022). Exploring the barriers to using assistive technology for individuals with chronic conditions: A meta-synthesis review. *Disability and Rehabilitation. Assistive Technology, 17*(4), 390–408. https://doi.org/10.1080/17483107.2020.1788181.

Hutchinson, C., Berndt, A., Cleland, J., Gilbert-Hunt, S., George, S., & Ratcliffe, J. (2020). Using social return on investment analysis to calculate the social impact of modified vehicles for people with disability. *Australian Occupational Therapy Journal, 67*(3), 250–259. https://doi.org/10.1111/1440-1630.12648.

Jenkins, D. J., & Holston, E. C. (2015). Conceptualizing the CHOICE of driving retirement by older adults. *Topics in Geriatric Rehabilitation, 31*(2), 90–97. https://doi.org/10.1097/TGR.0000000000000053.

Ji, M., Zhou, Y., Liao, J., & Feng, F. (2015). Pilot study on the Chinese version of the Life Space Assessment among community-dwelling elderly. *Archives of Gerontology and Geriatrics, 61*(2), 301–306. https://doi.org/10.1016/J.ARCHGER.2015.06.012.

Justiss, M. D., Mann, W. C., Stav, W. B., & Velozo, C. A. (2006). Development of a behind-the-wheel driving performance assessment for older adults. The older driver, Part 2. *Topics in Geriatric Rehabilitation, 22*(2), 121–128.

Kabátová, O., Puteková, S., Martinková, J., Súkenníková, M., Mavole, J. N., Hospital, M. B., Lou, M., & Sudan, S. (2016). Analysis of psychometric features of the Mini-Mental State Examination and the Montreal Cognitive Assessment methods Reviewers. *Clinical Social Work and Health Intervention, 7*(2).

Knoefel, F., Wallace, B., Goubran, R., Sabra, I., & Marshall, S. (2019). Semi-autonomous vehicles as a cognitive assistive device for older adults. *Geriatrics, 4*(4). https://doi.org/10.3390/geriatrics4040063.

Korner-Bitensky, N. A., Mazer, B. L., Sofer, S., Gelina, I., Meyer, M. B., Morrison, C., Tritch, L., Roelke, M. A., & White, M. (2000). Visual testing for readiness to drive after stroke: a multicenter study. *American Journal of Physical Medicine & Rehabilitation, 79*(3), 253–259. http://www.ncbi.nlm.nih.gov/entrez/query.fcgi?cmd=Retrieve&db=PubMed&dopt=Citation&list_uids=10821311.

Kowalski, K., Tuokko, H., & Tallman, K. (2010). On-road evaluation: Its use for the identification of impairment and remediation of older drivers. *Physical & Occupational Therapy in Geriatrics, 28*(1), 75–85. https://doi.org/10.3109/02703180903237861.

Langereis, B., Semeniuk, S., Kristalovich, L., & Mortenson, W. Ben (2022). Identifying current driver rehabilitation practices for clients with physical impairments. *British Journal of Occupational Therapy, 85*(8), 570–576. https://doi.org/10.1177/03080226211067432/ASSET/IMAGES/LARGE/10.1177_03080226211067432-FIG2.JPEG.

Liddle, J., Fleming, J., McKenna, K., Turpin, M., Whitelaw, P., & Allen, S. (2011). Driving and driving cessation after traumatic brain injury: Processes and key times of need. *Disability and Rehabilitation, 33*(25–26), 2574–2586. https://doi.org/10.3109/09638288.2011.582922.

Lindsay, S. (2020). Accessible and inclusive transportation for youth with disabilities: exploring innovative solutions. *Disability and Rehabilitation, 42*(8), 1131–1140. https://doi.org/10.1080/09638288.2018.1517194.

Liu, L. (2018). Occupational therapy in the Fourth Industrial Revolution. *Canadian Journal of Occupational Therapy, 85*(4), 272–283. https://doi.org/10.1177/0008417418815179/ASSET/IMAGES/LARGE/10.1177_0008417418815179-FIG10.JPEG.

Lorenzo, T. (2008). "We are also travellers": An action story about disabled women mobilising for an accessible public transport system in Khayelitsha and Nyanga, Cape Metropole, South Africa. *Journal of Occupational Therapy South African Journal of Occupational Therapy, 38*(1).

Lowans, C., Furszyfer Del Rio, D., Sovacool, B. K., Rooney, D., & Foley, A. M. (2021). What is the state of the art in energy and transport poverty metrics? A critical and comprehensive review. *Energy Economics, 101*, 105360. https://doi.org/10.1016/J.ENECO.2021.105360.

Maclachlan, J., Phenix, A., & Valavara, K. (2019). Can occupational therapy assessments be culturally safe? A critical exploration. In *Canadian Association of Occupational Therapists Conference, Niagara Falls, ON*.

Mazer, B. L., Korner-Bitensky, N. A., & Sofer, S. (1998). Predicting ability to drive after stroke. *Archives of Physical Medicine and Rehabilitation, 79*(7), 743–750. http://search.epnet.com/login.aspx?direct=true&db=cin20&an=1999001408.

McCrone, A., Smith, A., Hooper, J., Parker, R. A., & Peters, A. (2019). The life-space assessment measure of functional mobility has utility in community-based physical therapist practice in the United Kingdom. *Physical Therapy, 99*(12), 1719–1731. https://doi.org/10.1093/PTJ/PZZ131.

Peruzzi, M., Sanasi, E., Pingitore, A., Marullo, A. G., Carnevale, R., Sciarretta, S., Sciarra, L., Frati, G., & Cavarretta, E. (2020). An overview of cycling as active transportation and as benefit for health. *Minerva Cardioangiologica, 68*(2). https://doi.org/10.23736/S0026-4725.20.05182-8.

Pojani, D., & Stead, D. (2018). Policy design for sustainable urban transport in the global south. *Policy Design and Practice, 1*(2), 90–102. https://doi.org/10.1080/25741292.2018.1454291.

Portegijs, E., Iwarsson, S., Rantakokko, M., Viljanen, A., & Rantanen, T. (2014). Life-space mobility assessment in older people in Finland; Measurement properties in winter and spring. *BMC Research Notes, 7*(1), 1–9. https://doi.org/10.1186/1756-0500-7-323/TABLES/3.

Remillard, E. T., Campbell, M. L., Koon, L. M., & Rogers, W. A. (2022). Transportation challenges for persons aging with mobility disability: Qualitative insights and policy implications. *Disability and Health Journal, 15*(1). https://doi.org/10.1016/J.DHJO.2021.101209.

Restall, G., & Egan, M. (2022). Canadian occupational inter-relational practice process (COTIPP) framework. In G. Restall, & M. Egan (Eds.), *Promoting occupational participation: Collaborative rleationship-focused occupational therapy* (p. 122). Canadian Association of Occupational Therapists.

SAE International Taxonomy and Definitions for Terms Related to Driving Automation Systems for On-Road Motor Vehicles. SAE Standard J3016_202104, Rev. April. 2021.

Sangrar, R., Mueller, A. S., Gish, J., Griffith, L., Letts, L., & Vrkljan, B. (2018). Older drivers' use of rear view camera systems: Examining technology adoption in the high-tech automobile. *Gerontechnology, 17*(2), 90–101. https://doi.org/10.4017/GT.2018.17.2.003.00.

Sangrar, R., Mun, J., Cammarata, M., Griffith, L. E., Letts, L., & Vrkljan, B. (2019). Older driver training programs: A systematic review of evidence aimed at improving behind-the-wheel performance. *Journal of Safety Research, 71*, 295–313. https://doi.org/10.1016/J.JSR.2019.09.022.

Schofield, K., Kean, B., Oprescu, F., Downer, T., & Hardy, M. (2023). A systematic review and meta-synthesis of the complex and interconnected factors that influence planning for driving retirement. *Journal of Safety Research, 85*, 42–51. https://doi.org/10.1016/j.jsr.2023.01.005.

Schultheis, M. T., Weisser, V., Ang, J., Elovic, E., Nead, R., Sestito, N., Fleksher, C., & Millis, S. R. (2010). Examining the relationship between cognition and driving performance in multiple sclerosis. *Archives of Physical Medicine and Rehabilitation, 91*(3), 465–473. http://www.sciencedirect.com/science/article/B6WB6-4YM9T9C-X/2/39a43e2d91fca3348d43f63b51fae019.

Snih, S. Al, Peek, K. M., Sawyer, P., Markides, K. S., Allman, R. M., & Ottenbacher, K. J (2012). Life-space mobility in Mexican Americans aged 75 and older. *Journal of the American Geriatrics Society, 60*(3), 532–537. https://doi.org/10.1111/J.1532-5415.2011.03822.X.

Stav, W., Weidley, L. S., & Love, A. (2011). Barriers to developing and sustaining driving and community mobility programs. *The American Journal of Occupational Therapy, 65*(4), e38–e45. https://doi.org/10.5014/AJOT.2011.002097.

Stressel, D., Hegberg, A., & Dickerson, A. E. (2014). Driving for adults with acquired physical disabilities. *Occupational Therapy In Health Care, 28*(2), 148–153. https://doi.org/10.3109/07380577.2014.899415.

Stinchcombe, A., Gagnon, S., Kateb, M., Curtis, M., Bédard, M., Porter, M., & Polgar, J. (2017). Letting in-vehicle navigation lead the way: Older drivers' perceptions of and ability to follow a GPS navigation system. *Accident Analysis and Prevention, 106*. https://doi.org/10.1016/j.aap.2016.10.022.

Stinchcombe, A., Hopper, S., Mullen, N., & Bédard, M. (2021). Canadian older adults' perceptions of transitioning from driver to non-driver. *Occupational Therapy in Health Care, 38*(1), 110–130. https://doi.org/10.1080/07380577.2021.1936338.

Stock, S. E., Davies, D. K., Herold, R. G., & Wehmeyer, M. L. (2019). Technology to support transportation needs assessment, training, and pre-trip planning by people with intellectual disability.

Advances in Neurodevelopmental Disorders, 3(3), 319–324. https://doi.org/10.1007/S41252-019-00117-X/METRICS.

Supreme Court of Canada. (1999). *British Columbia (Superintendent of Motor Vehicles) v. British Columbia (Council of Human Rights).* https://scc-csc.lexum.com/scc-csc/scc-csc/en/item/1761/index.do

Transportation Research Board. (2016). Taxonomy and terms for stakeholders in senior mobility. In *Transportation Research Circular (Issue E-C211).* Transportation Research Board. http://onlinepubs.trb.org/Onlinepubs/circulars/ec211.pdf.

UK Driver and Vehicle Licensing Agency. (2021). *Assessing fitness to drive – a guide for medical professionals* (Issue March).

van Biljon, H., van Niekerk, L., Margot-Cattin, I., Adams, F., Plastow, N., Bellagamba, D., Kottorp, A., & Patomella, A. H. (2022). The health equity characteristics of research exploring the unmet community mobility needs of older adults: a scoping review. *BMC Geriatrics, 22*(1). https://doi.org/10.1186/S12877-022-03492-8.

Vander Veen, A., & Laliberte Rudman, D. (2022). Rethinking driving against medical advice: The situated nature of driving after stroke. *Canadian Journal of Occupational Therapy, 89*(4), 406–416. https://doi.org/10.1177/00084174221114670/ASSET/IMAGES/LARGE/10.1177_00084174221114670-FIG1.JPEG.

Veerhuis, N., Traynor, V., & Randle, M. (2022). '… It's hard to prepare yourself, it's like a death': Barriers and facilitators to older people discussing and planning for driving retirement. *Ageing and Society*, 1–27. https://doi.org/10.1017/s0144686x22001064.

Vrkljan, B. H., Myers, A. M., Blanchard, R. A., Crizzle, A. M., & Marshall, S. (2015). Practices used by occupational therapists and others in driving assessment centers for determining fitness-to-drive: A case-based approach. *Physical & Occupational Therapy in Geriatrics, 33*(2), 163–174. https://doi.org/10.3109/02703181.2015.1016647.

Windsor, T. D., Anstey, K. J., Butterworth, P., Luszcz, M. A., & Andrews, G. R. (2007). The role of perceived control in explaining depressive symptoms associated with driving cessation in a longitudinal study. *Gerontologist, 47*(2), 215–223.

Wolfe, M. K., McDonald, N. C., & Holmes, G. M. (2020). Transportation barriers to health care in the United States: Findings from the National Health Interview Survey, 1997-2017. *American Journal of Public Health, 110*(6), 815–822. https://doi.org/10.2105/AJPH.2020.305579.

REFLECTION

1. Describe why community mobility is a human right, even when driving is a government-regulated privilege.

2. What ethical tensions are likely to arise for an occupational therapist working in driving and community mobility?

3. What are the visual standards, licence renewal intervals and reporting requirements in your own practice jurisdiction? Becoming familiar with these will be essential to partner with individuals to address their driving needs.

4. What is the procedure to acquire a disability parking pass in your jurisdiction and what are the eligibility requirements?

35

MOVING AND POSITIONING OF PEOPLE

GILL CREIGHTON ■ SARAH ASH

Overview

The moving and positioning of people is a particular risk factor because of the unpredictable nature of the task. People vary in size, shape and physical/cognitive abilities and the adult human form is difficult to hold because of an uneven distribution of weight. The potential for uncooperative or aggressive behaviour increases the risk of injury for occupational therapists and carers. Additionally, the psychosocial impact of organisational and other work issues, such as high levels of demand, low levels of support or lack of control over workload, have been found to increase stress in employees, exacerbating symptoms of an existing musculoskeletal disorder or heightening awareness of musculoskeletal pain. Occupational therapists involved in moving and positioning risk assessments require an understanding of the biomechanics and ergonomic principles of safe moving and positioning, and the equipment options available. Balanced decision making is essential to provide people with every opportunity to facilitate assisted or independent movement and maximise occupational engagement.

KEY POINTS

■ Understanding of biomechanics and normal human movement is essential in the analysis and safe facilitation of the moving and positioning of people.

■ Moving and positioning practice and policy must be underpinned by legislation and risk assessment.

■ Occupational therapists and all who assist people to move need to have an awareness of personal joint and back care and mechanisms of injury.

■ Independence in movement should be encouraged when possible, using rehabilitation or compensatory approaches or a combination of both.

■ Care moving and positioning and therapeutic moving and positioning can be used together.

- Active participation of individuals can be encouraged by the appropriate use of equipment; this also reduces the risk of injury to all involved.
- Balanced decision making in risk assessment must take account of the needs and protection of everyone involved in the moving and positioning task.

INTRODUCTION

Moving and positioning is much more than simply ensuring legal obligations are met. It is also concerned with how health professionals promote a balanced, proportionate approach to moving and positioning, ensuring that every opportunity is available for the people receiving health services to participate and be as involved as possible within their existing strengths and the challenges of their illness, injury or impairment.

Independent normal movement is taken for granted by most people. People do not think about how they are going to turn in bed or stand up, as all these movement patterns are learned at the preverbal stage of development in infancy. When mobility is restricted by illness, injury or impairment, the occupational therapist plays a key role in analysing the demands of daily occupations, assessing the abilities of individuals and identifying the physical, social, cultural, attitudinal and legislative factors that may enable or disable each person in their daily routines, and then modifying the activity or the environment to better support occupational participation (World Health Organization, 2012). Moving and positioning is an intrinsic part of this process and includes direct handling of an individual and guidance and instruction to carers (Health and Safety Executive (HSE), 2023) Understanding of normal movement and biomechanics is crucial when developing the most appropriate and safe interventions. When considering moving and positioning interventions with an individual, a balance must be maintained between the needs and human rights of that individual and the safety of those assisting the person to move (Mandelstam, 2021).

Moving and positioning, in this chapter, refers to any activity involving transporting, supporting, lifting, putting down, pushing, pulling, carrying or moving a person or load (HSE, 2023). Such activities may be carried out by hand or using body force, or in conjunction with moving and positioning equipment. It encompasses all aspects of assisting people to move any part of their body; therefore activities ranging from supporting a limb while splinting, through to hoisting a person from the floor, all require knowledge and skill to maintain safety for the occupational therapist and the individual concerned. Application of safe moving and positioning principles is essential if occupational therapists are to protect themselves and those with whom they are working. The application of safe moving and positioning principles will be illustrated by the practice story presented in this chapter (Box 35.1).

IMPACT OF MOVING AND POSITIONING ON THE BODY: RISKS TO THE OCCUPATIONAL THERAPIST

Musculoskeletal disorders (MSDs) are a group of painful disorders of muscles, tendons, joints and nerves. All parts of the body can be affected, although the upper limbs and back are the most common areas affected. MSDs arise from movements such as bending, straightening, gripping, holding, twisting, clenching, squatting, kneeling and reaching. While each of the movements is not harmful in themselves, the repetition, static loading and lack of sufficient time to recover between movements, contribute to the development of MSDs.

According to a study by Morabito et al. (2021) one in five occupational therapists with less than five years' experience in Australia, reported workplace musculoskeletal problems and one in three occupational therapy students experienced musculoskeletal disorders that impacted their activities of daily living. The findings of this study suggested that students and recently graduated occupational therapists are at high risk of work-related musculoskeletal disorders. The physically demanding nature of work tasks and practice demands of delivering hands-on interventions, the physical handling of loads and a culture of underreporting are believed to contribute to this high incidence of work-related MSD among occupational therapists and students. The moving and positioning of people is one of the major occupational risks for healthcare workers (Garzillo et al., 2020).

The Manual Handling Operations Regulations 1992 (amended 2016) made under the Health and Safety at Work Act came into force in the United Kingdom

BOX 35.1
CAROLINE

INTRODUCING CAROLINE

Caroline is 54 years old. She is in hospital after a fall. She has multiple sclerosis, is intermittently ambulant, is unable to work and lives in a two-bedroom house with her husband Jim, who works long week-day hours. The occupational therapist involved with Caroline is responsible for ensuring her safe discharge and continuing care in the community. Safe mobility and assistance with moving are key areas of concern for Caroline as she is alone for periods during the day and Jim is often exhausted when he finishes work. Her interests are gardening and painting and she wishes to continue with these for as long as possible.

Caroline's diagnosis and prognosis must be considered when determining interventions. Using the medical model to consider the future effects of the disease process signposts her potential medical needs; however, occupational therapists are also concerned with psychosocial and environmental effects on Caroline's occupational participation. Using the International Classification of Functioning, Disability and Health (ICF) (World Health Organization, 2012), social and environmental aspects of her lifestyle and surroundings must be assessed to establish what factors may enable or disable her in the immediate and longer term. The potential need for equipment or adaptation must be considered, in order to facilitate safe mobility for as long as possible.

Occupational participation analysis will be central to any interventions. Mobility and assistance with moving and positioning will have a significant impact on how Caroline manages her daily life and carries out her chosen occupations, and to facilitate these and protect her carers, the occupational therapist must understand:

- Normal movement for each task or activity
- Changes in Caroline's abilities that may affect how she carries out tasks
- Compensatory approaches used to enable her to carry out tasks
- Her priorities for task completion
- Structure, components and order of tasks
- Jim and other carers' ability to assist
- Equipment and resources available
- Skill levels required to assist her to move or to use equipment

BEGINNING TO IDENTIFY RISKS

For the safety of Caroline and her carers, the occupational therapist needs to be aware of the mechanisms of injury and how daily activities could increase the risk of injury. By listing Caroline's daily activities, when these occur and how they are prioritised, the occupational therapist can identify where risks may be higher; for example, needing physical assistance to move into bed. Moving and positioning activities such as this may place Jim at increased risk of musculoskeletal disorders as he is often exhausted after work and risks injury by trying to work beyond his physical capability at that time.

The occupational therapist needs to work collaboratively with the couple to prioritise where formal care or careful use of equipment is needed to protect Caroline and Jim from injury and to facilitate maximum participation and independence for Caroline. Once activities have been identified and prioritised, the occupational therapist needs to analyse Caroline's performance and identify fluctuations in her ability. Application of normal movement and biomechanical principles will help identify areas of risk for Caroline and her carers. From this, a more detailed risk assessment can be carried out to develop a personal handling profile.

CONSIDERING PRINCIPLES OF NORMAL MOVEMENT AND BIOMECHANICS

Caroline may have increased fatigue at the end of the day and so need more assistance.

By understanding the principles of normal movement and biomechanics, the occupational therapist can reduce the potential for injury for Caroline and her carers. When transferring from a wheelchair to the bed, Jim might use a controversial technique known as the 'bear hug' to help Caroline to stand but he may not be aware of his own body postures. By standing in front of her and grasping her around the waist, Jim reduces Caroline's ability to use normal movement by blocking her potential to lean forward. He becomes the effort force. Caroline's COG (resistance force) is a significant distance from her knees (axis). As a result, he will need to use extra effort to bring her COG towards the edge of her base of support, thus destabilising her enough to move. Through careful task analysis, the occupational therapist can offer training in alternatives, such as those described here:

- Use chair raisers to raise the height of the chair.
- Encourage Caroline to utilise normal movement to position herself ready to stand.
- Use a handling belt.
- Train the couple in the safe use of a transfer board

When assisting a person to move, a distinction is made between 'therapeutic handling' and 'care handling' (Table 35.2). The definition of people handling is explained as *"activities in which a person is physically moved, supported or restrained. People handling requires someone to use force in order to lift, lower, push, pull or slide another person"* (Worksafe.qld.gov.au, 2023).

NB: When implementing an intervention programme that involves specific methods of moving, handling and positioning, the occupational therapist is responsible for

Continued on following page

BOX 35.1
CAROLINE (*Continued*)

carrying out those handling techniques, and must not expect others to carry out therapeutic handling techniques with a person unless the occupational therapist has specifically trained and assessed the competence of individuals in methods specific to that person (HCPC, 2014).

DETAILED RISK ASSESSMENT

Regular assessment of Caroline's performance and needs is required as her abilities fluctuate. Equipment should not be introduced too early, as retaining as much independence as possible is important. Interprofessional collaboration will be key to enable Caroline to retain her abilities and the occupational therapist may be the coordinating professional, ensuring contact with statutory and voluntary services. Task analysis will enable the occupational therapist to identify elements of daily activities in which Caroline is independent, partially dependent or totally dependent. Maintenance of mobility through analysis of normal movement and application of biomechanical principles to tasks will enable Caroline to focus her energy on activities that are most important to her.

Having established Caroline's occupational participation preferences and identified those that may present a risk of injury, the application of the risk assessment filter will assist the occupational therapist to decide which occupations present risk significant enough to apply formal risk assessment. From here the occupational therapist must select the most appropriate tools to use. The **T**ask, **I**ndividual capacity, **L**oad, **E**nvironment and **O**ther factors (TILEO) assessment can initially be used to establish the presence of significant risk.

After performing manual handling risk assessments for all activities where assistance is required and where there may be a risk of injury the occupational therapist will be able to produce a handling management plan. This should detail how and when Caroline needs assistance with moving and positioning, methods to be used and equipment required, giving information on how and when equipment is to be used, what the criteria are for these and who is able to use it. Consent must be gained from Caroline for manual assistance and use of equipment.

Environmental issues such as access, circulation space for equipment and potential hazards must all be assessed, particularly with regard to any mobility aids used by Caroline. The occupational therapist must consider alternative approaches to be used at different times of the day and night to facilitate the safest practice for Caroline and anyone assisting Caroline with mobility. There must also be a clear indication of any specific therapeutic handling that takes place, when this happens and with whom.

The occupational therapist must provide or source appropriate training and assessment of competence for all carers in both techniques and equipment used to reduce the risk of musculoskeletal injury. Consideration of the Human Rights Act (1998) is necessary when recommending formal care or equipment. Balanced decision making (Mandelstam, 2011) is important to enable Caroline to feel an active participant rather than a passive recipient. This collaborative and respectful approach will help minimise the risk of triggers such as anxiety-induced muscle spasms or emotional rejection of recommendations that may affect both Caroline's and her carers' safety. Most importantly, the handling and positioning management plan and risk assessment must be regularly reviewed, adapted and signed, to account for changes in Caroline's or her carers' functional ability or needs.

APPLYING PRINCIPLES OF SAFER HANDLING

Consent, cultural awareness and clear communication are paramount if changes to Caroline's environment and routine are implemented, or equipment or alternative practices are introduced to ensure safer handling. The environment must be safe for carers to work in, and they must be sufficiently trained to enable them to apply safe handling principles when working with Caroline.

CONSIDERATION OF RELEVANT LEGISLATION

The occupational therapist will need to balance the wishes and needs of Caroline with their own safety and that of others involved in her care, taking into account relevant legislation. Central to this is adherence to the *Code of Ethics and Professional Conduct* (RCOT, 2021). Local policies and procedures related to moving and positioning and equipment provision must be available and applied in all moving and positioning situations. This applies to general care handling and, more specifically, to therapeutic handling protocols. Underpinning the occupational therapist's safe practice will be up-to-date training in person handling, either through local service provision or attendance at a nationally recognised course. It is imperative that the occupational therapist has experience and expertise in assessing for and recommending appropriate equipment and handling techniques if this is to be part of the intervention plan for Caroline. Along with this is the occupational therapist's responsibility to ensure adequate training, assessment of competence and documentation in the safe use of any equipment and specific handling techniques recommended for carers.

on 1st January 1993. Under the regulations, employers must seek to avoid manual handling where possible. Where this is not possible, which is certainly the case when involved in the moving and positioning of people as an occupational therapist, employers and employees are required to adopt an ergonomic approach to removing or reducing the risk of manual handling injuries through safe systems of work and a safe working environment. The ergonomic approach to moving and positioning takes into consideration a wide range of relevant factors including the nature of the task, the load, the working environment and individual capability.

With improved training programmes, policies and procedures now in place, occupational therapists are much better informed regarding best practices to avoid hazardous handling and improve safe handling techniques both for themselves and the people with whom they work. Not all tasks placing stress on the body involve straightforward direct lifts of people; awkward and static body postures, holding loads away from the body and repetitive movements increase the risk of musculoskeletal injury. Repositioning a person in a chair or bed, assisting a person to eat, or assisting with personal care are typical examples of activities that can cause muscular overload of ligaments and tendons. Occupational therapists must be aware of the risk exposure when undertaking these activities, especially when educating family members or carers.

PRINCIPLES OF MOVEMENT

It is not the remit of this chapter to discuss the neurophysiological principles of movement. However, to make decisions related to the moving or positioning of people it is necessary to understand how a person moves in the absence of physical limitations. In the context of moving and positioning a person, this is called normal movement. Put simply, it is the way that a person would normally move: the voluntary and automatic movements produced by the nerve pathways and action of muscles on bones and joints, which then achieve a movement task in an energy-efficient, coordinated way. Patterns of movement are sequences of movement for the achievement of a motor goal. Normal movement requires combinations of movement patterns.

If a whole year group of occupational therapy students were lying supine on a floor, arms by their sides, legs straight and on a given cue turned onto their right sides, there would be many common components to their methods of completing the task. Movement generally starts with the head – looking to the right in this instance. The left shoulder girdle will follow the rotation of the cervical spine, and the left arm reaches across the chest. For the body mass to move, it is likely that the left knee will bend, the foot will be placed on the floor, and the 'reach' with the arm and the 'push' with the foot will cause the body to roll onto its side. Fig. 35.1A–D illustrate this sequence of 'normal' movement for turning to the side from supine.

Variations will of course occur – because of previous injury, body shape, age, medical condition and so on – but because the human form is generally made up of the same component parts, movement patterns are somewhat predictable. If an occupational therapist asks a person to move, and perhaps give the person instructions to do so, it is important that the occupational therapist first understands how a person would normally achieve the task and then consider the most effective and efficient approach for each person.

The objective of the occupational therapist is usually to enable people to do as much for themselves as possible. Placing a person in an optimum starting position, making use of biomechanical advantage and giving the opportunity for recruitment of muscles and joints may be sufficient to enable the person to complete a moving task or help the occupational therapist to identify the missing components or which compensatory movements the person is using. To meet this objective, occupational therapists need to have a sound knowledge of anatomy and basic principles of biomechanics.

BIOMECHANICAL PRINCIPLES

Biomechanics is the study of movement, how forces are applied by the muscles and how gravity impacts the skeletal system. Essentially, biomechanics is the science behind how the human body moves. To look further into the safe moving and positioning of people, it is necessary to have an understanding of basic biomechanics (refer to Chapter 36).

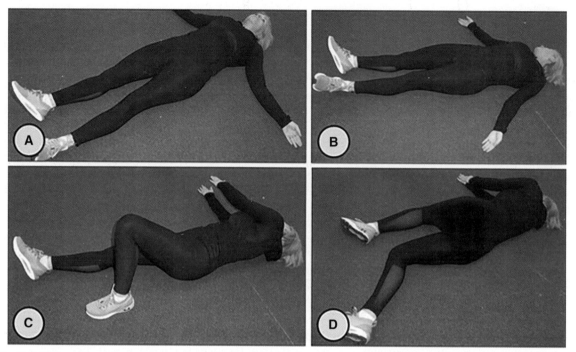

Fig. 35.1 ■ Normal movement sequence for turning onto the side from supine lying position. (A) Supine lying position. (B) Turning the head in the direction of the move. (C) Bending the knee and placing the foot flat on the floor while reading across the chest with the arm. (D) Reaching with the arm and pushing with the foot to turn onto the side.

Stability

The stability of an object is its ability to withstand external and internal forces and remain in its current position or shape. Stability in the human body can be thought of as how the body as an entirety, generates movement, uses or directs forces and encounters load (Elphinston, 2020). Stability is also dependent on other factors such as the base of support (BOS), location of the body (or body segment), the centre of gravity (COG) and, as a consequence, where the line of gravity (LOG) falls within the BOS. Stability is also affected to a degree by friction and internal and external forces acting on the body (Bunce et al., 2023).

Base of Support

The BOS is denoted by the contact points of an object or person with the ground and all the area inside those contact points, as illustrated in Fig. 35.2. A large BOS provides greater stability (Fig. 35.3). A small BOS means that the person is less stable (Fig. 35.4). Stability is also linked to the position of the COG and LOG relative to the BOS.

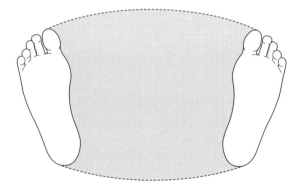

Fig. 35.2 ■ Base of support.

Centre of Gravity and Line of Gravity

Everything has a COG. This is the point at which the entire weight of an object is concentrated. As long as this point remains supported, it will remain in equilibrium. Unlike solid objects, bodies can alter their dimensions at will and in some circumstances, the changes in dimensions can be involuntary and unpredictable, due to dystonia or as a side effect of medications for

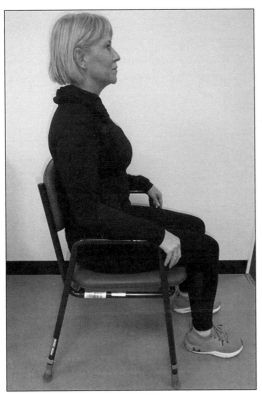

Fig. 35.3 ■ Large base of support from the back legs of the chair to the front of the person's feet.

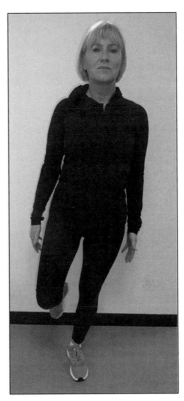

Fig. 35.4 ■ Small base of support denoted by one foot in contact with the ground.

instance. The COG in people changes constantly with each new position of the body.

The LOG is an imaginary line drawn vertically from the COG to the ground and helps to predict, at any time, where the COG is relative to the BOS. Knowing this information helps to estimate the stability of a person. The more central the COG and LOG are, within the BOS, the greater a person's stability (Fig. 35.5).

A low COG increases a person's stability. When a person is lying in prone or supine, they are at their most stable (Fig. 35.6).

In contrast, people are at their least stable when the COG is raised and the BOS is reduced, like standing on tiptoes on one leg. In this circumstance, it would not take much for the person to become unstable and fall.

Any shift in position of the COG, will more easily result in the LOG falling outside the BOS, thus destabilising the person. To maintain balance in this position of reduced stability, the person is dependent on the recruitment of appropriate muscle groups, vestibular and visual function and intact proprioception.

Friction

Another factor potentially affecting a person's ability to move, the effort required, and the quality of movement is friction. Where two objects are in contact with each other, friction will occur to a greater or lesser extent, depending on the type of surfaces in contact and the pressure between them. It is important to understand the effects of friction influences in different materials and their effects on movement. A surface with a high friction influence will resist movement across it; for example, a deep-pile wool carpet. Alternatively, a surface with a low friction influence will enable movement to occur more easily and reduce the degree of shearing forces on the moving object; for example, a slide sheet will lessen the friction, limiting and reducing the need

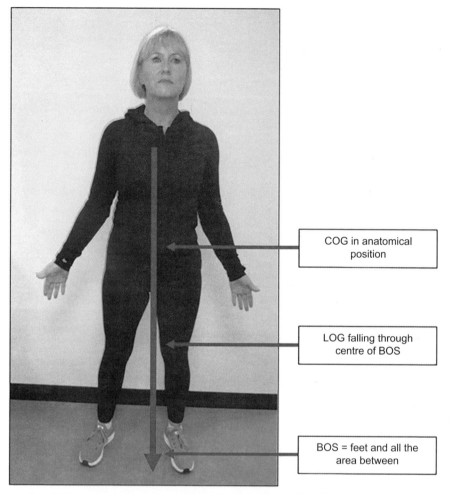

COG in anatomical position

LOG falling through centre of BOS

BOS = feet and all the area between

Fig. 35.5 ■ Centre of gravity in anatomical position and line of gravity falling within the centre of the base of support.

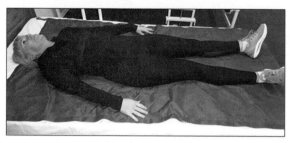

Fig. 35.6 ■ Large base of support with a low centre of gravity leads to maximum stability.

for undue effort from the occupational therapist or caregiver (Bunce et al., 2023)

Two types of friction exist, static and dynamic. Static friction resists movement. When a person sits still in a chair (Fig. 35.3), static friction between the thighs/buttocks and the chair seat prevents the person from slipping out of the chair. To overcome this static friction a person must create movement through internal or external forces. Once movement begins, dynamic friction occurs between the surfaces in contact with each other. For the occupational therapist and person, this can be either beneficial or a hindrance. If the person in Fig. 35.3 wishes to stand out of the chair, the high friction influence and his body weight will necessitate greater internal and external forces to enable them to move. Therefore a high friction influence will be beneficial in enabling them to stay in the chair but will make moving out of the chair more difficult. This is often the case when people are in bed (Fig. 35.6).

Static friction between the person's body and the bed means that they are very stable; however, when they need to move, the dynamic friction between the two surfaces increases the risk of shearing forces on their skin. The occupational therapist also has to exert much a greater external force to initiate movement, increasing their risk of a musculoskeletal injury. Using slide sheets, which have a very low friction influence, reduces the impact of shearing forces and requires less external force to create movement. This principle applies equally when people can sit up and move themselves on a bed. Using small slide sheets between the person and the bed reduces shearing forces and minimises the amount of effort required to move (Fig. 35.7).

Levers and Forces

To understand how people move, it is important to understand levers. A lever system comprises an axis, an effort force and a resistance force. In the human body the axis is commonly a joint. The effort force is denoted by the direction of movement of the body or body segment, and the resistance force opposes the movement. The process of standing from sitting neatly illustrates all these aspects and enables an analysis of why this activity can sometimes be difficult and how to make it easier. For this movement to be easy, the distance of the effort force from the axis should be equal to or greater than the distance of the resistance force, as the larger the distance of a force from an axis, the greater its mechanical advantage. The effort force in this case is the quadriceps muscles, which extend the knee. The axis is the knee joint, and the resistance force is the body weight, the central point of which is the COG. Fig. 35.8A and B illustrate that the distance of the resistance force from the axis is greater than the distance of the effort force, which is common, as muscle attachments cannot move and therefore are generally close to a joint.

When sitting upright in a chair, a person has a large BOS with the LOG falling through the centre of this support. The person is therefore very stable. To stand up, the person needs to destabilise the body. Fig. 35.8A and B illustrate the

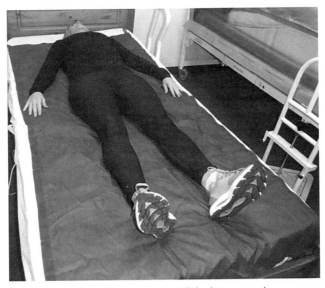

Fig. 35.7 ■ Reducing dynamic friction using slide sheets to make movement easier.

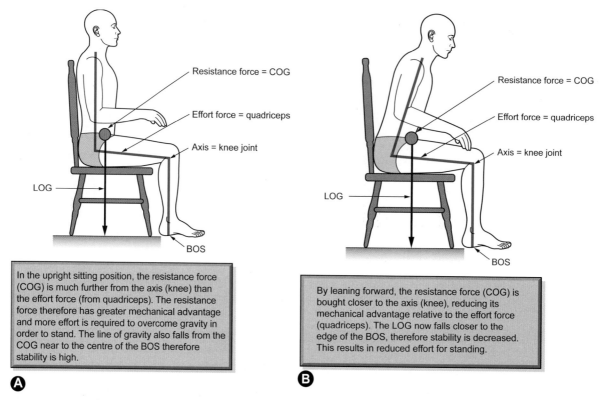

Resistance force = COG

Effort force = quadriceps

Axis = knee joint

LOG

BOS

In the upright sitting position, the resistance force (COG) is much further from the axis (knee) than the effort force (from quadriceps). The resistance force therefore has greater mechanical advantage and more effort is required to overcome gravity in order to stand. The line of gravity also falls from the COG near to the centre of the BOS therefore stability is high.

A

Resistance force = COG

Effort force = quadriceps

Axis = knee joint

LOG

BOS

By leaning forward, the resistance force (COG) is bought closer to the axis (knee), reducing its mechanical advantage relative to the effort force (quadriceps). The LOG now falls closer to the edge of the BOS, therefore stability is decreased. This results in reduced effort for standing.

B

Fig. 35.8 ■ Biomechanical principles related to upright sitting and preparation for standing.

biomechanical differences between static upright sitting and preparation for standing, and how changing the position of the body's COG facilitates standing with less effort.

To make standing even easier, occupational therapists can ask or assist the person to move their hips forward in the chair to bring the LOG closer to the edge of the BOS, thus destabilising them further. Additionally, by using chair raisers to increase the overall height of the chair, the angle at the hips and knees when sitting is decreased and the body's COG (resistance force) is automatically closer to the knees (axis). Its mechanical advantage is therefore decreased even further in relation to the quadriceps muscles (effort force).

Understanding the biomechanics and normal patterns of movement in an able-bodied adult of average body mass provides a working baseline from which it is possible to understand the impact of changes in tone (increased or decreased), body mass (increased or decreased, as in pregnancy or amputation) or joint function (pain, etc.) on movement. The application of this understanding of biomechanics and normal patterns of movement is illustrated in the practice story in Box 35.1.

For the most part, there is no single 'correct' way of moving a person to achieve a task. Most importantly, having a sound knowledge of biomechanics and human movement enables an accurate assessment of risk to achieve the completion of tasks while promoting maximum ability and facilitating occupational participation.

LEGISLATION

The legislation within this chapter refers to the UK context. Readers should refer to their local/relevant legislation to guide practice.

In the UK, legislation on the moving and positioning of people provides protection for both the handler and person, as well as meeting health and social care needs and observing human rights. The Manual Handling Operations Regulations 1992 (as amended) (HSE, 1992) are not in place to prohibit manual handling or endorse no-lifting policies, but to provide a flexible and balanced approach to risk ensuring that workers are not required to perform tasks that put them at unreasonable risk. All legislation relating to manual handling must be taken into consideration when assessing moving and positioning needs in any environment.

Key legislation relevant to moving and positioning in the UK, outlined in Table 35.1, allows for balanced decision making, when considering the needs of both the people being moved and those carrying out moving and positioning tasks (Mandelstam, 2011). Within civil law, occupational therapists have a duty of care to

TABLE 35.1
Summary of UK Legislation Relevant to Moving and Positioning

HEALTH & SAFETY AT WORK ACT (HSE 1974)

"It shall be the duty of every employer to ensure, so far as is reasonably practicable, the health, safety and welfare of all employees."

Employers

- Have a general duty to ensure the health safety and welfare of all employees.
- Protect people, other than those at work against risks to their health & safety arising out of work activities.
- Must provide instruction, supervision and training.

Employees

- Are responsible for their own health and safety and that of others who may be affected by their actions.
- Must make full and proper use of any system of work provided in the reduction of risk.
- Must use equipment in accordance with any training and instruction provided by the employer.

Management of Health & Safety at Work (Amendment) Regulations (MHSAW 2006)

- Explains the circumstances in which risk assessment should be undertaken in the workplace.
- Explains the process a workplace risk assessment should follow.
- Sets out the criteria as to when employers should undertake health and safety training.

Manual Handling Operations Regulations (MHOR 1992) (updated 2016)

- Defines manual handling.
- Explains the employer's responsibility with regard to hazardous manual handling in the workplace.
- Sets out the requirement for risk assessment for hazardous manual handling activities in the workplace.

Lifting operations & lifting equipment regulations (LOLER 1998) (updated 2014)

- Explains what lifting equipment (includes patient hoists and attachments for hoists) is and when it is used for work.
- Details the criteria by which lifting equipment should be inspected and the frequency of inspections.
- Sets out the criteria for staff training and supervision when using lifting equipment.

Provision & Use of Work Equipment Regulations (PUWER 1998)

- Details the criteria by which work equipment (including handling equipment) should be used only for its intended purpose.
- Details the criteria by which work equipment should be maintained in an efficient state and in good repair and working order.
- Sets out the criteria for staff training and supervision when using work equipment.

Reporting of injuries, diseases & dangerous occurrences Regulations (RIDDOR 2013)

- Sets out the criteria when workplace fatalities, injuries, diseases and dangerous occurrences should be reported to the authorities.
- Includes 'near misses'.

Equality Act 2010

- Aims to address issues of inequality in society on a wide range of subjects including disability.
- Defines disability.
- Defines discrimination of a person with a disability including types of discrimination and the environments in which a person should not be discriminated against.

Human Rights Act 1998

- Aims to encourage 'balanced decision making' for all parties to ensure human rights are maintained (e.g. when deciding how a person might be handled to not endanger themselves or their handlers).
- Provides the criteria in which a person's human rights might be breached, including being subjected to inhuman or degrading treatment or feeling their security has been breached.

Mental Capacity (Amendment) Act (MCA 2019)

- Aims to empower and protect people who may lack capacity including giving people choices about their care (e.g. how they wish to be handled if/when their mobility is compromised).
- Explains that a person's choices can only be deprived following a strict set of legal processes focussing on their best interest (e.g. that they are only handled safely and humanely).
- Sets out the criteria when restraint might be used on a person whose mobility is reduced (e.g. This might impact on chair selection or seating positioning for a person and/or the use of bed rails).

anyone who may be affected by an occupational therapist's actions or omissions. Therefore occupational therapists should aim to reduce the risk of injury to the lowest level reasonably practicable, considering the needs and rights of the person.

To ensure best practice, interprofessional collaboration is essential and the occupational therapist should work closely with other professionals to assess risks and develop realistic and safe moving and positioning protocols. The consideration of legislation in relation to the moving and positioning of a person is illustrated in the practice story in Box 35.1.

RISK ASSESSMENT

There are many factors to consider when moving and positioning a person, including:

- Weight distribution,
- Asymmetrical body mass,
- Unpredictable behaviour,
- Spasms/contractures,
- Loss of spatial awareness,
- Visual impairment and
- Attachments, e.g., percutaneous endoscopic gastrostomy (PEG) tube or catheter.

The level of risk may change depending on the intervention and the level of assistance required. In addition, environmental considerations must be considered, such as:

- Confined spaces,
- Attitude,
- Knowledge and frequency of the task, and
- Trip hazards.

Avoiding injury is a concern for all those involved in moving and positioning. As previously noted, under health and safety legislation employers must take measures to eliminate tasks that put staff at risk. If the elimination of risks is not possible, risks must be assessed and reduced to the lowest level that is reasonably practicable; regular review is essential.

When carrying out risk assessments occupational therapists need to consider the potential benefits to the person against the risk of injury to the handler (Johnson, 2011). For the handler, risks will be high where active rehabilitation (therapeutic moving and positioning) is happening. The occupational therapist will be testing the boundaries of the person's abilities to improve their occupational performance. Professional judgement will enable the occupational therapist to decide what is reasonable in terms of risk and balance this with the potential benefit to the person. In care moving and positioning situations the occupational therapist will make detailed assessments of the everyday needs of each individual to ensure the safest practice. These two approaches form the basis of the care–therapy handling continuum, which is illustrated in Table 35.2.

Risk assessment involves identifying hazards within a given situation and deciding whether these pose a risk of injury to those carrying out tasks. Risk assessment should be undertaken where any moving and positioning task is considered to present a health risk to those involved (HSE, 2015). Risk assessments may be *generic*, or *individual/task specific*.

Generic risk assessments cover all common tasks carried out within an area, including people and inanimate load handling. These assessments aim to establish key hazards and control measures associated with general locations, events or activities. For example, in a residential setting, profiling beds may be recommended to replace divan beds. Increasing a resident's independent movement on the bed reduces the need for manual assistance from staff for activities such as sitting up in bed, resulting in reduced risk of musculoskeletal injury for everyone involved (Fergusson Burt, 2007). *Generic risk assessments* are important tools as they can provide the basis for prioritising funds for additional resources. The stages of generic risk assessment are summarised in Box 35.2.

Individual risk assessments refer to specific moving and positioning and/or complex needs that fall outside generic protocols, and handling management plans providing more detail about processes, equipment, numbers and skills of handlers and type of assistance required for each task are developed. These plans should consider the individual's wishes and needs (Human Rights Act, 1998; Mandelstam, 2011), their fluctuating ability, plus the physical and psychosocial influences on all those involved in the tasks (HSE, 2013).

To facilitate decisions when risk assessment of inanimate handling tasks that cannot be avoided is required,

TABLE 35.2	
Types of Person Moving and Positioning	
Therapeutic moving and positioning	**Care moving and positioning**
Occurs within a structured setting or therapy session, usually by an occupational therapist in a department, hospital ward or within a person's home.	Occurs in wards, residential settings, a person's home, a school or other day facilities.
Short sessions, including active/passive moving, equipment use or positioning with a specific goal.	May be carried out a number of times a day, includes active/passive moving, use of equipment use and positioning of the person.
Requires cooperation from the individual.	Cooperation is encouraged, though may not involve active participation from the person because of limitations in physical or cognitive ability.
Improves or maintains performance.	Maintains performance, with or without the use of equipment, and may help improve overall mobility and quality of life. Can involve compensatory approaches.
Involves highly trained qualified staff.	Involves formal/informal carers, family members, school assistants, etc., who have received appropriate training.
Involves calculated risks to improve performance. Requires professional reasoning and expertise and completion of risk assessment documentation to support this. Needs to take account of required performance in a variety of environments.	Requires detailed risk assessments and a handling management plan to assist with essential activities of daily living.

the HSE published Lifting and Lowering Guidelines (COT, 2006) can be referred to. These guidelines apply to objects, not people and the guideline weights are for infrequent operations where the pace of work is not forced, adequate pauses to rest or use different muscles are possible, and the load is not supported by the

handler for any length of time. The guidelines form a useful tool to indicate whether further detailed assessment of each task is necessary. The individual risk assessment process is summarised in Box 35.3.

TILE(O) is a simple acronym to identify the main components of a moving and positioning assessment (HSE, 2004), it stands for **T**ask, **I**ndividual capacity, **L**oad, **E**nvironment and **O**ther factors (Box 35.4). An ergonomic approach to risk assessment requires analysis of all these components. A more detailed

---

BOX 35.2
STAGES OF GENERIC RISK ASSESSMENT

1. Identify risks associated with hazards or routine tasks.
2. Prioritise risks for action and identify who is at risk when carrying out the tasks.
3. Identify existing risk management measures.
4. Complete and record the risk assessments for identified tasks.
5. Establish further risk management/reduction measures for those tasks such as detailing specific ways in which handling activities should be carried out or where specific equipment is to be used (College of Occupational Therapists (COT), 2006).
6. Regularly review the risk assessments particularly if circumstances change.

Modified from Health and Safety Executive. (2008). *Risk management*. http://www.hse.gov.uk/risk/fivesteps.htm.

BOX 35.3
SUMMARY OF INDIVIDUAL RISK ASSESSMENT PROCESS

1. Identify potential hazards/hazardous activities.
2. Decide whether these pose a risk of injury to people who are moving or to those assisting them (using an assessment filter).
3. Identify existing measures to reduce risks of injury.
4. Complete risk assessment on those activities considered to present a risk of injury.
5. Identify further measures to reduce risks of injury while moving, lifting or carrying a load or assisting somebody to move.

Modified from Health and Safety Executive. (2008). *Risk management*. http://www.hse.gov.uk/risk/fivesteps.htm.

BOX 35.4
TILEO ASSESSMENT TOOL HANDLING OF PEOPLE

Task	What is the task? (Object): e.g. lifting a box (Person) e.g. personal care and standing transfers Does it need to be done? What does it entail (twisting, stooping, pushing, pulling, carrying long distances, sudden movements, prolonged effort, insufficient recovery periods)? Are there risks to the handler or others from carrying out the task?
Individual *(Handler)*	Do they have correct/sufficient skills and training? Are they in an at-risk group for injury? Are they wearing the correct clothing and footwear?
Load *(Person/ inanimate)*	What is the weight and distribution of the load? Is it bulky, difficult to grasp, unstable? If it is a person: What is their ability/diagnosis? What clothing are they wearing? What are the effects of their present condition? Are they cooperative? Can they weight bear? How much assistance do they need? Can they communicate? What is their skin condition? Are there behavioural concerns? Are there cultural issues? Do they have any splints, catheters, orthoses, PEG?
Environment	What are the levels of lighting, ambient temperature and humidity and do these enable safe handling? Are there any slip or trip hazards, inanimate or otherwise? Is the floor or ground surface safe for moving on? What are the space constraints on posture?
Other	Is the load in a dangerous or unsafe environment required to be moved? Is personal protective equipment (PPE) or other specialised clothing required? Does this specialised clothing cause any hindrance to movement or visibility? Is there an absence of the correct/suitable PPE? Are there personal factors between the person and handler? Is appropriate equipment available? Is the equipment well maintained, serviced and appropriate for the task? Is the equipment accessible? Have handlers been trained in its use?

description of the individual elements of a TILE(O) risk assessment can be found in *The Guide to the Handling of People* (6th ed.) (Smith, 2011).

Additionally, occupational therapists must consider potential *triggers* for adverse behaviour particularly when moving and positioning people with complex needs or challenging behaviour as these factors can increase the risk of injury. Triggers may include:

- Fear of equipment,
- Previous experiences of pain from poor moving and positioning procedures,
- Physiological responses, such as muscle spasms and
- Behaviour responses, such as aggression.

There is no legal maximum weight limit. The Manual Handling Operations Regulations guidance provides guidelines for lifting and lowering that indicate when a more detailed risk assessment should be completed and places the duty of care on employers to manage or control risk. Control measures will vary depending on the situation; considerations include:

- The strength, fitness and underlying physical and mental health conditions of the handler,
- The weight to be lifted and distance to be carried,
- The nature of the load and
- The postures to be adopted or the availability of equipment to facilitate the lift.

Having completed the risk assessment, all identified risks must be reduced to the lowest level reasonably practicable and clearly recorded in the risk reduction steps in a Handling Management Plan or Safe System of Work. These plans must be dated and signed and indicate a timescale for review or be reviewed whenever there is a significant change in a person's or carer's circumstances (HSE, 2020). There is no legal requirement for review at specific intervals; however, The British Safety Council advise that assessment should be reviewed periodically, proportionate to the level of risk involved, if the current assessment is no longer valid and there has been any change to the specific activity or task. Assessments should also be reviewed following accident, injury or ill health (British Safety Council, 2023).

BOX 35.5

EXAMPLES OF QUALITATIVE AND QUANTITATIVE RISK ASSESSMENT

- Rapid Entire Body Assessment (REBA) (Hignet & McAtamney, 2000)
- Finnish Work Ability Index (Ilmarinen, 1998)
- Ergonomic Workplace Analysis (Ahonen et al., 1989)
- Benner Scale (Benner, 1984)
- Functional Independence Measure (FIM) (Granger et al., 1993)
- Manual Tasks Risk Assessment Tool (ManTRA) (Straker et al., 2004)
- Rapid Upper Limb Assessment (RULA) (McAtamney & Corlett, 1993)
- NIOSH equation for lifting tasks (NIOSH, 1991)
- Manual Handling Assessment Chart (MAC) (HSE, 2003)
- Ovako Working Posture Assessment System (OWAS, 2007)

In complex moving and positioning situations, a more detailed assessment may be needed with risk filters used to establish which assessment tools would be appropriate to complete a formal assessment.

A range of possible assessments are listed in Box 35.5.

Handling Management Plan or Safe System of Work: This document outlines and explains the steps required to complete moving and handling tasks safely. Photographs or drawings can be used alongside the Handling Management Plan or Safe System of Work plan for increased clarity to reduce the impact of communication barriers. Written instructions should be clear, avoid the use of jargon and should include:

- Contact details of the occupational therapist's organisation,
- The contact details to report broken or faulty equipment,
- Points of safe use and basic maintenance arrangements and
- Manufacturer's instructions (COT, 2006).

Additional risk assessment tools are described in *The Guide to the Handling of People* (6th ed.) (Smith, 2011). The risk assessment process is illustrated in the practice story in Box 35.1.

PRINCIPLES OF SAFER MOVING AND POSITIONING

There is no single correct way to move a person or load (HSE, 2014). Each situation will demand a different approach, so basic principles are important to ensure optimum safety for everyone.

A balanced approach to moving and positioning tasks includes:

- Ensuring the rights of the person,
- Ensuring the handler's safety,
- Encouraging cooperation, and
- Reducing the risk of adverse reactions and injury (COT, 2006).

The application of a balanced approach is illustrated in the practice story in Box 35.1.

Equipment Provision and Use

Frequently, specialist moving and positioning equipment can improve productivity, enhance comfort, reduce costs and increase a person's independence (Sturman-Floyd, 2011). Task analysis and risk assessment should be used prior to equipment provision to address any mobility/movement issues and establish the person's abilities while encouraging as much active participation as possible. Equipment must meet relevant safety standards as defined by the Medical and Health Care Products Regulations Agency (MRHA) (2021), or safety standards relevant to a location, and must be compatible with the environment, appropriate to the task, and the handler must be trained and competent in its use (COT, 2006).

Legislation, organisational policies and best practices exist to protect people and their handlers. Occupational therapists who carry out moving and positioning tasks have a high risk of injury even when proper body mechanics are used (Frost & Barkley, 2012). However, opinion exists within rehabilitation settings that the use of moving and positioning equipment may impede a person's recovery (Waters & Rockefeller, 2010). In contrast, Arnold et al. (2011) and Darragh et al. (2013) found that using moving and position equipment enabled people to mobilise earlier and decreased their length of hospital stay. Examples of equipment are listed in Table 35.3.

Number of Handlers Required

There is no legal ruling regarding the number of handlers needed to use a hoist. The National Minimum Standards Regulations for Domiciliary Care (Department of Health (DOH), 2003), states 'two people fully trained in current safe handling techniques and the equipment to be used are always involved in the provision of care *when the need is identified* from the manual handling risk assessment'. This has been interpreted over the years to mean that two people are always required; however, this is not the case, and the number of handlers is always based on risk assessment.

Training

Employers have a legal responsibility to provide a safe system of work and to provide adequate training to meet the health and safety requirements of their employees (HSE 2012).

Training in principles of safe moving and positioning techniques and equipment provision is essential to ensure a safe system of work. However, evidence shows that often the principles learned during training are not applied in the workplace. More effective training strategies include making training workplace specific and with the equipment that is normally used (Clemes et al., 2010; Rose, 2011). Many organisations have adopted specific moving and positioning practical training supplemented with the theory of safe moving and positioning. Effective training always needs to work alongside appropriate levels of workplace supervision. Ensuring that staff are identified as competent and compliant with instruction and that this is maintained throughout their people-handling activities in the workplace is essential to minimise the risk of injury (Phillips et al., 2014).

There is no prescriptive guidance on what moving and positioning training courses should include or how long training should last, simply that training should be suitable for the individual, the tasks and the environment involved and should last long enough to cover all relevant information. The need to update training on a regular basis is strongly advised (National Back Exchange (NBE), 2010).

The NBE has produced professional standards and guidelines to ensure compliance with the law, meet requirements of best practice, meet continuing

TABLE 35.3
Example Equipment to Aid in Moving and Positioning

Handling Belt
A wide padded belt with handholds, a buckle and an adjustable strap that fits around the waist.
Used to help stabilise a user on standing, with transfers and to assist walking.

Hand Blocks
Plastic blocks with a handhold and slip-resistant base used singly or in pairs to lengthen arm reach and assist in moving on a bed.

Transfer Board
Flat wooden or plastic board, used to bridge gaps for transfers between seated surfaces.

One way glide
Padded cushion with an anti-slip base that allows movement in one direction only. Used to prevent slipping forward in a chair.

Flat slide sheet
A pair of flat sheets made of very low friction material, which when placed on top of one another become very slippery. Used to move a person on a flat surface, and for easier sling insertion.

In situ slide sheets
Fitted satin base sheet with cotton edge and top drawer sheet with satin on one side that remains in place on the bed for easier bed mobility.

Automated repositioning system
Electrically operated poles attached to either side of the bed. Slide sheet fitted to the mattress and a cotton top sheet attached to each pole and is rolled onto the pole as they turn. Both poles can turn to the left or right allowing the sheet to be rolled up or unrolled and enables the person lying on the sheet to be moved or turned passively. Used for repositioning, sling insertion and turning for personal care.

Manual stand turner
Foot plate with swivel function, height adjustable post with a handhold, foot brake, shin pad(s). For standing pivot transfers between seated surfaces.

Alternatively:

Base platform with 3 or 4 wheels, brakes, height adjustable frame with handholds and shin pads.
For transfers between seated surfaces
Support strap available in different sizes

Stand hoist
Mobile, battery-operated hoist with footplate, handhold and adjustable width legs designed to fit under and around chairs for supported standing transfers.

Seated transfer aids
Manual mobile transfer aid with pivoting/folding divided seat, adjustable knee brace and adjustable leg width to fit around furniture for transfers between seated surfaces.

Mobile electric hoists
Battery-operated wheeled base with brakes with adjustable legs, vertical mast and spreader bar with hooks or clips to allow a sling to be attached to transfer a person with no or limited weight-bearing ability.

Gantry/Two post hoists
Two freestanding posts or two telescopic posts that block against the ceiling, with track attached and hoist, suitable for lateral transfers.

Ceiling track hoist
Permanently mounted ceiling track, either straight track for lateral transfers, or Y/H track.

Slings
Fabric support cradle that is attached to a hoist spreader bar with either loop or clip fasteners.

Repositioning sheets
Large sheet with multiple loops along both sides to attach to hoist spreader bar used for repositioning in bed and transfers between flat surfaces.

Rigid oval boards
Pair of low-friction flexible boards used to insert slings.

Emergency lifting chair
Inflatable cushions with a compressor or metal frame with a seat and electronic control inserted under/around a fallen person to lift into a sitting position.

professional development (CPD) requirements and promote national consistency (NBE, 2010).

Providing Instruction to Others

If there is doubt about the occupational therapist's level of experience or expertise, they should not train others or delegate tasks related to moving and positioning or use of equipment. Principles of delegation and guidance to others in moving and positioning are discussed in *Accountability and Delegation* (Royal College of Nursing, 2023) and in *the Professional Standards for Occupational Therapy Practice, Conduct and Ethics* (Royal College of Occupational Therapy (RCOT), 2021). Providing instructions and information on the safe use of equipment is crucial in establishing safe working systems and is a legal responsibility. Failure to provide instructions has resulted in liability, for example, *Colclough v Staffordshire County Council,* 1998, cited in Mandelstam (2009).

CONCLUSION

Moving and positioning people, ranging from facilitating independent movement to maximise occupational engagement, through assisted movement to enable the completion of essential activities of daily living, to the use of specialist techniques and equipment to move the more dependent person, has been addressed in this chapter. Introduction of the Manual Handling Operations Regulations and other guidance has focused on reducing risks to professionals and carers who assist in the moving and positioning of people. Later, the introduction of the Human Rights Act (1998) has encouraged more balanced decision making (Mandelstam, 2011) in terms of the rights of both occupational therapists and carers and the people who require their services and has encouraged a more collaborative approach between occupational therapists and those receiving therapy or care. To provide occupational therapists with a 'toolbox' of principles with which to analyse moving and positioning tasks and establish appropriate levels of intervention across the continuum from care handling to treatment and therapeutic handling, the principles of risk assessment, legislation and safe handling along with principles of normal movement and biomechanics have been covered. Occupational therapists are reminded that there is no one correct way to move or position a person and because of this moving and positioning should be guided by sound principles and collaborative decision making, to establish safe approaches within the boundaries of professional practice and expertise. Task and activity analysis forms the basis of occupational therapy practice, and this should always be applied in the field of people moving and positioning to guide decision making and enable the best outcome for individuals and occupational therapists and carers.

Acknowledgement

The authors would like to thank the previous author of this chapter Tess Whitehead. As this chapter is based on her work.

REFERENCES

Ahonen, M., Launis, M., & Kuorinka, T. (1989). *Ergonomic workplace analysis* (Transl. G. Oja) (p. 33). Ergonomics Section Finnish Institute of Occupational Health.

Arnold, M., Radawiec, S., Campo, M., & Wright, L. R. (2011). Changes in functional independence measure ratings associated with a safe patient handling and movement program. *Rehabilitation Nursing, 36,* 138–144.

Benner, P. (1984). From novice to expert: Excellence and power in clinical nursing practice. Addison-Wesley. Cited by Crumpton, E. & Johnson, C. (2005). In J. Smith (Ed.), *The Guide to the Handling of People* (5th ed.). BackCare and Royal College of Nursing.

British Safety Council. (2023). *Risk assessment: What they are, why they're important and how to complete them.* https://www.britsafe.org/training-and-learning/find-the-right-course-for-you/informational-resources/risk-assessment/.

Bunce, E., Willlis, J., & Gibson, F. (2023). *The Great Ormond Street hospital manual of children and young people's nursing practices* (2nd ed.). John Wiley and Sons Ltd.

Clemes, S. A., Haslam, C. O., & Haslam, R. A. (2010). What constitutes effective manual handling training? A systematic review. *Occupational Medicine, 60,* 101–107.

College of Occupational Therapists (COT). (2006). *Manual handling guidance 3.* College of Occupational Therapists.

Darragh, A. R., Campo, M. A., Frost, L., Miller, M., Pentico, M., & Argulis, H. (2013). Safe-patient handling equipment in therapy practice: Implications for rehabilitation. *American Journal of Occupational Therapy, 67,* 45–53.

Department of Health. (2003). *Domiciliary care national minimum standards.* http://www.housingcare.org/downloads/kbase/2553.pdf.

Elphinston, J. (2020). *Sport, stability and performance movement.* Lotus Publishing.

Fergusson Burt, L. (2007). The potential benefits of the introduction of electric profiling beds in preference to manually height-adjustable Kings Fund beds within the NHS: A literature review. *Column, 19*(2), 12–15.

Frost, L., & Barkley, W. M. (2012). Patient handling methods taught in occupational therapy curricula. *American Journal of Occupational Therapy, 66*, 463–470.

Garzillo, E. M., Monaco, M. G. L., Corvino, A. R., D'Ancicco, F., Feola, D., Della Ventura, D., Miraglia, N., & Lamberti, M. (2020). *International Journal of Environmental Research and Public Health, 17*(14), 4971. https://www.ncbi.nlm.nih.gov/pmc/articles/PMC7399987/. Accessed 27.03.2023.

Granger, C. V., Hamilton, B. B., Linacre, J. M., Heinemann, A. W., & Wright, B. D. (1993). Performance profiles of the functional independence measure. *American Journal of Physical Medicine & Rehabilitation, 72*, 84–89. Cited by Crumpton, E., & Johnson C. (2005). In J. Smith (Ed.), The guide to the handling of people (5th ed.). BackCare and Royal College of Nursing.

Health Care professions Council. (2014). https://www.hcpc-uk.org/globalassets/resources/reports/professionalism-in-healthcare-professionals.pdf – accessed on 07.06.2023.

Health and Safety Executive. (1974). *Health and Safety at Work Act.* http://www.healthandsafety.co.uk/haswa.htm.

Health and Safety Executive. (1992). *Workplace (health safety and welfare) regulations. A short guide for managers.* http://www.hse.gov.uk/pubns/indg244.pdf.

Health and Safety Executive. (2003). *Manual handling assessment charts (MAC).* HSE.

Health and Safety Executive. (2004). *Manual handling operations regulations 1992 (as amended): Guidance on regulations.* L23. HMSO.

Health and Safety Executive. (2008). *Risk management.* http://www.hse.gov.uk/risk/fivesteps.htm.

Health and Safety Executive. (2012). *Manual handling at work: A brief guide.* http://www.hse.gov.uk/pubns/indg143.htm.

Health and Safety Executive. (2013). *Ergonomics and human factors at work: A brief guide.* http://www.hse.gov.uk/pubns/indg90.htm.

Health and Safety Executive. (2015). *What you need to do: Moving and positioning.* http://www.hse.gov.uk/healthservices/moving-handling-do.htm.

Health and Safety Executive. (2020). *Manual handling at work: A brief guide.* https://www.hse.gov.uk/pubns/indg143.pdf.

Health and Safety Executive. (2023) *Moving and positioning in health and social care.* Retrieved June 20, 2023, from https://www.hse.gov.uk/healthservices/moving-handling.htm.

Hignet, S., & McAtamney, L. (2000). Rapid entire body assessment. *Applied Ergonomics, 31*, 201–205.

Health Care professions Council. (2014). Retrieved June 7, 2023, from https://www.hcpc-uk.org/globalassets/resources/reports/professionalism-in-healthcare-professionals.pdf.

Human Rights Act. (1998). http://www.opsi.gov.uk/ACTS/acts1998/19980042.htm.

Ilmarinen, J. (1998). *Work ability index.* Finnish Institute of Occupational Health.

Johnson, C. (2011). Manual handling risk management. In J. Smith (Ed.), *The guide to the handling of people* (6th ed.). BackCare.

Mandelstam, M. (2009). *Community care practice and the law* (4th ed.). Jessica Kingsley.

Mandelstam, M. (2011). Manual handling: Legal framework and balanced decision making. In J. Smith (Ed.), *The guide to the handling of people* (6th ed.). BackCare.

Mandelstam, M. (2021). *Manual handling in health and social care* (2nd ed.). Jessica Kingsley Publishers.

McAtamney, L., & Corlett, E. N. (1993). RULA: A survey method for the investigation of work-related upper limb disorders. *Applied Ergonomics, 24*, 91–99.

Morabito, J., Penkala, S., & Coxon, K. (2021). Workplace musculoskeletal problems in occupational therapy students. *BMC Public Health.* Retrieved April 1, 2023, from. https://bmcpublichealth.biomedcentral.com/articles/10.1186/s12889-021-10653-8.

National Back Exchange. (2010). *Standards in manual handling: Taining guidelines.* http://www.nationalbackexchange.org/files/training_guidelines/training_guidelines.pdf.

NIOSH. (1991). *National Institute for Occupational Safety and Health: Safe Patient Handling and Movement (SPHM).* http://www.cdc.gov/niosh/index.htm.

OWAS (WinOWAS). (2007). *A computerized system for the analysis of work postures.* http://turva1.me.tut.fi/owas/index.html.

Phillips, J., Mellson, J., & Richardson, N. (2014). *It takes two? Exploring the manual handling myth.* Prism Medical: UK. https://prismmedical.co.uk/wp-content/uploads/.../Does-it-Take-Two.pdf.

Rose, P. (2011). Manual handling risk management. In J. Smith (Ed.), *The guide to the handling of people* (6th ed.). Middlesex: BackCare.

Royal College of Nursing. (2023). *Accountability and delegation.* https://www.rcn.org.uk/professional-development/accountability-and-delegation.

Royal College of Occupational Therapists. (2021). *Professional standards for occupational therapy practice, conduct and ethics.* College of Occupational Therapists.

Smith, J. (Ed.). (2011). *The guide to the handling of people* (6th ed.). Middlesex: BackCare/Royal College of Nursing.

Straker, L., Burgess-Limerick, R., Pollock, C., & Egeskov, R. (2004). A randomized and controlled trial of a participative ergonomics intervention to reduce injuries associated with manual tasks: Physical risk and legislative compliance. *Ergonomics, 47*(2), 166–188.

Sturman-Floyd, M. (2011). *Reducing the incidence and risk of pressure sores, manual handling loading and carer costs using 'In-bed systems'.* http://www.communityequipment.org.uk/wp-content/uploads/SturmanFloyd-paper-2011-Complete-final-paper.pdf.

Waters, T. R., & Rockefeller, K. (2010). Safe patient handling for rehabilitation professionals. *Rehabilitation Nursing, 35*, 216–222.

Worksafe.qld.gov.au. *People handling.* Retrieved June 7, 2023, from https://www.worksafe.qld.gov.au/safety-and-prevention/hazards/hazardous-manual-tasks/guidance-for-high-risk-industries/people-handling#:~:text=People%20handling%20relates%20to%20workplace,pull%20or%20slide%20another%20person.

World Health Organization. (2012). *International classification of functioning, disability and health.* www.who.int/classifications/icf/en.

REFLECTION

1. Describe what risk assessment procedures an occupational therapist should conduct before moving and positioning a person.

2. Explain why it is important, when involved in moving and position a person, to have an understanding of the biomechanical principles of based of support, location of body, centre of gravity, friction, and internal and external focuses acting on the body.

3. Indentify the differences between a standing hoist, mobile floor hoist and ceiling track hoist, and provide reasons why you would choose to use each type of hoist.

4. When providing training to a person requiring any moving and positioning procedure (e.g. assistance to stand from sitting down, turning in a bde or use of a hoist) and that person's family or carers, describe how you would ensure the person, family and carers are competent in implementing the procedure.

36

BIOMECHANICAL STRATEGIES TO INITIATE AND SUSTAIN OCCUPATIONAL PARTICIPATION

DANIEL CEZAR DA CRUZ ■ ANGELA M. MURPHY

CHAPTER OUTLINE

Overview

Biomechanics is the study of motion and the effect of force on motion, and biomechanical principles are intrinsic to everyone's occupations. Key concepts of biomechanics include kinetics, kinematics, anatomical planes of movement, joint range of motion, strength and endurance. In occupational therapy, knowledge of biomechanics is important when describing how movement is executed to ensure that appropriate assessments and interventions that suit an individual's capabilities are selected. The implementation of the biomechanical strategies of prevention, restoration and compensation involves consideration of joint range of motion, strength and endurance; and must be applied to obtain occupational participation outcomes. Biomechanical strategies applied in occupational therapy practice while implementing an occupational approach is the focus of this chapter. To illustrate the use of biomechanical principles in practice, a practice story of George and Louisa is presented.

KEY POINTS

- Biomechanics refers to the study of motion and the effect of focus on motion, and biomechanical principles are intrinsic to occupational participation.

- Key biomechanical concepts include kinetics, kinematics, anatomical planes of movement, joint range of motion, strength and endurance.

- Occupational therapists use biomechanical strategies to facilitate the occupational participation of individuals who experience limitations due to muscle weakness, inadequate range of motion or lack of endurance that can impact participation in daily life.

- Occupational therapists should use their professional reasoning to determine when assessment of biomechanical capacity is required and consider how any limitations impact a person's occupational participation.

- Impairment-focused assessments may be utilised alongside occupation-centred assessments to assist with co-designing occupational participation goals, interventions and outcomes.

- There are three biomechanical interventions: prevention, restoration and compensation.
- An occupation-focused approach ensures that biomechanical interventions are used to achieve occupational participation goals.

INTRODUCTION

Biomechanics can be described as the study of motion and the effect of force on motion. The concept of biomechanics is often confused with kinesiology, which can be described as the study of functional anatomy, consisting of musculoskeletal systems, movement efficiency from the anatomical standpoint and the actions of joints and muscles during simple and complex movement (Hamill et al., 2015). Nowadays, some aspects of kinesiology are incorporated into the biomechanics curriculum to serve as a qualitative introduction to human movement, although biomechanics is generally quantitative in nature.

In occupational therapy, knowledge of biomechanics is important when describing how movement is executed to ensure that appropriate assessments and interventions that suit an individual's capabilities are selected. For instance, because of a transhumeral amputation of a dominant arm due to a motor vehicle accident, a teacher is unable to drive his car to school and states that being able to do this is a priority. To regain abilities and occupational participation, the occupational therapist works with the teacher to enhance the function of the teacher's remaining arm (e.g. muscle power, muscle endurance, eye-hand coordination) through driving-related activities (e.g. steering manoeuvres, hand controls), as well as car modifications to suit the teacher's needs. The application of biomechanical principles is crucial for safe driving, as well as to prevent any long-term health consequences as a result of improper body mechanics.

Occupational therapists use biomechanical strategies to facilitate the occupational participation of individuals who experience limitations in physical performance, such as muscle weakness, inadequate range of motion or lack of endurance that can significantly affect participation in daily life. The focus of this chapter is to explain biomechanical principles to provide an overview of assessment of biomechanical

limitation and then to present how the biomechanical strategies of prevention, restoration and compensation are used by occupational therapists to promote occupational participation.

BIOMECHANICAL CONCEPTS

Kinetics

Kinetics is the study of the effect of force on motion and is founded on Newton's three laws (Rasdi, 2017):

a) *First Law of Inertia*: A body stays at rest or in motion in its current state unless acted upon by an external force. For instance, a person using a walker will not start moving until they put force on the equipment to start walking.

b) *Second Law of acceleration* (force/mass): The acceleration of a body is directly related to the force magnitude and the direction. To illustrate, someone who is playing ten-pin bowling might exert enough force to make the bowling ball roll with the right speed towards the pins.

c) *Third Law of Reaction*: When a body applies a force to another body, the second body reacts with equal force on the first body. For example, to stand up from the toilet seat, a person needs to apply force on the ground with their feet, allowing the ground force reaction to facilitate their movement.

Kinematics

Kinematics is the study of movement regardless of the causes of the movement (e.g. mass, force). The characteristics of the movement can be described in terms of displacement (change in position), velocity (rate of change in displacement) and acceleration (rate of change in velocity) in linear and angular movements. When a body is moving in a straight line (linear motion) in only one plane, the movement is described as one-dimensional (e.g. sitting on a train that is moving in a straight direction). When a body is moving in a curved path, the movement is described as two-dimensional (e.g. bending and extending the trunk while sitting). Finally, when a body is moving in space in all three planes, the movement is described as three-dimensional (e.g. swimming in a pool).

Occupational therapists use kinematic principles to observe and analyse how a person performs their occupations. An example of this is when an occupational therapist uses a goniometer to measure angular displacement (i.e. two-dimensional movement) that occurs at each joint (range of motion).

Anatomical Planes of Movement

Movement of the body and body parts occurs in three *anatomical planes* (Greene & Roberts, 2005):

1. Sagittal plane divides the body in right and left; for example, flexion-extension of the shoulder, elbow and wrist occur in the parallel sagittal plane.
2. Frontal or coronal plane divides the body into front and back; for example, adduction and abduction of the hip, shoulder and wrist.
3. Transverse or horizontal plane divides the body into upper and lower; for example, internal and external rotation of shoulder and hip joints.

Joint Range of Motion

Joints are connections between bones composed of connective tissues (ligaments) and muscles that allow different types of movement according to their structure and the soft tissues and skin that surround them (Grice, 2021; Kielhofner, 2009):

- Hinge joints allow movement in one plane; for example, the joint between the proximal and distal interphalangeal joints of the fingers that allows flexion and extension movements when writing and sewing.
- Ball and socket joints allow movement in more than one plane (coronal, sagittal and transverse); for example, volleyball player might flex, extend, abduct, adduct and externally and internally rotate their shoulder joints when playing a game. Due to the range and complexity of movements, ball and socket joints are more unstable as compared to hinge joints and are commonly more susceptible to injuries.

Active range of movement or motion (AROM) refers to the amount of movement of a joint caused by voluntary contraction of muscles (Flinn et al., 2008); for instance, when a person actively lifts their arm to reach items on a supermarket shelf.

Passive range of movement or motion (PROM) describes the amount of joint movement caused by external or outside forces (Flinn et al., 2008) and is exemplified when an occupational therapist flexes and extends a person's wrist and fingers through their full range of motion.

Muscular Strength

Muscular strength is the amount of force a person can exert or the amount of weight a person can lift in one single maximal isometric contraction (Flinn et al., 2008; Grice, 2021; Jacobs & Simon, 2020). Muscular strength is essential to allow movement and stability when skeletal muscles act on the joints. Movement is possible when muscles provide the force needed to stabilise and move parts of the body in different anatomical planes (Grice, 2021). The tension produced in the muscles can stabilise or move joints (Kielhofner, 2009). For example, when a person is writing, the proximal muscles, such as trapezius and deltoids, stabilise the arm while intrinsic muscles of the hand, such as thenar, hypothenar, interossei and lumbrical, allow the movement in the hand during handwriting (Almeida et al., 2013). When muscles produce forces with equal tension from all directions where the joint can move, they stabilise joints.

Endurance

Sustaining muscle effort or force for extended periods of time is about endurance (Grice, 2021). Moreover, beyond the normal capacity of the muscle and its condition, endurance is affected by the cardiovascular and pulmonary systems of a person (Grice, 2021).

There are two types of endurance:

a) Muscle endurance is the ability of a muscle or group of muscles to repeatedly contract against a force for a period of time without fatigue; for example, a person lifting tins of food repeatedly to organise a cupboard after shopping.
b) Cardiorespiratory endurance refers to the ability of the circulatory and respiratory (cardiorespiratory) systems to supply oxygen to muscles during continuous physical activity; for example, a person running a marathon (Kielhofner, 2009; Rowe & Zeiner, 2021).

Muscular and cardiorespiratory endurance are essential to occupational participation which is why occupational therapists refer to it as activity tolerance. The focus on how an individual can continue doing specific occupations is a focus of occupational therapy when addressing endurance (Rowe & Zeiner, 2021).

THE BIOMECHANICAL FRAME OF REFERENCE AND CONCEPTUAL MODELS OF PRACTICE

The Biomechanical Frame of Reference (BFoR) has long been part of occupational therapy practice. It underpinned occupational therapy practice during the 1950s and 1960s when occupational therapists embraced the medical model and applied a range of interventions such as splinting, exercises focused on muscle strength, endurance, range of movement and other biomechanical approaches to remediate physical injuries and impairments (Kielhofner, 2009; Yerxa, 2000) (refer to Chapter 8). During this period, occupational therapists used activities including exercise to improve and maintain musculoskeletal function;

however, there was little focus on occupational participation outcomes (Greene & Roberts, 2005). According to Greene and Roberts (2005), a biomechanical focus emphasises the mechanics of the musculoskeletal system; it does not address the cognitive, emotional and social aspects of human occupation. In addition, it does not consider performance in context within the environments in which an individual participates.

When using the BFoR in occupational therapy practice, a holistic view of individuals regarding what they want, need or are expected to do must be considered to ensure that biomechanical strategies facilitate occupational participation. Although the BFoR in itself is focused on the able-body and the biomedical model, occupational therapists add this frame of reference into their practice with an occupational lens; they choose a Conceptual Model of Practice that is occupation-centred and designed to explain the process and practice of occupational therapy (Duncan, 2021).

Occupational therapy interventions are complex (Creek, 2009; Yerxa, 1988) because occupational therapists utilise a range of resources and shift their intervention focus from skills to adapting the occupation

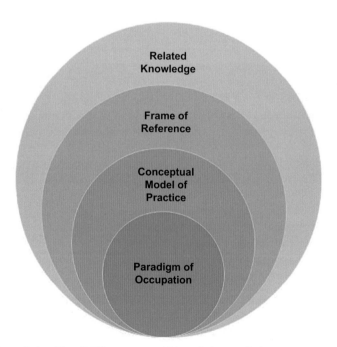

Fig. 36.1 ■ The overlapping relationship of different types of knowledge applied to occupational therapy practice. (From Kielhofner, G. (2009). *Conceptual foundations of occupational therapy practice* (4th ed.). F.A. Davis.)

and/or the environment to suggest alternative options that will facilitate occupational participation. Occupational therapists work collaboratively with individuals using knowledge that informs the values, nature, aim and scope of occupational therapy practice to understand and work with a person to achieve their occupational participation goals (Kielhofner, 2009). The overlapping relationship of the different types of knowledge that occupational therapists can utilise is illustrated in Fig. 36.1.

Occupational therapists can draw on a range of Conceptual Models of Practice to facilitate occupation-centred practice. Some examples of Conceptual Models of Practice include the the Kawa (River) Model (Turpin & Iwama, 2011), the Model of Human Occupation (MOHO) (Taylor et al., 2024), the Occupational Therapy Intervention Process Model (OTIPM) (Fisher & Marterella, 2019), the Person-Enviorment-Occupation (PEO) (Law et al., 1996), the Person- Environment-Occupation-Performance (PEOP) (Christiansen et al., 2015) and the Canadian Model of Occupational Participation (CanMoP) (Egan & Restall, 2022). In this chapter, the CanMOP was chosen to demonstrate how biomechanical strategies can be used to obtain occupational participation outcomes. A practice story (Box 36.1) is presented to illustrate the application of the biomechanical approach using the CanMOP as a Conceptual Model of Practice.

BIOMECHANICS AS PART OF HUMAN OCCUPATION

Ana Elisa is a singer (Fig. 36.2). When preparing for recitals, she practices techniques that include breathing, concentration, rest and being in a quiet environment. When singing, Ana's vocal cords work to produce sound according to each note. Moreover, her body posture and muscles are recruited at varying levels and contractions to allow stability, movement and endurance during her performance; her ability to do this is explained by the principles of biomechanics.

While biomechanics can explain body function, an occupational perspective informs another history. Ana Elisa is a professional singer. She has been singing since age 10. Exploring Ana's past occupational participation as a musician explains how she accessed or had opportunities to study music, how she

initiated her participation and how she sustained singing throughout her life. Understanding her occupational participation requires more than the knowledge of biomechanical principles for singing. Exploring Ana's history and relationships in occupational participation needs to address the context of why (purpose), where, when and with whom (meaning) she defines occupational participation (Egan & Restall, 2022). For example, the stage is always exciting: lights, every single moment, the audience, absorption and applauses are part of Ana's meaningful and valued occupational participation. Ana reflected,

> At the time of the performance, I feel the adrenaline of the expectation that everything will go well. I feel nervous because I am afraid of forgetting, especially the text. Nowadays, when I make a mistake, I don't sacrifice myself as much because I have learned, over time, to overlook certain unforeseen events and learn from them. There is the time to 'undress', give myself to the music and the public, and have fun! I feel like a warm wave that passes through my body controlled by my thoughts and transmitted by my voice. An invisible painting that I create in that moment through sound and words. My mind is focused on everything my instrument does that I can't see, just feel inside me. Posture, breathing, movement of the body, hands, facial expression, the voice working, the words coming out of my mouth, the sound of mine, the combination with other instruments, the attention to the maestro and the other singers, where my gaze goes, directs. Everything happens with a mix of expectation, adrenaline, and emotion. With or without errors, with or without those problems of the day that I mentioned before. And one presentation is never like another: each one is unique.

Ana Elisa's reflection on her occupational participation illustrates that biomechanical principles are intrinsic to what people do. A professional surfer might find it exciting to maintain balance, muscle strength and endurance while surfing a challenging wave during a competition; another person experiencing fatigue and pain while running might persist inspired by the commitment to complete their first marathon and a waiter might effortlessly manipulate

BOX 36.1
PRACTICE STORY: GEORGE AND LOUISA

George was referred to occupational therapy by his community nurse who had observed a decline in his occupational participation and mood. He lived with his wife, and they had one son and one grandchild, living nearby. George had a diagnosis of multiple sclerosis (relapsing-remitting) and a history of myocardial infarction (5 years ago). He was struggling to access, initiate and sustain his participation in his occupations as he had weakness in his lower limbs and reduced range of movement in his right hand. His meaningful relationship with his wife meant he was increasingly concerned about how much she was having to do at home, and he wanted to help with household tasks but was unable to stand for sufficient time to do this.

George had been the main wage earner for his family, on which he based his competence. Now that he was no longer employed, he wanted to help more around the home. He had enjoyed his job in a local factory, priding himself on the fact that he took very little sick leave. He retired at age 65 and looked back fondly at his employment; however, he was unhappy that he was now spending most of his time watching television. He had taken part in his local community and had lots of friends, but these friendships had drifted since his retirement. He hoped to be able to rekindle some of his old friendships and to help around the home, as well as go out with his wife. However, his concerns about regularly needing to go to the toilet meant that he tended to stay at home. George considered himself to have working class values, believing things should be done properly and fairly.

The occupational therapist collaborated with George and his wife Louisa to establish their priorities surrounding how to access, initiate and sustain his occupational participation. On observation, the occupational therapist could see that George struggled with an unsteady, one-sided sit-to-stand, positioned his feet too far forward to enable him to stand up from a seated position safely, had a weak and unsteady walking gait, was only able to stand for a short period of time and had difficulty opposing his right thumb.

The occupational therapist talked with George and Louisa about multiple sclerosis and the impact relapses and remission could have on occupational participation. George's pattern of relapse and remission had included infrequent relapses, and he was hoping his multiple sclerosis would continue in a similar pattern. However, he experienced anxiety about future relapses and the long-term progression of multiple sclerosis. George acknowledged that he experienced fatigue and felt that this inhibited his occupational participation.

The occupational therapist also explored whether George could be experiencing deconditioning and low mood from his reduced occupational participation and how a graded approach to building tolerance through participating in his valued occupations could be helpful. George identified that his continence issues were significantly concerning him, and he had stopped going out of the home as he was too embarrassed to see his friends.

To clearly identify the biomechanical approach/strategies used with George, these are stated in the [] brackets following each intervention.

Co-design priorities, goals, outcomes and plans with George and Louisa

Together George, Louisa and the occupational therapist agreed on the following goals. For George to be able to:
1. Complete a small number of kitchen occupations such as washing up on a sustained regular basis (at least once a day).
2. Reduce the number of times he was required to go to the toilet on a typical day.
3. Consider seeing friends and going out of the home with Louisa, once feeling stronger and the continence issue managed.
4. Explore occupations which were achievable on days when George was in relapse.
5. Explore ways of managing feelings of anxiety.

The occupational therapist assessed the home environment, which was small and had limited space in most areas.

In the beginning, the compensatory approach was considered, with possible equipment solutions discussed with George. A wheeled walker, perching stool, adapted cutlery, riser-recliner chair [assistive technology], through floor lift (local council did not provide stair lifts to people with multiple sclerosis) and downstairs toilet were considered [environmental adaptation]. The space was too limited for a perching stool in the kitchen. He agreed that adapted cutlery may be helpful but preferred to first work on establishing whether restoration of hand function, strength and range of movement to enable occupational participation in the kitchen was possible [remediation/restoration].

George agreed that a wheeled walker may be of benefit, but he wanted to become stronger so perceived this as a short-term solution with the hope of soon not requiring it. He aimed to be able to move from sit-to-stand more effectively and safely, have improved stamina for walking and standing and manipulate objects more effectively to complete valued occupations.

Referrals were sent to a physiotherapist and the continence specialist teams with his permission.

The occupational therapist demonstrated and supported George to adapt his occupational performance by practicing strategies to enable safe and effective sit-to-stand. It was agreed that George would practice using both upper limbs to enable him to push up from the chair and actively recruit his muscles in both lower limbs while standing, always checking and aiming for midline as well as positioning his feet in the appropriate position and aiming to have his 'nose over toes as he rose' [remediation and adapting occupational performance].

A plan for gradual increase in time spent standing was agreed [adapting occupational performance]. George agreed to practice standing and walking at least once an hour. He was encouraged to use the walker to reduce the risk of falls [assistive technology]. George identified that his main purpose for this was to gain strength to enable his participation in more meaningful occupations.

Some easy food preparation tasks were identified, such as making tea for his wife, making toast and chopping vegetables [using adapted cutlery/assistive technology] while sitting at the kitchen table [adapting occupational performance].

Some simple breathing exercises were taught along with education about the symptoms of anxiety in order that George could recognise and counteract symptoms caused by the sympathetic nervous system by initiating the parasympathetic nervous system [remediation]. A referral to a psychologist was also recommended but George declined.

Initiating occupational participation

George chose to begin by washing up two small items in the kitchen sink and built this to more items as he grew stronger and more accustomed to standing [restoration and adapting occupational performance]. He integrated planned midway rests when needed and practiced abdominal breathing when resting. George discussed with the occupational therapist how using his hands to complete more varied occupations would be beneficial for overall hand function and rather than avoiding to use his right hand, to aim to use it as much as possible, even if it meant

spending a few more seconds on the occupation and/or adapting how it might be completed [restorative and adaptive]. Together, they identified occupations requiring thumb opposition, such as holdi3ng a cup, holding crockery while washing up and playing cards and other games with his wife and grandson. He also identified how meaningful it would be to think creatively about games he could play with his grandson and that having fun with his grandson, wife and friends was important to him.

Sustaining occupational participation

Once George could see progress, he felt motivated to carry on and worked hard to practice regular sit-to-stand, walking, standing and performing a variety of occupations involving thumb opposition and abdominal breathing. In addition, he identified that abdominal breathing was helping and was interested in exploring more ways of relaxing and some easily accessible occupations for what he referred to as bad days [adapting occupational performance].

After 8 weeks and once his continence was being managed, he was able to complete a full load of washing up, standing for 10-minute intervals, involving a safe sit-to-stand and walk to the kitchen. He had become involved in quite a few other occupations around the home and had enjoyed his contributions to meal preparation.

He was then happy to discuss the possibility of going out with his wife and inviting friends to his home to play cards. Gradually, his confidence and motivation for leaving the home also increased so that he felt more able to go out for coffee and shopping with Louisa as well as to begin spending time with friends. He had details of the specialist multiple sclerosis relapse service so that he could quickly access treatment when he experienced a relapse. He was also informed that he could refer himself back to occupational therapy if required at any point in future.

---

a tray while clearing plates, glasses and cutlery from the table. All these occupations involve biomechanics and illustrate how biomechanical principles are part of each person's occupational participation.

APPLYING BIOMECHANICAL KNOWLEDGE

The knowledge and application of biomechanics can prevent harm, promote comfort and improve occupational participation. For example, biomechanical strategies can be used to:

- Ensure that a person is not in a supine position in a hospital bed when drinking liquid as this will place the person at risk of choking and aspirating fluids into the lungs (refer to Chapter 35).
- Position a person with multiple sclerosis with the right degree of seating tilt and recline in the wheelchair and with a specialist cushion to reduce the risk of pressure injuries in the buttocks (Mendes et al., 2019) (refer to Chapter 33).
- Teach a person with a complete level C6 spinal cord injury to extend the wrist to practice picking up and holding objects (e.g. a slice of bread or

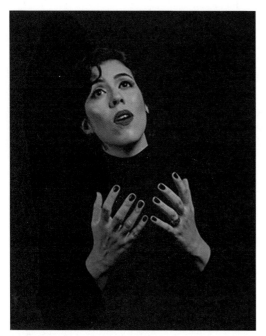

Fig. 36.2 ■ When Ana Elisa sings, biomechanics principles are needed for her occupational participation.

a mobile phone) using the passive tenodesis and a splint to stabilise the second metacarpophalangeal in a flexed position to facilitate the grasp (Fig. 36.3) (Jung et al., 2018) (refer to Chapter 40).

■ Understanding that prolonged oedema in the hands can be detrimental to the range of motion,

strength and soft tissues, impacting the use of the hands and occupational participation in daily activities (Miller et al., 2017) (refer to Chapter 40).

■ Recommend assistive technology devices to assist individuals to do a range of everyday activities, such as a thermoplastic device for a person to use the computer after a spinal cord injury (Tetraplegia C5) (Fig. 36.4) (refer to Chapter 31).

Occupational therapists use their knowledge of biomechanics to guide their professional decision-making in collaboration with the person receiving occupational therapy services (refer to Chapter 9). Biomechanical principles influence, for example, the correct height adjustment of assistive devices such as a raised toilet seat (Fig. 36.5). Increasing the height and angle of the toilet seat can result in diminished activity in the muscles of the trunk and legs, affecting the sway to stand up (Kim et al., 2015; Lee et al., 2016). Moreover, increasing the height of toilet seats for short elderly individuals can generate discomfort because they might not be able to have their feet on the floor, reducing stability and, therefore risks of falls (Lee et al., 2016) and hampering the ability to empty bowels.

ASSESSMENTS OF BIOMECHANICAL CAPACITIES

Occupational therapists can use the knowledge of biomechanics for assessment, intervention and evaluation

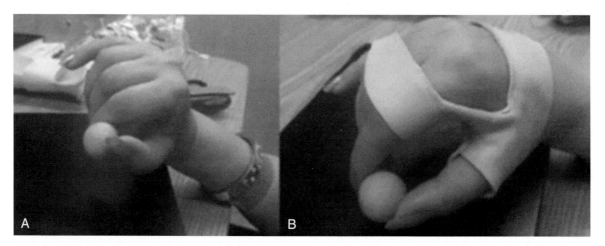

Fig. 36.3 ■ Tenodesis grip. (A) Grasping an object using tenodesis unassisted. (B) Grasping an object using tenodesis assisted by splint to stabilise joints.

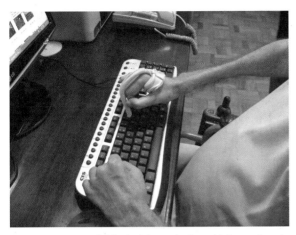

Fig. 36.4 ▪ An individual with a spinal cord injury using the computer with a splint to assist with pressing the keys of the keyboard.

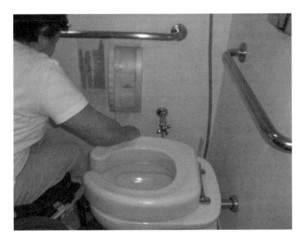

Fig. 36.5 ▪ Raised toilet seat can be used to make it easier to sit down and stand up from the toilet.

of the impact of limitations of movement, strength, endurance or a combination of these on a person's occupational participation (Grice, 2021; McMillan, 2021).

A comprehensive, detailed biomechanical assessment is widely published in occupational therapy books (see e.g. Flinn et al., 2008; Grice, 2021; Rowe & Zeiner, 2021) and is not a specific focus of the chapter.

Standardised and non-standardised assessments of biomechanical capacity (impairment-based) might be helpful in some settings where occupational therapists work. However, occupational therapists should use their professional reasoning to analyse when this type

of assessment is needed according to the population they work with and the agreed occupational participation outcomes. Results of these assessments do not fully capture how a person is experiencing difficulties in their occupational participation in everyday life. Hence, when occupational therapists assess range of motion, strength and endurance, they must also consider how any limitations impact the person's occupational participation. This approach requires a holistic assessment of occupational participation considering the history and relationships of an individual, their purpose and meaning, the context (micro, meso and macro) where occupational participation takes place and how the person is experiencing difficulties in accessing, initiating and sustaining the occupational participation (Egan & Restall, 2022). Therefore observation and interviews should also be used to determine a person's subjective perceptions of their capabilities and to identify what is important to them.

Examples of some assessments that may be used to identify biomechanical capacity are presented in Table 36.1. Suggested questions to capture the subjective experience of individuals regarding their biomechanical capabilities are presented in Table 36.2 where suggested questions exemplify how to adapt communication:

As mentioned before, measuring joint range of motion, endurance or strength can be important for specific health conditions and settings where occupational therapists work because the outcomes can provide evidence and feedback on a person's progress. Additionally, due to the complexity of intervention in health care, occupational therapists may need to consider and assess how pain, fatigue, oedema, spasticity, contractures, sensorimotor and other consequences of illness, injury or impairment might influence movement and stability of posture (Grice, 2021). However, focusing only on these components does not necessarily improve occupational participation since the person's occupational participation needs are not necessarily considered (Rasdi, 2017).

Occupation-focused assessments can contribute to occupational therapists remaining occupation-centred (refer to Chapter 13). The Canadian Occupational Performance Measure- COPM is an outcome measure widely researched that demonstrates clinical utility, validity and reliability in supporting meaningful goal formulation and measuring occupational outcomes on performance, satisfaction and can be utilised in

TABLE 36.1

Examples of Assessments That Can be Used to Identify a Person's Biomechanical Capacity

Assessment Focus	Example Assessments
Occupational participation	Model of human occupational screening tool (MOHOST) (Pakinson et al., 2006).
Occupational performance	Canadian Occupational Performance Measure (COPM) (Law et al., 1999) (refer to Chapter 16)
Occupational skills	Assessment of motor and process skills (Fisher & Jones, 1999); Dynamic performance analysis (refer to Chapter 18)
Environmental assessments	Home assessments, work assessments, assistive technology provision (Rasdi, 2017). (refer to Chapter 15)
Simulated functional tasks	Jebsen Taylor hand function (Jebsen et al., 1969)
Impairment-based: body function and structures	Range of motion: Active range of motion (AROM); Passive range of motion (PROM); Goniometry, Manual muscle testing (MMT); tip pinch, the lateral pinch and the palmar pinch and grip strength (Dynamometer), dynamic and static endurance (Flinn et al., 2008; Rowe & Zeiner, 2021)

different settings and populations (Colquhoun et al., 2017) (refer to Chapter 16).

BIOMECHANICAL INTERVENTIONS

A person's biomechanical capacities contribute to their ability to access, initiate and sustain occupational participation. When a person has had an injury, illness or impairment that is either impacted by or may impact on, their range of motion, strength and endurance, three intervention approaches are commonly used: preventative, restorative and compensatory (Kielhofner, 2009; McMillan, 2021).

When implementing these three intervention approaches, an occupational therapist must always work collaboratively with the person to understand their valued occupations within meaningful relationships and contexts (Egan & Restall, 2022).

TABLE 36.2

Example Questions and Prompts to Inform how the Range of Motion, Strength and Endurance Impact a Person's Occupational Participation

Biomechanical Components	Occupation-Focused Questions
Range of movement	How do you reach items on the top shelf of your kitchen cupboards? How do you feel you can change that?
	[Prompt: Reach for an object in the cupboard or clothes in your wardrobe]
	Can you tell me the things you cannot reach during your day-to-day occupations?
	What do you do to accomplish your tasks?
	[Prompt: Ask someone to help you, use a specific tool (e.g. Reacher) or create strategies to complete your activities]
Strength	What activities do you feel too weak to complete during your routine?
	What body parts do you feel need more strength to complete your activities?
	[Prompt: For example, arm, leg, trunk, right or left-hand-side?].
	What activities are you finding difficult to do?
	[Prompt: bake a cake, mop the floor, stand up from bed or toilet seat].
	Do you have any strategy to help you do these things?
Endurance	Are there any activities you start to do but find difficult to complete because you feel tired?
	[Prompt: cooking a meal, going to the grocery store, gardening]
	Are there any activities you do over the week or at weekends that are difficult to do and related to your heart?
	[Prompt: lifting a basket of clothes and walking, carrying supermarket bags, running, going up and down stairs]
	Tell me how you overcome these difficulties.

Preventative Approach

The preventative approach involves strategies that focus on eliminating or restricting the effect of predicted difficulties and complications. The rationale for this approach is that if individuals have muscles that can contract voluntarily and move joints, they should be encouraged to actively use these muscles and move the joints while participating in occupations to maintain their capacities. However, some individuals might face difficulties in moving parts of the body or the entire body due to injury or impairment, and in these cases, joints can be moved passively by another person or technology to maintain the joint range of motion. Orthosis or splints can also keep the integrity and alignment of joints, contributing to preventing joint deformity or stiffness (Kielhofner, 2009) (refer to Chapter 40).

Preventative approaches using biomechanical strategies can involve environmental adaptation. For example, a person's workspace, including a workstation, can be set up to reduce the risk of work-related injuries such as back pain or repetitive strain injury (refer to Chapters 26 and 29). The preventative approach can also be applied within schools, care homes, hospitals or any other places where occupational therapists work.

Preventative approaches can reduce the risk of secondary complications following an illness, injury or impairment. For example, a person who has had a spinal cord injury (Fig. 36.6A and B) requires supportive seating and positioning in the wheelchair to prevent scoliosis, kyphosis and other impairments that may impact their occupational participation.

Restorative Approach

The restorative approach focuses on improving a person's ability to do activities through remediation, restoration or establishment of skills. Remediation, restoration or establishment can directly address the impairment, using activities so that a person can recover lost skills or attain new skills. The focus is on identifying facilitators and barriers to performance and then designing strategies that restore, maintain, develop and/or improve the person's abilities required for occupational participation. These activities may be considered preliminary to being able to participate in meaningful occupation and may include exercises,

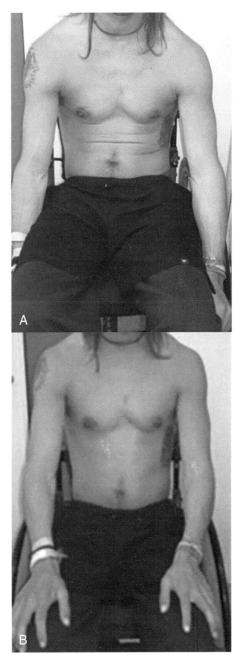

Fig. 36.6 ■ Wheelchair seating to enable support to reduce the risk of scoliosis, kyphosis and other impairments. (A) Posture before supportive seating provided. (B) Posture after supportive seating provided.

facilitation and inhibition techniques, positioning and transfers.

The restorative approach aims to increase or improve an individual's capacity to move and sustain posture for occupational participation. Therapeutic occupations can be used to restore muscle strength, range of movement and endurance (Kielhofner, 2009). Occupational therapists should work with a person to identify what their needs and priorities are and what meaning and purpose are associated with the gain of movement and posture. For example, a person recovering from an ulnar head fracture might have difficulty supinating their forearm (Fish & Palazzo, 2022). This person may want to be able to open doors, use eating utensils, turn on the shower and knead dough. An occupational therapist could work with this person and their family using graded exercises to restore the joint's range of movement, strength and endurance to enable them to return to being able to do the occupations they identified as important for them to participate in.

Compensatory Approach

The compensatory approach is directed at adapting the environment or the occupation to match a person's abilities. These strategies include those not focused on changing the person or adapting the environment but on making the best person–environment fit. In this case, the focus is on matching the abilities of the person with the environment or occupation that is most enabling. The main focus of this approach is to prevent or reduce occupational performance issues that may result from an impairment and limit/impact occupational participation. When using a compensation approach, changes may be made to how the occupation is done, the tools required to do the occupation and/or the environment.

This approach focuses on compensation for the lack of range of movement, strength or endurance due to illness, injury or impairment. A compensatory approach may comprise strategies such as:

1. *Assistive technology:* Devices such as splints or orthosis to stabilise joints or allow residual movement with more quality. For example, an orthosis that stabilises the wrist and allows the grasp of a fork or a pencil (Fig. 36.7) or a three-point ring to stabilise a lipstick. In case of individuals with amputations, prostheses can replace parts of the body to support walking, reaching, grasping and releasing objects as part of occupational participation (refer to Chapter 40).

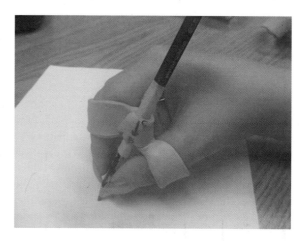

Fig. 36.7 ■ A customised splint to hold a pen for a person with a weak grasp.

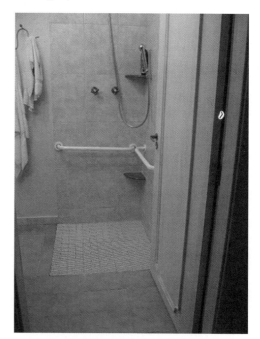

Fig. 36.8 ■ Adapted shower.

2. *Adapting the physical environment:* Modifications of the physical spaces, including ramps, grab bars, step-less showers (Fig. 36.8), toilet seats (Fig. 36.5), environmental control systems and reorganisation of the environment to facilitate access and initiation of occupational participation. Universal design principles can facilitate inclusive environments for people with different needs (refer to Chapter 29).

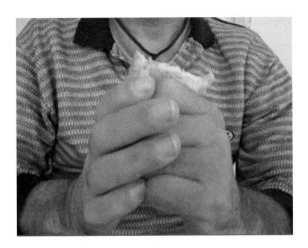

Fig. 36.9 ■ A person can use tenodesis grip to handle objects such as bread when eating.

3. *Adapting the way a person performs an occupation*: Modifications to the way a person performs an activity; for example, dressing using only one hand, using both hands to grasp a cup or using a tenodesis grip and both hands to hold a sandwich (Fig. 36.9).

The three compensation strategies can be combined. For example, a person who had a traumatic brain injury can go to the beach using a wheelchair designed specifically for that purpose (assistive technology), an accessible route to the beach (physical environment) and the support of friends and family to swim (adapting way person performs an occupation).

CONCLUSION

Knowledge of biomechanics is important to occupational therapy practice as biomechanical principles are intrinsic to the occupations people do. Occupational therapists can implement biomechanical strategies for people whose occupational participation is impacted by limitations of muscle weakness, reduced range of motion and/or decreased endurance. When assessing biomechanical capacity, occupational therapists consider using impairment-focused assessments alongside occupation-centred assessments to assist with co-designing occupational participation goals, interventions and outcomes. The implementation of the biomechanical strategies of prevention, restoration and compensation must be integrated with an occupation-centred practice to ensure that a person's occupational participation goals are the key outcomes of occupational therapy intervention.

REFERENCES

Almeida, P. H. T. Q., Cruz, D. M. C., Magna, L. A., & Ferrigno, I. S. V. (2013). An electromyographic analysis of two handwriting grasp patterns. *Journal of Electromyography and Kinesiology: Official Journal of the International Society of Electrophysiological Kinesiology, 23*(4), 838–843. https://doi.org/10.1016/j.jelekin.2013.04.004.

Christiansen, C. H., Baum, C. M., & Bass, J. D. (Eds.). (2015). *Occupational therapy: Performance, participation and well-being* (4th ed.). Slack Incorporated.

Colquhoun, H., Hunt, A. W., & Murchison, J. F. (2017). Canadian occupational performance measure. In M. Curtin, & M. A. Egan (Eds.), *Occupational therapy for people experiencing illness, injury or impairment: Promoting occupation and participation* (7th ed., pp. 185–191). Elsevier.

Creek, J. (2009). Occupational therapy defined as a complex intervention: A 5-year review. *British Journal of Occupational Therapy, 72*(3), 105–115. https://doi.org/10.1177/030802260907200304.

Duncan, E. A. S. (2021). Foundations for Practice in Occupational Therapy. 6th Edition. Elsevier: Edinburgh.

Egan, M., & Restall, G. (2022). Canadian model of occupational participation: Collaborative relationship-focused occupational therapy. In M. Egan, & G. Restall (Eds.), *Promoting occupational participation: Collaborative relationship-focused occupational therapy*. Canadian Association of Occupational Therapists.

Fish, M. J., & Palazzo, M. (2024). Distal Ulnar Fractures. [Updated 2023 Nov 22]. In: StatPearls [Internet]. Treasure Island (FL): StatPearls Publishing; Jan-. Available from: https://www.ncbi.nlm.nih.gov/books/NBK580565/.

Fish, M. J., & Palazzo, M. (2023). *Distal ulnar fractures*. StatPearls Publishing. https://www.ncbi.nlm.nih.gov/books/NBK580565/.

Fisher, A. G., & Marterella, A. (2019). *Powerful practice: A model for authentic occupational therapy*. Center for Innovative OT Solutions.

Flinn, N. A., Latham, C. A. T., & Podolski, C. R (2008). Assessing abilities and capacities: Range of motion, strength, and endurance. In M. V. Radomski, & C. A. T. Latham (Eds.), *Occupational therapy for physical dysfunction* (6th ed, pp. 91–185). Wolter Kluwer/Lippincott Williams & Wilkins.

Greene, D. P., & Roberts, S. L. (2015). *Kinesiology – e-book: Movement in the context of activity*. Elsevier Health Sciences.

Grice, K. O (2021). The biomechanical frame of reference. In D. P. Dirette, & S. A. Gutman (Eds.), *Occupational therapy for physical dysfunction* (8th ed., pp. 673–684). Wolters Kluwer.

Hamill, J., Knutzen, K. M., & Derrick, T. R. (2015). *Biomechanical basis of human movement* (4th ed.). Wolters Kluwer.

Jacobs, K., & Simon, L. (2020). *Quick reference dictionary for occupational therapy* (7th ed.). SLACK, Incorporated.

Jebsen, R., Taylor, N., Trieschmann, R., Trotter, M., & Howard, L. (1969). An objective and standardized test of hand function. *Archives of Physical Medicine and Rehabilitation, 50*, 311–319.

Jung, H. Y., Lee, J., & Shin, H.I. (2018). The natural course of passive tenodesis grip in individuals with spinal cord injury with preserved wrist extension power but paralyzed fingers and thumbs. *Spinal Cord. 56*(9): 900–906. https://doi.org/10.1038/s41393-018-0137-4. Epub 2018 May 22. PMID: 29789707.

Kielhofner, G. (2009). *Conceptual foundations of occupational therapy practice* (4th ed.). F.A. Davis.

Kim, B. J., Lee, S. K., Lee, J. H., & Kwon, H. Y. (2015). The effects of lower limb and trunk muscle activation on seat angle and height during sit to stand and stand to sit. *Journal of the Korean Society of Physical Medicine, 10*, 107–112.

Law, M., Cooper, B., Strong, S., Stewart, D., Rigby, P., & Letts, L. (1996). The person–environment–occupation model: A transactive approach to occupational performance. *Canadian Journal of Occupational Therapy, 63*, 9–23.

Lee, S. K., & Lee, S. Y. (2016). The effects of changing angle and height of toilet seat on movements and ground reaction forces in the feet during sit-to-stand. *Journal of Exercise Rehabilitation, 12*(5), 438–441. https://doi.org/10.12965//jer.1632700.350.

McMillan, I. R. (2021). The biomechanical frame of reference. In E. A. S Duncan (Ed.), *Foundations for practice in occupational therapy* (6th ed., pp. 152–164). Elsevier.

Mendes, P. V. B., Gradim, L. C. C., Silva, N. S., Allegretti, A. L. C., Carrijo, D. C. M., & Cruz, D. M. C. (2019). Pressure distribution analysis in three wheelchairs cushions of subjects with spinal cord injury. Disability and rehabilitation. *Assistive Technology, 14*(6), 555–560. https://doi.org/10.1080/17483107.2018.1463399.

Miller, L. K., Jerosch-Herold, C., & Shepstone, L. (2017). Effectiveness of edema management techniques for subacute hand edema: A systematic review. *Journal of Hand Therapy: Official Journal of the American Society of Hand Therapists, 30*(4), 432–446. https://doi.org/10.1016/j.jht.2017.05.011.

Rasdi, H. F. M (2017). Biomechanical strategies. In M. Curtin, M. Egan, & A. Jo (Eds.), *Occupational therapy for people experiencing illness, injury or impairment: Promoting occupation and participation*. Elsevier.

Rowe, V. T., & Zeiner, T. L. (2021). Motor function assessment: Range of motion, strength, and endurance. In D. P. Dirette, & A. G. Sharon (Eds.), *Occupational therapy for physical dysfunction* (8th ed., pp. 197–267). Wolters Kluwer.

Taylor, R. R., Bowyer, P., & Fisher, G. (Eds.). (2024). *Kielhofner's model of human occupation* (6th ed.). Lippincott.

Turpin, M., & Iwama, M. (2011). Kawa (River) model. In M. Turpin, & M. Iwama (Eds.), *Using occupational therapy models in practice: A field guide*. Churchill Livingstone Elsevier.

Yerxa, E. (1988). Oversimplification: The hobgoblin of theory and practice in occupational therapy. *Canadian Journal of Occupational Therapy, 55*(1), 5–7. https://doi.org/10.1177/000841748805500101.

Yerxa, E. J. (2000). Confessions of an occupational therapist who became a detective. *British Journal of Occupational Therapy, 63*(5), 192–199. https://doi.org/10.1177/030802260006300502.

REFLECTION

1. Why are biomechanical strategies considered to be the most common strategy used by occupational therapists working in the field of physical rehabilitation?

2. Why is the use of an occupation-based conceptual model of practice important when implementing biomechanical strategies?

3. Why should occupational therapists use their professional reasoning to determine whether to conduct assessments of biomechanical capacity?

4. Describe the three biomechanical intervention approaches – preventative, restorative and compensatory. Provide occupational therapy examples that illustrate the use of each approach.

5. Explain the purpose of gradation and adaption in relation to biomechanical strategies.

37 MANAGING FATIGUE

ANGELA M. MURPHY ■ MARIA DENISE PESSOA SILVA

CHAPTER OUTLINE

Overview

Fatigue is a common and often complex phenomenon that has a high prevalence across many populations and can be caused by multiple conditions. In this chapter, the prevalence, causes, consequences, assessments and interventions to manage fatigue are described and discussed. An occupational perspective of fatigue is presented to provide an understanding of how to support people living with fatigue to gain control of their lives and to promote occupational participation. Practical tips and resources for working with people who experience fatigue are presented.

KEY POINTS

■ Fatigue is a subjective sense or tiredness or exhaustion, which is often described as persistent and distressing. It is often disproportional to recent activity and does not necessarily respond to usual strategies of energy restoration, such as sleep and rest. Fatigue affects occupational participation and can be measured objectively using a plethora of validated assessments.

■ Fatigue is highly prevalent, not only as a primary complaint within the general population, but also as the primary or secondary symptom to many other prevalent health conditions such as chronic fatigue syndrome, myalgic encephalomyelitis, myalgic encephalopathy, cancer, stroke, multiple sclerosis and long COVID.

■ The causes of fatigue are multidimensional and transdiagnostic, and the precise mechanism through which it manifests is not clearly understood in all conditions. However, while aetiologies may vary or not be completely elucidated, fatigue is broadly experienced in similar ways. Therefore the focus of occupational therapy interventions should be to facilitate occupational participation, taking into account each person's experience and individual needs.

■ A comprehensive occupational therapy assessment is vital to understand how fatigue impacts an individual and hinders normal participation in occupations that matter to them.

■ Occupational therapists can use numerous strategies to educate and empower individuals living with fatigue, as well as to assist them in managing this symptom. These include providing education and advice, helping individuals to plan, prioritise and pace themselves during activities, suggesting and trialling ergonomic positions to promote energy conservation during activities and advising and prescribing equipment and adaptations where appropriate.

THE CONCEPT OF FATIGUE

Fatigue is often described as a subjective sense of tiredness, exhaustion, diminished energy and an increased need to rest, characterised as persistent and distressing (Mota & Pimenta, 2006). Additionally, fatigue is described as disproportionate to changes in activity level or as a symptom that is not relieved by common strategies of energy restoration, such as rest. It is described as interfering with usual functioning and affecting an individual's well-being, participation, engagement and independence (Berger et al., 2010; Mitchell & Berger, 2006).

The experience of fatigue can vary in duration and intensity; it can be defined as recent (lasting less than a month), prolonged (lasting between 1 and 6 months) or chronic (lasting 6 months or more) (Cornuz et al., 2006). There is a distinction between what is considered normal tiredness and pathological fatigue. Healthy individuals will often experience tiredness following physical or mental effort or overexertion, and this usually resolves after rest (Loge et al., 1998). Pathological fatigue is not related to how much a person has done. There may or may not be a clear physiological reason for the fatigue a person is experiencing (Reid et al., 2000).

Fatigue is often experienced as part of a cohort of symptoms, associated with a diagnosis or factor that may determine its cause or physiological mechanism. Examples of diagnoses that may be associated with fatigue include cancer, brain injury and Parkinson's disease. Examples of other factors that may be associated with fatigue include the use of medications and side effects of treatments, such as radiotherapy and chemotherapy. However, fatigue can be idiopathic and unexplained when experienced as a stand-alone symptom and when other diagnoses or factors are ruled out (Reid et al., 2000).

Chronic fatigue can present as a syndrome even when unexplained and is often accompanied by other symptoms, such as difficulties in sleeping, focusing and concentrating, as well as musculoskeletal pain, mood changes, and headaches (Reid et al., 2000). Chronic fatigue syndrome, also known as myalgic encephalomyelitis, is a diagnosis classified by the International Classification of Diseases under code *8E49 Post viral fatigue syndrome*, within Chapter 8: Diseases of the Nervous System (WHO, 2019).

Fatigue can be a secondary symptom, for example, resulting from the side effects of medication, infection, poor sleep, nutrition, or deconditioning (Fox, 2010). Physical deconditioning can result from avoidance of participating in occupations (often to avoid experiencing fatigue), and over time, this can lead to muscle weakness and decreased aerobic capacity (Evans & Lambert, 2007; Fox, 2010). Experiencing fatigue can be distressing, as it impedes the ability of affected people to do the things they need and want to do (Egan & Restall, 2022). It can impede a person's ability to participate in meaningful social interactions, preventing social participation, and influencing physical and mental health and well-being.

Prevalence

Only a small number of studies have investigated the prevalence of fatigue, as an isolated symptom, in the general population (Galland-Decker et al., 2019; Lerdal et al., 2005; Loge et al., 1998). Galland-Decker et al. (2019) assessed the prevalence of fatigue among 2,848 individuals living in Lausanne, Switzerland, aged between 45 and 86 years old. These individuals were assessed with the fatigue severity scale (FSS), which measures fatigue on a scale ranging from 1 to 7 points, 1 being the lowest fatigue experienced and 7 being the highest. They found that 22.1% scored ≥4 in the FSS, whereas 10.9% scored ≥5. Lerdal et al. (2005) assessed a population of 1,893 Norwegians aged 19–81 years old and found that 46.7% scored ≥4 in the FSS, whereas 23.1% scored ≥5. Galland-Decker et al. (2019) attribute this difference to the wider age range that Lerdal et al. (2005) included in their sample. Loge et al. (1998) also studied the prevalence of fatigue in the Norwegian population and found this to be 22% among 2,323 individuals they assessed using the Chalder Fatigue Scale (Chalder et al., 1993).

In chronic fatigue syndrome/myalgic encephalomyelitis, where fatigue is the central symptom, studies of fatigue prevalence are redundant as fatigue is the main determinant in this syndrome. However, the prevalence of chronic fatigue syndrome/myalgic encephalomyelitis in the general population has been studied. A systematic review, which incorporated 1,085,976 participants across 1,291 articles found that the prevalence of chronic fatigue syndrome in the general population is 0.89% (Lim et al., 2020). When participants in the studies included in the systematic review were separated into three different population groups, chronic fatigue syndrome prevalence presented as follows: 1.45% in the general population, 1.62% in specific populations (e.g. nurses and war veterans) and 0.89% in children and adolescents.

There are multiple studies that have investigated the prevalence of fatigue in several conditions, such as cancer, multiple sclerosis, stroke and long COVID. The prevalence of fatigue in each of those conditions is presented in Table 37.1.

Causes

The causes of fatigue are multidimensional and transdiagnostic. Causes for conditions such as chronic fatigue syndrome/myalgic encephalomyelitis are yet to be determined, but consideration is given to genetic, environmental and immunological factors, as well as possible alterations in the neuroendocrine system (among others) (Sapra & Bhandani, 2022). For other conditions, such as multiple sclerosis, stroke and head injury, fatigue is considered to be a primary chronic symptom (Alghamdi et al., 2021; Asano & Finlayson, 2014; Schonberger et al., 2017).

Menting et al. (2018) conducted a study to determine the variance in fatigue severity across chronic diseases. These authors suggest fatigue can be explained by transdiagnostic factors, meaning that individuals may benefit from transdiagnostic approaches, which, instead of focusing on the disease itself, centre on a person's individual needs. Okkes et al. (2002) found that the cause of fatigue was not identified in at least one-third of people who attended primary care with a complaint of fatigue. The remaining two-thirds were ultimately found to have diagnoses ranging between viral illnesses, respiratory tract infections, iron deficiency anaemia, adverse effects of medications, and mental health diagnoses (Okkes et al., 2002).

Despite awareness of pathological causes and the research that has been conducted, fatigue is a subjective experience and often cannot be measured or explained sufficiently in medical terms. Understanding the biological mechanisms that may underlie fatigue is important, as this may contribute to assessment and intervention decisions. However, much of the research on biological mechanisms is still in its infancy.

TABLE 37.1
Prevalence of Fatigue in Different Health Conditions

Type of Study	Health Condition	Sample Size	Fatigue Prevalence	References
Systematic review	Cancer	129 studies with 71,568 individuals	11%–99%[a]	Al Maqbali et al. (2021)
Systematic review	Multiple Sclerosis	54 studies with 22,723 individuals	36.5%–78%	Oliva Ramirez et al. (2021)
Systematic review	Stroke	66 studies with 11,697 individuals	46.79%	Zhan et al. (2022)
Systematic review	Stroke	35 studies with 6,851 individuals	48%	Alghamdi et al. (2021)
Systematic review	Stroke (7 years post stroke)		80%	Pedersen et al. (2022)
Systematic review	Long COVID	52 studies with 127,117 individuals	45.2%	Salari et al. (2022)

[a]The authors attribute the heterogeneity of these figures to the diversity in assessment scales, as well as unique features and treatment options for each cancer type. The overall prevalence was found to be 49%, and in people with advanced cancer, the prevalence of fatigue was 60.6%. Individuals with gastrointestinal cancer, breast cancer and lymphoma presented fatigue prevalence of 50%, 49.7% and 43.3%, respectively.

From Al Maqbali, M., Al Sinani, M., Al Naamani, Z., Al Badi, K., & Tanash, M. I. (2021). Prevalence of fatigue in patients with cancer: A systematic review and meta-analysis. *Journal of Pain and Symptom Management, 61*(1), 167–189.e14. https://doi.org/10.1016/j.jpainsymman.2020.07.037.

Schonberger et al. (2017) carried out a cross-sectional study with people experiencing fatigue resulting from traumatic brain injury to investigate neurological correlates of subjective fatigue and objective fatigability using magnetic resonance imagery (MRI), the FSS and a vigilance task. They found that subjective fatigue did not correlate with measures of brain lesions. However, changes in decision time were significantly predicted by lesions in the right frontal lobe, suggesting decreased functional connectivity of attentional networks. They propose that this can result in increased effort to complete cognitive tasks, influencing a person's energy and fatigue levels. They concluded that the disparate nature of subjective experience and objective measures requires further investigation.

While there may be various aetiologies, there are many similarities in how fatigue is experienced and described (Fox, 2010). Therefore the focus of occupational therapy should be on facilitating occupational participation rather than establishing causative factors.

Consequences of Fatigue

As people strive to live good lives, consistent with their needs, values and aspirations (Egan & Restall, 2022), fatigue can provide a barrier to occupational participation. It can impact people and their families emotionally, socially, mentally, vocationally, physically and spiritually (Van Heest et al., 2017). Fatigue can affect a variety of life domains, including employment, education, personal care, home care, leisure and social relationships (Kos et al., 2015).

Fatigue can be a serious debilitating primary symptom of many conditions and diseases. It can be experienced cognitively and physically, and can have a significant impact on mental and physical health and well-being as an often hidden, invisible and debilitating symptom (Kos et al., 2015). It is often accompanied by other symptoms, including pain, headaches, sleep disturbance, cognitive difficulties, sore throat and swollen glands (NICE, 2021; Pemberton & Berry, 2014).

Fatigue severity may outweigh the severity of the identified or assumed primary cause. For example, a person with mild head injury or multiple sclerosis may experience severe fatigue (Raina et al., 2022). Therefore as with any other condition, gathering the person's narrative descriptions (alongside relevant assessment and outcome measures) is essential to establishing a clear understanding.

Fatigue can significantly impede occupational participation as people can feel overwhelmed at initiating even the smallest task. Therefore fatigue can be a barrier to the person developing their occupational potential and identity (Asaba & Wicks, 2010; Markus & Nurius, 1986; Murphy & Stevenson, 2018).

ASSESSMENT

The first meeting between an occupational therapist and the person experiencing fatigue signals the beginning of the therapeutic relationship. The occupational therapist needs to gain an understanding of the person's history, relationships and contexts (micro, meso and macro) (Egan & Restall, 2022), as well as how fatigue may be limiting occupational participation. An important aspect of this is to establish a rapport and to ensure that the person's experiences are validated, as fatigue is often invisible and misunderstood (Fox, 2010). This stage is an opportunity to provide validation and understanding of the person's experiences and initiate a collaborative relationship.

Hocking and Hammell (2017) state that assessment is a collaborative process, which provides occupational therapists with the necessary knowledge to 'take appropriate action to address people's occupational needs' (p. 171). Potentially because of its multifaceted nature and association with numerous diagnoses, there are many fatigue assessments available (Whitehead, 2009). A number of these assessments are designed for specific diagnoses, and others focus on fatigue as a normal occurrence in life, irrespective of pathological conditions. Fatigue assessments focus on assessing fatigue severity, duration of fatigue and/or the impact of fatigue on everyday activities. Assessments that focus on one single factor, typically the severity of fatigue, are named unidimensional, whereas multi-dimensional assessments aim to measure the intensity of fatigue, as well as its duration, pattern and impact on several domains of a person's life, such as cognition, behaviour and social participation (Whitehead, 2009). Some concerns have been raised about fatigue assessments which rely on memory-based responses, as it is proposed that the outcomes of these types of

TABLE 37.2
Fatigue Assessments

Fatigue Assessments	Domains	Items	Scale Type	Target Population
Fatigue Severity Scale (FSS) Krupp et al. (1989)	Activities of daily living, life participation and sleep	9 items	7-point Likert scale	Multiple sclerosis, chronic fatigue syndrome
Brief Fatigue Inventory (BFI) Groenvold et al. (2000)	Severity and impact	9 items	5-point Likert scale	Cancer, multiple sclerosis and chronic fatigue syndrome
Fatigue Symptom Inventory (FSI) Jason et al. (1999)	Severity, impact, duration	13 items	5-point Likert scale	Cancer General population
European Organization for the Research and Treatment of Cancer - Quality of Life Questionnaire (EORTC QLQ-C30: Fatigue subscale) Aaronson et al. (1993)	Fatigue	4 items	4-point Likert scale	Cancer
Fatigue Scale for Motor and Cognitive Functions (FASMCF) Larun et al. (2006)	Motor and cognitive fatigue	20 items	5-point Likert scale	Multiple sclerosis
Fatigue Impact Scale (FIS) Fisk et al. (1994)	Physical, cognitive and psychosocial	36 items	5-point Likert scale	Multiple sclerosis, fibromyalgia, chronic fatigue syndrome, rheumatoid arthritis and cancer
Multidimensional Fatigue Inventory (MFI-20) Smets et al. (1995)	General fatigue, mental, physical, reduced motivation, reduced activity	20 items	7-point Likert scale	Chronic fatigue syndrome, cancer and other conditions
Brief Mental Fatigue Questionnaire (BMFQ) Kim and Kim (2011)	Mental	9 items	5-point Likert scale	Physical or psychiatric diagnoses
Functional Assessment of Chronic Illness Therapy – fatigue Subscale (FACIT-F) Sklar et al. (1997)	Impact and severity	13 items	5-point Likert scale	Chronic conditions

assessments may misrepresent the construct being measured (Juengst et al., 2019; Lenaert et al., 2022; Van den Bergh & Walentynowicz, 2016).

A set of parameters and characteristics have been identified to assist with determining which fatigue assessment to use. An evaluation of fatigue assessments should include (Kirkova et al., 2006; Shields et al., 2006):

- Scale usability, i.e. whether the instrument is easy to understand and complete;
- Clinical/research utility, i.e. sensitivity and specificity of assessment to discriminate between cases and non-cases;
- Sensitivity to measure changes; and
- Robust psychometric properties, i.e. precision, reproducibility and accuracy.

There is a wide variety of fatigue assessments frequently and broadly used in practice. They each focus on different criteria and domains of fatigue, and have been developed for use within various populations and for specific conditions of which fatigue is a symptom. A selection of fatigue assessments is presented in Table 37.2.

FATIGUE APPROACHES AND INTERVENTIONS

As with any intervention, fatigue management must also be person-centred (Bakker et al., 2019). The individuality of each person who is experiencing fatigue and their micro, meso and macro contexts must always be considered to inform the co-design of the occupational therapy process (Egan & Restall, 2022) (refer to Chapter 11). Occupational therapists must always check for contraindications of strategies that are specific to the condition the person has, as well as examine and explore up-to-date research to inform professional reasoning.

This section presents several interventions for fatigue management, providing strategies for establishing occupational balance, gaining control over fatigue and aiming for more meaningful occupational participation. Strategies are presented in no specific order. The order used in practice is multifactorial and relies upon the co-creation of goals and discussion of the required conditions for success (Egan & Restall, 2022).

Establishing occupational balance tends to be an earlier requirement of the therapy process, as monitoring and then adjusting occupational participation can be easier to execute than challenging thoughts and feelings. Many of the strategies and interventions are strength-based, problem-solving approaches that rely on core occupational therapy skills.

Establishing Occupational Balance

Wagman et al. (2012) define occupational balance as 'the experience of having the right amount of occupations and the right variation between occupations in the right occupational pattern' (p. 326). The environmental pressures placed on individuals can be overwhelming, leading to occupational imbalance, ill health and sickness (Håkansson et al., 2009). Håkansson et al. (2009) investigated the experiences of participation in daily occupations and their association with health and well-being. They found that a person's perception of manageability, personal meaning and balance were indicators of a person's occupational balance and feelings of health and well-being. They stated that 'experiencing manageability means perceiving that the demands of the occupational pattern do not exceed the personal and contextual resources the individual is able to mobilise' (p. 111). In the context of managing fatigue, this means establishing a pattern of occupation that does not exceed personal resources.

Achieving an occupational balance can be quite complex and is not merely focusing on balancing different occupations into equal portions. Rather, it is a concept that focuses on need satisfaction, levels of meaningfulness, types of occupation (Håkansson

et al., 2020) and manageability (Håkansson et al., 2009). It can be seen as a match between actual and desired occupational participation (Matuska, 2012), with high levels of meaningful occupational participation in tandem with low levels of unmet occupational needs (Eakman, 2015), as well as a balance between types of occupation, abilities, resources, and meeting personal needs and those of others (Dür et al., 2014).

Occupational therapists can support people with fatigue to establish occupational balance. The Occupational Balance Questionnaire (Wagman & Håkansson, 2014) can provide some insights into what may be impacting a person's occupational balance. For example, asking about the balance of activities completed for self and others allows exploration of where a person's energy may be focused. Asking how meaningful occupations are may assist with establishing satisfaction and consideration of the balance obtained between occupations that are perceived to be energy giving compared to energy taking. Perception of energy as a commodity that needs protection or conservation can help build awareness, analogies, and metaphors that can be useful aids to support understanding. Occupational Participation Schedules (Pemberton & Berry, 2014) can also help establish a person's occupational participation through identifying whether they have access to, and can initiate and sustain the occupations that they find meaningful and purposeful (Egan & Restall, 2022). It is, therefore, proposed that fatigue management can support a person to access, initiate and sustain their occupational participation.

Occupational Participation Schedules

Occupational Participation Schedules are used to gather the information that an occupational therapist and the person experiencing fatigue can collaboratively analyse. The patterns to observe relate to:

1. how the person's fatigue presents;
2. areas of satisfaction;
3. areas of dissatisfaction; and
4. areas of possible change/adaptation.

The occupational therapist would usually demonstrate how to use the Occupational Participation Schedules and then ask the person to regularly record their participation. The Schedules provide an occupation-focused method of information gathering where individuals can record their occupational participation and ascribe a score to their fatigue (10 = the worst it has ever been and 0 = no fatigue).

It should be noted that the use of Occupational Participation Schedules relies on motivation and the ability to be organised and engage cognitively. The completion of the Schedules may be supported by a carer or family member who knows the person, if the person has difficulty in writing. It is advisable to discuss whether this is a realistic method for the person in question, and if not, explore alternative methods of understanding their fatigue and its impact. For example, audio recording or picture communication symbols to record occupational participation and fatigue levels may work for some.

The Occupational Participation Schedules can assist a person to understand the impact of fatigue and consider how to manage their fatigue levels. By supporting the person to plan, pace and grade their participation, the Occupational Participation Schedules can identify how control is being gained, and thereby contribute to increasing a person's occupational participation.

Analysing and Modifying Occupations to Establish a Baseline

A combined rehabilitative approach that includes education and exercise has been found to be an effective way to manage fatigue (Asano & Finlayson, 2014; Kim et al., 2022; Kos et al., 2015; Salome et al., 2019). When referring to aerobic exercise, the occupations include walking, swimming, cycling and dancing.

The CanMOP (Egan & Restall, 2022) encourages occupational therapists to look beyond performance and towards participation, which is defined as 'having access to, initiating and sustaining valued occupations within meaningful relationships and contexts' (Egan & Restall, 2022, p. 76) (refer to Chapter 11). However, a challenge for many people living with fatigue is that they themselves compare how life is in the present with how life was in the past, and this then impacts their perceptions of how they believe life may be in the future. This may lead to loss of motivation and, in turn, influence daily occupational participation, so the person either tries to do as much as they used to do in the past (boom), leading to increased symptoms, or they avoid participation (slump), sometimes believing the occupation may cause harm and/or additional symptoms, which in the long-term can lead to occupational deprivation. Often a boom/slump pattern of occupational participation slowly evolves (Pemberton & Berry, 2014), adding to the confusion of onlookers who are unable to understand why something was possible one day and not another.

A common response to feeling fatigued and limited in energy is to do as much as possible when there is the slightest hint of energy. Therefore it is helpful to begin to think of energy as a commodity. Using analogies, such as how a mobile telephone battery works, can be helpful. For example, how it responds when it is completely flat, requiring a longer time to recharge, compared to one that is regularly topped up, can be used to explain how having regular rests can be helpful.

Once the impact of fatigue is understood, collaborative problem-solving can identify new and adapted ways of promoting occupational participation. A common approach to this is the self-management advice, commonly referred to as the 5 Ps (Cooper, 2006):

1. Planning (making a list, scheduling and allocating rest periods);
2. Prioritising (what do they want and need to do?);
3. Pacing (slowing down, taking breaks and doing one thing at a time);
4. Positioning (choosing a posture that will help them save energy) and
5. Permission (self-permission to ask others for help and to take rests).

An advice sheet on the 5 Ps and how they can be used for advice and self-management for people experiencing fatigue is presented in Box 37.1.

Once the person with fatigue has practised balancing their occupations within a baseline of not too much and not too little, occupational participation can be gradually increased. However, fatigue caused by some conditions may require careful monitoring, as grading too fast may result in payback (worsened fatigue). Payback fatigue (Parslow et al., 2018) often occurs later (after participation) and is perceived to occur because of participating in occupations excessively. Therefore ceasing participation before energy levels have depleted too far through establishing good patterns of rest can be helpful within the process of establishing a baseline.

BOX 37.1
FATIGUE MANAGEMENT ADVICE SHEET FOR PEOPLE EXPERIENCING FATIGUE – THE 5 Ps

Fatigue can affect people in many ways. It most commonly presents as physical exhaustion, but it can also be manifested as emotional and cognitive tiredness, affecting all areas of daily life.

Here are some self-management strategies that may help manage fatigue, commonly named 'The 5 Ps': Planning, Prioritising, Pacing, Positioning and Permission.

PLANNING

Planning means, in fact, writing up a plan of the occupations that are intended to be accomplished on a given day. When writing the occupations down, it is useful to try to identify which ones are likely to demand more energy. It is helpful to think that occupations that include standing up when cooking, moving around when cleaning a house or maintaining concentration for long periods of time, such as reading and sending emails are the ones that demand more energy. Keeping an occupational diary to identify when you feel more energised can also help. It is important to know when you feel more energised so that you can plan activities around these times and optimise the use of energy.

PRIORITISING

There is no secret about this one. Prioritising means choosing the most important occupation from your plan, the things you must accomplish. This means focusing on the most important tasks and identifying the ones that may be postponed or delegated for someone else to do or help with. For example, you may decide paying a bill is more important than washing up, or doing something fun with a loved one may have higher importance than cleaning the house.

PACING

Pacing has two different aspects in fatigue management. One of them is not rushing and allowing time to complete an activity; it is also understanding that it is acceptable to do tasks more slowly, and to not complete a certain task as quickly as other people or as fast as you used to do in the past. The second aspect of pacing is introducing regular breaks and time for recovery, especially during longer activities, such as going out to the park for a long walk.

POSITIONING

Positioning is about being aware of which position you adopt when performing a certain occupation, and opting for positions that involve sitting down rather than standing up, and those which offer support to other areas of the body, such as the back and arms. When you adopt supportive positions for a certain task, you can focus more energy on the task itself, rather than wasting energy trying to maintain your posture. If you want to bake a cake, for example, it is a good idea to set up a table with all ingredients within your reach. This way, you can bake while sitting and focus your energy on the activity, rather than wasting energy standing up and walking around the kitchen to fetch ingredients. Your occupational therapist can help you identify which equipment might benefit you and help you save energy in everyday activities, such as cooking, showering and dressing.

PERMISSION

Permission has two different aspects as far as energy conservation is concerned. One of them is understanding that it is acceptable to ask for help. This means asking and allowing other people to help, as well as giving yourself permission to delegate tasks. The other aspect of permission is respecting your own limits, allowing yourself to rest and to choose not to do something when you are running out of energy to do so.

How we Think Influences What we do and how we Adapt to Change

Moss-Morris et al. (2021); Van Kessel et al. (2008) and Mohr et al. (2003) found that a cognitive approach to managing fatigue in multiple sclerosis was effective, and White et al. (2011) found cognitive behavioural therapy (CBT) effective for people with chronic fatigue syndrome/myalgic encephalomyelitis. Occupational therapists assist people to understand the impact that thoughts and feelings can have on occupational participation and vice versa. The reciprocal interaction between thoughts and feelings and occupational participation has been found to be beneficial for fatigue management (Asano & Finlayson, 2014). Occupational therapists can help people with fatigue identify any unhelpful thoughts that perpetuate unhelpful patterns of occupational participation, such as doing too little, leading to deconditioning, or doing too much, leading to extreme fatigue.

Automatic thoughts are common, and thoughts that begin with words such as 'I should' 'I must' and 'I can't' can be barriers to managing fatigue, perpetuating a boom/slump pattern. For example, '*I should always put 100% into what I do*' prevents balance and facilitates forcing occupational participation beyond a person's capacity (Moore & Redmond, 2014). Similarly, negative thoughts, such as '*I'm useless if I can't do this*' can lead to negative feelings and have a negative impact on occupational participation. Some of these types of thoughts come from personal assumptions that work as guides to how a person behaves, and some link also to core beliefs, which are often about how a person feels about themselves or others (Moore & Redmond, 2014). Often these types of thoughts are based on assumptions rather than facts. Occupational therapists can support people with fatigue to challenge unhelpful assumptions, and the thoughts that accompany them through exploring together the impact they have on occupational participation. Working collaboratively with the person to identify the impact that thoughts have on occupational participation can be done through thought diaries and building self-awareness around motivations for occupational participation.

How to Manage Cognitive Fatigue

There is emerging evidence confirming a high prevalence of cognitive dysfunction in individuals experiencing fatigue originating from chronic medical conditions. In their systematic review, Menzies et al. (2021) found significant correlations between fatigue and cognitive dysfunction in studies with individuals diagnosed with cancer, chronic fatigue syndrome and multiple sclerosis. The association between fatigue and cognitive difficulties, regardless of whether the former is the cause or consequence of the latter, can be particularly detrimental to a person's ability to participate in personal and practical activities of daily living and actively engage in occupations, such as leisure and work.

The interventions proposed for memory rehabilitation are compensatory and include the use of memory aids, strategies for paying attention, minimising distractions and teaching people alternative ways of processing, storing and retrieving information. These management techniques, which involve training and repetition of cognitive tasks, are believed to activate neural networks, although the exact mechanism through which cognitive rehabilitation occurs is still imprecise (Taylor et al., 2021).

Interventions commonly applied to improve the cognitive function of people with multiple sclerosis have been shown to be effective (das Nair et al., 2012; Rosti-Otajärvi & Hämäläinen, 2014; Taylor et al., 2021). Cancer-related fatigue has been described as containing cognitive, physical and emotional dimensions. The cognitive difficulties presented by people with cancer have been named 'chemo brain' or 'brain fog' and more formally defined as 'cancer-related cognitive impairment' (CRCI). This has been reported to affect as many as 75% of people with gynaecologic cancer receiving chemotherapy (Craig et al., 2014), with a prevalence of between 17% and 33% across all people with cancer who are receiving chemotherapy (Huehnchen et al., 2020).

CRCI can be characterised by difficulties affecting an individual's memory, attention and concentration, processing speed and executive functions (Lange & Joly, 2017). These difficulties can hamper an individual's ability to concentrate, multitask and remember words and names. Ultimately, these difficulties have the potential to diminish a person's quality of life and affect their occupational participation. These symptoms usually subside within 6 to 12 months following chemotherapy completion; however, there are reports of persistent cognitive impairment lasting as long as 20 years post chemotherapy (Koppelmans et al., 2012; Yamada et al., 2010).

Fatigue education and management are often deployed as a therapeutic approach in practice to help people manage cognitive difficulties arising from cancer and cancer treatment. Other interventions for CRCI include compensatory strategies, presential or web-based cognitive rehabilitation programmes, physical activities, and relaxation programmes (Joly et al., 2019; Liang et al., 2019).

The management of cognitive impairments for people with chronic fatigue syndrome focuses on strategies, including cognitive pacing (focusing on one task at a time), sleep hygiene, use of caffeine or short-acting stimulants (if well tolerated), minimising sensory input, such as noise and light, by using earplugs and eye masks, and use of simple memory aids, such as note-taking and calendar reminders (Bateman et al., 2021; US ME/CFS Clinician Coalition, 2021).

The practice story in Box 37.2 illustrates how an occupational therapist can work with a person experiencing fatigue.

BOX 37.2
BARBARA

Occupational Participation: Barbara is a 76-year-old lady who describes fatigue that is generalised and fluctuates in severity throughout the day. Barbara's occupational participation involves making all meals and completing household tasks. She also enjoys shopping, socialising, reading and gardening.

History and Relationships: Barbara is a wife, mother, friend, colleague and sister. She worked in a bakery and a college canteen until her fatigue prevented her from continuing. She enjoys meeting with friends during shopping trips. She has two daughters who live locally.

Possibilities, access, initiate, sustain: Barbara is finding her usual routines and habits increasingly difficult to access, initiate and sustain. Her occupational participation tends to take on a boom/slump pattern. She expresses frustration at her daily limitations and would like to gain greater control. She has access to support from her daughters and can afford to pay for help around the home.

Context – micro, meso, macro: Barbara and her family live in an industrial city, where there have been historically high levels of unemployment. The city she has lived in her whole life was bombed almost beyond recognition during World War II. Her formative years were spent at local state schools, while her father worked in shipyards and her mother was a housekeeper. There were very few expectations of Barbara from an academic perspective as a white working-class female. Similarly, resources were limited, leading to lifetime frugality.

Canadian Occupational Therapy Inter-Relation Practice Process (Restall et al., 2022) (refer to Chapter 12)

Seek understanding and define purpose: The beginning of the therapeutic relationship focused on co-creating the conditions for how Barbara and the occupational therapist would work together. This is informed by the collaborative relationship-focused occupational therapy (Restall & Egan, 2022) and involves hearing Barbara's narrative and lived experience of living with fatigue and its impact on occupational participation within the context of her cultural surroundings. The occupational therapist, aware of her own culturally informed perspectives, asked questions relating to contextual factors to identify Barbara's cultural values, priorities and potential barriers. The occupational therapist found that Barbara identified asking for help and resting as challenging, feeling she should be allocating 100% of her energy to her valued occupations. It was agreed that the aim of occupational therapy would be to support Barbara to access, initiate and sustain meaningful occupational participation. Through discussion it was also established that some barriers to changing some aspects of occupational participation related to her own and others' beliefs. This reflective discussion acknowledged Barbara's entitlements to make decisions for herself. The Functional Assessment of Chronic Illness Therapy – Fatigue Subscale (FACIT-F) (Sklar et al., 1997) was used as part of the initial assessment with Barbara to provide a rating of her fatigue. Barbara scored 30/52, indicating moderate-to-severe impact of fatigue on occupational participation.

Explore occupational participation: Barbara's occupational participation was discussed and observed while she carried out her prioritised occupations. She then described how she found the participation process. She was often overambitious with planning which occupations to participate in, and was frustrated and disappointed when fatigue became a barrier to sustainability of doing occupations.

Co-design priorities, goals, outcomes and plans: A plan with the general aim of 'enjoying life despite fatigue' was established with a specific goal of Barbara wishing to explore options for fatigue management, including understanding fatigue, grading, pacing and adapting her occupations to establish whether any strategies could help in managing her fatigue to establish a better occupational balance and, therefore, gain what could be perceived as control over her fatigue. Barbara's goal in her words was 'I would like to gain some control over my fatigue, rather than it controlling me. This will mean spending more quality time with my family and friends and doing the things I love, such as gardening and reading'.

Trial the plan, explore change and refine the plan: The occupational therapist discussed with Barbara, how to use occupation schedules; how to pace, grade and adapt occupations to enable occupational participation without resulting in severe fatigue. Barbara trialled the schedules, discussed her findings with her occupational therapist, and tried altering how she performed her valued occupations, according to her subjective experiences of fatigue during and after occupational participation and perceived acceptable alterations to her occupational patterns.

The schedules identified that severe fatigue occurred after preparing meals and carrying out household tasks, resulting in frustration at having less energy for her prioritised pleasurable occupations. Therefore Barbara decided to delegate household tasks, prioritise and carefully plan time with her family and use pre-prepared meals (her daughter offered to batch cook meals which could be easily prepared). She set targets for reading and gardening for a maximum amount of time doing both, which could be gradually increased or decreased, depending on what felt appropriate. Barbara tried listening to an audio book, used some light, long-handled equipment for gardening and decided upon rest periods (having established what a rest could meaningfully entail). Barbara began to plan carefully how days out with her family could be managed realistically by identifying good venues, using a wheelchair for anything involving long walks, setting time limits of what was realistic and reasonable, while still allowing enjoyment and sustainability of her valued occupations.

Plan for transition: Once Barbara felt more in control of her fatigue and was able to access, initiate and sustain her occupational participation with greater enjoyment and satisfaction, the process of discharge was discussed. Barbara completed the FACIT-F (Sklar et al., 1997) as a follow-up assessment and was pleased to see that her score had changed from 30/52 to 41/52. She now found it easier to start and complete tasks, felt less frustrated, and enjoyed her social occupations more.

CONCLUSION

Fatigue is described as a subjective sense of tiredness, exhaustion, diminished energy and increased need to rest, characterised as persistent, distressing (Mota & Pimenta, 2006) and disproportionate to occupational participation (Berger et al., 2010; Mitchell & Berger, 2006).

Its prevalence is high among many long-term conditions such as stroke, multiple sclerosis, head injury, cancer and chronic fatigue syndrome/myalgic encephalomyelitis. It can be a primary or secondary symptom which has debilitating effects on accessing, initiating and sustaining occupational participation and, therefore, leads to further decline in health and well-being.

There are numerous assessments used to assess fatigue. Occupational therapy interventions can involve firstly understanding the fatigue and its impact, establishing occupational balance through planning, prioritising and managing occupations, resulting in empowerment and greater sustainability of meaningful and purposeful occupational participation. This leads to gaining control, which empowers and facilitates access, initiation and sustainability of occupational participation and engagement (Egan & Restall, 2022) for those whose lives it affects.

Ultimately it is essential that occupational therapists are aware of the skills and value they can add to the lives of people who experience the debilitating effects of fatigue. Occupational therapists play a pivotal role in supporting people who experience fatigue to lead more fulfilling and productive lives through meaningful management of fatigue.

REFERENCES

Aaronson, N. K., Ahmedzai, S., Bergman, B., Bullinger, M., Cull, A., Duez, N. J., Filiberti, A., Flechtner, H., Fleishman, S. B., & de Haes, J. C. (1993). The European Organisation for Research and Treatment of Cancer QLQ-C30: A quality-of-life instrument for use in international clinical trials in oncology. *Journal of the National Cancer Institute, 85*(5), 365–376.

Al Maqbali, M., Al Sinani, M., Al Naamani, Z., Al Badi, K., & Tanash, M. I. (2021). Prevalence of fatigue in patients with cancer: A systematic review and meta-analysis. *Journal of Pain and Symptom Management, 61*(1), 167–189.e14. https://doi.org/10.1016/j.jpainsymman.2020.07.037.

Alghamdi, I., Ariti, C., Williams, A., Wood, E., & Hewitt, J. (2021). Prevalence of fatigue after stroke: A systematic review and meta-analysis. *European Stroke Journal, 6*(4), 319–332. https://doi.org/10.1177/23969873211047681.

Asaba, E., & Wicks, A. (2010). Occupational terminology. *Journal of Occupational Science, 17*(2), 120–124. https://doi.org/10.1080/14427591.2010.9686683.

Asano, M., & Finlayson, M. L. (2014). Meta-analysis of three different types of fatigue management interventions for people with multiple sclerosis: Exercise, education, and medication. *Multiple Sclerosis International*, 798285. https://doi.org/10.1155/2014/798285.

Bakker, K., Steultjens, E., & Price, L. (2019). The lived experiences of adults with a visual impairment who experience fatigue when performing daily activities. *British Journal of Occupational Therapy, 82*(8), 485–492. https://doi.org/10.1177/0308022619841491.

Bateman, L., Bested, A. C., Bonilla, H. F., Chheda, B. V., Chu, L., Curtin, J. M., Dempsey, T. T., Dimmock, M. E., Dowell, T. G., Felsenstein, D., Kaufman, D. L., Klimas, N. G., Komaroff, A. L., Lapp, C. W., Levine, S. M., Montoya, J. G., Natelson, B. H., Peterson, D. L., Podell, R. N., … Yellman, B. P. (2021). Myalgic encephalomyelitis/chronic fatigue syndrome: Essentials of diagnosis and management. *Mayo Clinic Proceedings, 96*(11), 2861–2878. https://doi.org/10.1016/j.mayocp.2021.07.004.

Berger, A. M., Abernethy, A. P., Atkinson, A., Barsevick, A. M., Breitbart, W. S., Cella, D., Cimprich, B., Cleeland, C., Eisenberger, M. A., Escalante, C. P., Jacobsen, P. B., Kaldor, P., Ligibel, J. A., Murphy, B. A., O'Connor, T., Pirl, W. F., Rodler, E., Rugo, H. S., Thomas, J., & Wagner, L. I. (2010). NCCN clinical practice guidelines cancer-related fatigue. *Journal of the National Comprehensive Cancer Network, 8*(8), 904–931. https://doi.org/10.6004/jnccn.2010.0067.

Chalder, T., Berelowitz, G., Pawlikowska, T., Watts, L., Wessely, S., Wright, D., & Wallace, E. P. (1993). Development of a fatigue scale. *Journal of Psychosomatic Research, 37*(2), 147–153. https://doi.org/10.1016/0022-3999(93)90081-P.

Cooper, J. (2006). *Occupational therapy in oncology and palliative care* (2nd ed). Wiley Appendix 15.

Cornuz, J., Guessous, I., & Favrat, B. (2006). Fatigue: A practical approach to diagnosis in primary care. *Canadian Medical Association Journal, 174*(6), 765–767. https://doi.org/10.1503/cmaj.1031153.

Craig, C. D., Monk, B. J., Farley, J. H., & Chase, D. M. (2014). Cognitive impairment in gynecologic cancers: A systematic review of current approaches to diagnosis and treatment. *Supportive Care in Cancer, 22*(1), 279–287. https://doi.org/10.1007/s00520-013-1961-8.

das Nair, R., Ferguson, H., Stark, D. L., & Lincoln, N. B. (2012). Memory rehabilitation for people with multiple sclerosis. *Cochrane Database of Systematic Reviews*, (3), CD008754. https://doi.org/10.1002/14651858.CD008754.pub2.

Dür, M., Steiner, G., Fialka-Moser, V., Kautzky-Willer, A., Dejaco, C., Prodinger, B., Stoffer, M. A., Binder, A., Smolen, J., & Stamm, T. A. (2014). Development of a new occupational balance-questionnaire: Incorporating the perspectives of patients and healthy people in the design of a self-reported occupational balance outcome instrument. *Health and Quality of Life Outcomes, 12*, 45. https://doi.org/10.1186/1477-7525-12-45.

Eakman, A. M. (2015). The meaningful activity wants and needs assessment: A perspective on life balance. *Journal of Occupational*

Science, 22(2), 210–227. https://doi.org/10.1080/14427591.2013.7
69405.

Egan, M., & Restall, G. (2022). Canadian model of occupational participation: Collaborative relationship-focused occupational therapy. In M. Egan, & G. Restall (Eds.), *Promoting occupational participation: Collaborative relationship-focused occupational therapy* (pp. 76–82). Canadian Association of Occupational Therapists.

Evans, W. J., & Lambert, C. P. (2007). Physiological basis of fatigue. *American Journal of Physical Medicine and Rehabilitation, 86*(1 Suppl), S29–S46. https://doi.org/10.1097/phm.0b013e31802ba53c.

Fisk, J. D., Ritvo, P. G., Ross, L., & Hauser, S. L. (1994). The fatigue impact scale: Validation of a new measure of the impact of fatigue on patients with multiple sclerosis. *Clinical Rehabilitation, 8*(4), 356–364.

Fox, K. (2010). *Fatigue management in chronic illness: Implications for use in a one: one occupational therapy session*. University of Illinois-Chicago: Department of Occupational Therapy.

Galland-Decker, C., Marques-Vidal, P., & Vollenweider, P. (2019). Prevalence and factors associated with fatigue in the Lausanne middle-aged population: A population-based, cross-sectional survey. *BMJ Open, 9*(8), e027070. https://doi.org/10.1136/bmjopen-2018-027070.

Groenvold, M., Aaronson, N. K., Bjordal, K., Hagen, R., Kaasa, S., & Aass, N. (2000). Fatigue in cancer patients who participated in phase III trials—The development and psychometric properties of a brief fatigue inventory (BFI). *Journal of Pain and Symptom Management, 20*(2), 113–123.

Håkansson, C., Lissner, L., Björkelund, C., & Sonn, U. (2009). Engagement in patterns of daily occupations and perceived health among women of working age. *Scandinavian Journal of Occupational Therapy, 16*(2), 110–117. https://doi.org/10.1080/11038120802572494.

Håkansson, C., Wagman, P., & Hagell, P. (2020). Construct validity of a revised version of the Occupational Balance Questionnaire. *Scandinavian Journal of Occupational Therapy, 27*(6), 441–449. https://doi.org/10.1080/11038128.2019.1660801.

Hocking, C., & Hammell, K. W. (2017). Process of assessment. In M. Curtin, J. B. Molineux, & M. Supyk-Mellson (Eds.), *Occupational therapy for people experiencing illness, injury or impairment* (7th ed., pp. 171). Elsevier.

Huehnchen, P., van Kampen, A., Boehmerle, W., & Endres, M. (2020). Cognitive impairment after cytotoxic chemotherapy. *Neuro Oncology Practice, 7*(1), 11–21. https://doi.org/10.1093/nop/npz052.

Jason, L. A., Richman, J. A., Rademaker, A. W., Jordan, K. M., Plioplys, A. V., Taylor, R. R., Johnson, J. S., & Plioplys, S. (1999). A brief fatigue inventory for primary care. *Journal of Psychosomatic Research, 47*(1), 91–100.

Joly, F., Lange, M., Dos Santos, M., Vaz-Luis, I., & Di Meglio, A. (2019). Long-term fatigue and cognitive disorders in breast cancer survivors. *Cancers (Basel), 11*(12), 1896. https://doi.org/10.3390/cancers11121896.

Juengst, S. B., Terhorst, L., Kew, C. L., & Wagner, A. K. (2019). Variability in daily self-reported emotional symptoms and fatigue

measured over eight weeks in community dwelling individuals with traumatic brain injury. *Brain Injury, 33*(5), 567–573. https://doi.org/10.1080/02699052.2019.1584333.

Kim, H., & Kim, Y. (2011). Development and validation of the brief mental fatigue questionnaire. *Journal of Clinical Neurology, 7*(2), 103–110.

Kim, S., Xu, Y., Dore, K., Gewurtz, R., Larivière, N., & Letts, L. (2022). Fatigue self-management led by occupational therapists and/or physiotherapists for chronic conditions: A systematic review and meta-analysis. *Chronic Illness, 18*(3), 441–457. https://doi.org/10.1177/17423953211039783.

Kirkova, J., Davis, M. P., Walsh, D., Tiernan, E., O'Leary, N., LeGrand, S. B., Lagman, R. L., & Russell, K. M. (2006). Cancer symptom assessment instruments: A systematic review. *Journal of Clinical Oncology, 24*(9), 1459–1473.

Koppelmans, V., Breteler, M. M., Boogerd, W., Seynaeve, C., Gundy, C., & Schagen, S. B. (2012). Neuropsychological performance in survivors of breast cancer more than 20 years after adjuvant chemotherapy. *Journal of Clinical Oncology, 30*(10), 1080–1086. https://doi.org/10.1200/JCO.2011.37.0189.

Kos, D., Inge van Eupen, J., Meirte, J., Van Cauwenbergh, D., Moorkens, G., Meeus, M., & Nijs, J. (2015). Activity pacing self-management in chronic fatigue syndrome: A randomised controlled trial. *American Journal of Occupational Therapy, 69*(5), 6905290020p1–6905290020p11. https://doi.org/10.5014/ajot.2015.016287.

Krupp, L. B., LaRocca, N. G., Muir-Nash, J., & Steinberg, A. D. (1989). The fatigue severity scale: Application to patients with multiple sclerosis and systemic lupus erythematosus. *Archives of Neurology, 46*(10), 1121–1123.

Lange, M., & Joly, F. (2017). How to identify and manage cognitive dysfunction after breast cancer treatment. *Journal of Oncology Practice, 13*(12), 784–790. https://doi.org/10.1200/JOP.2017.026286.

Larun, L., Wilhelmsen-Langeland, A., Ekeland, A. G., Vøllestad, N. K., & Stanghelle, J. K. (2006). The fatigue scale for motor and cognitive functions (FASMCF): Reliability and construct validity. *Clinical Neurophysiology, 117*(6), 1217–1222. https://doi.org/10.1016/j.clinph.2006.01.010.

Lenaert, B., van Kampen, N., van Heugten, C., & Ponds, R. (2022). Real-time measurement of post-stroke fatigue in daily life and its relationship with the retrospective fatigue severity scale. *Neuropsychological Rehabilitation, 32*(6), 992–1006. https://doi.org/10.1080/09602011.2020.1854791.

Lerdal, A., Wahl, A. K., Rustøen, T., Hanestad, B. R., & Moum, T. (2005). Fatigue in the general population: A translation and test of the psychometric properties of the Norwegian version of the fatigue severity scale. *Scandinavian Journal of Public Health, 33*(2), 123–130. https://doi.org/10.1080/14034940410028406.

Liang, M. I., Erich, B., Bailey, C., Jo, M. Y., Walsh, C. S., & Asher, A. (2019). Emerging from the Haze: A pilot study evaluating feasibility of a psychoeducational intervention to improve cancer-related cognitive impairment in gynecologic cancer survivors. *Journal of Palliative Care, 34*(1), 32–37. https://doi.org/10.1177/0825859718796794.

Lim, E. J., Ahn, Y. C., Jang, E. S., Lee, S. W., Lee, S. H., & Son, C. G. (2020). Systematic review and meta-analysis of the prevalence of chronic fatigue syndrome/myalgic encephalomyelitis (CFS/ME). *Journal of Translational Medicine, 18*(1), 100. https://doi.org/10.1186/s12967-020-02269-0.

Loge, J. H., Ekeberg, O., & Kaasa, S. (1998). Fatigue in the general Norwegian population: Normative data and associations. *Journal of Psychosomatic Research, 45*(1), 53–65. https://doi.org/10.1016/S0022-3999(97)00291-5.

Markus, H., & Nurius, P. (1986). Possible selves. *American Psychologist, 41*(9), 954–969. https://doi.org/10.1037/0003-066X.41.9.954.

Matuska, K. (2012). Description and development of the life balance inventory. *OTJR Occupation Participation & Health, 32*(1), 220–228. https://doi.org/10.3928/15394492-20110610-01.

Menting, J., Tack, C. J., Bleijenberg, G., Donders, R., Droogleever Fortuyn, H. A., Fransen, J., Goedendorp, M. M., Kalkman, J. S., Strik-Albers, R., van Alfen, N., van der Werf, S. P., Voermans, N. C., van Engelen, B. G., & Knoop, H. (2018). Is fatigue a disease-specific or generic symptom in chronic medical conditions? *Health Psychology, 37*(6), 530–543. https://doi.org/10.1037/hea0000598.

Menzies, V., Kelly, D. L., Yang, G. S., Starkweather, A., & Lyon, D. E. (2021). A systematic review of the association between fatigue and cognition in chronic noncommunicable diseases. *Chronic Illness, 17*(2), 129–150. https://doi.org/10.1177/1742395319836472.

Mitchell, S., & Berger, A. (2006). Cancer related fatigue: The evidence base for assessment and management. *Cancer Journal, 12*, 374–387. https://doi.org/10.1097/00130404-200609000-00007.

Mohr, D. C., Hart, S. L., & Goldberg, A. (2003). Effects of treatment for depression on fatigue in multiple sclerosis. *Psychosomatic Medicine, 65*, 542–547.

Moore, S., & Redmond, C. (2014). Thoughts and feelings. In S. Pemberton, & C. Berry (Eds.), *Fighting fatigue: A practical guide to managing the symptoms of CFS/ME* (pp. 114–149). Hammersmith Books.

Moss Morris, R., Harrison, A. M., Safari, R., Norton, S., van der Linden, M. L., Picariello, F., Thomas, S., White, C., & Mercer, T. (2021). Which behavioural and exercise interventions targeting fatigue show the most promise in multiple sclerosis? A systematic review with narrative synthesis and meta-analysis. *Behaviour Research and Therapy, 137*, 103464. https://doi.org/10.1016/j.brat.2019.103464.

Mota, D. D. C. F., & Pimenta, C. A. M. (2006). Self-report instruments for fatigue assessment: A systematic review. *Research and Theory for Nursing Practice, 20*(1), 49–78. https://doi.org/10.1891/rtnp.20.1.49.

Murphy, A., & Stevenson, J. (2018). Occupational potential and possible selves of masters level healthcare students with dyslexia: A narrative inquiry. *Journal of Occupational Science, 26*(1), 18–28. https://doi.org/10.1080/14427591.2018.1517387.

National Institute for Clinical Excellence (NICE). (2021). Myalgic encephalomyelitis (or encephalopathy)/chronic fatigue syndrome: Diagnosis and management, NICE Guideline 206. Retrieved 23rd May 2023, from https://www.nice.org.uk/guidance/ng206.

Okkes, I. M., Oskam, S. K., & Lamberts, H. (2002). The probability of specific diagnoses for patients presenting with common symptoms to Dutch family physicians. *Journal of Family Practice, 51*, 31–39.

Oliva Ramirez, A., Keenan, A., Kalau, O., Worthington, E., Cohen, L., & Singh, S. (2021). Prevalence and burden of multiple

sclerosis-related fatigue: A systematic literature review. *BMC Neurology, 21*(1), 468. https://doi.org/10.1186/s12883-021-02396-1.

Parslow, R. M., Anderson, N., Byrne, D., Shaw, A., Haywood, K. L., & Crawley, E. (2018). Adolescent's descriptions of fatigue, fluctuation and payback in chronic fatigue syndrome/myalgic encephalopathy (CFS/ME): Interviews with adolescents and parents. *BMJ Paediatrics Open, 2*(1), e000281. https://doi.org/10.1136/bmjpo-2018-000281.

Pedersen, A., Almkvist, E., Holmegaard, L., Lagging, C., Redfors, P., Blomstrand, C., Jood, K., Samuelsson, H., & Jern, C. (2022). Fatigue 7 years post-stroke: Predictors and correlated features. *Acta Neurologica Scandinavica, 146*(3), 295–303. https://doi.org/10.1111/ane.13665.

Pemberton, S., & Berry, C. (2014). *Fighting fatigue: A practical guide to managing the symptoms of CFS/ME*. Hammersmith Books.

Raina, K., Morse, J., Chisholm, E., Whyte, E., & Terhorst, L. (2022). An internet-based self-management intervention to reduce fatigue among people with traumatic brain injury: A pilot RCT. *American Journal of Occupational Therapy, 76*(4), 1–8. https://doi.org/10.5014/ajot.2022.048587.

Reid, S., Chalder, T., Cleare, A., Hotopf, M., & Wessely, S. (2000). Chronic fatigue syndrome. *BMJ, 320*, 292–296. https://doi.org/10.1136/bmj.320.7230.292.

Restall, G., & Egan, M. (2022). Key Characteristics of relationship-focused practice. In M. Egan & G. Restall (Eds.), *Promoting occupational participation: Collaborative relationship focused occupational therapy* (pp. 101). Canadian Association of Occupational Therapists.

Restall, G., Egan, M., Valavaara, K., Phenix, A., & Sack, C. (2022). Canadian occupational therapy inter-relational practice process. In M. Egan & G. Restall (Eds.), *Promoting occupational participation: Collaborative relationship-focused occupational therapy* (pp. 124–139). Canadian Association of Occupational Therapists.

Rosti-Otajärvi, E. M., & Hämäläinen, P. I. (2014). Neuropsychological rehabilitation for multiple sclerosis. *Cochrane Database of Systematic Reviews*, (2), CD009131. https://doi.org/10.1002/14651858.CD009131.pub3.

Salari, N., Khodayari, Y., Hosseinian-Far, A., Zarei, H., Rasoulpoor, S., Akbari, H., & Mohammadi, M. (2022). Global prevalence of chronic fatigue syndrome among long COVID-19 patients: A systematic review and meta-analysis. *Biopsychosocial Medicine, 16*(1), 21. https://doi.org/10.1186/s13030-022-00250-5.

Salome, A., Sasso, T., Franchini, G., Valter, S., & Paolucci, T. (2019). Occupational therapy in fatigue management in MS: An umbrella review. *Multiple Sclerosis International, 2019*, 2027947. https://doi.org/10.1155/2019/2027947.

Sapra, A., & Bhandari, P. (2022). *Chronic fatigue syndrome*. StatPearls Publishing. https://www.ncbi.nlm.nih.gov/books/NBK557676/.

Schönberger, M., Reutens, D., Beare, R., O'Sullivan, R., Rajaratnam, S., & Ponsford, J. (2017). Brain lesion correlates of fatigue in individuals with traumatic brain injury. *Neuropsychological Rehabilitation, 27*(7), 1056–1070. https://doi.org/10.1080/09602011.2016.1154875.

Shields, A., Gwaltney, C., Paty, J., & Shiffman, S. (2006). FDA: Documentation of PRO instruments to meet contemporary FDA standards. White Paper. Food and Drug Administration.

Sklar, M., Burish, T. G., & Cook, K. F. (1997). Development and validation of the functional assessment of chronic illness therapy fatigue scale. *Quality of Life Research, 6*(6), 535–542. https://doi.org/10.1023/A:1026413210664.

Smets, E. M., Garssen, B., Bonke, B., & De Haes, J. C. (1995). The Multidimensional Fatigue Inventory (MFI) psychometric qualities of an instrument to assess fatigue. *Journal of Psychosomatic Research, 39*(3), 315–325. https://doi.org/10.1016/0022-3999(94)00125-O.

Taylor, L. A., Mhizha-Murira, J. R., Smith, L., Potter, K. J., Wong, D., Evangelou, N., Lincoln, N. B., & das Nair, R. (2021). Memory rehabilitation for people with multiple sclerosis. *Cochrane Database of Systematic Reviews, 10*(10), CD008754. https://doi.org/10.1002/14651858.CD008754.pub4.

US ME/CFS Clinician Coalition. (2021, February 20). ME/CFS treatment recommendations. https://mecfscliniciancoalition.org/mecfs-clinician-coalition-treatment-recs-v1.

Van den Bergh, O., & Walentynowicz, M. (2016). Accuracy and bias in retrospective symptom reporting. *Current Opinion in Psychiatry, 29*(5), 302–308. https://doi.org/10.1097/YCO.0000000000000267.

Van Heest, K., Mogush, A., & Mathiowitz, V. (2017). Effects of a one-to-one fatigue management course for people with chronic conditions and fatigue. *American Journal of Occupational Therapy, 71*(4), 7104190040p1–7104190040p9. https://doi.org/10.5014/ajot.2017.023226.

Van Kessel, K., Moss-Morris, R., Willoughby, E., Chalder, T., Johnson, M. H., & Robinson, E. (2008). A randomised controlled trial of cognitive behaviour therapy for multiple sclerosis fatigue. *Psychosomatic Medicine, 70*, 205–213.

Wagman, P., & Håkansson, C. (2014). Introducing the Occupational Balance Questionnaire (OBQ). *Scandinavian Journal of Occupational Therapy, 21*(3), 227–231. https://doi.org/10.3109/11038128.2013.876148.

Wagman, P., Håkansson, C., & Björklund, A. (2012). Occupational balance as used in occupational therapy: A concept analysis. *Scandinavian Journal of Occupational Therapy, 19*(4), 322–327. https://doi.org/10.3109/11038128.2011.596219.

White, P. D., Goldsmith, K. A., Johnson, A. L., Potts, L., Walwyn, R., DeCesare, J. C., Baber, H. L., Burgess, M., Clark, L. V., Cox, D. L., Bavinton, J., Angus, B. J., Murphy, G., Murphy, M., O'Dowd, H., Wilks, D., McCrone, P., Chalder, T., & Sharpe, M., PACE trial management group. (2011). Comparison of adaptive pacing therapy, cognitive behaviour therapy, graded exercise therapy, and specialist medical care for chronic fatigue syndrome (PACE): A randomised trial. *Lancet, 377*(9768), 823–836. https://doi.org/10.1016/S0140-6736(11)60096-2.

Whitehead, L. (2009). The measurement of fatigue in chronic illness: A systematic review of unidimensional and multidimensional fatigue measures. *Journal of Pain and Symptom Management, 37*(1), 107–128. https://doi.org/10.1016/j.jpainsymman.2007.08.019.

World Health Organization. (2019). *ICD-10: International statistical classification of diseases and related health problems. 10th revision (ICD-10).* WHO. https://icd.who.int/browse10/2019/en.

Yamada, T. H., Denburg, N. L., Beglinger, L. J., & Schultz, S. K. (2010). Neuropsychological outcomes of older breast cancer survivors: Cognitive features ten or more years after chemotherapy. *Journal of Neuropsychiatry and Clinical Neurosciences, 22*(1), 48–54. https://doi.org/10.1176/jnp.2010.22.1.48.

Zhan, J., Zhang, P., Wen, H., Wang, Y., Yan, X., Zhan, L., Chen, H., Xu, N., & Lu, L. (2023). Global prevalence estimates of poststroke fatigue: A systematic review and meta-analysis. *International Journal of Stroke, 18*(9), 1040–1050. https://doi.org/10.1177/17474930221138701.

REFLECTION

1. Explain why fatigue is more likely to be successfully managed with a multi-dimensional and person-centred approach.

2. In Barbara's practice story (Box 37.2) the Canadian Occupational Therapy Inter-Relation Practice Process (Restall et al., 2022) is applied. Why might this be a relevant Process to use with Barbara?

3. In Barbara's practice story (Box 37.2), the occupational therapist refers to considering their own culturally informed perspectives. How might this influence the relationship between Barbara and the occupational therapist? What influences your own culturally informed perspectives and how does this influence you and your work?

4. Why is it important to hear a person's narrative?

38

MANAGING PAIN

JENNY STRONG ■ KATIE ROBINSON ■ LUCIANA BUIN

Overview

Chronic pain is a health condition which can dramatically impact the lives and occupational participation of people who have this condition. This complex condition affects people across the lifespan. Occupational therapy can play an essential role in enhancing the lives of individuals with chronic pain. Occupational therapists should be alert to the presence of pain and be able to utilise their core occupational therapy skills to enable individuals to identify and attain their important occupational participation goals.

In this chapter, the contextual background for working with individuals with chronic pain is provided. Some of the many difficulties people face in their everyday lives living with chronic pain are highlighted as their lived experiences are important to understand when working with them. Three practice stories are presented to illustrate how occupational therapists can contribute to the occupational participation and the resultant quality of life of people who live with chronic pain.

KEY POINTS

■ Occupational therapists make an important contribution to assisting people living with chronic pain achieve their occupational participation goals.

■ Occupational therapists may meet people living with chronic pain in many practice settings.

■ The biopsychosocial model of pain 'assesses the integrated "whole person", with both mind and body together as interconnected entities, recognising biological, psychological and social components of pain and illness'.

■ Occupational therapists seek to understand the important past, present and future imagined life roles of individuals and identify barriers to the person's ability to participate in these relevant life roles.

■ Participating in occupations is a determinant of health and well-being and can alleviate anxiety, discomfort and pain.

■ Occupational therapists work in partnership with individuals with chronic pain (and their families as relevant) to identify important occupational participation goals and to equip them with ways to meet these goals.

INTRODUCTION

Occupational therapists have the privilege of working with individuals and their families across many stages of the lifespan. This connection may occur in a variety of settings such as residential aged care facilities, children's hospitals, community centres, schools and adult hospitals. The fundamental concern occupational therapists have is to work collaboratively with people and their families to meet their personally relevant occupational participation goals (Ochoa & Skubik-Peplaski, 2023).

Pain is 'an unpleasant sensory and emotional experience associated with or resembling that associated with actual or potential tissue damage' (Raja et al., 2020, p. 1976). It is multidimensional and is one of the most frequent reasons for seeking health services. It can be classified based on its duration as acute or chronic (lasting more then three months) (Treede et al., 2015) or its physiological mechanism as nociceptive (related to the activation of nociceptors), neuropathic (dysfunction of the nervous system somatosensorial) or nociplastic (from altered nociception despite any clear evidence of factual or threatened tissue damage) (IASP, 2017; Kosek et al., 2021). More information on the three types of pain is provided in Table 38.1.

Pain is a natural process, essential for survival, an alert mechanism that could indicate to the body the presence of tissue damage so that the defence mechanisms are activated, guaranteeing protection; however, if the pain becomes chronic, it ceases to be an alert mechanism and becomes unnecessary (Fuchs & Cassapian, 2012). Pain is not synonymous with injury. The physiological component of pain is called nociception. Nociception is the phenomenon of the encoding and processing of stimuli (Bausbaum et al., 2009). Pain is the unpleasant emotional experience that usually accompanies nociception (Patel, 2010).

One of the barriers people may face in meeting their occupational participation goals is chronic or persistent pain (van Griensven & Strong, 2023). Worldwide, epidemiological data from the United Kingdom, Canada, China, Japan, Australia, New Zealand and the United States suggest that the prevalence of chronic pain ranges from 20% to 50% (Canadian Pain Taskforce Report, 2020; Deloitte Access Economics, 2019; Dominick et al., 2011; Fayaz et al., 2016; Gaskin & Richard, 2012; Inoue et al., 2015; Kuehn, 2018; Yongjun et al., 2020). Chronic pain is not just a symptom; it is recognised as a disease/health condition in its own right (PainUK, 2014). Although pain may not bring an obvious risk of death, it causes critical occupational participation difficulties and high costs in the health system. Within the International Classification of Diseases (ICD-11), chronic pain is considered more than a symptom; it is classified as a disease. The World Health Organization (WHO) recognises it as a public health problem worldwide. According to the International Association for the Study of Pain (IASP), one-third of the population experiencing chronic pain is less able to sustain occupational participation while in pain (Dueñas et al., 2016).

An elderly person with peripheral neuropathy may find it an indeterminable struggle to move around and complete their daily personal occupations. A young female may find the intractable pain of endometriosis is a barrier to them participating in their studies and social occupations with their peers. A young mother with fibromyalgia may find their parenting occupational roles impacted. A middle-aged person with chronic back pain after a workplace injury may experience disruption to their worker role, with cascading impacts on their family relationships and financial security.

TABLE 38.1

Types of Pain, Physiological Cause and Examples

Type of Pain	Physiological Cause	Description of Pain	Example of Condition
Nociceptive pain	Damage to non-neural body tissue such as skin, muscle, viscera	Throbbing, aching	Tennis elbow
Neuropathic pain	Damage to peripheral nerves or central nervous system caused by a lesion or disease	Shooting, burning	Trigeminal neuralgia
Nociplatic pain	Altered nociception with central nervous system sensitisation despite any clear evidence of injury or disease	Aching, burning, throbbing, pain hypersensitivity, allodynia	Fibromyalgia

THE IMPACT OF CHRONIC PAIN ON OCCUPATIONAL PARTICIPATION

Chronic pain has a profound impact on occupational participation. The mechanisms through which pain impacts occupation participation are complex and include both the limitations imposed by pain and the fear of activity increasing or triggering pain. A central feature of the experience of chronic pain is unpredictability. Across several qualitative studies, people with chronic pain have described difficulty controlling or predicting pain, leading to vigilance and calculation of the risk of participating in occupations (Crowe et al., 2017).

Chronic pain negatively affects the quality of life, occupational participation and relationships (Hadi et al., 2019). Sleep disturbance and sleep disorders are prevalent among people with chronic pain (Mathias et al., 2018). Adults with chronic pain report challenges participating in physical activity, with diverse factors influencing their participation, including pain, fatigue, perceived risks, motivation, other health conditions and lack of support for physical activity or exercise (Vader et al., 2021). There is a large volume of literature describing the challenges people with chronic pain face in sustaining employment including the specific adversarial struggle that they face to maintain their credibility at work (Toye et al., 2016). A meta-synthesis of studies of the experience of low back pain identified the stressful financial implications of sick leave due to pain and challenges maintaining productivity for those who remain at work (MacNeela et al., 2015).

People living with chronic pain describe implications that the condition has on their relationships, including diminished trust and mutual understanding in spousal relationships and increasing social withdrawal due to challenges maintaining friendships and other affiliations (MacNeela et al., 2015). People with chronic pain also experience significant sexual dysfunction including lack of interest in sexual activity and low levels of satisfaction within their sex lives (Flegge et al., 2023).

The occupational participation consequences of chronic pain extend beyond the person living with pain to informal caregivers and families of people with chronic pain. A study of Spanish informal caregivers identified that they described their experience of caring for a person with chronic pain as 'becoming a secondary actor in one's own life' (De Sola et al., 2023, p. 409). This theme describes how being an informal caregiver to a person with chronic pain becomes the most important role in the caregiver's life to the point of overshadowing the caregiver's own needs (De Sola et al., 2023).

Chronic pain is highly prevalent among older adults (Larsson et al., 2017). Older adults report that pain has a detrimental impact on their sleep and participation in valued occupations and relationships (Gillsjö et al., 2021). Musculoskeletal pain in older adults is associated with lower activity levels, disability, increased occurrence of falls, depression and anxiety symptoms (Blyth et al., 2017). Older people rarely experience chronic pain in the absence of other health conditions. Health research and policy have repeatedly called for a shift away from focusing on single diseases in older adults to focusing on co-occurring conditions. Multiple studies across international contexts have repeatedly identified common patterns of health complaints in older adults, including a 'musculoskeletal pattern' (Prados-Torres et al., 2014), where conditions such as arthritis commonly co-occur with other conditions such as depression and obesity.

Management of musculoskeletal pain in older adults continues to be a major healthcare challenge due to several factors including polypharmacy (Reid et al., 2015) and pharmacokinetic and pharmacodynamic considerations for this population when prescribing medication (Schwan et al., 2019). Older adults with chronic pain and other chronic conditions are vulnerable to polypharmacy and potentially inappropriate prescribing. Further barriers to the management of chronic pain in older adults include a limited evidence base to guide treatment and concerns about treatment-related harm (Reid et al., 2015).

MODELS OF PRACTICE

Chronic pain interferes with different aspects of the person's life, limiting their occupational participation and decreasing their quality of life. It negatively affects their daily routine, physical and mental health, personal and family relationships and work interactions (Dueñas et al., 2016). It is a multidimensional and complex experience the most efficient treatment of which is multidisciplinary rehabilitation, involving doctors, nurses, nutritionists, psychologists, social workers, physiotherapists and occupational therapists (Hesselstrand et al., 2015). The biopsychosocial model of pain is the most cited and is more effective than unimodal treatments (Nicholas, 2022). The biopsychosocial model of pain 'assesses the integrated "whole person", with both mind and body together as interconnected entities, recognising biological, psychological and social components of pain and illness' (Bevers et al., 2016, p. 99).

The philosophy, models and frameworks of a number of occupational therapies are consistent with the Biopsychosocial Model (American Occupational Therapy Association, 2021), including the Person–Environment–Occupational Performance (PEOP) Model, the Model of Human Occupation (MOHO) and the Canadian Model of Occupational Participation (CanMOP) (Egan & Restall et al., 2022) (refer to Chapter 11).

As part of their assessment of the person living with chronic pain, occupational therapists seek to understand the important life roles of individuals (past, present and future imagined life roles). Then, barriers to the person's ability to participate in these relevant life roles are identified. The occupational therapist directs their attention to an individual's performance, habituation and volitional systems, as all three are fundamental to their rehabilitation outcomes (Andrews, 2023; Strong, 1996). Utilising assessment tools such as the Occupational Performance History Interview (OPHI-I; OPHI-II) and the Canadian Occupational Performance Measure (COPM), the occupational therapist works with each individual to identify personally relevant role performance goals and then develops treatment protocols (Andrews, 2023; Kielhofner & Henry, 1988; Kielhofner et al., 2001; Law et al., 1990; Strong, 1996). A wide range of other outcome measures and/or assessments can also potentially be employed depending on the individual's personally relevant occupational participation goals. These assessments could be focused on the individual, occupation or environment (e.g. the Pain Catastrophising Scale (Sullivan et al., 1995), Tampa Scale for Kinesiophobia (Swinkels-Meewisse et al., 2003), Pittsburgh Sleep Quality Index (PSQI) (Buysse et al., 1989), the Worker Role Interview (Braveman et al., 2005), the Assessment of Motor and Process Sills (Fisher & Jones, 2013) or assessment of

the workplace and work participation via a workplace visit (Coole et al., 2014)). Occupational therapy has shown promising results in reducing pain and returning to work (Bosy et al., 2010; Hesselstrand et al., 2015). Occupational therapists have the knowledge, skill and expertise to assess how pain interferes with the person's physical, social and spiritual life domains and understand the full complexity of the impact of pain on the individual's life (Lagueux et al., 2018). Occupational therapists offer tools for pain management in everyday life, with interventions such as adaptations of a person's daily occupations (Skjutar et al., 2010). Among the possible interventions occupational therapists may use are occupation management (which includes occupational analysis, skill development, occupational adaptation, problem solving, prioritisation, planning and pacing of occupations to avoid imbalance between rest and activity), ergonomics, communication skills, coping, relaxation strategies, stress management, setting and achieving goals through graded activities, use of assistive technology such as orthoses and assistance in returning to work (Andrews, 2023; Hill, 2016).

UNDERSTANDING THE EXPERIENCES OF THREE PEOPLE WITH CHRONIC PAIN AND ILLUSTRATING THE OCCUPATIONAL THERAPIST'S CONTRIBUTION

In this section, three practice stories (Boxes 38.1–38.3) are presented to illustrate how occupational therapists work in collaboration with people experiencing chronic pain to enable them to attain the occupational participation goals that are important to them. It is important during the initial meeting to learn what the person values. Occupational therapists will draw on strategies to support and enable the person to meet their occupational participation goals. Given that the goals and circumstances of each individual may differ, the strategies enacted in occupational therapy practice with people with chronic pain vary. These strategies may include physical rehabilitation for the person such as training in somatic awareness and muscle relaxation, education, environmental strategies such as home and job task modifications and strategies such as pacing, along with psychological rehabilitation (Hesselstrand et al., 2015; Ochoa & Skubik-Peplaski, 2023; Robinson et al., 2011).

BOX 38.1
SELMA

Selma is an 82-year-old Irish female living alone on a farm with her pet dog. Her husband passed away 6 months ago, and a neighbour has been helping her with the farm since then. She has osteoarthritis in several joints and had a left total hip replacement 5 years ago. Selma drives to the local village every day to attend mass, go to the shops and sometimes visits friends. In the past few months, she has visited her doctor almost weekly as she is struggling with pain in both hips and knees. Pain is affecting her ability to sleep and has led to her reducing her participation in many occupations. She no longer goes for walks or completes heavier household occupations such as cleaning windows or washing floors. She is nervous of falling and is worried about maintaining her independent lifestyle if the pain progresses. Her doctor referred her to a community occupational therapist, Liz, noting that Selma had a 10 year+ history of osteoarthritis for which she takes paracetamol regularly and was also taking anticoagulant medication and digoxin for atrial fibrillation and a calcium channel blocker for hypertension.

Liz visited Selma at home and spent their first meeting conducting a narrative-style interview where Liz learned about Selma's valued occupations and routines, how her occupational roles and routines have changed since her husband passed away and how her osteoarthritis is impacting her occupational participation. Throughout the initial meetings, Liz was attuned to how Selma described her osteoarthritis pain and noted that Selma expressed extreme negativity about the prospect of managing her pain. Liz asked Selma to maintain an activity diary for a week and to record a daily narrative account of her pain and how it affected her.

Together they reviewed the diary a week later and negotiated three occupational participation goals. Selma wanted to:

1. Improve her sleep quality and quantity
2. Comfortably walk outdoors daily with her dog
3. Safely participate in light household activities and identify a cleaner to assist with heavier activities.

Liz implemented a range of interventions including cognitive behaviour therapy to address Selma's overly negative beliefs about her pain. This involved the use of a diary to record thoughts and beliefs, the use of mantras and coping statements and behavioural challenges. With Selma's agreement, Liz made a series of minor modifications to the home environment to facilitate continued safe participation in daily activities such as rearranging storage to eliminate the need to use a step to reach high places and the installation of a series of grab rails to reduce the risk of falls in the bathroom and at the front door. Liz implemented a sleep hygiene programme and meditation regime with Selma to address sleep quality and quantity. Finally, Liz worked with Selma over a 6-week period to gradually increase her walking distance and then supported Selma to join a local Nordic walking group of older adults.

BOX 38.2
MÁRCIA

Márcia, a 72-year old females, sought occupational therapy at the request of her daughter Joana. Márcia had tried several treatments previously but without the success she had hoped for. She was already seeing a physiotherapist and attending Pilates classes twice a week.

Three years ago, Márcia began to feel severe pain in her lumbar spine, making it difficult for her to do household chores and her favourite occupation, dancing. Then, one night, when she turned over in bed, she felt what she called a 'trigger' just above her buttocks, causing her to fear movement during the night and worsening her sleep quality.

In the initial interview, Márcia told the occupational therapist, Pat, that the orthopaedic doctor advised her, after checking imaging tests of her spine to do low-impact physical exercises, such as Pilates and hydro gymnastics and forbade her to perform household chores. This caused her family to become hyper-vigilant about Marcia's activities. Her husband and daughters asked her to stop doing household chores, not to carry any weight or perform bending or squatting movements. In her interview, Márcia vented: 'I feel useless, and my house is a mess; I like to take care of my things. They will not let me do anything else, and I'm afraid to try, and the pain will get worse'.

During the first session with Marcia, Pat listened actively and empathetically, letting her talk about her journey up to attending the appointment. Pat was able to gather essential information about her occupational identity, routine, beliefs and expectations. Márcia was an active female, married for a long time and had an excellent supportive relationship with her family. She had three children and five grandchildren. She liked to take care of and play with her grandchildren and participate in occupations with her husband, including dancing, which was very important to her. In addition, Márcia was an exemplary homemaker who liked to sweep the floor and clean the furniture every day.

Continued on following page

BOX 38.2
MÁRCIA—(Continued)

She rated the level of her low back pain 7/10 on the numeric pain scale and said that it made her sad, irritable and frustrated that she could not do the things she liked to do. The medications prescribed by the doctor did not successfully manage the intensity of the pain. During the physical examination and based on the communication with Márcia's other healthcare providers, Pat identified no red flags (indicators of serious pathology e.g. malignancy or fracture) related to Márcia's back pain. While observing Márcia during the initial assessment, Pat also noticed that she appeared tense during movements. Márcia explained: 'I'm afraid to sit down and get up from the sofa or lower chairs and to turn over in bed while I sleep. I also cannot play on the floor with my granddaughter or carry her in my arms. I'm terrified of triggering worsening of the pain with any sudden or jarring movement'.

Pat conducted a few assessments with Márcia, including the Canadian Occupational Performance Measure (COPM), the Tampa Scale for Kinesiophobia and the Pittsburgh Sleep Quality Index (PSQI). These were done to inform Pat's professional reasoning and collaborative goal setting. The assessment results indicated that the key occupational participation problems were difficulties performing household chores, especially cleaning the floor, completing activities related to being a grandmother and enjoying her hobby (dancing). The assessments also identified that Márcia had poor sleep quality and a low degree of kinesophobia.

Márcia and Pat together determined that her occupational participation goals were being able to sit without fear or pain, playing with her grandchildren, dancing with her husband and doing all the housework tasks with satisfaction.

The intervention started with body awareness techniques to enable Márcia to identify muscle tension and muscle relaxation exercises, breathing exercises and meditation techniques.

Education on the neuroscience of pain was provided, including an explanation of the functioning of the lumbar spine, differences between nociception and pain and the use of metaphors and images to understand the presence and worsening of pain.

Due to Márcia's fear of moving, the occupational therapist enabled her to have gradual exposure to more challenging/feared movements and activities. Everyday activities were simulated and practiced such as the task of sitting in different contexts and environments and lying down and rolling over in different planes of movement.

For household tasks and activities related to her role as a grandmother, self-management strategies including pacing, energy conservation and joint protection were implemented. Márcia identified her priorities as a homemaker and set short- and medium-term goals to enable her to return to doing activities that were important to her and that met her level of satisfaction.

As Márcia's management of her pain improved, she felt more confident moving around, and her mood and sleep improved. Her family members were provided with education about pain to correct their erroneous beliefs regarding spine care and hypervigilance. The family was provided with information about the self-management strategies that Márcia was learning and implementing to achieve her goals.

Márcia began to perform a wider range of occupations and was able to achieve her occupational goals to a level she was satisfied with.

She continued doing her physical exercises, using the coping and pacing strategies and was even able to return to dancing eventually. According to Joana, her daughter, Márcia had a sparkle in her eyes again.

BOX 38.3
REBECCA

Rebecca was 17 years old when she was referred to the occupational therapist by a gynaecologist that she had starting seeing 5 months ago. She attended her appointment with her mum, Susan. Rebecca appeared tired, and when she and her mum sat down, she looked tense and said: 'I've never heard of an occupational therapist before; what can you do for me?' Before Alison could respond, Susan said: 'Beccy, just give the lady a chance. Dr Smithfield said it would help'.

Alison gave Rebecca a welcoming smile and said: 'Good morning Rebecca. My name is Alison. I identify as female and love how much I learn from young people in my work as an occupational therapist. My role is to work with you to help you get back to doing the things that you want to do in your life. The things that are important to you'.

'So you can't take my pain away then?' she asked. 'That's what's important to me!'

'Well, Rebecca, some of the strategies I suggest may help to both minimise your pain and to do things. If it is okay with you, I would really like to learn more about you and your story. I appreciate you've told this to so many people already, but I would like to understand how it's been for you. Would you mind if I make a few notes while you are talking?' Note – Rebecca identified as she/her.

Continued on following page

BOX 38.3
REBECCA—(*Continued*)

Rebecca was the only child born to teacher parents, Susan and Damien. She did well at school and had positive social connections. She was an active child and loved the water. From swimming lessons as a baby, she graduated to swim club and serious training. She was winning her club age championship until she turned 12 when she started menstruating and the excruciating pain began. It gradually worsened until she was incapacitated for 3–5 days each month. Nothing seemed to help, not the Panadol, not the hot packs. She could not swim; she could not go to school. Her doctor suggested taking the contraceptive pill, and despite her parents' misgivings, they agreed. Several pills were trialled, each for 3 months, so her whole school year in grade 8 was impacted. This absenteeism left her feeling rejected by her school friends, and she no longer wanted to socialise with her swimming friends. Finally, when she was 14, she was referred to a gynaecologist, who did a laparoscopy but found 'nothing'. He suggested some stronger medications, which helped a bit.

She felt such despair, saying, 'if there was no biological reason, why was I in agony every month?' She fell behind in her schoolwork; she put on weight because she could not swim anymore; she missed doing things with her friends and became increasingly isolated. Sometimes it seemed it was just her and mum against the world. She tried herbal medicine, but that made her nauseous and did not take the pain away. Sometimes it became so bad that her mum took her up to the local hospital emergency department, where she was given Endone. Her teenage years dragged on, in this cycle of despair.

Worried about her mood, her doctor suggested that she should see a child psychiatrist, but Rebecca refused. 'I am not making this pain up' she said. 'It's in my pelvis, not my head.' Her mum suggested that she should see a different gynaecologist, who did scans and suggested another laparoscopic surgery to investigate. She readily agreed and endometriosis was detected and treated. She and her mum were relieved but also angry that it had not been detected earlier. The pain had not gone completely, but it seemed more bearable, most of the time. Her gynaecologist suggested that she would bring in the multidisciplinary team to help.

As Alison listened to Rebecca's story, the catalogue of occupational participation losses she had faced over the past 5 years became clear. Alison thought, 'No wonder Rebecca was not interested in seeing me'.

'You have had to deal with so many things, Rebecca' Alison said. 'All that uncertainty, that pain, and how it has interfered with the things that you enjoy, like swimming, school and seeing friends. What I would like to do now is to reframe things a bit and get you to think about what are the most important things you want to be able to do with your life right now. We'll use an assessment called the Canadian Occupational Performance Measure (COPM)' (Law et al., 1990).

Rebecca's most pressing occupational participation goal was to return to school and to finish her exams. Rebecca said that she wanted to do well enough to get into university and a health science course. She was not sure exactly what, but she hoped she could do something that would help others who suffered like she had done. This was important to her. Rebecca and Alison then explored the barriers she was facing. She found sitting for long periods uncomfortable. She had difficulties in concentrating, and she became fatigued by lunchtime. She was self-conscious about being 'fat' and worried that the other girls would laugh at her. She became anxious. She was also highly sensitive to touch (Alison asked Rebecca to complete the Sensory Profile 2 [Dunn, 2014]). She also described difficulties she had with her teachers who just did not understand what she was experiencing. One of her teachers had intimated that she never had period pain, and she doubted that it really was as bad as Rebecca was saying.

One of the important strategies that occupational therapists teach people with pain is pacing. There is growing evidence of the effectiveness of this strategy (Andrews et al., 2012, 2018). Alison suggested to Rebecca that they tackle return to school by first doing a thorough task analysis of the activities and routines required of her, and then apply the strategy of pacing. This needed to be in parallel with meetings with teachers and providing them with contemporary pain information. Expecting Rebecca to return to school full time straight away was unrealistic. They negotiated with the school for Rebecca to begin a modified return to school programme, starting part-time with fewer subjects for a term and building up to full time.

Rebecca (and her mum) learnt about the pain and stress cycle, and ways she could calm herself and minimise pain. She learnt how to use relaxation techniques, and she trialled a weighted lap pad for when she was sitting.

In parallel, Rebecca saw a dietician to assist her with her diet and weight concerns, a physiotherapist who tried to increase her core strength and fitness and a psychologist who worked with her on her mood and self-esteem. All of Rebecca's health team kept in regular contact, and monthly tele-meetings were held with Rebecca and her mum and the multidisciplinary team.

As can be seen in the cases of Selma, Márcia and Rebecca, the occupational therapist begins by developing a partnership that is focused on the occupational participation goals that are important for each person. Once these goals are identified – beyond the goal of 'taking my pain away' – the occupational therapist will conduct a thorough assessment of contributing factors, which may include physical factors such as sensory sensitivity or low muscle strength to psychological factors such as fear of movement and environmental factors such as attitudes of others such as teachers or family members or workplace barriers. A broad range of management strategies may be used, including education about the neurophysiology of pain, cognitive behavioural therapy, graded activity and re-engagement, advocacy and relaxation techniques (Andrews, 2023; Hesselstrand et al., 2015; Ochoa & Skubik-Peplaski, 2023; Robinson et al., 2011; van Griensven & Strong, 2023). These strategies are always tailored to the needs of each individual.

EXAMPLES OF EVIDENCE-BASED STRATEGIES FOR PEOPLE WITH CHRONIC PAIN

The use of occupation in the intervention of people with chronic pain is well-reported in the literature. Participating in occupations is a determinant of health and well-being and can alleviate anxiety, discomfort and pain (Weinstock-Zlotnick & Mehta, 2019). Studies suggest that occupational participation is a potential mediator in the experience of pain, physically, psychologically and socially altering this process (Lagueux et al., 2018).

In a systematic review of the ways individuals approach their daily activities (either by avoiding participating in their activities or by overactivity where the person will persist in doing their activities despite the pain), it was found that avoiding participating in occupations was associated with poorer functioning outcomes (Andrews et al., 2012). The relationship between persisting with activities (overactivity) and functional outcomes was less clear; persisting with activities seemed to be a useful coping strategy for people until people persisted to the point where the pain was greatly aggravated (Andrews et al., 2012). The review also found that while a person's use of pacing approaches to do their activities was linked with better

psychological functioning, it was associated with more pain and disability (Andrews et al., 2012).

Given the sensory hypersensitivity associated with many pain conditions (Kosek et al., 2021), some occupational therapists have begun to look at implementing sensory approaches to help with the modulation of pain (see Bar-Shalita et al., 2019). Meanwhile, Meredith et al. (2021) recently demonstrated that the proprioceptive input from weighted blankets helped individuals cope better with pain.

Occupational therapists use graded activities, workplace trials and participatory ergonomics with people who want to return to work (Anema et al., 2007; Fishbain et al., 2016, Hadjistavropoulos & Clark, 2001; Hesselstrand et al., 2015; Peters, 2023) have been encouraging, showing enhanced work capacity (Ibrahim et al., 2019) and lower sick leave (Lambeek et al., 2010).

The recommended approach to managing pain in later life involves a multidisciplinary team of healthcare providers and addresses the depression, isolation and disability that pain can cause (Reid et al., 2015). The role of occupational therapy with this population includes individual education, coaching older adults to enable participation in occupations, environmental adaptations and cognitive behavioural therapy (Zimmerman, 2003). A systematic review and meta-analysis of 22 studies found that for older adults, psychological interventions that used cognitive behavioural modalities were associated with small but significant improvements in pain, catastrophising beliefs and improved self-efficacy for managing pain (Niknejad et al., 2018). Pain catastrophising has received major focus in pain research in recent decades and refers to a tendency to hold overly negative responses to pain or pain-related cues (Sullivan et al., 1995, 2001). For example, the person living with chronic pain may believe things like 'Because I have this pain, I am never going to be able to hold down a job' or 'My life is over now that I have pain'. The occupational therapist will work with the person using task analysis skills to demonstrate how the individual is able to participate in personally meaningful occupations despite pain.

CONCLUSION

In this chapter, the impact chronic pain can have on people's lives has been explained. Occupational therapists may find themselves working with such individuals across the lifespan. Core occupational therapy principles around assessment and management are important regardless of setting. As illustrated in the practice stories, occupational therapists work in partnership with individuals with chronic pain (and their families as relevant) to identify important occupational participation goals and to equip them with ways to meet these goals. Equipped with an appropriate practice model, occupational therapists guide and support people to meet their goals.

REFERENCES

American Occupational Therapy Association. (2021). Role of occupational therapy in pain management. *The American Journal of Occupational Therapy, 75*(Supplement_3), 7513410010. https://doi.org/10.5014/ajot.2021.75S3001.

Andrews, N. E., Strong, J., & Meredith, P. J. (2012). Activity pacing, avoidance, endurance, and associations with patient functioning in chronic pain: A systematic review and meta-analysis. *Archives of Physical Medicine and Rehabilitation, 93*(11), 2109–2121.e7. https://doi.org/10.1016/j.apmr.2012.05.029.

Andrews, N. E. (2023). Participating in life roles through self-management. In H. van Griensven & J. Strong (Eds.), *Pain a textbook for health professionals* (3rd ed., pp. 137–143). Elsevier.

Andrews, N. E., Strong, J., Meredith, P. J., & Brandjerporn, G. S. (2018). Approach to activity engagement and differences in activity participation in chronic pain: A five-day observational study. *Australian Occupational Therapy Journal, 65*, 575–585. https://doi.org/10.1111/1440-1630.12516.

Anema, J. R., Steenstra, I. A., Bongers, P. M., de Vet, H. C., Knol, D. L., Loisel, P., & van Mechelen, W. (2007). Multidisciplinary rehabilitation for subacute low back pain: Graded activity or workplace intervention or both? A randomized controlled trial. *Spine, 32*(3), 291–300. https://doi.org/10.1097/01.brs.0000253604.90039.ad.

Bar-Shalita, T., Granovsky, Y., Parish, S., & Weissman-Fogel, I. (2019). Sensory modulation disorder (SMD) and pain: A new perspective. *Frontiers in Integrative Neuroscience, 13*, 27. https://doi.org/10.3389/fnint.2019.00027.

Basbaum, A. I., Bautista, D. M., Scherrer, G., & Julius, D. (2009). Cellular and molecular mechanisms of pain. *Cell, 139*(2), 267–284.

Bevers, K., Watts, L., Kishino, N. D., & Gachtel, R. J. (2016). The biopsychosocial model of the assessment, prevention, and treatment of chronic pain. *US Neurology, 12*, 98–104. https://doi.org/10.17925/USN.2016.12.02.98.

Blyth, F. M., & Noguchi, N. (2017). Chronic musculoskeletal pain and its impact on older people. *Best Practice & Research Clinical Rheumatology, 31*(2), 160–168. https://doi.org/10.1016/j.berh.2017.10.004.

Bosy, D., Etlin, D., Corey, D., & Lee, J. W. (2010). An interdisciplinary pain rehabilitation programme: Description and evaluation of outcomes. *Physiotherapy Canada. Physiotherapie Canada, 62*(4), 316–326. https://doi.org/10.3138/physio.62.4.316.

Braveman, B., Robson, M., Velozo, C., Kielhofner, G., Fisher, G., Forsyth, K., & Kerschbaum, J. (2005). *A user's guide to Worker Role Interview (WRI): Version 10.0.* University of Illinois.

Buysse, D. J., Reynolds 3rd, C. F., Monk, T. H., Berman, S. R., & Kupfer, D. J. (1989). The Pittsburg Sleep Quality Index: a new instrument for psychiatric practice and research. *Psychiatry Research, 28*(2), 193–213. https://doi.org/10.1016/0165-1781(89)90047-4.

Canadian Pain Taskforce (2020). Canadian Task Force Report: October 2020. Working together to better understand, prevent and, manage chronic pain: What we heard. Government of Canada, 1–75. ISBN:978-0-660-36395-0.

Coole, C., Birks, E., Watson, P. J., & Drummond, A. (2014). Communicating with employers: Experiences of occupational therapists treating people with musculoskeletal conditions. *Journal of Occupational Rehabilitation, 24*, 585–595.

Crowe, M., Whitehead, L., Seaton, P., Jordan, J., Mccall, C., Maskill, V., & Trip, H. (2017). Qualitative meta-synthesis: The experience of chronic pain across conditions. *Journal of Advanced Nursing, 73*(5), 1004–1016. https://doi.org/10.1111/jan.13174.

Deloitte Access Economics. (2019). *The cost of pain in Australia.* https://www2.deloitte.com/au/en/pages/economics/articles/cost-pain-australia.html.

De Sola, H., Failde, I., Estalella, I., & Maquibar, A. (2023). Becoming a secondary actor of one's own life: A qualitative study of the experiences of informal caregivers in the care of people with chronic pain. *Health Expectations, 26*(1), 409–418. https://doi.org/10.1111/hex.13671.

Dominick, C., Blyth, F., & Nicholas, M. (2011). Patterns of chronic pain in the New Zealand population. *The New Zealand Medical Journal, 124*(1337), 63–76.

Dueñas, M., Ojeda, B., Salazar, A., Mico, J. A., & Failde, I. (2016). A review of chronic pain impact on patients, their social environment and the health care system. *Journal of Pain Research, 9*, 457–467. https://doi.org/10.2147/JPR.S105892.

Dunn, W. (2014). Sensory Profile 2. Pearson Assessments. https://www.pearsonassessments.com.

Egan, M., & Restall, G. (Eds.). (2022). *Promoting occupational participation: Collaborative relationship-focused occupational therapy; 10th Canadian occupational therapy guidelines; guidelines for occupational therapy in Canada.* Canadian Association of Occupational Therapists.

Fayaz, A., Croft, P., Langford, R. M., Donaldson, L. J., & Jones, G. T. (2016). Prevalence of chronic pain in the UK: A systematic review and meta-analysis of population studies. *BMJ Open, 6*(6), e010364. https://doi.org/10.1136/bmjopen-2015-010364.

Fishbain, D. A., Gao, J., Lewis, J. E., & Zhang, L. (2016). At completion of a multidisciplinary treatment program, are psychosocial variables associated with a VAS improvement of 30% or more, or an absolute VAS score improvement of 1.5 cm or more? *Pain Medicine, 17*, 781–789. https://doi.org/10.1093/pm/pnv006.

Fisher, A. G., & Jones, K. B. (2013). *Assessment of motor and process skills. Vol. II: user manual* (8th ed., p. 354). Three Star Press, Inc., Fort Collins, Colorado.

Flegge, L. G., Barr, A., & Craner, J. R. (2023). Sexual functioning among adults with chronic pain: Prevalence and association with pain-related outcomes. *Pain Medicine, 24*(2), 197–206.

Fuchs, M., & Cassapian, M. R. (2012). A Terapia Ocupacional e a dor crônica em pacientes de Ortopedia e Reumatologia: Revisão bibliográfica [Occupational therapy and chronic pain with orthopedics and rheumatology patients: A literature review]. *Cadernos Brasileiros De Terapia Ocupacional, 20*(1), 107–119. https://www.cadernosdeterapiaocupacional.ufscar.br/index.php/cadernos/article/view/554.

Gaskin, D. J., & Richard, P. (2012). The economic costs of pain in the United States. *The Journal of Pain, 13*(8), 715–724. https://doi.org/10.1016/j.jpain.2012.03.009.

Gillsjö, C., Nässén, K., & Berglund, M. (2021). Suffering in silence: A qualitative study of older adults' experiences of living with long-term musculoskeletal pain at home. *European Journal of Ageing, 18*, 55–63. https://doi.org/10.1007/s10433-020-00566-7.

Hadi, M. A., McHugh, G. A., & Closs, S. J. (2019). Impact of chronic pain on patients' quality of life: A comparative mixed-methods study. *Journal of Patient Experience, 6*(2), 133–141. https://doi.org/10.1177/2374373518786013.

Hadjistavropoulos, H. D., & Clark, J. (2001). Using outcome evaluations to assess interdisciplinary acute and chronic pain programs. *The Joint Commission Journal on Quality Improvement, 27*(7), 335–348. https://doi.org/10.1016/s1070-3241(01)27029-1.

Hesselstrand, M., Samuelsson, K., & Liedberg, G. (2015). Occupational Therapy Interventions in Chronic Pain–A Systematic Review. *Occupational Therapy International, 22*(4), 183–194. https://doi.org/10.1002/oti.1396.

Hill, W. (2016). The role of occupational therapy in pain management. *Anaesthesia and Intensive Care Medicine, 17*(9), 451–453. https://doi.org/10.1016/j.mpaic.2016.06.008.

Ibrahim, M. E., Weber, K., Courvoisier, D. S., & Genevay, S. (2019). Recovering the capability to work among patients with chronic low Back pain after a four-week, multidisciplinary biopsychosocial rehabilitation program: 18-month follow-up study. *BMC Musculoskeletal Disorders, 20*(1), 439. https://doi.org/10.1186/s12891-019-2831-6.

Inoue, S., Kobayashi, F., Nishihara, M., Arai, Y. C., Ikemoto, T., Kawai, T., Inoue, M., Hasegawa, T., & Ushida, T. (2015). Chronic pain in the Japanese Community – Prevalence, characteristics and impact on quality of life. *PLoS One, 10*(6), e0129262. https://doi.org/10.1371/journal.pone.0129262.

International Association for the Study of Pain. (2017). IASP terminology. https://www.iasp-pain.org/Education/Content.aspx?ItemNumber=1698.

Kielhofner, G., & Henry, A. (1988). Development and investigation of the occupational performance history interview. *American Journal of Occupational Therapy, 42*, 489–498.

Kielhofner, G., Mallison, T., Forsyth, K., & Lai, J. S. (2001). Psychometric properties of the second version of the occupational performance history interview (OPHI-II). *American Journal of Occupational Therapy, 55*, 260–267.

Kosek, E., Clauw, D., Nijs, J., Baron, R., Gilron, I., Harris, R. E., Mico, J. A., Rice, A. S., & Sterling, M. (2021). Chronic nociplastic pain affecting the musculoskeletal system: Clinical criteria and grading system. *Pain, 162*(11), 2629–2634. https://doi.org/10.1097/j.pain.0000000000002324.

Kuehn, B. (2018). Chronic pain prevalence. *Journal of American Medical Association, 320*(16):1632. https://doi.org/10.1001/jama.2018.16009.

Lagueux, É., Dépelteau, A., & Masse, J. (2018). Occupational therapy's unique contribution to chronic pain management: A scoping review. *Pain Research & Management, 2018*, 5378451. https://doi.org/10.1155/2018/5378451.

Lambeek, L. C., van Mechelen, W., Knol, D. L., Loisel, P., & Anema, J. R. (2010). Randomised controlled trial of integrated care to reduce disability from chronic low back pain in working and private life. *British Medical Journal, 340*, c1035. https://doi.org/10.1136/bmj.c1035.

Larsson, C., Hansson, E. E., Sundquist, K., & Jakobsson, U. (2017). Chronic pain in older adults: Prevalence, incidence, and risk factors. *Scandinavian Journal of Rheumatology, 46*(4), 317–325. https://doi.org/10.1080/03009742.2016.1218543.

Law, M., Bapiste, S., McColl, M., Opzoomer, A., Polatajko, H., & Pollack, N. (1990). The Canadian occupational performance measure: An outcome measure for occupational therapy. *Canadian Journal of Occupational Therapy, 57*, 82–87.

MacNeela, P., Doyle, C., O'Gorman, D., Ruane, N., & McGuire, B. E. (2015). Experiences of chronic low back pain: A meta-ethnography of qualitative research. *Health Psychology Review, 9*(1), 63–82. https://doi.org/10.1080/17437199.2013.840951.

Mathias, J. L., Cant, M. L., & Burke, A. L. J. (2018). Sleep disturbances and sleep disorders in adults living with chronic pain: A meta-analysis. *Sleep Medicine, 52*, 198–210. https://doi.org/10.1016/j.sleep.2018.05.023.

Meredith, P. J., Andrews, N. E., Thackeray, J., Bowen, S., Poll, C., & Strong, J. (2021). Can sensory- and attachment-informed approaches modify the perception of pain? *Journal of Pain and Symptom Management, 2021*, 1–8. https://doi.org/10.1155/2021/5527261.

Nicholas, M. K. (2022). The biopsychosocial model of pain 40 years on: Time for a reappraisal? *Pain, 163*(Suppl 1), S3–S14. https://doi.org/10.1097/j.pain.0000000000002654.

Niknejad, B., Bolier, R., Henderson, C. R., Jr, Delgado, D., Kozlov, E., Löckenhoff, C. E., & Reid, M. C. (2018). Association between psychological interventions and chronic pain outcomes in older adults: A systematic review and meta-analysis. *JAMA Internal Medicine, 178*(6), 830–839. https://doi.org/10.1001/jamainternmed.2018.0756.

Ochoa, L., & Skubik-Peplaski, C. (2023). Occupational Therapists' Beliefs and Experiences Managing Chronic Pain, Wellness, and Occupational Performance. *OTJR: Occupational Therapy Journal of Research, 44*(1), 139–147. https://doi.org/10.1177/15394492231164945.

Pain UK. (2014). Chronic pain is a 'disease in its own right': Pain UK. [online] Available at: https://painuk.org/blog/2014/12/chronic-pain-is-a-disease-in-its-own-right/ [Accessed 18 Aug. 2023].

Patel, N. B. (2010). Physiology of pain. Em Guide to pain management in low-resource settings. In A. Kopf & N. B. Patel (Eds.), *International Association for the Study of Pain*, 13–17. Seattle.

Peters, S. E. (2023). Workplace Rehabilitation. In H. van Griensven & J. Strong (Eds.), *Pain a textbook for health professionals* (3rd ed., pp. 273–296). Elsevier.

Prados-Torres, A., Calderón-Larrañaga, A., Hancco-Saavedra, J., Poblador-Plou, B., & van den Akker, M. (2014). Multimorbidity patterns: A systematic review. *Journal of Clinical Epidemiology, 67*(3), 254–266. https://doi.org/10.1016/j.jclinepi.2013.09.021.

Raja, S. N., Carr, D. B., Cohen, M., Finnerup, N. B., Flor, H., Gibson, S., Keefe, F. J., Mogil, J. S., Ringkamp, M., Sluka, K. A., Song, X. J., Stevens, B., Sullivan, M. D., Tutelman, P. R., Ushida, T., & Vader, K. (2020). The revised international association for the study of pain definition of pain: Concepts, challenges, and compromises. *Pain, 161*(9), 1976–1982. https://doi.org/10.1097/j.pain.0000000000001939.

Reid, M. C., Eccleston, C., & Pillemer, K. (2015). Management of chronic pain in older adults. *British Medical Journal, 350*, 532. https://doi.org/10.1136/bmj.h532.

Robinson, K., Kennedy, N., & Harmon, D., (2011). Is occupational therapy adequately meeting the needs of people with chronic pain? *The American Journal of Occupational Therapy, 65*(1), 106–113. https://doi.org/10.5014/ajot.2011.09160.

Schwan, J., Sclafani, J., & Tawfik, V. L. (2019). Chronic pain management in the elderly. *Anesthesiology Clinics, 37*(3), 547–560.

Skjutar, A., Schult, M. L., Christensson, K., & Müllersdorf, M. (2010). Indicators of need for occupational therapy in patients with chronic pain: Occupational Therapists' Focus groups. *Occupational Therapy International, 17*(2), 93–103. https://doi.org/10.1002/oti.282.

Strong, J. (1996). *Chronic pain, the occupational therapist's perspective*. Churchill Livingstone.

Sullivan, M. J., Bishop, S. R., & Pivik, J. (1995). The pain catastrophizing scale: Development and validation. *Psychological Assessment, 7*(4), 524.

Sullivan, M. J., Thorn, B., Haythornthwaite, J. A., Keefe, F., Martin, M., Bradley, L. A., & Lefebvre, J. C. (2001). Theoretical perspectives on the relation between catastrophizing and pain. *The Clinical Journal of Pain, 17*(1), 52–64.

Swinkels-Meewisse, E. J., Swinkels, R. A., Verbeek, A. L., Vlaeyen, J. W, & Oostendorp, R. A. (2003). Psychometric properties of the Tampa Scale for kinesiophobia and the fear-avoidance beliefs questionnaire in acute low back pain. *Manual Therapy, 8*(1):29–36.

Toye, F., Seers, K., Allcock, N., Briggs, M., Carr, E., & Barker, K. (2016). A synthesis of qualitative research exploring the barriers to staying in work with chronic musculoskeletal pain. *Disability and Rehabilitation, 38*(6), 566–572. https://doi.org/10.3109/0963 8288.2015.1049377.

Treede, R. D., Rief, W., Barke, A., Aziz, Q., Bennett, M. I., Benoliel, R., Cohen, M., Evers, S., Finnerup, N. B., First, M. B., Giamberardino, M. A., Kaasa, S., Kosek, E., Lavand'homme, P., Nicholas, M., Perrot, S., Scholz, J., Schug, S., Smith, B. H., … Wang, S. J. (2015). A classification of chronic pain for ICD-11. *Pain, 156*(6), 1003–1007. https://doi.org/10.1097/j.pain.0000000000000160.

Vader, K., Doulas, T., Patel, R., & Miller, J. (2021). Experiences, barriers, and facilitators to participating in physical activity and exercise in adults living with chronic pain: A qualitative study. *Disability and Rehabilitation, 43*(13), 1829–1837. https://doi.org/10.1080/09638288.2019.1676834.

van Griensven, H., & Strong, J. (2023). Introduction to pain. In H. van Griensven & J. Strong (Eds.), *Pain Textbook for Health Professionals* (3rd ed., pp. 1–5). Elsevier.

Weinstock-Zlotnick, G., & Mehta, S. P. (2019). A systematic review of the benefits of occupation-based intervention for patients with upper extremity musculoskeletal disorders. *Journal of Hand Therapy, 32*(2), 141–152. https://doi.org/10.1016/j.jht.2018.04.001.

Yongjun, Z., Tingjie, Z., Xiaoqiu, Y., Zhiying, F., Feng, Q., Guangke, X., Jinfeng, L., Fachuan, N., Xiaohong, J., & Yanqingj, L. (2020). A survey of chronic pain in China. *Libyan Journal of Medicine, 15*(1), 1730550.

Zimmerman, B. (2003). The Occupational Therapist's Role in the Management of Persistent Pain in Older Adults. *World Federation of Occupational Therapists Bulletin, 48*(1), 13–35. https://doi.org/1 0.1080/20566077.2003.11721148.

USEFUL WEBSITES AND RESOURCES FOR STUDENTS

https://europeanpainfederation.eu.

www.iasp-pain.org.

https://www.iasp-pain.org/education/curricula/iasp-curriculum-outline-on-pain-for-occupational-therapy/.

www.paininmotion.be.

www.pesquisaemdor.com.br.

https://www.painaustralia.org.au/.

REFLECTION

1. You are an occupational therapist working in a vocational rehabilitation facility. Describe the approach you would take when meeting a new client – a 43 year old man who has been off work for 4 months now due to a back injury.

   Model answer: task analysis of his job, physical assessment of his capacity, determining match between task requirements and his capabilities, consider modifying work tasks or environment.

2. How can an occupational therapist help promote the occupational participation of people with chronic pain in physical activities and leisure?

   Answer: knowing the client's identity and occupational routine and encouraging them to perform pleasurable activities that fit into their routine.

39

IMPROVING ARM FUNCTION AFTER ACQUIRED BRAIN IMPAIRMENT

ANNIE MCCLUSKEY ■ NATASHA A. LANNIN ■ KARL SCHURR ■ SIMONE DORSCH ■ LAUREN J. CHRISTIE

CHAPTER OUTLINE

Overview

This chapter provides a framework for optimising motor performance in adults who have a brain impairment. Conditions such as stroke and brain injury are the main focus; however, the chapter content can also apply to adults with other neurological conditions. Skills and knowledge required by occupational therapists are identified, including knowledge of motor behaviour, essential components of reaching to grasp and reaching in sitting, ways to identify compensatory strategies and develop and test movement hypotheses to enhance participation. Factors that enhance skill acquisition are discussed, including task specificity, practice intensity and timely feedback. Suggestions for effective coaching and training that are task specific and help optimise people's motor learning are presented. Finally, a summary of evidence-based interventions to improve motor performance is provided.

KEY POINTS

■ Essential knowledge in neurological rehabilitation includes an understanding of normal biomechanics and skill acquisition.

■ A person's motor performance can be observed and compared with expected performance. Hypotheses about the causes of observed movement differences can then be made and tested.

■ Paralysis, weakness and loss of coordination affect upper limb motor performance. To improve motor performance after brain impairment, therapists should primarily focus on improving strength and coordination.

■ To teach people motor skills, therapists need to develop competent coaching skills.

■ Motor performance to enable occupational participation can be improved using evidence-based strategies such as high-intensity, repetitive, task-specific training, mirror therapy, mental practice, electrical stimulation and constraint-induced movement therapy.

INTRODUCTION

Upper motor neuron lesions typically cause impairments such as paralysis, weakness and loss of sensation. These impairments can limit occupational participation in everyday tasks and activities such as grasping a cup, eating, sitting safely on the toilet and dressing. Occupational therapists and physiotherapists work together to retrain motor and sensory impairments that interfere with doing everyday tasks and activities. This chapter provides a framework to systematically observe, analyse and measure motor impairments. Targeted evidence-based interventions will be described. Therapists need to proactively seek and train muscle activity and not just teach compensatory one-handed techniques or wait for recovery.

ESSENTIAL SKILLS, KNOWLEDGE AND ATTITUDES FOR IMPROVING MOTOR PERFORMANCE

Therapists can think of themselves as 'movement scientists' (Carr et al., 1987; Refshauge et al., 2005). A movement scientist uses specialist knowledge from basic science (e.g. neuroplasticity, muscle biology), applied science (e.g. biomechanics of normal movement and motor control), education and adult learning (e.g. coaching strategies, feedback and practice) to inform analysis and training. Analysis should focus on the person's preferred roles and occupations, what they need and want to be able to do such as holding a grandchild's hand, changing a baby's nappy or typing

emails. Focusing on these roles and occupations at all stages of recovery can help to engage and motivate people. Valid, reliable instruments are used to measure changes in performance and to evaluate the effectiveness of an intervention. Systematic reviews and randomised controlled trials are critically appraised, and their clinical implications are used to guide treatment. The first step in this process involves movement analysis, where therapists identify missing or decreased essential components. Next, therapists can hypothesise about which impairments may be the cause of the movement problems and compensatory strategies and make these impairments the focus of intervention.

ANALYSING MOVEMENT

Movement analysis involves observing a person as they attempt a task, then comparing their attempt with typical movement. Therefore therapists need to understand the biomechanics of normal movement, including kinematics and kinetics. The biomechanics of reaching to grasp a glass or cup will be described to illustrate the process of movement analysis.

Normal Reaching to Grasp

The kinematics and kinetics of reaching to grasp have been described elsewhere (Alt Murphy & Häger, 2015). *Kinematics* refers to what can be seen (i.e. angular displacements, velocity and acceleration). For example, when a person reaches for a glass or cup, as shown in Fig. 39.1, shoulder flexion and thumb abduction movements can be observed. The *kinetics* (or forces) that cause these displacements can be inferred but not directly observed. In the example shown, the anterior deltoid and thumb abductor muscles, respectively, cause the angular displacements observed at the shoulder and thumb.

Normal reaching to grasp can be divided into three phases: transport, preshaping and grasp (Table 39.1). Each phase involves essential components that are necessary for efficient performance (Carr & Shepherd, 2010).

Transport refers to movement of the arm and hand forward to the cup. Essential components include shoulder flexion, protraction and external rotation to move the arm forward, with varying degrees of elbow flexion and extension, depending on reach height and

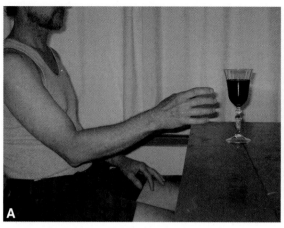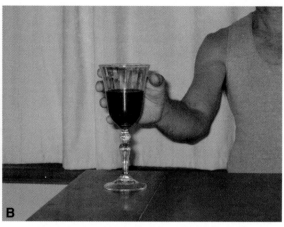

Fig. 39.1 ■ Transport, preshaping, grasp.
(A) Transport: The hand is transported to the glass using shoulder forward flexion and external rotation, elbow flexion then extension. Preshaping: The forearm aligns the hand in the correct orientation for the glass, combined with wrist extension, finger MCP extension and thumb abduction, making the required space for the glass.
(B) Grasp: Rotation of the CMC joint of the thumb and palmar cupping of the hand enable opposition of the thumb and finger pads. Flexion of finger MCP joints and thumb enables grasp.

TABLE 39.1		
Essential Components of Reaching to Grasp a Glass: A Framework for Analysis		
Phase	**Essential Components**	**Primary Muscles**
Transport:	External rotation	■ Infraspinatus, supraspinatus, teres minor, posterior deltoid
	Shoulder flexion	■ Anterior deltoid, pectoralis major and minor, coracobrachialis, biceps brachii
	Protraction	■ Serratus anterior, pectoralis major
	Elbow flexion and extension	■ Biceps brachialis, brachialis, triceps brachii, brachioradialis
Preshaping:	Ulnar or radial deviation	■ Flexor and extensor ulnaris, flexor and extensor carpi radialis
	Supination	■ Supinator, biceps brachii
	Wrist extension	■ Extensor carpi radialis longus, extensor ulnaris
	Thumb abduction	■ Abductor pollicus longus and brevis
	Thumb conjunct rotation (opposition)	■ Opponens pollicus (thumb abduction and flexion at the carpometacarpal thumb joint enabling pulp-to-pulp opposition of the thumb to the fingers)
	Metacarpophalangeal extension	■ Extensor digitorum, extensor indicus (index finger), extensor digiti minimi (little finger)
	Interphalangeal flexion	■ Flexor digitorum superficialis, flexor digitorum profundus
	Finger abduction	■ Dorsal interossei; abductor digit minimi
Grasp:	Metacarpophalangeal flexion	■ Lumbricals; flexor digitorum profundus
	Interphalangeal flexion	■ Flexor digitorum superficialis (PIP joint), flexor digitorum profundus
	Adduction and flexion of thumb	■ Adductor pollicus, first dorsal interossei, flexor pollicus longus and brevis, opponens pollicus

distance. When reaching for a cup that is equal to or greater than an arm's length away, the hips flex to transport the trunk and arm towards the cup. Trunk displacement via hip flexion is observed earlier in the movement sequence when people reach for objects farther away. The elbow may not fully extend at the end of reach (Fig. 39.1) unless that is the only way to reach the object (Fig. 39.2).

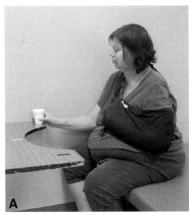

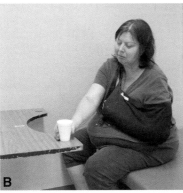

Fig. 39.2 ■ Reaching when sitting.
(A) Within arm's length: No hip or trunk displacement is required. Minimal shoulder flexion with some elbow extension.
(B) At arm's length and across to the affected side: Hip and shoulder flexion with elbow extension help this person reach for the cup.

Preshaping of the hand, fingers and thumb begins almost simultaneously with transport of the arm. Preshaping involves anticipating and making the shape and size of the cup. The forearm in Fig. 39.1 is midway between supination and pronation; the wrist is extended and the thumb abducted, with sufficient metacarpophalangeal (MCP) extension for the fingers to fit around the object. The interphalangeal joints of the fingers remain curved, replicating the shape of the wineglass shown. The fingers may also be slightly abducted to conform to the shape of the object.

Grasp begins when the fingers and thumb touch the object. MCP and finger flexion, thumb adduction and conjunct rotation of the thumb and fingers enable grasp and apply an equal force from either side of the

cup to keep the cup upright in preparation for drinking. If any of these essential components are missing, a person will need to use compensatory strategies to reach, preshape and grasp.

When reaching for an object, the brain automatically selects the most appropriate hand trajectory, decides when to begin forming the appropriate shape and anticipates how much grip force to use based on experience and visual input. There is initial acceleration of the hand followed by deceleration before grasp. The proportion of time allocated to acceleration and deceleration will vary depending on the nature of the object (e.g. a glass vs. a mug) and the intent of the person (e.g. picking up a knife to cut food or placing the knife in the sink). Adaptations to these anticipated forces may also need to be made at the point of grasp. Grasp is based on the *intrinsic* properties of the object, such as the shape, size and perceived fragility as well as factors such as distance from the object and the fact whether the person is sitting or standing.

This timing and synchronisation of reaching require careful, systematic observation if differences are to be recognised, compared with the expected essential components. For example, in healthy adults, transport of the arm and hand preshaping begin almost simultaneously (van Vliet, 1998), although the arm begins to move slightly before the thumb and fingers open.

Reaching to grasp in children has been investigated (e.g. Zoia et al., 2006) and compared with adult reaching. If object size and distance reached are varied, adults and 5-year-old children show very similar reaching strategies. The major differences are longer movement duration and deceleration times and a larger hand aperture in 5-year-old children. People with sensory impairments who are uncertain about their grasp may also reach with a larger than necessary aperture.

In summary, when reaching forward for a cup, the arm begins to move slightly before the hand opens. When reaching for close objects, the elbow typically remains flexed, with shoulder flexion and external rotation helping to transport the hand forward. When reaching for distant objects, hip flexion helps transport the hand forward together with shoulder flexion, external rotation and elbow extension. These features are the 'essential components' of reaching (Carr & Shepherd, 2010).

Postural Adjustments in Sitting

In the next section, a summary is provided of the adjustments needed to maintain sitting when reaching for an object and features to observe when analysing sitting. Analysing and training sitting and leg extensor activation can help prevent falling and leaning when a person reaches; this motor control problem is often erroneously thought to result from 'trunk weakness'. Other features including *base of support, reaching distance* and *direction* will be discussed. These features can be manipulated during analysis and training to make seated reaching easier or more challenging.

When reaching in sitting, the motor control system anticipates which muscles are necessary to maintain balance and avoid falling. These postural adjustments are required, for example, during dressing and toileting. The base of support and the direction and speed of reaching – all influence the muscle activity required when reaching in sitting (Dean et al., 1999a, b). The *base of support* comprises the feet and thighs when sitting with both feet on the floor (see Fig. 39.2A and B). When reaching forward, the leg muscles are critical for maintaining sitting (Dean et al., 1999a, b). For example, when reaching for an object at 140% of arm's length, tibialis anterior contracts before anterior deltoid in the arm. Soleus, quadriceps and biceps femoris muscles contract soon after to control the forward movement of our body mass (Crosbie et al., 1995; Dean et al., 1999a) see Fig. 39.3.

If thigh support is reduced when reaching forward, the contribution of the leg muscles increases (Dean et al., 1999b). If both feet are off the floor, the base of support now comprises only the thighs (Fig. 39.3F). Consequently, postural adjustments cannot be made using the large muscles that cross the knees and ankles, and the feet cannot be stabilised on the floor. Instead, with this smaller base of support, only the muscles around the hip maintain sitting and prevent falling. In this way, reaching distance is significantly reduced when both feet are off the ground.

Reaching direction also influences leg muscle activity, so reaching for an object on the right side results in increased right leg extensor activation (Dean et al., 1999b). Therapists can apply the research on normal seated reach when training people who have difficulty staying upright after experiencing a stroke. For example, reaching forward will be easiest when there is maximal thigh support and both feet are on the floor. The person will be more successful if they are first asked to reach to a target within arm's length. This practice will allow the person to learn to control hip flexion and forward movement of the trunk as they reach, before being expected to reach beyond arm's length.

Feedback also helps to increase learning. If they are unable to generate sufficient extensor force through the affected leg, they may need feedback about whether the leg muscles are working or not. Bathroom scales can provide feedback about force being generated through the affected leg and whether the leg muscles are pushing at the appropriate time or not (i.e. anticipating the transfer of weight forward) to prevent the person falling. This type of practice can improve reaching in sitting (Dean et al., 2007; Dean & Shepherd, 1997). Training seated reach typically starts with reach to the nonaffected side and forward, gradually increasing the distance reached, then reaching across the midline towards the affected side. If a person can contract their leg extensors in anticipation of weight transference to the affected side, they are more likely to be able to sit safely and perform reaching tasks.

In summary, seated reach can be progressed by gradually increasing the distance and changing the direction of reach (i.e. to the unaffected side, then forward, then to the affected side) and decreasing the amount of thigh support.

Focus on Negative not Positive Impairments

Impairments after a stroke or brain injury can be classified as either *negative* or *positive* (Ada & Canning, 2005). *Negative* impairments refer to the *loss* of function and include paralysis (inability to activate muscles), weakness (loss of muscle strength), loss of coordination and loss of sensation. *Positive* impairments are 'added' features and may include abnormal postures and exaggerated reflexes which may lead to spasticity. The *negative* impairments, particularly weakness, limit people with neurological conditions from moving in the way they need to function efficiently. There is a strong relationship between negative impairments (specifically loss of strength) and activity limitations after a stroke; however, positive impairments (such as spasticity) do not show a consistent

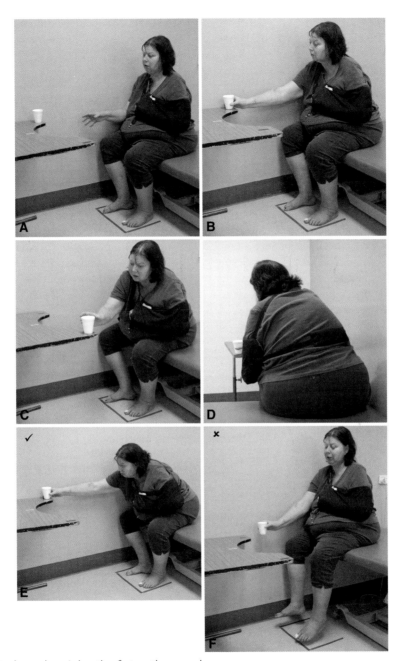

Fig. 39.3 ■ Reaching beyond arm's length – feet on the ground.
(A) Preshapes the hand at the beginning of reach.
(B) This person is pressing down on the floor for support and flexes at the hips to help reaching.
(C) Reaching beyond arm's length to the affected side. This task requires greater leg extensor activity on the affected left leg.
(D) Viewed from behind. Note the weight shift forward and to the left.
(E) Practising reaching well beyond arm's length to load the leg extensor muscles. As leg strength improves, the cup can be placed further across to the affected left side to increase the demand on the affected leg.
(F) Feet off the ground. Unable to reach forward greater than arm's length because the leg extensor muscles cannot contribute.

relationship with activity limitations (Ada et al., 2006; Dorsch et al., 2021; Harris & Eng, 2007; Zackowski et al., 2004).

Despite this evidence, therapy textbooks (e.g. Brashear, 2015) and experienced therapists often focus on the identification and management of positive impairments such as spasticity. However, research outcomes question this emphasis on positive impairments because interventions that target spasticity such as botulinum toxin do not improve upper limb function or participation (Andringa et al., 2019; Lannin et al., 2020). Examples of interventions that focus on loss of strength and coordination (the negative impairments) along with supporting evidence are provided in this chapter. Improving negative impairments is more likely to improve outcomes for people who have experienced a stroke.

A final note about analysing and labelling motor impairments – therapists sometimes erroneously use the terms *spasticity* or *high tone,* when describing soft tissue stiffness, or muscle overactivity which may be compensating for weak muscles. It is important to distinguish between contracture, stiffness and spasticity in order to plan appropriate interventions. Unfortunately, commonly used measurement scales of spasticity such as the Modified Ashworth Scale (MAS) do not distinguish between the mechanical and neural properties of muscle. Consequently, the incidence of spasticity after stroke, as measured using the MAS, is often overestimated. Fortunately, the Tardieu Scale does distinguish between the mechanical and neural properties of a muscle because it measures the response of a muscle to a fast or slow stretch (Patrick & Ada, 2006). The Tardieu Scale, not the MAS, should be used to identify and measure spasticity.

Contractures

Changes in the mechanical-elastic properties of muscles and connective tissue can limit joint range of movement. When analysing movement, a contracture can be recognised by loss of joint range (Ada & Canning, 2005). Resistance to movement is typically due to peripheral changes in muscle fibres and connective tissue (Pandyan et al., 2003), not due to central nervous system changes or spasticity.

Contractures are undesirable for many reasons, particularly the limitations they can have on

movement. The incidence of contracture post-stroke is surprisingly high. A contracture had developed at one or more joints in 52% of 200 consecutive people who experienced a stroke by their 6-month follow-up (Kwah et al., 2012). A person with contractures of pectoralis major, biceps brachii, wrist or finger flexor muscles may be unable to reach forward or preshape their hand during grasp. Efforts are required to actively prevent muscle contractures using motor retraining. To date, serial casting is the only intervention that has been shown to effect transient increases in the range of motion in the upper limb elbow flexors (Moseley et al., 2008). No effective treatments for prevention or longer-term management of contractures have yet been found (Harvey et al., 2017). Short-duration stretch methods such as passive ranging of joints and external devices such as hand splints do not reverse contractures (Lannin et al., 2007). Strategies to elicit muscle contractions and initiate movement early after stroke are required and are discussed later in this chapter.

In summary, muscles adapt quickly to altered positions and immobilisation. Sarcomeres and connective tissue can undergo structural changes resulting in loss of joint range of motion and resistance to movement, which can be measured during analysis. As yet, there are no demonstrated interventions that prevent or reverse contractures.

Recognising Compensatory Strategies

When analysing performance, therapists can learn to recognise compensatory strategies that a person is using due to abnormal muscle activity (Carr & Shepherd, 2010). Compensations may be due to muscle weakness, contracture or both. For example, a person with weak shoulder forward flexion who is asked to reach for a cup may compensate by using hip flexion and/or shoulder abduction to reach forward. These patterns of muscle contraction or 'abnormal synergies' were believed to be part of normal recovery, but there is no neurophysiological explanation for them. Rather, this compensatory muscle activity probably represents the best biomechanical option available to a person who cannot activate their muscles appropriately (Carr & Shepherd, 2010).

The more a person practises using compensations, the more difficult it is to change those compensations. Therapists can help people learn how to contract

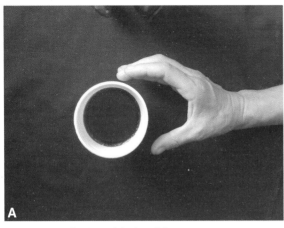
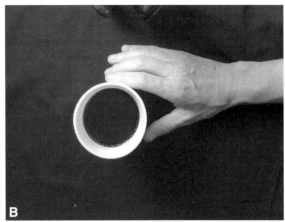

Fig. 39.4 ■ Preshaping of the hand for a cup.
(A) Normal. Forearm and hand form the appropriate shape in preparation to grasp the cup: forearm mid position, wrist extension, thumb abduction and rotation, MCP extension with some IP flexion.
(B) Decreased thumb abduction (thumb in extension). Note compensations: forearm pronation, decreased wrist extension, increased MCP extension.
    It is important to train wrist extension combined with thumb abduction for preshaping to pick up a glass or cup.

muscles more appropriately. When observing reach to grasp, the kinematics should be compared with normal movement. For example, a person usually opens their hand and abducts the thumb at the beginning of reach. Thumb abduction and finger extension are essential for making space to accommodate an object. Typically, people who cannot abduct their thumb and/or extend their fingers and wrist may compensate by extending their thumb, flexing their wrist, pronating their forearm and/or abducting the shoulder (Carr & Shepherd, 2010) See Fig. 39.4. These strategies may help place the hand but are inefficient and inflexible in the long term.

When a person transports their arm towards a cup within arm's reach, it can be observed whether or not they are using their shoulder flexors and external rotators or excessive shoulder elevation, internal rotation or abduction. The latter three compensatory movements may suggest weakness of their shoulder flexors and/or external rotators. Alternatively, these three shoulder movements may compensate for an absence of essential components and weakness at the wrist, thumb or fingers. If a person can extend but not abduct their thumb, they may pronate their forearm, abduct and internally rotate their shoulder to make an aperture for the cup as shown in Fig. 39.4B.

In summary, compensatory strategies are a common result of the loss of essential components. Therapists need to analyse performance, identify missing essential components, hypothesise about the causes of the observed compensations and then test these hypotheses systematically. Interventions should aim to minimise compensations to enable the person who has experienced a stroke to learn to move efficiently without compensating.

Hypothesising About Compensatory Strategies

The final step when analysing movement is to develop and test hypotheses about the causes of missing essential components to help plan interventions. One hypothesis might be that the shoulder muscles are too weak to lift the arm against gravity. That hypothesis can be tested by assessing muscle strength (i.e. manual muscle testing). If a person cannot easily reach forward, muscles to check include anterior deltoid and infraspinatus. Consequently, strength training of these muscles may then be required.

A second hypothesis could be that internal rotators, elbow, wrist and finger flexors are stiff. This hypothesis can be tested by checking the passive range of external rotation, forward flexion, elbow, wrist and finger extension and thumb abduction. Loss of range will reduce the ability to reach for a cup.

A third hypothesis is that the person may be using excessive force in their finger and wrist flexors when reaching. The biceps muscle may contract to compensate for anterior deltoid weakness. This hypothesis can be tested by setting up a practice task that minimises effort. For example, reaching with the arm supported on a table and a piece of paper under the hand to reduce friction.

A fourth hypothesis might be that the task or environmental set-up is too challenging. The cup may be too far away or the table too high. Test these hypotheses by placing the cup closer or lowering the table. Tape a lightweight cup into their hand to decrease task demands and the need for preshaping. The person can concentrate on transporting the cup, not preshaping. Each movement hypothesis can be tested systematically.

Assuming the person's movement problems have been correctly analysed, missing essential components and compensations identified and hypotheses tested, the next step is to design an intervention programme to improve performance. This programme will need to address motor learning.

TEACHING MOTOR SKILLS

Therapists need to use effective coaching and provide training that is task specific to optimise people's motor learning.

Making Training Task Specific

Task-specific training is the intentional practice of a specific skill or task (Bayona et al., 2005), for example, practising reaching to grasp a cup, handwriting or using cutlery or chopsticks. This term does not refer to the practice of nonspecific tasks, for example, lifting the arm for no reason, touching the head or nose or stacking cones. People learn what they practise. If a person wants to improve drinking from a cup, they should practise reaching for and drinking from a cup, not a cone that vaguely resembles a cup. If the person has no active hand movement, modify the task by taping a light plastic cup in their hand and sliding the cup forward on the table. Context-specific training involves incorporating different environmental constraints that influence that task, for example, reaching for cups of different shapes, textures and weights in different locations. Increasing demands in this way can

assist learners to problem solve and understand the rules underlying task performance (Magill & Anderson, 2021). However, adding such demands in the early stages of learning is not appropriate when task demands need to be reduced to maximise the person's ability to practise. In summary, training should replicate the skill or task that a person wants to learn. Valuable time should not be wasted on nonspecific practice.

Maximising Practice and Repetitions

There is a dose-response relationship between amounts of practice and outcomes after stroke (Schneider et al., 2016). In studies that provide evidence of definitive changes in functional magnetic resonance imaging, massed practice and hundreds of repetitions of practice have been done (Carey et al., 2002). Therapists need to use specific strategies to help people achieve large amounts of practice. Setting a repetition target can dramatically increase practice. In one study (Waddell et al., 2014), 15 participants post stroke completed an average of 2956 repetitions of upper limb tasks during their hospital admission and averaged 289 repetitions per hour (95% CI, 280 to 299). To enable more time for practice, therapists need to find ways for people to practise independently or in a semi-supervised group and not rely only on one-to-one practice with a therapist.

Effective Instructions and Feedback

Effective coaching requires instructions to be limited to critical features and have an external, rather than an internal focus. Providing too many instructions and/ or instructions with an internal focus will overload the learner's attentional capacity and interfere with motor learning (Magill & Anderson, 2021). An internal focus instruction brings attention to the movement or muscles that produce the movement, as opposed to an external focus instruction which brings attention to the outcomes of the movement. An example of internal focus is: 'Lift your arm up with the elbow straight'. Environmental set-up can provide an external focus to instructions, for example, when practice is set up, the instruction can be: 'Lift the cup and place it on the target'.

Extrinsic feedback is critical to the teaching and learning of motor skills and can be classified into knowledge of performance and knowledge of results (Kilduski & Rice, 2003).

Knowledge of performance refers to the information about the movement process or attempt, for example, 'You are placing the cup to the left of the target'. This feedback is helpful to learners, particularly concerning corrections that are needed during subsequent attempts (Kernodle & Carlton, 1992). *Knowledge of results* refers to the information about the movement outcome, for example, 'You picked up the cup 10 times in 20 seconds'. This type of feedback can be used to quantify what someone has achieved during a training session, providing clear evidence that performance is changing with practice. A practice task involving feedback is illustrated in Fig. 39.5. Concurrent knowledge of results – that is, feedback provided during performance – can negatively influence learning. Providing summary or average feedback after task completion is more likely to benefit learning (van Vliet & Wulf, 2006). For example, 'The 10 repetitions took 1:30 mins the first time but only 1:10 mins the second time' and 'Of the 10 repetitions completed, you spilt water twice during the first set and only once during the second set'. In summary, therapists should use a small number of simple instructions with an external focus and provide structured feedback during sessions.

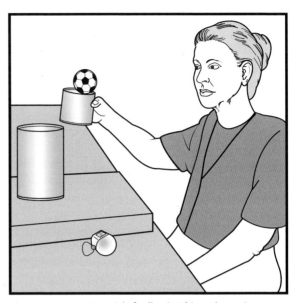

Fig. 39.5 ■ Practice with feedback. This task requires accurate shoulder forward flexion and external rotation, wrist extension with control of radial deviation for successful placement of the can from the table to the target. The mini-football rolls off if coordination is poor. Note the counter on the table to count repetitions.

EVALUATING CHANGES IN PERFORMANCE

Therapists need to re-evaluate motor and occupational performance by using objective measures before and during training. Ideally, a review of performance and goals will occur at every session, for example, picking up a pen to write a word legibly, carrying a shopping bag or opening the thumb and fingers wide enough to grasp a small cup. Outcome measures that focus on roles and participation – what a person needs and/or wants to be able to do – are needed to motivate and remind people, including the treating therapist, why specific practice has been prescribed. One example of such an outcome measure is the Canadian Occupational Performance Measure (Law, 2014). If performance is not changing, the problem may lie with the therapist rather than the learner. Common reasons for lack of improvement include unclear instructions, feedback and goals. If instructions are unclear, the learner may not understand the expected goal. Similarly, if feedback is unclear (or absent), the person may

not understand how to change the next movement attempt to achieve success.

If the task is too difficult (or too easy), progress may not be seen. When re-measurement of performance shows little or no progress, it is vital to reflect on the possible reasons. If the movement hypotheses are correct, therapists can then critically appraise their teaching skills. Alternatively, if a different movement hypothesis is made, new training strategies will be needed.

EVIDENCE-BASED INTERVENTIONS TO IMPROVE UPPER LIMB MOTOR PERFORMANCE AND SENSATION

In adult rehabilitation, interventions found to improve performance of upper limb motor control commonly involve high intensity of practice and repetitions and task-specific training (Pollock et al., 2014). Task-specific training involves the active use of the arm without the therapist's facilitation of movement. A systematic review found that Bobath therapy, where the therapist's facilitation of movement is fundamental, is less effective than task-specific training for improving arm activity outcomes (standardised mean difference –1.07, 95% CI, –1.59 to –0.55, 5 trials) and Fugl-Meyer scores (mean difference –7.84, 95% CI, –12.99 to –2.69, 3 trials) (Dorsch et al., 2023). People need to spend as much time as possible actively practising without facilitation of movement, although enabling active practice can be challenging. Setting targets such as 300 repetitions per session, and recording and reviewing repetitions helps to increase practice intensity (Birkenmeier et al., 2010; Waddell et al., 2014).

With greater recognition that intensive practice can improve outcomes, many therapists prescribe homework. Homework may be individually tailored or involve the use of 'off-the-shelf' programmes such as the Graded Repetitive Arm Supplementary Programme (GRASP; Harris et al., 2009), which has been shown to significantly improve arm recovery compared with usual therapy alone.

In the following section, evidence supporting individual interventions is reported. To keep up to date with new research and practice guidelines, therapists should access national guidelines in their country. Guideline recommendations in English are updated regularly online in Canada (Heart and Stroke Foundation of Canada, 2022), Australia and New Zealand (Stroke Foundation, 2022) and the United Kingdom and Ireland (Intercollegiate Stroke Working Party, 2023).

Strength Training for Paralysed and Very Weak Muscles

Some people may be unable to produce any muscle force (paralysis) or adequate amounts of force. Strength training that involves effortful, repetitive practice improves strength and function and, importantly, does not increase spasticity as many therapists believe (Ada et al., 2006; Harris & Eng, 2010).

Interventions that can help increase strength in people with very weak muscles such as wrist and finger extensors include robotic therapies (Hayward et al., 2010), electrical stimulation (Nascimento et al., 2014) and functional electrical stimulation (FES) applied during activity (Howlett et al., 2015), assistive

---

BOX 39.1
PRACTICE STORY: MARY AND LEO

Leo is an occupational therapist in a large district hospital in rural Australia who has provided an example of a training programme for Mary, a person who has experienced a stroke and wanted to return to her roles as a homemaker and gardener. Her occupational goals included preparing a meal, using a knife in her right hand, tying her shoelaces and gardening.

When I saw Mary there was recovery in the arm muscles, but significant overactivity, compensations at the shoulder and poor hand control. For example, when reaching for a cup, I observed shoulder elevation and abduction, finger clenching, elbow flexion with the body moving forward instead of the arm and hand. Compensations for poor shoulder flexion and loss of external rotation and thumb abduction included shoulder elevation and abduction and excessive finger and wrist flexor activity. It was hard work for Mary.

Training sessions targeted shoulder flexion and anterior deltoid muscle strength in lying, to reduce the demands of gravity. Mary was asked to rest the right hand on her forehead with the elbow flexed, and to control anterior deltoid in that position. When Mary could hold the hand unaided in supine, the next progression was sliding the right hand actively from forehead to pillow and crown of the head, to control anterior deltoid. Mary then progressed to reach further to a target on the wall. Supine was chosen because Mary could not lift the right arm up against gravity in sitting without compensating. Other practice tasks focused on shoulder external rotation, elbow, wrist and finger extension and thumb abduction. Each component was brought together, to eventually work on functional reaching in sitting (Fig. 39.6).

Mary practiced for approximately two hours daily for three months (unsupervised for some of the time), then one hour daily for another three months, then about three hours a week for the last three months. Overall Mary took 36 weeks before functional grasp and release were achieved. In the first six weeks Mary completed 12,810 repetitions, with an average of 427 repetitions per session, and 85 per exercise. After 36 weeks, a score of 16/57 was recorded on the Action Research Arm Test, compared with 2/57 at the beginning, a 14-point change. With a combination of task-specific training, intensive practice, objective measurement and feedback, Mary's hand function slowly improved. She could pick up and hold a knife, prepare simple meals and garden using both hands, but still lacked advanced hand coordination. Without persistence and practice, and a focus on her goals, I don't think these outcomes would have been achieved.

To enable practise between sessions, Leo used practice records with photographs. The rehabilitation team ran a cross-disciplinary upper limb group several times a week. Therapy assistants and relatives also helped supervise practice using homework books with instructions, goals and illustrations by the therapist.

technologies such as the SMART arm device (Barker et al., 2008), dynamic hand orthoses such as Saeboflex (Alexander et al., 2021) and modified task-specific practice (de Sousa et al., 2018). Examples of task-specific practice that may increase muscle strength are shown in Figs. 39.7–39.12.

Practice Story: Mary and Leo (Box 39.1) describes the application of an upper limb training programme

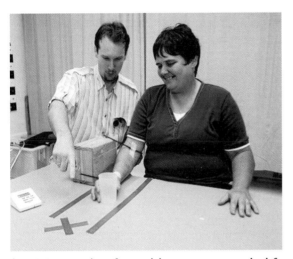

Fig. 39.6 ■ Practice of essential components required for reaching (forward flexion and external rotation) and drinking from a cup. Post-stroke M had limited opportunities to engage in occupations such as drinking from a cup with her dominant right hand. Weak shoulder flexors and external rotators and an inability to open the thumb or fingers to pre-shape correctly prevented the use of the hand and arm. The occupational therapist is helping M practice shoulder flexion and external rotation – essential components of reaching – while maintaining wrist extension and forearm in supination. In this photograph, M is sliding the cup forward while staying inside the lines (electrical tape stuck to the table).

Two drinking straws have been applied to the arm, one to the inner elbow and another to the back of the wrist. The straws acted as visual cues, reminding M to maintain shoulder external rotation (the straw stays in contact with the wooden block) and wrist extension (the knuckles stay in contact with the flexible straw). The practice environment demands external rotation, wrist extension and supination to be successful. This set-up gives immediate visual feedback if internal rotation and abduction occur when reaching forward as the hand will move outside the lines, or the elbow straw will lose contact with the box.

M is learning to monitor their performance, which is important for practice outside of therapy sessions. Notice the timer/counter near the therapist's right hand, to record practice time and repetitions.

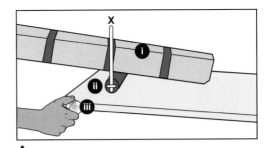

A

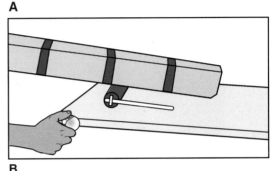

B

Fig. 39.7 ■ Strategy to train protraction. When a person is very weak, this exercise can be used to seek muscle activity with minimal force required. The person is seated with a table close, to support the weight of the arm. The goal is active protraction by moving the straw to touch the target. The target distance and height can be changed depending on the person's ability.
(A)
  i. Cardboard cylinder secured with tape to hold the arm straight
  ii. Cylinder to minimise friction
  iii. Straw taped to the cylinder
  iv. Target
  v. Counter
(B) Protraction - straw touches the target. Goal achieved. The person can count their repetitions on the counter.

for Mary, who has experienced a stroke and wants to be able to prepare a meal, use a knife in her right hand, tie her shoelaces and look after her garden.

Electrical Stimulation

Electrical stimulation can produce a muscle contraction and improve strength and activity outcomes in people who are very weak. One systematic review found a moderate effect from cyclical electrical stimulation on *strength* outcomes from 11 trials and a small effect on *activity* from 6 trials (Nascimento et al., 2014). The authors concluded that electrical stimulation increased arm movement more than conventional

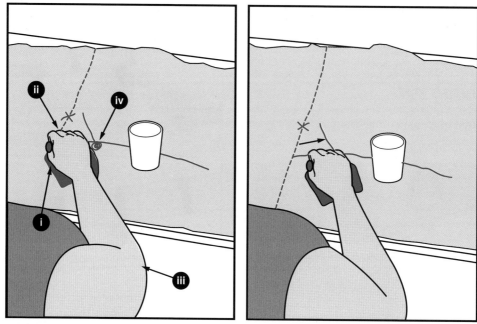

Fig. 39.8 ■ Eliciting external rotation – home practice example.
i. Cloth under the hand to reduce friction
ii. Dotted line indicates starting position – aligned with the navel
iii. Small cylinder held between the right elbow and body (not visible)
iv. The goal – without dropping the cylinder

(A) This person is practising external rotation. There is a large sheet of paper on the table which the person can take home. The pen marks show the start position for their right hand, with dotted line indicating the navel. Their arm is supported on the table. There is a small cylinder between the elbow and body, to give feedback if there is any shoulder abduction or extension (which are compensations). The goal is to slide to touch the line, following the arc drawn on the paper (this arc was drawn with assistance from the therapist using a pen held in the person's hand). If the hand does not follow the arc, the arm is not externally rotating.

(B) They have externally rotated their shoulder and covered the target line without dropping the cylinder. Goal achieved. Progress is recorded on the sheet as the range improves.

therapy. Another systematic review found a large effect from FES on upper limb activity (standardised mean difference 0.69, 95% CI, 0.33 to 1.05) (Howlett et al., 2015). In summary, electrical stimulation and FES can be used with people who have very weak muscles to improve both strength and activity level outcomes.

Mirror Therapy

Mirror therapy uses visual illusion to trick the brain and promote motor recovery. A person watches a mirror reflection of their intact hand while performing repetitive movements. The mirror gives the illusion that the affected arm can move. This therapy is used with people who have moderate to severe weakness

to improve motor function. A Cochrane review of 62 trials concluded that mirror therapy can improve motor function and performance of daily activities after stroke (Thieme et al., 2018). Most of the included trials provided 15 to 60 minutes of supervised mirror therapy daily for 2 to 8 weeks. Although improvements in some trials were small, mirror therapy is inexpensive to deliver and can be completed in a hospital or at home.

Reducing Muscle Force During Grasp

Some individuals contract too many or incorrect muscles when grasping objects. This behaviour is characteristic of early skill acquisition, and importantly, is

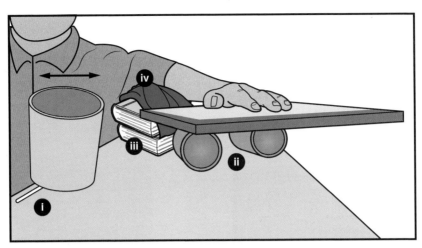

Fig. 39.9 ▪ Eliciting elbow flexion and extension.
i.   Straw taped underneath the container, which allows the container to rock (in the direction of the arrows) when pushed lightly
ii. Cylinders under the board to minimise friction
iii. Books or box to raise the shoulder to horizontal
iv. Slidesheet to reduce friction and allow the arm to move more easily
After set up by therapist or carer, this person can practice unaided. The goal is to flex the elbow, tip the container and return to the start position.

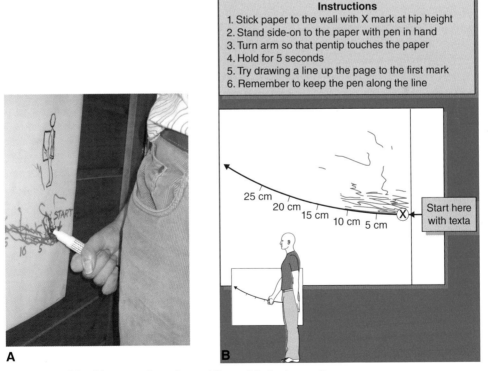

Fig. 39.10 ▪ Practice of shoulder external rotation and forward flexion in standing.
(A) The person is holding a pen in the photo and attempting to forward flex while keeping the pen in contact with the paper. If the shoulder internally rotates the pen will no longer touch the paper. This task is difficult; consequently, there is excessive muscle activity when holding the pen. As the task becomes easier, excessive muscle activity should decrease.
(B) Progress can be measured on the paper. The short-term goal initially is to keep the pen tip touching the X mark for 5 seconds x 3 times in a row. The next goal is to draw a line to the 5-cm mark.

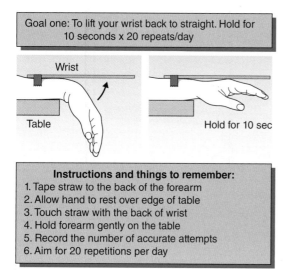

Fig. 39.11 ■ Wrist extension example. Wrist extension is essential for most grasping tasks such as picking up a cup or glass. This page from a practice book shows the exercise, goal and things to remember. The goal is to lift the wrist back to touch the straw and hold for 10 seconds.

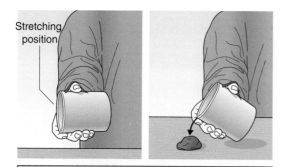

Fig. 39.12 ■ Supination practice. Practice book showing the practice in the learner's own words: 'After a short stretch, turn the cup over to touch pink blob; hold for a count of 10'. The goal is to turn the cup over, touch the pink blob and hold there for 10 seconds.

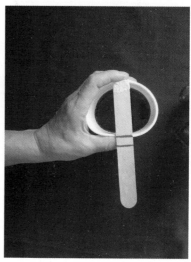

Fig. 39.13 ■ Force regulation practice. The cup provides immediate feedback about the force applied. The goal is to hold the cup without deforming it. The paddlepop stick provides immediate feedback. Once a person can hold the cup without deforming it, the goal might be to transport the cup (e.g. from the table to their mouth) without deforming it.

not spasticity. One focus of therapy is to teach people to contract the right muscles at the right time and reduce excessive effort in other muscles. Changing task demands and the environment can reduce effort, for example, by asking a person to lift a light plastic cup off the table instead of a glass, or slide rather than lift a cup. If a person is unable to preshape while reaching, taping a cup into their hand can reduce task demands and help them focus on reaching. If too much force is applied, use a disposable cup that deforms easily when grasped to provide feedback about force production (see Figs. 39.13 and 39.14). No trials of these interventions have been published to date.

Different instructions may also help a person to become more self-aware and learn to contract some muscles while relaxing others or producing less force in other muscles. For example:

'When you grasp the cup, don't press so hard. Keep the round shape'.

'If you press too hard, the water will come up above the marked line'.

'Try not to squash the cup. Use light pressure on the sides of the cup'.

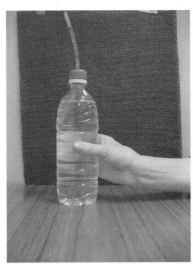

Fig. 39.14 ■ Force regulation practice.

How to make this feedback device:
1. Find a plastic water bottle with a lid that fits well so that no water or air escapes when the bottle is squeezed.
2. Drill a small hole in the lid that allows plastic tubing to be pushed through but no air entry (it is essential that no air enters between the tube and lid of the bottle).
3. Fill the bottle with water. Screw on the cap.
4. Draw two lines on the tubing as targets.
5. Squeeze the bottle so that water moves between the two lines without squirting out the tubing.

Individual goals can be established depending on how a person uses feedback and their individual skill acquisition. For example: How many times can they accurately move the water between the targets? Can they lift the bottle and maintain the water at a target level?

Coordination Training

Some individuals can grasp and pick up but not manipulate objects such as a knife or fork. Training in advanced hand functions involves more than cutting up bread or copying writing. Analysis and training demand careful observation and problem solving so that therapists can identify essential components that are missing or altered. Tasks requiring advanced skill performance (and analysis) include handwriting and use of cutlery and chopsticks.

With small objects, training of grip force during lift-off and manipulation will be required. Healthy adults typically apply a force slightly higher than the minimum required to prevent object slippage (Nowak & Hermsdorfer, 2003) but not so much that a fork or knife rotates. People who have experienced a stroke

apply significantly greater mean grip forces at lift-off (≥39%) compared with healthy adults (Blennerhassett et al., 2006; Quaney et al., 2005). Impaired sensation is likely to compound these problems; however, task-specific training strategies are likely to be similar for people with and without sensory impairment. If a person has difficulty using cutlery or a pen, they need to engage in part-practice and force control training with these objects. Picking up an object precisely without rotating the handle, cutting food and writing are tasks that require appropriate force production and accurate opposing forces of the thumb and fingers to be successful. See Figs. 39.15 and 39.16 for two examples.

Mental Practice

Mental practice is used routinely in sports training to improve skill acquisition and can be used to promote motor recovery. In rehabilitation, a person can mentally rehearse a task, for example, imagining the transport and preshaping actions of picking up a cup, without physically attempting them. Two recent systematic reviews of mental practice involving people who have experienced a stroke (Barclay et al., 2020; Stockley et al., 2021) found positive short-term effects for arm and hand function and activities of daily living, particularly early after stroke and for people with more severe weakness. Mental practice requires discipline and has the potential to improve arm function when used as an adjunct to therapy.

Constraint-Induced Movement Therapy

Constraint-induced movement therapy (CIMT) improves movement and use of the affected hand and promotes neuroplasticity (Corbetta et al., 2015). CIMT involves three active components delivered intensively over two weeks: (1) task-specific repetitive practice involving 1:1 shaping with feedback and progression, for 3 to 6 hours a day; (2) a restraint such as a mitt worn for 90% of waking hours; and (3) a transfer-of-training package involving home practice (Taub et al., 2013). The restraint is used to discourage the use of the unaffected hand and greater use of the affected hand, but the restraint does not appear to be essential (Krawczyk et al., 2012). It is probably the intensive task-specific practice and coaching that promote neuroplasticity

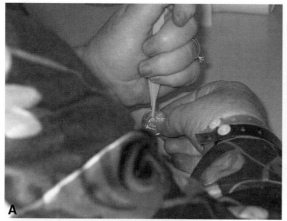
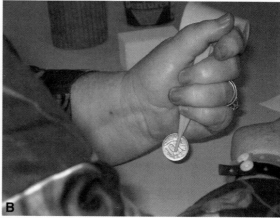
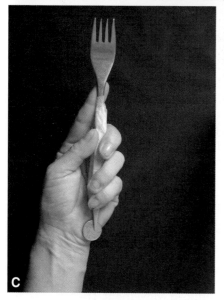

Fig. 39.15 ▪ Practice strategies for fork use.

This person was unable to hold the fork in their hand because the ring and little fingers were unable to generate sufficient force when the wrist flexed to press into food. This is a common problem: insufficient rotation of the ring and little fingers across the palm of the hand (palmar cupping), combined with insufficient flexor force in inner range of the ring and little finger flexors. Consequently, the fork (or knife) becomes unstable in their hand.

Below are some ideas for training which engages the learner:

(A and B) Force generation within the ring and little fingers, using plastic tweezers while holding a coin. The coin will drop out if there is insufficient force from the ring and little fingers. A larger object can be used if a coin is too difficult (e.g. two coins taped together or small wooden block). Once the coin can be held successfully, the person can progress to pronating their hand (where they can no longer see the coin), then gradually increase the amount of wrist flexion. (C) Practising index finger MCP flexion with IP extension, while holding tweezers and the coin. The tweezers are taped onto the fork handle. Practice can now move on to using food while attempting to maintain a flexion force in the ring and little fingers, keeping the coin in place and the fork stable.

and change arm function. Eligible participants in trials typically have active wrist and finger extension at study commencement. For a detailed description of CIMT eligibility criteria and procedures, see Taub et al. (2013).

Trials conducted in acute care settings early post-stroke report significantly better improvements in arm function, immediately following the intervention for participants who received CIMT, (Kwakkel et al., 2016; Thrane et al., 2015). However, between-group differences were not maintained at follow-up. The collective research shows a moderate effect of CIMT on upper limb motor performance (Corbetta et al., 2015).

Sensory Retraining

Therapists can use passive and active approaches to address sensory impairments. Passive approaches include electrical stimulation, thermal stimulation (heat or cold), and pressure or movement by a therapist to increase sensory awareness of the limb such as via intermittent pneumatic compression. More trials have evaluated the effect of passive than active approaches (Serrada et al., 2019); passive techniques typically involve little or no active exploration by the person. Passive approaches vary greatly in intensity and intervention duration and whether or not therapy was combined with another intervention (such as mirror therapy or electrical stimulation).

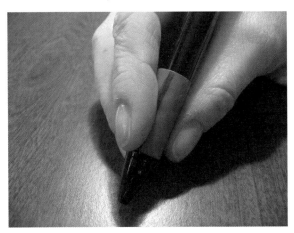

Fig. 39.16 ▪ **Pen use.** Example of part-practice for pen control.
Goal: To rotate the line on the pen in both directions x 5 times. To be successful, the opposition force of the thumb and fingers need to be maintained while the pen is rotated. This exercise involves the extrinsic flexor and intrinsic muscles of the hand to maintain opposition of thumb and fingers.
Reminders:
- Try to rotate the pen gently.
- Count the number of repetitions before losing control of the pen.
- Practice with different-sized pens or pencils.
- Aim to practice three times daily x 5 minutes.

Active approaches focus on somatosensory discrimination and recognition tasks, such as texture discrimination, tactile object recognition, limb position, and object recognition using mirror therapy and mental practice (Arya et al., 2022). Tasks gradually progressed in discrimination difficulty and feedback provided (Turville et al., 2019). Somatosensory discrimination retraining improves arm sensation after stroke, but the impact on function is less clear. Although further rigorous trials are needed to replicate the SENSe trial (Carey et al., 2011), the SENSe retraining programme can be implemented by therapists with fidelity using a manual and DVD (Carey, 2012). SENSe is available at https://sensetherapy.net.au/.

PREVENTING AND MANAGING SECONDARY IMPAIRMENTS

Contractures

Loss of shoulder external rotation range of movement is common after experiencing a stroke. In one study (n = 52), the majority of people who had a stroke experienced a loss of external rotation range greater than 60 degrees (Lindgren et al., 2012), with some participants unable to attain neutral (0 degrees). This loss of range correlated with shoulder pain (Lindgren et al., 2012) and will affect the performance of self-care tasks. Therefore therapists need to anticipate and help prevent contractures by proactively seeking muscle activity.

Muscle stretching has been a popular intervention for managing muscle length changes and contracture, in addition to strengthening opposing muscles. Some years ago, animal studies suggested that 30-minute stretches prevented the development of contractures (Goldspink & Williams, 1990; Williams, 1990). Unfortunately, the changes observed in animal muscles were not reproduced in human stretching studies. For a review of stretching research, see Harvey and colleagues (2017). Disappointingly, high-quality trials have not found statistically or clinically worthwhile benefits from prolonged stretches in people after a stroke or brain or spinal cord injury.

Sustained stretches have also been applied using serial casts to immobilise muscles in their stretched positions. Serial casts produce transient changes in the range of motion at the elbow in adults with traumatic brain injury; however, these improvements were not sustained after cast removal (Moseley et al., 2008).

A hand splint worn nightly for 4 weeks to prevent contracture after experiencing a stroke or brain injury found no difference in wrist extensibility compared with control participants who did not wear a splint (Lannin et al., 2007). Nor did an overnight thumb web-space splint worn for 3 months reduce contractures in people with a neurological condition (Harvey et al., 2006). Disappointingly, electrical stimulation used while a wrist extension splint was worn did not prevent the development of contractures postABI (Leung et al., 2012).

The current evidence strongly suggests that therapists should not routinely apply stretches or splints during rehabilitation. There is uncertainty about whether stretch interventions are effective in the longer term, and if so, how often stretches should be administered and how long they should be held.

Shoulder Pain

Shoulder pain can limit a person's participation in activities. The causes of shoulder pain are still uncertain but may include impingement of tissues around the shoulder joint, trauma from pulling on the arm and loss of external rotation. A Cochrane systematic review (Ada et al., 2005a) found that shoulder strapping with adhesive tape delayed the onset of shoulder pain but did not reduce pain once it had developed. Other randomised controlled trials have confirmed the benefits of strapping for preventing and delaying the onset of shoulder pain (Appel et al., 2011; Griffin & Bernhardt, 2006; Pandian et al., 2013).

Electrical stimulation can also reduce shoulder pain when applied to the supraspinatus, posterior and middle deltoid and trapezius muscles (Koog et al., 2010; Viana et al., 2012).

Shoulder Subluxation

Shoulder slings and supports have not been well-researched despite their frequent use in practice. Expert opinion is that external supports such as wheelchair and chair attachments are needed to support the weight of the arm (Foongchomcheay et al., 2005). Triangular slings can reduce a shoulder subluxation, but slings that do not support the arm will probably not reduce a subluxation (Ada et al., 2005b).

Electrical stimulation can stimulate muscle contractions around the shoulder joint in people with little or no muscle activity. A meta-analysis of 10 trials of electrical stimulation to prevent or reduce subluxation in the first 6 months after experiencing a stroke found that stimulation reduced subluxation by an average of 4.9 mm (95% CI, 3.3–6.6 mm) (Vafadar et al., 2015).

Improving Movement in People with Spasticity

For people with spasticity that interferes with function, the most common medical intervention is chemodenervation using botulinum toxin type A or BoNT-A (Sheean et al., 2010). Results from a meta-analysis found that BoNT-A reduced spasticity (Andringa et al., 2019) but did not improve functional outcomes. The large BoTULS study (Shaw et al., 2010) evaluated the addition of BoNT-A to an upper limb therapy programme. No between-group differences were reported in upper limb function. So although BoNT-A may temporarily reduce spasticity, it is unlikely to improve hand function.

The InTENSE trial (Lannin et al., 2020) combined intensive evidence-based motor retraining and BoNT-A to determine if together they improved upper limb activity more than BoNT-A plus an exercise handout. After 3 months, there was no between-group difference in goal attainment or blocks moved using the affected hand or in any secondary outcome except strength in favour of the experimental group. Participants in that study had limited active movement at the start of therapy, which may have influenced the outcomes.

In summary, people who have experienced a stroke or brain injury usually want improved hand use, not just less spasticity. Evidence-based interventions recommended in this chapter have greater potential to improve function than BoNT-A. Therapists should focus on negative impairments such as loss of strength, rather than focusing on reducing spasticity.

FUTURE DIRECTIONS

The earlier rehabilitation begins, the better the recovery following a stroke or brain injury. Greater intensity of treatment translates into better outcomes. Therapists are now moving away from 'hands-on' therapies towards evidence-informed interventions that apply motor learning theory and promote neuroplasticity. One-on-one therapy is being supplemented with homework and group programmes where people practise together.

Telerehabilitation has increased post-COVID-19. This mode of delivery can reduce travel time and may reduce costs, with some sessions provided face-to-face and some by telephone and using the Internet. The 2020 Cochrane review (Laver et al., 2020) reported on outcomes from 22 trials and found that people who received telerehabilitation post-stroke had similar outcomes for activities of daily living to those receiving face-to-face therapy or no telerehabilitation.

The need for increased intensity of practice has led to the testing of novel rehabilitation techniques such as virtual reality and robotic therapy. Virtual reality enables people to practise independently or semi-supervised. When virtual reality was used in addition to conventional upper limb therapy (providing more time in therapy), there was a statistically significant difference between groups (standardised mean difference

0.49, 95% CI, 0.21–0.77) based on 10 studies and 210 participants (Laver et al., 2017).

Robotic therapy allows some of the labour-intensive training to be performed by automated devices, increasing repetitions, upper limb function and activities of daily living post-stroke (Mehrholz et al., 2012; Pollock et al., 2014). Although improvements are similar to those achieved with dose-matched intensive task-specific training (Norouzi-Gheidari et al., 2012), a robotic device allows individuals to practise semi-supervised.

As the evidence grows in support of more intensive therapy, interventions such as CIMT, virtual reality and robotics will be used more often because they increase practice opportunities, and CIMT in particular has been shown to improve outcomes. Technologies continue to improve. Consequently, it is not possible to predict what advances will become routine practice in the future. The important message for therapists is to remain abreast of current scientific evidence.

CONCLUSION

This chapter has focused on the process of analysing and retraining motor performance and sensation in adults with brain impairment. The content is necessarily impairment-focused because much of upper limb rehabilitation, particularly in hospital settings, focuses on eliciting muscle activity and strength training before the return of functional grasp. Therapists need to remind themselves and the people they are working with of the occupational engagement and participation goals of training – for example, eating a meal with family members using cutlery in both hands. Once a person can grasp and manipulate objects, tasks and goals become more obvious. Although the overall goal may be to increase engagement in occupations, therapists should not ignore impairment-focused interventions.

REFERENCES

Ada, L., & Canning, C. (2005). Changing the way we view the contribution of motor impairments to physical disability after stroke. In K. Refshauge, L. Ada, & E. Ellis (Eds.), *Science-based rehabilitation: Theories into practice* (pp. 87–106). Elsevier Butterworth Heinemann.

Ada, L., Dorsch, S., & Canning, C. (2006). Strengthening interventions to increase strength and improve activity after stroke: A systematic review. *Australian Journal of Physiotherapy, 52*, 241–248.

Ada, L., Foongchomcheay, A., & Canning, C. (2005). Supportive devices for preventing and treating subluxation of the shoulder after stroke. *Cochrane Database of Systematic Reviews, 1*, CD003863.

Ada, L., O'Dwyer, N., & O'Neill, E. (2006). Relation between spasticity, weakness and contracture of the elbow flexors and upper limb activity after stroke: An observational study. *Disability & Rehabilitation, 28*, 891–897.

Alexander, J., Dawson, J., & Langhorne, P. (2021). Dynamic hand orthoses for the recovery of hand and arm function in adults after stroke: A systematic review and meta-analysis of randomised controlled trials. *Topics in Stroke Rehabilitation, 29*(2), 114–124.

Alt Murphy, M. A., & Håger, C. K. (2015). Kinematic analysis of the upper extremity after stroke: How far have we reached and what have we grasped? *Physical Therapy Reviews, 20*(3), 137–155.

Andringa, A., van de Port, I., van Wegen, E., Ket, J., Meskers, C., & Kwakkel, G. (2019). Effectiveness of Botulinum Toxin treatment for upper limb spasticity poststroke over different ICF domains: A systematic review and meta-analysis. *Archives of Physical Medicine & Rehabilitation, 100*(9), 1703–1725.

Appel, C., Mayston, M., & Perry, L. (2011). Feasibility study of a randomized controlled trial protocol to examine clinical effectiveness of shoulder strapping in acute stroke patients. *Clinical Rehabilitation, 29*(9), 833–843.

Arya, K. N., Pandian, S., Joshi, A. K., Chaudhary, N., & Agarwal, G. G. (2022). Active sensory therapies enhancing upper limb recovery among poststroke subjects: A systematic review. *Annals of Neurosciences, 29*(2–3), 104–115.

Barclay, R. E., Stevenson, T. J., Poluha, W., Semenko, B., & Schubert, J. (2020). Mental practice for treating upper extremity deficits in individuals with hemiparesis after stroke. *Cochrane Database of Systematic Reviews, 5*, CD005950.

Barker, R., Brauer, S., & Carson, R. (2008). Training of reaching in stroke survivors with severe and chronic upper limb paresis using a novel non-robotic device: A randomized clinical trial. *Stroke, 29*, 1800–1807.

Bayona, N. A., Bitensky, J., Salter, K., & Teasell, R. (2005). The role of task-specific training in rehabilitation therapies. *Topics in Stroke Rehabilitation, 12*, 58–65.

Birkenmeier, R. L., Prager, E. M., & Lang, C. E. (2010). Translating animal doses of task-specific training to people with chronic stroke in 1-hour therapy sessions: A proof-of-concept study. *Neurorehabilitation and Neural Repair, 24*(7), 620–635.

Blennerhassett, J. M., Carey, L. M., & Matyas, T. A. (2006). Grip force regulation during pinch grip lifts under somatosensory guidance: Comparison between people with stroke and healthy controls. *Archives of Physical Medicine and Rehabilitation, 87*, 418–429.

Brashear, A. (Ed.). (2015). *Spasticity diagnosis and management* (2nd ed.). Demos Medical.

Carey, J. R., Kimberley, T. J., Lewis, S. M., Auerbach, E. J., Dorsey, L., Rundquist, P., & Ugurbil, K. (2002). Analysis of fMRI and finger tracking training in subjects with chronic stroke. *Brain, 125*(4), 773–788.

Carey, L. (2012). *SENSe: Helping stroke survivors regain a sense of touch. A manual for therapists.* Florey Neuroscience Institute.

Carey, L., Macdonell, R., & Matyas, T. A. (2011). SENSe: Study of the effectiveness of neurorehabilitation on sensation: A randomized controlled trial. *Neurorehabilitation and Neural Repair, 25*(4), 304–313.

Carr, J. H., & Shepherd, R. B. (2010). Reaching and manipulation. In *Neurological rehabilitation: Optimizing motor performance* (2nd ed. pp. 123–162). Churchill Livingstone Elsevier.

Carr, J. H., Shepherd, R. B., Gordon, J., Gentile, A. M., & Held, J. M. (1987). *Movemement science: Foundations for physical therapy in rehabilitation.* Aspen.

Corbetta, D., Sirtori, V., Castellini, G., Moja, L., & Gatti, R. (2015). Constraint-induced movement therapy for upper extremities in people with stroke. *Cochrane Database of Systematic Reviews, 10,* CD004433.

Crosbie, J., Shepherd, R., & Squire, T. (1995). Postural and voluntary movement during reaching in sitting: The role of the lower limbs. *Journal of Human Movement Studies, 28,* 103–126.

Dean, C., & Shepherd, R. (1997). Task related training improves performance of seated reaching tasks after stroke: A randomised controlled trial. *Stroke, 28,* 722–728.

Dean, C., Channon, E., & Hall, J. (2007). Sitting training early after stroke improves sitting ability and quality and carries over to standing up but not to walking: A randomised controlled trial. *Australian Journal of Physiotherapy, 53,* 97–102.

Dean, C., Shepherd, R., & Adams, R. (1999a). Sitting balance 1: Trunk and arm coordination and the contribution of the lower limbs during self-paced reaching in sitting. *Gait and Posture, 10,* 135–146.

Dean, C., Shepherd, R., & Adams, R. (1999b). Sitting balance 11: Reach direction and thigh support affect the contribution of the lower limbs when reaching beyond arm's length in sitting. *Gait and Posture, 10,* 147–153.

DeSousa, D., Harvey, L., Dorsch, S., & Glinsky, J. (2018). Interventions involving repetitive practice improve strength after stroke: A systematic review. *Journal of Physiotherapy, 64,* 210–221.

Dorsch, S., Ada, L., Sorial, T., & Fanayan, E. (2021). The relationship between strength of the affected leg and walking speed after stroke varies according to the level of walking disability: A systematic review. *Physical Therapy, 101*(12), pzab233. https://doi.org/10.1093/ptj/pzab233.

Dorsch, S., Carling, C., Cao, Z., Fanayan, E., Graham, P. L., McCluskey, A., Schurr, K., Scrivener, K., & Tyson, S. (2023). Bobath therapy is inferior to task-specific training and not superior to other interventions in improving arm activity and arm strength outcomes after stroke: A systematic review. *Journal of Physiotherapy, 69*(1), 15–22. https://doi.org/10.1016/j.jphys.2022.11.008.

Foongchomcheay, A., Ada, L., & Canning, C. (2005). Use of devices to prevent subluxation of the shoulder after stroke. *Physiotherapy Research International, 10,* 134–145.

Goldspink, G., & Williams, P. (1990). Muscle fibre and connective tissue changes associated with use and disuse. In L. Ada & C. Canning (Eds.), *Key issues in neurological physiotherapy* (pp. 197–218). Butterworth Heinemann.

Griffin, A., & Bernhardt, J. (2006). Strapping the hemiplegic shoulder prevents development of pain during rehabilitation: A randomized controlled trial. *Clinical Rehabilitation, 20,* 287–295.

Harris, J. E., & Eng, J. J. (2007). Paretic upper-limb strength best explains arm activity in people with stroke. *Physical Therapy, 87,* 88–97.

Harris, J. E., & Eng, J. J. (2010). Strength training improves upper limb function in people with stroke. A meta-analysis. *Stroke, 41,* 136–140.

Harris, J. E., Eng, J. J., Miller, W. C., & Dawson, A. S. (2009). A self-administered graded repetitive arm supplementary program (GRASP) improves arm function during inpatient stroke rehabilitation: A multi-site randomized controlled trial. *Stroke, 40,* 2123–2128.

Harvey, L., de Jong, I., Goehl, G., & Mardwedel, S. (2006). Twelve weeks of nightly stretch does not reduce thumb web-space contractures in people with a neurological condition: A randomised controlled trial. *Australian Journal of Physiotherapy, 52,* 251–258.

Harvey, L. A., Katalinic, O. M., Herbert, R. D., Moseley, A. M., Lannin, N. A., & Schurr, K. (2017). Stretch for the treatment and prevention of contractures. *Cochrane Database of Systematic Reviews, 2017*(1), CD007455. http://doi.org/10.1002/14651858.CD007455.pub3. Accessed 13 August 2024.

Hayward, K., Barker, R., & Brauer, S. (2010). Interventions to promote motor recovery in stroke survivors with severe paresis: A systematic review. *Disability and Rehabilitation, 32,* 1973–1986.

Heart and Stroke Foundation of Canada. (2022). *Canadian stroke best practice recommendations (CSBPR)* (7th ed.). Heart and Stroke Foundation of Canada. https://www.strokebestpractices.ca/recommendations.

Howlett, O. A., Lannin, N. A., Ada, L., & McKinstry, C. A. (2015). Functional electrical stimulation improves activity after stroke: A systematic review with meta-analysis. *Archives of Physical Medicine & Rehabilitation, 96*(5), 934–943.

Intercollegiate Stroke Working Party. (2023). *National clinical guideline for stroke for the United Kingdom and Ireland.* Intercollegiate Stroke Working Party. https://www.strokeguideline.org/contents/.

Kernodle, M. W., & Carlton, L. G. (1992). Information feedback and the learning of multiple-degree-of-freedom activities. *Journal of Motor Behaviour, 24,* 187–196.

Kilduski, N. C., & Rice, M. S. (2003). Qualitative and quantitative knowledge of results: Effects on motor learning. *American Journal of Occupational Therapy, 57,* 329–336.

Koog, Y. H., Jin, S. S., Yoon, K., & Min, B. (2010). Interventions for hemiplegic shoulder pain: Systematic review of RCTs. *Disability and Rehabilitation, 32*(4), 282–291.

Krawczyk, M., Sidaway, M., Radwanska, A., Zaborska, J., Ujma, R., & Cztonkowska, A. (2012). Effects of sling and voluntary constraint during constraint-induced movement therapy for the arm after stroke: A randomized, prospective, single-centre, blinded observer rater study. *Clinical Rehabilitation, 26,* 990–998.

Kwah, K. L., Harvey, L. A., Diong, J. H., & Herbert, R. D. (2012). Half of the adults who present to hospital with stroke develop at least one contracture within six months: An observational study. *Journal of Physiotherapy, 58,* 41–47.

Kwakkel, G., Winters, C., van Wegen, E. E. H., Nijland, R. H. M., van Kuijk, A. A. A., Visser-Meily, A., & on behalf of the EXPLICIT-Stroke Consortium. (2016). Effects of unilateral upper limb training in two distinct prognostic groups early after stroke: The EXPLICIT-Stroke randomized clinical trial. *Neurorehabilitation & Neural Repair, 30*(9), 804–816.

Lannin, N. A., Cusick, A., McCluskey, A., & Herbert, R. D. (2007). Effects of splinting on wrist contracture after stroke: A randomized controlled trial. *Stroke, 38,* 111–116.

Lannin, N. A., Ada, L., English, C., Ratcliffe, J., Faux, S. G., Palit, M., Gonzalez, S., Olver, J., Cameron, I., Crotty, M., & on behalf of the InTENSE Trial Group. (2020). Effect of additional rehabilitation after Botulinum Toxin-A on upper limb activity in chronic stroke: The InTENSE trial. *Stroke, 51*, 556–562.

Laver, K. E., Adey-Wakeling, Z., Crotty, M., Lannin, N. A., George, S., & Sherrington, C. (2020). Telerehabilitation services for stroke. *Cochrane Database of Systematic Reviews, 1*, CD010255. https://doi.org/10.1002/14651858.CD010255.pub3.

Laver, K. E., Lange, B., George, S., Deutsch, J. E., Saposnik, G., & Crotty, M. (2017). Virtual reality for stroke rehabilitation. *Cochrane Database of Systematic Reviews, 11*(11), CD008349. https://doi.org/10.1002/14651858.CD008349.pub4. Accessed 13 August 2024.

Law, M. C. (2014). *Canadian occupational performance measure* (5th ed.). Canadian Association of Occupational Therapists (CAOT) Publications ACE.

Leung, J., Harvey, L. A., & Moseley, A. M. (2012). Electrical stimulation and splinting were not clearly more effective than splinting alone for contracture management after ABI: An RCT. *Journal of Physiotherapy, 58*, 231–240.

Lindgren, I., Lexell, J., Jonsson, A. C., & Brogardh, C. (2012). Left-sided hemiparesis, pain frequency, and decreased passive shoulder range of abduction are predictors of long-lasting poststroke shoulder pain. *Physical Medicine and Rehabilitation, 4*, 561–568.

Magill, R. A., & Anderson, D. (2021). *Motor learning and control: Concepts and applications* (12th ed.). McGraw-Hill Education.

Mehrholz, J., Hadrich, A., Platz, T., Kugler, J., & Pohl, M. (2012). Electromechanical and robot-assisted arm training for improving generic activities of daily living, arm function and arm muscle strength after stroke. *Cochrane Database of Systematic Reviews, 6*, CD006876. https://doi.org/10.1002/14651858.CD006876.pub3.

Moseley, A. M., Hassett, L. M., Leung, J., Clare, J. S., Herbert, R. D., & Harvey, L. A. (2008). Serial casting versus positioning for the treatment of elbow contractures in adults with traumatic brain injury: A randomized controlled trial. *Clinical Rehabilitation, 22*(5), 406–417.

Nascimento, R., Michaelsen, S. M., Ada, L., Polese, J. C., & Teixeira-Salmela, L. F. (2014). Cyclical electrical stimulation increases strength and improves activity after stroke: A systematic review. *Journal of Physiotherapy, 60*, 22–30.

Norouzi-Gheidari, N., Archambault, P. S., & Fung, J. (2012). Effects of robot-assisted therapy on stroke rehabilitation in upper limbs: Systematic reviews and meta-analysis of the literature. *Journal of Rehabilitation Research and Development, 49*(4), 479–496.

Nowak, D. A., & Hermsdorfer, J. (2003). Selective deficits of grip force during object manipulation in patients with reduced sensibility of the grasping digits. *Neuroscience Research, 47*, 65–72.

Pandian, J. D., Kaur, P., Arora, R., Vishwambaran, D. K., Toor, G., Mathangi, S., Vijaya, P., Uppal, A., Kaur, T., & Arima, H. (2013). Shoulder taping reduces injury and pain in stroke patients: Randomized controlled trial. *Neurology, 80*(6), 528–532.

Pandyan, A. D., Cameron, M., Powell, J., Stott, D. J., & Granat, M. H. (2003). Contractures in the post-stroke wrist: A pilot study of its time course of development and its association with upper limb recovery. *Clinical Rehabilitation, 17*(1), 88–95.

Patrick, E., & Ada, L. (2006). The Tardieu Scale differentiates contracture from spasticity whereas the Ashworth Scale is confounded by it. *Clinical Rehabilitation, 20*, 173–182.

Pollock, A., Farmer, S. E., Brady, M. C., Langhorne, P., Mead, G. E., Mehrholz, J., & van Wijck, F. (2014). Interventions for improving upper limb function after stroke. *Cochrane Database of Systematic Reviews, 2014*(11), CD010820. https://doi.org/10.1002/14651858.CD010820.pub2.

Quaney, B. M., Perera, S., Maletsky, R., Luchies, C. W., & Nudo, R. J. (2005). Impaired grip force modulation in the ipsilesional hand after unilateral middle cerebral artery stroke. *Neurorehabilitation and Neural Repair, 19*, 338–349.

Refshauge, K. M., Ada, L., & Ellis, E. (Eds.). (2005). *Science-based rehabilitation: Theories into practice*. Elsevier Butterworth-Heinemann.

Schneider, E. J., Lannin, N. A., Ada, L., & Schmidt, J. (2016). Increasing the amount of usual rehabilitation improves activity after stroke: A systematic review. *Journal of Physiotherapy, 62*(4), 182–187.

Serrada, I., Hordacre, B., & Hillier, S. L. (2019). Does sensory retraining improve sensation and sensorimotor function following stroke: A systematic review and meta-analysis. *Frontiers in Neuroscience, 13*, 402.

Shaw, L., Rodgers, H., Price, C., van Wijck, F., Shackley, P., Steen, N., Barnes, M., Ford, G., Graham, L., & BoTULS investigators. (2010). BoTULS: A multicentre randomised controlled trial to evaluate the clinical effectiveness and cost effectiveness of treating upper limb spasticity due to stroke with botulinum toxin type A. *Health Technology Assessment, 14*(26), 1–113.

Sheean, G., Lannin, N. A., Turner-Stokes, L., Rawicki, B., Snow, B. J., & Cerebral Palsy Institute. (2010). Botulinum toxin assessment, intervention and aftercare for upper limb hyper tonicity in adults: International consensus statement. *European Journal of Neurology, 17*, 74–93.

Stockley, R. C., Jarvis, K., Boland, P., & Clegg, A. J. (2021). Systematic review and meta-analysis of the effectiveness of mental practice for the upper limb after stroke: Imagined or real benefit? *Archives of Physical Medicine and Rehabilitation, 102*(5), 1011–1027.

Stroke Foundation. (2022). *Clinical guidelines for stroke management*. Stroke Foundation. https://informme.org.au/guidelines/living-clinical-guidelines-for-stroke-management.

Taub, E., Uswatte, G., Mark, V. W., Morris, D. M., Barman, J., Bowman, M. H., Bryson, C., Delgado, A., & Bishop-McKay, S. (2013). Method for enhancing real-world use of a more affected arm in chronic stroke: Transfer package of constraint-induced movement therapy. *Stroke, 44*, 1383–1388.

Thieme, H., Morkisch, N., Mehrholz, J., Behrensc, J., Borgetto, B., & Dohle, C. (2018). Mirror therapy for improving motor function after stroke. *Cochrane Database of Systematic Reviews, 7*(7), CD008449. https://doi.org/10.1002/14651858.CD008449.pub3.

Thrane, G., Askim, T., Stock, R., Indredavik, B., Gjone, R., Erichsen, A., & Anke, A. (2015). Efficacy of constraint induced movement therapy in early stroke rehabilitation: A randomized controlled multisite trial. *Neurorehabilitation & Neural Repair, 29*(6), 517–525.

Turville, M. L., Cahill, L. S., Matyas, T. A., Blennerhassett, J. M., & Carey, L. M. (2019). The effectiveness of somatosensory retraining for improving sensory function in the arm following stroke: a systematic review. *Clinical Rehabilitation, 33*(5), 834–846.

Vafadar, A. K., Côté, J. N., & Archambault, P. S. (2015). Effectiveness of functional electrical stimulation in improving clinical outcomes in the upper arm following stroke: A systematic review and meta-analysis. *BioMed Research International, 2015*, 729768.

van Vliet, P. M., & Wulf, G. (2006). Extrinsic feedback for motor learning after stroke: What is the evidence? *Disability and Rehabilitation, 28*, 831–840.

van Vliet, P. M. (1998). An investigation of reaching movements following stroke. University of Nottingham. PhD thesis.

Viana, R., Pereira, S., Mehta, T., Miller, T., & Teasell, R. (2012). Evidence for therapeutic interventions for hemiplegic shoulder pain during the chronic stage of stroke: A review. *Topics in Stroke Rehabilitation, 19*(6), 514–522.

Waddell, K. J., Birkenmeier, R. L., Moore, J. L., Hornby, T. G., & Lang, C. E. (2014). Feasibility of high-repetition, task-specific training for individuals with upper-extremity paresis. *American Journal of Occupational Therapy, 68*, 444–453.

Williams, P. (1990). Use of intermittent stretch in the prevention of serial sarcomere loss in immobilised muscle. *Annals of Rheumatological Disease, 49*, 316–317.

Zackowski, K. M., Dromerick, A. W., Sahrmann, S. A., Thach, W. T., & Bastian, A. J. (2004). How do strength, sensation, spasticity and joint individuation relate to the reaching deficits of people with chronic hemipareis? *Brain, 127*, 1035–1046.

Zoia, S., Pezzetta, E., Blason, L., Scabar, A., Carrozzi, M., Bulgheroni, M., & Castiello, U. (2006). A comparison of the reach-to-grasp movement between children and adults: a kinematic study. *Developmental Neuropsychology, 30*(2), 719–738.

REFLECTION

1. Describe the essential components of reaching for a glass (i.e. transporting the hand forwards, and pre-shaping the hand) in healthy adults, both when a glass is within comfortable arms reach, then beyond comfortable arms reach.

2. Describe common compensations that may be observed when a person with upper limb impairments reaches for a cup.

3. Provide some examples of positive and negative impairments of the upper limb after brain impairment. Discuss the importance of addressing negative impairments as a therapist.

4. List and describe the physical set-up of three interventions that you could use with a person who is very weak after a stroke (i.e. someone that cannot lift their arm up onto a table) in the inpatient hospital setting.

5. Discuss strategies that you might use to retrain force generation or control, when a person uses too much force to (a) pick up a cup, and (b) manipulate a fork.

40

HAND THERAPY AND ORTHOTICS

KATIE O'DONNELL ■ YELIZ PRIOR

Overview

The chapter on hand therapy and orthotics delves into the specialised domain of occupational therapy dedicated to aiding individuals whose upper limbs may be impacted by a spectrum of factors, including traumatic injuries, degenerative conditions, inflammatory diseases, neurological issues and postoperative conditions. Concurrently, the practice of orthotics involves the art of crafting, adapting and fitting orthoses, tailored to enhance the hand and wrist's structural attributes and subsequently elevate occupational performance. Within this comprehensive exploration, the chapter examines the pertinent anatomical and pathophysiological aspects relating to the hand, prevalent hand ailments and injuries, as well as the strategic interventions encompassing occupational therapy and orthotics. The overarching objective remains the optimisation of occupational engagement, underscoring the pivotal role played by therapeutic approaches and orthotic interventions.

KEY POINTS

- Hand therapy interventions must be based on sound anatomical knowledge, an understanding of the healing and inflammatory process and the consideration of the unique occupational participation needs of each person.

- Assessments should incorporate standardised outcome measures, including functional and person-reported assessments to gauge the progress and effectiveness of interventions.

- While considering the severity of the hand injury or condition is important, the primary focus should centre on how the hand condition impacts the individual's life, aiming to optimise occupational participation.

- Orthoses serve as adjunctive interventions utilised either to establish or restore an individual's skills or to prevent the occurrence or development of secondary complications.

- Given the inconsistent evidence of a superior orthosis design, fabrication or wearing regimen, the orthosis selected should maximise occupational participation.

'Your hand opens and closes, opens and closes. If it were always a fist or always stretched open, you would be paralysed. Your deepest presence is in every small contracting and expanding, the two as beautifully balanced and coordinated as birds' wings'.

Jelaluddin Rumi (1207–1273)

INTRODUCTION

The hand is a delicate and sophisticated structure that is capable of a vast array of intricate skills and plays an integral role in many functional tasks. It is part of the human body incorporating strength, sensation and dexterity; it is strong enough to carry the entire weight of a human body on a few fingertips yet nimble enough to manipulate a grain of rice between two fingertips with precision. The hand's rich and complex sensory innervation enables people to anticipate extreme temperatures, discriminate between textures and shapes and adapt their grip to manipulate tools.

Hands are used to support communication; hands can be used to draw attention by raising one in class, enhance a listener's understanding of a story through gestures, provide visual cues to verbal directions and are the foundations of sign language (Perniss et al. 2020). Hands are such an integral part of communication that congenitally blind individuals, who have never witnessed gesturing, have been observed to move their hands when they talk (Iverson & Goldin-Meadow, 1998).

Hands are visible to the person and the public and so, for many, a hand injury has more than just physical consequences; a change in the appearance of the hands can result in a significant psychological impact (Dunpath et al., 2015). One study found that one in three people with a hand injury had high depression and posttraumatic stress disorder (PTSD) scores (Richards et al., 2011). Chown et al. (2017) found that participants reported 'PTSD, work avoidance, appearance and body image issues, sleep disturbance, pain and psychosocial and marital functional difficulties'. Additionally, concerns around aesthetics and social desirability impacted social participation and reduced adherence to hand orthoses worn in long-term conditions such as rheumatoid arthritis (Prior et al., 2022).

Hand therapy is the art and science of rehabilitation of the upper limb, which includes the hand, wrist, elbow and shoulder girdle (HTCC, 2020). Hand therapy may be practised by either a registered occupational therapist or physiotherapist, although it is estimated that approximately 70% of hand therapists are occupational therapists (Ewald, 2015). Hand therapists use specialised skills for assessment, planning and treatment to provide therapeutic interventions to prevent dysfunction and restore a person's ability to complete tasks and fully participate in life. The International Federation of Societies for Hand Therapy (IFSHT) supports the development of hand therapy worldwide, and its member countries have their own national societies. Many countries have a recognition programme to become an accredited hand therapist, which may consist of a formal examination, diplomas and/or portfolio programme.

While hand therapy is a subspecialty within occupational therapy, the upper limb and its function must be considered by all occupational therapists, regardless of their area of practice. An inability of a person to use their hands can lead to occupational deprivation across a wide spectrum of activities. Hands are used in the most basic of self-care tasks to complex activities required for work, leisure and caregiving. For example, hands are used to plait children's hair, to undertake spiritual worship, for eating and dressing and to create moments of intimacy. Occupational therapists must have an overarching awareness of the basic anatomy of the upper limb with its key biomechanical and sensory features and an understanding of common hand conditions and injuries to conduct a thorough assessment and design interventions that will meet the person's needs and support them to achieve their occupational participation goals.

HAND ANATOMY

Bones are the framework of the hand. They provide a stable base for soft tissues like tendons and ligaments to anchor to and are largely responsible for the overall shape of the hand. The bones of the hand can be grouped into the carpal bones, including eight small bones which make up the wrist, the base of the hand, and the digits which include the metacarpals

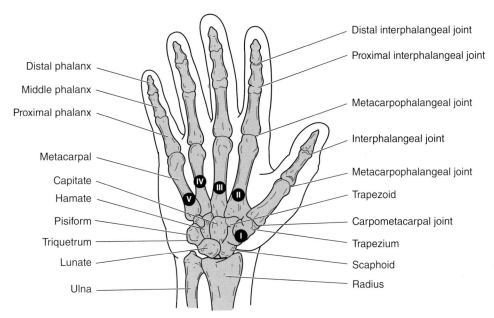

Distal interphalangeal joint
Proximal interphalangeal joint
Metacarpophalangeal joint
Interphalangeal joint
Metacarpophalangeal joint
Trapezoid
Carpometacarpal joint
Trapezium
Scaphoid
Radius

Distal phalanx
Middle phalanx
Proximal phalanx
Metacarpal
Capitate
Hamate
Pisiform
Triquetrum
Lunate
Ulna

Fig. 40.1 ■ Anatomical features of the hand.

and the phalanges. The carpal bones are arranged in two rows, the proximal row of the scaphoid, lunate, triquetrum and pisiform which articulates with the radius and ulna to make up the wrist and the distal row of the trapezium trapezoid, capitate and hamate which articulates distally with the metacarpals (Fig. 40.1).

The bony architecture of each digit is essentially the same, except for the thumb. The long bones of the metacarpals form the palm of the hand and create the metacarpophalangeal joint (MCP) with the proximal phalange, followed by the medial and distal phalanges which create the proximal (PIP) and distal (DIP) interphalangeal joints. The MCP joint is a condyloid joint which facilitates movement in two planes through flexion/extension and abduction/adduction of the fingers while the interphalangeal joints are hinge joint for flexion and extension only. The thumb differs from the other digits as there are only two phalanges which make up an interphalangeal joint. The carpometacarpal joint of the thumb is a flattened saddle shape, which articulates with the trapezium to facilitate opposition, one of the unique movements of the thumb. Each digit of the hand can move independently of, as well as work in unison with, the other digits to manipulate objects and perform a variety of grips.

Each joint is supported by ligaments. These are collagenous fibres that interconnect two bones. Ligaments are pliable and flexible to allow joint movement but strong enough to prevent injuries such as dislocations.

Muscles drive the movement of the hand (Fig. 40.2). Small intrinsic muscles are located within the hand and are responsible for many of the smaller fine motor movements. Larger, extrinsic muscles originate in the forearm. The muscles are inserted into the hand's skeleton by tendons.

Three main nerves supply the sensory and motor aspects of the hand: the median, ulnar and radial nerves (Figs. 40.3–40.5). The median nerve travels through the carpal tunnel at the proximal palmar aspect of the wrist and innervates the thumb, index and middle finger and the radial aspect of the ring finger. The ulnar nerve innervates the little and ring finger, and the radial nerve innervates the dorsal proximal aspect of the thumb, ring and middle finger and the radial aspect of the ring finger. Arterial supply of blood to the hand is from the radial and ulnar arteries.

The skin in the hand is mobile on the dorsal aspect to allow for free mobility of the hand joints while the palmar aspect of the skin is thicker and can create

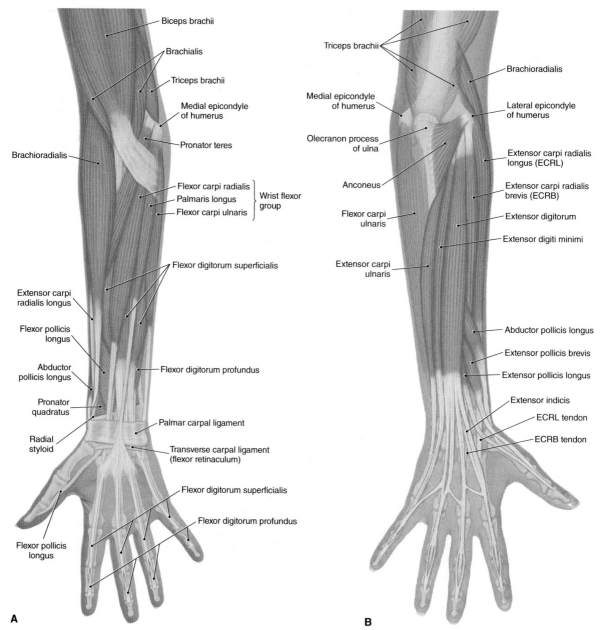

Fig. 40.2 ■ Muscles of the forearm and hand. (A) Anterior, (B) Posterior.

tension to facilitate different grip patterns. The skin, bones and soft tissue structure of the hand determine the shape of the hand and create three arches in the hand (Fig. 40.6). The longitudinal arch, which runs along the fingers and metacarpals, the proximal transverse arch across the distal carpal row and the distal transverse arch at the level of the metacarpal heads. These arches are the basis of the flexibility of the hand and allow movement which supports prehension and manipulation of movement.

MEDIAN NERVE

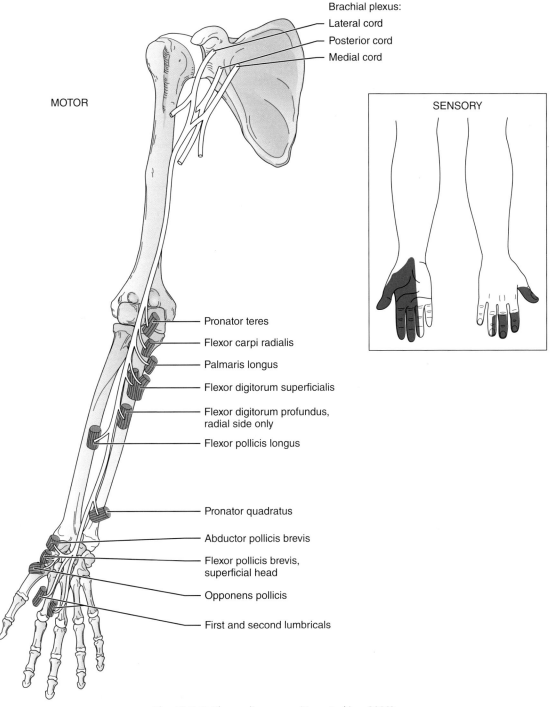

Brachial plexus:
Lateral cord
Posterior cord
Medial cord

MOTOR

SENSORY

Pronator teres

Flexor carpi radialis

Palmaris longus

Flexor digitorum superficialis

Flexor digitorum profundus, radial side only

Flexor pollicis longus

Pronator quadratus

Abductor pollicis brevis

Flexor pollicis brevis, superficial head

Opponens pollicis

First and second lumbricals

Fig. 40.3 ■ The median nerve. (From Jenkins, 2009)

ULNAR NERVE

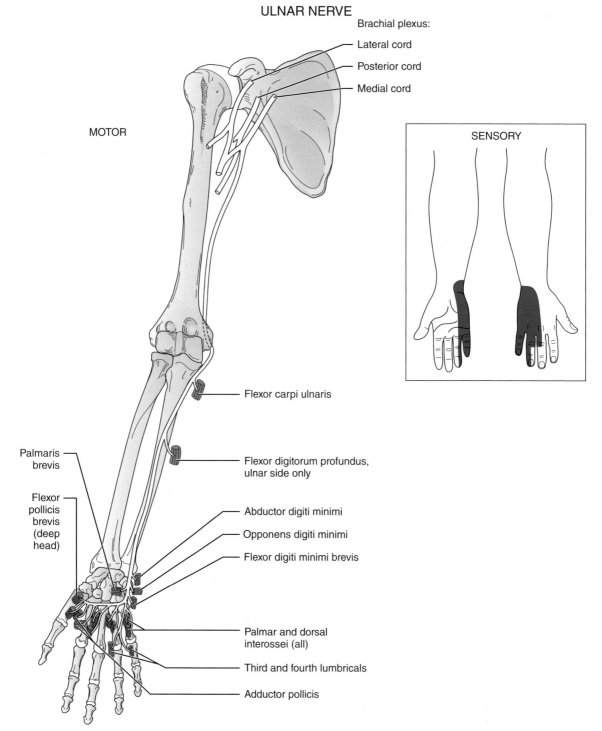

Brachial plexus:
— Lateral cord
— Posterior cord
— Medial cord

MOTOR

SENSORY

— Flexor carpi ulnaris

— Flexor digitorum profundus, ulnar side only

Palmaris brevis

Flexor pollicis brevis (deep head)

— Abductor digiti minimi

— Opponens digiti minimi

— Flexor digiti minimi brevis

— Palmar and dorsal interossei (all)

— Third and fourth lumbricals

— Adductor pollicis

Fig. 40.4 ■ The ulna nerve. (From Jenkins, 2009).

RADIAL/AXILLARY NERVES

MOTOR

SENSORY

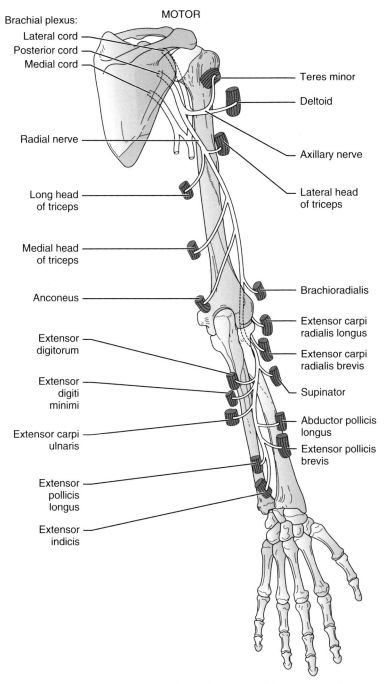

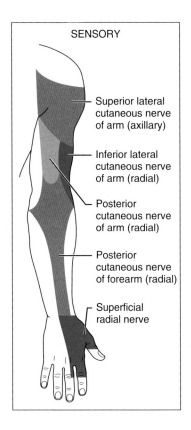

Brachial plexus:
Lateral cord
Posterior cord
Medial cord

Radial nerve

Long head
of triceps

Medial head
of triceps

Anconeus

Extensor
digitorum

Extensor
digiti
minimi

Extensor carpi
ulnaris

Extensor
pollicis
longus

Extensor
indicis

Teres minor

Deltoid

Axillary nerve

Lateral head
of triceps

Brachioradialis

Extensor carpi
radialis longus

Extensor carpi
radialis brevis

Supinator

Abductor pollicis
longus

Extensor pollicis
brevis

Superior lateral
cutaneous nerve
of arm (axillary)

Inferior lateral
cutaneous nerve
of arm (radial)

Posterior
cutaneous nerve
of arm (radial)

Posterior
cutaneous nerve
of forearm (radial)

Superficial
radial nerve

Fig. 40.5 ■ The radial nerve. (From Jenkins, 2009).

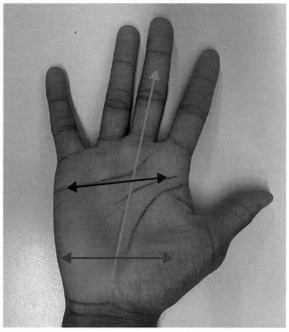

Longitudinal Arch

Distal Transverse Arch

Proximal Transverse Arch

Fig. 40.6 ■ The arches of the hand.

HAND INJURIES

Hand trauma is a common occurrence, and the prevalence has increased in recent years, perhaps due to an ageing population (Manley et al., 2019). Fractures can account for up to 50% of hand injuries, followed by soft tissue injuries such as tendon and nerve lacerations (Manley et al., 2019). Men of working age (15–59 years) are disproportionately affected by hand injuries, which can lead to significant physical, economic and psychological implications (de Putter et al., 2012). Understanding the healing process for fractures, soft tissue and wounds is essential when creating a hand therapy programme. Occupational therapists must also consider the person's specific occupational participation goals and demands to develop a programme that improves the hand condition while protecting the healing structures and promoting recovery. Interventions are guided by stages of healing, which are outlined in the next section:

Fracture Healing

The process of fracture healing can be characterised by three overlapping stages: inflammation, reparative and remodelling.

(i)   *Inflammation:* Immediately after a fracture occurs, a haematoma is generated from the blood vessels that supply the bone and periosteum. This haematoma coagulates in between and around the fracture ends. This creates a template for the soft callus formation of the reparative stage. This inflammation peaks at 24 hours and lasts up to 7 days. The end of this stage often coincides with a reduction in pain and swelling.

(ii) *Reparative:* Around day 5, a soft callus replaces the haematoma which provides some structure for the fracture, although it is not stable enough for the person to use. Soft callus can easily bend or deform if the fracture is not supported. Over time the soft callus reorganises into hard callus by osteoblasts, which can take several weeks.

(iii) *Remodelling:* This is the longest phase, often starting around 6 weeks and may last for months to several years. During this stage, the hard callus responds to activity, external forces, functional demands and growth. During this stage, regular bone replaces the hard callus, and it remodels until it looks like how it looked prior to the fracture.

Most bones take 4 to 6 weeks to heal; however, some of the smaller bones of the hand like the phalanges can take as little as three weeks.

Wound Healing

Wound healing is a dynamic process that covers the initial injury, to wound closure, to reorganisation of scar tissue. It can be described in four distinct but overlapping stages (Myers, 2020).

Stage 1: Haemostasis: Blood from the damaged vessels comes into contact with exposed collagen. The platelets from the blood activate the release of clotting factors. These clots help stop the bleeding at the vessel. This stage can last up to 24 hours.

Stage 2: Inflammation (Fig. 40.7A): Neutrophils enter the site and begin debriding injured tissue and bacteria. This process can create warmth and redness at the wound site, swelling and pain from increased pressure from the oedema for the injured person. This lasts between 4 and 6 days.

Stage 3: Proliferation: Fibroblasts create new tissue through collagen synthesis, which gives the healing wound structure and creates tensile strength. This causes tissue granulation, which contracts the wound and pulls the margins closer together. This process begins between day 2 and 5 and ends between days 14 and 28.

Stage 4: Maturation (Fig. 40.7B): The collagen structure crosslinks resulting in increased strength to the tissue. The scar begins to shrink and remodel as tissue contracts. This process starts around day 21 but can last up to 2 years.

All soft tissue structures such as tendons and nerve tissue heal in a similar fragile and complex fashion (Fig. 40.8). Healing times are influenced by many local factors such as foreign bodies, infection and wound care management and systemic factors such diabetes and cardiovascular disease, nutrition, the use of certain medication such as steroid and the age of the affected person as older skin can cause the dermal layer to be thin and less resistance to shearing forces.

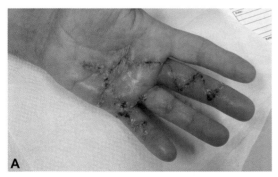

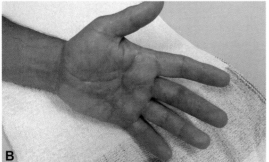

Fig. 40.7 ■ Inflammatory and remodelling stages of wound healing. (A) Inflammatory stage of wound healing, (B) Remodelling stage of wound healing.

HAND CONDITIONS

Hand therapy can be provided to people with reduced upper limb function from non-traumatic circumstances such as musculoskeletal and neurological conditions, fine motor dysfunction such as dyspraxia as well as congenital hand differences.

Occupational therapists who work in hand therapy may work with individuals who are affected by osteoarthritis (OA) and/or rheumatoid arthritis (RA), which are prevalent rheumatic and musculoskeletal conditions known to impact the hands. OA is a degenerative joint disease that commonly affects the hand and causes pain, structural changes to the joints and reduced grip strength and function (Di Nicola, 2020). OA commonly affects individuals aged 45 years and over. RA is an autoimmune disease that initially affects the small joints of the hand, progressing to larger joints. Often the bone and cartilage of joints are destroyed and tendons and ligaments are weakened (Bullock et al., 2019), causing pain, stiffness, swelling

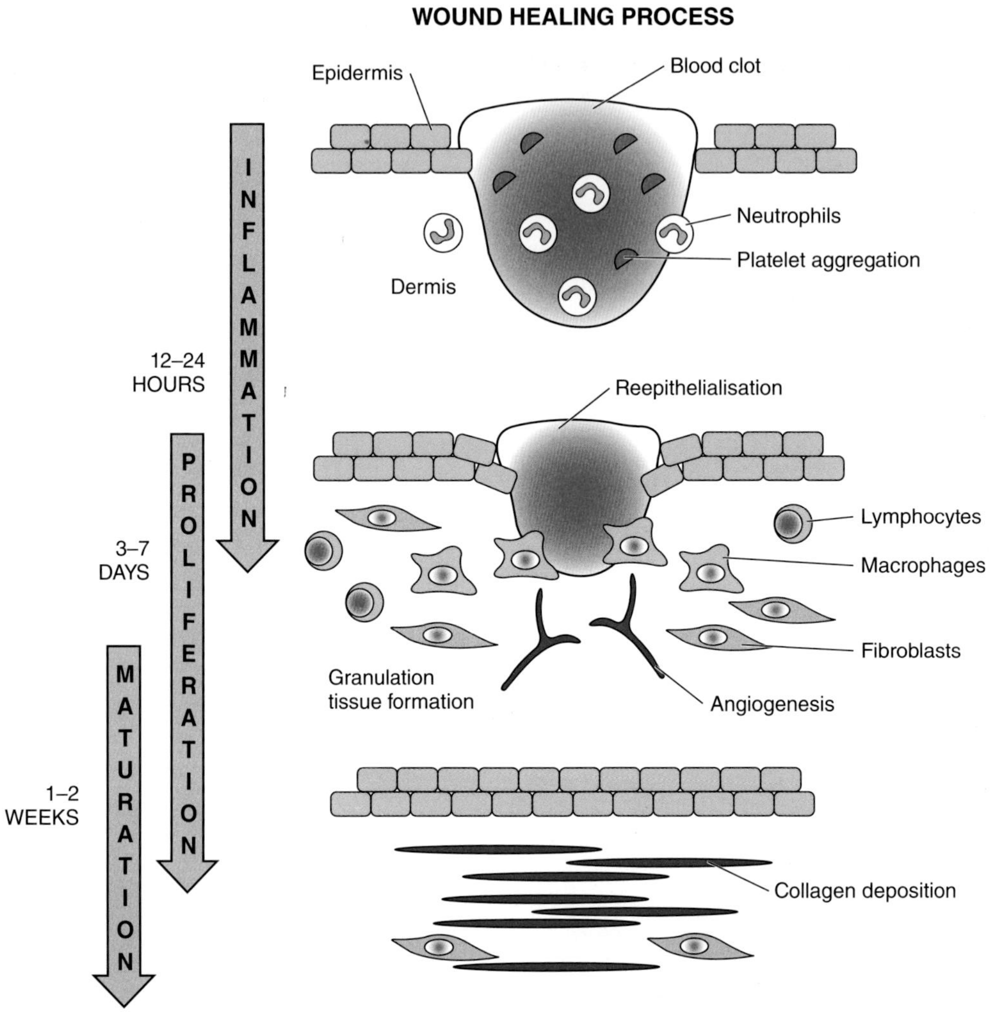

WOUND HEALING PROCESS

Fig. 40.8 ■ Schema of skin-wound healing. (From Kondo & Ishida, 2010).

and loss of function (Horsten et al., 2010). Although the onset of RA is commonly around the ages of 35 to 60 years, it can affect people at any age; for example, children before the age of 16 years may experience juvenile idiopathic arthritis (JIA). Hand therapy plays a vital role in the conservative management of these conditions and can involve the provision of education on ergonomics, activity modification, joint protection, adaptive equipment, orthoses and hand exercises (Hammond et al., 2020; Siegel et al., 2017).

Neurological conditions such as stroke, cerebral palsy and multiple sclerosis (MS) may impact the hands by causing pain and altered motor patterns with high or low muscle tone. Hand therapy can involve the provision of orthotics to reduce the risk of contractures in people with spasticity or provide support to maximise upper limb function through exercise or adaptive techniques.

ASSESSMENT OF THE HAND

Assessment is typically the first contact an occupational therapist will have with a person and is a key part of the occupational therapy process. Assessments should be centred on occupational participation in life roles (RCOT, 2021). It should be undertaken responsibly, according to professional standards and with appropriate knowledge. An assessment should be appropriate to the individual person, in-depth and thorough to obtain all the necessary information regarding the impact of the person's hand condition on their occupational participation. This is essential to create a personalised and collaborative intervention programme to optimise outcomes as most hand therapy approaches promote self-management.

When providing hand therapy, occupational therapists must have a knowledge of wound and fracture healing timeframes for people recovering from hand trauma to protect healing structures and optimise physical recovery. Likewise, in hand conditions such as RA and OA, occupational therapists must understand the disease process. Hence, the hand assessment harmonises elements from the medical model, a perspective frequently woven into the biopsychosocial framework by hand therapists. In this context, biological factors are thoughtfully examined alongside psychosocial considerations, aligning with the approach advocated by Burley et al. (2018). This approach ensures that the assessment of occupational participation is underpinned by individuals' psychosocial requirements, placing their goals squarely at the core of the intervention. Consequently, assessments manifest as multi-faceted processes, encompassing the collection of both subjective and objective data.

History Taking

Gathering a full, detailed history is an essential part of the subjective assessment and should be completed before any physical examination. It allows the person an opportunity to lead the conversation and explain what they feel is most relevant about themselves and their journey to date. History taking should take a narrative approach. Occupational therapists must listen empathetically, taking into consideration the person's lived experience and how their hand impairment may be impacting their life. It also helps establish the person's perceptions, expectations, wants and needs in the early stages of the therapeutic relationship (O'Brien, 2012) so that these can be explored and incorporated into the plan collaboratively.

The occupational therapist must collect all the basic information, for example, age, past medical history, living and social circumstances, occupation and interests. Information specific to the hand is also required, such as hand dominance, use of hands in meaningful occupation and the impact of the hand condition on these. A detailed account of the mechanism of injury in trauma cases can help indicate what structures may be involved for diagnostic purposes and what complications an occupational therapist should be on the lookout for. The occupational therapist should establish the educational needs of a person to understand reasons behind activity limitations, knowledge and skills to adopt ergonomic approaches to reduce pain, fatigue and joint strain, as well as hand and upper limb range of movement, muscle strength and endurance to inform assessment, goal setting and intervention planning (Hammond et al., 2020) (Refer to the Chapter 22).

The Assessment Process

Physical Assessment

The assessment process in hand therapy typically involves observation, palpation and then movement. Using this information along with the history discussed with the person gathers a well-rounded evaluation and provides the foundation for successful therapy.

> *Observation:* The observation component begins while a person is in the waiting room to see if and how they are using their hand/s as it can be beneficial to see spontaneous function rather than a formalised assessment. The occupational therapist can note if the person is holding the arm in a protective, guarding posture and/or whether they are using it to hold their phone or push up from the chair to observe behavioural patterns. It is also a good opportunity to observe other nonverbal communication such as facial expressions and body language. The physical condition of the hand can be observed, noting any wounds or scars, muscle atrophy, oedema, skin colour changes, nail changes or anatomical deformity.
>
> *Palpation:* Palpation of the person's hand is an essential part of the assessment process, but it must be done with their consent and a considered, gentle approach with an awareness of any discomfort they may experience to touch. The occupational

therapist can feel if the hand is excessively sweating and check the skin moisture or dryness. It is also important to check subjective signs such as their hand sensation, pain levels and patterns, joint stability and stiffness and check the scar for the presence of any tethering or adherence. For people who have RA, palpation is an important part of the physical examination to identify soft tissue swelling caused by synovitis. This typically affects the proximal interphalangeal, metacarpophalangeal and wrist joints, whereas the distal interphalangeal joints are most affected by OA. The 'squeeze test' is performed by squeezing the hand around the MCP joints to ascertain if this is overly painful and is used to identify the possibility of arthritis in at least one of the joints compressed.

Movement: Careful attention must be paid to the movement of the entire arm, checking the hand and all other necessary joints. The occupational therapist will be considering any joint stiffness, reports of pain on movement and the passive and active range of movement of each joint with the person's informed consent.

Assessment of Occupational Participation

It is important to consider the impact of hand impairment on a range of occupations including eating, dressing, washing, sexual activities, shopping, housework, gardening, caring, driving, communication, work and leisure (Hammond et al., 2020; Prior et al., 2018).

Assessment of the Social and Psychological Status

Pain and function are determined and mediated by psychological status. Occupational therapists should not solely rely on physical and functional assessment of the hand and upper limb but draw on their psychological and counselling skills to assess the person's mood, attitude and self-efficacy to appraise their status (Hammond et al., 2020). Demographic or lifestyle factors including age, gender, living status, employment status and work status have been found to predict hand pain and functional limitations (Green et al., 2016) and therefore require special attention.

The use of Standardised Outcome Measures

Once the initial information has been gathered, the occupational therapist should select one or more outcome measures to identify pertinent issues to inform goal setting. Outcome measures can help to determine the baseline functional status of a person's hand, measure the effectiveness of interventions, detect change and can help motivate a person to actively participate in self-management. They can be used to benchmark against other services and add to the body of clinical effectiveness. It is also important for professional credibility that occupational therapists can demonstrate clinical effectiveness of their interventions.

A wide variety of outcome measures have been proposed for upper limb extremity conditions, including those for the evaluation of wrist and hand function. Any outcome measure chosen by the occupational therapist must be comprehensive, valid and reliable to adequately measure the effectiveness of the intervention (Cantero-Tellez et al., 2019). There is an established collection of outcome measures within hand therapy that are considered to meet these criteria, including goniometry for measuring range of movement, dynamometry for measuring strength, Semmes Weinstein monofilaments for measuring sensation and volumetry for measuring oedema (MacDermid et al., 2015).

Historically, outcome measures in hand therapy predominantly focused on objective measures. However, there is a growing focus on using Patient Reported Outcome Measures (PROM) to assess the impact of hand impairment from the affected person's perspective to gain a greater understanding of the impact on their well-being and quality of life. These include PROMs culturally adapted and psychometrically tested within specific populations to demonstrate validity and reliability in conditions such as RA, for example, the Disabilities of the Arm, Shoulder and Hand (DASH) questionnaire (Hammond et al., 2018) and the Measure of Activity Performance of the Hand (MAP-Hand) Questionnaire (Prior et al., 2018), which can help capture the functional improvements that are not possible to identify by objective measures.

The wider impact of hand pain and problems on daily activities could be measured by using the Evaluation of Daily Activity Questionnaire (EDAQ), which provides a large scale of daily activities across 14 domains, which can be used separately (i.e. per activity domain) or combined to arrive at two scores across self-care and mobility (Hammond et al., 2015, 2017). Additionally, there are other PROMs that measure self-efficacy (e.g. Arthritis Self-Efficacy Scale (Hewlett et al., 2001), psychological status (Hospital Anxiety and Depression Scale (Smarr & Keefer, 2011)) and self-management education needs (e.g. Educational Needs Assessment Tool (Ndosi et al., 2011)) to support goal setting and evaluation of interventions in hand therapy.

The evaluation process is cyclical throughout the occupational therapy process and the intervention outcomes are reevaluated to reveal new findings by which to target interventions so that appropriate modifications and updates to the initial therapy goals can be made (Klein, 2020). At the end of the therapeutic process, interventions and progress must be evaluated to determine whether the individual's functional and therapeutic goals have been reached and whether the interventions have been effective.

GOAL SETTING AND INTERVENTION PLANNING

The information gathered through a therapeutic dialogue, initial interview and assessments highlight the physical, social, environmental and psychological factors that may be influencing a person's ability to achieve their full occupational potential. The occupational therapist then works collaboratively with the person, using the information gathered to formulate objectives, usually discussed in the framework of goal setting. An intervention plan can then be created and agreed by both parties based on these identified goals.

Occupational therapists should create personalised intervention plans based on a person's occupational participation needs, choices and aspirations. Any intervention plan should support and empower a self-management approach, where possible (RCOT, 2020). This process should be underpinned by professional reasoning based on the best available evidence (American Occupational Therapy Association, 2021) and supported by collaborative, shared decision-making to encourage adherence to therapy to optimise outcomes.

Interventions are personalised to each individual and may include a wide array of options including advice, activity modification, ergonomics, education, onward signposting for relevant information, supporting self-efficacy to use self-management approaches

and job retention and/or to return to work or participation in other occupational activities.

Common Interventions

Oedema Management

Oedema is a normal physiological response to injury caused by damage to the tissues and capillaries, which impedes the effectiveness of the lymphatic system (Miller, 2017). Oedema also commonly occurs in long-term conditions such as psoriatic arthritis which can cause swelling of the entire digit (dactylitis) in RA causing swelling of the synovial membrane of joints, and in OA, when the disease process is active, individuals can have subtle or even inflamed joints (van Der Helm-van Mil, 2020).

If left untreated, oedema can persist and lead to chronic inflammation. This can affect joint and soft tissue mobility, function, pain and strength and result in deformity, affecting the aesthetic appearance of the hand and limiting a person's ability to remain or return to work (Ching & Prior, 2023; Hammond et al., 2023) and/or participate in meaningful occupations (Miller, 2022). Timely treatment of oedema is a key intervention in hand therapy and typically involves a multimodality approach, including elevation, motion and massage.

Elevation: Elevation of the hand above the heart, helps assist flow within the lymphatic system and reduces the interstitial pressure in the acute stages of injury. Ideally, the hand should be raised above the heart as much as possible (Miller, 2022), using pillow or slings for support if needed, until the inflammatory stage has passed.

Motion: Active movement contracts the muscles creating a pumping mechanism that can help move the oedema away from the site of injury (Miller et al., 2017). In certain circumstances, movement may be restricted due to the healing timeframes of delicate structures. In these scenarios, occupational therapists should support individuals to maintain active range of movement in all unaffected joints to assist with oedema management.

Massage: Massage can be used in the management of swelling, although there is ongoing debate about the type of pressure that should be applied and its effectiveness (Priganc et al., 2020). Some recommend firm retrograde massage, moving distally to proximally in the acute stages of recovery and lighter massage as part of 'manual oedema mobilisation,' which is more appropriate in more stubborn oedema (Miller, 2022).

Compression Gloves

Compression gloves or low-stretch bandages such as coban wrap lightly spiral layered on a finger are commonly used by occupational therapists to manage hand oedema caused by injury, rheumatological or neurological conditions. However, there is a paucity of research evidence to support this. Compression or arthritis gloves are widely prescribed to people with OA and RA for daytime wear to lessen hand pain and improve hand function and/or night-time wear to lessen pain, improve sleep and reduce morning stiffness. The most used compression gloves are three-quarter-finger length arthritis gloves as prescription of compression gloves has changed from the traditional full-length gloves to open-finger gloves in the last decade to allow the use of these gloves when people are engaged in their everyday occupations (Hammond & Prior, 2022).

Compression gloves are provided to people with arthritis for a wide range of reasons including reducing swelling pain. However, the evidence to support the effectiveness of compression gloves in the management of hand symptoms for people with RA and OA remains weak, and the main mechanism in operation to help relieve hand pain is thought to be the provision of warmth, rather than compression (Hammond et al., 2016, 2021; Prior et al., 2022). Consequently, prescription for arthritis gloves is not recommended for providing pressure for hand pain, function or stiffness. Instead, occupational therapists should advise people to consider the potential advantages offered by a loosely fitting, three-quarter finger length glove (which is commercially available in high streets shops) in terms of warmth, comfort and support (Hammond et al., 2021; Prior et al., 2022; RCOT, 2022).

Joint Stiffness

Joint stiffness is a common complication after a traumatic hand injury or surgery and is considered a clinical nemesis for hand therapists. An immobilised, injured joint is prone to contractures. Once movement restarts following an injury, pain and swelling may restrict the joint from moving through a full arc of movement. New collagen is then laid down in a shortened, disorganised pattern contributing to the restriction of range of movement as this can shorten the surrounding soft tissue structures such as the joint capsule and ligaments. If this is not addressed early, then the stiffness can become chronic and more challenging to treat. Exercise involving active and passive range of movement exercises and splinting are the most common interventions to counteract joint stiffness.

> *Exercise:* Movement is important in optimising joint mobility, improving gliding of the tendons and overcoming joint stiffness (Catalano et al., 2019). Exercises can be active, active assisted, passive or resistive. The type and frequency of exercise advised by an occupational therapist will be based on the healing timeframes of injured structures. In the early stages of rehabilitation, exercises may be advised to be completed on a 'little but often' approach to avoid exacerbated pain, oedema or inflammation. Exercises will also focus on the specific goals of the person and to help them to return to their required activities. For example, an electrician will require good wrist flexion with finger flexion to navigate into tight corners with a screwdriver, whereas a recreational gym-goer will require the ability to take weight onto a fully extended wrist to be able to do a push up. An additional benefit of exercise is that it can be taken away from the clinical environment and completed by the person at home. Passive and active exercises to maintain the mobility of the wrist are illustrated in Figs. 40.9 and 40.10, respectively.
>
> *Orthoses:* Orthoses can be used to progressively stretch the joint or soft tissue structures (Rongieres, 2018). These can be static, dynamic or progressive depending on the individualised needs and stage of recovery of the person. Occupational therapists may use orthoses to facilitate exercises, such as blocking off the PIP joint to encourage isolated DIP flexion. Further explanations on the use and benefit of orthoses are provided later in this chapter.
>
> *Functional Activity:* As range of movement improves, it is vital that this translates to meaningful occupational participation for individuals.

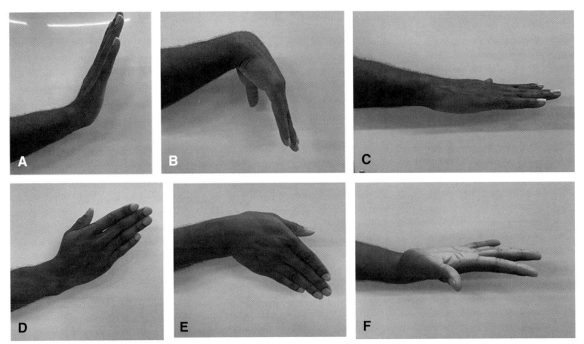

Fig. 40.9 ■ Active exercises of the Wrist Active exercises must exert a force by using muscles to move a body part. (A) Wrist extension, (B) Wrist flexion, (C) Pronation, (D) Radial deviation, E: Ulnar deviation, (F) Supination.

Therefore, occupation-based interventions within hand therapy are essential to support return to usual occupations (Valdes et al., 2021). The use of meaningful activities and occupations has been found to increase adherence to a rehabilitation programme (Cole et al., 2019). Occupation-based interventions embody occupational therapy practice and helps to strengthen professional identity (Henrichon & Toth-Cohen, 2022).

Arthritis

Exercise: Hand Exercise programme have shown to be beneficial in both OA (Østerås et al., 2017) and RA (Lamb et al., 2015). There is strong evidence hand exercise programmes of high intensity (i.e. daily with 30 repetitions of medium resistance exercises for 10–20 minutes, cumulatively) lead to significantly better outcomes in function, pain and grip strength than low intensity (Hammond & Prior, 2016). The SARAH trial is one such high-intensity, individually tailored, programme delivered using a health psychology approach with 1 x/week sessions over 6 weeks, plus a home programme continued during and after, leading to significant and clinically effective results after 12 months and is strongly recommended for clinical practice (Lamb et al., 2015). It is essential to regularly prompt people to continue hand exercises. Effectiveness decreases over time if exercise is not maintained (Williamson et al., 2017).

Ergonomic Education: Hand exercises should be taught alongside ergonomic education to optimise outcomes. Ergonomics approaches help to reduce pain and fatigue during activities. This can include altered movement patterns and the use of proper joint mechanics, restructuring activities, using ergonomic equipment and assistive technology and activity pacing, planning and problem solving to modify activities and routines (Hammond et al., 2020). Decreasing pain and fatigue through using ergonomic interventions and education can facilitate a person's ability to increase exercise frequency, function and grip strength (Niedermann et al., 2012).

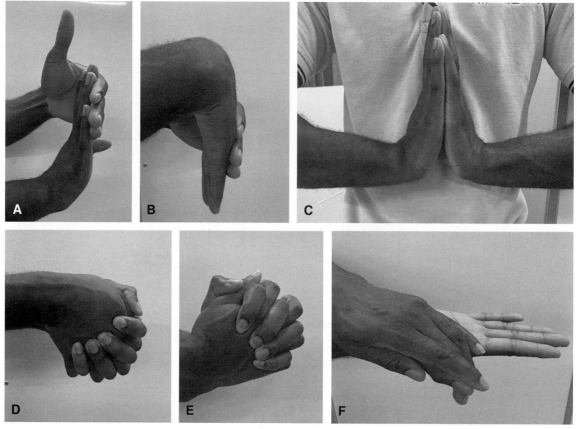

Fig. 40.10 ■ Passive exercises of the wrist. Passive exercises use an external force (e.g. their other hand or assistance from another person) to move a body part. (A) Passive wrist extension, (B) Passive wrist flexion, (C) Passive wrist extension through a 'Prayer Stretch', (D) Passive radial deviation, (E) Passive ulnar deviation, (F) Passive supination.

Scar Management

Scarring is a normal part of the wound-healing process caused by the formation and crosslinking of collagen. Wound healing is an individualised process, influenced by a person's genetic make-up, medical conditions, the severity and location of the wound and the care that scar receives (Quershi & Orgill, 2012). Cutaneous, superficial scars typically heal quickly and fade overtime, but deeper or more complex wounds can lead to excessive collagen formation causing contractures, adhesions and hypertrophic or keloid scarring.

Scarring can restrict movement, cause pain and disturb sleep and some may find them aesthetically unacceptable. People with scars are more likely to experience anxiety and depression, and scars can limit a person's ability to participate in social and work activities (Ngaage & Agius, 2018).

Because of the difficulty in objectively measuring scar progression and the individualised nature of scarring, evidence for therapeutic techniques remains limited (Yoshida et al., 2022). Commonly used strategies are outlined ahead:

Massage: Massage is frequently used in the management of scars (Duncan & Flowers, 2015). The mechanisms of its effectiveness are unclear, but it is thought to help soften tissues and maintain functional mobility by breaking down adhesions, realigning the collagen and flattening the superficial scar (Scott et al., 2022). Gentle but firm pressure can be applied in a circular motion with nonfragranced lotion to hydrate the scar and reduce friction.

Silicone: Silicone it often the first-line, gold standard for scar management (Tran et al., 2020). It can be applied to a closed wound in the form of gel sheets, as mouldable putty that can line splints or in topical gel form. Although the exact mechanisms are unclear, it is thought that silicone can contribute to keeping the scar hydrated and reduce a build-up of excess collagen, capillary activity and pigmentation (Wang et al., 2020). Gel sheets or mouldable silicone putty should be worn for at least 12 hours a day and may require weeks or months of use. They can be costly so may not be accessible to everyone.

Orthoses: Orthoses are often used in the early stages of wound healing and in acute burns to rest and immobilise the damaged tissue. Orthoses can be used in the remodelling stage of wound healing, to apply a slow, gentle, progressive stretch to the tissues (Parry et al., 2020). It is thought that this can modify and realign collagen formation increasing the pliability of scar tissue (Azad et al., 2000). Occupational therapists must consider the amount of pressure they apply with orthoses. If the force is too great, it can reactivate the inflammatory cycle and potentially exacerbate contractures.

Pain Management

Hand pain is common and a primary reason for referrals to hand therapy. Mechanisms of hand and wrist pain are complex and multifactorial, particularly as the hand and wrist consist of a web of different bones, muscles and ligaments that allow for a great number of movement and dexterity. In addition, pain is a subjective experience with a strong psychological component (Hoffman et al., 2020). Pain may be due to a primary condition (e.g. osteoarthritis), may result from an intervention (e.g. hand exercises and orthoses) or strenuous activities (e.g. repetitive use of hand, wrist and fingers in a manual job) or may be the primary complaint (e.g. fibromyalgia syndrome).

Common causes of hand pain are OA (pain, stiffness and deformity of finger joints or thumb CMC joint), carpal tunnel syndrome (tingling and numbness in median nerve distribution and reduced fine dexterity), ganglion cysts (a fluid-filled sac that forms as a herniation from a joint capsule or tendon sheath), tendinopathies (e.g. De Quervains, a thickening of the thumb extensor tendon sheath with tenosynovitis), trigger finger/thumb (flexor tendon nodule prevents smooth gliding within sheath and finger/thumb locks in flexion) and complex regional pain syndrome, in which the continued pain and sensitivity is disproportionate to a stimulus. Hand pain can also be caused by serious injury (e.g. likely fracture, dislocation, acute tendon rupture) infection (e.g. osteomyelitis) and inflammatory conditions (e.g. RA). In people with inflammatory conditions such as RA, pain-related functional limitations can persist even when the disease is controlled by disease-modifying antirheumatic drugs (dMARDs) (Nagy et al., 2021). Most have bilateral hand symptoms, resulting in difficulties with participating in occupations (Hammond et al., 2021).

Rehabilitation aims are to reduce hand symptoms such as pain, maintain hand function to support individual's occupational participation and increase quality of life. Effective pain management requires a comprehensive and personalised approach, which may require physical modalities such as occupation-based interventions, elevation, exercise and compression, psychological support and self- management strategies. It could also entail collaboration with the wider multidisciplinary team to optimise outcomes.

Hand Function

Historically, occupational therapists have used a reductionist, biomedical approach in the practice of hand therapy (Grice, 2015; Robinson et al., 2016), often with an emphasis on optimising objective measures like range of movement instead of functional outcomes. However, there has been a shift in recent years, with a growing focus on delivering occupational-focused practice (Henruchon & Toth-Cohen, 2022; Robinson et al., 2016).

Occupation-focused practice means participating in meaningful tasks as part of treatment. Participating in meaningful tasks can help engagement in rehabilitation, distract from any discomfort and use the body in more automatic movements that feel familiar (Weinstock-Zlotnick & Mehta, 2019). It can help avoid learned disuse of the hand and create a sense of satisfaction, accomplishment and enjoyment. This in turn may help engagement in rehabilitation and encourage self-management (Visser et al., 2021).

Hand function requires a sufficient range of movement, mobility, strength and dexterity. Occupational therapists need to consider the necessary grips and strength the person may need to return to their normal activities and incorporate these into their treatment plan. The most common hand grip positions are illustrated in Fig. 40.11.

Orthoses

An orthosis (plural orthoses) is a custom-made or prefabricated device, externally applied to any part of the body to restore or improve the functional and structural characteristics of the musculoskeletal and nervous systems. It is one of the most common

interventions used in hand therapy and is an integral part of rehabilitation (Keller et al., 2022). It can be used to promote healing of structures, relieve pain, stabilise joints, prevent or correct deformity and facilitate occupational participation.

Orthosis fabrication is not isolated to the care of acute injuries; it is often used with people diagnosed with arthritis or a neurological condition, in neonatal care and with many other people who many benefit from the additional support an orthosis can provide their upper limbs. Orthosis fabrication is often referred to as both an art and a science. Occupational therapists must have an appropriate level of knowledge of anatomy and physiology, biomechanics, occupational science and the mechanical properties of orthotic material and fabrication. This must be integrated with sound professional

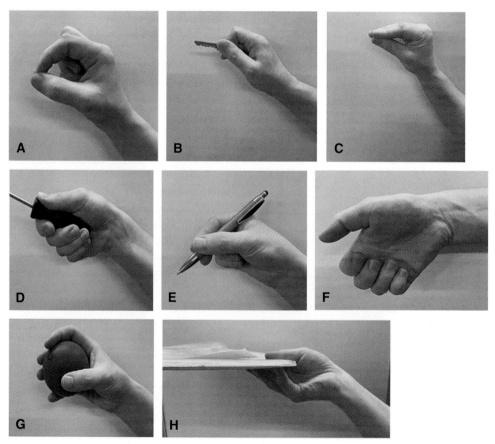

Fig. 40.11 ■ Common hand grip positions. (A) Pulp pinch, (B) Lateral (key pinch), (C) Five finger pinch, (D) Diagonal volar grip, (E) Tripod grip, (F) Transverse volar grip, (G) Spherical volar grip, (H) Extension grip.

reasoning, activity and task analysis and technical skills to create an orthosis that is fit for purpose and is beneficial to the person. An orthosis should be comfortable, felt to be beneficial by the person being prescribed the orthosis and should create little to no interference with daily function (O'Brien et al., 2010). The occupational therapist must also be able to clinically justify the purpose and value of the orthosis and communicate this clearly to the person to facilitate a collaborative, relationship-focused practice to optimise engagement with this treatment modality and support adherence.

The application and use of an orthosis are often based on the experience of the occupational therapist and orthoses may come in the form of compression garments, prefabricated splints and customised thermoplastic splints. Our understanding of the role of orthoses is continually evolving, driven by dynamic shifts in scientific knowledge and evidence. Simultaneously, the nature of orthoses and the materials used in their construction are also undergoing rapid transformations. Occupational therapists need to stay updated with emerging evidence and trends to provide optimal evidence-based care for individuals undergoing hand therapy. Often, professional bodies, such as the Royal College of Occupational Therapists in the UK, has published guidance to support practice (RCOT, 2022).

Hand orthoses are typically applied to either immobilise the hand or support mobilisation. Occupational therapists need to have clear professional justification to decide what type, if any, orthosis is best for the person. This should be a collaborative process between the occupational therapist and the person and can involve other relevant people (e.g. family, surgeon). Some of the most common reasons for splinting are outlined ahead:

Protection of Healing Structures: Orthoses can immobilise an injured area to prevent prolonging the inflammatory healing period. The normal inflammatory response to trauma responds well to a period of rest as this can assist with reducing the amount of oedema present in the surrounding tissues. Immobilisation periods should be as short as deemed safe, as any prolonged periods of immobilisation may lead to unnecessary stiffness and atrophy (Toeman & Midgley, 2010).

Controlled Motion: Certain healing structures such as flexor tendon repairs or dislocations may benefit from a splint to facilitate movement within a controlled range. This allows for optimal movement to prevent adherent scarring and joint stiffness but avoids unnecessary tension at end range, which could risk joint stability or ruptures to repaired tendons.

Pain Management: Removeable orthoses may be useful in acute injuries as an extra support to minimise pain. There is some evidence that orthoses can reduce the pain experienced in chronic conditions such as RA and OA (RCOT, 2022). However, orthoses should never be offered as an isolated intervention. It should be offered in combination with other interventions such as exercise and self-management advice (Adams et al., 2021).

Function: Orthoses can be used as a compensatory intervention to facilitate function when a person may have absent, weak or imbalanced muscles, nerve injuries or amputations. Although an orthosis cannot restore the affected movements, it can help support or stabilise a particular joint position such as wrist extension, which can assist in achieving a functional grip. Orthoses can also be used as adaptive aids, for example, to help people use cutlery, pens or mobile phones (Fig. 40.12).

Improving Joint Motion and Soft Tissue Glide: Immobilised joints, oedema and scarring can cause adhesions, which limit joint range of movement and soft tissue length. Prolonged positioning at the maximal end range of movement in a low load progressive stretch can help tissue remodelling and improve range and tendon gliding, in turn, minimising adhesions from scarring (Parry et al., 2020). There are a variety of types of orthoses that could be used to achieve this stretch, and these are outlined in the following section:

Position of Safe Immobilisation: The 'position of safe immobilisation' is obtained using a position of safe immobilisation (POSI) orthosis (Fig. 40.13). The POSI orthosis is commonly used to rest the hand during recovery from acute injury or surgery. It may also be referred to as intrinsic plus, Edinburgh or clam digger orthosis. The key characteristics are (Chen et al., 2019; Tang, 2019):

1. Wrist extension of 10–45 degrees
2. Maximum MCP joint flexion (typically 60–90 degrees)

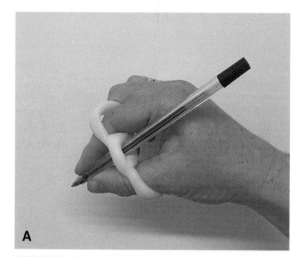

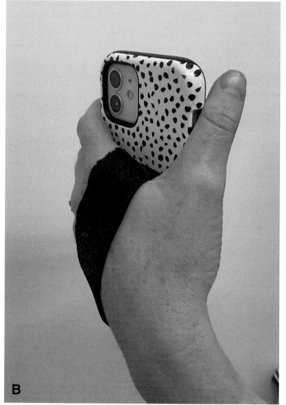

Fig. 40.12 ■ Adaptive Splints. (A) Adaptive pen splint, (B) Adaptive rigid hand strap with velcro attachment to phone to facilitate holding in when finger function impaired.

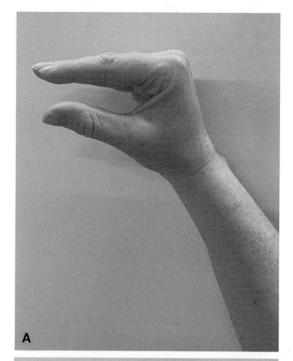

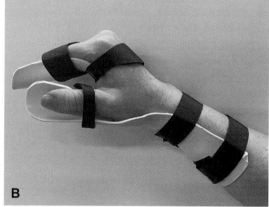

Fig. 40.13 ■ Position of safe immobilisation. (A) Position of safe immobilisation, (B) POSI splint.

3. Full interphalangeal joint extension (ideally in a neutral position)
4. Maintain the 1st web space or C-shape of the thumb

The MCP joints tend to contract into extension, while the interphalangeal joints, particularly the proximal interphalangeal joints, contract into a fixed flexed position. The POSI maintains the collateral ligaments of these joints at their optimal length to help avoid excessive stiffness. The slight extension at the wrist prevents compression or excessive stretch to the median nerve.

Types of Orthoses

While the American Society of Hand Therapists have published an Orthosis Classification System (Fess, 2005), there is no universally agreed classification system. Orthoses are often categorised into four different designs: static, serial static, dynamic and static progressive. Orthoses can be moulded or fabricated by occupational therapist or prefabricated splints (Fig. 40.14).

Static: A static orthosis or 'splint' can be fabricated from moulded thermoplastic material or a prefabricated 'off the shelf' device which is applied directly to the hand to maintain the hand in a specific position. This is often used to rest an injured hand, provide additional support or prevent a deformity such as ulnar drift from worsening. A static orthosis can be worn continuously or removed for periods of time, dependent on the purpose and the needs of the person.

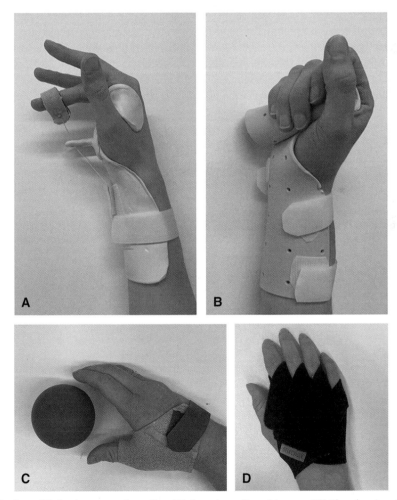

Fig. 40.14 ■ Types of splints. (A) Static progressive splint, (B) A resting splint with cone, (C) Thumb spica, (D) Prefabricated splint to prevent ulnar deviation.

Serial Static: Serial static orthoses are applied to keep the tissue at its maximal length and changed frequently to progressively increase this length. They are typically circumferential, nonremovable and made from plaster cast. They need to be changed on a regular basis, which can require frequent visits to clinic. This may be a challenge for occupational therapists if they have limited capacity and for people who may find it difficult to attend frequent appointments due to the potential time and economic implications.

Dynamic: Dynamic orthoses apply a constant force to the intended joint or digit. They have a static base, usually made from moulded thermoplastic and an outrigger attachment, which applies force through rubber bands, springs or neoprene. The tension is maintained even when the fingers are moved through their range of motion. This can provide a passively assisted range of movement (Glasgow et al., 2011) or be used as an active-resisted exercise modality against the line of pull (Jacobs & Austin, 2021).

Static Progressive: Static progressive orthoses apply low load force to the tissues at the end of their ROM. They are similar in structure to dynamic orthoses, with a base and outrigger support but the force is static, not dynamic. Once the joint position and optimal tension are pain and function for individuals with achieved, no further stress is applied. The force can only be adapted through progressive increments, often using Velcro or mechanical components (Jacobs & Austin, 2021).

CONCLUSION

Existing studies have demonstrated the effectiveness of hand therapy within small subgroups. Notably, techniques applied in hand therapy have shown improvements in pain and function for individuals with osteoarthritis and RA affecting their hands (Dziedzic et al., 2015; Lamb et al., 2015). Group hand therapy emphasising educational behavioural approaches has proven successful in enhancing self-management strategies and alleviating pain in those with inflammatory arthritis (Hammond, 2003). Moreover, optimal outcomes following hand joint implant surgery are achieved through concurrent hand therapy rehabilitation (Adams et al., 2012).

Hand therapists have pioneered postoperative orthotics and exercise regimes, leading to fewer ruptures and enhanced functional outcomes post-tendon repair surgery (Peck et al., 2014). Early hand therapy intervention, encompassing range of movement exercises and daily activity support, has been associated with superior upper limb function and grip strength compared to delayed or no intervention (Collis et al., 2020; Lee et al., 2023). However, while these insights highlight the role of hand therapy, its complete contribution within injury, disease and rehabilitation contexts remain a subject of ongoing investigation.

Robust randomised controlled trial evidence underscores the benefits of high-intensity hand exercise programmes, employing cognitive behavioural techniques for improved pain, function and grip strength outcomes (Hammond & Prior, 2016; Lamb et al., 2015). Notably, evidence supports two distinct types of wrist and hand orthoses: functional elastic wrist orthoses for daily activity support and swan neck deformity splints for enhanced hand dexterity (RCOT, 2020). While previous research has exhibited a biomedical bias, acknowledging the influence of the social context on long-term adherence to self-management strategies such as ergonomics, exercise programs and orthotic usage is crucial for moderating clinical outcomes (Ong et al., 2014).

The shift towards an occupation-based approach in hand therapy has gained momentum in recent years (Burley et al., 2018; Robinson et al., 2016; Visser et al., 2021). In this regard, occupational therapists are uniquely positioned to drive this approach through a collaborative relationship-focused occupational therapy, optimising occupational participation and aligning with holistic and functional perspectives (Hammond et al., 2020).

While further research is warranted to solidify the evidence base for hand therapy delivered by occupational therapists, their core skills harmonise seamlessly with the holistic and functional approach necessary to empower individuals in achieving occupational participation goals post-hand injury or while managing long-term health conditions. Rooted in anatomical understanding and healing principles, occupational therapists' professional reasoning, when coupled with collaborative decision-making and individualised goal setting, underscores the potential of hand therapy to promote recovery, alleviate pain, enhance function and foster overall well-being.

REFERENCES

Adams, J., Barratt, P., Rombach, I., et al. (2021). The clinical and cost effectiveness of splints for thumb base osteoarthritis: A randomized controlled clinical trial. *Rheumatology (Oxford, England), 60*(6), 2862–2877.

Adams, J., Ryall, C., Pandyan, A., Metcalf, C., Stokes, M., Bradley, S., & Warwick, D. J. (2012). Proximal interphalangeal joint replacement in patients with arthritis of the hand: a meta-analysis. *The Journal of Bone & Joint Surgery British, 94*(10), 1305–1312.

American Occupational Therapy Association. (2021). Occupational therapy scope of practice. *The American Journal of Occupational Therapy, 75*(Supplement_3).

Azad, S., Gerrish, J., & Dziewulski, P. (2000). Hypertrophic scars and keloids: An overview of the aetiology and management. *British Journal of Hand Therapy, 5*(1), 16–20.

Bullock, J., Rizvi, S. A., Saleh, A. M., Ahmed, S. S., Do, D. P., Ansari, R. A., & Ahmed, J. (2019). Rheumatoid arthritis: a brief overview of the treatment. *Medical Principles and Practice, 27*(6), 501–507.

Burley, S., Di Tommaso, A., Cox, R., & Molineux, M. (2018). An occupational perspective in hand therapy: A scoping review. *British Journal of Occupational Therapy, 81*(6), 299–318.

Cantero-Téllez, R., Naughton, N., Algar, L., & Valdes, K. (2019). Linking hand therapy outcome measures used after carpal tunnel release to the international classification of functioning, disability and health: A systematic review. *Journal of Hand Therapy: Official Journal of the American Society of Hand Therapists, 32*(2), 233–242.

Catalano, L. W., 3rd, Alton Barron, O., Glickel, S. Z., & Minhas, S. V. (2019). Etiology, evaluation, and management options for the stiff digit. *Journal of the American Academy of Orthopaedic Surgeons, 27*(15), e676–e684.

Chen, J., Chen, C., & Gong, K. (2019). Intrinsic plus position versus moderate metacarpophalangeal joint flexion for hand fractures. *The Journal of Hand Surgery, European Volume, 44*(9), 987–988.

Ching, A., & Prior, Y. (2023). Exploring the perceptions of how living with osteoarthritis affects employed people's work productivity. *Musculoskeletal Care, 21*(3), 683–693. https://doi.org/10.1002/msc.1739.

Chown, G., Beckwold, M., Chernosky, H., Lozoskie, J., & Yerkes, A. (2017). The use of Psychosocial services Post hand and upper Limb injury and Trauma: A pilot study. *HAND, 13*(5), 529–537.

Cole, T., Robinson, L., Romero, L., & O'Brien, L. (2019). Effectiveness of interventions to improve therapy adherence in people with upper limb conditions: A systematic review. *Journal of Hand Therapy, 32*(2), 175–183.

Collis, J., Signal, N., Mayland, E., & Clair, V. W.-S. (2020). A systematic review of how daily activities and exercises are recommended following volar plating of distal radius fractures and the efficacy and safety of early versus late mobilisation. *Hand Therapy, 25*(4), 139–151. https://doi.org/10.1177/1758998320967032.

de Putter, C., Selle, R., & Polinder, S. (2012). Economic impact of hand and wrist injuries: Health-care costs and productivity costs in a population-based study. *The Journal of Bone and Joint Surgery, 94*(9), e56.

Di Nicola V. (2020). Degenerative osteoarthritis a reversible chronic disease. *Regenerative therapy, 15*, 149–160. https://doi.org/10.1016/j.reth.2020.07.007.

Duncan, S., & Flowers, C. (2015). *Therapy of the hand and upper extremity: Rehabilitation protocols*. Springer.

Dunpath, T., Chetty, V., & Van Der Reyden, D. (2015). The experience of acute burns of–the hand – Patients perspectives. *Disability and Rehabilitation, 37*(10), 892–898.

Dziedzic, K., Nicholls, E., Hill, S., Hammond, A., Handy, J., Thomas, E., & Hay, E. (2015). Self-management approaches for osteoarthritis in the hand: a 2×2 factorial randomised trial. *Annals of the rheumatic diseases, 74*(1), 108–118. https://doi.org/10.1136/annrheumdis-2013-203938.

Ewald, S. (2015). Development of hand therapy as a specialty. *BMC Proceedings, 9*(Suppl 3), A108.

Fess, E. (2005). Classification and Nomenclature of Splints and Splint Components. In E. Fess, K. Gettle, C. Philips, & J. Janson (Eds.), *Hand and Upper Extremity Splinting* (3rd Ed.) (pp. 120–140). Philadelphia, PA: Mosby.

Glasgow, C., Tooth, L., Fleming, J., & Peters, S. (2011). Dynamic splinting for the stiff hand after trauma: predictors of contracture resolution. *Journal of Hand Therapy: Official Journal of the American Society of Hand Therapists, 24*(3), 195–206.

Green, D. J., Jordan, K. P., Protheroe, J., & van der Windt, D. A. (2016). Development of hand phenotypes and changes in hand pain and problems over time in older people. *Pain, 157*(3), 569–576. https://doi.org/10.1097/j.pain.0000000000000402.

Grice, K. O. (2015). The use of occupation-based assessments and intervention in the hand therapy setting–A survey. *Journal of Hand Therapy, 28*(3), 300–306.

Hammond, A. (2003). Patient education in arthritis: Helping people change. *Musculoskeletal Care, 1*(2), 84–97. https://doi.org/10.1002/msc.44.

Hammond, A., Adams, J., & Prior, Y. (2020). Chapter 26: Occupational therapy' in 'section 6: Non-drug treatments. In D. Scott, J. Galloway, A. Cope, A. Pratt, & A. Strand (Eds.), *Oxford textbook of rheumatoid arthritis* (5th Ed.), pp. 311–321. Oxford University Press.

Hammond, A., Jones, V., & Prior, Y. (2015). The effects of compression gloves on hand symptoms and hand function in rheumatoid arthritis and hand osteoarthritis: A systematic review. *Clinical Rehabilitation, 30*(3), 213–224. https://doi.org/10.1177/0269215515578296.

Hammond, A., Prior, Y., Adams, J., Firth, J., O'Neill, T., & Hough, Y. (2023). Perceptions of arthritis glove wear of patients with rheumatoid arthritis and persistent hand pain: A nested questionnaire study within the A-Gloves trial. *Musculoskeletal Care, 21*(2), 405–416. https://doi.org/10.1002/msc.1709.

Hammond, A., Prior, Y., Horton, M., Tenant, A., & Tyson, S. (2017). The psychometric properties of the evaluation of daily activity questionnaire in seven musculoskeletal conditions. *Disability and Rehabilitation, 40*(17), 2070–2080. https://doi.org/10.1080/09638288.2017.1323027.

Hammond, A., Prior, Y., & Tyson, S. (2018). Linguistic validation, validity and reliability of the British English versions of the disabilities of the arm, shoulder and hand (DASH) questionnaire and QuickDASH in people with rheumatoid arthritis. *BMC Musculoskeletal Disorders, 19*, 118. https://doi.org/10.1186/s12891-018-2032-8.

Hammond, A., & Prior, Y. (2016). A systematic review of the effectiveness of hand exercise interventions in rheumatoid arthritis. *British Medical Bulletin, 119*(1), 49–62. https://doi.org/10.1093/bmb/ldw024.

Hammond, A., & Prior, Y. (2022). Arthritis glove provision in rheumatoid arthritis and hand osteoarthritis: A survey of United Kingdom rheumatology occupational therapists. *Hand Therapy, 27*(1), 3–13. https://doi.org/10.1177/1758998321106020.

Hammond, A., & Prior, Y. (2021). Compression gloves for patients with hand arthritis (C-GLOVES): A feasibility study. *Hand Therapy.* https://doi.org/10.1177/1758998320986829.

Hammond, A., Prior, Y., Cotterill, S., et al. (2021). Clinical and cost effectiveness of arthritis gloves in rheumatoid arthritis (A-GLOVES): Randomised controlled trial with economic analysis. *BMC Musculoskeletal Disorders, 22*(1), 1–13. https://doi.org/10.1186/s12891-020-03917-8. https://rdcu.be/cdivP.

Hammond, A., Tennant, A., Tyson, S., Hawkins, R., Nordenskiold, U., & Prior, Y. (2015). The reliability and validity of the English version of the evaluation of daily activity questionnaire for people with rheumatoid arthritis. *Rheumatology, 54*(9), 1605–1615. https://doi.org/10.1093/rheumatology/kev008.

Hand Therapy Certification Commission. (2020). Definition of hand therapy and scope of practice of certified hand therapists. https://www.htcc.org/docs/default-source/about/htcc-definition-and-sop.pdf?Status=Master&sfvrsn=8371146_3.

Henrichon, K., & Toth-Cohen, K. (2022). Perspectives and influences on occupation based hand therapy. *Canadian Journal of Occupational Therapy, 89*(3), 294–306.

Hewlett, S., Cockshott, Z., Kirwan, J., et al. (2001). Development and validation of a self-efficacy scale for use in British patients with rheumatoid arthritis (RASE). *Rheumatology, 40*, 1221–1230.

Horsten, N., Ursum, J., Roorda, L., van Schaardenburg, D., Dekker, J., & Hoeksma, A. (2010). Prevalence of hand symptoms, impairments and activity limitations in rheumatoid arthritis in relation to disease duration. *Journal of Rehabilitation Medicine, 42*(10), 916–921.

Hoffman, H. G., Boe, D. A., Rombokas, E., et al. (2020). Virtual reality hand therapy: A new tool for nonopioid analgesia for acute procedural pain, hand rehabilitation, and VR embodiment therapy for phantom limb pain. *Journal of Hand Therapy, 33*(2), 254–262.

Iverson, J., & Goldin-Meadow, S. (1998). Why people gesture when they speak. *Nature, 396*, 228.

Jacobs, M., & Austin, N. (2021). *Fabrication process manual for orthotic intervention for the hand and upper extremity: Splinting principles and process* (3rd ed.). Wolters Kluwer Health.

Jenkins, D. (2009). Hollinshead's functional anatomy of the limbs and back [9th ed.]. Saunders.

Keller, J., Henderson, J., Landrieu, K., Dimick, M., & Walsh, M. (2022). The 2019 practice analysis of hand therapy and the use of orthoses by certified hand therapists. *Journal of Hand Therapy, 35*(4), 628–640. https://doi.org/10.1016/j.jht.2021.04.008.

Kondo, T., & Ishida, Y. (2010). Molecular pathology of wound healing. *Forensic science international, 203*(1-3), 93–98. https://doi.org/10.1016/j.forsciint.2010.07.004.

Klein, L. (2020). Evaluation of the Hand and Upper Extremity in Cooper's Fundamentals of Hand Therapy (3rd Ed.), St. Louis, Missouri. Mosby, pp. 46–65.

Lamb, S., Williamson, E., Heine, P., et al. (2015). Exercises to improve function of the rheumatoid hand (SARAH): a randomized controlled trial. *Lancet, 385*(9966), 421–429.

Lee, J. K., Yoon, B. H., Kim, B., Ha, C., Kil, M., Shon, J. I., & Lee, H. I. (2023). Is early mobilization after volar locking plate fixation in distal radius fractures really beneficial? A meta-analysis of prospective randomized studies. *Journal of Hand Therapy:*

Official Journal of the American Society of Hand Therapists, 36(1), 196–207. https://doi.org/10.1016/j.jht.2021.10.003.

MacDermid, J., Solomon, G., & Valdes, K. (Eds.). (2015). Clinical assessment recommendations. American Society of Hand Therapists.

Manley, O, Wormald, J., & Furniss, D. (2019). The changing shape of hand trauma: An analysis of hospital episode statistics in England. *Journal of Hand Surgery (European Volume), 44*(5), 532–536.

Miller, L., Jerosch-Herold, C., & Shepstone, L. (2017). Effectiveness of edema management techniques for subacute hand edema: A systematic review. *Journal of Hand Therapy, 30*(4), 432–446.

Miller, L., Jerosch-Herold, C., & Shepstone, L. (2022). How should interventions to treat hand oedema be delivered? An online Delphi Consensus. *Hand Therapy, 27*(2), 58–66.

Myers, B. (2020) Wound Management: Principles and Practices (3rd edition) New York. Pearson.

Nagy, G., Roodenrijs, N. M. T., Welsing, P. M., et al. (2021). EULAR definition of difficult-to-treat rheumatoid arthritis. *Annals of the Rheumatic Diseases, 80*(1), 31–35. https://doi.org/10.1136/annrheumdis-2020-217344.

Ndosi, M., Tennant, A., Bergsten, U., et al. (2011). Cross-cultural validation of the Educational Needs Assessment Tool in RA in 7 European countries. *BMC Musculoskelet Disord, 12*, 110.

Ngaage, M., & Agius, M. (2018). The psychology of scars: A mini-review. *Psychiatria Danubina, 30*(7), 633–638.

Niedermann, K., Buchi, S., Ciurea, A., et al. (2012). Six and 12 months' effects of individual joint protection education in people with rheumatoid arthritis: a randomized controlled trial. *Scandinavian Journal of Occupational Therapy, 19*, 360–369.

O'Brien, L. (2010). Adherence to therapeutic splint wear in adults with acute upper limb injuries: A systematic review. *Hand Therapy, 15*(1), 3–12.

O'Brien, L. (2012). The evidence on ways to improve patient's adherence in hand therapy. *Journal of Hand Therapy, 25*(3), 247–250.

Ong, B. N., Rogers, A., Kennedy, A., et al. (2014). Behaviour change and social blinkers? The role of sociology in trials of self-management behaviour in chronic conditions. *Sociol Health Illn, 36*, 226–238.

Østerås, N., Kjeken, I., Smedslund, G., et al. (2017). Exercise for hand osteoarthritis. *Cochrane Database Syst rev, 1*, CD010388. https://doi.org/10.1002/14651858.CD010388.pub2.

Parry, I., Schneider, J., Yelvington, M., et al. (2020). Systematic review and expert consensus on the use of orthoses (Splints and Casts) with adults and children after burn injury to determine practice guidelines. *Journal of Burn Care & Research, 41*(3), 503–534.

Perniss, P., Vinson, D., & Vigliocco, G. (2020). Making Sense of the Hands and Mouth: The Role of "Secondary" Cues to Meaning in British Sign Language and English. *Cognitive science, 44*(7), e12868. https://doi.org/10.1111/cogs.12868.

Peck, F., Roe, A., Ng, C., Duff, C., McGrouther, D., & Lees, V. (2014). The Manchester short splint: A change to splinting practice in the rehabilitation of zone II flexor tendon repairs. *Hand Therapy. 19*(2), 47–53. https://doi.org/10.1177/1758998314533306.

Priganc, V., Reese Walter, J., & Sublett, S. (2020). Edema assessment and management practice patterns among hand therapists: Survey research. *Journal of Hand Therapy, 33*(3), 378–385.

Prior, Y., Bartley, C., Adams, J., Firth, J., Culley, J., O'Neill, T. W., & Hammond, A. (2022). Does wearing arthritis gloves help with hand pain and function? A qualitative study nested within an RCT. *Rheumatology Advances in Practice, 6*(1), rkac007. https://doi.org/10.1093/rap/rkac007.

Prior, Y., Tenant, A., Tyson, S., Kjeken, I., & Hammond, A. (2018). Measure of activity performance in the hand (MAP-Hand) questionnaire: Linguistic validation, cultural adaptation and psychometric testing in people with rheumatoid arthritis (RA) in the UK. *BMC Musculoskeletal Disorders, 19*(1), 1–12. https://bmcmusculoskeletdisord.biomedcentral.com/articles/10.1186/s12891-018-2177-5.

Qureshi, A., & Orgill, D. (2012). Pathophysiology of post-operative scars. *European Surgery, 44*, 68–73.

Richards, T., Garvert, D. W., McDade, E., Carlson, E., & Curtin, C. (2011). Chronic psychological and functional sequelae after emergent hand surgery. *The Journal of Hand Surgery, 36*(10), 1663–1668. https://doi.org/10.1016/j.jhsa.2011.06.028.

Robinson, L. S., Brown, T., & O'Brien, L. (2016). Embracing an occupational perspective: Occupation-based interventions in hand therapy practice. *Australian Occupational Therapy Journal, 63*(4), 293–296.

Rongieres, M. (2018). Management of posttraumatic finger contractures in adults. *Hand Surgery and Rehabilitation, 37*(5), 275–280.

Royal College of Occupational Therapists. (2020). *Hand and wrist orthoses for adults with rheumatological condition* (2nd ed.). RCOT.

Royal College of Occupational Therapists. (2021). Professional standards for occupational therapy practice, conduct and ethics. RCOT.

Royal College of Occupational Therapists. (2022). *Addendum to Hand and wrist orthoses for adults with rheumatological conditions: Practice guideline for occupational therapists* (2nd ed.). RCOT.

Scott, H., Stockdale, C., Robinson, A., Robinson, L., & Brown, T. (2022). Is massage an effective intervention in the management of post-operative scarring? A scoping review. *Journal of Hand Therapy, 35*(2), 186–199.

Siegel, P., Tencza, M., Apodaca, B., & Poole, J. (2017). Effectiveness of occupational therapy interventions for adults with rheumatoid arthritis: A systematic review. *American Journal of Occupational Therapy, 71*(1) 7101180050p1–7101180050p11.

Smarr, K., & Keefer, A. (2011). Measures of depression and depressive symptoms: Beck depression inventory-II (BDI-II), center for epidemiologic studies depression scale (CES-D), geriatric depression scale (GDS), hospital anxiety and depression scale (HADS), and patient health questionnaire-9 (PHQ-9). *Arthritis Care & Research, 63*(Suppl 11), S454–S466.

Tang, J. (2019). On the safe position for hand immobilization. *The Journal of Hand Surgery, European, 44*(9), 993–995.

Toeman, A., & Midgley, R. (2010). Hand therapy management of metacarpal fractures: An evidence-based patient pathway. *Hand Therapy, 15*(4), 87–93.

Tran, B., Wu, J., Ratner, D., & Han, G. (2020). Topical scar treatment products for wounds: A systematic review. *Dermatologic Surgery: Official Publication for American Society for Dermatologic Surgery, 46*(12), 1564–1571.

Valdes, K., Naughton, N., Cantero Tellez, R., & Szekeres, M. (2023). The use of occupation-based interventions and assessments in hand therapy: A cross-sectional survey. *Journal of Hand Therapy, 36*(1), 214–220.

Valdes, K., Naughton, N., Cantero Tellez, R. and Szekeres, M. (2021) The use of occupation-based interventions and assessments in hand therapy: A cross-sectional survey. Journal of Hand Therapy. S0894-1130(21)00157-5.

van Der Helm-van Mil, A. (2020). Clinical Features of Rheumatoid Arthritis in Oxford textbook of rheumatoid arthritis. In D. Scott, J. Galloway, A. Cope, A. Pratt, V. Strand (5th Ed.) (pp. 109–120). Oxford University Press.

Visser, E., de Klerk, S., Jacobs-Nzuzi Khuabi, L.-A., & Joubert, M. (2021). Occupation-based intervention in therapy for upper limb musculoskeletal conditions: A systematic review. *Hand Therapy, 26*(4), 146–158.

Wang, F., Li, X., Wang, X., & Jiang, X. (2020). Efficacy of topical silicone gel in scar management: A systematic review and meta-analysis of randomised controlled trials. *International Wound Journal, 17*(3), 765–773.

Weinstock-Zlotnick, G., Mehta, S. P. (2019). A systematic review of the benefits of occupation-based intervention for patients with upper extremity musculoskeletal disorders. *Journal of Hand Therapy, 32*(2), 141–152. https://doi.org/10.1016/j.jht.2018.04.001.

Williamson, E., McConkey, C., Heine, P., et al. (2017). Hand exercises for patients with rheumatoid arthritis: An extended follow-up of the SARAH randomized controlled trial. *BMJ Open, 7*, e013121. https://doi.org/10.1136/bmjopen-2016-013121.

Yoshida, A., Yamamoto, M., Li-Tsang, C., Iwatsuki, K., & Hirata, H. (2022). A systematic review assessing the effectiveness of hand therapy programmes in adults with burns using the international classification of functioning, disability and health framework. *Nagoya Journal of Medical Science, 84*(4), 689–704.

REFLECTION

1. Name some of the common outcome measures used within hand therapy. Describe the ways in which you could consider occupational participation within the assessment process.

2. Describe the four stages of wound healing. What complications can arise from the wound healing process? What treatment modalities can be issued to help improve this?

3. Why might an orthosis be used as a treatment modality? What are some of the potential limitations of using an orthosis?

4. You work in an outpatient clinic and have been referred a 42-year-old female with joint stiffness, pain and swelling due to rheumatoid arthritis. She is a mother of two, works part-time in an office role and enjoys crafting. Describe your assessment process and the interventions that may be beneficial.

41

WORKING WITH PEOPLE LIVING WITH VISION IMPAIRMENT

CARLIA RIX ■ AMY MATHEWS

CHAPTER OUTLINE

Overview

Promoting occupational participation for people living with vision impairment is within the role of occupational therapy across a broad spectrum of generalist and specialist practice settings. Vision impairment has a high prevalence throughout the world and across all ages of the human lifespan and frequently presents as a comorbidity in nonvision specialist settings. People living with vision impairment benefit from adaptive strategies and techniques based on brighter, bigger, bolder principles to achieve their goals. The incorporation of accessibility features within mainstream technologies is improving access to print and participation in a variety of meaningful occupations. A collaborative approach that acknowledges an individual's occupational goals and utilises the occupational therapist's knowledge ensures a co-designed intervention plan that will improve occupational participation. For a person with a vision impairment, the most appropriate functional assistive technology and techniques focus on light adaptation, increased contrast, magnification and developing compensatory skills by enhancing touch, smell, hearing, taste senses and visual memory within their environments and performance contexts.

KEY POINTS

- Occupational therapists work with people with vision impairment across a broad spectrum of generalist and specialist practice settings.

- Occupational therapists working with an ageing population will encounter a high prevalence of people requiring support to adapt to living with low vision and vision impairment.

- Occupational therapy programmes and enabling strategies for people living with vision impairment are based on brighter, bigger, bolder principles, overlayed with compensatory and adaption techniques.

- Low-vision assistive devices require prescription by members of a low-vision multidisciplinary team, including occupational therapists to ensure optimum functionality, promotion of eye health, value for money, education on ergonomics and safety of use to achieve maximum participation.

INTRODUCTION

Vision is the primary part of the sensory system responsible for processing sensory information. Vision and visual perception involve motor, cognitive, communicative and emotive functions that allow for the rapid assimilation of details from the environment to enable decision-making (Zolton, 2007). Vision enables people to see the beauty of the world, such as sunset across the ocean, observe body language, such as making eye contact and nodding to indicate interest during a conversation and to notice hazards in the environment and negotiate around obstacles, such as overhanging branches at head height or objects on a path.

Conditions that impact vision occur in people of all ages with young children and older people particularly affected. It is estimated that 2.2 billion people worldwide have a visual impairment caused by congenital conditions, ageing, disease, trauma, brain injury or infections (World Health Organization [WHO], 2019). Data predictions of vision impairment suggest that by 2050, 1 in 6 people over the age 65 years will be vision impaired due to an increasingly ageing population. Compared to their counterparts in higher-income countries, people living in low- and middle-income countries are more likely to experience preventable vision impairment, with unaddressed presbyopia, cataract and uncorrected refractive errors being the main causes of vision impairment (WHO, 2022).

Occupational therapists work with people who have a vision impairment at any stage of their lifespan to facilitate achievement of their occupational participation goals. This work may occur in a low-vision setting or other generalist settings. Using professional skills (either advanced low vision or basic first responder) and knowledge of occupational theory, paired with vision rehabilitative or compensatory techniques, occupational therapists work collaboratively with the person to maximise functional vision, strengthen other influencing factors to achieve an individual's goals and facilitate occupational participation (Whittaker et al., 2016). Often this work is carried out by a multidisciplinary team in a hospital, clinic or community setting to ensure a holistic service is co-designed and implemented to meet the needs of the individual.

This chapter aims to introduce specific knowledge, skills, strategies, equipment and resources essential for an occupational therapist to consider the systems, barriers and solutions when working with people who have a vision impairment. A practice story will provide an example of how an occupational therapist and person with a vision impairment can collaborate to co-design solutions to strengthen the individual's occupational participation. Additional resources to support further learning in this area of practice are offered at the end of the chapter.

The Visual System

To understand the many reasons why vision loss can occur, it is important to understand the basic anatomy and physiology of the eye and visual system (Fig. 41.1). The visual pathway begins with light rays reflecting from an object and entering the eye through the clear, outer layer known as the cornea. The light rays pass through the pupil and lens, which is behind the iris (coloured part of the eye). The cornea and the lens focus the light rays onto the retina at the back of the eye. The photoreceptor cells in the retina consist of rods and cones. Rods are in the periphery of the retina and offer high sensitivity in low-light situations, although the acuity is poor. Cones are concentrated in the macula, the area responsible for detailed and colour vision and are active in light providing good visual acuity. Photoreceptor cells in the retina pick up the light signals, change them into nerve impulses and convey these to the brain via the optic nerve and optic chiasm (the junction where nerve fibres cross to join other nerve fibres), where they can be perceived and understood as a visual image by the visual cortex in the occipital lobe (Fig. 41.2).

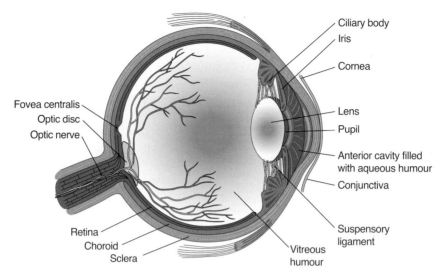

Fig. 41.1 ■ Basic anatomy and physiology of the eye and visual system.

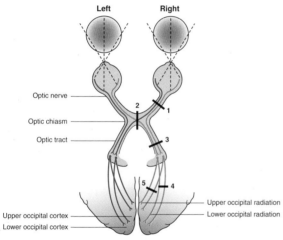

Fig. 41.2 ■ Visual pathway: optic nerve, optic chasm, optic tract.

Vision Impairment

The World Health Organization (WHO) uses the term *visual impairment* to collectively describe distance (including blindness) or near vision impairment. Within these two groups, WHO further defines categories of mild, moderate, severe, near vision impairment or blindness. These categories provide a functional description regarding the impact of visual acuity. In practical terms, *low vision* refers to a level of vision that cannot be corrected to a visual acuity close to 6/6 with glasses, contact lenses or medical treatment. Vision impairment can present as a reduction in visual acuity, visual field loss or a combination of both. It may remain stable or deteriorate over time. There are many conditions that cause vision impairment that a person can be born with, acquire or develop later in life. The common visual conditions and their functional implications occupational therapists may encounter when working with older adults in Western populations are listed in Table 41.1.

Measuring Vision

The degree of vision impairment is determined by a person's visual acuity, visual field loss or both. Visual acuity determines how well the central retina is functioning and refers to the ability to see fine detail up close (near visual acuity) and at a distance (distance visual acuity). Near visual acuity is measured using modified charts made of letters, words, numbers or symbols to determine a comfortable and functional level for reading. It is often referred to as N (scale) with a number (e.g. N12). Distance visual acuity is often assessed by measuring the smallest letters a person can see on a standardised eye chart from six metres (20 feet) (WHO, 2022).

Normal visual acuity is recorded as 6/6 (20/20), meaning a person with normal vision can see the letters on the standardised chart from six metres. The larger the bottom number of the fraction, the more impaired is a person's visual acuity. For example, if a

TABLE 41.1
Common Vision Conditions in Adults (Western Population)

Condition	Definition	Functional Implications
Albinism	A hereditary condition in which there is a lack of pigment (melanin), either throughout the entire body or within the eyes.	Reduced visual acuity Sometimes nystagmus Photophobia and glare sensitivity
Cataracts	Lens of the eye becomes cloudy. Onset can be congenital or develop later in life.	Blurred vision Depth perception issues Colour vision dulled Glare sensitivity
Charles Bonnet syndrome	When people with vision problems see things that they know are not real; sometimes called visual hallucinations.	May cause emotional distress, resulting in anxiety and social isolation All kinds of forms, from simple patterns of straight lines to detailed pictures of people or buildings may be seen.
Cerebral visual impairment (CVI)	A lifelong brain-based visual impairment caused by impaired functioning in parts of the brain that process vision. Sometimes misdiagnosed as an emotional or psychological disorder.	Struggle with visual attention and visual recognition Visually preceiving something but frequently being unable to identify or see certain parts of what is in front of them in cluttered spaces or with moving scenes. Difficulty recognising faces and finding missing items. Poor hand-eye coordination
Diabetic retinopathy	Bleeding or blocking up of blood vessels within retina causing vision loss. Total blindness may result.	Vision-loss dependent on extent and location of damage in eye
Glaucoma	An imbalance in the internal pressure within the eye relative to the ability of the nerve tissue to resist pressure. Total blindness may occur if not detected and treated. Drops, tablets or surgery are used to control the pressure and prevent further sight loss.	Progressive peripheral vision loss Reduced depth perception Glare sensitivity Reduced contrast perception
Hemianopia	The absence of half of the visual field, occurring on opposite sides or on the same side in one or both eyes.	Peripheral vision difficulties Neglect/not seeing objects on affected side
Keratoconus	A bulging forward of the central cornea (clear front surface of the eye) with thinning and scarring as a result. Treated by way of hard contact lenses, which aim to reduce the growth of the cornea as well as provide clearer vision. In extreme cases, a corneal transplant may be performed.	Progressive vision loss Possible glare sensitivity Distorted vision makes seeing details difficult
Macular degeneration (MD)	Progressive central vision deterioration and loss. Treatments in the form of antiangiogenic drugs and laser therapy are available that may slow or pause the progression of the degeneration.	Reduced visual acuity and visual distortion Colour vision becomes dull Poor depth perception Reduced contrast sensitivity
Nystagmus	Rapid, continual, involuntary movement of one or both eyes.	Reduced visual acuity and difficulty finding a focal point Effects may be reduced by the adoption of a compensatory head posture (Be aware of ergonomics as neck/shoulder issues from awkward postures to stabilise eye movement
Quadrantanopia	Visual field loss where there is a loss of one-quarter of the visual field in one or both eyes.	See Hemiopia
Retinitis pigmentosa (RP)	A hereditary condition with progressive degeneration of light-sensitive cells and pigment layer of the retina. Total blindness may result.	Restricted field of vision (i.e. tunnel vision) from progressive peripheral vision loss Loss of night vision Visual acuity decreases

(From National Eye Institute/National Institutes of Health [NEI/NIH]. [2022]. *Eye Conditions and Diseases*. National Eye Institute. Www.nei.nih. gov. https://www.nei.nih.gov/learn-about-eye-health/eye-conditions-and-diseases.)

person's visual acuity were 6/24, the person would be able to see a line of letters on the chart at six metres that a person without visual impairment would be able to see from 24 metres. The number indicates the size of the objects that can be seen comfortably. Tables 41.2 and 41.3 provide examples of the terms given to measure visual acuity levels (WHO, 2022).

The visual field is the total area a person sees without turning their head or eyes. A full visual field with both eyes open is approximately 190 degrees horizontally and 135 degrees vertically. A central visual field loss includes the area immediately surrounding the spot on which the person is focusing as opposed to a peripheral field loss beyond and surrounding the central field. Visual field loss can be a result of damage anywhere along the visual pathway from the retina to the visual cortex and is described functionally as what cannot be seen. Visual field loss can be described in halves (and quarters) using anatomical reference points – for example, binasal hemianopia (half field loss on both sides of the nasal side of the eye), bitemporal hemianopia (half field loss on both sides of the temporal side of the eye) or right homonymous hemianopia (half field loss on the right side of each eye) (Fig. 41.3).

A total peripheral visual field loss with central field maintained will result in tunnel vision. If the central field is lost and the peripheral field maintained, vision requiring detail, such as reading, is lost. A visual field of less than 60 degrees will start to significantly affect a person's ability to move about within the environment. A person usually requires at least 120 degrees of visual field horizontally to drive a vehicle. A visual field of less than 10 degrees in the least affected eye will result in a person being deemed legally blind.

Visual Perception

During an assessment, it may sometimes become apparent that neither a person's visual acuity nor visual field is the cause for the visual impairment; rather the visual impairment may be a result of a perception issue. Visual perception difficulties may be diagnosed on eye report as Cerebral Vision Impairment (CVI) (National Eye Institute/National Institutes of Health, 2022). Visual perception is the process whereby a raw image from a person's eyes is taken by their brain to organise, associate and provide a context from memory to interpret what is being seen (Zoltan, 2007). The

TABLE 41.2
Impact of Visual Acuity Levels

Visual Acuity Level	Description
6/6	Normal vision
6/12	Reduced vision (Australian legal driving limit)
6/18	Low vision (World Health Organization definition)
<6/60	Legal blindness (eligible for various entitlements)

(From World Health Organization. [2022]. *Blindness and Vision Impairment.* World Health Organization. https://www.who.int/news-room/fact-sheets/detail/blindness-and-visual-impairment.)

TABLE 41.3
Terms Used to Indicate That Vision Is Too Reduced to See a Chart

Term	Description
Count fingers (CF)	Count fingers at distance specified
Hand movements (HM)	Can see a hand moving at a close distance in front of the eyes
Light perception (LP)	Can perceive light and dark but no detail
No light perception (NLP)	Totally blind

(From Warren, M., & Barstow, E. A. [2011]. *Occupational therapy interventions for adults with low vision.* Aota Press.)

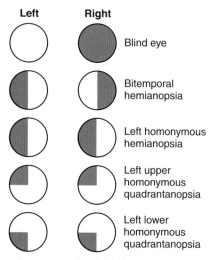

Fig. 41.3 ■ Visual field loss terminology.

visual image therefore becomes understandable and meaningful to the person.

Visual perceptual processing or visual information processing is a set of higher cognitive skills used to gather visual information and integrate it with other senses to create understanding and meaning from what is being experienced. This process allows the development of schemes to derive meaning from what is seen. Broadly, these skills can be divided into three groups:

- *Visual spatial skills*: observing the object, then accurately reporting its relationship in space relative to the person viewing the object.
- *Visual analysis skills*: identify, sort organise, store and recall information.
- *Visual integration skills*: combine the information with other senses or with other visual information (Zoltan, 2007).

The *Hierarchy of Vision Perception* by Mary Warren (1993) provides a developmental framework to illustrate that higher levels of vision cognition and adaptation are built upon the lower levels of oculomotor control, visual fields and visual acuity. Referral to a specialist low vision service is essential to optimise participation for a person with any form of visual perceptual issue.

For more detail on Visual Perceptual Processing Skills refer to Table 41.4.

MULTIDISCIPLINARY TEAM MEMBERS IN VISION REHABILITATION

The provision of services for people with vision impairment varies between countries; there is no standard model of service delivery and funding. In addition, the funding available will differ among health, social and voluntary sectors. In the World Report on Vision, WHO (2019) emphasised the need for person-centred collaboration between individuals, groups and specialists. Occupational therapists specialising in vision impairment usually work within coordinated multidisciplinary teams of vision rehabilitation professionals who may include but are not limited to (Wallace et al., 2020):

- Ophthalmologists: doctors/surgeons who diagnose and treat disease;
- Optometrists: diagnose and monitor eye disease. Prescribe glasses/contact lenses;
- Orthoptist: assess functional vision, prescribe visual enhancement aids and suggest adaptive techniques;
- Orientation and Mobility Specialists: assess and train in the use of mobility aids, mobility concepts/techniques and teach carers about guiding a person with low vision;
- Assistive Technology Consultants: assess, train and prescribe use of technologies to access various formats of information such as computer, mobile and print;
- Well-being/psychology services: emotional adjustment to living with VIP;
- Case managers/Support Coordinators: connect people to services and manage funding to access support required.

ASSESSMENT OF PERSON WITH VISION IMPAIRMENT

Occupational therapists should strive to promote occupational possibilities that are important to the person through a strength and rights-based approach (Egan & Restall, 2022). In their guide to low-vision rehabilitation, Whittaker et al. (2016) suggested the four components of occupational therapy low-vision evaluation assessment include:

1. Developing an occupational profile;
2. Evaluation of functional vision;
3. Determination of specific goals and
4. Evaluation of capabilities.

To inform a collaborative relationship-focused approach of striving for sustained and meaningful occupational participation, occupational therapists can use the domains of the Canadian Occupational Therapy Inter-Relational Practice Process (COTIPP) to guide interactions and the assessment process (Restall et al., 2022) (refer to Chapter 12). The COTIPP is not necessarily sequential, but a typical sequence for low-vision service is explained in Table 41.5 alongside the application of COTIPP to a person who has low vision as illustrated in Marj's story (Box 41.1).

TABLE 41.4	
Visual Perception Processing Skills	

Visuospatial Skills	**OBSERVING AN OBJECT, THEN ACCURATELY REPORTING ITS RELATIONSHIP IN SPACE RELATIVE TO THE PERSON VIEWING THE OBJECT**	
	Visuospatial skill	**Difficulties with reduced visuospatial skill**
	Dyspraxia	Poor coordination and balance
	Left/right discrimination	Inability to determine left and right direction and the difference between the two
	Bilateral integration	Inability to cross the midline; inability to use both hands at the same time
	Dysgraphia	Reversing numbers or letters when writing
	Spatial integration/scanning	Difficulties reading horizontally or vertically
	Position in space/spatial awareness	Difficulties observing an object, then accurately reporting its relationship in space relative to the person viewing the object
Visual Analysis Skills	**IDENTIFY, SORT, ORGANISE, STORE AND RECALL INFORMATION**	
	Visual Analysis Skill	**Difficulties with reduced visual analysis skill**
	Figure ground	Difficulty attending to or searching for a specific form or item while ignoring irrelevant information
	Form constancy	Difficulty discriminating the differences and consistencies in forms including shape, size, colour and orientation
	Visual closure	Difficulty using clues to determine the appearance of the final image or object
	Visuospatial memory	Difficulty recalling the spatial location of an object
	Visual sequential memory	Difficulty viewing and then recalling a sequence of letters/numbers/objects in order
	Visual agnosia	Difficulties recognising objects visually despite objects being familiar to them; objects may be recognised using other senses
Visual Integration	**COMBINE INFORMATION WITH OTHER SENSES OR WITH OTHER VISUAL INFORMATION**	
	Visual Integration Skill	**Difficulties with reduced visual integration skill**
	Visualisation or visual-visual integration	Difficulties matching a written word with an image in the mind or vice versa
	Visual-motor integration	Inability to coordinate visual information with gross motor and fine motor (e.g. threading a needle and catching a ball)
	Visual-auditory integration	Inability to coordinate visual information with auditory information (e.g. seeing a word and saying it out loud)

(From Zoltan, B. [2007]. *Vision, perception, and cognition: A manual for the evaluation and treatment of the adult with acquired brain injury.* Slack.)

ENABLING SKILLS AND STRATEGIES

Drawing on assessment information and the established goals, strategies to maximise functional vision including modifying the environment to accommodate a person's visual needs, introducing visual aids or equipment and adapting the occupation to achieve goals can be implemented. The unique aspects of interventions for people with vision impairment include focusing on decreasing the visual demands of a desired occupation, increasing the visibility of the environment and developing the other senses to restore or promote occupational participation (Gilbert & Baker, 2011).

In a systematic review by Arbesman et al. (2013) evidence was found that multicomponent occupational therapy programmes improve occupational participation for older adults with low vision. Key components of positive outcomes included person-directed goals, education and exchange of information about low vision, training in problem-solving skills, relaxation techniques and instruction in the use of low-vision assistive technologies. Using a multidisciplinary

TABLE 41.5

Canadian Occupational Therapy Inter-Relational Practice Process Framework

COTIPP Stage	Description When Working with a Person with Visual Impairment	Applying the COTIPP with Marj
Connect	Prior to initial connection, the occupational therapist gathers and reviews available referral information including eye reports, past assessments and case notes to commence development of an occupational profile. The occupational therapist should be conscious of the considerations for working with a person with visual impairment listed in Box 41.2. When explaining available services and collaborative processes the occupational therapist aims to build trust to understand the person, their history and goals they wish to achieve. Using active listening and an Occupational Performance Coaching approach (refer to Chapter 27) the occupational therapist identifies any contextual considerations unique to the person, including funding sources, timeframes, personal economic considerations and comorbidities that may impact service delivery (Graham et al., 2021).	As her occupational therapist, Sally reviewed the case notes from Marj's initial consultation and the ophthalmologist referral letter (See Box 41.3). Sally telephoned Marj to introduce herself, clarify the reason for the referral and inform her about the occupational therapy role and service. Sally confirmed that Marj prefers the use of pronouns she/her. Sally used a coaching approach and listened as Marj shared her occupational narrative, including her hopes and expectations for services and her life. Sally adopted the key characteristics of collaborative relationship-focused occupational therapy practice (Restall & Egan, 2022) by defining the collaborative working relationship between therapist and Marj. Consent was obtained to authorise an agency file be created for the purposes of retaining any relevant information and giving consent for the agency to obtain and exchange relevant information to and from other professionals, including Marj's ophthalmologist and optometrist.
Seek to understand and define purpose	The occupational therapist seeks to understand the person holistically including factors influencing participation. Mohler et al. (2015) suggested the occupational therapist can build trust by clarifying a person's: ■ Goals and reason for accessing occupational therapy services; ■ History (e.g. occular condition, visual acuities, medical, social situation); ■ Context (physical and social), strengths, supports, previous occupational participation history; ■ Psychological factors of confidence, motivations, grief and loss and ■ Level of functional vision All vision conditions may vary in presentation and symptom severity. Functional vision or residual vision, refers to the individual way a person uses their remaining vision to perform routine tasks. A Functional Vision Evaluation (FVE) is recommended to add detailed functional visual and ocular history to the occupational profile (Whittaker et al., 2015). This information can determine visual barriers to participation, suggest enabling strategies for optical and nonoptical techniques to improve functional vision and assist realistic goal setting. FVE is performed by a low-vision specialist (either optometrist or orthoptist) and includes a variety of assessments to determine visual acuity, contrast sensitivity, visual fields and neurological functions. Where FVE cannot be completed, the occupational therapist can elicit this information by: ■ Using tele-health to facilitate interaction with a low-vision specialist.	From reading the first contact notes and throughout this conversation, Sally began to create an occupational profile of Marj including her support networks and daily occupations. Sally explained the organisation's approach of collaborative relationship-focused practice and goal-directed care. Sally subsequently scheduled an initial centre-based appointment to work with Marj to identify her goals. Sally confirmed that the preferred format for providing information to Marj was via large print. Sally provided information on the organisation's requirements and policies, which included information on privacy, consent, safety and confidentiality, complaints and suggestions for improvement, rights and responsibilities and the use of an advocate. Sally offered opportunities for Marj to ask any questions, raise concerns and any additional considerations to ensure safety for both parties.

Continued on following page

	TABLE 41.5	
	Canadian Occupational Therapy Inter-Relational Practice Process Framework—(*Continued*)	
COTIPP Stage	**Description When Working with a Person with Visual Impairment**	**Applying the COTIPP with Marj**
	■ Identifying, defining and educating about known symptoms reported and mitigation techniques for participation and/or support referral. ■ Completing functional tests, for example, with regards to understanding visual field deficits after a neurological event, a basic confrontational visual field screening test (Box 41.4) can be completed to evaluate visual factors. As part of understanding the person, the occupational therapist should explore psychological factors, specifically grief and loss and provide education to support acceptance of their changed circumstances. A meta-analysis by Zheng et al. (2017) found that 25% of people with eye conditions also reported depressive symptoms, and thus referral to a mental health specialist should be prioritised when symptoms impact participation in daily activities or continue for extended periods.	
Explore occupational participation	Continuing with a collaborative approach the occupational therapist and person with a vision impairment together explore and evaluate barriers and opportunities for participation. Whittaker et al. (2016) suggested that this stage may include use of the following: 1. Indirect assessment 2. Direct assessment **Indirect Assessment** Building on previous domains, standardised assessments can determine the specific areas where direct assessment is needed or aid in determining priorities when setting goals. Attention to the options already explored (including techniques, aids and equipment) is important at this stage. For people living with blindness or low vision, Whittaker et al. (2016) recommended the use of a formal standardised low-vision visual functioning questionnaire that contains a self-report of current capabilities. One relevant assessment is the Impact of Vision Impairment – Very Low Vision (IVI-VLV) questionnaire (Finger et al., 2014). The results of this assessment highlight daily activities that are frequently considered to require very little physical or cognitive effort but have unique barriers when vision is limited. The Montreal Cognitive Assessment (MoCA)- BLIND may be used if there are concerns about a person's cognition (Wittich et al., 2010) **Direct assessment** The occupational therapist may ask the person to participate in a functional assessment so that activity demands, performance skills and behaviour patterns in the environment in which the task is completed to understand the specific vision-related requirements can be observed.	During the initial centre-based appointment, Sally continued a coaching conversation, informed by the Canadian Model of Occupational Participation to explore specifics and develop a fuller understanding of Marj's occupational participation goals. Sally completed indirect assessments, including completing the Impact of Vision Impairment (IVI-VLV) form where Marj achieved a score indicating her vision loss was having a moderate impact on daily living, mobility, safety and emotional well-being. Together, Marj and Sally explored Marj's occupational participation goals (Restall & Egan, 2021). Sally reflected on the contextual factors, structures and supports around Marj that could be engaged to Marj to achieve her goals. Marj was referred to an orthopist who completed a Functional Vision Evaluation (direct assessment) to explore ways to maximise functional vision to read labels on price tickets, and additionally labels on ingredients to support her goal of cooking. The orthoptist provided a summary of the assessment results (see Table 41.6.) to Marj and the team, which identified the need for good lighting to compensate for her reduced contrast sensitivity; Marj was also prescribed a 3.5 × LED handheld magnifier to assist with reading small print. As part of a collaborative approach to service delivery, Sally arranged for the Orientation and Mobility (O&M) specialist to meet Marj and the orthoptist. The O&M sought to understand the orthoptic assessment outcomes relevant to refining and reviewing the approach for service and to assist with planning interventions that would assist in achieving Marj's mobility goals.

TABLE 41.5

Canadian Occupational Therapy Inter-Relational Practice Process Framework—(*Continued*)

COTIPP Stage	Description When Working with a Person with Visual Impairment	Applying the COTIPP with Marj
	Whittaker et al. (2016) recommended a vision-specific environmental assessment includes a focus on the following factors: ■ Environmental lighting, specifically light source type and position. ■ Luminosity (brightness) and glare. ■ Outdoor light sources and window coverings. ■ Environmental layout and arrangement. Including organisation, placement and storage. ■ The ergonomic position when performing tasks, including the positioning of reading stands and tables to maximise functional vision. ■ Environmental hazards, prevention techniques and emergency responses to risks. The Low Vision Home Assessment (Barstow, 2015; Bennett et al., 2014) and the Home Environment Lighting Assessment (Perlmutter, 2013; Perlmutter et al., 2013) are examples of assessments that can be used by occupational therapists to improve environmental conditions in homes.	
Co-design priorities	The occupational therapist will facilitate a joint conversation to review the occupational profile information and reflect on assessment findings with the person. Areas of reduced occupational participation and the person's ratings of their perceived level of current performance and satisfaction are identified and prioritised with the person. The occupational therapist's experience and knowledge combined with visual acuity information (from eye report) inform limitations of functional vision to ensure realistic expectations of what the individual perceives as their rehabilitation potential. For example, reading a standard newspaper may not be realistic, but text-to-speech devices may provide a person with a level of independence in accessing the content.	Sally organised the information she collected using Canadian Occupational Performance Measure (COPM) (Law et al., 2014) (refer to Chapter 16). Marj listed the following occupational performance areas as the most important for her: ■ Difficulties preparing Sunday roast dinner for the family. ■ Misreading tickets (price tags) when volunteering at the local charity shop. ■ Insufficient skills to travel independently to meet friends at the local coffee shop and to attend her volunteer work. In a collaborative discussion, Sally used a coaching approach empowering Marj to define her occupational participation goals in SMART (Specific, Measurable, Achievable, Realistic and Timely) format. Marj rated her current performance and satisfaction and prioritised those goals for therapy. Understanding the meaning, history and context of these occupations assisted the conversation and process of rating. The following goals were developed *Goal 1: I will be independent making the weekly Sunday roast dinner for my family by the end of the year – Importance: 10; Performance: 5; Satisfaction: 5* *Goal 2: I will be independent reading the labels on price tickets by the end of the year – Importance: 7; Performance: 1; Satisfaction: 1* *Goal 3: I will be independent mobilising from my home to the coffee and charity shops by the end of the year – Importance: 8; Performance: 4; Satisfaction: 4*

Continued on following page

TABLE 41.5

Canadian Occupational Therapy Inter-Relational Practice Process Framework—(*Continued*)

COTIPP Stage	Description When Working with a Person with Visual Impairment	Applying the COTIPP with Marj
Plan, trial plan, explore change, refine plan	Collaborative sharing of perspectives, concerns and solutions from the person, the occupational therapist, family members and the broader low-vision team will allow a plan of action to be created. The plan will be based on the person's SMART (Specific, Measurable, Achievable, Realistic and Timely) goals and will also include the agreed period for trial and review (Bovend'Eerdt et al., 2009). SMART goals are a standardised way of writing goals in rehabilitation. The occupational therapist offers this information to the person in their preferred accessible format. As part of the planned trial, regular sharing of perspectives is essential to monitor unforeseen challenges and explore the changes and effectiveness of intervention. For example, to understand how the task ended the way it did due to the lack of visual information, the occupational therapist may articulate their observations to the person, who may not identify their own near misses or unseen dangers.	The following plan was agreed by Marj and Sally: ■ Sally would complete a functional cooking assessment at Marj's home to support identification of options to strengthen participation, performance and safety in the task of preparing a roast meal. ■ Marj would meet the O&M at Marj's home to explore her community access goal, beginning with building low-vision mobility skills. Further O&M sessions would focus on skill development and training using public transport for Marj to develop independence getting from her home to the coffee and charity shops by the end of the year. In preparation, Sally considered safety and subsequently completed the home risk assessment to determine potential hazards and risks prior to visiting the property. The risk assessment identified that Marj had two small indoor dogs. On Sally's request, it was agreed the dogs were to be restricted to the laundry during the home visit. Sally conducted a direct functional cooking assessment in Marj's kitchen to assess her performance in a familiar environment (refer to Chapters 17 and 18). This assessment involved coaching through an activity analysis, breaking down tasks to ascertain the skills required to address Marj's goal to be able to prepare a Sunday roast dinner for her family (Table 41.7). After this assessment, Sally and Marj explored the areas Marj perceived as challenging and explored solutions. Sally reassured Marj that she was there to support her to achieve her occupational participation goals. She coached Marg to explore, identify and trial her own solutions. With Marj's permission, Sally contributed suggestions based on her experience and assessment observations that Marg could adapt to suit her unique situation. It was Marj's decision regarding which techniques/modifications/adaptions would be implemented as part of exploring change and refining plan. To refine the plan, Sally and Marj agreed upon the following techniques to achieve the goal of hosting Sunday roast for the family: ■ Enhance lighting and contrast to increase viability of all nearby tasks ■ Use a magnifier for several tasks ■ Reduce clutter ■ Educate her family on organisational strategies ■ Explore adaptive techniques and/or equipment to compensate for low vision Sally scheduled another home visit to implement the agreed objectives within meal preparation to *review and refine* further to achieve goal. Enabling strategies explored to support participation in cooking are presented in Table 41.7.

	TABLE 41.5	
	Canadian Occupational Therapy Inter-Relational Practice Process Framework—(*Continued*)	
COTIPP Stage	**Description When Working with a Person with Visual Impairment**	**Applying the COTIPP with Marj**
		The next session held at Marj's home reviewed her approach to meal preparation using the purchased adaptations and modifications completed by the family. Marj reflected on her progress, reviewed both the adaptions and modifications implemented, identified reasons why they were effective or ineffective and refined these based on feedback. Marj acknowledged that to sustain her level of participation in tasks, she would need to continue adapting the way she completes the task including accepting offers from family to support task. Sally listened to understand the significance of these changes.
		During this time, the O&M continued to worked with Marj, advising Sally that she had prescribed Marj with an ID cane to assist compensating for her reduced depth perception when negotiating steps in unfamiliar environments. After being educated on local public transport systems Marj was now feeling confident that she could use a combination of walking and public transport to mobilise to the coffee shop and charity shop.
Plan for transition	The occupational therapist must support transition out of the service by first supporting a conversation to critically review the goals established earlier in service delivery to measure outcomes. This includes conversation exploring the factors that might disrupt long-term independence and participation, along with strategies to mitigate future barriers. The occupational therapist must ensure the person has understood the techniques, aids or assistive technology to enable them to problem solve to find solutions that achieve their occupational participation now and into the future. The occupational therapist may offer to provide materials in their preferred format for future reference. Post low-vision service supports including organisations and self-directed learning are provided in the resources section of this chapter and may be offered to the person.	After the completion of the previous interventions, Sally had a centre-based appointment with Marj to collaboratively review her goals and re-administer the COPM. *Goal 1: I will be independent making the weekly Sunday roast dinner for my family by the end of the year – Importance: 10; Performance: 8; Satisfaction: 8* *Goal 2: I will be independent reading the labels on price tickets by the end of the year – Importance: 7; Performance: 9; Satisfaction: 9* *Goal 3: I will be independent mobilising from my home to the coffee and charity shops by the end of the year – Importance: 8; Performance: 8; Satisfaction: 8* Marj discussed her hopes and aspirations for the future, such as returning to work at charity shop; however, she did not want to pursue this at this time. Sally acknowledged with Marj that her condition was degenerative and that she would require further occupational therapy services in the future. Marj was provided with information about aids, equipment and techniques discussed with the various professionals whom Marj worked with and details for accessing their low-vision service as required in future. Sally provided Marj with a variety of resources for ongoing support, including links to websites, podcasts, online videos, support groups and eye-health organisations.

BOX 41.1
MARJ'S STORY

Marj, is a 71-year-old lady, who lives at home with her husband. She has two daughters and five grandchildren. Marj has always prioritised her family and has a matriarch type role, including babysitting and hosting Sunday roasts for her family. She was passionate about helping others and volunteered at a local charity shop. Every week, she enjoyed meeting her friends for a coffee at a local cafe and would often drive to a friend.

Four months ago, while volunteering at her local charity shop, Marj experienced some difficulty reading the labels, reading other items and gave incorrect change to a customer. She decided to book an appointment at her local eye clinic to review her bifocal glasses. As part of the assessment, her optometrist identified an abnormal blood vessel leaking into the region of the macula and referred Marj to an ophthalmologist. At this specialist appointment, Marj was diagnosed with wet age-related macular degeneration. Marj underwent eye injections to prevent further damage and to reduce the swelling. She was advised that she no longer met the minimum legal standard to drive a motor vehicle. Marj was also told her vision loss was permanent and could not be rectified with stronger prescription

glasses. She was referred to the local blindness and low-vision community service. Marj was devastated that she could not regain her lost vision, she could no longer drive and she could not obtain a stronger prescription for the lens in her glasses.

Marj did not return to her duties at the charity shop and declined invitations to go out with friends for a coffee. She was concerned about becoming dependent on others but eventually followed up the referral to her local blindness and low-vision community service. Upon arrival at the low-vision provider, Marj was seen by a senior clinician for initial assessment, which was conducted as an informal conversation. Marj was informed of the range of services available and completed the Impact of Vision Impairment – Very Low-vision (IVI-VLV) (Finger et al., 2014) screening tool. During their collaborative discussion, Marj determined her priorities were reading, identifying money, accessing the community and daily tasks around the home. She was then referred to an orthoptist, occupational therapist and orientation and mobility specialist. Sally was assigned as Marj's occupational therapist from the blindness and low-vision community service.

---

approach, the occupational therapist may suggest training sessions with an Orientation and Mobility Specialist or an Orthoptist Assessment. Multiple training sessions have been found to facilitate the development of independence in daily activities (Arbesman et al., 2013).

When working with people with vision impairment, occupational therapists use the principles of 'brighter, bigger, bolder'. Additionally, occupational therapists need to determine whether a person's other senses could be used to compensate for the vision loss. These strategies can often make occupational participation easier by capitalising on functional vision and the other senses and should be implemented before exploring more complex solutions (Whittaker et al., 2016).

Brighter: Is There Enough Light?

The visual system depends on light to operate; therefore, appropriate lighting is the most important aid to vision (Smallfield & Kaldenberg, 2020). As people age, their contrast sensitivity along with dark and light adaptation diminishes because less light reaches the retina in an ageing eye. It is also difficult for an ageing visual system to adapt quickly to dramatic changes in

brightness, for example walking inside to a dark house from being outside on a bright sunny day. The occupational therapist or orthoptist can help a person determine their lighting preferences.

Recommending lighting changes in response to vision impairment depends on the needs and context of an individual, and there is no single lighting solution. There are two types of lighting to consider: general and task lighting.

General lighting refers to both artificial light and daylight. There are many visual and health reasons to maximise use of natural daylight. General lighting improves distance vision tasks such as mobilising safely around the home (Whittaker et al., 2016). Example recommendations to maximise general lighting can be found in Box 41.5.

Task lighting is light focused on a particular area where a task is being performed (such as reading, drawing, sewing or playing board games). By moving the light source closer to the viewed object, the intensity of light is increased. When you reduce the distance of the light source from the viewed object by half, the intensity of light on the object is increased four times. The light can be placed as close as 15 cm (5.9 inches)

BOX 41.2

CONSIDERATIONS FOR WORKING WITH A PERSON WITH VISUAL IMPAIRMENT

GUIDING A PERSON WITH VISION IMPAIRMENT

- People with vision impairment may find it helpful to be guided by another person, particularly in an unfamiliar environment. To do this safely, respectfully and efficiently, the following sighted guide techniques can be used (Vision Australia, 2023):
  - Ask the person if assistance is required. The person with vision impairment may hold the elbow of the person guiding. The person guiding should have a relaxed, slightly bent arm and describe the environmental landmarks and general travel direction to the person with vision impairment. Not all people with little or no sight will use this method, so it is important to ask what specific assistance they require.
  - If the person with vision impairment uses a mobility aid (e.g. a walking stick), advise the person to use this aid. Also encourage the use of grab rails where available.
  - Walk at a comfortable pace for the person with vision impairment, who should be approximately one pace behind the guide.
  - When required, offer to guide the hand of the person with vision impairment to the grab rail, car door or other object.
  - If the guide must leave, ensure that the person with vision impairment is aware of the location (verbally describe) and is in a comfortable position.
  - Refer to the following video on guiding for more information: https://visionau.canto.com/b/L6PEG

COMMUNICATING EFFECTIVELY WITH A PERSON WITH VISION IMPAIRMENT

Strategies to assist communicating effectively include the following (Vision Australia, 2023):

- Address the person with vision impairment by name and introduce yourself before commencing a conversation.
- Use accurate and specific language when giving directions; for example, 'The door is on your left' rather than 'It's over there'.
- Use specific language when describing the person's surroundings; for example, specify the features of a building, such as the waiting area drink fountain and identify the people present when entering a room.
- Identify what is making a particular sound when required, such as a cart travelling down a corridor.
- Inform the person with vision impairment when you are leaving and when other people have left the room or conversation.
- In a dangerous situation, say STOP (rather than 'look out').

Note: It is generally acceptable to use everyday language with words such as 'blind', 'look', 'see' and 'watch' during conversations with a person with vision impairment. These concepts and words are part of everyday language and do not need to be adjusted when communicating with a person with vision impairment.

---

from the item the person is looking at. If the light is too bright or glare is reflecting into the person's eyes, the lamp should be repositioned or dimmed. The best position for an adjustable lamp is between the person and the item being looked at, directed at the task and below eye level. This positioning ensures that excess light shines away from the person's eyes; therefore, reflections will not be a problem and the proximity of the light source on the task will provide maximum illumination (Fig. 41.4).

For most people with low vision, lighting is a very useful tool for enhancing functional vision. However, it is equally important to remember that not all people benefit from additional lighting because of glare sensitivity (e.g. people diagnosed with cataracts, keratoconus). The challenge is to provide enough light without creating glare or shadows. If glare is a problem, venetian blinds, vertical blinds, sheer blinds, curtains or tinted windows can be used to reduce discomfort from glare. Reflective glare can be reduced by placing a dark-coloured cloth or tea towel on a shiny object, sink, bench or table that is causing the reflection.

Bigger: Can the Detail Be Made Bigger?

Big objects are generally easier to see than small objects for most people. This can be achieved in many ways, both simple and complex, depending on individual needs. The process of enlarging an image on the retina is known as magnification (Whittaker et al., 2016). Magnification devices come in many shapes, forms and strengths, including hand magnifiers (Fig. 41.5), stand magnifiers and pocket magnifiers. Some magnifiers have built-in lights to enhance illumination of the item. It is helpful to think of magnification devices as tools for a specific use such as reading mail, seeing menus at a restaurant, watching a football game

BOX 41.3
MARJ'S REFERRAL LETTER

Eye Specialist Services
1 Vision Rd
Vision Town, 1234

10/01/2023
To whom it may concern at Low Vision and Blindness Services,
   Re: Marj Person
   DOB: 01/01/1952
   Address: 123 Country Road
   Vision Town, 1234
Please accept this referral for Marj, who is living with low vision as described ahead. She has been undergoing injections to stabilise her vision. She has recently discontinued driving and reports difficulties with daily living tasks in addition to immobility.

Last Attendance:	10/01/2023	
Condition:	Age-Related Macular Degeneration	
Acuities:	LE: 6/18	RE: 6/95
Visual Fields:	Not assessed	
Prognosis:	Permanent	
Does this person meet Legally Blind Status?	Yes	**No**
Next Attendance:	10/03/2023 (recommended attendance every 8 weeks)	

Sincerely

Dr Robert Robertson
Ophthalmologist

BOX 41.4
CONFRONTATIONAL VISUAL FIELD TEST

A basic confrontational field test can be used by occupational therapists to screen if a person has a visual field loss. This test requires sound observations but minimal equipment (Zolton, 2007).

Note: To have a direct comparison, the occupational therapist conducting a confrontational visual field test will be testing their own visual field at the same time.

If the occupational therapist does not have a normal visual field, this test will not be appropriate.

1. The occupational therapist and person with vision impairment should be facing each other and positioned 50 cm (1.6 ft) apart.
2. The occupational therapist then asks the person to close/cover one eye; the occupational therapist then closes/covers their opposite eye (i.e. if the person closes/covers their left eye, then the occupational therapist should cover/close their right eye).
3. The occupational therapist then asks the person to stare at the occupational therapist's open eye, and the occupational therapist stares at the person's open eye.
4. Starting in the top outer quadrant the occupational therapist slowly moves a finger/pen/object into their visual field, asking the person to indicate when they see the finger/pen/object. The occupational therapist compares where the person indicated the finger/pen/object was seen to when they saw the finger/pen/object entering their visual field.
5. The occupational therapist repeats this process with each quadrant, ensuring the object starts from outside their own visual field.
6. Once all four quadrants have been assessed for one eye, the occupational therapist assesses the person's other eye in the same manner.
7. If the occupational therapist detects a visual field loss (i.e. the person's visual field does not match the occupational therapist's visual field), the person should be referred on for formal testing by an orthoptist and optometrist.

		TABLE 41.6		
		Marj's Orthoptic Assessment Results		
Vision Distance (With Correction)	Vision Near (With Correction)	Refraction	Magnification	Contrast Sensitivity – Melbourne Edge Test
RE 6/95 + (EF) LE 6/18	N12 at 25 cm with focal light	RE + 1.00/–0.50 × 70 LE –0.50 DS Add: + 4.00 for reading	N6 with a 3.5 × LED handheld magnifier (This device was purchased during the assessment.)	10 dB (with refraction correction and focal lighting) 5 dB without lighting

DS, Diopter sphere; *EF,* eccentric fixation; *LE,* left eye; *RE,* right eye.

		TABLE 41.7
		Marj's Kitchen Skills Assessment and Suggested Practical Strategies
Task Analysis	Observations	Practical Enabling Strategies to Support Participation in Cooking
Food Collection and Reading		
Collecting food items	Difficulty locating items in cupboards and drawers. Reduced contrast within pantry between shelving and products. Food items stored inconsistently within pantry and fridge. Assistance needed to verify or identify objects as randomly selected.	Marj identified the following techniques: ■ Reduce the clutter by moving the nonessential items into a different storage location of the house and remove any out of date products or products that are not used in daily cooking. ■ Use available small baskets to group similar items together in small plastic baskets. When an item from a group is required, pick up the small plastic basket containing this item and place it on a bench in good light for easier selection. ■ Stick to the same brands Marj is familiar with so that they are easier to identify and differentiate. Sally encouraged these techniques and with Marj's permission offered additional low-vision strategies as follows: ■ Continue using existing sensory modalities and proprioceptive feedback when collecting food items, highlighting the way Marg was already using touch, size/weight, shape, texture and smell and develop this awareness. ■ Education provided on increasing overall kitchen organisation and reduce clutter, such as the following: ■ Decide where items belong and return the items to the same place. ■ Insert frequently used items in the most accessible cupboards and drawers. ■ Painting the insides of cupboards white to maximise the brightness and contrast so that items were easier to find.
Reading food labels/ use-by date/ directions on packaging	Incorrectly identified spice jars and salt/pepper, condiments, prompted by occupational therapist to use sense of smell.	Marj tried using her prescribed magnifier to read labels on food items. Marj felt frustrated picking up her magnifier to read each product. Sally suggested the following: ■ Large-print labels using white sticker and thick black text attached to items, enabling Marj to read the labels just wearing her glasses. A rubber band round the salt condiments to assist identifying using sense of touch.
Reading recipes	Unable to read recipe book wearing reading glasses.	Marj used her prescribed magnifier to read recipes from her cookbook. Marj found this to be comfortable for familiar recipes as the magnifier was positioned in the same place as her recipe books and was used to spot identify ingredients as prompts. Marj stated that an alternative solution may be needed for more complex recipes.
Food Preparation		

Continued on following page

	TABLE 41.7	
	Marj's Kitchen Skills Assessment and Suggested Practical Strategies—(*Continued*)	
Task Analysis	**Observations**	**Practical Enabling Strategies to Support Participation in Cooking**
Chopping, slicing, peeling techniques	Cutting self when collecting knives from drawer. Difficulty slicing vegetables in even portions; unable to identify where the skin has been removed when peeling vegetables. When Marj is positioned at bench, the main central light casts a shadow at this area. Marj felt frustrated with excess of time taken and injuries sustained while completing these tasks.	Marj identified the following techniques: ■ Stabilising the chopping board. ■ Removing or cutting a section of food to provide a flat surface for stability when cutting or slicing. ■ Continuing to store knives separately in a knife block. ■ Place dirty knives in a safe location, that is, rear of the sink until cleaning. ■ Trial using multisize slicer (Mandolin) to slice. Sally offered the following: ■ Wash knives immediately following their use, dried and returned. Sally suggested the following slicing techniques to try: ■ Use a contrast chopping board when preparing vegetables; for example, use a dark board when slicing light-coloured onions and potatoes. ■ Throughout task, reorientate the food continually to provide a flat, stable base for cutting. Slow down and take time to do the slicing. ■ Where possible, maintain contact of the knife blade tip with the board when slicing. ■ Once a section is sliced, do not remove the knife blade from the 'main' food source but continue to slice the next piece. ■ Use the index finger of opposing hand to judge slice thickness (this finger can also be used to butt knife edge against before slicing). ■ Consider using a peeler as an alternative; for example, vegetable peelers work well for slicing cheese/shaving chocolate. Sally suggested the following peeling techniques to try: ■ Avoid washing vegetables before peeling so that the different surface texture changes can be used as a guide. ■ Use a chopping board to stabilise 'long' food such as carrots, courgette and cucumber and peel downwards towards the board. ■ Peel using a systematic method, such as top to bottom, left to right. ■ Peel over a sink to contain peelings to avoid mess. ■ Use unwashed potatoes, as the dirt and dark skin make identifying missed patches easier (do not wash potatoes beforehand). Focal lighting was successfully trialled during these tasks. This resulted in Marj installing an undercabinet LED light to illuminate the counter area.
Pouring techniques	Difficulty identifying water level in mug. Kettle positioned in shadowed corner on the bench on the opposite side of kitchen from the sink. Excess spillage on bench after task.	Marj identified the following techniques: ■ Pour liquid over a sink area to ensure any spills are contained in the sink area. ■ Use of hearing to listen to water level rising. Sally made the following suggestions: ■ Use adequate lighting to highlight the cup as much as possible; the undercabinet fluorescent light provided Marj with efficient lighting. ■ Connect the lip of the kettle or jug with the cup to ensure that water flows into the centre of the cup. ■ Detect the level of the liquid being poured into the cup by listening for changes in water pitch as the cup fills. ■ Use a white or lightly coloured cup to provide colour contrast to dark liquids such as tea or coffee and assist in determining the level of liquid. Add the milk last. ■ Marj successfully trialled a liquid level indicator and purchased this to assist in preparing a cup of coffee.

TABLE 41.7
Marj's Kitchen Skills Assessment and Suggested Practical Strategies—(*Continued*)

Task Analysis	Observations	Practical Enabling Strategies to Support Participation in Cooking
Use of utensils (e.g. can opener)	Difficulty locating utensils and bowls as numerous items stored on top of one another. Independent using can opener.	Marj identified the following techniques: ■ Reduce the number of items in the drawer. ■ Hanging frequently used utensils on hooks placed at eye level near the space where they are used. ■ Purchase different coloured utensils for higher contrast and discrimination. Sally suggested the following: ■ Drawer dividers and organisational aids. Objects be stored only one row deep (not stacked) to reduce visual clutter.
Measurement of ingredients	Difficulty identifying the correct measuring cups; unable to read measurement on scales with glasses, difficulty managing pouring from packets and scooping from narrow-mouthed containers.	Marj identified the following techniques: ■ Marj used her magnifying aid to assist in reading the kitchen scales. Sally suggested the following: ■ Label individual measuring cups with Polymark paint to create raised tactile marker to identify the different levels. ■ Converting liquid measurements to cups as it is easier to read measuring cups. ■ Using talking weighing scales. ■ Transfer packets of dry food into wide-mouth storage containers to allow Marj to scoop out contents using measuring cups with greater stability and ease. ■ Filling measuring cup then running knife over top to ensure it is full and level. ■ Clearly label and organisation containers.
Appliance use		
Use of stovetop	Independent setting low-high temperature. Set and adjusted temperature accordingly throughout task. Difficulty locating the dial indicator to identify when the stove is off. When Marj is positioned at stove, the central light casts a shadow, inhibiting ability to read the dials and controls.	Marj identified the following techniques: ■ Use magnifier over the dial. ■ Most frequently used setting is 180 degrees. Sally applied raised tactile paint (Polymark paint) onto dial indicators with contrasting colours, enabling Marj to easily identify the dial settings. ■ An additional undercabinet LED light was installed to illuminate the dials and food cooking on the stove. Sally recommended to turn off dials before removing food as a safety precaution.
Use of oven	Unable to identify temperature settings on oven dial, relied on memory.	Marj identified the following techniques: ■ Use magnifier over the dial. Sally applied tactile paint in contrasting colour onto dial indicators and frequently used temperature settings.
Use of other appliances (toaster, sandwich makers, rice cooker, etc.)	Difficulty locating numbers and determining controls on the microwave.	Marj successfully trialled large-print number stickers.
Monitoring cooking process	Used wall clock in lounge room to monitor time, unable to read watch.	Marj identified the following techniques: ■ Apply tactile marker to existing timer to identify cooking intervals of 5 minutes. Sally trialled large-print watches and timers to assist Marj in monitoring cooking time. Marj purchased a large-print watch as she felt this had multiple uses.
Identifying cooked food	Difficulty identifying sautéed garlic/onions to her liking. Cooked vegetables and meat accordingly to time specifications. Fearful of transferring hot items from the oven or undercooking meats.	Marj identified the following techniques: ■ Prepare area on bench to rest hot items near the oven before transferring foods. Sally demonstrated safe techniques to remove hot items from oven, which included the following: ■ Wearing elbow-length oven mitts to prevent injuries on forearm. These mitts were purchased by Marj.

Continued on following page

TABLE 41.7

Marj's Kitchen Skills Assessment and Suggested Practical Strategies— (Continued)

Task Analysis	Observations	Practical Enabling Strategies to Support Participation in Cooking
		▪ As Marj was right-handed, it was suggested she stands at the left side of the oven, placing her nondominant hand on the counter next to the oven for balance support. Then she could use her right hand to find the oven door handle and open the oven door. ▪ Locate the oven rack and pull it out a little. ▪ With two hands, place the item to be baked on the oven rack and push the rack back in. ▪ With her right hand, close the oven door. To determine whether the chopped onions had sautéed, it was suggested Marj uses a sensory approach to smell and hear the changes in cooking progress. Marj also thought timing this process helped, as well as a talking thermometer to be certain roast meat was cooked through.
Clean-up		
Washing dishes/using dishwasher	Missed grime on plate when washing plates. Experiences glare in the late afternoon. Window gets full afternoon sun. Marj was required to pull down block-out blind, which prevented natural light from entering.	Marj identified the following techniques: ▪ To reduce the impact of glare at the kitchen sink, avoid completing tasks when the glare was most intense. ▪ Allow dishes to soak at high glare times and return when natural light is more comfortable. Sally suggested the following: ▪ Placing a tea towel over one shoulder to allow Marj to easily dry her hands and wipe spillages. ▪ Fill her sink and clean as you go, using water for cleaning hands and placing dirty dishes in as they are used. ▪ Consider inserting translucent blinds to maximise the natural light entering while also controlling the impact of glare. Run her fingertips lightly over object surfaces to locate food residue or areas requiring special attention and use her spare hand to locate a free/open space before placing dishes in the rack.
Cleaning sink, bench	Careful to wipe down bench.	Sally suggested using a systematic approach when wiping down the bench; for example, begin in the far right corner of the table surface, working from the far edge to the front edge using small circular movements and overlapping strokes.

Additional Comments

Assessment session

Lighting levels were recorded between 92 lux at sink and 85 lux at stove area with one central luminaire (8-Watt warm LED, 3000 Kelvin – warm light). When Marj is positioned at stove, the central light casts a shadow, inhibiting ability to read the dials and controls. Measurements of illumination (lux) levels were taken using a light metre with the lights switched on and daylight blocked out as much as possible to experience lighting levels that Marj would regularly be exposed to in evenings when cooking. Australian Standards recommend that illumination levels should be around 550–600 lux for task lighting in kitchens.

Hypotheses/Plausible Explanation

Reduced ability to read fine detail without appropriate levels of magnification and lighting. Increased clutter is causing visual confusion and increasing time delay in identification of items. Without organization, unable to rely on visual memory to differentiate between grouped items. Consider audible options

Practical strategy session

Before finalising the session, Marj asked about other techniques and assistive technologies she should consider that may assist her to be able to independently cook. Sally suggested that a common strategy used by people with vision impairment was to use the voice-commanded audio options on their mobile phones to:

▪ Set timers using voice
▪ Read out recipes
▪ Respond to questions such as conversions of quantities from millilitres or grams to cups or options to substitute an ingredient for an available alterative in the pantry or fridge.

Sally suggested that this option could potentially assist in other areas of Marj's life, such as advising of a new email or text and reading it out.

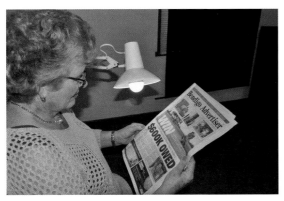

Fig. 41.4 ■ A woman applying task lighting to assist with reading the newspaper. The lamp is approximately 20 cm (7.8 inches) away and angled at approximately 45 degrees to the paper. She is also using her reading glasses at a working distance of 30 cm.

or reading street signs. A person diagnosed with low vision requires assessment, prescription and education in the use of appropriate magnification aid by an eye-health specialist. Incorrect magnification aids can be detrimental to the person, as they can lead to eye strain and fatigue. Purchasing unsuitable aids can be costly and lead to abandonment (Şahlı & İdil, 2019).

It is important for occupational therapists to be aware that the magnification device does not replace the vision that has already deteriorated; however, it will maximise a person's remaining vision when engaging in specific tasks.

Magnification can be achieved using four different methods: relative size magnification, relative distance magnification, angular magnification and electronic magnification.

- *Relative size magnification* refers to enlarging the object. For example, accessing large-print calendars, clocks, phones (Fig. 41.6), books, crosswords, sheet music and cooking recipes can make these objects visually easier to see and read.
- *Relative distance magnification* refers to moving the object closer or moving closer to the object. For example, when a person moves the lounge chair closer to the television or brings a book closer to the eyes, the retinal image of the television or book becomes larger, making it visually easier to see. When this occurs, a magnifier or optical lens should be considered to achieve maximum capacity of optimal functional vision. Ensuring correct magnification when completing tasks will reduce eye strain.
- *Angular magnification* is the magnification experience when a person looks through an optical device (e.g. telescope or a binocular) that creates an image which is larger than the actual object. This method is effective in producing magnification for distance objects while allowing the person to stay at his or her chosen distance from the object. For example, viewing a theatre production with a binocular or using a binocular to read the signs within the supermarket aisle will magnify the object of interest.
- *Electronic magnification* refers to the use of electronic equipment with the capability to enlarge or adapt the colour of near items (newspaper or letter) or distance items (television or stage at a theatre) (Fig. 41.7). For safety, it is recommended that a person is stationary when using both options. A simple and available option to many people is use of camera and zoom function on smartphones.

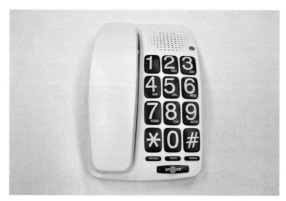

Fig. 41.5 ■ Relative size magnification: large numbers and buttons on a telephone; a tactile marker inserted on the speaker function is also illustrated.

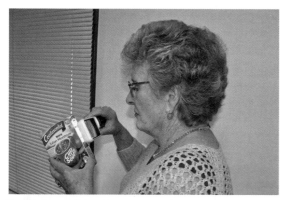

Fig. 41.6 ■ Relative distance magnification: handheld illuminated magnifier to read a jar label.

Bolder: Is There Enough Contrast?

Light/dark contrast is created by the amount of light that is reflected from different surfaces. The greater the contrast between the object and the object's background, the easier it is to see the differences. Black-on-white or white-on-black produces the best contrast for many people, but sometimes putting light colours against dark backgrounds is enough to see objects more clearly. Examples for using colour contrast to assist people with vision impairment include:

- Using a black felt-tipped pen for writing, instead of a ballpoint pen or pencil.
- White potatoes are difficult to see on a white chopping board or plate, instead trial using a darker board.

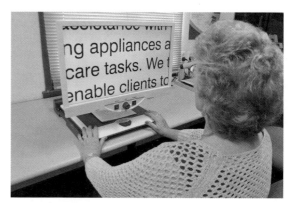

Fig. 41.7 ■ Electronic magnification: a desktop closed circuit television (CCTV).

- Using a white plate on a dark-coloured placemat.
- Painting the edge of stairs with a wide strip of contrasting colour paint.

Bolder is a highly effective strategy for most eye conditions and easily implemented using existing items within a person's home. This strategy is particularly relevant for supporting people with vision loss in nonspecialist settings.

Incorporating the Use of Other Senses

Techniques that promote the use of sensory functions such as hearing, touch, smell and taste can provide people with visual impairments with additional information about the environment and the performance of a task. Often the information provided by the senses supplements and supports information being received visually (Gilbert & Baker, 2011). Sensory exercises can help people increase their overall sensitivity and abilities and assist them to gain trust in the information they receive from their remaining senses.

Hearing

Hearing can provide auditory awareness of a person's environment, such as the sound of a door being opened, a car driving past, a cup being filled, water boiling and the click of switches as appliances are turned on and off. For people with vision impairment, the use of audible devices can reduce unnecessary eye strain or ease of functionality such as the use of talking clocks and kitchen scales. Most computers, tablets or mobile phones have built-in audio screen readers to access information using touch or verbal gestures that audibly read the information, thus reducing unnecessary visual fatigue. Smart home devices provide access to information in a nonvisual way, for example, asking for the weather, news reports or other information that require researching the Internet.

Touch

Touch is an extremely important means for a person with visual impairment to receive information about the environment. For example, a person with vision impairment may rely on touch to find switches, identify coins by their individual shape, size and milling or the orientation of clothes when dressing.

The 'bolder' contrast principle can be transferred to incorporate tactile components by creating a textured or tactile mark making an item or object (e.g. a button on a microwave) stand out from its background when touched. As an example, a tactile marker has been attached to the speaker button on the phone in Fig. 41.5 to assist a person to identify this button on the phone. Tactile markings such as Polymark paint or Velcro can be put onto appliances to assist with determining the various settings. Tactile symbol systems and braille have also been designed to assist with communication and literacy.

Touch is also critical in techniques used for moving around the community. When using a mobility cane or other mobility device (Fig. 41.8), the person will learn to identify the differences in surfaces (rough or smooth surface, tactile ground indictors), obstacles and judge depths or distances. People may also use a travel technique called trailing, in which they lightly press the walls using the back of their hand as they walk to guide direction and gain tactile information of their route.

Smell and Taste

Using the senses of smell and taste can provide information on the freshness of fruit and vegetables, alert an individual to food burning in the oven and assist in differentiating between different flavours such as salt or sugar, herbs and spices. Aromas can also provide a useful guide to assist with orientation to a particular area, for example within the home, identifying the scent of flowers in the living room, baking aromas in the kitchen and detergent in the laundry room. In external environments, smell can aid orientation by

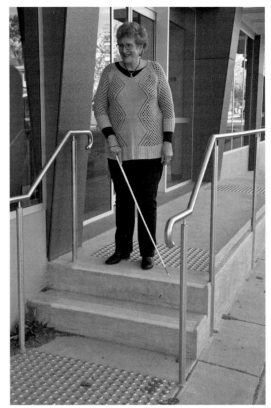

Fig. 41.8 ■ A person using an ID cane to identify hazards and depth perception; tactile ground surface indicators (TGSIs) and contrast marking are also presented in this figure.

providing feedback on proximity for example to a bakery by identifying direction of the scent. Learning to heighten awareness of smell and taste can compensate for visual impairment by providing information that would otherwise be obtained visually.

Using Visual Memory

In addition to the senses, a person who has developed vision impairment can use visual memory to consciously form accurate mental pictures of people, places and everyday objects. A person can create an accurate mental picture of a space or object by recalling the vast storehouse of visual memories accumulated throughout a lifetime, combined with description. In low-vision settings, the saying 'a place for everything and everything in its place' is commonly heard and is one of the most effective strategies to support identifying items using organisation and memory.

ADAPTIVE TECHNOLOGY AND VISION IMPAIRMENT

Accessing print material for people with vision impairments or who have a print impairment such as dyslexia has improved in recent years due to advances in technologies. Historically, alternative format consisted of braille, audiobooks or Optical Character Recognition (OCR) devices exclusive to reading print material, with angular magnification via the use of monocular or binocular the best option for distance text-like street signs. Wallace et al. (2020) emphasised how adaptive technology has become more accessible (both physically and financially) and is now more compatible with mainstream devices such as computers, smartphones (built-in accessibility and phone apps for people with vision impairment), smart watches, tablets and wearable devices that can read any text from street signs, pamphlets, information booklets, maps and documents sent via regular mail including handwritten notes.

Smart technologies are considered a key enabler for vision impaired and blind people to access information and digital services and thus should be explored through both demonstration and education (Şahlı & İdil, 2019). These technologies dramatically influence participation in and access to written communication, mobility and many other areas of daily life.

There are four main types of technology described ahead:

1. Magnification (as covered in the bigger subsection earlier)
2. Audio
3. Text-to-speech
4. Braille

Audio formats are readily available through mainstream technologies and through legislation and are no longer used exclusively by people with vision impairment. Examples of audio formats include audio recordings of books, audio narration of text (such as reading aloud a text message or email) and descriptive services, for example, audio description on films, television shows and the theatre. Low-vision equipment suppliers offer a range of equipment options to increase ease of access with built-in audible functions, such as talking microwaves or talking calculators. Many electronic magnifiers offer the ability to enlarge the text and read aloud.

Text-to-speech is also being used in mainstream in form of voice commands or listening to body of text. Common examples include smart technologies where a question can be asked and the device will search the Internet and provide a response or dictation of text or email converted from audio to text. Screen-reading software is available on mobile apps, for example, to scan and read a menu at a restaurant or to access complex computer functions of text, navigate computer programmes and describe an image. Distance text-to-speech is available in the form of wearable devices that can read street signs, train platform signs and bus timetables.

Braille users have range options of portable devices compatible with laptops including refreshable braille displays and braille embossers (printers).

In choosing adaptive technology options for a person, consideration should be given to the usability of the technology. Comprehensive training and support for the technology is also required to ensure successful integration of the technology into the everyday life of the person with vision impairment. Thorough assessment to determine the most suitable and versatile aid to meet a person's needs is essential to reduce abandonment and optimise participation.

For more information about these products, the Australian Disability Clearinghouse on Education and Training provides further information on these inclusive technologies for people who are blind or vision impaired (refer to resources section for additional information).

ERGONOMICS AND VISION IMPAIRMENT

Visual ergonomics is a significant consideration for occupational therapists when adaptive technology and assistive aids are prescribed. The use of devices may require a person to adopt a forward-leaning posture to create a specific working distance to maximise functional vision. It is essential for occupational therapists to review how the prescribed aid is used in the environment. For example, for a person who has been prescribed a magnifier and enjoys reading in their favourite lounge chair, there is a need to assess the use of the magnifier (focal distance) and the person's posture when in the lounge chair. A lap tray or reading tilt table may be introduced to minimise muscle strain and to ensure the person is comfortable when using the magnifier for reading (Kaldenberg, 2019). When using electronic devices, such as CCTV, computer or e-reader, assessing the aid within the environment and providing education regarding screen time, environmental glare, eye breaks, screen height, font size, contrast and brightness is essential to ensure eye health is maintained and to optimise functional vision and occupational participation (Schieman et al., 2016).

FALLS PREVENTION AND VISION IMPAIRMENT

Occupational therapists play a key role in assisting people with vision impairment to remain safe and independent in their homes and communities. Falls prevention education and techniques are essential for people with vision impairment as they are significantly more likely to fall compared with a person without vision impairment (Burton et al., 2021). They are also likely to limit their occupational participation because of a fear of falling as a result of the perceived risk due to reduced vision (Wang et al., 2012). Visual information is used to balance and coordinate movement and avoid obstacles and hazards. Visual field loss, reduced contrast sensitivity, diplopia, multifocal optical lenses and a general fear of falling – all increase the risk of falls (Şahlı & İdil, 2019). There are many factors that can place people with vision impairment at risk of a fall; some of these include general health, balance and proprioception, vision loss, medications and the physical environment (Burton et al., 2021). Further details about falls prevention strategies can be found in Chapter 32.

CONCLUSION

Working with people living with vision impairment is a specialised area of occupational therapy practice. Where possible, referral to low-vision specialist services will lead to improved outcomes for people who have low vision or blindness (Wallace et al., 2020). The basic principles of assessment and intervention can be incorporated into practice when access to specialised services is limited. The assessment of a person with vision impairment can be direct or indirect using formal, informal and observational techniques; ideally, assessment and intervention should involve a multidisciplinary team collaborating with the person to understand the functional impact of vision loss and the subsequent impact on the person's occupational participation. Enabling strategies can be simple (bigger, bolder and brighter) or complex (adaptive technology, equipment and intensive therapy focusing on developing compensatory skills by enhancing touch, smell, hearing, taste senses and visual memory). Ongoing critical reflection is essential for the occupational therapist to explore any changes and identify possible solutions to define plans to meet an individual's occupational participation goals. Finally, consideration of resources, supports and training for transitioning out of service will promote long-term participation and lifelong independence.

Acknowledgement

Special thanks and gratitude to the original authors of this chapter in the 7th edition of this book, Kirsty Stewart and Alexandra Lonsdale.

RESOURCES

Globally, there are many agencies and organisations that provide support to people in the low-vision and blindness community.

- American Foundation for the Blind (AFB): www.afb.org
- Blind Foundation: http://blindfoundation.org.nz
- Guide Dogs Australia: http://www.guidedogsaustralia.com
- National Eye Institute https://www.nei.nih.gov/
- National Federation of the Blind: https://nfb.org
- Royal Blind: www.royalblind.org
- Royal National Institute of Blind People (RNIB): http://www.rnib.org.uk
- Royal London Society for Blind People (RLSB): http://www.rlsb.org.uk
- Royal Society for the Blind: http://www.rsb.org.au
- Texas School for the Blind and Visually Impaired: http://www.tsbvi.edu

- The Hadley School for the Blind: https://hadley.edu/
- Thomas Pocklington Trust: http://www.pocklington-trust.org.uk
- VisAbility: http://www.visability.com.au
- Vision Australia: www.visionaustralia.org

Textbooks
- Whittaker, S., Schieman, M., & Sokol-McKay, D. (2016). *Low vision rehabilitation: A practical guide for occupational therapists.* Slack Incorporated.
- Warren, M., & Barstow, E. A. (Eds.). (2011). *Occupational therapy interventions for adults with low vision.* American Occupational Therapy Association Press.
- Dickinson, C., Hernandez Trillo, A., & Crossland, M. (2023). *Low vision: Principles and management.* Elsevier.

Vision-Specific Occupational Therapy Assessments
- Montreal Cognitive Assessment (Blind/Telephone Version) https://mocacognition.com/
- The Impact of Vision Impairment – Very Low Vision (IVI-VLV) questionnaire (IVI-VLV) (Finger et al., 2014) https://www.cera.org.au/pro-questionnaires/
- Perlmutter M. (2013). *Home environment lighting assessment (HELA).* https://www.ot.wustl.edu/about/resourcesut/assessments-388
- Veterans Affairs Low-Vision Visual Functioning Questionnaire (VA LV VFQ-48)

YouTube Channels
Professionals and agencies also use YouTube as a platform to deliver information. The following YouTube channels provide additional learning, including assessments and the application of low-vision principles:

- AFB channel: https://www.youtube.com/user/afb1921/videos
- Guide Dogs (UK): https://www.youtube.com/user/GuideDogsUK/videos
- Optometry Today: https://www.youtube.com/user/OTMultimedia
- Perkins Vision: https://www.youtube.com/user/PSB1829/videos

- RNIB: https://www.youtube.com/user/rnibuk/videos
- Vision Australia product demonstrations: https://www.youtube.com/@VisionAustralia/videos.

Low-Vision Products
For high-cost or optical equipment, proper assessment and prescription is recommended. For low-cost items, these can be quick and easy solutions to overcome many daily-living challenges. The links below offer information about both high-cost and low-cost products.

- Australian Disability Clearinghouse on Education and Training https://www.adcet.edu.au/inclusive-technology/blind-and-vision-impaired
- Vision Australia Product Shop https://shop.visionaustralia.org/
- American Printing House for the Blind https://www.aph.org/shop/
- RNIB https://shop.rnib.org.uk/

TEDx talks
TED talks provide inspirational speakers from individuals with lived experiences https://www.ted.com/search?q=vision+impaired

Podcasts
- Hadley Audio Podcasts https://hadley.edu/podcasts
- Vision Australia, https://radio.visionaustralia.org/podcasts
- VisAbility https://www.visability.com.au/podcasts/
- Apple Podcasts Low Vision Moments https://podcasts.apple.com/ca/podcast/low-vision-moments/id1536469789
- Blind Citizens Australia https://www.bca.org.au/podcasts/

REFERENCES
Arbesman, M., Lieberman, D., & Berlanstein, D. R. (2013). Methodology for the systematic reviews on occupational therapy interventions for older adults with low vision. *American Journal of Occupational Therapy, 67*(3), 272–278. https://doi.org/10.5014/ajot.2013.007021.

Barstow, B. A., Warren, M., Thaker, S., Hallman, A., & Batts, P. (2015). Client and therapist perspectives on the influence of low vision and chronic conditions on performance and occupational therapy intervention. *American Journal of Occupational Therapy, 69*(3). 6903270010p1. https://doi.org/10.5014/ajot.2015.014605.

Bovend'Eerdt, T. J., Botell, R. E., & Wade, D. T. (2009). Writing SMART rehabilitation goals and achieving goal attainment scaling: A practical guide. *Clinical Rehabilitation, 23*(4), 352–361. https://doi.org/10.1177/0269215508101741.

Burton, M. J., Ramke, J., Marques, A. P., Bourne, R. R. A., Congdon, N., Jones, I., Tong, B. A. M. A., Arunga, S., Bachani, D., Bascaran, C., Bastawrous, A., Blanchet, K., Braithwaite, T., Buchan, J. C., Cairns, J., Cama, A., Chagunda, M., Chuluunkhuu, C., Cooper, A., … Faal, H. B. (2021). The Lancet Global Health Commission on Global Eye Health: Vision beyond 2020. *The Lancet Global Health, 9*(4), e489–e551. https://doi.org/10.1016/S2214-109X(20)30488-5.

Dickinson, C., HernandezTrillo, A., & Crossland, M. (2023). *Low vision: Principles and management*. Elsevier.

Egan, M., & Restall, G. (2022). *Promoting occupational participation: Collaborative relationship-focused occupational therapy*. Canadian Association of Occupational Therapists.

Finger, R. P., Tellis, B., Crewe, J., Keeffe, J. E., Ayton, L. N., & Guymer, R. H. (2014). Developing the impact of vision impairment–very low vision (IVI-VLV) questionnaire as part of the LoVADA protocol. *Investigative Opthalmology & Visual Science, 55*(10), 6150. https://doi.org/10.1167/iovs.14-14731.

Gilbert, M. & Baker, S. (2011). Evaluation and intervention for basic and instrumental activities of daily living. In M. Warren & E. Bartow (Eds.), *Occupational therapy interventions for adults with low vision* (pp. 227–268). Bethesda, MD: Bethesda American Occupational Therapy Association.

Graham, F., Kennedy-Behr, A., & Ziviani, J. (2021). *Occupational performance coaching: A manual for practitioners and researchers*. Routledge.

Kaldenberg, J. (2019). Low vision rehabilitation services: Perceived barriers and facilitators to access for older adults with visual impairment. *British Journal of Occupational Therapy, 82*(8), 466–474. https://doi.org/10.1177/0308022618821591.

Law, M., Baptiste, S., Carswell, A., McColl, M. A., Polatajko, H. J., & Pollock, N. (2014). *Canadian occupational performance measure* (5th ed.). Canadian Association of Occupational Therapists (CAOT) Publications.

Mohler, A. J., Neufeld, P., & Perlmutter, M. S. (2015). Factors affecting readiness for low vision interventions in older adults. *American Journal of Occupational Therapy, 69*(4), 6904270020p1. https://doi.org/10.5014/ajot.2015.014241.

National Eye Institute/National Institutes of Health (NEI/NIH). (2022). *Eye Conditions and Diseases*. Courtesy: National Eye Institute, National Institutes of Health (NEI/NIH). https://www.nei.nih.gov/learn-about-eye-health/eye-conditions-and-diseases.

Perlmutter, M. S., Bhorade, A., Gordon, M., Hollingsworth, H., Engsberg, J. E., & Baum, M. C. (2013). Home lighting assessment for clients with low vision. *American Journal of Occupational Therapy, 67*(6), 674–682. https://doi.org/10.5014/ajot.2013.006692.

Restall, G. J., & Egan, M. Y. (2021). Collaborative relationship-focused occupational therapy: Evolving lexicon and practice. *Canadian Journal of Occupational Therapy, 88*(3), 220–230. https://doi.org/10.1177/00084174211022889.

Restall, G., Egan, M., Valavaara, K., Phenix, A., & Sack, C. (2022). Canadian occupational therapy inter-relational practice process framework. In M. Egan & G. Restall (Eds.), Promoting occupational participation: collaborative relationship-focused occupational therapy (pp. 120–149). Canadian Association of Occupational Therapists.

Şahlı, E., & İdil, A. (2019). Common approach to low vision: Examination and rehabilitation of the patient with low vision. *Turkish Journal of Ophthalmology, 49*(2), 89–98. https://doi.org/10.4274/tjo.galenos.2018.65928.

Smallfield, S. & Kaldenberg, J. (2020). Occupational therapy interventions to improve reading performance of older adults with low vision: A systematic review. *The American Journal of Occupational Therapy : Official Publication of the American Occupational Therapy Association, 74*(1), 7401185030p1–7401185030p18. https://doi.org/10.5014/ajot.2020.038380.

Vision Australia. (2023). *Tips on communicating to patients with vision loss*. Vision Australia Blindness and Low Vision Services. https://www.visionaustralia.org/news/tips-communicating-patients-vision-loss.

Wallace, S., Alao, R., Kuper, H., & Jackson, M. L. (2020). Multidisciplinary visual rehabilitation in low- and middle-income countries: A systematic review. *Disability and Rehabilitation, 44*(8), 1164–1175. https://doi.org/10.1080/09638288.2020.1794063.

Wang, M. Y., Rousseau, J., Boisjoly, H., et al. (2012). Activity limitation due to a fear of falling in older adults with eye disease. *Investigative Ophthalmology & Visual Science, 53*(13), 7967–7972.

Warren M. (1993). A hierarchical model for evaluation and treatment of visual perceptual dysfunction in adult acquired brain injury, Part 1. *The American Journal of Occupational Therapy : Official Publication of the American Occupational Therapy Association, 47*(1), 42–54. https://doi.org/10.5014/ajot.47.1.42.

Warren, M., & Barstow, E. A. (2011). *Occupational therapy interventions for adults with low vision*. Aota Press.

Whittaker, S., Scheiman, M., & Sokol-Mckay, D. A. (2016). *Low vision rehabilitation: A practical guide for occupational therapists* (2nd ed.). Slack Incorporated.

Wittich, W., Phillips, N., Nasreddine, Z. S., & Chertkow, H. (2010). Sensitivity and specificity of the montreal cognitive assessment modified for individuals who are visually impaired. *Journal of Visual Impairment & Blindness, 104*(6), 360–368. https://doi.org/10.1177/0145482x1010400606.

World Health Organization. (2019). *World report on vision*. World Health Organization. Www.who.int: https://www.who.int/publications/i/item/9789241516570.

World Health Organization. (2022). *Blindness and Vision Impairment*. World Health Organization. https://www.who.int/news-room/fact-sheets/detail/blindness-and-visual-impairment.

Zheng, Y., Wu, X., Lin, X., & Lin, H. (2017). The prevalence of depression and depressive symptoms among eye disease patients: A systematic review and meta-analysis. *Scientific Reports, 7*(1). https://doi.org/10.1038/srep46453.

Zoltan, B. (2007). *Vision, perception, and cognition: A manual for the evaluation and treatment of the adult with acquired brain injury*. Slack.

REFLECTION

1. As a Occupational Therapist working for a low-vision service, you have received a new referral. The eye report states this person has a diagnosis of age-related macular degeneration, for which the person attends regular eye health checks, and wears bifocal glasses that are more than two years old. During the initial phone contact the person reports difficulties with near tasks such as reading labels of food packaging, preparing a hot drink, using the telephone, and reading mail. What low-vision service would you prioritise first and why?

2. As an occupational therapist you are working on a rehabilitation ward with a man who has diabetes, a history of falls and a recently fractured neck of femur and is preparing for discharge back to his home within the next week. He is attending the balance clinic, where he discloses that he also has glaucoma. What information relating to his vision could you provide that may assist in preventing another fall?

3. As an occupational therapist, you are working in a transitional care unit with a 28-year-old woman who has a diagnosis of ideopathic intercranial hypertension, which has resulted in optic nerve damage. Her vision has been assessed as light perception only. She is currently 1000 km away from her home and is reliant on her smartphone to communicate with friends and family. What strategies could you put in place to assist her with maintaining communication with her friends and family?

42

COGNITION AND PERCEPTION

JUDY L. RANKA ■ CHRISTINE J CHAPPARO ■ MELISSA THERESE NOTT

Overview

Cognition and perception are central to participation in occupational performance. Historically, occupational therapists have focused on identifying and treating cognitive and perceptual impairments. Contemporary approaches assess impairment as a person carries out specific everyday tasks. Interventions increasingly incorporate principles of instruction and task training methods. Rather than impairment as the primary focus, this chapter describes the place of cognition and perception in occupational therapy which aims to support occupational participation. In doing so, an information processing view of cognition is described and used to explain how cognition and perception contribute to occupational participation. One occupational therapy assessment and intervention approach, the Perceive, Recall, Plan and Perform System of Task Analysis is described. This approach is grounded in information-processing theory framed by person-specific occupational needs and aspirations and focuses on the effectiveness of cognitive strategy use during occupational participation. Examples are given, which demonstrate how constructs from the assessment can be used to observe cognitive strategy application during occupational participation and how cognitive strategy application strengths and difficulties impacting occupational participation can be addressed through intervention. A practice story of a man who experiences difficulties with occupational participation as a consequence of a stroke is provided to illustrate the use of the System.

KEY POINTS

■ Safe, effective, ethical and satisfying occupational performance and participation depend on the integrity of a person's cognitive and perceptual functions.

■ Contemporary information processing theory provides an inclusive model of cognition where attention, perception, memory, thinking, response generation and executive control are parts of a continuum of information flow in the brain.

- The Perceive, Recall, Plan and Perform (PRPP) System of Task Analysis is a collaborative, rights-based, strengths-oriented and ecologically valid assessment and intervention approach to functional cognition that is based on information processing theory and grounded in occupational performance.

- The PRPP System focuses on how people use information processing (cognitive) strategies to stop, attend, sense, recall, figure out, initiate and sustain occupational participation.

- Although this System is an Occupational Performance Model (Australia) approach, the principles, processes and constructs align with collaborative, relationship-focused occupational therapy described in the Canadian Model of Occupational Participation.

INTRODUCTION

In occupational therapy, occupational participation has been defined as, 'having access to, initiating and sustaining valued occupations within meaningful relationships and contexts' (Egan & Restall, 2022a, p. 76). Mental functions of the brain are critical to a person's ability to carry out activities and participate in the wider community (World Health Organization, 2001). These functions comprise cognition, the 'mental action or process of acquiring knowledge and understanding through thought, experience and the senses' (Oxford University Press, 1989). Cognition gives people the capacity to learn and remember occupational participation experiences, assign meaning to those experiences and construct a personal occupational participation history.

Historically, occupational therapists have transitioned through approaches to addressing cognition in practice with adults, beginning with a *functional approach* where cognition was rarely considered, and therapy focused on teaching people how to do activities of daily living. The publication of seminal works in neuroscience (Critchley, 1954; Luria, 1962) raised awareness of cortical functions and led to the development of neuropsychological tests. Similarly, in occupational therapy ways to observe and label perceptual and cognitive impairment emerged (Siev et al., 1986) as part of an approach commonly referred to as *impairment focused*. Numerous assessments used by occupational therapists evolved, for example, Addenbrooke's Cognitive Evaluation III (ACE-III) (Hodges

& Larner, 2017), Lowenstein Occupational Therapy Cognitive Assessment (LOTCA) (Katz et al., 1989), Montreal Cognitive Assessment (MoCA) (Nasreddine et al., 2005) and the Kimberley Indigenous Cognitive Assessment (KICA) (LoGiudice et al., 2006). Many more are described elsewhere (Al-Heizan & Edwards, 2019; American Occupational Therapy Association, 2019; Edwards et al., 2019).

An *impairment-focused* approach provides occupational therapists with ways to measure deficits and terminology to describe these deficits; however, test administration is limited to people who have the cognitive and language capacity to follow instructions. Assessments of this type usually do not account for educational level or allow for cultural, contextual or temporal nuances and their ability to predict performance and participation in everyday life is questionable. The negative effects of an impairment or deficit discourse on participation rights and opportunities are reported (Fogarty et al., 2018). Some people may be stigmatised with unsubstantiated labels such as 'dementia' or 'neglect'. Others may be denied opportunities for independence or financial services, such as insurance coverage. Direction is provided for occupational therapy intervention from these assessment findings. Typically, therapy activities that resemble test items are practised with the assumption that gains in cognitive capacity will generalise to improvement in occupational participation. Occupational therapists and others have come to understand the limitations of procedures which measure impairment in isolation from a person's participation needs and desires (Burgess et al., 2006; Heaton & Pendleton, 1981; Kingstone et al., 2008; Tupper & Cicerone, 1990) and therapy outcomes that fail to generalise outside of the therapy context (Bayley et al., 2014).

A second approach available to occupational therapists and others focuses on identifying the level of *cognitive functioning* in people experiencing cognitive impairment, typically from traumatic brain injury. Health professionals using this approach monitor and document cognitive recovery, predict the direction of behavioural change and support functional improvement. Recovery scales of cognitive functioning used with people following traumatic brain injury include the Rancho Los Amigos Scale–Revised [RLAS-R] (Ng & Chua, 2005), Wessex Head Injury Matrix (Shiel et al., 2000) and the Coma Recovery Scale–Revised [CRS-R]

(Giacino & Kalmar, 2004). Items on these scales range from identifying the person's initial responsiveness to sensory stimulation from a comatose state to the ability to participate in community life. In mental health, occupational therapists may use the Allen Cognitive Level Screen leather lacing test item (Allen Cognitive Group, 2022) to identify a person's global cognitive processing capacities, learning potential and problem-solving skills and use findings to determine the feasibility of community living and the level and type of supports required to optimise occupational participation.

A shift in practice has occurred towards establishing *functional cognition* as the domain of occupational therapy (American Occupational Therapy Association, 2013, 2019). *Functional cognition* refers to the 'cognitive ability to perform daily life tasks, incorporating metacognition, executive function, other domains of cognitive functioning, motor performance skills and performance patterns' (Giles et al., 2020, p. 2). Simply, it is the use of cognitive processes in the context of performing everyday activities and occupations (Wesson & Giles, 2019).

Assessments that align with *functional cognition* are consistent with the measurement property of ecological validity. Contemporary use of this term refers to the 'representativeness' of a task (the extent to which an assessment corresponds in form and context to an everyday situation) and the 'generalisability' of test results (the degree to which poor performance is predictive of everyday problems) (Burgess et al., 2006; Kingstone et al., 2008). Assessments of this type are classed as performance assessments (World Health Organization, 2001). They provide information about what a person does or perceives to do in everyday life contexts. Such assessments measure performance against specific criteria rather than an expected norm. Examples developed by occupational therapists include: the Executive Function Performance Test (EFPT) (Baum & Wolf, 2013); the ADL-Focused Occupation-Based Neurobehavioural Evaluation (A-ONE) (Árnadóttir, 1990, 2011); Kettle Test (Maeir et al., 2009) and the occupation-embedded assessment of online awareness (Doig et al., 2017). Others are described in Wolf et al. (2019).

Most tests of functional cognition assess specific dimensions of cognition as a person performs predetermined, standardised tasks within controlled contexts. The impact of limitations in functional cognition on occupational participation is inferred. Some recommend supplementing these assessments with self-report goal achievement scales such as the Canadian Occupational Performance Measure (COPM) (Law et al., 2023) or the Goal Attainment Scale (GAS) (Turner-Stokes, 2009) to measure real-life impact (American Occupational Therapy Association, 2019). Others suggest inclusion of assessments of cognitive impairment to confirm findings about deficits discovered through assessment of functional cognition (Wolf & Baum, 2019). Information obtained from assessments of functional cognition is used to choose from intervention approaches that address the identified cognitive impairments within a skills training or compensation framework (Barco et al., 2019). These approaches include, for example, the Neurofunctional Approach (Clark-Wilson et al., 2014); the Cognitive Orientation to Daily Occupational Performance (CO-OP) (Polatajko & Mandich, 2004); and the Multi-context Approach (Toglia, 2018).

The contribution of a *functional cognition* approach to the profession has been to integrate occupational therapy practice which targets cognition with occupation as a core construct of occupational therapy. However, limitations exist when the occupations assessed are fixed, the assessment context is pre-determined, the performance expectations have been standardised, results are obtained from self-report only and multiple assessments are required. For some people, the list of 'test' occupations may not be ones that are needed or desired by the person or collective, leading to an assessment situation that is interpreted as contrived. People who have significant cognitive or language impairment, such as those emerging from coma or with aphasia, may not comprehend the instructions. Some people may misunderstand the performance expectations or feel threatened by test protocols, resulting in unsafe healthcare delivery. Self-report statements may not reflect reality. The feasibility of conducting multiple assessments within time constraints is questioned (Prinsen et al., 2016) and many cannot be used for re-test purposes. Particular issues arise with their use in cross-cultural contexts (Mushquash & Bova, 2007) and with First Nations peoples (Dingwall et al., 2014, 2017; Jacklin et al., 2020) who may not perceive the assessment tasks or context as being culturally safe (Smith et al., 2023).

For these reasons, ecological approaches to addressing functional cognition are needed that adopt a collaborative relationship-focused approach (Restall & Egan, 2022) to assessment where personally meaningful and culturally safe occupations are identified and performance is assessed in relevant, person-specific home, community or health care participation contexts (refer to Chapter 12). This requires a shift in focus from diagnosing cognitive impairment, monitoring cognitive recovery or addressing limitations in functional cognition to more authentic ways of identifying how people use cognition to meet the participation demands of everyday life. Such an approach would allow for idiosyncratic ways of doing things, which may be individually or collectively chosen or common to a group, culturally determined, historically or contextually shaped and are flexible in terms of how much is done. For some people, completion of a whole task independently may be a realistic and desired outcome. For others who are unable to complete a whole task, assessing how well a person carries out parts of a task or does so with the support of another person may be the focus. Research has demonstrated that being able to initiate and sustain engagement in something meaningful and satisfying is associated with perceptions of a high quality of life (Erikkson et al., 2012; Yerxa, 1998). For example, some people may find that being able to groom a dog or finish the last steps of preparing a meal are more fulfilling than putting on a shirt or paying a bill. Approaches with high ecological validity are truly 'representative' of authentic occupational participation requirements, and the findings 'generalise' directly to everyday life.

Understanding how cognition and perception contribute to occupational participation requires a deeper exploration of what is meant by these terms. In this chapter, an information processing model of cognition is described which views cognition and perception as interrelated parts on a continuum of brain function (Michel, 2020). The elements of information processing theory as they relate to occupational participation are explained, followed by a description of one approach to assessment of functional cognition and intervention that is grounded in occupational performance and information processing theory, the *Perceive, Recall, Plan and Perform System of Task Analysis (PRPP System)*. Examples are provided, which describe how the PRPP System can be used to observe effective and ineffective information processing during occupational performance and how information processing required for occupational participation can be supported in occupational therapy practice.

INFORMATION PROCESSING AND COGNITIVE STRATEGIES

Contemporary information processing theory provides an inclusive model of cognition where attention, perception, memory, thinking, response generation and executive control are parts of a continuum of information flow in the brain. An information processing view of cognition focuses on abilities (Huitt, 2003). It is not a model of cognitive or other impairment. Information processing theory can be used to explain how people use cognition in everyday life (Cambridge Cognition, 2023) and the difficulties anyone may experience in meeting the cognitive demands of occupations and contexts. Principles derived from information processing theory can be used to design intervention which aims to enhance occupational participation by building a person's autonomy and competence using strategies required to process and respond to information from occupations and contexts more effectively.

Models of information processing such as the one illustrated in the central boxes of Fig. 42.1 trace the staged flow of information from initial input and reception, through several internal processing operations, to the final output response and subsequent feedback loop (Eysenck & Keane, 2020; Friedenberg & Silverman, 2011). The human brain or information processor takes in information (sensory input, registration), interprets, stores, relocates and remembers it for use (memory), manipulates and organises information, plans and evaluates ideas, allocates attention, regulates overall processing (metacognition, executive control), initiates, monitors and controls output responses (actions, behaviour) and processes internal and external feedback about responses. The flow of information is not linear. Recursive arrows between stages of processing illustrate the dynamic and interdependent nature of information processing.

Despite the remarkable power and flexibility of the human brain, its capacity to process information is limited (Marois & Ivanoff, 2005). What is processed and

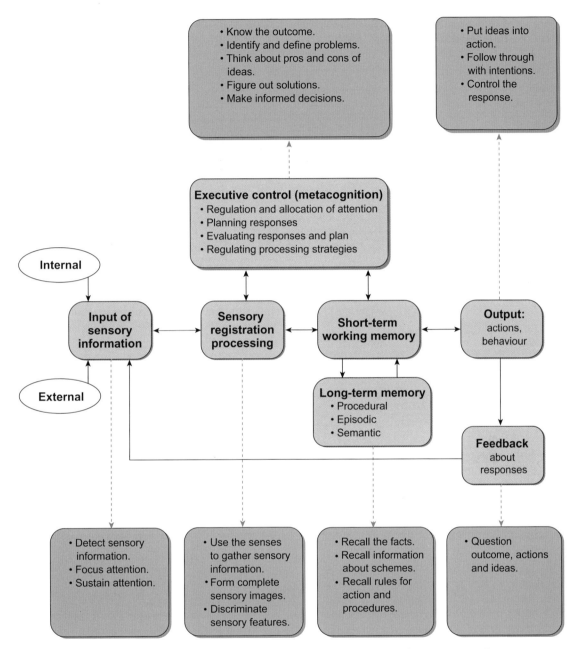

Fig. 42.1 ◼ Information processing model with examples of associated cognitive strategies.

the quality of processing throughout the whole system is controlled by an executive system that monitors and regulates these processes in order to organise thinking, change thinking or evaluate decisions and outcomes when processing or performance is not going smoothly (Diamond, 2013). This has been referred to as 'meta-strategic control' in people's abilities to apply the thinking strategies that process information (Couchman et al., 2010; Demetrious & Kazi, 2006; Fox & Christoff, 2014). Metastrategic control assists people to cope with the many problems of performance that arise during everyday participation allowing them to not just 'do what they know' but to figure out the most effective way to perform under specific and variable conditions. Information processing (cognitive) strategies are goal-oriented thinking strategies that people use to do the following: identify important or difficult information; understand and retain information; retrieve information from memory; apply relevant information to what has to be done; plan responses; and simultaneously cope with internal and external distractions during performance of a task (Siegler, 2007).

Cognitive strategies have been defined as being either externally or internally generated. *External* cognitive strategies are external sources used by people to support the 'thinking' aspects of task performance (Katz et al., 2011), for example, electronic devices to assist memory for the timing of daily activities or calendars as reminders of dates. *Internal* cognitive strategies are mental strategies that are part of the process of thinking through task performance (Siegler, 2007; Toglia et al., 2012). These strategies include, for example, using visualisation to imagine performance, making face-name associations or using mental rehearsal. The internal cognitive strategies discussed in this chapter are the internally generated thinking strategies that people use to allocate attention, take in sensory information, form sensory perceptions, interpret, store, remember information, plan, problem solve, decide and initiate, sustain and monitor output action as they meet occupational participation demands. Many of these strategies are observable behaviours a person uses during task performance. Examples of these cognitive strategies are in the outer boxes in Fig. 42.1.

It has been suggested that to offset a limited capacity to process information, people use a general set of cognitive strategies across occupations or situations (Siegler, 2007). Research during the early development of the Perceive, Recall, Plan and Perform Assessment (Occupational Performance Network, 2023) confirmed that people use the same set of internal cognitive strategies to solve problems of everyday life but apply them differently depending on salient conditions (e.g. perceived importance, skill expected, time factors, safety risks, presence of disability). Cognitive strategy use is the application of internally generated 'thinking' strategies in the 'here and now' and entails choosing and applying the 'best' strategies to fit a particular situation.

Cognitive strategies used to process information during occupational participation are determined by the demands of the occupation and context and the processing capacity of the person. At times of illness, fatigue or emotional distress, anyone can experience difficulties using cognitive strategies needed to meet these demands. People may, for example, have difficulty staying focused on the task, miss critical sensory signals, forget key information, lose a train of thought or have difficulty following through with intentions. Although for most people this is temporary, many people experience persistent difficulties in cognitive strategy use. These may be people who have neurological, psychological, developmental or emotional disorders, who live with chronic conditions such as pain and fatigue, who have significant physical impairment or who experience overwhelming pressure from contextual factors. The nature of the disorder is not viewed as a deficit in cognition but a difficulty in applying cognitive strategies required for safe, effective, ethical and satisfying occupational participation.

ADDRESSING COGNITIVE STRATEGY APPLICATION DURING PARTICIPATION

One evidence-based example of an approach that addresses the specific and particular participation needs of people is the *Perceive, Recall, Plan and Perform System of Task Analysis (PRPP System)* (Chapparo & Ranka, 1997b, 2010; Chapparo et al., 2017b). The PRPP System is a dynamic *assessment* and *intervention* approach in which the assessment process seeks to (1) measure a person's occupational performance skill and cognitive strategy application strengths and (2) use the results to inform intervention that focuses on improving occupational participation by simultaneously addressing occupational performance mastery and cognitive strategy application requirements. The PRPP System evolved out of the Occupational Performance Model (Australia) (OPM[A]) (Chapparo & Ranka, 1997a; Chapparo et al., 2017a; Turpin & Iwama, 2011) and aligns closely with the key concepts of collaborative relationship-focused occupational therapy (Egan & Restall, 2022b) (refer to Chapter 12).

The PRPP Assessment

The PRPP Assessment (PRPP-A) was built on concepts proposed by (Romiszowski, 1984) and developed through multiple research phases commencing in 1990 (Occupational Performance Network, 2023). It is a standardised, criterion-referenced, authentic and ecologically valid assessment of *applied cognition* that is strengths-oriented, occupation-embedded, performance-focused and contextually situated. The PRPP-A can be used with anyone; it is inclusive of all life stages, genders, diagnoses and cultures (Aubin et al., 2014; Burrows et al., 2022; Juntorn et al., 2017; Ranka & Chapparo, 2010; Sproats et al., 2013; Sturkenboom et al., 2020), including with First Nations Peoples in Australia (Smith et al., 2023) and with people who have minimal to significant difficulty processing information (Bootes & Chapparo, 2010; Lewis et al., 2016; Nott & Chapparo, 2008, 2020; White et al., 2020). It is also used as a framework for understanding and explaining dimensions of practice reasoning and decision-making in occupational therapy (Chapparo & Ranka, 2019). The PRPP-A is administered in two stages.

PRPP-A Stage One: Occupational Performance Mastery

Stage One embeds the assessment in occupations that are personally and culturally meaningful. This part of the assessment allows for the individuality of occupational participation to be considered. Administration of Stage One begins with the occupational therapist, person and/or relevant role partners working in collaboration to identify and prioritise everyday occupations of importance, including the meaning ascribed to them, significance they hold, future possibilities, cultural relevance and where and how the occupations typically are or will be carried out. Through this process, the priorities and goals are determined. Unique to the PRPP-A is that *any* occupation can be used as the assessment task/s, ranging from looking when asked to do so, holding a spoon, playing a game, fishing, travelling in the community or managing business routines.

Occupational therapists observe the person performing a sample of occupations from the prioritised list and determine whether performance is effective compared with that person's expectations of performance or the expectations of significant role partners in the collective. Procedural task analysis methods

(Johassen et al., 1989) are used to break down the sample of occupations into roles, routines, tasks, steps, skill sets or do/say social interactions depending on the purpose of the assessment. The occupational therapist judiciously sets the performance criterion from all these data. This differs from other norm- or criterion-referenced assessments where the criteria are set by the test developers and described in test administration protocols. Performance is observed and scored using a standardised rubric of error types. Stage One yields a Total Mastery Score expressed as a percentage of the performance the person has mastered. This forms the basis for measuring person-specific occupational participation outcomes, provides objective information about occupational participation concerns to share with the person and/or role partners and guides intervention that aims to improve mastery.

PRPP-A Stage Two: Cognitive Strategy Application

Stage Two focuses on identifying strengths in cognitive strategy use while also identifying the cognitive strategy application reasons for any errors observed in Stage One. Stage Two is grounded in information processing theory which is reflected in Stage Two Conceptual Model (Fig. 42.2). At the centre are four processing quadrants: Perceive (attention, sensory perception), Recall (learning, memory, recall), Plan (planning, decision making, judgement) and Perform (initiating and sustaining action, monitoring responses, controlling and adjusting output). Multidirectional, recursive arrows mirror the multi-staged flow of information in Fig. 42.1.

The four central *quadrants* are further divided into 12 *subquadrants* that represent information processing operations. These appear in the middle ring of Fig. 42.2. Key descriptive words, *descriptors*, are used to name and frame the cognitive strategies assessed during task performance. Descriptors form the outer ring of the system. Each descriptor is an observable behaviour that has been operationally defined for assessment purposes. These same descriptors are targeted in the intervention.

The goal of assessing cognitive strategy application is to determine whether people are able to process information required by particular person-specific occupations in particular person-specific contexts in order to participate optimally. In other words, accurate

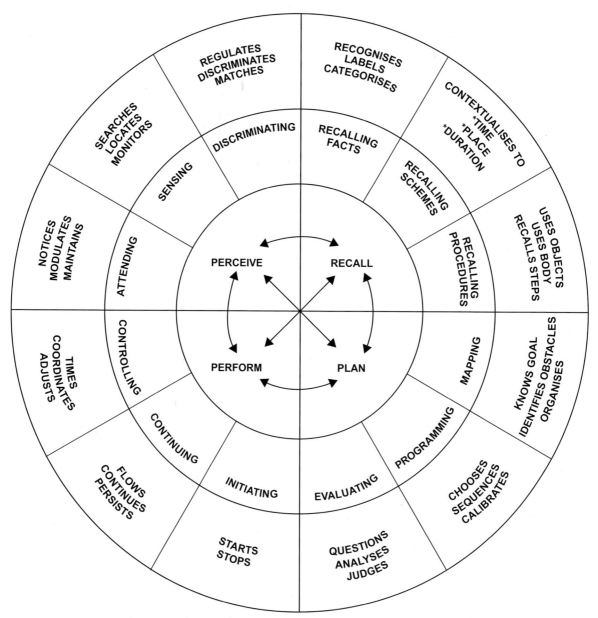

Fig. 42.2 ■ The PRPP System of Task Analysis Stage Two Conceptual Model.

assessment is referenced to particular person-specific criteria that are determined by the nature and complexity of the cognitive demands posed by the occupation and the context and the cognitive capacity of the person to meet those demands. This approach acknowledges the contextually and temporarily nuanced relationship between the occupational therapist and the person and differs from most approaches to cognitive assessment that specifies one standard of performance against which everyone's cognitive capacities are measured. Applied cognitive task analysis methods (Schraagen et al., 2000) support this part of the assessment. Occupational therapists administering Stage Two of the PRPP-A engage in a series of practice reasoning questions that guide quality and ethical practice. Occupational therapists ask themselves:

- What cognitive strategies does this occupation demand?
- What cognitive strategies does the participation context demand?
- Is the person applying the cognitive strategies needed for safe, effective, ethical performance in context?

The rubric for reliable scoring taught in PRPP-A training courses specifies criteria for assigning a 3-2-1 score for each *descriptor* relative to whether that behaviour aided or interfered with Mastery on Stage One. Stage Two yields a Total Subquadrant Strategy Application Score expressed as a percentage of the strategies applied for each of the 12 information processing operation subquadrants. These scores yield a cognitive strategy application profile and are used to measure person-specific outcomes. Stage Two guides occupational therapy intervention decisions about how to improve Stage One Mastery. Identified strengths in cognitive strategy application are supported and needed behaviours for improved mastery strengthened. Compensations are suggested for behaviours that will not change.

PRPP Intervention

The PRPP Intervention (PRPP-I) was first conceptualised and disseminated in 1994 by Chapparo and Ranka at occupational therapy conferences and elsewhere in that decade (Chapparo & Ranka, 1996, 1999) and effectiveness demonstrated with children and adults (Challita et al., 2019; Lindstad et al., 2023; Nott & Chapparo, 2008, 2020; Occupational Performance Network, 2023). It is an occupation-embedded approach that relies on findings from task analysis and seeks to improve occupational performance and participation mastery by simultaneously addressing *applied cognition*. PRPP-I is built on principles of instruction recommended by many (Barco et al., 2019; Snell, 1987); however, the instructional cues and prompts used in this intervention are guided by the information processing theoretical foundation of the PRPP System. PRPP-I is an extension of the 'Stop, Think, Do' programme developed for use with children and adolescents (Beck & Horne, 1992; Murphy & Cooke, 1999) and the 'Goal, Plan, Do and Review' programme

developed for adults with traumatic brain injury (Ylvisaker et al., 1998). Core principles of PRPP-I are outlined in Box 42.1.

PRPP-I involves teaching people to apply cognitive strategies (descriptor behaviours) during occupational participation practice attempts by using a combination of '*Stop, Attend, Sense, Think, Do*' meta-prompts. These meta-prompts align with dimensions of information processing reflected in the PRPP Stage Two Conceptual Model (Fig. 42.2) and are depicted in the PRPP Intervention Conceptual Framework (Fig. 42.3).

Effective performance may require that a person can *Stop* (stop themselves from making mistakes or stop/pause to learn something else), *Attend* (focus on important information), *Sense* (perceive sensory information relevant to the situation), *Think to recall* (learn, store and retrieve information), *Think to plan* (figure out, problem solve, plan a response, evaluate performance) and *Do* (implement the plan, monitor output). Each Stop, Attend, Sense, Think, Do meta-prompt encapsulates a group of PRPP descriptors that are used to individualise intervention. One or two descriptor behaviours from two or more Stop, Attend, Sense, Think, Do meta-prompts are selected from PRPP Assessment findings and ordered as a sequence of cognitive strategies that are then prompted or modelled by the occupational therapist. The order may vary depending on the information processing sequence that is the target of intervention; for example, Attend-Sense-Do, Stop-Recall-Do, Think-Sense-Recall, Do-Think-Do.

Occupational therapists using the PRPP Intervention act as *cognitive mediators* in providing instruction, and are themselves, an integral part of the relational context of therapy. They connect the person's thinking to the occupation being performed in context. This is a dynamic process that occurs through specific *Stop, Attend, Sense, Think, Do* occupational cues and added prompts that may be gestural, verbal, visual, tactile or physical. Cues and prompts align with the type of information each PRPP Quadrant processes: Perceive (sensory); Recall (information-giving/retrieval); Plan (figuring out/checking out); Perform (action/stop action) and are delivered 'in the moment' a particular cognitive strategy is required. The occupational therapist's role as a cognitive mediator fades as the person begins to internalise and apply the strategies without prompts, assuming greater autonomy. For some people, prompts may always be needed to optimise

BOX 42.1
CORE PRINCIPLES OF PRPP INTERVENTION

Principle	Definition
Intervention goal is occupational performance mastery	■ The expected outcome is improved performance of everyday occupations (routines, tasks, steps, skill sets, social interactions) required by the person's occupational roles and context. ■ Intervention success is therefore measured by increased occupational performance mastery.
Application of evidence-based principles of systematic instruction	■ The goal of intervention is clear to person. ■ Prompt hierarchies are used. ■ Multiple opportunities for practice of the task and target cognitive strategies are offered. ■ Performance errors are prevented. ■ Learning occurs across occupations and natural contexts to promote generalisation. ■ Feedback is specific to performance mastery and the cognitive strategy that is the target of intervention.
Target descriptors (cognitive strategies) are operationally defined and measurable behaviours	■ Descriptors required for occupational performance (Fig. 42.2, outer ring) are identified using the PRPP Assessment and their effectiveness measured before and throughout the intervention.
'Chunking' of descriptors across multiple PRPP quadrants is planned	■ Usually starting with 'Stops' to correct errors, at least one or two descriptors from two or more processing quadrants of 'Attend/Sense' (Perceive quadrant), 'Think to remember' (Recall quadrants), 'Think to figure out/evaluate' (Plan quadrant) and 'Do' (Perform quadrant) are chosen. ■ Training in single descriptors is not used. ■ A line of processing required for effective performance mirrors the direction of arrows in the centre of the PRPP Stage Two Conceptual Model (Fig. 42.2).
Focus of intervention is on application of cognitive strategies (descriptors) to everyday participation requirements	■ The cognitive strategies required for effective performance are taught using gestural, verbal, visual or physical prompts given during performance and supplemented with strategy application modelling by the therapist if required. ■ The person is taught to self-instruct (internalise) strategies for subsequent self-direction, if possible.

performance and are embedded as permanent cues in the occupational participation context. PRPP Intervention provides a framework for explaining to others involved who provide care or support to a person that cues and/or prompts are needed, the type of cues/prompts to use and how to place or deliver them.

OBSERVING COGNITIVE STRATEGY APPLICATION

The PRPP-A and PRPP-I are accessed internationally by occupational therapists through structured training courses taught by members of the international PRPP Instructors group.

The constructs of the PRPP-A are used to structure questionnaires, frame interview questions and observe (sometimes without scoring) occupational performance and participation. Examples of some observations of Stage Two cognitive strategy application made by an occupational therapist using the PRPP-A are provided below along with a synopsis of the information processing foundation to these observations. The practice story in Box 42.2 provides specific examples of observations made and the focus of PRPP-I.

Perceive: Observing Attending and Sensory Processing Strategies During Occupational Participation

During occupational participation, people continually receive sensory information from the context and their bodies. Not all sensory information is meaningful and much is discarded. Sensory information that

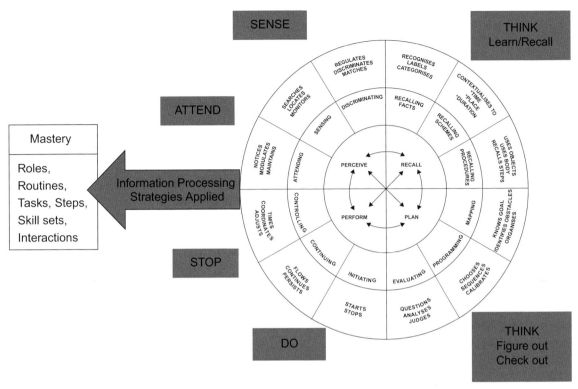

Fig. 42.3 ■ PRPP Intervention Conceptual Framework.

makes an impact is noticed. The person focuses on it, perhaps only momentarily, and then either keeps paying attention to it or decides to shift the focus of their attention to something else. Sensory information that has captured the person's attention is processed more deeply and, if tolerated, details of the information are registered (Slavin, 2020). People use registered sensory information to create multisensory pictures of their bodies and the sensory characteristics of occupations and contexts (Wolpert et al., 2011). These sensory processing operations contribute to the creation of a sensory history or memory for sensory events.

Occupational therapists observing cognitive strategy application look for signs that people are aware of and attending to important sensory information, purposefully using their sensory systems to get more sensory information, forming complete sensory images, finding locations of sensory information in space, tolerating sensory inputs and differentiating between the sensory details of occupations, contexts and themselves as required for the specific occupational

participation situation. Fig. 42.2 illustrates the *Attend*, *Sense* and *Discriminate* behaviours considered. These behaviours are the *Attend/Sense* cognitive strategies addressed in the intervention.

Recall: Observing Information Storage and Retrieval Strategies During Occupational Participation

In the Recall stage of information processing, incoming sensory images are transferred to short-term working memory, the temporary information processing storage facility (Baddeley et al., 2002). Working memory is a type of short-term memory where new experiences are compared with past learning and is activated when a person pays deeper attention to sensory input or a thought that 'comes to mind'. Working memory has a limited capacity, so incoming information continually replaces information that is already in this short-term storage. Information that is not placed into long-term storage for later use fades (Baddeley, 2002; Baddeley & Hitch, 1974; Nee et al., 2013). Long-term memory

BOX 42.2
WILLIAM'S STORY

William's story is used to illustrate how observations of occupational performance and participation can be interpreted using the PRPP Assessment constructs. Although the PRPP approach is not specific to any diagnosis or age group, a practice story of a man who lives with the consequences of a cerebrovascular accident (CVA) was chosen to link concepts of applied cognition presented in this chapter to a person who has specific cognitive impairment.

WILLIAM

William is a 60-year-old man who sustained a right hemisphere cerebrovascular accident (CVA). He was found in bed by his son with a dense left hemiparesis, slurred speech and left-sided facial droop. Medical assessment revealed a right frontoparietal haemorrhage that was surgically evacuated. William spent three weeks in an inpatient rehabilitation unit prior to being transferred to a transitional living unit (TLU) where he is currently receiving rehabilitation. William presents with a mild left upper limb (L-UL) hemiparesis but has active arm placement in all directions and isolated finger control except when fatigued. L-UL protective sensation is intact, but there is a mild discriminative sensory impairment in his fingers. There are obvious signs of left-sided body and spatial inattention confirmed by provocative testing. Language is unimpaired. William walks short distances with a cane, left ankle-foot orthosis (AFO) and near supervision. He requires stand-by assistance for showering and dressing. At this stage in his recovery, William experiences significant fatigue in the TLU and when on weekend leave at home.

The processes used to implement the PRPP approach with William align with the foundational processes and action domains of the Canadian Occupational Therapy Inter-relation Practice Process (COTIPP) (Restall et al.,

2022) (refer to Chapter 12). After an initial meeting with William in which the occupational therapist focused on connecting and initiating the therapeutic relationship, William, his wife, teenage son and the therapist worked in collaboration to establish priorities and co-create a plan to optimise occupational participation. Together they acknowledged that William desired to return to live at home with his family, but his return to work as a bus driver was uncertain at this stage. He hoped to keep working part time as a groundskeeper and occasional short-order cook at his local lawn bowling club, and this was confirmed as a possibility by the club managers. An initial plan was agreed where William would make a grilled cheese and tomato sandwich in the TLU kitchen, and therapy would aim to assess and improve his occupational performance mastery. Subsequently, and on critical reflection by the occupational therapist, this plan was modified to include more tasks and routines that William wished to do at home and in his own yard as he transitioned to community living. Future plans included pursuing a role at the bowling club, and occupational therapy shifted in this direction.

OBSERVATION FINDINGS AND INTERVENTION IMPLICATIONS FOR WILLIAM

William's ability to apply cognitive strategies to what he does is presented in Box 42.3 by PRPP Quadrant to emphasise his difficulties in ease of linking concepts presented in this chapter to his story. Occupational therapists who are trained in the use of the PRPP System blend assessment findings into a cohesive whole and design a 'fluid' and dynamic intervention approach where priorities change as the person begins to process and respond to information more effectively.

---

storage is where people store their wealth of occupational participation experience (history), bringing pertinent information back into working memory when required (Nee et al., 2013; Sodorow & Rickabaugh, 2005). Each person has a unique occupational participation knowledge base, an *internal functional reference system* or frame of reference that gives meaning and purpose to occupational participation and serves as a platform from which information is retrieved for quick and automatic performance.

Memory for occupational participation involves two important information processing operations: recognition, the identification of an experience as familiar; and retrieval, the capacity to regain stored

memories about that experience. Both recognition and retrieval are dependent on adequate prior processing of sensory information, successful storing of information and purposeful use of strategies that allow a person to access stored information.

Research during the early development of the PRPP Assessment revealed three broad categories of memories used during occupational participation: factual or declarative memory; schematic or episodic memory; and procedural memory (Chapparo & Ranka, 1997b). Collectively these memories form a knowledge base that reflects what a person has learned, how they have interpreted sensory perceptions and what they know or believe to be 'true'

BOX 42.3
PRPP OBSERVATION FINDINGS AND INTERVENTION IMPLICATIONS

Perceive: Attending, Sensing, Discriminating

As William made the sandwich, he was observed to have difficulty:
- noticing incoming sensory information on his left-hand side, especially when fatigued.
- changing the focus of his attention from small details in front of him (one object in the pantry) to the 'big picture' of the context (kitchen, cane, general layout of the environment).
- maintaining attention for the duration of the task.
- searching for and finding the objects he needed (systematically searching for the knife, chopping board, sandwich press, bread and ingredients).
- monitoring the use of his left hand (position in space), his cane and doors left open.

Implications: Attend, Sense

Successful participation requires that William learn to:
- shift the focus of his attention from the small details to the broader context and back as he proceeds through the task.
- look for and find things he needs and keep up to date with where his body and cane are relative to objects (doors) in the kitchen.

William was prompted to:
- change the field of attention,
- use his eyes to look, use his skin and joints to feel his left arm,
- keep up to date with sensory information,
- think about and tell himself to focus and look.

Therapy included:
- placing enhanced sensory cues in the context.
- using gestural prompts to signal how and where to shift attention and search for information.
- using verbal and tactile prompts to supplement gestures for where to focus, shift focus and search for information.

Recall: Recalling Facts, Recalling Schemes, Recalling Procedures

As William made the sandwich, he was observed to have difficulty:
- remembering where to find things in this familiar kitchen, where to position himself and where he placed his cane.
- knowing that time was passing and how long the task was taking compared to the time available.
- remembering how long to leave the sandwich in the press.
- remembering to use his (body) left hand and to keep it involved in what he was doing.
- remembering the steps for this familiar task. He forgot to pre-heat the press, unwrap/add cheese (positioned to the left side) and add tomato (positioned to the right).

Implications: Think to Recall

William knew the facts, but effective participation required him to:
- think about and recall information about schemes, that is, where things are likely to be found, how long things typically take and where his left arm is.
- think about and recall information about using his left hand.
- think about and recall the known steps for the task he was doing.

Simply practising 'doing' a variety of occupations would not help William. Effective participation required that he remind himself to apply these strategies.

William was prompted to:
- store and retrieve information from his internal reference system and use that knowledge to guide performance across multiple tasks and contexts.

Therapy included:
- incorporating the familiar (e.g. known people, places and things).
- directive and explicit forms of instruction (e.g. do this and like this).
- reflection and retrieval questions (e.g. get a picture from inside your head, tell me about and tell yourself).
- repetition and mental practice (e.g. do it again, think about doing it and record it in your head).
- application of principles of errorless learning to ensure the correct way was learned.

Continued on following page

BOX 42.3
PRPP OBSERVATION FINDINGS AND INTERVENTION IMPLICATIONS—(*Continued*)

Plan: Mapping, Programming, Evaluating

As William made the sandwich, he was observed to have difficulty:

- identifying obstacles for task completion (inattention to left body and space, left hand weakness, position of the cane and plastic wrapping on the cheese).
- organising his thoughts, equipment and ingredients and 'getting ready' to complete the task (he started doing the task without thinking it through first).
- preplanning and constructing a logical sequence that factored in obstacles and included steps to address these.
- figuring out or choosing where to do the task (at a table, on the kitchen bench, near power point) and how to position himself and his cane relative to the bench.
- analysing potential risks.
- choosing the best strategy for place, procedures and use of objects and his left hand.
- making the best judgments leading to safety concerns with appliance use and the potential for falls.

Implications: Think to Figure Out, Check Out

William knew the goal and had some knowledge that he could use as a platform for performance, but effective participation required that he:

- learnt that when conditions change, existing knowledge is insufficient.
- thought about the changed conditions and identified obstacles that might or do get in the way,
- weighed the pros and cons of ideas and played situations out in his mind to figure out what might work,
- made informed decisions and had alternative methods as back-up plans to choose from if his original choices are ineffective.

Rather than simply direct or tell William what to do, effective performance required that he engaged in the thinking required to plan and problem solve.

William was prompted to:

- use thinking strategies by asking himself questions across tasks and contexts.

Therapy included:

- verbal prompts in the form of targeted questions (e.g. 'What do you have to do? What do you have to think about? What might get in the way? What are the options? What will you do first? Are there any risks?').
- gestural prompts to indicate 'thinking'.
- think-it-through together methods.
- ideas generation.
- modelling thinking (e.g. 'when I think about...').

Perform: Initiating, Continuing, Controlling

Perform difficulties are cognitive in nature; they do not exist independent of other Perceive, Recall and Plan strategies. William's Perform difficulties are the consequences of previously described difficulties. As he made the sandwich, William was observed to have difficulty:

- starting and restarting after distractions.
- keeping his performance flowing – there were long pauses between task steps as he stopped to think about next steps.
- continuing through the task – attempted to give up and stop on two occasions.
- adjusting his body in the correct position relative to objects or contextual features (e.g. doors and the table).

Perform Implications: Do, Stop

Intervention addressed those Perceive, Recall and Plan strategies described above together with Perform prompts.

William was prompted to:

- tell himself stop/start/resume now, adjust his hand position and slow down to better monitor and control his own performance.

Therapy included:

- use of gestural, verbal, visual, touch and physical prompts to teach self-start, self-stop, keep going, change actions and slow down strategies.

about themselves and their bodies, other people and their bodies, objects and parts of the whole object, equipment and parts, materials and pieces, contexts, actions and behaviours. This knowledge, gained across the lifespan, reflects the person's and collective's histories, cultures and understanding of the world. During occupational participation, this knowledge base helps a person answer the following questions:

- *'Do I know what...'? 'Do I know who...'?*
- *'Do I know when...'? 'Do I know where...'? 'Do I know how long...'?*
- *'Do I know how to use...'? 'Do I know how to do...'?*

The purpose of occupational therapy assessment of (PRPP) Recall strategies is, in part, to determine what people have learned (know), how their knowledge is constructed and how useful it is for everyday living. Occupational therapists look for signs that people have correctly stored and interpreted and are retrieving facts about what/who, schematic information about when/where/how long and procedural knowledge about how to use known objects and body parts and the order of known steps as needed for the specific here and now occupational participation situation. Fig. 42.2 illustrates the *Recalling Facts, Recalling Schemes* and *Recalling Procedures* behaviours considered. These behaviours are the *Think to recall* cognitive strategies addressed in intervention.

Plan: Observing Goal Setting, Planning and Evaluating Strategies During Occupational Participation

The ability to plan occupational participation experiences requires thinking strategies such as organisation, problem solving, decision making and self-awareness (Eysenck & Keane, 2020; Fox & Christoff, 2014). These operations are referred to as metacognition within the information processing system and are managed by executive control (Fig. 42.1). This dimension of processing can be thought of as the stage where the 'metacognitive rules' are applied to problem solve, analyse information and make decisions. The rules are not linked to any particular type of information or ability but are applied to all information that must be organised for use. Executive control operations govern processing; they ensure that attention remains focused

on important details and that thinking remains goal focused (Diamond, 2013).

Every day, people use their metacognition and executive control functions to apply thinking strategies to what they do. The thinking that is involved in planning is most apparent when people are required to make a choice, figure out ways of engaging or participating by themselves, create new routines, combine familiar routines in different ways or cope with the unexpected (Meltzer, 2018). Examples range from choosing what to order for dinner or wear to a party, to creating new family routines, arranging international travel, figuring out what to do when there is an electrical power outage or operating complex workplace plant and equipment. When people are doing familiar occupations in usual contexts or are given explicit instructions for what and how to do something, as happens during administration of most standardised tests, planning capacities may be masked.

Planning operations are different to mere memory retrieval. They involve figuring out extensions or elaborations to habitual ways of doing and judging the risks and benefits of decisions made. People who engage in planning, problem solving and self-evaluation construct and evaluate their own action plans with reference to a particular goal, an idea or an understanding of what is to happen. The goal focus of planning triggers executive operations that control processing throughout the system to ensure that the goal remains forefront in thinking and preparing plans for action (Fox & Christoff, 2014).

Specific observations associated with the (PRPP) Plan stage of information processing involve looking for signs that the people are engaging in the thinking required to plan, problem solve, make decisions and self-evaluate as they engage in novel, difficult or complex occupational participation situations. Occupational therapists observe to see if the person knows the endpoint or goal, is aware of obstacles to overcome, gets thoughts, body, other people and/or context organised, makes best choices, constructs precise action sequences and engages in critical thinking and reflection. Fig. 42.2 illustrates the *Mapping, Programming* and *Evaluating* behaviours considered. These behaviours are the *Think to figure out/check out* cognitive strategies addressed in the intervention.

Perform: Observing Output and Performance Monitoring Strategies During Occupational Participation

The Perform stage of information processing focuses on the use of thinking strategies to follow through with decisions and carry out procedures to act or speak. Perform behaviours are dependent on the formation of an adequate plan (Plan), having and accessing an internal reference system of experience (Recall) and rapid and accurate processing of changing body and contextual sensory details (Perceive) as required for occupational participation. Researchers have linked reduced thinking strategies and reduced speed of processing to inefficient response control and timing (Schmidt & Wrisberg, 2008). Perform responses generate further sensory input into the information processing system which enables self-monitoring and contributes to determinations of success or efficacy (Wolpert et al., 2011).

Occupational therapists observing (PRPP) Perform aspects of occupational participation look for signs that people are initiating the necessary starting, stopping and re-starting responses, generating the effort needed to sustain performance, changing the speed of performance according to demands and modifying action patterns when required. Fig. 42.2 illustrates the *Initiating, Continuing* and *Controlling* behaviours considered. These behaviours are the *Do/Stop* cognitive strategies addressed in intervention.

CONCLUSION

This chapter described how an information processing model of cognition can be used as a framework to examine the effectiveness of cognitive strategy application during occupational participation. One example of an authentic, collaborative, ecologically valid and strengths-oriented approach to working with people, the *Perceive, Recall, Plan and Perform (PRPP) System of Task Analysis Assessment and Intervention,* was described. This approach adopts a capabilities perspective. It represents a shift away from a focus on deficits and extends contemporary views of functional cognition to examining how people apply cognitive strategies to achieve person-specific participation goals in person-specific contexts. Examples of how the PRPP Assessment can be used to structure informal

observations of cognitive strategy application during occupational participation were given, and William's story illustrated how findings from these observations informed PRPP Intervention that aimed at enhancing occupational participation. Links to the key characteristics of collaborative relationship-focused occupational therapy and the Canadian Occupational Therapy Inter-relational Practice Process were highlighted.

REFERENCES

Al-Heizan, M., & Edwards, D. F. (2019). Cognitive domain-specific testing to support interpretation of performance assessment. In T. J. Wolf, D. F. Edwards, & G. M. Giles (Eds.), *Functional cognition and occupational therapy: A practical approach to treating individuals with cognitive loss* (pp. 161–176). AOTA Press.

Allen Cognitive Group. (2022). https://allencognitive.com/2023/05/.

American Occupational Therapy Association. (2013). Cognition, cognitive rehabilitation, and occupational performance. *American Journal of Occupational Therapy, 67,* S9–S31. https://doi.org/10.5014/ajot.2013.67S9.

American Occupational Therapy Association. (2019). Cognition, cognitive rehabilitation, and occupational performance. *American Journal of Occupational Therapy, 73*(Supplement 2), 1–25. https://doi.org/10.5014/ajot.2019.73S201.

Árnadóttir, G. (1990). *Brain and behaviour: Assessing cortical dysfunction through activities of daily living (ADL).* Mosby.

Árnadóttir, G. (2011). Impact of neurobehavioral deficits on activities of daily living. In G. Gillen (Ed.), *Stroke rehabilitation: A function-based approach* (3rd ed., pp. 456–500). Elsevier/Mosby.

Aubin, G., Lamoureaux, J., Gélinas, I., Chapparo, C., Stip, E., & Rainville, C. (2014). Daily task performance and information processing among people with schizophrenia and healthy controls: A comparative study. *British Journal of Occupational Therapy, 77*(9), 466–474. https://doi.org/10.4276/0308207541117.

Baddeley, A. D. (2002). *Your memory: A user's guide.* Carlton Books.

Baddeley, A. D., & Hitch, G. J. (1974). Psychology of learning and motivation. In G. A. Bower (Ed.), *Handbook of memory disorders* (pp. 47–89). Academic Press.

Baddeley, A. D., Kopelman, M. D., & Wilson, B. A. (Eds.). (2002). *Handbook of memory disorders* (2nd ed.). Wiley.

Barco, P. P., Gillen, G., & Wolf, T. J. (2019). Intervention selection: Learning and concepts of transfer. In T. J. Wolf, D. F. Edwards, & G. Gillen (Eds.), *Functional cognition and occupational therapy: A practical approach to treating individuals with cognitive loss* (pp. 177–188). AOTA Press.

Baum, C. M., & Wolf, T. J. (2013). *Executive Function Performance Test manual.* Washington University in St. Louis.

Bayley, M. T., Tate, R., Douglas, J. M., Turkstra, L. S., Ponsford, J., Stergiou-Kita, M., Kua, A., & Bragge, P. (2014). INCOG guidelines for cognitive rehabilitation following traumatic brain injury: Methods & Overview. *Journal of Head Trauma Rehabilitation, 29*(4), 290–306. https://doi.org/10.1097/HTR.0000000000000070.

Beck, J., & Horne, D. (1992). A whole school implementation of the stop, think, do! social skills training program. In B. Willis & J.

Izard (Eds.), *Student behavior problems: Directions, perspectives and expectations*. Australian Council for Educational Research.

Bootes, K., & Chapparo, C. (2010). Difficulties with multitasking on return to work after TBI: A critical cases study. *Work, 36*(2), 207–216. https://doi.org/10.3233/WOR-2010-1021.

Burgess, P. W., Alderman, N., Forbes, C., Costello, A., Coates, L. M.-A., Dawson, D., Anderson, N. D., Gilbert, S., Dumontheil, I., & Channon, S. (2006). The case for the development and use of 'ecologically valid' measures of executive function in experimental and clinical psychology. *Journal of the International Neuropsychological Society, 12*(2), 194–209. https://doi.org/10.1017/S1355617706060310.

Burrows, W., Hocking, C., & Chapparo, C. (2022). Learning, translating, and applying the perceive, recall, plan, perform system of task analysis assessment to practice: Occupational therapists' experiences. *British Journal of Occupational Therapy, 85*(7), 496–504. https://doi.org/10.1177/03080226211042264.

Cambridge Cognition. (2023). *What is cognition?* Cambridge University. Retrieved March 31, 2023, from https://www.cambridgecognition.com/.

Challita, J., Chapparo, C., Hinitt, J., & Heard, R. (2019). Effective occupational therapy intervention with children demonstrating reduced social competence during playground interactions. *British Journal of Occupational Therapy, 82*(7), 433–442. https://doi.org/10.1177/0308022619832467.

Chapparo, C., & Ranka, J. (1996). *The perceive, recall, plan & perform system of task analysis – training manual for NSWAOT continuing education*. Occupational Performance Network.

Chapparo, C., & Ranka, J. (1997a). Occupational performance model (Australia): A description of constructs and structure. In C. Chapparo & J. Ranka (Eds.), *The occupational performance model (Australia) monograph 1*. Total Print Control. www.occupationalperformance.com/monograph.

Chapparo, C., & Ranka, J. (1997b). The perceive, recall, plan and perform system of task analysis. In C. Chapparo & J. Ranka (Eds.), *Occupational performance model (Australia) monograph 1* (pp. 189–198). Total Print Control. www.occupationalperformance.com/monograph.

Chapparo, C., & Ranka, J. (1999). *Improving cognition through application of systematic instruction: The PRPP system intervention (Postgraduate Master Class)*. University of Sydney.

Chapparo, C., & Ranka, J. (2010). Occupation analysis: Cognition and acquired brain impairment. In L. Mackenzie & G. O'Toole (Eds.), *Occupation analysis in practice* (pp. 147–162). Wiley-Blackwell.

Chapparo, C., & Ranka, J. (2019). Clinical reasoning in occupational therapy. In J. Higgs, M. A. Jones, S. Loftus, & N. Christensen (Eds.), *Clinical reasoning in the health professions* (4th ed., pp. 265–278). Butterworth Heinemann.

Chapparo, C., Ranka, J., & Nott, M. (2017a). Occupational performance model (Australia): A description of constructs, structure and propositions. In M. Curtin, M. Egan, & J. Adams (Eds.), *Occupational therapy for people experiencing illness, injury or impairment* (7th ed., pp. 134–147). Elsevier.

Chapparo, C., Ranka, J., & Nott, M. (2017b). Perceive, recall, plan and perform system of task analysis and intervention. In M. Curtin, M. Egan, & J. Adams (Eds.), *Occupational therapy for people experiencing illness, injury or impairment* (7th ed., pp. 243–257). Elsevier.

Clark-Wilson, J., Giles, G. M., & Baxter, D. M. (2014). Revisiting the neurofunctional approach: Conceptualizing the core components for the rehabilitation of everyday living skills. *Brain Injury, 28*, 1646–1656. https://doi.org/10.3109/02599052.2014.946439.

Couchman, J. J., Coutinho, M. V. C., Beran, M. J., & Smith, J. D. (2010). Beyond stimulus cues and reinforcement signals: A new approach to animal metacognition. *Journal of Comparative Psychology, 124*(4), 356–368. https://doi.org/10.1037/a0020129.

Critchley, M. (1954). *The parietal lobes*. Edward Arnold and Co.

Demetrious, A., & Kazi, S. (2006). Self-awareness in g (with processing efficiency and reasoning). *Intelligence, 34*(3), 297–317. https://doi.org/10.1016/j.intell.2005.10.002.

Diamond, A. (2013). Executive functions. *Annual Review of Psychology, 64*, 135–168. https://doi.org/10.1146/annurev-psych-113011-143750.

Dingwall, K., Gray, A. O., McCarthy, A., Delima, J. F., & Bowden, S. C. (2017). Exploring the reliability and acceptability of cognitive tests for Indigenous Australians: A pilot study. *BMC Psychology, 5*(1), 26. https://doi.org/10.1186/s40359-017-0195y.

Dingwall, K., Lindeman, M. A., & Cairney, S. (2014). 'You've got to make it relevant': Barriers and ways forward for assessing cognition in Aboriginal clients. *BMC Psychology, 2*(13), 1–11. https://doi.org/10.1186/2050-7283-2-13.

Doig, E., Fleming, J., Ownsworth, T., & Fletcher, S. (2017). An occupation-based, metacognitive approach to assessing error performance and online awareness. *Australian Occupational Therapy Journal, 62*(2), 137–148. https://doi.org/10.1111/1430-1630.12322.

Edwards, D. F., Al-Heizan, M., & Giles, G. M. (2019). Baseline cognitive screening tools. In T. J. Wolf, D. F. Edwards, & G. M. Giles (Eds.), *Functional cognition and occupational therapy: A practical approach to treating individuals with cognitive loss* (pp. 53–64). AOTA Press.

Egan, M., & Restall, G. (2022a). Canadian model of occupational participation (CanMOP). In M. Egan & G. Restall (Eds.), *Promoting occupational participation: Collaborative relationship-focused occupational therapy*. Canadian Association of Occupational Therapists.

Egan, M., & Restall, G. (2022b). *Promoting occupational participation: Collaborative relationship-focused occupational therapy*. Canadian Association of Occupational Therapists.

Erikkson, G., Aasnes, M., Tistad, M., Guidetti, S., & von Koch, L. (2012). Occupational gaps in everyday life one year after stroke and the association with life satisfaction and impact of stroke. *Topics in Stroke Rehabilitation, 19*(3), 243–255. https://doi.org/10.1310/tsr1903-243.

Eysenck, M. W., & Keane, M. T. (2020). *Cognitive psychology: A student's handbook* (8th ed.). Psychology Press.

Fogarty, W., Lovell, M., Langenberg, J., & Heron, M.-J. (2018). Deficit discourse and strengths-based approaches: Changing the narrative of aboriginal and torres strait islander health and wellbeing. The Lowitja Institute and the National Centre for Indigenous Health Research, Australian National University.

Fox, K., & Christoff, K. (2014). Metacognitive facilitation of spontaneous thought processes: When metacognition helps the wandering mind find its way. In S. M. Fleming & C. D. Frith (Eds.), *The cognitive neuroscience of metacogntion* (pp. 293–319). Springer. https://doi.org/10.1007/978-3-642-45190-4_12.

Friedenberg, J., & Silverman, G. (2011). *Cognitive science: An introduction to the study of mind.* SAGE Publicaitons.

Giacino, J. T., & Kalmar, K. (2004). *Coma recovery scale – revised (CRS-R).* Solaris Health System.

Giles, G. M., Edwards, D. F., Baum, C., Furniss, J., Skidmore, E., Wolf, T., & Leland, N. E. (2020). Making functional cognition a professional priority. *American Journal of Occupational Therapy, 74*(1), 1–6. https://doi.org/10.5014/ajot.2020.741002.

Heaton, R. K., & Pendleton, M. G. (1981). Use of neuropsychological tests to predict adult patients' everyday functioning. *Journal of Consulting and Clinical Psychology, 49*(6), 807–821. https://doi.org/10.1037/0022-006X.49.6.807.

Hodges, J. R., & Larner, A. (2017). Addenbrooke's cognitive examinations: ACE, ACE-R, ACE-III, ACEapp, and M-ACE. In A. J. Larner (Ed.), *Cognitive screening instruments* (pp. 109–137). Springer. https://doi.org/10.1007/978-3-319-43775-9_6.

Huitt, W. (2003). *The information processing approach to cognition.* Educational Psychology Interactive. Retrieved March 31, 2023, from http://www.edpsycinteractive.org/topics/cognition/infoproc.html.

Jacklin, K., Pitawanakwat, K., Blind, M., O'Connell, M. E., Walker, J., Lemieux, A. M., & Warry, W. (2020). Developing the Canadian Indigenous cognitive assessment for use with Indigenous older Anishinaabe adults in Ontario, Canada. *Innovation in Aging, 4*(4), igaa038. https://doi.org/10.1093/geroni/igaa038.

Johassen, D.A., Hannum, W.H., & Tessmer, M. (1989). *Handbook of task analysis procedures.* Praeger.

Juntorn, S., Sriphetcharawut, S., & Munketvit, P. (2017). Effectiveness of information processing strategy training on academic task performance in children with learning disabilities: A pilot study. *Occupational Therapy International, 2017,* 6237689. https://doi.org/10.1155/2017/6237689.

Katz, N., Baum, C. M., & Maeir, A. (2011). Introduction to cognitive intervention and cognitive functional evaluation. In N. Katz (Ed.), *Cognition, occupation and participation across the lifespan: Neuroscience, neurorehabilitation and models of intervention in occupational therapy* (3rd ed., pp. 3–12). AOTA Press.

Katz, N., Itzkovich, M., Overmuch, S., & Elazar, B. (1989). Lowenstein occupational therapy cognitive assessment (LOTCA) battery for patients: Reliability and validity. *American Journal of Occupational Therapy, 42,* 184–192. https://doi.org/10.5014/ajot.43.3.184.

Kingstone, A., Smilek, D., & Eastwood, J. D. (2008). Cognitive ethology: A new approach for studying human cognition. *British Journal of Psychology, 99*(2), 317–340. https://doi.org/10.1348/000712607X251243.

Law, M., Baptiste, S., Carswell, A., McColl, M. A., Polatajko, H., & Pollock, N. (2023). *Canadian Measure of Occupational Performance (CMOP).* Retrieved March 31, 2023, from https://www.thecopm.ca/.

Lewis, J., Chapparo, C., Mackenzie, L., & Ranka, J. (2016). Work after breast cancer: Identification of cognitive difficulties using the perceive, recall, plan and perform (PRPP) system of task analysis. *British Journal of Occupational Therapy, 79*(5), 323–332. https://doi.org/10.1177/0308022616639983.

Lindstad M. Ø., Obstfelder, A. U., Sveen, U., & Stigen, L. (2023). Feasibility of the perceive, recall, plan and perform system of intervention for persons with brain injury in community-based rehabilitation: A pilot for a multiple-baseline design study. *British Medical Journal Open, 13,* 1–11. https://doi.org/10.1136/bmjopen-2022-067593.

LoGiudice, D., Smith, K., Thomas, J., Lautenschlager, N. T., Almeida, O. P., Atkinson, D., & Flicker, L. (2006). Kimberley indigenous cognitive assessment tool (KICA): Development of a cognitive assessment tool for older indigenous Australians. *International Psychogeriatrics, 18*(2), 269–280. https://doi.org/10.1017/S1041610205002681.

Luria, A. R. (1962). *Higher cortical functions in man.* Basic Books, Inc.

Maeir, A., Hagit, H., & Katz, N. (2009). Kettle test–A brief measure of cognitive functional performance: Reliability and validity in stroke rehabilitation. *American Journal of Occupational Therapy, 63*(5), 592–599. https://doi.org/10.5014/ajot.63.5.592.

Marois, R., & Ivanoff, J. (2005). Capacity limits of information processing in the brain. *Trends in Cognitive Sciences, 9*(6), 296–305. https://doi.org/10.1016/j.tics.2005.04.010.

Meltzer, L. (2018). *Executive function in education: From theory to practice* (2nd ed.). The Guilford Press.

Michel, A. (2020). *Cognition and perception: Is there really a distinction?* Association for Psychological Science. Retrieved July 4, 2023, from https://www.psychologicalscience.org/observer/cognition-and-perception-is-there-really-a-distinction.

Murphy, D. P., & Cooke, J. (1999). Traffic light lessons: Problem solving skills with adolescents. *Community Practitioner, 72*(10), 322–324.

Mushquash, C. J., & Bova, D. L. (2007). Cross-cultural assessment and measurement issues. *Journal on Developmental Disabilities, 13*(1), 53–65.

Nasreddine, Z. S., Phillips, N. A., Bedirian, V., Charbonneau, S., Whitehead, V., Collin, I., Cummings, J. L., & Chertkow, H. (2005). *Montreal Cognitive Assessment (MoCA).* APA PsycTests. https://doi.org/10.1037/t27279-000.

Nee, D. E., Brown, J. W., Askren, M. K., Berman, M. G., Demiralp, E., Krawitz, A., & Jonidas, J. (2013). A meta-analysis of executive components of working memory. *Cerebral Cortex, 23*(2), 264–282. https://doi.org/10.1093/cercor/bhs007.

Ng, Y. S., & Chua, K. S. (2005). States of severely altered consciousness: Clinical characteristics, medical complications and functional outcome after rehabilitation. *NeuroRehabilitation, 20*(2), 97–105.

Nott, M. T., & Chapparo, C. (2008). Measuring information processing in a client with extreme agitation following traumatic brain injury using the perceive, recall, plan and perform system of task analysis. *Australian Occupational Therapy Journal, 55*(3), 256–263. https://doi.org/10.1111/j.1430-1630.2007.00685.x.

Nott, M. T., & Chapparo, C. (2020). Cognitive strategy use in adults with acquired brain injury. *Brain Injury, 1*(7), 508–514. https://doi.org/10.1080/02699052.2020.1725837.

Occupational Performance Network. (2023). *PRPP instrument development.* Retrieved March 31, 2023, from www.occupationalperformance.com.

Oxford University Press. (1989). *Oxford English dictionary* (2nd ed.). Oxford University Press.

Polatajko, H., & Mandich, A. (2004). *Enabling occupation in children: The cognitive orientation to daily occupational performance [CO-OP] Approach*. Canadian Association of Occupational Therapists.

Prinsen, C. A. C., Vohra, S., Rose, M. R., Boers, M., Tugwell, P., Clarke, M., Williamson, P. R., & Terwee, C. B. (2016). How to select outcome measurement instruments for outcomes included in a 'core Outcome Set' – a practical guideline. *Trials, 17*(1), 439. https://doi.org/10.1186/s13063-016-1555-2.

Ranka, J., & Chapparo, C. (2010). Assessment of productivity performance in men with HIV associated neurocognitive disorder (HAND). *Work, 36*(2), 193–206. https://doi.org/10.3233/WOR-2010-1020.

Restall, G., & Egan, M. (2022). Collaborative relationship-focused occupational therapy. In M. Egan & G. Restall (Eds.), *Promoting occupational participation: Collaborative relationship-focused occupational therapy* (pp. 97–117). Canadian Association of Occupational Therapists.

Restall, G., Egan, M., Valavaara, K., Phenix, A., & Sack, C. (2022). Canadian occupational therapy inter-relational practice process (COTIPP). In M. Egan & G. Restall (Eds.), *Promoting occupational participation: Collaborative relationship-focused occupational therapy* (pp. 119–150). Canadian Association of Occupational Therapists.

Romiszowski, A. (1984). *Designing instructional systems*. Kogan Page.

Schmidt, R. A., & Wrisberg, C. A. (2008). *Motor learning and performance: A situation-based learning approach* (4th ed.). Human Kinetics.

Schraagen, J., Chipman, S., & Shalin, V. (2000). *Cognitive task analysis*. Lawrence Erlbaum Associates.

Shiel, A., Horn, S. A., Wilson, B. A., Watson, M. J., Campbell, M. J., & Mclellan, D. L. (2000). The Wessex head injury matrix (WHIM) main scale: A preliminary report on a scale to assess and monitor patient recovery after severe head injury. *Clinical Rehabilitation, 14*(4), 408–416. https://doi.org/10.1191/0269215500cr326oa.

Siegler, R. S. (2007). Cognitive variability. *Developmental Science, 10*(1), 104–109. https://doi.org/10.1111/j.1467-7687.2007.00571.x.

Siev, E., Freishtat, B., & Zoltan, B. (1986). *Perceptual and cognitive dysfunction in the adult stroke patient: A manual for evaluation and treatment*. Slack.

Slavin, R. E. (2020). *Educational psychology: Theory and practice* (13th ed.). Pearson.

Smith, R. L., Ranka, J., & Nott, M. (2023). Using the perceive, recall, plan and perform assessment of cognitive strategy use with Aboriginal and Torres Strait Islander peoples: Initial exploration of clinical utility. *Australian Occupational Therapy Journal, 70*(4), 446–459. https://doi.org/10.1111/1430.1630.12866.

Snell, M. (1987). *Systematic instruction of persons with severe handicaps*. Charles E. Merrill Publishing Co.

Sodorow, L. M., & Rickabaugh, C. A. (2005). *Psychology* (6th ed.). Atomic Dog Publishing.

Sproats, M., Ranka, J., & Nott, M. T. (2013). Addressing cognitive load in upper limb prosthetic training using the perceive, recall, plan & perform (PRPP) Intervention: A critical case study. *Australian Occupational Therapy Journal, 60*(Supp. 1), 89.

Sturkenboom, I. H. W. M., Nott, M. T., Bloem, B. R., Chapparo, C., & Steultjens, E. M. J. (2020). Applied cognitive strategy behaviours in people with Parkinson's disease during daily activities: A cross-sectional study. *Journal of Rehabilitation Medicine, 52*(1), 1–9. https://doi.org/10.2340/16501977-2635.

Toglia, J. P. (2018). The dynamic interactional model and the multicontext approach. In N. Katz & J. P. Toglia (Eds.), *Cognition, occupation and participation across the lifespan: Neuroscience, neurorehabilitation and models for intervention in occupational therapy* (4th ed., pp. 355–383). AOTA Press.

Toglia, J. P., Rodger, S. A., & Polatajko, H. (2012). Anatomy of cognitive strategies: A therapist's primer for enabling occupational performance. *Canadian Journal of Occupational Therapy, 79*(4), 225–236. https://doi.org/10.2182/cjot.2012.79.4.4.

Tupper, D. E., & Cicerone, K. D. (1990). *The neuropsychology of everyday life: Assessment and basic competencies*. Kluwer Academic Publishers.

Turner-Stokes, L. (2009). Goal attainment scaling (GAS) in rehabilitation: A practical guide. *Clinical Rehabilitation, 23*, 362–370. https://doi.org/10.1177/0269215508101742.

Turpin, M., & Iwama, M. K. (2011). *Using occupational therapy models in practice: A field guide*. Churchill Livingstone/Elsevier.

Wesson, J., & Giles, G. M. (2019). Understanding functional cognition. In T. J. Wolf, D. F. Edwards, & G. M. Giles (Eds.), *Functional cognition and occupational therapy: A practical approach to treating individuals with cognitive loss* (pp. 7–20). AOTA Press.

White, J., Nott, M. T., Barr, C., Chapparo, C., & George, S. (2020). Stroke survivors' occupational performance and cognitive strategy use: A pilot exploration of strengths and difficulties using the perceive recall plan perform system of task analysis. *British Journal of Occupational Therapy, 83*(11), 701–709. https://doi.org/10.1177/0308022620951028.

Wolf, T. J., & Baum, C. M. (2019). Occupational profile: The anchor of functional-cognitive assessment. In T. J. Wolf, D. F. Edwards, & G. M. Giles (Eds.), *Functional cognition and occupational therapy* (pp. 47–52). AOTA Press.

Wolpert, D. M., Diedrichsen, J., & Flanagan, J. R. (2011). Principles of sensorimotor learning. *Nature Review Neuroscience, 12*(12), 739–751. https://doi.org/10.1038/nrn3112.

World Health Organization. (2001). *The international classification for functioning, disability and health (ICF)*. World Health Organization. Retrieved March 31, 2023, from https://www.who.int/classifications/icf/en/.

Yerxa, E. J. (1998). Health and the human spirit for occupation. *The American Journal of Occupational Therapy, 52*(6), 412–418. https://doi.org/10.5014/ajot.52.6.412.

Ylvisaker, M., Szekeres, S., & Feeney, T. (1998). Cognitive rehabilitation: Executive functions. In M. Ylvisaker (Ed.), *Traumatic brain injury rehabilitation: Children and adolescents* (2nd ed., pp. 240–254). Butterworth-Heinemann.

REFLECTION

1. Compare and contrast the strengths and limitations of an impairment-focused approach, cognitive recovery levels approach and a functional cognition approach to practice.

2. Discuss the concept of ecological validity as it relates to person/people-centred practice.

3. Draw and describe elements of an information processing theoretical framework of cognition and discuss its application to occupational participation.

4. Explain how a person's use of cognition can be observed during occupational participation using the PRPP Assessment constructs.

5. Discuss how these observations guide intervention using the PRPP Intervention model.

Section 5

PRACTICE STORIES – PROMOTING OCCUPATIONAL PARTICIPATION

SECTION OUTLINE

MRS TREMBLAY: CONTINUUM OF CARE FROM HOSPITAL TO COMMUNITY FOLLOWING A STROKE

KATRINE SAUVÉ-SCHENK ■ VALERIE METCALFE ■ DOROTHY KESSLER

CHAPTER OUTLINE

INTRODUCTION

Mrs Tremblay has experienced a stroke. This practice story presents her journey as she engages with occupational therapy services on the continuum of care from hospital to community using the Canadian Occupational Therapy Inter-Relational Practice Process Framework (COTIPP) (Restall et al., 2022) (refer to Chapter 12).

The COTIPP is an occupational therapy practice framework composed of six action domains that describe what occupational therapists do (connect, seek understanding and define purpose, explore occupational participation, co-design priorities goals outcomes and plans, trial the plan, explore change and refine plans, plan for transition). These action domains are centred around the essential underlying process of building and sustaining relationships with individuals, groups and communities and on three foundational processes: reflecting and reasoning, using justice, equity and rights-based lenses and seeking to understand the contexts (Restall et al., 2022) (refer to Chapter 12).

We begin by describing the foundational processes that are similar between three occupational therapy practice areas. This is followed by a detailed description of Mrs Tremblay's journey from acute care (with Katrine) to inpatient rehabilitation (with Dorothy) and finally to community rehabilitation (with Valerie). Throughout the process, we strive to implement collaborative relationship-focused practice (refer to Chapter 12), ensuring we reflect on our own biases and create a respectful relationship that considers Mrs Tremblay's context, emotional and physical safety and her right to make decisions regarding her care (Restall et al., 2022).

Build and Sustain Relationships

As regulated healthcare professionals, we will each build and sustain a relationship with Mrs Tremblay that is based on respect, choice, collaboration and trust while acknowledging the power structures that exist between us. To support this relationship, each of us is responsible for ensuring that Mrs Tremblay has provided her informed consent to participate in our service. Consent is an ongoing process, involving discussions between Mrs Tremblay and each of us at every encounter, but obtaining consent will only be clearly stated once in each of our stories.

Reflect, Critically Reflect and Reason

We each reflect and reason on the models, frameworks and practice guidelines that influence our day-to-day practice.

Across the acute care, inpatient rehabilitation and community rehabilitation practice settings, we use the Canadian Model of Occupational Participation (CanMOP) (Egan & Restall, 2022) to guide how we understand and support occupational participation (refer to Chapter 11); that is, we consider the importance of occupations identified by Mrs Tremblay and work towards finding solutions that will promote and sustain meaningful occupational participation in her contexts.

Our practice integrates evidence-informed guidelines and considers each person individually in deciding how to incorporate research evidence (Canadian Association of Occupational Therapists, 2009). We refer to the Canadian Stroke Best Practice Recommendations (CSBPR) when considering assessments and interventions (Heart and Stroke Foundation of Canada (HSFC), 2023). This document synthesises stroke research and classifies interventions according to varying levels of evidence for stroke care which we understand will evolve as research advances. Therefore it is our professional responsibility to keep up to date with

emerging evidence and to understand the implications of this to clinical practice. In this practice story, the Canadian best practices are flagged with the[B] symbol.

Use Justice-, Equity- and Rights-Based Lenses

We also recognise that we need to critically evaluate how our values, beliefs and contexts influence our practice and may create barriers to equitable access to occupational participation.

ACUTE CARE (KATRINE)

Seek to Understand the Practice, Occupational Therapist and the Individual or Collective Contexts

I am an occupational therapist on a 60-bed neuroscience unit in a Canadian acute care hospital. The average length of stay for people admitted to this unit is 7 days. All services are covered by the government health insurance plan. I work within an interdisciplinary team and typically provide services to individuals who have recently experienced a stroke. This medical condition often causes great changes to a person's occupational participation.

Seek Understanding and Define Purpose

I received a referral from the unit physician for Mrs Tremblay who was admitted 2 days ago with a diagnosis of ischaemic cerebrovascular accident (CVA) or stroke in the right middle cerebral artery. Before meeting with Mrs Tremblay, I reviewed her medical chart for information pertaining to her living and social situations, as well as her diagnosis, medical history and medical restrictions. Verifying the medical chart before every interaction with Mrs Tremblay was important for keeping her and myself safe. I ensured that the physician's orders indicated that she could tolerate activity and that there were no contraindications to mobilisation or therapy. The chart review revealed the information presented in Table 43.1.

Connect

I met Mrs Tremblay in her room and confirmed how she preferred to be addressed. I explained occupational therapy and my role on the unit. We discussed

TABLE 43.1
Mrs Tremblay's Chart Review

Mrs L. Tremblay, 72-Year-Old Woman

Diagnosis	Right cerebrovascular accident (CVA). Day 2 post-stroke.
	Was visiting a friend when she experienced symptoms of a stroke. Ambulance was called and she was brought to the local hospital. There she was diagnosed with a stroke, started on tissue plasminogen activator (tPA) and transferred to the regional acute care hospital, neurosciences floor.
Medical history	Knee osteoarthritis on right side, hypertension, osteoporosis, hyperlipidemia, atrial fibrillation.
Restrictions	Activity as tolerated, no other restrictions.
Social history	Lives alone in an apartment in a rural setting.
	Steps to access front door of apartment building.
Notes from other team members	Chart notes from the physiotherapist indicate that Mrs Tremblay requires the assistance of two people to roll her in bed and to sit at the edge of the bed. It was also noted that her left-hand function was affected. Nursing staff specified that she is still using a Foley catheter.

risks and benefits of occupational therapy services and the plan for our sessions together. She provided consent to proceed.

Seek Understanding and Define Purpose

We discussed events leading to and since her hospital admission. She said she was grateful her stroke happened while she was at her friend's house and not alone at home. Mrs Tremblay described her home environment and how she filled her days. Before her stroke, she did not need assistance to take care of herself or her apartment; she drove a car, enjoyed knitting and was active in her church community. Mrs Tremblay added that she had no children. She could rely on her friends and sister, as well as a nephew.

Mrs Tremblay said that since the stroke, her biggest concerns were fatigue and pain in her left arm that was affecting her sleep. She said that needing help to eat, to do her morning routine and to move around the room was distressing to her.

I noted that during our conversation, Mrs Tremblay had difficulty giving details about recent events. She was not sure how many days she had been in hospital nor which hospital she was in.

Explore Occupational Participation

Mrs Tremblay agreed that I would better understand her reported difficulties if I observed her doing those activities that could be completed in her room.

As Mrs Tremblay was already lying in bed, I began by addressing her concern of comfort in bed. She reported

feeling most comfortable in supine with support under her left shoulder. She required a moderate level of assistance to roll from side-to-side in bed and to move herself to a seated position at the edge of the bed. Mrs Tremblay had difficulty using the bed rails because she had limited reach and grasp with her left arm and hand. Although she had some movement in her left ankle, knee and hip, she could not independently move the left leg to the edge of the bed. Sitting at the edge of the bed, she required minimal assistance to maintain static sitting balance. I provided support for balance while I measured her to determine the size of wheelchair she would need.

During breakfast, I noted that Mrs Tremblay was able to bring food to her mouth using her right hand. She had insufficient functional movement in her left hand for bilateral tasks (e.g. opening containers). I set up Mrs Tremblay for oral care, during which she required assistance for bilateral tasks such as opening the toothpaste tube. She was able to brush her teeth, swish and spit water in the basin.

Throughout the assessment, I observed that she was having difficulties finding items on the left side of her table. When cued to look to the left, she could find what she was looking for. I also noticed that Mrs Tremblay was easily distracted by her roommates' conversations with visitors.

The nursing staff informed me that Mrs Tremblay required assistance with her sponge bath, as well as changing her gown and incontinence briefs. They confirmed that she did not have any areas of skin redness or breakdown.

Co-design Priorities, Goals, Outcomes and Plans

Mrs Tremblay experienced challenges participating in several activities (eating, grooming, dressing, toileting, transfers, functional mobility and sleeping) because of the

- decreased function in her left upper and lower extremities,
- poor sitting balance,
- left shoulder pain,
- fatigue,
- challenges with sustained attention,
- decreased visual attention to the left side,
- disorientation to time and place and
- poor short-term memory.

I determined that Mrs Tremblay was at high risk of developing skin breakdown and a pressure injury due to her decreased mobility; for example, her inability to reposition herself independently in bed is one of many risk factors for developing a pressure injury (Norton et al., 2017). Pressure injuries can cause pain and discomfort and lead to social isolation and reduced participation in daily activities (Gorecki et al., 2010). Prevention of pressure injuries is therefore an interprofessional priority (Norton et al., 2017).

Mrs Tremblay and I reviewed these findings. She stated that her main goal was to 'get better so I can go home'. Together, we agreed on the following goals that could be addressed in the acute care setting:

1. *Sleep:* Mrs Tremblay will be comfortably positioned in bed to facilitate sleep, manage shoulder pain and prevent skin breakdown.
2. *Functional mobility and seating*: Mrs Tremblay will be able to move about her room independently and sit up in a wheelchair that supports her participation in personal care and social activities for 3 × 1 hour per day.
3. *Grooming and eating:* Mrs Tremblay will complete eating and grooming tasks independently.

My reflection on priorities for Mrs Tremblay within the acute care setting is presented in Box 43.1.

I informed Mrs Tremblay that further cognitive assessments and treatment were recommended and that this would be addressed during her inpatient rehabilitation[B] (HSFC, 2023).

BOX 43.1
REFLECTION ON PRACTISE CONTEXT

While individuals have many concerns about their occupational participation after having a stroke, the acute-care setting prioritises specific occupational goals because of limited resources and the short-time individuals are in the unit. Goals that mitigate risks, facilitate recovery and lead to a discharge plan are prioritised.

Trial the Plan, Explore Change, and Refine the Plan

Goal 1. Bed Positioning

We trialled a foam positioning aid to support the left arm and shoulder in a neutral position, and I used Mrs Tremblay's feedback to find the most comfortable bed positions. We discussed how proper shoulder positioning can help manage pain following stroke[B] (HSFC, 2023). We reviewed how she could be repositioned in bed with staff assistance and the importance of repositioning frequently (alternating lying on her back and on her side) to prevent pressure injuries. With her consent, I posted positioning and repositioning instructions over her bed for staff information, with a reminder to place the call bell to her right side so that Mrs Tremblay could contact a staff member when she required repositioning.

During the first 4 days following her stroke, Mrs Tremblay made progress and was able to turn independently in bed and reposition herself using the bedside rail. She kept the positioning aid so that she could support her shoulder as she reported that the shoulder pain occasionally kept her awake at night.

Fortunately, no skin breakdown was reported.

Goal 2. Functional Mobility and Seating

Based on my assessment, I loaned Mrs Tremblay a manual 45 cm wide × 45 cm deep wheelchair with a left-side half-tray, contoured backrest, contoured foam cushion, positioning seat belt and two footrests from the hospital equipment pool (refer to Chapter 33). The wheelchair was adjusted, and I observed that this seating system provided adequate support for her to maintain good sitting balance and posture. Her left arm was positioned on the wheelchair's half-tray – she reported that she found this a comfortable position that also reduced the shoulder pain. We discussed safety, and Mrs Tremblay demonstrated how to fasten and undo the seat belt and apply and remove the brakes using her right hand.

I removed the right footrest, and Mrs Tremblay tried propelling with one hand and one foot. She agreed to have the rehabilitation assistant work with her to practice manoeuvring the wheelchair safely, using strategies to avoid bumping objects on her left side (e.g. scanning left, then right, then left again at regular intervals when mobilising).

I explained the benefits of sitting up in a wheelchair when participating in activities such as grooming and eating. I recommended she gradually increase her sitting time by 15 to 30 minutes every day if she could tolerate it. We agreed on a tentative sitting schedule for the next few days. I included this schedule in the nursing care plan.

Mrs Tremblay chose to sit up for 1 hour on the first day. Within 5 days, she progressed to sitting in her wheelchair for a total of 3 hours per day with breaks. She was able to propel herself short distances in her room and in the halls with the rehabilitation assistant.

Over the following week, Mrs Tremblay progressed to spending most of the day up in the wheelchair with one rest in the afternoon. She continued to manage shoulder pain by positioning her left upper extremity on the half-tray when sitting in the wheelchair. She was able to independently propel the wheelchair in her room using one foot and one hand.

On discharge from acute care, even though the physiotherapist informed me that Mrs Tremblay was starting to ambulate using a four-wheeled walker with assistance, Mrs Tremblay continued to use the wheelchair as her main method of moving around the unit.

Goal 3. Personal Care

I provided Mrs Tremblay with a piece of nonslip material to help stabilise items on her table and encouraged her to use her left arm/hand as much as possible during all activities. I explained visual inattention, and I taught her two visual scanning strategies[B] (HSFC, 2023):

1. Reminding herself to regularly 'look to the left' and

BOX 43.2
REFLECTION ON BUILDING A COLLABORATIVE RELATIONSHIP

My contact time with Mrs Tremblay was short, but I felt, we were able to move forward on small goals that were meaningful to her and respected her values and beliefs. Although not necessarily apparent in my charting, I spent a significant amount of time providing emotional support and encouragement and helping her adjust to the changes she was experiencing.

---

2. Using the visual cue (a left-pointing arrow sticker on her tabletop) when she could not find an item.

I informed the team about a possible left-sided neglect and encouraged them to use the same strategies with Mrs Tremblay.

Mrs Tremblay agreed to practice grooming tasks while up in her wheelchair with the support of the rehabilitation assistant. The rehabilitation assistant encouraged Mrs Tremblay to consistently use her left hand for stabilising items and cued her to use her visual scanning strategies.

On discharge from acute care, Mrs Tremblay participated in daily grooming tasks and eating while sitting up in her wheelchair. During oral care, she began using her left hand to stabilise items such as her toothbrush while applying toothpaste to it and dishes when eating. I noted that she also required fewer cues to locate items on her table.

Plan for Transition

While happy with her progress, Mrs Tremblay stated that she could not return home in a wheelchair. She expressed a desire to participate in a rehabilitation program. I discussed her progress with the team, and we referred her to the inpatient rehabilitation team – she was accepted 2 days later.

Mrs Tremblay was discharged from the acute care unit and transferred to inpatient stroke rehabilitation at another facility. Mrs Tremblay was pleased with the proposed transfer and the progress she had made in acute care. I completed all documentation and discharged her from my caseload and reflected on my relationship with Mrs Tremblay and the progress she had made (Box 43.2).

INPATIENT REHABILITATION (DOROTHY)

Context

I am an occupational therapist in a specialised stroke rehabilitation unit in a government-funded rehabilitation hospital. I work in an interdisciplinary team. People with stroke are admitted to our unit from acute care. The focus of our rehabilitation program is to promote neurological recovery and increase independence for discharge to home or to a location that can meet people's care needs.

Seek Understanding and Define Purpose

I begin my assessment by reviewing the medical chart, noting the objectives set and achieved with Mrs Tremblay in acute care.

Connect/Explore Occupational Participation

After reviewing the chart, the physiotherapist, nurse and I met with Mrs Tremblay. We introduced ourselves, asked her about her abilities and needs and explained our roles, what we wanted to assess, and the reasons for these assessments. Mrs Tremblay consented, and we completed the initial mobility assessment that included bed mobility, ability to transfer and wheelchair and seating needs. We also screened for fall risks[B] (HSFC, 2023) (refer to Chapter 32).

During the assessment, Mrs Tremblay was able to turn in bed using a half-bed rail and to transfer from her bed to a chair with the assistance of one person and a four-wheeled walker. I provided her with a hospital wheelchair that allowed propulsion with one foot and one hand, a contoured foam cushion to promote optimal hip and pelvic alignment and a lap half-tray to support her left upper extremity. She was able to propel the wheelchair but bumped into the left side of doorways. When I brought this to Mrs Tremblay's attention, she said she had been told that her stroke could be making her brain not pay attention to the left side. She described one of the strategies that she had been taught. We discussed continuing to work on this together.

I then met with Mrs Tremblay to identify occupational participation issues and learn more about her previous living situation, daily routine and occupational participation goals. I used both a top-down and bottom-up approach to identify occupational participation issues, determine what physical, cognitive, perceptual and communicative abilities might facilitate or hinder her performance and develop a therapy plan.

When asked about her occupational participation goals, Mrs Tremblay identified that she wished to return to live in her apartment and that this required that she be able to look after herself, including being able to wash and dress, walk, go up and down stairs and make her meals. Mrs Tremblay lived alone in a second-storey apartment in a rural village. There were 15 steps to access her apartment with no landing and a rail on the left side going down. Mrs Tremblay used to drive to buy her groceries at the small grocery store in the village and to the bank to withdraw money for groceries and other daily expenses. Her nephew assisted with other finances.

Mrs Tremblay's sister lived in the same community. She had several good friends who were willing to offer support, but she did not want to bother them. I also learned that Mrs Tremblay had grown up on a farm and valued 'hard work'.

Mrs Tremblay felt that she would currently have difficulty managing household tasks such as preparing meals and cleaning because of her inability to use her left arm and hand effectively and the need to walk with a walker.

During the interview, Mrs Tremblay communicated effectively, although for more complex discussions she needed time to process information. I explained to her that I usually assess a person's personal care abilities, arm and hand movement and sensation, cognition and perception related to everyday tasks. I explained that these are areas that can be affected after a stroke and this type of information can be helpful for planning intervention. Mrs Tremblay agreed to participate in these assessments.

Personal Care

The following morning, I met with Mrs Tremblay in her room to evaluate her ability to eat, wash, dress, groom and manage her toileting needs. I used Dynamic Performance Analysis (Polatajko et al., 2000) (refer to Chapter 18).

Mrs Tremblay was able to walk to and transfer onto the toilet using a four-wheeled walker and my assistance. She required help to manage her clothing and clean herself after going to the toilet.

Mrs Tremblay then moved to the sink to complete her care while sitting in her wheelchair. I encouraged her to do as much as possible on her own and explained that I would provide her with suggestions and assist her if necessary.

Mrs Tremblay was able to complete grooming tasks with the setup of needed items, verbal cueing to look to the left to find items in her left personal space and cueing to work out how to use her left hand to assist when putting toothpaste on the toothbrush. She was able to wash at the sink with reminders to use her left hand to assist when applying soap and wringing out the washcloth. She required assistance to wash her right arm and back and assistance to stand to wash her buttocks.

Mrs Tremblay started to dress by putting her right arm into her upper garment clothing first but then could not place her left arm in the appropriate sleeve. I guided her to problem solve how to put her shirt on and she was able to figure out that it was easier to start with her left arm. With a bit more guidance she applied a similar strategy of starting with her left leg to put on underpants and trousers. She was then able to complete all her dressing tasks with cueing to orient clothing and assistance to fasten her bra and raise and fasten her trousers. She had difficulty reaching her feet to put on her socks and shoes. I noticed that Mrs Tremblay was becoming quite tired and decided to help her finish dressing without introducing new techniques or assistive devices.

During the assessment, I noted that Mrs Tremblay took a long time to complete her personal care as she required time to process information and to plan her approach to tasks. She was also easily distracted by other activity that was happening in her room and in the hallway.

Next, I arranged a time to meet with Mrs Tremblay in the occupational therapy room to complete the assessment.

Sensorimotor Ability

I used the Chedoke-McMaster Stroke Assessment: Impairment Inventory stage of arm and hand as a formal assessment of upper extremity motor recovery (Gowland et al., 1993). Mrs Tremblay achieved Stage 4 recovery for her left arm (beginning to move out of synergistic patterns) and Stage 3 for her left hand (movement in synergistic patterns), with one item in the Stage 4 level.

I also assessed how Mrs Tremblay used her left arm and hand for daily tasks. I noted that she attempted tasks using only her right hand first. If she had difficulty, she occasionally used her left hand to assist. She was able to reach and grasp items at waist height using a gross grasp but had difficulty releasing them. I assessed sensation and found that Mrs Tremblay had intact sensation in her upper and lower extremities. Therefore, loss of sensation did not explain the lack of integration of the left upper extremity when completing daily activities. Mrs Tremblay might have body neglect in addition to the visual neglect already noted. Alternatively, her lack of use may be due to the effort required to use the left upper extremity. Regardless of the cause, I chose to focus on interventions that would encourage Mrs Tremblay to use her left upper extremity in bilateral tasks.

(Further information on skills and strategies for improving arm function and occupational participation after brain impairment can be found in Chapters 28 and 42).

Cognition and Perception

During performance-based assessments, I had observed that Mrs Tremblay had difficulty scanning to her left side, slowed processing speed and difficulty organising her clothing. I decided to formally assess her visuospatial attention using the Bells Test, a validated paper-and-pencil test which requires finding and crossing out of bells from an array of other shapes (Gauthier et al., 1989). Mrs Tremblay's results indicated a left-sided neglect of her near extra personal space. I also observed that she did not consistently use a structured scanning approach. This could affect her efficiency and accuracy when interpreting visual information and contribute to her slowed speed of processing and difficulty organising clothing during the personal care assessment.

(Further information on skills and strategies for cognition, perception and occupational participation can be found in Chapters 28 and 42).

Co-design Priorities, Goals Outcomes and Plans

Mrs Tremblay and I discussed the assessment findings. She was keen to work hard, so pacing would be important to prevent fatigue during occupational therapy. I felt there was good potential for her to be able to use her left arm and hand during daily activities, but we may need to explore adaptive approaches for some tasks. We would also need to explore the potential impact of her cognitive and perceptual difficulties on her ability to safely resume financial management and household tasks.

Mrs Tremblay and I talked about goals that could be achieved during inpatient rehabilitation, focusing on those that would be essential for her to return home. We agreed on the following goals:

1. *Personal care*: Mrs Tremblay will be able to complete washing, dressing, grooming and toileting independently using assistive devices as needed.
2. *Functional mobility and transfers*: Mrs Tremblay will be able to transfer to and from the toilet independently using grab bars, transfer to the bathtub using grab bars and a bath seat with hands on steadying assistance and walk indoors independently with a mobility device.
3. *Home management:* Mrs Tremblay will be able to prepare a simple two-dish meal independently and manage her medications, basic finances, cleaning and groceries with structure and support.

The overall goal was that Mrs Tremblay be discharged to her home with referrals to community supports and therapy services. Mrs Tremblay and I discussed and agreed on a plan to achieve these goals.

Trial Plan, Explore Change Refine Plans

Mrs Tremblay was seen daily for occupational therapy by the rehabilitation assistant or me to promote recovery and practice adaptive strategies related to her goals. Activities to promote use of the left upper extremity were planned to be novel, task-related and progressively graded, including repetitive bilateral activities[B], for example, folding towels and doing up buttons (HSFC, 2023). Therapeutic activities were also designed to practice functional balance (e.g. standing at counter to put items on a shelf) and scanning strategies[B] (e.g. use of natural anchors on the left such as the edge of the small therapy table) (HSFC, 2023).

Goal 1. Personal Care

I referred Mrs Tremblay to the rehabilitation assistant to support retraining in personal care activities (washing, dressing, grooming) once per week. I also asked the rehabilitation assistant to help Mrs Tremblay practice using a sock aid and long-handled shoehorn. Nursing staff also supported her to carry over her learning from day-to-day, as time permitted[B] (HSFC, 2023).

Mrs Tremblay attained her goal of being able to wash, dress, groom and toilet herself independently. She was able to reach her feet and to use her left hand sufficiently to be able to put on socks and shoes. Although she found it easier to use the sock aid and long-handled shoehorn, she preferred not to and noted that she would consider using these devices later if this task did not get easier.

Goal 2. Functional Mobility and Transfers

I consulted regularly with the physiotherapist to keep abreast of Mrs Tremblay's mobility status and adjusted the occupational therapy sessions that included walking and carrying items within the therapy room as needed. While walking, Mrs Tremblay practised scanning strategies such as locating items on both sides of her environment as well as strategies to promote safe mobility, such as slowing down when hallways were busy. Mrs Tremblay learned to walk using a four-point cane and scanning strategies to promote safety.

As Mrs Tremblay's mobility improved, I reassessed the equipment she needed to be able to complete toilet transfers and toileting safely. She regained her ability to transfer and toilet herself independently using a grab bar on her right side to steady herself while managing her clothing.

During occupational therapy sessions, we practiced 'dry' bathtub transfers and Mrs Tremblay learned to complete the transfer using a grab bar near the outside edge of the bathtub and light steadying assistance. She agreed that a bath seat would be useful when showering as she did not feel secure standing with her eyes closed. We transitioned to practicing in a real shower when Mrs Tremblay felt comfortable. I provided her with the information needed to purchase the recommended equipment and have it installed.

Goal 3. Home Management

Meal Preparation

Mrs Tremblay and I planned an evaluation of her ability to prepare a simple meal, identify safety concerns and find solutions to meal preparation difficulties.

Mrs Tremblay prepared soup and a ham and cheese sandwich. She required extra time and occasional cueing to find items in the kitchen when these were located on her left side. The kitchen was quiet with no distractions and Mrs Tremblay was able to focus on preparing the meal. She had difficulty with bilateral tasks that required an adapted grip, such as cutting, but was able to use her left hand effectively when washing dishes. I added kitchen-related tasks such as cutting and opening jars to her daily occupational therapy programme.

Mrs Tremblay learned to prepare a simple two-dish meal independently. We identified strategies to keep focused during meal preparation, such as not answering the phone when cooking. She was able to integrate use of her left hand to assist with most tasks but was still nervous when chopping. The use of assistive devices for meal preparation was discussed.

Medication, Financial and Household Management

Mrs Tremblay learned to manage taking her medications independently using a dosette.

During occupational therapy sessions, Mrs Tremblay and I chose basic financial management and household tasks to practice such as budgeting for groceries, putting items away and doing laundry. Following these tasks, Mrs Tremblay and I were not concerned about her ability to manage day-to-day tasks, but she preferred that her nephew continue to assist with other finances.

Plan for Transition

A discharge date was set for 5 weeks after admission. A meeting was arranged 2 weeks before this date. Mrs Tremblay invited her sister to attend and together, with the interdisciplinary team members, they discussed her current abilities and available support services in the community and home environment. Although everyone agreed that Mrs Tremblay would be able to manage within her apartment with support from community services and family, the team and Mrs Tremblay were concerned about safety going up and down the stairs to the apartment. Mrs Tremblay did not want to be isolated in her apartment and suggested that she could live with her sister, who lived in a bungalow, while waiting to get stronger. Therefore, the discharge destination was changed. A referral to community services for assistance with showering and home management tasks was made.

BOX 43.3
REFLECTION ON JUSTICE AND EQUITY 1

I was worried about Mrs Tremblay's ability to return to live on her own safely. I knew returning home was very important to her and thought that she might decide to accept the risks involved in doing this. If she had insisted on going home, it would have been difficult for me to reconcile my values of being person-centred and promoting safety. I noted that being comfortable and supporting people in making 'risky' decisions is an area for my own professional development (refer to Chapter 20).

The doctor told Mrs Tremblay that she should not drive for 3 months and should be reassessed at that point. As Mrs Tremblay wished to eventually return to live at home and wanted to return to driving, we discussed outpatient occupational therapy. She agreed that she would like to receive this service and I completed a referral.

I reflected on potential justice and equity issues in relation to Mrs Tremblay (Box 43.3).

PART 3: OUTPATIENT REHABILITATION (VALERIE)

Context

Mrs Tremblay was referred to me by the inpatient rehabilitation team. The centre where I work includes occupational therapists, physiotherapists, speech language pathologists in a community outpatient setting using an interprofessional team approach. An individual is seen for up to 20 sessions per profession and appointments are usually held at the clinic. Community visits are done as needed. My role at this stage of a person's recovery is to focus on barriers to participation in community living. Mrs Tremblay was waitlisted for 1 month until I was able to see her.

Connect

Before meeting with her, I reviewed the referral and accompanying documentation, including the inpatient rehabilitation occupational therapist's discharge summary.

During our first meeting, I presented what occupational therapy might look like in this outpatient context and how we would work together to identify and work towards her occupational goals. I talked about potential service constraints due to the limited number of visits allowed. I explained the interprofessional and student training nature of the clinic. Mrs Tremblay consented to participate in the occupational therapy service and an occupational therapy student's participation in her care. Then I listened. I wanted to learn about Mrs Tremblay beyond the information on the referral.

I let her tell her story, asking open-ended prompting questions. As she talked, I began to gather a more complete picture of who she was and her rehabilitation process thus far, as well as how she saw her future.

Seek Understanding and Define Purpose

We discussed how she had been managing since discharge and the challenges she experienced since moving to her sister's home. Several themes emerged: feelings of isolation, dependence and uselessness. After further discussion, I was able to determine that these feelings were originating from two sources.

Although able to do certain tasks like meal preparation, she was not participating in these tasks as she felt that she was not doing them well enough for her sister's approval. After exploring her leisure activities and social participation[B] (HSFC, 2023), I was able to discover the second source of her feeling of uselessness – loss of engagement in activities through which she was able to give to others, such as knitting hats for premature babies and serving at mass at her church. Now her activities revolved around her basic needs. She had few, if any, valued occupations.

Explore Occupations

Together we began the process of identifying what occupations might help her to regain her feelings of independence and usefulness. Using the Canadian Occupational Performance Measure (COPM) (Law et al., 2014) (refer to Chapter 16), she identified the following goals as most important:

1. Safely and independently climb the stairs to her own apartment so that she could return home.
2. Resume driving.
3. Complete a simple pattern using a straight-knit stitch.
4. Participate in serving at the mass service at her church. My reflection on this goal is presented in Box 43.4.

BOX 43.4
REFLECTION ON JUSTICE AND EQUITY 2

Mrs Tremblay is a member of a different faith community than I am. I take a moment to reflect on my beliefs and values to ensure that I will not be imposing my views on her. I am unsure of the tasks involved with serving mass at her place of worship and so make a mental note to be sure to be open to and listen carefully and respectfully as I gather more information to better understand and support her participation in this occupation.

For each of these goals, we followed the iterative COTIPP process of exploring occupational participation, co-design priorities, goals, outcomes and plans, trialling the plan, exploring changes and refining the plan. This process is described below for each goal.

Goal 1 Climb Stairs to her Apartment

Mrs Tremblay reported having a flight of 15 stairs with a right ascending railing to access her apartment. She said that within the 3 weeks of working with the outpatient rehabilitation physiotherapist, she was able to climb five steps with assistance. We talked about doing a stair-climbing assessment in her home environment, once she progressed to being able to climb 15 steps continuously at the clinic.

After 8 weeks, both Mrs Tremblay and the physiotherapist reported that she was able to climb 15 continuous steps. The occupational therapy session for the following week was scheduled at her home, where she demonstrated that she could climb up the steps to access her apartment safely. She had more difficulty descending, as the railing was on her stroke-affected side.

I recommended installing a railing on the other side of the stairway, but Mrs Tremblay was unsure if her landlord would agree. With her permission I wrote a letter to her landlord explaining my recommendation, the rationale, and advocating for safe accessibility not just for Mrs Tremblay, but all the tenants (refer to Chapter 21). The landlord agreed and the railing was installed 2 weeks later. After the installation of the railing, Mrs Tremblay spent the weekend in her own apartment. Her sister and nephew were present when she climbed or descended the steps. Mrs Tremblay reported being ecstatic about the accomplishment but realised that the effort of going up and down the stairs fatigued her greatly. She agreed to work on incorporating energy conservation strategies into her daily life to help manage her fatigue.

By discharge, she had made plans to move to her apartment permanently. She planned to temporarily have someone present when she climbed the stairs, and she reported feeling more confident each day.

Goal 2 Resume Driving

Mrs Tremblay showed me the letter she received from the Ministry of Transportation indicating that her driver's licence had been suspended because of her stroke. She talked about how driving gave her a sense of independence, especially because she lived alone in a rural community. She was aware that she could not safely drive because of the reduced movement of her left arm and leg but hoped that would change.

After reviewing the letter, I explained to Mrs Tremblay that a comprehensive driving evaluation was required[B] (HSFC, 2023) and that the clinic was not an accredited functional driving evaluation centre. Her goal of returning to driving was beyond the scope of this clinic (refer to Chapter 34).

We discussed how I could support her through the steps required to have her driving formally assessed, including practising some of the prerequisite skills to prepare for a formal evaluation and for potential return to driving. She agreed that preparing for the driving evaluation would be a good objective.

Mrs Tremblay consented to participate in several standardised perceptual and cognitive assessments[B] (HSFC, 2023) to help determine components that might affect her ability to resume driving. I also observed functional head and neck range of motion and completed standardised tests for the upper extremity post-stroke[B] (HSFC, 2023). Although not specifically linked to driving, these evaluations were chosen to provide more information on sub-skills necessary for controlling a car.

The results of these evaluations revealed that Mrs Tremblay had mild difficulties with dual attention, visual memory, visuospatial awareness and reaction time, which could affect her ability to safely operate a vehicle. Also, she demonstrated decreased grasp and mobility of her left arm, deficits that could limit her ability to control a regular steering wheel and to use

---

BOX 43.5

EXAMPLE OF A SESSION PLAN FOR MRS TREMBLAY DURING OUTPATIENT REHABILITATION

Mrs Tremblay's Treatment Session Plan – Week 4
1. Review progress in driving evaluation centre process – confirm her doctor filled out the required paperwork (2 mins)
2. Review homework from last week – 20 road sign questions, 20 rules of the road questions and home fine motor programme (13 mins)
3. Cognitive/perceptual stimulation – e-tablet with online games: *Trains* (movement tracking, anticipation and planning) and *Eagle Eye* (visual dual attention, simultaneous central and peripheral stimuli) games (15 mins)
4. Functional activity practice for setting up at church service – standing, carrying items two handed, one step. Reinforce body mechanics (15 mins)
5. Mirror therapy (Harris et al., 2009) – pronation/supination, wrist flex/extension, finger gross flex/extension and individual tapping (10 mins)
6. Knitting with student (5 mins)

---

the signal indicator. Her right foot and arm function were intact; therefore, she would be able to use the accelerator and brake and operate other controls in the car such as window wipers, radio and control the steering wheel with that hand. She also displayed adequate trunk control and head and neck movement.

We planned that intervention sessions would incorporate activities to stimulate cognitive-perceptual skills (refer to Chapter 42) and motor components for her left upper extremity (refer to Chapters 28 and 39). We would also review the process to resume driving and the rules of the road.

During sessions, Mrs Tremblay participated in therapeutic activities designed to improve cognitive, perceptual and motor abilities. These were graduated in difficulty as her performance improved. We also practised task-specific activities about rules of the road, environmental scanning and simulated mirror-checking activities[B] (HSFC, 2023). See Box 43.5 for a sample session plan. A home programme was provided to augment the in-person sessions.

By discharge, Mrs Tremblay reported feeling confident about the rules of the road and had shown progress in her perceptual and cognitive skills. Her grasp improved so that she could hold a steering wheel; however, the motor control in her left arm was not adequate for steering. We discussed that she would likely require vehicle adaptations for one-handed driving. Her functional driving evaluation appointment was scheduled in 1 month. Mrs Tremblay stated that she would continue to practice the skills while waiting.

Despite her progress, Mrs Tremblay was aware of the possibility that she might not pass the evaluation. She expressed that she would be disappointed but could function with the support of her sister and friends. In case of need, I provided her with contact information for a community organisation that provided transportation to medical appointments for a nominal fee.

I reflected on the interventions that I provided in relation to return to driving (Box 43.6).

Goal 3 Resume Knitting

Using Mrs Tremblay's own knitting project brought from home, I completed a Dynamic Performance Analysis (DPA) (Polatajko et al., 2000) (refer to Chapter 18). She was neither able to maintain a functional grasp nor able to manipulate her wrist to position the left needle. She could explain the steps of what needed to be done but could not complete the task. She became visibly upset by her inability to accomplish this task and ended by throwing the needles on the table. Mrs Tremblay had the required knowledge and cognitive skills to complete this task; however, the fine motor control in her left hand was a limitation, and she became quite frustrated even attempting the task.

To mitigate Mrs Tremblay's frustration and promote success experiences, I proposed we focus initially on her left-hand function rather than directly on practicing the activity.

During the DPA, I learned that my occupational therapy student did not know how to knit. I asked Mrs Tremblay if she would be interested in teaching the student to knit; that way she could be involved in the activity without the frustration of being confronted with her lost function. She agreed.

I provided Mrs Tremblay with activities to stimulate motor recovery and fine motor return in session and at home[B] (HSFC, 2023). See session treatment plan in Box 43.5.

When working with the student on knitting, Mrs Tremblay became fully engaged in the knitting activity and did not express any frustration. As motor recovery improved in her left hand and forearm, Mrs Tremblay began to participate more in the teaching sessions with the student and at times demonstrated to the student how to knit. By the end of the student's six-week placement, Mrs Tremblay had developed a strategy to stabilise her wrist and maintain grasp long enough to knit several stitches consecutively, and she had successfully taught the student a simple pattern. We replaced her time teaching the student with task-specific practice, and by the end of the interventions, she had completed a dishcloth. She was adequately satisfied with the results that she had begun to knit a baby hat at home.

Goal 4 Resume Roles in Religious Service

Mrs Tremblay was able to clearly describe the steps and tasks required in the different roles she had performed at her church. Mrs Tremblay had the knowledge and cognitive skills to perform these tasks. Activity tolerance, motor recovery to her left upper extremity and mobility were limitations to her being able to participate in this occupation.

For this goal, I chose to use an Occupational Performance Coaching approach (refer to Chapter 27). Mrs Tremblay and I engaged in a process to identify her preferred performance, options and strategies to achieve her goal. Mrs Tremblay wondered whether the energy conservation strategies (refer to Chapter 37) she had learned were applicable in this activity. She proposed a few ideas of how she might modify some of the tasks involved.

On the day of the home visit, we also went to Mrs Tremblay's church. There, we were able to practice some of the tasks we had tried at the clinic (Box 43.5) as well as discuss possible task modifications with the priest. The priest said that he and the community would support accommodations. Mrs Tremblay was initially hesitant to have the processes changed to accommodate her. As we discussed further, she agreed that it would be a first step in the goal of resuming her previous roles at the church.

By the end of sessions at the clinic, she had set up the altar before the beginning of mass on two occasions and had taken up the collection once with minimal assistance. Mrs Tremblay was very happy with the resumption of these roles and was determined to continue improving and trying new ones.

Transition

At the end of her 20 sessions, Mrs Tremblay's scores on the COPM had increased by at least two points on each of the evaluation scales indicating a clinically important change (Eyssen et al., 2011). Her energy level continued to be a challenge, but she had learned how to plan out her days to manage her fatigue. She had a programme of home activities that she continued to do to maintain her gains and prepare for her appointment at the functional driving evaluation centre. She and I agreed that she had achieved her goals within the context of the clinic's scope and that discharge was appropriate. We discussed options for what she could do should she encounter further occupational participation challenges. She identified that she could use a process similar to the one we used for her return to serve at mass. Also, information on occupational therapy services through the local public Home and Community Care Support Services were provided.

On discharge, Mrs Tremblay reported being more confident. She was involved in her community and engaged in her life rather than just surviving day-to-day. Despite her initial resistance to having anyone in the community adjust to her needs, I hoped that the experiences and strategies she learned through our interventions would help her in the future when she came across other problems.

Mrs Tremblay's file in occupational therapy at the clinic was closed.

REFERENCES

Canadian Association of Occupational Therapists. (2009). *Joint position statement on evidence-based occupational therapy (1999 reviewed for currency 2009)*. Canadian Association of Occupational Therapists. https://caot.ca/document/3697/J%20-%20Joint%20Position%20Statement%20on%20Evidence%20based%20OT.pdf.

Egan, M., & Restall, G.(2022). The Canadian model of occupational participation. In M. Egan & G. Restall (Eds.). *Promoting occupational participation: Collaborative relationship-focused occupational therapy, 10th Canadian Occupational Therapy Guidelines*, (pp. 73–95). Canadian Association of Occupational Therapists.

Eyssen, I. C. J. M., Steultjens, M. P. M., Oud, T. A. M., Bolt, E. M., Maasdam, A., & Dekker, J. (2011). Responsiveness of the Canadian occupational performance measure. *Journal of Rehabilitation Research and Development, 48*(5), 517–528.

Gauthier, L., Dehaut, F., & Joanette, Y. (1989). The bells test: A quantitative and qualitative test for visual neglect. *International Journal of Clinical Neuropsychology, 11*(2), 49–54.

Gorecki, C., Lamping, D. L., Brown, J. M., Madill, A., Firth, J., & Nixon, J. (2010). Development of a conceptual framework of health-related quality of life in pressure ulcers: A patient-focused approach. *International Journal of Nursing Studies, 47*, 1525–1534.

Gowland, C., Stratford, P., Ward, M., Moreland, J., Torresin, W., Van Hullenaar, S., Sanford, J., Barreca, S., Vanspall, B., & Plews, N. (1993). Measuring physical impairment and disability with the Chedoke-McMaster stroke assessment. *Stroke, 24*, 58–63.

Harris, J. E., Eng, J. J., Miller, W. C., & Dawson, A. S. (2009). A self-administered graded repetitive arm supplementary program (GRASP) improves arm function during inpatient stroke rehabilitation: A multi-site randomized controlled trial. *Stroke, 40*(6), 2123–2128.

Heart and Stroke Foundation of Canada (HSFC). (2023). *Recommendations*. Canadian Stroke Best Practices. https://www.strokebestpractices.ca/recommendations.

Law, M., Baptiste, S., Carswell, A., McColl, M. A., Polatajko, H., & Pollock, N. (2014). *Canadian occupational performance measure* (5th ed.). CAOT Publications ACE.

Norton, L., Parslow, N., Johnston, D., Ho, C., Afalavi, A., Mark, M., O'Sullivan-Drombolis, D., Moffatt, S. (2017). *Best practice recommendations for the prevention and management of pressure injuries. In: Foundations of best practice for skin and wound management. A supplement of Wound Care Canada*. WoundsCanada. https://www.woundscanada.ca/docman/public/health-care-professional/bpr-workshop/172-bpr-prevention-and-management-of-pressure-injuries-2/file.

Polatajko, H. J., Mandich, A., & Martini, R. (2000). Dynamic performance analysis: A framework for understanding occupational performance. *American Journal of Occupational Therapy, 54*(1), 65–72.

Restall, G., Egan, M., Valvaara, K., Phenix, A., & Sack, C. (2022). Canadian occupational therapy inter-relational practice process framework. In M. Egan, & G. Restall (Eds.), *Promoting occupational participation: collaborative relationship-focused occupational therapy, 10th occupational therapy guidelines* (pp. 121–150). CAOT.

MR FITCH: WORK RETENTION VOCATIONAL REHABILITATION

YELIZ PRIOR

INTRODUCTION

This practice story takes place in the context of a rheumatology occupational therapy department within a National Health Service (NHS) hospital in the United Kingdom (UK). Occupational therapists in rheumatology are considered 'specialists' who work within a multidisciplinary team (MDT) of rheumatologists, rheumatology nurse specialists and other allied health professionals (AHP) specialising in rheumatology (e.g. physiotherapists, podiatrists and pharmacists) to provide vital support to people with rheumatic and musculoskeletal conditions.

The practice story depicts the journey of a person with a rheumatic condition receiving a job retention vocational rehabilitation (JRVR) intervention from a rheumatology occupational therapist using the Canadian Model of Occupational Participation (CanMOP) (Egan & Restall, 2022) (refer to Chapter 11). The role of occupational therapists in collaborating with people to facilitate participation in work is further explored in Chapter 26, emphasising the importance of a proactive approach to assessment and intervention to minimise work disability.

The occupational therapy process described in this practice case story is mapped to the six action domains

of the Canadian Occupational Therapy Inter-relationship Practice Process (COTIPP) (Restall et al., 2022) to illustrate the practical application of this approach (refer to Chapter 12). Foundational processes and actions for promoting occupational participation are based on the COTIPP (Restall et al., 2022) to highlight the relational aspects of the interactions between the occupational therapist and the individual in the practice story, integrating the model, approach and framework in occupational therapy practice.

REFERRAL TO OCCUPATIONAL THERAPY

Referrals are accepted from a range of healthcare professionals within the rheumatology department. Some services also accept referrals from primary care practitioners (e.g. general practitioners (GP)), community-based services and self-referrals from individuals known to the service. These referrals are thoughtfully prioritised, with an emphasis on promptly identifying who requires urgent occupational therapy intervention to mitigate potential risks. Concurrently, those with less urgent needs are scheduled for routine appointments.

Referral Letter

I hope this message finds you well. I am writing to request an occupational therapy assessment for Mr Fitch, a 35-year-old individual diagnosed with axial spondyloarthritis and joint hypermobility. Mr Fitch is currently employed as a warehouse worker and has been experiencing significant challenges at work due to pain, sleep disturbance and fatigue. Given the nature of his work and the physical demands it entails, his ability to perform his job effectively has been compromised. His AS-WIS[1] score is 19, indicating medium to high work instability and need for vocational rehabilitation. We believe that an occupational therapy assessment and intervention could be instrumental in addressing these concerns and enhancing his self-management strategies.

We greatly appreciate your prompt attention to this referral and look forward to collaborating with you to provide Mr Fitch with the comprehensive care and support he needs to regain control over his health and work-related challenges.

Please do not hesitate to contact us if you require any additional information or if you would like to discuss this case further.

THE SIX ACTION DOMAINS OF THE CANADIAN OCCUPATIONAL THERAPY INTER-RELATIONSHIP PRACTICE PROCESS (COTIPP)

Connect

The first meeting is akin to laying the cornerstone of trust upon which the therapeutic relationship is constructed. Individuals often arrive with a degree of uncertainty, perhaps even apprehension. How the occupational therapist engages during this initial

interaction profoundly influences the degree of trust that can be fostered. This trust forms the basis for future collaboration and empowers the person to share their concerns, struggles and aspirations openly.

This is the time when the occupational therapist begins to understand the individual's unique circumstances. It involves listening attentively to their narrative, learning about their life roles and comprehending the impact of health conditions on their daily existence. It is a process of gathering insights that will inform subsequent interventions. The first meeting allows both parties to set clear expectations for the therapeutic journey. It is a space to articulate goals, discuss potential challenges and establish a shared vision of what success looks like. Clarity in these areas is essential for aligning efforts effectively.

Beyond the clinical aspects, the first meeting also enables the formation of an emotional connection. It is about conveying empathy, compassion and a genuine commitment to the individual's well-being. This emotional bond underpins the therapeutic alliance, fostering a sense of safety and comfort. As such, it holds immense potential and significance in collaborative relationship-focused occupational therapy (Egan & Restall, 2022).

Background

History

Mr Fitch is a 35-year-old male recently diagnosed with Axial Spondyloarthritis (AxSpA). He has a history of multiple joint problems, including low back pain, knee pain, shoulder and neck pain, spanning five years and impacting his ability to work. Initially, his symptoms were managed by his general practitioner under the diagnosis of joint hypermobility. Currently, he is under the care of a rheumatology consultant and has been referred to physiotherapy, awaiting evaluation.

Clinical Symptoms

Mr Fitch presents with persistent but intermittent low back pain, occasionally radiating to the posterior of his hips. His pain is rated on the Pain Visual Analogue

---

[1]**Ankylosing Spondylitis Work Instability Scale (AS-WIS)** is a 20-item questionnaire, which identifies individuals thought to be at low (<11 points), moderate (11–18 points) or high (>18 points) risk of work instability. Cucos, I., Dadoun, S., Jacquemin, C., Kreis, S., Fabre, S., Hudry, C., Pertuiset, E., Fautrel, B., & Gossec, L. (2021). Prediction of work impact in axial spondyloarthritis by the work instability scale: A prospective cohort study of 101 patients. *The Journal of Rheumatology, 48*(7), 1002–1006. https://doi.org/10.3899/jrheum.191397.

Scale (VAS)[2] with a best score of 5/10 and a worst score of 8/10. He describes the pain as an intermittent dull ache with sharp pain upon movement. These symptoms have significantly impacted his sleep quality.

In addition to low back and hip pain, Mr Fitch experiences significant fatigue, sometimes more debilitating than his musculoskeletal symptoms. He reports early morning stiffness, lasting approximately 20 to 30 minutes. Pain tends to worsen towards the end of the day, particularly after prolonged periods of standing, which is an inherent aspect of his occupation. There are no signs of any joint swelling, eye problems, bowel issues, heel pain or skin rashes, which could present with AxSpA.

Clinical Examination

Range of Movement (ROM): Mr Fitch exhibits full ROM at the lumbar spine, hips and neck.

Skin Elasticity: No notable abnormalities in skin elasticity.

Scarring: Absence of widened atrophic scars.

Bruising: Mr Fitch does not report bruising easily.

Bloods: Normal inflammatory blood tests, erythrocyte sedimentation rate (ESR) and C-reactive protein (CRP) recorded on multiple occasions.

Noteworthy Medical History

Mr Fitch's past includes a background as a talented gymnast during his school years. However, he discontinued gymnastics at the age of 14 due to recurrent ankle sprains, initially on the left side and subsequently on the right side.

Family History

Father has osteoarthritis, no other family history of note.

---

[2]**Pain Visual Analogue Scale (VAS)** is a tool commonly used in rheumatology occupational therapy to measure and assess the intensity or severity of a person's pain. It provides a simple and straightforward way for individuals to self-report the level of pain they are experiencing. The scale typically consists of a horizontal line that is either 10 or 100 millimetres in length, with 'no pain' at one end (usually the left) and 'worst pain imaginable' at the other end (usually the right). Individuals asked to indicate their pain level by making a mark or drawing a line on the scale. The position of the mark or line along the scale is used to quantify the pain intensity. This is a subjective measure as it relies on the patient's self-reported perception of their pain.

Medical Management

Mr Fitch has been prescribed a nonsteroidal antiinflammatory drug (NSAID), which is used to treat mild to moderate pain and helps to relieve symptoms of AxSpA, including inflammation, swelling, stiffness and joint pain. This is taken daily with a proton-pump inhibitor (PPI) to prevent upper gastrointestinal complications associated with long-term use of NSAIDS (Gwee et al., 2018). Occasional use of paracetamol and ibuprofen over the counter; reports that the ibuprofen tends to be the more effective of these two options in relieving the back and hip pains.

Relationships and Interests

Mr Fitch is married and has a 15-year-old son from a previous relationship who lives 2 hours away. Additionally, he has two young children, aged 1 and 2 years, with his current partner. His partner is not currently employed. Mr Fitch enjoys spending quality time with his young family and playing computer games remotely with his older son. However, his persistent back and hip pain have significantly impacted his ability to enjoy one of his favourite pastimes: extended hours of gaming while seated comfortably on his gaming chair, an activity he once used to indulge in without discomfort.

Education and Work Status

Mr Fitch left school at 16 and worked in retail since. For the last couple of years, he has been employed as a warehouse worker at a well-known, large online retail company. His work schedule comprises 38 hours a week, and he is also expected to work overtime as needed. His shifts are on a rotating basis, either from 7:30 am to 3:30 pm or from 12:30 pm to 8:30 pm.

His primary responsibilities include unloading deliveries and transferring them to an in-house storage system, packing orders and operating a forklift when required. It is a fast-paced working environment, and Mr Fitch is entitled to a 30-minute meal break, along with a 5-minute break in the first and second half of his shift. Mr Fitch is granted 4 weeks of holiday entitlement per year.

Recently, he faced some work-related challenges and took one week of annual leave to rest and recuperate. It is important to note that he is hesitant about taking sickness absence due to his limited number of days available, which is a result of his relatively short tenure with the company. In terms of commuting, Mr Fitch relies on a moped to cover the five-kilometre journey across town to reach his workplace from his home.

Seek Understanding and Define Purpose

Understanding Mr Fitch's Context: A Collaborative Approach

Within COTIPP, context is not merely a set of external circumstances, it is a holistic and interrelated web of influences. It appreciates the intricate dance where various aspects of context influence and are influenced by each other (Restall et al., 2022). Understanding the unique context of each individual is a multifaceted effort that requires a dynamic, contextual and temporal perspective.

At the heart of this collaborative journey lies the imperative for the occupational therapist to discern, from Mr Fitch's viewpoint, the essential elements that he deems vital within the therapeutic relationship. It is about comprehending what occupational therapy means to him, what he seeks to achieve and the outcomes that resonate with his unique life story. In essence, it involves seeing the world through his eYes , experiencing his challenges and embracing his aspirations. This process is inherently contextual, rooted in the recognition that occupational therapy is not a one-size-fits-all venture. Mr Fitch's needs, goals and expectations are distinctly his own, shaped by his lived experiences, his family, his job and the intricacies of his health condition. To embark on this collaborative journey effectively, the occupational therapist must navigate this intricate landscape of individuality and contextuality, charting a course that aligns with Mr Fitch's desires for his own well-being.

Moreover, variability in individual and contextual factors significantly shapes the collaborative landscape. Every individual brings a unique set of characteristics, preferences and circumstances to the therapeutic table. These factors encompass not only his health condition but also the intricate interplay of psychological,

social and environmental elements. In essence, building collaborative relationships are about recognising the nuances of his context, appreciating the ups and down of his journey and tailoring the therapeutic experience to align seamlessly with his evolving needs and aspirations.

Delayed Diagnosis: Navigating Comorbidities

Mr Fitch's diagnostic journey has not been straight forward. His initial diagnosis of joint hypermobility obscured the presence of AxSpA, delaying early diagnosis and access to treatment. This delay was also attributed to the physical nature of his job, which may have exacerbated the severity of his pain and fatigue.

One condition, AxSpA, is characterised by axial skeleton stiffness, while the other, joint hypermobility, manifests as a wider range of peripheral joint movements. The coexistence of these seemingly paradoxical disorders introduces an element of confusion and a conundrum in terms of self-management. Delayed diagnosis not only prolongs the uncertainty for individuals like Mr Fitch but also casts a shadow on their quality of life, as they grapple with pain from the early stages and face joint damage in the long term (Pinto et al., 2017).

Here, the occupational therapist's role extends to appreciating the multidimensional nature of AxSpA as only a minority of individuals living with AxSpA manifest ongoing inflammation via inflammatory marker blood tests such as ESR or CRP. This revelation, though more pronounced in the early stages of the disease, remains a significant facet even in Mr Fitch's case, where five years have elapsed since symptom onset. A staggering 50% to 60% of individuals with AxSpA consistently exhibit normal CRP levels, despite experiencing ongoing disease activity (Landewé et al., 2018). This discrepancy between objective markers and subjective experience of persisting symptoms such as pain and fatigue is a hallmark of AxSpA and underscores the necessity of a comprehensive, collaborative relationship-focused approach in understanding the full impact of Mr Fitch's condition on his life.

Navigating the Impact: Pain, Fatigue and Their Ripple Effects

The impact of pain and fatigue (refer to Chapters 37 and 38) reverberates through the various domains of

Mr Fitch's life. It infiltrates his work environment, casting shadows on his ability to remain in work. As indicated by the AS-WIS score of 19, he falls within the category of high risk for work disability. This classification carries profound implications, especially considering that he is the primary wage-earner for his family. The weight of this responsibility can undoubtedly lead to heightened stress levels, further complicating his health journey.

Additionally, the far-reaching effects of pain and fatigue extend into his personal life, diminishing his ability to partake in a favourite pastime activity. This activity is not merely a leisure pursuit; it serves as a conduit for connecting with his older son, who resides two hours away. The inability to engage in this cherished bonding experience due to his condition is emotionally taxing and accentuates the need for a more nuanced understanding of the psychological and social facets of his condition.

Holistic Exploration: The Multifaceted Landscape

Beyond medical indicators, it is crucial to delve deeper into Mr Fitch's context. Occupational therapists are uniquely positioned to navigate the complex interplay of job-related factors, psychological well-being and condition-specific factors to assess, plan and deliver work rehabilitation interventions (Prior et al., 2015). This holistic exploration paves the way for a tailored intervention that not only addresses the physical aspects of his condition but also attends to the intricacies of his work-life balance, emotional well-being and family dynamics.

Explore Occupational Participation

Occupational participation lies at the heart of occupational therapy, and it is a dynamic process that unfolds through a collaborative journey between the occupational therapist and the individual.

Co-Creation of Conditions

The process begins with the co-creation of conditions for exploring occupational participation. It is a deliberate and thoughtful endeavour where the occupational therapist and Mr Fitch collaborate to establish an environment conducive to open dialogue and reflection. This involves setting the stage for trust, respect

and mutual understanding. The occupational therapist cultivates this environment through active listening, empathy and nonjudgemental attitude, respecting Mr Fitch's autonomy, maintain strict confidentiality and communicate clearly about the therapy process. By doing so, they create a safe space where Mr Fitch feels comfortable sharing concerns, hopes and uncertainties regarding his difficulties at work and daily life.

Identifying Occupational Concerns

Within this nurturing environment, Mr Fitch is encouraged to express his current occupational participation concerns. These concerns span a wide spectrum, from difficulties in performing his manual duties at work (e.g. load movement, reach and driving) to anxiety about job stability, struggling to engage in meaningful leisure activities with his family. The occupational therapist listens attentively, seeking to gain a comprehensive understanding of how these concerns impact Mr Fitch's overall well-being. Emotional support and coping strategies are provided when needed, and clear professional boundaries are established. Given the importance of work to the male gender role, the occupational therapist continuously reflects on their own biases and self-awareness to ensure the creation of a safe space that promotes trust, respect and empowerment in the therapeutic relationship.

Use of Work Patient Reported Outcome Measures (Work PROMs)

Support within the workplace, whether from managers, colleagues or employers, plays a critical role in aiding individuals like Mr Fitch to help sustain their employment. This support extends beyond practical assistance and encompasses the creation of an inclusive workplace culture that prioritises accessibility (Gignac et al., 2009). It also entails providing the psychological support necessary to navigate the unique challenges associated with disabilities in the workplace (Li et al., 2006).

Given Mr Fitch's circumstances, the occupational therapist decides to utilise Work Patient Reported Outcomes (Work PROMs) to gain further insights into Mr Fitch's perception of his abilities, limitations and well-being, which may not be fully captured by clinical or objective assessments alone. PROMs assist occupational therapists in tailoring plans to the specific needs and goals of each individual. By understanding how an individual perceives their condition and its impact, occupational therapists can design interventions that align with the individual's priorities. PROMs serve as valuable tools for tracking changes in an individual's progress over time. Occupational therapists can use them to measure the effectiveness of interventions, identifying areas of improvement and areas that may require further attention or modification. PROMs also facilitate shared decision-making between occupational therapists and individuals by involving them in the assessment process and considering their perspectives. Occupational therapists can collaborate more effectively with individuals to set treatment goals and make informed choices about their care. When self-reported outcomes are documented and shared, it can highlight the impact of specific conditions and the value of occupational therapy in addressing these issues.

Perceived Workplace Support Scale (PWSS) (Box 44.1) is a Work PROM, which comprises three distinct subscales measuring support from managers, co-workers and the organisation itself (Gignac et al., 2007; Hammond et al., 2023). Another Work-specific PROM is the Workplace Accommodations, Benefits, Policies and Practices Scale (WABPPS) (Gignac et al., 2015; Hammond et al., 2023) (Box 44.2) which not only evaluates formal accommodations provided by employers but also considers the informal support accessed by workers. The PWSS includes 19 items each scored 0 = strongly disagree to 4 = strongly agree: Part 1 Manager Support (four items, range 0–16), Part 2 Co-worker Support (eight items, range 0–32) and Part 3 Organisational Support (seven items, range 0–28), with higher scores indicating better perceptions of workplace support (Hammond et al., 2023). The WABPPS has two parts. Part 1 consists of 16 work accommodations, policies or benefits, with four related questions about need for, use, availability and, if used, helpfulness. Items can be considered individually, or the total number of items needed, available and used are summed (score range for each question is 0–16). Items can be used to explore whether work needs are met, unmet or exceeded, with those scoring 0–1 having low, 2–4 medium and 5 or more high need/use (Hammond et al., 2023).

Research has indicated that individuals facing greater limitations due to their condition and experiencing elevated job-related stress are more likely to require and utilise such work accommodations (Hammond et al., 2023). These scales have been rigorously tested for their psychometric validity for individuals with AxSpA in the UK, affirming their applicability in this population. Therefore, these tools aid occupational therapists in comprehensively assessing and addressing the multifaceted dimensions of workplace support, an essential component of Mr Fitch's journey towards managing his condition effectively while sustaining his employment.

Mr Fitch's scores for the PWSS were calculated as a sum for each of the three subscales (Part 1 (Manager Support): 7/16; Part 2 (Co-worker Support): 18/32; Part 3 (Organisational Support): 12/28) – higher scores indicating greater levels of support (Box 44.1). Completing this questionnaire, which asks detailed questions about his perception of the managerial and organisational attitudes and behaviours made him realise that the support was available to him, but he was reluctant to access it, partly due to his relatively short tenure, and partly because he may have been making assumptions that use of available support could paint a negative picture of him in the eYes of his colleagues and manager. He did not feel able to talk to his co-workers about personal matters because he did not have a chance to develop a type of relationship with them to allow this. However, he acknowledged that they were mostly supportive of others when people needed help, and if he did needed support, he would probably get it. He was aware that some of his colleagues had worked together longer, and socialised outside of work (e.g. going to pub after work), but although he was invited to these outings, his pain and fatigue levels stopped him taking part. Also, he would rather spend his free time with his family. He recognised the need to invest into these relationships, but this had not been a priority until now. He thought the company frowned on employees who cut back on their hours of work for personal reasons but also acknowledged that this might be his perception rather than a fact as his assumptions were based on a previous experience at another retail company, which was a smaller business compared to his current employer and did not have as many staff as the current company did. Thus, there were more opportunities to

BOX 44.1
BRITISH-ENGLISH PERCEIVED WORKPLACE SUPPORT SCALE (PWSS)

For All Parts: If you have more than one job, answer thinking about your <u>main</u> job.

PART 1: YOUR MANAGER OR SUPERVISOR

These statements ask if you feel your manager or supervisor considers the **personal needs,** <u>including health needs,</u> of others. Please **tick** the box that indicates how much you agree or disagree with each statement.

- **If you are self-employed** <u>and do not have</u> **a manager or supervisor, please:** tick this box ☐ and go to Part 2.

Part 1: These statements are about your manager or supervisor

	Strongly Disagree	Disagree	Do Not Agree or Disagree	Agree	Strongly Agree
1. My manager does not understand that there are times when employees' personal needs have to come before their work.	☐	☒	☐	☐	☐
2. In organising meeting times or work hours, my manager shows little concern for employees' personal needs.	☐	☒	☐	☐	☐
3. My manager does what she or he can to make things easier when employees are having personal difficulties.	☐	☒	☐	☐	☐
4. My manager does things to help employees balance their work and their personal life.	☐	☐	☒	☐	☐

PART 2: YOUR CO-WORKERS

These statements ask if you feel your co-workers consider the **personal needs,** <u>including health needs,</u> of others. Please **tick** the box that indicates how much you agree or disagree with each statement.

- **If you are self-employed and/or** <u>do not have</u> **any co-workers, please:** tick this box ☐ and go to Part 3.

Part 2: These statements are about your co-workers

	Strongly Disagree	Disagree	Do Not Agree or Disagree	Agree	Strongly Agree
5. I cannot talk about personal matters with my co-workers.	☐	☒	☐	☐	☐
6. My co-workers do not really care about how things are going for me personally.	☐	☒	☐	☐	☐
7. My co-workers do not pitch in and help me out in practical ways.	☐	☐	☐	☒	☐
8. I cannot depend on my co-workers for practical help.	☐	☐	☒	☐	☐
9. If I have to miss work for part of the day, there **are** co-workers who would fill in for me as much as they could.	☐	☐	☐	☒	☐
10. I have co-workers who go out of their way to help me at work.	☐	☐	☒	☐	☐

Continued on following page

BOX 44.1
BRITISH-ENGLISH PERCEIVED WORKPLACE SUPPORT SCALE (PWSS)—(*Continued*)

Part 2: These statements are about your co-workers

	Strongly Disagree	Disagree	Do Not Agree or Disagree	Agree	Strongly Agree
11. If I were having difficulties of a personal nature, there are co-workers who would show concern for me.	☐	☒	☐	☐	☐
12. I have co-workers who would support me through difficult personal issues.	☐	☐	☐	☒	☐

PART 3: THE COMPANY, BUSINESS, OR ORGANISATION YOU WORK FOR

These statements ask if you feel that the company, business, or organisation you work for considers the **personal needs**, including health needs, of its employees.

Please tick the box that indicates how much you agree or disagree with each statement.

■ **If you are self-employed** and consider this section is not applicable, **please tick this box** ☐

Part 3: These statements are about your company, business, or organisation

In general.......	Strongly Disagree	Disagree	Do Not Agree or Disagree	Agree	Strongly Agree
13. People with personal needs do **not** do as well in this company	☐	☐	☒	☐	☐
14. This company frowns on employees who cut back on their hours of work for personal reasons.	☐	☐	☐	☒	☐
15. To succeed in this company employees must put their personal needs second.	☐	☒	☐	☐	☐
16. This company believes that employees who take a leave of absence for personal needs are not serious about their jobs.	☐	☐	☒	☐	☐
17. This company gives out a message that employees should not allow their personal needs to interfere with their work.	☐	☐	☒	☐	☐
18. This company has a way of showing that it supports people who have personal needs.	☐	☒	☐	☐	☐
19. This company tries to help employees make work arrangements that suit their personal needs.	☐	☒	☐	☐	☐

SCORING

Items are scored 0 (strongly disagree) to 4 (strongly agree). Higher scores indicate greater levels of support. Items are summed for each of the three sub-scales. Sub-scale scores should be reported separately. A total scale score for all three sub-scales **cannot** be created.

    Part 1: 4 items. **Items 1 and 2** must be reverse scored. Score range is 0–16.

    Part 2: 8 items. **Items 5, 6, 7,and 8** must be reverse scored. Score range is 0–32.

    Part 3: 7 items. **Items 13, 14, 15, 16 and 17** must be reversed scored. Score range is 0–28.

    Missing or non-applicable items: one missing item only is allowed in each sub-scale and can be replaced with the mean or median score of the remaining items (as appropriate).

accommodate individuals' need for working part-time. He also reflected that the current employer did not openly show the support for his personal needs, but then again, he never clearly expressed his needs to his manager or colleagues either.

In terms of the WABPPS questionnaire, Part 1 items were summarised for subscales (workplace accommodations, workplace policies and workplace benefits) to explore whether work needs were met, unmet or exceeded, with those scoring 0–1 having low, 2–4 medium and 5 or more high need/use. The WABPSS scores suggested that Mr Fitch has high unmet workplace accommodation needs (i.e. needs were greater than use) (Box 44.2). Again, completing this questionnaire also made him realise that he did not know the answer to some of the questions as to whether the policy/benefit was available at his workplace (e.g. allow employees to have more breaks and rest periods) because although he needed it, he never asked, or it was not openly discussed. When the policy/benefit was available (e.g. flexi time/flexible working), he did not use it because he wanted to make a good impression and did not want to come across demanding. He was aware of the sickness absence policy, but he chose not to use this and instead used his annual leave for some respite because he did not want to have a 'sick record'. In Part 2, he acknowledged that his current employed did not refuse any work modifications, adjustments, policies or benefits. Although he never asked for such accommodations, he knew that his employer had policies in place to offer access if requested. This demonstrates that the WABPPS can be used to play a part in activating people by prompting them to identify the presence of work accommodations, benefits and policies (Hammond et al., 2023).

Armed with this deeper understanding, the occupational therapist collaborates with Mr Fitch to develop a job retention vocational rehabilitation (JRVR) programme. This programme aims to empower Mr Fitch to remain in his current job by addressing physical, psychological and environmental factors. In doing so, the occupational therapist leverages their familiarity with current work legislation, statutory and third-sector employment support services and employee rights, all with the goal of enhancing Mr Fitch's confidence in his ability to continue working effectively. This collaborative approach exemplifies the essence of collaborative relationship-focused practice, where the person and the occupational therapist co-create the conditions for exploring and addressing current occupational participation concerns, aspirations, perceived possibilities, desires for change and the essential relationships that influence the journey towards improved well-being and sustained employment (Restall et al., 2021).

Exploring Aspirations and Possibilities

Occupational therapy is not just about addressing limitations; it is equally focused on nurturing aspirations and uncovering possibilities. Within this collaborative process, the occupational therapist engages in a dialogue with Mr Fitch to delve into his occupational aspirations. As trust builds between Mr Fitch and the occupational therapist, he candidly shares his

BOX 44.2
BRITISH-ENGLISH WORKPLACE ACCOMMODATIONS, BENEFITS, POLICIES AND PRACTICES SCALE (WABPPS)

Part 1: We are interested in learning about any policies, benefits or job modifications/reasonable adjustments at your workplace which might help you to manage your work and any health needs you may have. If you have more than one job, think about your <u>main job.</u>

<u>Thinking about your health needs over the last 12 months</u>, please indicate for each option if:

Q1) you <u>needed</u> it; **Q2)** it was/is <u>available</u> to you (even if you've not used it); **Q3)** you <u>used</u> it; and **Q4)** if Yes, if <u>helpful</u>. Please **tick** the appropriate answer. <u>ALWAYS ANSWER QUESTIONS 1 and 2.</u>

Are you self-employed (including business owner)?   Yes ☐   No ☒   *If Yes, self-employed*

Please <u>always</u> answer Questions 1 and 2. If any are **not** available to you, please **tick** "No" for Question 2. Please still answer Question 1 about whether you needed it (even if it was/is not available to you).

Part 1:	Q1 Have you ever <u>needed</u> this policy/benefit/ modification?	Q2 Is it <u>available</u> at your workplace? *If no, continue to the next question below...*	Q3 <u>If Yes:</u> Have you <u>used</u> this policy/benefit/ modification?	Q4 If Yes, was this <u>helpful</u> in managing your health or work needs?				
				Not at all	A Little	Somewhat	Quite a bit	A great deal
a. Flexi time or flexible working.	Yes ☒ No ☐	Yes ☒ No ☐ Don't know ☐	Yes ☐ No ☒	☐	☐	☐	☐	☐
b. Extended health benefits (e.g., private health care/insurance, eye tests, physiotherapy, occupational health).	Yes ☒ No ☐	Yes ☒ No ☐ Don't know ☐	Yes ☐ No ☒	☐	☐	☐	☐	☐
c. Special leave or leave of absence (paid or unpaid), e.g., for medical and rehabilitation appointments.	Yes ☒ No ☐	Yes ☒ No ☐ Don't know ☐	Yes ☐ No ☒	☐	☐	☐	☐	☐
d. Part-time work with same rights as full-time workers, but some benefits are pro-rata, e.g., annual leave allowance, bonus payments.	Yes ☐ No ☒	Yes ☒ No ☐ Don't know ☐	Yes ☐ No ☐	☐	☐	☐	☐	☐
e. Allow you more breaks and rest periods.	Yes ☒ No ☐	Yes ☐ No ☐ Don't know ☒	Yes ☐ No ☐	☐	☐	☐	☐	☐

BOX 44.2

BRITISH-ENGLISH WORKPLACE ACCOMMODATIONS, BENEFITS, POLICIES AND PRACTICES SCALE (WABPPS) —(Continued)

Part 1:	Q1 Have you ever needed this policy/benefit/ modification?	Q2 Is it available at your workplace? If no, continue to the next question below...	Q3 If Yes: Have you used this policy/benefit/ modification?	Q4 If Yes, was this helpful in managing your health or work needs?				
				Not at all	A Little	Somewhat	Quite a bit	A great deal
f. Help you learn new skills (e.g., work-related training).	Yes ☒ No ☐	Yes ☒ No ☐ Don't know ☐	Yes ☒ No ☐	☐	☐	☒	☐	☐
g. Special equipment for your work (e.g., adapted computer keyboard, adjustable chair, assistive devices, adapted tools).	Yes ☒ No ☐	Yes ☒ No ☐ Don't know ☐	Yes ☒ No ☐	☐	☐	☐	☒	☐
h. Modified work duties (e.g., give up or change work tasks that are difficult).	Yes ☒ No ☐	Yes ☐ No ☐ Don't know ☒	Yes ☐ No ☐	☐	☐	☐	☐	☐
i. Altered your hours of work to give you more flexibility (e.g., compressed work week; job sharing; altered shifts).	Yes ☒ No ☐	Yes ☐ No ☐ Don't know ☒	Yes ☐ No ☐	☐	☐	☐	☐	☐
j. Made changes to your workstation (e.g., closer to lift, toilet, staff/coffee room).	Yes ☐ No ☒	Yes ☐ No ☐ Don't know ☒	Yes ☐ No ☐	☐	☐	☐	☐	☐
k. Changed your work environment (e.g., changed door handles, provided accessible parking).	Yes ☐ No ☒	Yes ☐ No ☐ Don't know ☒	Yes ☐ No ☐	☐	☐	☐	☐	☐

Continued on following page

BOX 44.2

BRITISH-ENGLISH WORKPLACE ACCOMMODATIONS, BENEFITS, POLICIES AND PRACTICES SCALE (WABPPS) —(Continued)

	Q1 Have you ever _needed_ this policy/benefit/modification?	Q2 Is it _available_ at your workplace? (If no, continue to the next question below...)	Q3 _If Yes:_ Have you _used_ this policy/benefit/modification?	Q4 If Yes, was this _helpful_ in managing your health or work needs? (Not at all / A Little / Somewhat / Quite a bit / A great deal)
l. Allowed you to work from home on occasions or for part of the week.	Yes ☐ No ☒	Yes ☐ No ☒ Don't know ☐	Yes ☐ No ☐	☐ ☐ ☐ ☐ ☐
m. Arranged for others to help you with work tasks.	Yes ☒ No ☐	Yes ☐ No ☐ Don't know ☒	Yes ☐ No ☒	☐ ☐ ☐ ☐ ☐
n. Health and Wellbeing programmes (e.g., exercise facilities or subsidised/paid gym membership, healthy eating advice, flu jabs).	Yes ☒ No ☐	Yes ☒ No ☐ Don't know ☐	Yes ☒ No ☐	Not at all ☐ A Little ☐ Somewhat ☒ Quite a bit ☐ A great deal ☐
o. Employee Assistance Programme (EAP) (i.e., confidential assistance/support with personal/family problems affecting work).	Yes ☐ No ☒	Yes ☐ No ☐ Don't know ☒	Yes ☐ No ☐	☐ ☐ ☐ ☐ ☐
p. Sickness absence management policy for people with long-term health conditions (disability leave).	Yes ☒ No ☐	Yes ☐ No ☒ Don't know ☐	Yes ☐ No ☒	☐ ☐ ☐ ☐ ☐

BOX 44.2
BRITISH-ENGLISH WORKPLACE ACCOMMODATIONS, BENEFITS, POLICIES AND PRACTICES SCALE (WABPPS) —(*Continued*)

Part 2:

Please **tick** the appropriate answer:

1. Has your current employer, in your **main** job, refused any work modifications, adjustments, policies or benefits (listed in the table above: i.e., options a to p) that you have <u>asked</u> for?

☐ Yes , my employer has refused

☒ No, my employer has or will provide them

☐ Not applicable: I've not needed any of these work modifications, adjustments, policies or benefits

2. **If you answered Yes to question 1**: what reason(s) did your employer give for refusing those work modifications, adjustments, policies, or benefits to your work? (*Please tick all that apply*)

☐ Too expensive

☐ Not practical or possible for this type of job

☐ Can't provide to only one person, would have to provide to others (favouritism)

☐ Would inconvenience others

☐ Impact on team performance

☐ Not available in this workplace

☐ On a waiting list

☐ Employer or supervisor refused (no reason given)

☐ No reply from employer

☐ Other (please specify) _____

Scoring Instructions:

Note: All respondents are asked if they have needed the policy/benefit in the past 12 months, regardless of availability. This allows assessment of unmet need. The time period is specified as 12 months, rather than "currently need." Many respondents with episodic/intermittent problems may not "currently need" to use a workplace benefit/accommodation, **but** during times of more intense symptoms or other difficulties, they have needed it.

The timeframe of 12 months could be shortened to six months. However, some accommodations (e.g., modifications to the work environment) are relatively rare and can be overlooked within a shorter time frame.

Part 1: Items can be examined on an individual level, or "Yes" answers summed to identify the total number of workplace accommodations, benefits, and policies:

■ Needed (Yes = 1; No = 0),

■ Available (Yes = 1; No = 0; with the number of "Don't Know" items separately identified, and/or recoded to 0 to allow a sum to be created. If the person does not know about availability, it is effectively, at the time of completion, not available for them. This situation could change with investigation about availability in their own workplace and/or education about employment rights.

■ and Used (Yes = 1; No = 0).

■ How helpful each item is considered is summarised by item (for those using the item).

Findings can also be used to examine issues of: unmet workplace accommodation needs (i.e., needs > use), accommodation needs met (i.e., needs = use), and accommodation needs exceeded (i.e., needs < use).

Continued on following page

BOX 44.2
BRITISH-ENGLISH WORKPLACE ACCOMMODATIONS, BENEFITS, POLICIES AND PRACTICES SCALE (WABPPS) —(*Continued*)

All items could be potentially needed by respondents, but the availability of workplace benefits and policies is influenced by, for example: the size of the organisation worked for, as smaller companies may not have these benefits or written policies. This is also often the case for the self-employed, unless they work as sub-contractors to another organisation, in which case the employer's benefits and policies may also apply to them.

- **Items e through m:** workplace accommodations for employees with long-term conditions or disabilities.
- **Items b, n, and o:** workplace benefits, which may only be available in larger organizations.
- **Items a, c, d, and p:** workplace policies, as well as workplace accommodations that can be requested by employees with long-term conditions or disabilities.

Items could also be examined separately for workplace accommodations (nine items), workplace policies (four items), and workplace benefits (three items), if required.

Parts Two and Three: frequency of responses is presented.

A WORK-PROM study manual with further details will be available at: https://usir.salford.ac.uk/view/authors/10108.html – search Monographs.

© Hammond A, Tennant A, Prior Y, Gignac M. 2023.

Total Scores for Mr Fitch's Assessment

Part 1	Needed	Available	Used
Workplace accommodations	6	2	2
Workplace policies	3	3	0
Workplace benefits	2	2	1

trepidations about discussing his difficulties with his manager to ask for work accommodations. Mr Fitch grapples with self-doubt stemming from a previous bad experience with a manager at another company, where he felt undermined and not appreciated for his work ethic. He expressed that he takes pride in not just pulling his weight but going above and beyond the requirements of his job to show commitment to his work. He really appreciated his place of work as it was closer to home and paid better than a previous employer, and he also had some company benefits such as access to training courses to develop further skills, access to flu/COVID-19 immunisations and discounts at various retailers as a staff benefit.

Desire for Change

Occupational participation often involves a desire for change. Understanding the desire for change is essential as it fuels the commitment and determination needed to obtain positive outcomes from the intervention. The occupational therapist collaboratively explores Mr Fitch's readiness for change using the Stages of Change Model (Prochaska & Norcross, 2002) (refer to Chapter 22) and realising that he is at the 'contemplation' stage (ambivalent about change) discusses the pros and cons of changing his negative beliefs towards accessing job accommodations with him. The occupational therapist helps Mr Fitch to identify specific reasons for contemplating change (e.g. improving his pain and fatigue levels to allow him to spend quality time with his family and work colleagues) and any perceived barriers to making this change (e.g. his manager and colleagues may see him in a negative light for getting a special treatment). Mr Fitch's desire for change is fuelled by a profound need for pain alleviation and improved management of his condition. The prospect of a less physically demanding role offers a glimmer of hope for enhanced well-being and quality of life. However, it is not just about pain mitigation; Mr Fitch's need for change signifies a longing for need to make more quality time for his family and increasing the likelihood for remaining at work until retirement by preventing work disability.

Important Relationships

Occupations are intricately linked to a person's relationships – with themselves and with others. In this context, the occupational therapist explores the significance of important relationships in Mr Fitch's life. These relationships can either support or hinder occupational participation. By recognising these dynamics, the person and the occupational therapist can work collaboratively to enhance the individual's social and interpersonal skills, fostering a more enriching and supportive social network. Mr Fitch has a close relationship with his partner, who is understanding and supportive to him. At work, he has a good relationship with his line manager and colleagues, but they are unaware of his struggles. He is reticent about asking for help as he does not like the idea of his colleagues taking on the burden of his workload.

Co-Design Priorities, Goals, Outcomes and Plans

As Mr Fitch better understands the need for change and moves from the contemplation stage to the preparation stage (change is planned within the coming month), the occupational therapist and Mr Fitch engage in a collaborative process to jointly establish priorities, define goals and outcomes and formulate plans (refer to Chapter 19). The occupational therapist helps him identify specific, achievable goals (e.g. using SMART goals), provides information on strategies for change and offers resources to support for developing an action plan.

Strategies to reduce the difficulty Mr Fitch experiences staying in work include:

- Education concerning AxSpA and condition management (refer to Chapter 22)
- Advice on current work legislations, the employee's rights to facilitate increased confidence in their ability to work (refer to Chapter 26)
- Education about load movement – assess weights handled and their frequency, assess method of storage of goods, assess method of order picking, assess use of assistive devices (refer to Chapters 31 and 35)
- Fatigue management through energy conservation and graded activity/pacing (refer to Chapter 37)

- Discuss disclosure so that he can discuss need to change work practices
- More rest breaks and appropriate restroom facilities
- Educate about working postures – FLT driving, picking, sitting, reaching
- Assess for footwear
- Stress management through increasing self-efficacy (refer to Chapters 24 and 37)
- Relaxation training
- Discuss shift patterns/start times – negotiate later start if possible

Trial the Plan, Explore Change and Refine the Plan

In the context of COTIPP, implementation is the crucial phase where the occupational therapist collaboratively puts into action a tailored plan with Mr Fitch, with a focus on enhancing occupational well-being and work participation.

An essential starting point is providing Mr Fitch with comprehensive education about AxSpA and its management (refer to Chapter 22). This knowledge empowers him to understand his condition better, recognise early warning signs and make informed decisions about his health. Understanding work legislations and employee rights is vital (refer to Chapter 26). This knowledge equips him with the confidence to advocate for himself in the workplace, ensuring that he receives the necessary accommodations and support. A detailed assessment of the demands of his job (e.g. weights handled, their frequency and methods of goods storage) helps identify potential stressors in his work environment, allowing for adjustments to reduce strain on his body. Techniques such as energy conservation and graded activity, as well as pacing, are introduced to help Mr Fitch manage his energy levels effectively throughout the workday (refer to Chapter 37). By understanding when and how to disclose his condition, he can work collaboratively with his employer to adapt work practices as needed, fostering a supportive work environment. The plan includes provisions for more frequent rest breaks and ensuring that appropriate rest facilities are available. These adjustments aim to reduce the physical demands of Mr Fitch's job, allowing him to recover during work hours. Mr Fitch's work postures are assessed, considering aspects such as forklift driving, order picking, sitting and reaching. Ergonomic recommendations are made to optimise his workstations for greater comfort and reduced strain. Footwear is evaluated to ensure it provides the necessary support and comfort for Mr Fitch during his work shifts. Proper footwear can significantly impact his physical well-being. Stress management techniques are incorporated into the plan. These include strategies to increase self-efficacy and resilience, which can help Mr Fitch cope with the emotional challenges of managing a chronic condition while working. Techniques for relaxation and stress reduction are introduced (refer to Chapters 24 and 37). These practices can be applied during work breaks or at home to alleviate tension and promote overall well-being. Discussions around shift patterns and start times are initiated, with a focus on negotiating for a later start, if possible. This accommodation can provide Mr Fitch with additional time to manage his condition in the mornings, when he experiences morning stiffness.

Each of these strategies is implemented with the active involvement and collaboration of Mr Fitch. The occupational therapist ensures that the strategies align with his preferences and priorities, emphasising the person-centred nature of the intervention. Additionally, regular communication and feedback loops are established to assess the effectiveness of these strategies in practice.

Plan for Transition

Key Objective: To facilitate a seamless transition from occupational therapy by actively engaging Mr Fitch in the planning process and addressing his concerns and goals.

The occupational therapist initiates an open and empathetic dialogue with Mr Fitch regarding his thoughts and feelings about transitioning from occupational therapy. Ensuring that he understands the purpose of this transition phase. During this, the occupational therapist explores their expectations for the transition period by asking 'what does he hope to achieve or maintain as he moves forward'? to ensure that the person's goals align with their long-term well-being and work participation.

This involves a review of Mr Fitch's progress and accomplishments throughout his occupational therapy journey. The occupational therapist celebrates Mr Fitch's achievements and acknowledges his resilience in managing AxSpA while sustaining employment. To address unresolved concerns, the occupational therapist actively listens to any concerns or uncertainties Mr Fitch may have about ending occupational therapy. At this stage, it is important to ensure that any lingering challenges or unanswered questions are addressed comprehensively.

Mr Fitch is provided with additional resources and information on self-management strategies specific to working with AxSpA (e.g. National Axial Spondyloarthritis Society's (NASS) Guide to Managing my axial SpA (AS) at work – available at https://nass.co.uk/resource/nass-guide-to-managing-your-axial-spa-as-at-work/ – as it is important to empower him with the tools and knowledge needed to continue managing his condition effectively.

The occupational therapist also discusses relevant community resources, support groups or local services that Mr Fitch can access after transitioning from occupational therapy. This can include continued access to educational materials or workshops available through the National Axial Spondyloarthritis Society (NASS): https://nass.co.uk/managing-my-as/.

This is followed by collaborating on a timeline for the gradual transition. This may involve reducing the frequency of occupational therapy sessions while ensuring that Mr Fitch feels confident in his ability to apply what he has learned independently. The occupational therapist also establishes a feedback mechanism to encourage Mr Fitch to share his thoughts and experiences during the transition. This helps to regularly assess his comfort level with the process and address any emerging concerns during this transitional period.

During this time, the occupational therapist ensures that all relevant information and progress reports are documented and shared with Mr Fitch to serve as a reference for his future self-management.

The overarching principle guiding this transition plan is shared decision-making and empowerment. Mr Fitch is at the centre of the transition process, actively participating in setting goals, addressing concerns and making choices about his future self-management. The occupational therapist's role is to facilitate this process, providing guidance, information and support as needed.

The transition process will be gradual, with a timeline tailored to Mr Fitch's preferences and readiness.

It will include ongoing discussions and evaluations to ensure a smooth and successful transition.

The success of this transition plan will be measured by Mr Fitch's ability to effectively manage his AxSpA, sustain his employment and maintain an improved quality of life independently. Additionally, his feedback and comfort level with the transition process will be key indicators of success.

CONCLUSION

By actively listening to and seeking to understand Mr Fitch's perspective about transitioning from occupational therapy, the aim is to empower him with the confidence, skills and resources needed to continue his journey towards well-being and work participation. This collaborative approach aligns with the principles of COTIPP, emphasising a holistic and person-centred transition process.

REFERENCES

Egan, M., & Restall, G. (2022). Canadian model of occupational participation: Collaborative relationship-focused occupational therapy. In M. Egan, & G. Restall (Eds.), *Promoting occupational participation: Collaborative relationship-focused occupational therapy*. Canadian Association of Occupational Therapists.

Gignac, M. A., & Cao, X. (2009). 'Should I tell my employer and coworkers I have arthritis'? A longitudinal examination of self-disclosure in the work place. *Arthritis and Rheumatism, 61*(12), 1753–1761. https://doi.org/10.1002/art.24889.

Gignac, M. A., Cao, X., & McAlpine, J. (2015). Availability, need for, and use of work accommodations and benefits: Are they related to employment outcomes in people with arthritis? *Arthritis care & Research, 67*(6), 855–864. https://doi.org/10.1002/acr.22508.

Gignac, M. A., Sutton, D., & Badley, E. M. (2007). Arthritis symptoms, the work environment, and the future: Measuring perceived job strain among employed persons with arthritis. *Arthritis and Rheumatism, 57*(5), 738–747. https://doi.org/10.1002/art.22788.

Gwee, K. A., Goh, V., Lima, G., & Setia, S. (2018). Coprescribing proton-pump inhibitors with nonsteroidal anti-inflammatory drugs: Risks versus benefits. *Journal of Pain Research, 11*, 361–374. https://doi.org/10.2147/JPR.S156938.

Hammond, A., Tennant, A., Ching, A., Parker, J., Prior, Y., Gignac, M. A. M., Verstappen, S. M. M., & O'Brien, R. (2023). Psychometric testing of the British-English Perceived Workplace Support Scale, Work Accommodations, Benefits, Policies and Practices Scale, and Work Transitions Index in four rheumatic and musculoskeletal conditions. *Musculoskeletal Care. 21*(4), 1261–1278. https://doi.org/10.1002/msc.

Landewé, R., Nurminen, T., Davies, O., & Baeten, D. (2018). A single determination of C-reactive protein does not suffice to declare a patient with a diagnosis of axial spondyloarthritis 'CRP-negative., *Arthritis Research & Therapy, 20*(1), 209. https://doi.org/10.1186/s13075-018-1707-8.

Li, X., Gignac, M. A., & Anis, A. H. (2006). Workplace, psychosocial factors, and depressive symptoms among working people with arthritis: A longitudinal study. *The Journal of Rheumatology, 33*(9), 1849–1855.

Pinto Carneiro, J. B., Pinto de Souza, T., Antunes de Oliveira, T. M. L., & Euzébio Ribeiro, S. L. (2017). Coexistence of spondyloarthritis and joint hypermobility syndrome: Rare or unknown association? *Reumatismo, 69*(3), 126–130. https://doi.org/10.4081/reumatismo.2017.993.

Prior, Y., Amanna, E. A., Bodell, S. J., & Hammond, A. (2015). A qualitative evaluation of occupational therapy-led work rehabilitation for people with inflammatory arthritis: Perspectives of therapists and their line managers. *The British Journal of Occupational Therapy, 78*(8), 467–474. https://doi.org/10.1177/0308022615581312.

Prochaska, J. O., & Norcross, J. C. (2002). Stages of Change. In J. C. Norcross (Ed.), *Psychotherapy relationships that work: Therapist contributions and responsiveness to patients* (pp. 303–313). Oxford University Press.

Restall, G., Egan, M., Valavaara, K., Phenix, A., & Sack, C. (2022). Canadian occupational therapy inter-relational practice process. In M. Egan, & G. Restall (Eds.), *Promoting occupational participation: Collaborative relationship-focused occupational therapy*. Canadian Association of Occupational Therapists.

ARTHUR: PROMOTING OCCUPATIONAL PARTICIPATION OF A PERSON WITH A LIFE-LIMITING ILLNESS

DANIEL LOWRIE

CHAPTER OUTLINE

This practice story is based around my time working with a 76-year-old male named Arthur. Arthur had a diagnosis of prostate cancer with bone metastases. My occupational therapy role involved coverage of an inpatient cancer care ward and shared responsibility of inpatient and community palliative care caseload. Minor features of this practice story have been altered to reflect contemporary practice contexts and to ensure anonymity.

PALLIATIVE CARE AND OCCUPATIONAL THERAPY

The World Health Organisation (2020) describes palliative care as an approach that improves the quality of life and prevents and reduces symptoms and complications experienced by people with life-threatening illness and their families. This is achieved through the early identification, correct assessment and treatment of pain and other problems, whether physical, psychosocial or spiritual and also encompasses the provision of support with practical needs and bereavement counselling. In doing so, palliative care offers a support system to help people live as well as possible until death.

Contemporary palliative care practice has its historical roots in the development of the modern hospice movement in the 1960s. The modern hospice movement arose out of concerns that the medicalisation of dying had resulted in it becoming 'gruesome, lonely, dehumanised and mechanical' (Kübler-Ross, 1977, p. 6) and hidden from the view of the majority of the population including, quite often, the individual who was dying (Glaser & Strauss, 1965, 1968). In response to this, the modern hospice movement set out to provide care that addressed individuals' psychosocial and spiritual needs as well as their physical symptoms (Saunders, 1965). To some extent, the modern hospice movement and, in turn, contemporary palliative care services have been successful in achieving these aims, with evidence suggesting that these services play a critical role in promoting improved end-of-life care outcomes among people with life-limiting illness and their caregivers (Higginson et al., 2011; Temel et al., 2010).

It should be noted, however, that although palliative care is recognised as a fundamental element of the human right to health, it is estimated that only 14% of people in need of palliative care go on to receive it (World Health Organisation, 2020). Access to formalised palliative care services varies markedly across the world, with unmet needs being particularly prominent in low- and middle-income countries (Sallnow et al., 2022; World Health Organisation, 2020). Furthermore, when it comes to the provision of care and support with end-of-life needs, many argue that only illness-related dying receives attention from healthcare services, resulting in considerable unmet needs among those dying as a result of poverty, dementia, incarceration or social conflict (Kellehear, 2009).

A common misconception about palliative care is that it is only provided to people in the last days and weeks of life. Although palliative care services frequently do provide support to people during these latter phases of dying, their involvement with people with life-limiting illness[1] will often commence months or even years before this time. Improvements in medical management of dying mean that people live with a dying diagnosis[2] for considerably longer than in historical times (Ashby, 2009). In many ways, this lengthening of life might be regarded as a positive outcome. However, the opportunities stemming from the lengthening of life are also accompanied by challenges associated with the protracted period of time in which an individual is living with a dying diagnosis.

During this time, for example, people with life-limiting illness often seek to maintain valued roles and occupations but can find it increasingly difficult to do so due to the progression of symptoms and loss of function. On top of this, people who are dying (and their families) find themselves needing to navigate the complex interface between the dual states of 'living while dying' and 'dying while living'. Sometimes,

this involves a focus on living, founded on a desire for normalcy and stability during a time of significant physical, psychosocial and spiritual change. At other times, practical, personal and relational features of the dying role may be prioritised so as to enable preparation for death (Brose et al., 2023; Bye, 1998; Hammill et al., 2019; Jacques & Hasselkus, 2004; Lowrie et al., 2019; Park Lala & Kinsella, 2011). In the face of this complexity, there is a need to ensure, in so far as is possible, that people with life-limiting illness and those who matter to them are supported in spending their time in a way that meaningfully reflects their dynamic and evolving goals, aspirations and needs. If practised well, occupational therapy can play an important part in achieving this end (Mills & Payne, 2015).

The scope of occupational therapy in palliative care is broad. Position statements on occupational therapy in palliative and end-of-life care from the World Federation of Occupational Therapy and professional occupational therapy associations in the USA, Canada and Australia collectively detail a wide range of roles including optimising quality of life, promoting occupational performance and adaptation in valued occupational roles, supporting capacity to attend to affairs and develop legacy, assisting in symptom management, assisting people with life-limiting illness to remain in their preferred place of care, providing expert assessment and intervention to ensure safety and participation within the home and community and providing support and education to informal caregivers. Importantly, these documents discuss the occupational therapy role as extending to the support of persons with life-limiting illness as well as their family and friends in a manner that attends to their needs and respects the autonomy of all parties (American Occupational Therapy Association, 2016; Canadian Occupational Therapy Association, 2017; Occupational Therapy Australia, 2015; World Federation of Occupational Therapy, 2016).

Despite the potential scope and value of occupational therapy in palliative and end-of-life care, questions have been raised as to the extent to which practice in this field genuinely aligns with the occupational philosophy underpinning the profession. Keesing and Rosenwax (2011) identified a range of structural barriers that compromise the fulfilment of occupation-centred practice in palliative care, including the misunderstanding of the occupational therapy role, workload

---

[1] The term 'person with a life-limiting illness' has been used in this chapter to refer to individuals who have been diagnosed with an incurable illness that they are likely to die of at some point in the future.

[2] The phrase 'dying diagnosis' has been included to reflect the complicated experience of living with a life-limiting illness while also managing the emotional and social responses that often accompany the dying status.

pressures, late and/or reactive referrals and the dominance of the medical model within acute-care settings. They found that these barriers contributed to missed opportunities to meaningfully address important end-of-life occupational issues such as role loss and role change, occupational deprivation and role imbalance and isolation among caregivers. More recent literature has echoed these findings, arguing that a lack of occupational orientation in palliative care occupational therapy can compromise the opportunities for people with life-limiting illness to engage in meaningful experiences in the time left available to them (Mills & Payne, 2015).

To a large extent, these concerns regarding unfulfilled occupational therapy potential in palliative care are justified. Qualitative research exploring occupation at end-of-life has found it to yield numerous benefits. For example, occupation can provide a medium to nurture existential reflection, support the enrichment of relationships, enable end-of-life preparations, accommodate adaptation to change, assert normality and enhance a person with life-limiting illness' sense of normality and self-worth (Brose et al., 2023; Jacques & Hasselkus, 2004; Lyons et al., 2002; Park Lala & Kinsella, 2011; Svidén et al., 2010). It follows, therefore, that failure to adequately consider and support occupational engagement in palliative and end-of-life care can result in considerable unmet need and, arguably, potential harm.

However, in evaluating these practice limitations, it is important that the role of occupational therapy in undertaking activities that, at face value, may not seem occupationally rich (such as discharge planning and assistive technology prescription) are not inadvertently undervalued. Helping people to return to and remain in their homes matters. For many people, home serves as the foundation for their most valued occupational roles and routines. It can be a place where habitual patterns of behaviour within a familiar environment become slowly etched into an individual's sense of being and, in doing so, shape the meaning attached to an individual's occupational roles and relationships. Indeed, it is common for simple and seemingly mundane occupations to be highly valued by people with life-limiting illness, due to the sense of connection, familiarity and competence that accompanies them (Park Lala & Kinsella, 2011; Svidén et al., 2010).

Occupational therapists may not always see the broader occupational value of the efforts that they make towards assisting a person with life-limiting illness to return home in a timely and safe manner. However, just because these benefits are unseen does not mean that they do not occur. As such, quality occupational therapy in palliative and end-of-life care can take many forms. Sometimes, this will involve actions that seem occupationally rich, with a clear orientation towards meaning making. At other times, an occupational therapist's input might centre around efforts to assist a person with life-limiting illness to be in a place where they feel safe and supported, thereby nurturing the foundational conditions needed for occupational engagement. Provided they are undertaken well, both of these forms of practice may be of considerable value to people with life-limiting illness.

CONNECT

My practice with Arthur began with the receipt of an urgent phone call referral from the hospital radiation therapy department. The radiation therapist requested assessment of Arthur due to difficulties in safely transferring him from a hospital bed to a wheelchair as needed to transport him for his treatment.

In palliative care practice, it is very important that occupational therapists take the time to ensure they develop a solid background understanding of an individual's medical condition, past and current treatments, likely prognosis and social situation prior to their first meeting with them. This ensures that the occupational therapist is well prepared for the initial conversations and reduces the need for the individual and/or their caregivers to repeat information unnecessarily. Unfortunately, due to the urgent nature of this referral, I was not afforded the opportunity to prepare myself for my meeting with Arthur in the way that I normally would. Having received the referral, a physiotherapy colleague and I attended the radiation therapy department to assist. A review of Arthur's notes indicated that he had a recent diagnosis of prostate cancer with bone metastases. Prostate cancer is the second most diagnosed form of cancer among males and is also the fifth leading cause of death from cancer in males (Ferlay et al., 2015). Arthur was attending the hospital for a course of external beam radiation therapy. This is a form of cancer treatment that kills cancer cells by delivering a controlled dose of radiation that destroys genetic material needed for cell division (Roy & Spratt, 2022).

In a discussion with the radiation therapists, we were told that Arthur had stated that he needed to use the toilet but, when trying to get out of bed, had been in a lot of pain and was not able to safely stand. We then proceeded to assess Arthur's transfers. On our arrival, we found Arthur sat on the edge of his bed using his upper limbs to support himself in the seated position. We asked Arthur about his recent mobility, and he indicated that he had been experiencing some numbness and mild weakness in his lower limbs over recent days accompanied by pain around his lumbar region. Arthur stated that the pain and weakness had increased over recent hours such that he was now unable to stand. He said that he had assumed that these symptoms had occurred because of his treatment. Based on Arthur's physical presentation and reports of his recent symptoms, both the physiotherapist and I became concerned that Arthur might be experiencing metastatic spinal cord compression (MSCC).

Metastases to the spine are thought to occur in approximately 3 to 5% of people with cancer but are more common in prostate, breast and lung cancer, with incidence as high as 15% to 20% among these diagnostic groups (National Institute for Health and Care Excellence, 2008). MSCC is a complication that can occur due to pathological vertebral body collapse or tumour growth that causes compression of the spinal cord or cauda equina, leading to irreversible neurological damage such as paraplegia or tetraplegia (Al-Qurainy & Collis, 2016). MSCC is an oncological emergency and, once suspected, urgent action needs to be taken to minimise weight-bearing through the spine by lying the individual flat (or with partial elevation) in a supine position if symptoms allow until formal diagnostic assessment of spinal stability can be completed (National Institute for Health and Care Excellence, 2023).

The physiotherapist and I carefully transferred Arthur into a supine position on his bed. We asked him to remain in this position until further assessment of his spine could be completed, indicating that we were concerned about his spinal stability. We also stated that we needed to speak with his treating medical team

so that further assessment could be organised. We arranged an urgent conversation with the radiation oncologist who was overseeing Arthur's care. In this conversation, we discussed Arthur's presenting symptoms and expressed concern that he may be experiencing MSCC. The radiation oncologist agreed with this concern and arranged an medical resonance imaging (MRI) of Arthur's spine. This investigation revealed widespread lumbosacral metastases that had resulted in vertebral body collapse and MSCC.

Arthur was informed of his diagnosis of MSCC in a meeting with his radiation oncologists at which I was not present. In this meeting, his treating team discussed that the extent of his disease progression meant his prostate cancer had advanced further than they thought and suggested that his expected prognosis was approximately 6 months. This is profoundly challenging news to come to terms with, particularly when coupled with the prospect of permanent and sudden disability resulting from MSCC (Eva, 2009). Essentially, Arthur was confronted simultaneously with both a dying diagnosis and the likelihood of paraplegia. Evidence suggests that people with MSCC and their families often experience considerable distress associated with the rapid loss of mobility and independence associated with the condition, with this distress further compounded by the uncertainty about their future (Eva, 2009; Warnock & Tod, 2014). Arthur's treating team assessed surgical intervention to be inappropriate based on the extent and nature of his disease progression. They recommended Arthur undergo five fractions of radiation therapy and a course of corticosteroids (oral dexamethasone) with the aim of reducing his neurological symptoms, inflammation and pain. With Arthur's consent, they also referred him to the specialist palliative care team.

Seek Understanding and Define Purpose

As Arthur's occupational therapist, it was important that I remained mindful of the impact that the news of his disease progression, prognosis and functional and occupational changes may have had upon him. Moreover, I also needed to be cognisant of the fact that my only interaction with Arthur up to this point had been brief and, most likely, challenging for him. In my next meeting with Arthur, I made sure that I was well prepared and had ample time available to spend with him. I reintroduced myself and explained the purpose and function of my professional role as an occupational therapist, particularly in relation to enabling his safe return home and in working with him towards the attainment of his occupational goals. I also took time to find out a little more about his life history and current priorities. In this conversation, I learned that Arthur lived, with his wife, in a town approximately 10 kilometres away from the hospital in which he was being treated. Arthur had an adult daughter who had two young children (Arthur's grandchildren). Family seemed very important to Arthur and returning home was a high priority for him. Arthur went on to tell me about his professional history. Although he had been retired for almost ten years, Arthur had worked as a university lecturer for much of his career. When Arthur was speaking with me about this, I garnered a sense that he felt it helpful to project this part of his identity as a means of countering the near-constant focus upon his medical and functional deterioration that he had experienced over recent days. In essence, he was resisting an unwanted focus upon a dying identity and dying roles (Lowrie, 2020). I took time to listen to Arthur's stories of his working life. Doing so came from a genuine interest in Arthur as a person as well as my recognition that speaking about his past was an important element of Arthur's efforts to reconcile his present circumstances.

During our conversation, I asked Arthur about his understanding of his condition and the impact on him. It was clear in his response that Arthur was not ready to accept any suggestion that the functional losses he had experienced over recent days might be permanent. This is neither atypical nor unreasonable. Although the likelihood of achieving the functional return needed to walk or complete standing transfers was low, it remained a possibility at this point. Evidence suggests that, although improvements in performance status in people in palliative care tend to be rare, variability around recovery exists and, hence, premature assumptions about likely rehabilitation outcomes can be problematic (Runacres et al., 2016). Furthermore, even if improvements in mobility were not to occur, it is common for people with MSCC to retain a positive outlook on their likely functional recovery and ability to cope (Warnock & Tod, 2014). In her study of the constructions of disability among people with MSCC,

Eva (2009) describes what, at face value, appears to be inconsistent attitudes towards recovery, whereby individuals resisted the idea of themselves as disabled while also acknowledging a future need to accommodate changed circumstances. Individuals managed the tension between these two positions through a process of 'twin-tracking' whereby they gradually adjusted to change while asserting normality where possible, thereby allowing the gradual reordering and restructuring of their lives (Eva, 2009, p. 134).

The lessons from this research are important for occupational therapists working in palliative care settings. My clinical experience in working with people with MSCC made me aware that Arthur was unlikely to regain the ability to ambulate. However, Arthur was not at a point at which he recognised this for himself. Although initiating processes towards enabling Arthur to return home was important at this stage, it was also critical that any conversations or planning that I engaged in did not disrupt Arthur's sense of identity. Hence, I aimed to approach discussions with Arthur honestly but tentatively in a way that promoted his hope and positive perception of self, while also looking ahead towards his future goals and likely needs. This can be a difficult balance to strike and only Arthur would know the extent to which I managed this in a way that reflected his evolving wishes and priorities. For my part, I tried to remain reflectively aware of the importance of carefully considered communication and endeavoured, where possible, to ensure that all conversations were collaborative and constructive.

Adjusting to a dying diagnosis can be difficult for many individuals. This is, perhaps, not surprising when consideration is given to the social expectations that surround illness roles, particularly for those with a cancer diagnosis. Societal discourse and associated expectations surrounding cancer and its treatment are often marked by the need for an individual to battle and fight against the disease, with this fight framed as a form of heroic struggle (Seale, 2001). Paradoxically, however, once a dying diagnosis is confirmed, expectations of the individual rapidly shift from the need to fight or battle a disease to the need to come to a place of acceptance and peace with their dying status (Zimmerman, 2012). Sometimes, when this does not occur, well-meaning health professionals respond to this perceived 'denial of death' with attempts to gently cajole the individual towards a state of acceptance (Li & Arbor, 2006). This can be problematic as it imposes a somewhat homogenised perspective of 'the good death' upon the dying person and restricts their opportunity to adjust to change in a manner and pace that best reflects their individual circumstances and preferences.

EXPLORE OCCUPATIONAL PARTICIPATION

Arthur's main goal at this time was to continue to work towards independence in standing, standing transfers and walking. The first step required careful assessment of graded sitting (by gradually elevating the head of Arthur's hospital bed) so as to monitor his neurological symptoms and pain (National Institute for Health and Care Excellence, 2023). Once this assessment was safely completed, Arthur was assisted to sit on the edge of his bed by supporting himself with his upper limbs. Arthur had very limited lower limb power which was assessed as being between 1 and 2 out of 5 on the Oxford grading scale in various muscle groups (Clarkson, 2000). Although he remained focused on the goals of standing and walking, Arthur was willing to be provided with a wheelchair to assist with his mobility and a pressure cushion to reduce the likelihood of pressure sore development. When setting Arthur up with this equipment, I advised him of the critical importance of performing pressure-relieving manoeuvres or weight shifts approximately every 20 minutes to relieve pressure through his ischial tuberosities, sacrum/coccyx and greater trochanters (Bae et al., 2022; Sprigle et al., 2019).

Despite experiencing weakness and fatigue resulting from his condition and treatment, Arthur was able to slowly self-propel in his wheelchair independently for short distances. Due to his lack of lower limb power, a decision was made not to pursue sliding board transfers with Arthur due to the risk of falls and overall physical burden upon him. This meant that Arthur needed to be hoisted in and out of his bed to a wheelchair, wheeled shower commode or high-backed armchair on the ward. The physiotherapist continued to work with Arthur over several days on improving his bed mobility and sitting balance, while monitoring for signs of functional return in his lower limbs. I

periodically assisted with these sessions and also spent time with Arthur on increasing his confidence and tolerance in wheelchair use. This time was valuable for a few reasons. Firstly, and most obviously, safety and independence in bed and wheelchair mobility would be important for Arthur's future return home. Secondly, Arthur was motivated to participate in this rehabilitation and his continued engagement will have assisted in curtailing deconditioning and associated functional decline (Bae et al., 2022). Furthermore, continued engagement in occupations of importance to individuals with life-threatening illness is known to promote a feeling of competence and self-worth, while also supporting a graded adjustment to change (Lyons et al., 2002; Svidén et al., 2010). Finally, working with Arthur towards his rehabilitation goals helped his physiotherapist and me to better understand his priorities, motivations and likely needs, while establishing a sense of partnership and trust in his ongoing therapeutic relationship with us. We worked with Arthur in this way over three weeks. Unfortunately, however, his power and control in his lower limbs did not improve during this time.

With the realisation that Arthur's goals of returning to standing and walking were now likely to be unachievable, an important conversation to inform him of our concerns became necessary. Although Arthur might have had insight into his lack of progress in this area, having this confirmed by his physiotherapist accompanied by the suggestion that no further gains were likely to be made, seemed hard for him to accept. Therapists in these situations find themselves in ethically challenging territory. Veracity is needed when working with individuals like Arthur so that they can consolidate plans for return home (or elsewhere) against the backdrop of a relatively short prognosis. However, communicating news of this nature can lead to a degree of distress and, in some instances, be viewed as taking hope away from the individual in question. I spent time with Arthur after this conversation to answer questions that he had and listen to his fears and concerns. During this discussion, I asked Arthur whether he would like me to arrange a psychologist or counsellor to speak with him; however, he did not wish to pursue this referral. In partnership with the physiotherapist, we agreed to continue with rehabilitation efforts as we had been doing over recent weeks while also advancing plans for home. As part of this plan, we suggested arranging a family meeting to discuss next steps. Arthur was agreeable to this idea.

CO-DESIGN PRIORITIES, GOALS, OUTCOMES AND PLANS

Family meetings in palliative care can be valuable in facilitating important discussions with people with life-limiting illness and their caregivers and offer a forum through which they can share their care preferences, future goals, values and concerns. Such discussions can help in promoting consensus, reducing caregiver stress, identifying unmet needs and directing future plans concerning community care (Hudson et al., 2009). Family meetings in palliative care are often attended by a range of health professionals, although consideration should be given to which professionals need to attend in order to prevent unintentionally presenting a professional power imbalance. Family meetings should not only be well organised but also run flexibly to ensure that the thoughts, goals and questions of the person with life-limiting illness and those they have invited to attend can be adequately heard and addressed (Glajchen et al., 2022).

Arthur's family meeting was attended by his wife (Jane) and his daughter (Kyla). The meeting was chaired by Arthur's palliative care consultant. A range of useful, contemporary guidelines exist to support the structure of family meetings (see, for example, Widera et al. [2020]). Arthur's family meeting followed a similar broad format in which all attendees introduced themselves and briefly explained their roles. The palliative care consultant then asked Arthur and his family to describe their understanding of Arthur's illness and prognosis and provided an opportunity for them to ask questions about this. As had been the case with Arthur, it was evident that news of Arthur's prognosis and likely limited functional recovery were difficult to process for his family. Arthur became visibly upset during this discussion as did his wife. Arthur spoke of his professional and academic achievements in his life and stated he could not believe that his life had been reduced to what it had now become.

The meeting then progressed to a phase of planning, whereby next steps could be collaboratively discussed and agreed upon. Arthur expressed a clear wish

to return home. Jane indicated that she was supportive of this wish. Kyla also expressed in principle support but expressed concern about how her parents would manage at home. As Arthur's occupational therapist, I agreed to explore these concerns further and collaborate with Arthur and his family on co-designing a plan of action. After the family meeting, I spoke to Arthur and Jane and discussed the possibility of undertaking an access visit to their home. They both thought that this would be a good idea, so I arranged for a visit to occur the next day, with Jane in attendance.

This visit proved to be very useful. Although I had gathered information about Arthur's home setup in early conversations with him, having the ability to see his home helped to better understand his likely needs. Arthur had a small step on the entrance to his home, which I ascertained could be managed through the provision of a portable wheelchair threshold ramp. The inside of the house was spacious, and there was level access to all rooms, as needed to accommodate a self-propelled wheelchair. There was also sufficient space in the living room to place a high-backed armchair and good turning space for a mobile hoist.

Based on Arthur's description of his home, I had concerns about potential problems with his bedroom setup. Unfortunately, these concerns proved to be well founded. I knew that Arthur's bedroom would require a minimum turning circle of approximately 1.2 m^2 to allow for safe hoist transfers between his bed and a wheelchair or wheeled toilet and shower commode (Australian Building Codes Board, 2019). This space was not available. Jane identified that there was a spare bedroom that she and her daughter could empty that would offer more room for hoist transfers. I measured this room and determined that it would be large enough for safe hoist transfers to occur. However, this would also mean that Arthur could no longer sleep in his own bedroom. Recommending a change of this nature needs to be approached with caution. I knew that Arthur wanted to return home; however, altering the room and bed in which he sleeps might inadvertently change the meaning of home to him and/or alter the nature of his relationship with his wife (Lowrie, 2020; Morgan et al., 2022). It later turned out, though, that Arthur was willing for this change of bedroom to occur if it meant a return home was possible. This averted a potential challenge to our plans.

Arthur's bathroom was large with good access to the toilet for his wheeled toilet and shower commode. Access to the shower was level but hindered by a screen door that would most likely need to be removed. I was concerned that arranging for this to occur might result in a significant delay to Arthur's return home. However, when I discussed this concern, Jane informed me that their neighbour was a self-described handyman and might be able to assist.

TRIAL THE PLAN, EXPLORE CHANGE AND REFINE THE PLAN

With the home visit complete, I discussed the findings and various recommendations with Arthur and Jane, both of whom were keen to proceed. I was able to arrange the required assistive technology via a local equipment supplier using a palliative care equipment hire scheme. This funding scheme had been established to ensure rapid access to assistive technology provision so as to enable timely discharge home for people with life-limiting illness. The assistive technology that I ordered included a hospital bed and pressure mattress, over bed table, self-propelled wheelchair and pressure cushion, mobile hoist, high-backed armchair, wheeled toilet and shower commode and portable threshold ramp. The hospital social worker arranged community carers to visit twice daily to assist with hoisting Arthur into and out of bed and to help in managing his toileting and showering.

The assistive technology (mentioned above) was delivered approximately a week later. I made another visit to Arthur's home to check on the setup and provide education to Jane and Kyla on safe use of the mobile hoist and other items of equipment. I was pleased to find that Arthur's neighbour had removed the shower screen and also installed a shower curtain in its place. Jane told me that when she spoke with her neighbour and his wife about the need for modifications in the bathroom, they had been more than happy to help. Beyond this, they had offered to sit with Arthur during the times when Jane needed to leave the house for shopping or other administrative tasks and also to assist with other jobs such as mowing the lawn or managing the garden.

Arthur's neighbours' actions proved to be a highly valuable part of his successful return home. They also reflect what can be a crucial, and often missing, element of end-of-life care, namely the involvement of the community. In recent times, there has been a growing push towards the engagement of 'compassionate communities' in the care and support of people with life-limiting illness and their caregivers. Proponents of the 'compassionate communities' movement argue that the involvement of informal networks of community care (such as neighbours, friends and others) benefits people with life-limiting illness and their caregivers as well as the community itself (Abel, 2018; Aoun et al., 2022; Kellehear, 2013). Given the statistics cited earlier in this chapter concerning global unmet need in palliative care, this argument seems to have considerable merit. Certainly, for Arthur and Jane, the involvement of their neighbours made a significant difference in assisting Arthur to remain at home during his last months of life.

Arthur returned home via ambulance a few days later. I visited Arthur and Jane again to check that the environment setup remained suitable and that no unexpected difficulties had arisen. When discussing this with Arthur something seemed wrong. When I asked him about this, he revealed to me that although the home setup was generally good, prior to his admission to hospital he had spent most of each day sitting in his shed at the back of his yard where he would smoke his pipe and read or paint. He further stated that he would like to start doing this again and, in particular, wanted to paint a picture to give to his grandchildren to remember him by. This was clearly an important request. I was aware that, for many people, the creation and/or passing on of artefacts to future generations is an important part of the transmission of self and nurturing of legacy at end-of-life (Hunter, 2008; Pollard, 2006). This left me with a challenging situation. Due to their being a small step into his shed, accessing this environment would require another portable threshold ramp. Furthermore, in order to paint, Arthur would likely need a tiltable wheelchair tray table so as to prevent him from having to lean forward to a canvas and risk losing balance in his chair. Although spending time in his preferred outdoors environment and creating an artistic work of legacy were undoubtedly worthy occupational goals (Jacques & Hasselkus, 2004), I was concerned that based on the established funding criteria, if I were to request provision of these items, there was a solid chance that my application would be refused. I decided to pursue the application anyway. I framed my argument transparently and honestly, pointing out that provision of these items, although not essential, would make a major difference to Arthur's quality of life. The application for the portable threshold ramp was approved but, unfortunately, the tiltable wheelchair tray was declined. I phoned Arthur to let him know. Although he was disappointed, he told me that his neighbour had already suggested to him that he might be able to make him an easel that could be positioned over his wheelchair and that he would now pursue this option. I felt very pleased to hear this news, knowing how important the painting seemed to be to Arthur.

PLAN FOR TRANSITION

The application and subsequent installation of the ramp into Arthur's shed constituted my last point of contact with Arthur. Arthur remained at home for a few months before his condition further deteriorated, and he was admitted to the palliative care centre for end-of-life care. I was on leave at the time when Arthur was admitted and, therefore, did not have an opportunity to see him in his last days. A curious feature of palliative care occupational therapy is that the individuals whom occupational therapists work with will often remain on their caseloads up until (and sometimes beyond) the point of their death. Hence, although much of the professional role of palliative care occupational therapists involve assisting a person with life-limiting illness and their caregivers in planning for and managing life's final transition, a formal transition out of the occupational therapy service often does not occur until after the person has died.

Due to the fact that I was on leave at the time of Arthur's death, a colleague arranged collection of Arthur's assistive technology on my behalf. I did see Jane again a few months later, when she was attending the hospital to visit a friend. I spoke to her briefly and expressed my condolences. Jane indicated that the last few months had been hard but, with the support of family, she was slowly starting to make sense of life without Arthur. She had been offered bereavement support from the palliative care team but decided to decline the offer. I took comfort in hearing that Jane

was starting to do okay but recognised that grief can be as unpredictable as it is unique (Kübler-Ross & Kessler, 2005).

I chose not to ask Jane whether Arthur completed the painting for his grandchildren or whether the time spent at home and in his shed had been as meaningful to him as he had wished. For my part I hope that it was and that his final months of life were both manageable and rewarding. I enjoyed working with both Arthur and Jane and felt proud of the sense of connection that we managed to achieve through a very difficult time in their lives. For some palliative care therapists, reflecting on the relationships and connections that they establish with a person with life-limiting illness with whom they work can play an important role in supporting closure and managing professional grief (Treggalles & Lowrie, 2018). I find that this is often the case for me. Indeed, it is the capacity to make such connections with people and assist them at a very precious time of their lives that makes palliative care occupational therapy such a rewarding field of practise. It is a privilege to be able to play a part, however small, in contributing to the sense of manageability and meaningfulness of someone's end-of-life journey. I hope that my part in Arthur's journey helped in achieving this end.

REFERENCES

Abel, J. (2018). Compassionate communities and end-of-life care. *Clinical Medicine (London, England), 18*(1), 6–8. https://doi.org/10.7861/clinmedicine.18-1-6.

Al-Qurainy, R., & Collis, E. (2016). Metastatic spinal cord compression: Diagnosis and management. *British Medical Journal, 353*, i2539. https://doi.org/10.1136/bmj.i2539.

American Occupational Therapy Association. (2016). The role of occupational therapy in end-of-life care. *American Journal of Occupational Therapy, 70*, 1–12. http://dx.doi.org/10.5014/ajot.2017.706S2RACCreview.

Aoun, S. M., Richmond, R., Gunton, K., Noonan, K., Abel, J., & Rumbold, B. (2022). The compassionate communities connectors model for end-of-life care: Implementation and evaluation. *Palliative Care and Social Practice, 16*. 26323524221139655. https://doi.org/10.1177/26323524221139655.

Ashby, M. (2009). The dying human: A perspective from palliative medicine. In A. Kellehear (Ed.), *The study of dying: From autonomy to transformation*. Cambridge University Press.

Australian Building Codes Board. (2019). National construction code. In *Volume 1, amendment 1: Specification F2.9 Accessible adult change facilities*. Australian Building Codes Board. https://ncc.abcb.gov.au/editions/2019-a1/ncc-2019-volume-one-amendment-1/section-f-health-and-amenity/specification-f29.

Bae, C. R., Gelvosa, M. N., & Jeon, J. Y. (2022). Rehabilitation in advanced cancer patients with bone metastases and neural compromise: Current status and future directions. *Current Oncology Reports, 24*(8), 1023–1033. https://doi.org/10.1007/s11912-022-01229-9.

Brose, J. M., Willis, E., & Morgan, D. D. (2023). The intentional pursuit of everyday life while dying: A longitudinal qualitative study of working-aged adults living with advanced cancer. *Palliative Medicine, 37*(8), 1210–1221. https://doi.org/10.1177/02692163231180911.

Bye, R. A. (1998). When clients are dying: Occupational therapists' perspectives. *The Occupational Therapy Journal of Research, 18*(1), 3–24.

Canadian Occupational Therapy Association. (2017). CAOT Position statement: Occupational therapy and end-of-life care. https://caot.ca/document/6130/PS_EndofLife.pdf.

Clarkson, H. M. (2000). *Musculoskeletal assessment: Joint range of motion and manual muscle strength.* Lippincott Williams & Wilkins.

Eva, G., Paley, J., Miller, M., & Wee, B. (2009). Patients' constructions of disability in metastatic spinal cord compression. *Palliative Medicine, 23*(2), 132–140. https://doi.org/10.1177/0269216308099959.

Ferlay, J., Ferlay, J., Soerjomataram, I., Dikshit, R., Eser, S., Mathers, C., Rebelo, M., Parkin, D. M., Forman, D., & Bray, F. (2015). Cancer incidence and mortality worldwide: Sources, methods and major patterns in GLOBOCAN 2012. *International Journal of Cancer, 136*(5), E359–E386. https://doi.org/10.1002/ijc.29210.

Glajchen, M., Goehring, A., Johns, H., & Portenoy, R. K. (2022). Family meetings in palliative care: Benefits and barriers. *Current Treatment Options in Oncology, 23*(5), 658–667. https://doi.org/10.1007/s11864-022-00957-1.

Glaser, B. G., & Strauss, A. L. (1965). *Awareness of dying.* Aldine Transaction.

Glaser, B. G., & Strauss, A. L. (1968). *Time for dying.* Aldine Transaction.

Hammill, K., Bye, R., & Cook, C. (2019). Occupational engagement of people living with a life-limiting illness: Occupational therapists' perceptions. *Australian Occupational Therapy Journal, 66*(2), 145–153. https://doi.org/10.1111/1440-1630.12557.

Higginson, I. J., Costantini, M., Silber, E., Burman, R., & Edmonds, P. (2011). Evaluation of a new model of short-term palliative care for people severely affected with multiple sclerosis: A randomised fast-track trial to test timing of referral and how long the effect is maintained. *Postgraduate Medical Journal, 87*(1033), 769–775. https://doi.org/10.1136/postgradmedj-2011-130290.

Hudson, P., Thomas, T., Quinn, K., & Aranda, S. (2009). Family meetings in palliative care: Are they effective? *Palliative Medicine, 23*(2), 150–157. https://doi.org/10.1177/0269216308099960.

Hunter, E. G. (2008). Legacy: The occupational transmission of self through actions and artifacts. *Journal of Occupational Science, 15*(1), 48–54. https://doi.org/10.1080/14427591.2008.9686607.

Jacques, N. D., & Hasselkus, B. R. (2004). The nature of occupation surrounding dying and death. *OTJR: Occupational Therapy Journal of Research, 24*(2), 44–53. https://doi.org/10.1177/153944920402400202.

Keesing, S., & Rosenwax, L. (2011). Is occupation missing from occupational therapy in palliative care? *Australian Occupational Therapy Journal, 58*(5), 329–336. https://doi.org/10.1111/j.1440-1630.2011.00958.x.

Kellehear, A. (2009). *The study of dying: From autonomy to transformation.* Cambridge University Press.

Kellehear, A. (2013). Compassionate communities: End-of-life care as everyone's responsibility. *QJM: Monthly Journal of the Association of Physicians, 106*(12), 1071–1075. https://doi.org/10.1093/qjmed/hct200.

Kübler-Ross, E. (1977). *On death and dying.* Tavistock Pub.

Kübler-Ross, E., & Kessler, D. (2005). *On grief and grieving: Finding the meaning of grief through the five stages of loss.* Scribner.

Li, S., & Arber, A. (2006). The construction of troubled and credible patients: A study of emotion talk in palliative care settings. *Qualitative Health Research, 16*(1), 27–46. https://doi.org/10.1177/1049732305284022.

Lowrie, D. (2020). *An examination of role change at end of life in a contemporary, regional Australian context.* Doctoral dissertation. James Cook University.

Lowrie, D., Ray, R., Plummer, D., & Yau, M. (2019). Examining the transitions between living and dying roles at end-of-life. *Death Studies, 43*(10), 601–610. https://doi.org/10.1080/07481187.2018.1504836.

Lyons, M., Orozovic, N., Davis, J., & Newman, J. (2002). Doing-being-becoming: Occupational experiences of persons with life-threatening illnesses. *The American Journal of Occupational Therapy, 56*(3), 285–295. https://doi.org/10.5014/ajot.56.3.285.

Mills, K., & Payne, A. (2015). Enabling occupation at the end of life: A literature review. *Palliative & Supportive Care, 13*(6), 1755–1769. https://doi.org/10.1017/S1478951515000772.

Morgan, D. D., Willis, E., Sweet, K., Roe, P., Rabaçal, J., & Currow, D. C. (2022). The Complexities of prescribing assistive equipment at the end of life–Patient and caregivers' perspectives. *Healthcare (Basel), 10*(6), 1005. https://doi.org/10.3390/healthcare10061005.

National Institute for Health and Care Excellence. (2008). *Metastatic spinal cord compression: Diagnosis and management of patients at risk of or with metastatic spinal cord compression.* Full guideline. www.nice.org.uk/guidance/cg75/evidence/full-guideline-242052589.

National Institute for Health and Care Excellence. (2023). *Spinal metastases and metastatic spinal cord compression.* National Institute for Health and Care Excellence. https://www.nice.org.uk/guidance/ng234.

Occupational Therapy Australia. (2015). *Position paper: Occupational therapy in palliative care.* Occupational Therapy Australia. https://otaus.com.au/publicassets/6d5829df-2503-e911-a2c2-b75c2fd918c5/Occupational%20Therapy%20and%20Palliative%20Care%20(August%202015).pdf.

Park Lala, A., & Kinsella, E. A. (2011). A phenomenological inquiry into the embodied nature of occupation at end of life. *Canadian Journal of Occupational Therapy (1939), 78*(4), 246–254. https://doi.org/10.2182/cjot.2011.78.4.6.

Pollard, N. (2006). JOS comment: Is dying an occupation? *Journal of Occupational Science, 13*(2–3), 149–152. https://doi.org/10.1080/14427591.2006.9726508.

Roy, S., & Spratt, D. E. (2022). Radiotherapy for advanced prostate cancer. In K. L. Stratton, & A. K. Morgans (Eds.), *Urologic oncology.* Springer.

Runacres, F., Gregory, H., & Ugalde, A. (2016). Restorative care for palliative patients: A retrospective clinical audit of outcomes for patients admitted to an inpatient palliative care unit. *BMJ Supportive & Palliative Care, 6*(1), 97–100. https://doi.org/10.1136/bmjspcare-2014-000774.

Sallnow, L., Smith, R., Ahmedzai, S. H., Bhadelia, A., Chamberlain, C., Cong, Y., Doble, B., Dullie, L., Durie, R., Finkelstein, E. A., Guglani, S., Hodson, M., Husebø, B. S., Kellehear, A., Kitzinger, C., Knaul, F. M., Murray, S. A., Neuberger, J., O'Mahony, S., … Wyatt, K. (2022). Report of the *Lancet* commission on the value of death: Bringing death back into life. *The Lancet (British Edition), 399*(10327), 837–884. https://doi.org/10.1016/S0140-6736(21)02314-X.

Saunders, C. (1965). The last stages of life. *The American Journal of Nursing, 65*(3), 70–75. https://doi.org/10.1097/00000446-196503000-00026.

Seale, C. (2001). Sporting cancer: Struggle language in news reports of people with cancer. *Sociology of Health & Illness, 23*(3), 308–329. https://doi.org/10.1111/1467-9566.00254.

Sprigle, S., Sonenblum, S. E., & Feng, C. (2019). Pressure redistributing in-seat movement activities by persons with spinal cord injury over multiple epochs. *PloS One, 14*(2), e0210978. https://doi.org/10.1371/journal.pone.0210978.

Svidén, G. A., Tham, K., & Borell, L. (2010). Involvement in everyday life for people with a life threatening illness. *Palliative & Supportive Care, 8*(3), 345–352. https://doi.org/10.1017/S1478951510000143.

Temel, J. S., Greer, J. A., Muzikansky, A., Gallagher, E. R., Admane, S., Jackson, V. A., Dahlin, C. M., Blinderman, C. D., Jacobsen, J.,

Pirl, W. F., Billings, J. A., & Lynch, T. J. (2010). Early palliative care for patients with metastatic non–small-cell lung cancer. *The New England Journal of Medicine, 363*(150), 733–742. https://doi.org/10.1056/NEJMoa1000678.

Treggalles, K., & Lowrie, D. (2018). An exploration of the lived experience of professional grief among occupational therapists working in palliative care settings. *Australian Occupational Therapy Journal, 65*(4), 329–337. https://doi.org/10.1111/1440-1630.12477.

Warnock, C., & Tod, A. (2014). A descriptive exploration of the experiences of patients with significant functional impairment following a recent diagnosis of metastatic spinal cord compression. *Journal of Advanced Nursing, 70*(3), 564–574. https://doi.org/10.1111/jan.12215.

Widera, E., Anderson, W. G., Santhosh, L., McKee, K. Y., Smith, A. K., & Frank, J. (2020). Family meetings on behalf of patients with serious illness. *New England Journal of Medicine, 383*(11), e71. https://doi.org/10.1056/NEJMvcm1913056.

World Federation of Occupational Therapy. (2016). Occupational therapy in end-of-life care. https://wfot.org/resources/occupational-therapy-in-end-of-life-care.

World Health Organisation. (2020). *Palliative care–Key facts*. World Health Organisation. https://www.who.int/news-room/fact-sheets/detail/palliative-care.

Zimmermann, C. (2012). Acceptance of dying: A discourse analysis of palliative care literature. *Social Science & Medicine (1982), 75*(1), 217–224. https://doi.org/10.1016/j.socscimed.2012.02.047.

PERSON-CENTRED RISK ASSESSMENT AND PLANNING

MICHELLE VILLENEUVE

INTRODUCTION

Disability Inclusive Disaster Risk Reduction (DIDRR) is about increasing the safety and well-being of people with disability in emergency situations. It requires partnerships between people and the services that support them working together with government and emergency services to make sure that people with disability have the same opportunity to access emergency preparedness information, to participate in emergency preparedness programs in their community and to be included as a valuable stakeholder in local community disaster risk reduction. Approaches used to develop DIDRR must emphasise doing with, not for people with disability (Casey-Lockyer & Myers, 2017).

In this practice story, the role occupational therapists can play in increasing the safety and well-being of the people with disabilities that they support in preparing for disasters is presented. As person-centred practitioners[1] occupational therapists enable people with disabilities to assess their own preparedness and develop emergency plans tailored to their specific support needs and risk situation.

In contemporary times, a growing number, intensity and duration of disasters are being witnessed and experienced. Emergency events, such as bushfires, floods, cyclones, extreme heat and pandemics have caused significant fatalities, injuries and financial loss across the world (Dietz et al., 2020), with a disproportionate impact on people with disability (Stough & Kelman, 2018).

People with disability have often been excluded when it comes to planning for disasters triggered by natural hazards and other emergencies (e.g. house fires, pandemic). The growing body of literature shows that people with disability are the most neglected people during disaster events (Twigg et al., 2018). People with disability are two to four times more likely to die in a disaster than the general population (Fujii, 2015). They struggle to obtain the help they need resulting in higher risk of injury and loss of property (Alexander, 2015), greater difficulty with evacuation (Malpass et al., 2019) and sheltering (Twigg et al., 2011) and have more intensive health and social services needs during and after disaster events (Phibbs et al., 2015). There is a range of contributing factors including stigma and discrimination that marginalise people with disability

---

[1]In this book the term 'person-centred' has been replace with 'collaborative relationship focused practice' (refer to Chapter 12). The term person-centred is retained in this chapter due to the name of the approach being presented: Person-Centred Emergency Preparedness (P-CEP).

from mainstream social, economic and cultural participation (Villeneuve et al., 2021). Multiple categories of social vulnerability intersect with disability consequently amplifying risk during emergencies.

Personal emergency preparedness saves lives (Fuse & Yakota, 2012). Despite the importance of being adequately prepared, studies have found that people with disability and chronic conditions are less likely to engage in preparedness behaviours due to individual and social barriers (Gershon et al., 2013; Phibbs, 2015; Villeneuve et al., 2020). People with disability may need additional support, resources or advocacy to enable their emergency preparedness. One proposed way of facilitating this is to leverage the roles of service providers like occupational therapists who have routine interactions with the people they support (Subramaniam & Villeneuve, 2019). Research has recognised the interdependence of people at greatest disaster risk and their support networks in achieving safety and well-being before, during and after disaster (Pyke & Wilton, 2020; Villeneuve et al., 2021), acknowledging the important role that community, health and disability service providers can play in enabling person-centred emergency preparedness (Subramaniam & Villeneuve, 2019).

PERSON-CENTRED APPROACH

A person-centred approach is widely used and prominent across many helping professions. It comes with specific expectations for how professionals should work with people receiving their services. Person-centredness refers to a way of interacting with people that meets their needs, gives them choice and control and engages them as active agents so that they have ownership over decisions and actions. It has a focus on discovering what people value and finding ways to bridge gaps between opportunities and achievement of valued functioning (e.g. safety and well-being in emergencies). Person-centred planning should result in actions that reflect what is possible, not just what is available (Sanderson, 2013). Using person-centred approaches to help people access and engage with risk information and emergency preparedness is an important support role occupational therapists must play when enabling effective planning with people who have additional support needs in emergencies.

Relationships are the cornerstone of person-centred planning and support. Establishing relationships and

negotiating person-centred goals is challenging but rewarding work. It requires emotional investment. Quite often, the tools (assessments, outcome measures) and the contexts of service planning and delivery (time constraints, travel distances, administrative support or lack of it) undermine efforts to be truly person-centred. Occupational therapists build rapport when working in a person-centred manner. The trust formed within the therapeutic relationship can empower people with disability to consider their emergency preparedness. By using a person-centred approach occupational therapists can support people to take steps to be more prepared to handle various emergencies caused by natural hazards and other unforeseen events like housefires or pandemics.

The United Nations Convention on the Rights of Persons with Disability (UNCRPD) (United Nations, 2006) recognises that while people with disability may have additional support needs that increase their vulnerability to disasters, their rights to protection and safety must remain uncompromised in situations of risk which includes natural hazard emergencies (Article 11). The UNCRPD outlines that inclusivity and accessibility are fundamental components of any programme contributing to empowerment and participation of people with disabilities. This must include access to personal emergency preparedness for people with disability. A person-centred approach to disaster preparedness and risk reduction should focus on two things: (a) ensuring all people are safe in disasters and (b) making sure that people with disability receive the help they need to prepare, respond and recover from disasters (Abbott & Porter, 2013; Villeneuve, 2019). These ideas are supported by the Sendai Framework for Disaster Risk Reduction (SFDRR) 2015–2030, which called for a more person-centred approach to disaster risk reduction (UNISDR/UNDRR, 2015).

ENABLING EMERGENCY PREPAREDNESS

A small number of scoping studies have been published that provide initial direction for occupational therapists to consider their role and responsibilities in emergency preparedness, disaster response and recovery (Habib et al., 2013; Jeong et al., 2016; Parente et al., 2017; Scaffa et al., 2006). The World Federation of Occupational Therapists (WFOT) (2022) Disaster Preparedness and

Risk Reduction Manual outlines principles and elaborates potential roles that occupational therapists can play at different levels (e.g. micro, meso and macro – refer to Chapter 11). At the micro level, the WFOT Manual reminds occupational therapists that they are expected to prepare in their personal lives for disasters by having a plan and communicating and practising the plan with their immediate contacts. Indeed, everyone needs to be ready and know how they will respond in a disaster.

With its emphasis on disaster management and climate changes adaptation, the WFOT Manual primarily focuses on ways that occupational therapists can work with communities in response to disaster events. However, it does not mention how occupational therapists can use their core expertise in person-centred planning as part of their regular work to help improve the safety and well-being of the people they support, especially before disasters happen. The Person-Centred Emergency Preparedness (P-CEP) framework and process tool were created to be used by various service providers, including occupational therapists. This tool assists people to prepare themselves for emergencies and guides others in doing the same. The P-CEP starts with the individual (micro) and enables the identification of factors at the organisational (meso) and community (macro) levels that either facilitate or impede emergency preparedness. The process elements of the P-CEP support multi-stakeholder collaborative action to identify and remove barriers that increase disaster risk by enabling the identification and removal of barriers at each level, micro, meso and macro. The knowledge and skills that occupational therapists bring to this process can increase safety and well-being outcomes for the people they support when disasters strike.

PERSON-CENTRED EMERGENCY PREPAREDNESS (P-CEP)

The P-CEP framework and process tool were developed through a co-design process involving multiple stakeholders, including people with disability and their supporting services (i.e. community, health, allied health and disability service providers), government and emergency personnel (Villeneuve, 2022) (refer to Chapter 19).

P-CEP conceptualises emergency preparedness as a person-centred developmental process involving multiple stakeholders working together to expand opportunities for people with disability to access information and resources and convert those resources into preparedness actions that optimise self-reliance and planful reliance on others. The aim is to increase safety and well-being of people with disability before, during and after emergencies (Villeneuve, 2022). The P-CEP takes an all-hazards approach by incorporating self-assessment and tailored preparedness for disasters triggered by natural hazard events and other emergencies (e.g. house fire, health emergencies). In short, P-CEP helps match emergency planning to the support people need for their health and safety in emergencies. Enabling an optimal fit between people and their environments so that they can achieve their valued occupational participation goals is the foundation of occupational therapy practice.

The P-CEP framework and process tool has three components:

a. A *capability framework* consisting of eight elements to support self-assessment of strengths and support needs (refer to Chapters 10 and 31);
b. *Principles* guiding the joint effort of multiple stakeholders to enable tailored emergency preparedness planning; and
c. Four *process steps* enabling the developmental progression of preparedness actions and facilitating linkages between people with disability, their support services and emergency managers.

A. P-CEP Capability Framework

The P-CEP breaks the self-assessment and emergency planning process down into eight areas familiar to occupational therapists: communication, personal support, social connectedness, transportation, assistive technology, assistance animals, management of health and living situations (Villeneuve, 2019).

The P-CEP framework or 'capability wheel' is used to facilitate emergency planning conversations (Fig. 46.1), allowing the person to lead and direct the planning process by considering what their support needs are and how they routinely manage those supports. Focusing on how people manage in the context of their everyday lives enhances conversations about roles, responsibilities and capabilities. This builds broader understanding about the opportunities and choices that people have and expands dynamic consideration of factors that influence their choices (positively or negatively) in emergency situations.

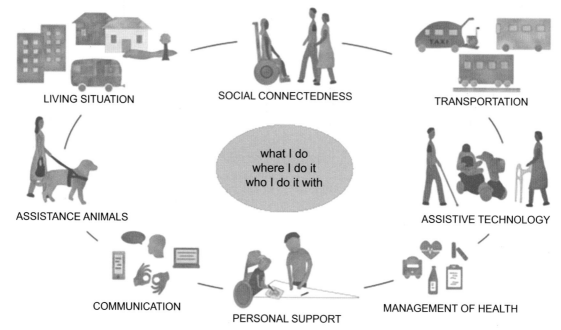

LIVING SITUATION   SOCIAL CONNECTEDNESS   TRANSPORTATION

what I do
where I do it
who I do it with

ASSISTANCE ANIMALS   ASSISTIVE TECHNOLOGY

COMMUNICATION   PERSONAL SUPPORT   MANAGEMENT OF HEALTH

Fig. 46.1 ■ P-CEP Capability Framework. (From Villeneuve (2022) [Collaborating4Inclusion www.collaborating4inclusion.org]).

An important goal of involving people in co-designing their own emergency planning is to make sure they are included in deciding what they can do for themselves and what they need support for during emergencies. Researchers like Bokarjova and colleagues (2009) have said that emergency plans should help people feel confident, handle changes and judge situations, all while making them feel empowered about their capability to adapt in situations of uncertainty. Subramaniam and Villeneuve (2019) pointed out how important it is for people to take an active role in emergency planning to make sure their safety and well-being are considered. They suggested that planning tools should focus on enabling and including everyone. The P-CEP approach builds on the idea of planning that is centred around the person (Towell & Sanderson, 2004) to make these goals happen.

Person-centredness ensures meaningful inclusion in emergency preparedness by acknowledging the individual as the expert in their lives. When occupational therapists act in a person-centred way, they learn about a person's experiences, abilities and what kind of help they need. Occupational therapists can use that knowledge to respond in ways that increase opportunities for people with disability to achieve safety and well-being in emergencies. For instance, occupational therapists might provide information about local risks, steps to get ready or community help that can be useful in planning for emergencies. Planning can also include using new understandings about the function-based support needs of people with disability to inform community-level planning to protect and support people during disasters (e.g. helping governments make evacuation shelters more accessible). Alternatively, it could involve mobilising local community resources to overcome gaps in preparedness (e.g. advocating for accessible transportation needed to evacuate safely). Person-centred interactions, facilitated with the right tools, can lead to a cascade of actions that expand opportunities and promote equity for people with disability.

The effectiveness of the P-CEP Capability Framework in empowering individuals to take control of their own personal emergency preparedness planning is illustrated in Box 46.1. It highlights how occupational therapists can seamlessly integrate the P-CEP into their regular assessments, aiding individuals in identifying key areas to enhance their personal emergency preparedness.

BOX 46.1
EFFECTIVENESS OF P-CEP CAPABILITY FRAMEWORK

During early development of the P-CEP, the research team accompanied allied health service providers on their home visits to people who receive disability, health and aged care services. These service providers were early adopters when it came to adding natural hazard disasters to their routine risk assessment and intake processes. For example, the manager of one health service developed a one-page (12-item) risk assessment and trained staff to complete it with every person at initial referral and during their six monthly reviews.

This 12-item risk assessment tool had been in use for approximately 12 months when the first draft of the P-CEP was ready for trial. To better understand how the P-CEP could be embedded into practice, the research team first observed the use of the 12-item assessment. The following observations were made about the risk assessment and its administration:

- The form contained only closed-ended (yes/no) questions (e.g. Are you aware of the possible natural hazards that could affect you, in your local area? Do you have anyone able to assist you in case of an Emergency or Natural Disaster?)
- The service provider was required to pass judgement on the nature, type or degree of risk based on what they knew or understood about the person, their situation or their exposure to hazard risks (e.g. Is the person cognitively impaired? Does the person live in a high-risk area? Is the person identified as vulnerable?).
- The service provider did most of the talking. Their tone was sombre. The person did not ask any questions.
- The service provider completed the form without showing or sharing it with the person or their family.
- Once completed, the form remained with the service provider.
- In every instance of review, the person's emergency contact, who was identified during the initial assessment, was no longer a reliable contact (e.g. they had died, moved away, did not live in the same city).

The following day, the P-CEP approach was workshopped with this same group of service providers who then trialled it with other people. The following was observed when implementing P-CEP:

- The capability wheel (Fig. 46.1) was placed in front of the person and one open-ended question was asked (Tell me about your capabilities and how you manage your support needs. Think about the everyday: what you do, where you do it and who you do it with. Start where you like and skip the areas that don't apply to you).

- The person used the capability wheel as a prompt. They shared relevant information about their capabilities and management of support needs.
- Service providers used what they learned from the person to prompt discussion about how they might manage their support needs in the event of an evacuation and shelter-in-place scenarios.
- The person did most of the talking. They were animated and the conversation included moments of humour. With a sense of humility, the service providers shared information about their own preparedness planning. Together they discussed local risks. Sometimes questions were asked that neither the service provider or the person could answer. They brainstormed where they could find answers and made a plan to do so (e.g. council; local fire brigade).
- The person asked questions and engaged in active problem solving (e.g. What do people pack in their emergency kit? I suppose I should make sure I have extra catheters and bags. My power wheelchair is important to me, I need to figure out how to take it and my manual wheelchair with me if I have to leave; housefire is my biggest risk, I need to think about alternate exits from my home because only one door is accessible).
- The conversation (typically lasting 20 minutes) was unfinished and service providers made plans to continue the conversation on future visits. They continued with other matters before bringing the visit to a close.
- The P-CEP was left with the person who was encouraged to continue the conversation with their family, friends and neighbours.
- The conversation prompted modest but immediate changes to some care plans (e.g. When the garden and indoor plants do not need tending or there are no groceries to put away, the support worker could assist the person with gathering and making digital copies of important documents, pictures and information; emergency contact details were replaced with the names of good friends and nearby neighbours).

In the debrief, all service providers reported learning more about each person in that 20-minute P-CEP conversation than they had in many weeks, months or even years of working with the people they support. This experience gave the group pause to consider the potential of the P-CEP Capability Framework in directing how they interact with people in a person-centred way and the power of embedding emergency preparedness conversations into routine assessment and care.

B. P-CEP Principles

The P-CEP offers a conversational process to motivate, sustain and support emergency preparedness. Person-centred emergency planning is best enabled when the facilitator (or conversation partner) fully embraces its principles. Consistent with person-centred planning approaches (Sanderson, 2013), the conversation should be directed by individuals and enable them to lead their own preparedness actions. However, emergency planning places high demands on people with disability – particularly when they rely on others to assure their safety and well-being when faced with disasters and other emergencies. It can be overwhelming to sustain emergency preparedness when there are obstacles. Occupational therapists can start by making their own emergency plans using the P-CEP. This helps them to know the tool and learn how to use it for their own personal and household emergency plan. This makes it easier to understand how others could also use it to plan for their unique support needs and risks. The P-CEP process steps reinforce the importance of talking about emergency preparedness with family, friends and neighbours because they make up our essential support network during emergencies.

In addition to principles of person-centred planning, P-CEP is underpinned by the Capability Approach (refer to Chapters 10 and 31) and the Transtheoretical (Stages of Change) Model (refer to Chapter 22). The Capability Approach, introduced by Sen in 1992, is a person-centred framework for understanding how things like environments, personal traits and the way things are organised, all come together to affect a person's ability to make decisions that matter to them. For example, having an emergency plan tailored to their personal support needs, receiving early warnings through accessible communication channels, evacuating to a safe location with accessible facilities, contributing to decision making about local emergency management planning and being supported by people you trust (Villeneuve et al., 2021). The P-CEP focuses attention on individual strengths or capabilities (Villeneuve et al., 2018), including:

a. The opportunities and choices people have to access information, learn about their disaster risk and take steps to increase their preparedness and
b. The factors that enable or limit those choices.

The step-wise approach to P-CEP builds on the Stages of Change model (Prochaska et al., 1993) (refer to chapter 22). This model outlines that people move through different stages of action when they change their behaviour (Table 46.1). People getting ready for emergencies will be in different stages of change (Bockarjova et al., 2009). The P-CEP recognises that getting prepared for emergencies is something that is worked on over time, not just once. It is more than just understanding the help that might be required during emergencies. It involves truly considering how likely certain risks are in places where people live, work and play and how prepared each person is at any given moment. The aim is to keep getting better at preparing for emergencies and to keep checking and updating plans as things change. This is particularly important for people with disabilities because their support needs may change frequently over time and will be influenced by the availability of supports.

TABLE 46.1		
Stages of Preparedness		
Stage	**Description**	**Reflective Questions**
Precontemplation	Individuals have no intention to change behaviour in the near future; they may not be aware that change is needed.	Have you thought about planning for emergencies? Have you experienced a natural hazard or other emergency?
Contemplation	Individuals are aware that a problem exists and are seriously thinking about overcoming it, but they have not yet made a commitment to take action.	Have you tried to learn or find more information about how to prepare for emergencies? Do you know what steps you need to take?
Preparation	Individuals intend to take action and have started to make some changes.	Do you have an emergency kit? Have you gathered supplies or considered evacuation routes? Do you know where to turn for information and support?

	TABLE 46.1	
	Stages of Preparedness—(*Continued*)	
Stage	**Description**	**Reflective Questions**
Action	Individuals modify their behaviour or environment to overcome problems and reach certain goals.	Have you taken action to make a plan for yourself, family or household? Have you tailored the plan to your unique support needs? What does that look like for you? Who else does your plan involve?
Maintenance	Individuals maintain behaviour changes for at least six months or more.	Have you updated your emergency plans, discussed your plan with others or re-stocked your supplies for emergencies in the past 3 to 6 months? What contingencies have you developed?

From Villeneuve, M., Sterman, J., & Llewellyn, G. (2018). *Person-centred emergency preparedness: A process tool and framework for enabling disaster preparedness with people with chronic health conditions and disability*. Centre for Disability, Research and Policy, University of Sydney, NSW 2006.

C. P-CEP Process Steps

As a process tool, the P-CEP breaks planning down into four steps:

1. *Identify* your strengths and support needs in everyday life.
2. *Know* your level of emergency preparedness and *learn* about your disaster risk.
3. *Plan* for how you will manage your support needs in an emergency.
4. *Communicate* the plan with your support network and address gaps through collaboration.

It is helpful to think of these steps as a series of planning conversations that connect people with disability to others who have roles and responsibilities in emergency management and disaster risk reduction (e.g. emergency services personnel, community engagement and resilience staff of local governments).

Occupational therapists are adept at using step-by-step approaches to support people to thoroughly assess their own capabilities and support needs. Consequently, occupational therapists can play a vital leadership role in facilitating P-CEP by starting the conversation from a position of strength, working together with people to talk about their daily supports and how they will handle things if there are disruptions during disasters.

The P-CEP guides this step-wise process so that people can take specific actions to enhance their personal emergency preparedness. This approach assures that the plans people make are customised to their specific support requirements and risks. Using P-CEP, occupational therapists can play a pivotal role in enabling people with disabilities to have emergency plans matched to their support needs. The P-CEP Workbook (Villeneuve et al., 2020) provides information, tools and direction to facilitate each step. It also has real stories and advice from people with disability, which gives a realistic and positive view, based on their own experiences of getting ready for emergencies. Video-based resources, case studies and guidance material are available to help you get started at https://collaborating4inclusion.org/pcep/.

Occupational therapists also bring specific skills in understanding how illness, injury and impairments interact with environments to increase vulnerability. They have in-depth knowledge about the function-based support needs of the people they work with and an understanding of the individual's support network. With their expertise in assessing the fit between people and their environments (refer to Chapters 7 and 15), occupational therapists are optimally placed to assess people and their environments to establish their needs, risks, resources and level of emergency preparedness. As person-centred practitioners, occupational therapists can support people with disabilities to take the lead when it comes to self-assessing the type and level of support they may need and to begin planning for how they will respond together with their support network in an emergency.

Occupational therapists form a crucial member of a person's support networks and can help to link people to information and supports they may need to make an emergency plan. For example, they can work with the person to determine if they rely on electrical devices, medication or medical treatments and put strategies in place to ensure these forms of assistance continue without interruption during disasters (Subramaniam & Villeneuve, 2019). Taking a collaborative approach can help people with disabilities to consider the suitability of their existing plan in a range of scenarios and assist them to make their plans more specific. For example, if the person needs support to evacuate, occupational therapists can prompt the person to identify who will provide this support and communicate this plan to them. As an advocate, occupational therapists can play an instrumental role needed to:

- Identify the gaps that perpetuate disaster risks for the people they support and
- Work in partnership with others (e.g. other service providers from the community, healthcare and disability sectors; local government; emergency services) to address barriers to safety and well-being in emergencies.

SUMMARY

P-CEP recognises emergency planning as a continuous process of generative learning, focused on multi-stakeholder learning and actions that lead to better outcomes for everyone in the community. In this way, person-centredness in emergency preparedness builds systems learning (from the micro to the meso and macro-levels) among multiple stakeholders, each having different roles, knowledge, networks and capabilities. P-CEP conversations can enable transformation towards community-level DIDRR by creating a virtuous spiral of positive change that shapes how others in the community (e.g. government and emergency services) enact their roles and responsibilities to ensure that nobody is left behind when disasters strike.

Skilled person-centred practitioners, like occupational therapists, are an important ally in using P-CEP and embedding it into their routine interactions with people. By initiating conversations about P-CEP and working in partnership with people with disability, occupational therapists are optimally placed to identify and address factors that increase vulnerability disaster. Using the P-CEP capability framework, principles and process steps along with their deep understanding of individuals and their approach to collaboratively managing illness, injuries and impairments, occupational therapists will empower those they assist to be aware, capable and prepared for emergencies. P-CEP responds to a significant knowledge gap regarding how occupational therapists can effectively enhance emergency preparedness in partnership with the people they support.

REFERENCES

Abbott, D., & Porter, S. (2013). Environmental hazard and disabled people: From vulnerable to expert to interconnected. *Disability & Society, 28*(6), 839–852.

Alexander, D. (2015). Disability and disaster: An overview. In I. Kelman & L. M. Stough (Eds.), *Disability and Disaster*. Disaster Studies. Palgrave Macmillan, London. https://doi.org/10.1057/9781137486004_2.

Bockarjova, M., van der Veen, A., & Geurts, P. A. T. M. (2009). A Flood disaster in the Netherlands: a trade-off between paying for protection and undertaking action? In *56th North American REgional Science Association International Conference 2009.* https://research.utwente.nl/en/publications/a-flood-disaster-in-the-netherlands-a-trade-off-between-paying-fo.

Casey-Lockyer, M., & Myers, S. (2017). Disability integration throughout the disaster cycle of prepare, respond and recover. *Journal of Business Continuity & Emergency Planning, 10*(3), 249–258.

Dietz, T., Shwom, R. L., & Whitley, C. T. (2020). Climate change and society. *Annual Review of Sociology, 46*(1), 135–158. https://doi.org/10.1146/annurev-soc-121919-054614.

Fujii, K. (2015). *The great East Japan earthquake and persons with disabilities affected by the earthquake – Why is the mortality rate so high? – Interim report on JDF support activities and proposals.* Paper presented at the Report on the Great East Japan Earthquake and Support for People with Disabilities, Japan Disability Forum (JDF).

Gershon, R. R., Kraus, L. E., Raveis, V. H., Sherman, M. F., & Kailes, J. I. (2013). Emergency preparedness in a sample of persons with disabilities. *American Journal of Disaster Medicine, 8*(1), 35–47.

Habib, M. M., Uddin, M. J., Ur Rahman, S., Jahan, N., & Akter, S. (2013). Occupational therapy role in disaster management in Bangladesh. *World Federation of Occupational Therapists Bulletin, 68*(1), 33–37.

Jeong, Y., Law, M., DeMatteo, C., Stratford, P., & Kim, H. (2016). The role of occupational therapists in the contexts of a natural disaster: A scoping review. *Disability and Rehabilitation, 38*(16), 1620–1631. https://doi.org/10.3109/09638288.2015.1106597.

Malpass, A., West, C., Quaill, J., & Barker, R. (2019). Experiences of individuals with disabilities sheltering during natural disasters: An integrative review. *Australian Journal of Emergency Management, 34*(2), 60–65.

Parente, M., Tofani, M., De Santis, R., Esposito, G., Santilli, V., & Galeoto, G. (2017). The role of the occupational therapist in disaster areas: Systematic review. *Occupational Therapy International, 2017*(1), 6474761. https://doi.org/10.1155/2017/6474761.

Phibbs, S., Good, G., Severinsen, C., Woodbury, E., & Williamson, K. (2015). Emergency preparedness and perceptions of vulnerability among disabled people following the Christchurch earthquakes: Applying lessons learnt to the Hyogo Framework for action. *Australasian Journal of Disaster and Trauma Studies, 19*, 37–46.

Prochaska, J. O., DiClemente, C. C., & Norcross, J. C. (1993). In search of how people change: Applications to addictive behaviors. *Addictions Nursing Network, 5*(1), 2–16.

Pyke, C., & Wilton, R. (2020). Planning for inclusion? An assessment of Ontario's emergency preparedness guide for people with disabilities. *International Journal of Disaster Risk Reduction, 51*, 101888.

Sanderson, H. (2013). Person centred planning. In *People with Profound & Multiple Learning Disabilities* (pp. 130–145). David Fulton Publishers.

Scaffa, M. E., Gerardi, S., Herzberg, G., & McColl, M. A. (2006). The role of occupational therapy in disaster preparedness, response, and recovery. *The American Journal of Occupational Therapy, 60*(6), 642. https://doi.org/10.5014/ajot.60.6.642.

Sen, A. (1992). *Inequality reexamined*. Oxford University Press.

Stough, L. M., & Kelman, I. (2018). People with disabilities and disasters. In L. M. Stough & I. Kelman (Eds.), *Handbook of disaster research* (pp. 225–242). Springer.

Subramaniam, P., & Villeneuve, M. (2019). Advancing emergency preparedness for people with disabilities and chronic health conditions in the community: A scoping review. *Disability and Rehabilitation, 42*(22), 3256–3264. https://doi.org/10.1080/09638288.2019.1583781.

Towell, D., & Sanderson, H. (2004). Person-centred planning in its strategic context: Reframing the mansell/beadle-brown critique. *Journal of Applied Research in Intellectual Disabilities, 17*(1), 17–21. https://doi.org/10.1111/j.1468-3148.2004.00177.x.

Twigg, J., Kett, M., Bottomley, H., Tan, L. T., & Nasreddin, H. (2011). Disability and public shelter in emergencies. *Environmental hazards, 10*(3–4), 248–261. https://doi.org/10.1080/17477891.2011.594492.

Twigg, J., Kett, M., & Lovell, E. (2018). *Briefing note: Disability inclusion and disaster risk reduction*. Overseas Development Institute.

United Nations. (2006). *Convention on the rights of persons with disabilities*. United Nations.

United Nations Office for Disaster Risk Reduction (UNISDR/UNDRR). (2015). *Sendai framework for disaster risk reduction 2015–2030*. UNISDR.

Villeneuve, M. (2019). Increasing involvement of people with disability. *Australian Journal of Emergency Management, 34*(4), 16–17.

Villeneuve, M. (2022). Disability-inclusive emergency planning: Person-centered emergency preparedness. In *Oxford Research Encyclopedia of Global Public Health*.

Villeneuve, M., Abson, L., Pertiwi, P., & Moss, M. (2021). Applying a person-centred capability framework to inform targeted action on disability inclusive disaster risk reduction. *International Journal of Disaster Risk Reduction, 52*, 101979. https://doi.org/10.1016/j.ijdrr.2020.101979.

Villeneuve, M., Abson, L., Yen, I., & Moss, M. (2020). *Person-centred emergency preparedness (P-CEP) workbook*. Centre for Disability Research and Policy, The University of Sydney, NSW 2006. https://collaborating4inclusion.org/wp-content/uploads/2020/08/2020-08-19-Person-Centred-Emergency-Preparedness-P-CEP-WORKBOOK_FORM_FINAL.pdf.

Villeneuve, M., Sterman, J., & Llewellyn, G. (2018). *Person-centred emergency preparedness: A process tool and framework for enabling disaster preparedness with people with chronic health conditions and disability*. Centre for Disability, Research and Policy, University of Sydney, NSW 2006.

World Federation of Occupational Therapists (WFOT). (2022). *Disaster preparedness and risk reduction manual*. WFOT. www.wfot.org.

DISASTER PREPAREDNESS AND RISK REDUCTION

R LYLE DUQUE ■ PEÑAFRANCIA E. CHING

CHAPTER OUTLINE

INTRODUCTION

Disasters cause serious disruptions to the everyday functioning of communities and people within those communities (International Federation of Red Cross and Red Crescent Societies, n.d.; World Federation of Occupational Therapists, 2022). Disasters are caused by natural, man-made or technological hazards that may result in the loss of life or injury, property damage, social and economic disruption or environmental degradation. Hazards may be natural, human-induced/technological or biological (International Federation of Red Cross and Red Crescent Societies, n.d.; United Nations Office for Disaster Risk Reduction, 2007). Some examples of each type of hazard are provided in Table 47.1.

Hazards are ubiquitous, and several of them may be present at any given point in time in a community, area or region. The probability of hazards resulting in disasters is determined by the interaction between a community's exposure, vulnerability and capacity to adapt to or resist existing or potential hazards. This probability is known as *disaster risk* (International Federation of Red Cross and Red Crescent Societies, n.d.).

Disaster risk is increased by a community's *exposure* to hazards over longer periods of time. This risk is compounded by the community's *vulnerability* or susceptibility to the adverse effects of hazards. The vulnerability of communities is determined by certain physical, social, economic and environmental factors or processes. Some examples of factors that increase

TABLE 47.1
Examples of Different Types of Hazards

Natural Hazards	Human-Induced Hazards	Biological Hazards
Earthquakes	Nuclear plant accidents	Epidemics
Typhoons/cyclones	Oil/chemical spills	Plagues
Volcanic eruptions	Industrial plant accidents	Pandemics
Wildfires	Environmental degradation	
Drought		
Heatwaves		

the vulnerability of certain communities include lack of access to health and social care, poverty and residence in hazardous geographic locations. Some examples of vulnerable people within communities include women, children, persons with disabilities, those with existing disorders or diseases (e.g. non-communicable diseases), displaced persons, economic, cultural or ethnic minorities and Indigenous peoples (United Nations Office for Disaster Risk Reduction, 2007; World Federation of Occupational Therapists, 2022).

In recent years, disasters have resulted in increasing damage to infrastructure, injuries, loss of lives and economic loss for people, communities and populations globally (International Federation of Red Cross and Red Crescent Societies, 2023a). Disasters have also become more complex and multi-layered, with multiple disasters simultaneously affecting parts of or even the entire world (Duque et al., 2012; International Federation of Red Cross and Red Crescent Societies, 2023b). This is best illustrated by the effects of the COVID-19 pandemic that have been amplified by local and regional disasters such as flooding (e.g. in the USA; Davies, 2023), armed conflict (e.g. war in Ukraine) or tsunami (e.g. in Tonga; British Broadcasting Corporation, 2023). Factors such as climate change, environmental degradation, unplanned urbanisation, poorly developed social and healthcare systems, geopolitical tensions and conflicts and global epidemics and pandemics increase the probability of disasters becoming more frequent and their impact longer lasting and of greater magnitude (United Nations Office for Disaster Risk Reduction, 2015).

DISASTER PREPAREDNESS AND RESPONSE

The global effort to address the effects of disasters can be traced to the establishment of the United Nations Disaster Relief Office (UNDRO) in 1971. Among its purposes were to study, prevent, control and predict natural disasters; encourage governments to improve national disaster warning systems and advise governments on disaster planning. In 1987, the UN General Assembly declared 1990–1999 as the International Decade for Natural Disaster Reduction. Its aim was to foster international cooperation in mitigating the effects of disasters on people. In 1994 the World Conference on Natural Disaster Reduction was convened in Yokohama, Japan. The conference produced the Yokohama Strategy and Plan of Action.

This document sets out the principles upon which disaster reduction strategies should be based, the plan of action to operationalise the principles and provide guidelines to follow up the outcomes from the implementation of the strategies (UNDRR, n.d.).

The result of the review of the outcomes from the Yokohama Strategy and Plan of Action culminated in the formulation of the Hyogo Framework for Action: 2005–2015 (HFA). This document provided a review of the implementation of the Yokohama Strategy and Plan of Action and identified *five areas requiring further attention:*

1. Governance;
2. Risk identification, assessment, monitoring and early warning;
3. Knowledge management and education;
4. Reduction of underlying risk factors and
5. Preparedness for effective response and recovery (United Nations Office for Disaster Risk Reduction, 2007).

The Sendai Framework for Disaster Risk Reduction 2015–2030 built upon the HFA, highlighting the progress made since the adoption of the HFA. The Sendai Framework sought to ensure continuity of the principles and actions initiated by the antecedent frameworks. The major thrusts of the Framework are:

- Emphasis on disaster risk management rather than disaster management;
- Identification of seven global targets;
- Disaster risk reduction as an outcome;
- Preventing new risks and reducing existing ones and
- Building resilience (United Nations Office for Disaster Risk Reduction, 2015).

An analysis of the evolution of these frameworks demonstrates ongoing learning and implementation of knowledge to reduce disaster risk and improve response to and management of disasters. More specifically, current disaster risk preparedness and response frameworks and strategies emphasise:

- Disaster risk reduction and preparedness, including prevention of new risks, with the recognition that disasters may be sudden or slow-onset;
- Disaster preparedness that is multi-hazard and considers the complexity of the effects of disasters;

- The importance of a multi-sectoral, inclusive and accessible approach to disaster preparedness and response;
- The intricate and intimate relationship between disasters, social justice and sustainable development;
- The importance of building resilience at all levels and
- Coordinated and integrated collaboration among stakeholders, particularly between developed and developing nations (United Nations Office for Disaster Risk Reduction, 2015; World Federation of Occupational Therapists, 2022).

DISASTERS AND OCCUPATIONS

Disasters adversely impact the occupational lives of individuals and communities and negatively affect health and well-being, cause damage to property and infrastructure, result in environmental destruction and disrupt the rhythm of daily life. Disasters can lead to injuries, illnesses, disability and loss of lives. Destruction of property and infrastructure results in and/or exacerbates the loss of livelihood, upending of relationships, poverty, stress on social and healthcare

systems and geopolitical conflicts (Sima et al., 2017; World Federation of Occupational Therapists, 2022). Ultimately, all these consequences may result in occupational disruption and deprivation, both in the short- and long-term.

Occupational therapists, with their unique knowledge and skill in understanding occupational participation, their skill in occupational and task analysis and their ability to remediate deficits, support, modify and adapt occupations and environments and advocate for progressive, just and inclusive policies and programmes, are in a position to engage in this practice area. Within this context, occupational therapists can influence the impact of disasters on an individual and collective level.

The three practice stories presented in Boxes 47.1–47.3 illustrate how occupational therapists can engage in disaster preparedness (see also Chapter 47) at different levels as well as participate in response and rehabilitation efforts following a disaster.

The practice stories show how the occupational lives of individuals and communities have been disrupted by a disaster and highlight how the unique skill sets of occupational therapists can be used to facilitate recovery and build resilience.

BOX 47.1
MARINA'S STORY

Marina was a 21-year-old lady. She was vibrant, filled with hopes and dreams for her family. She and her family lived in a community on the outskirts of Ormoc City, a coastal city in the province of Leyte, located in central Philippines. It had a population of 230,000 and was one of the hardest-hit places when super typhoon Haiyan struck the country in 2013.

Marina had just started work as a cashier in the city centre. She was to be married to her childhood boyfriend, Ruben, in five months' time. Her father, a farmer, was looking forward to working less in the field and looking after a future grandchild. Now that Marina had a job and was to marry, her family pinned their hopes on her and her future husband for a brighter future.

Their house was built on the hillside and was made from light materials such as thin planks of wood for the walls and galvanised iron sheets for roofing. Their community was made up of several families that worked as farmers. Their neighbours' houses were similarly made from light materials. Their community was economically challenged and low-resourced.

Super typhoon Haiyan struck Ormoc City on November 6, 2013. While there were government announcements

about how strong the typhoon was, no one anticipated its magnitude and impact. Overnight, rain poured and the winds swept through houses in the province and the region. Village leaders sounded the emergency alarm as a cue for people to evacuate. However, the howling wind drowned out the sound of the alarm. Marina looked out of the window and saw debris, including house parts hurled by the wind. As she shut the window, she suddenly felt a huge weight on her back. The last thing she recalled prior to losing consciousness was that she was pinned to the ground.

Marina was found under the rubble the following day. She was unable to move her legs and had difficulty lifting her arms. She was unable to feel below the level of her neck, and she experienced occasional involuntary stiffness of her extremities. She was brought to a nearby hospital and discharged after 4 to 5 weeks with a diagnosis of complete spinal cord injury C7 to C8 neurological level. Marina became depressed after her fiancé called off the wedding. There were several other casualties from her village.

The Philippine Academy of Occupational Therapists sent a group of volunteer occupational therapists to Ormoc to assist with the response and rehabilitation efforts seven weeks after the disaster. This team had training

Continued on following page

BOX 47.1
MARINA'S STORY—(*Continued*)

in psychosocial debriefing and coordinated with a local speech-language pathologist who connected them with the village chief. This connection with the village chief was crucial in understanding the local community, including how to access the community members band, identifying who would benefit from occupational therapy services. The village chief assigned community health workers to the group to assist the occupational therapists in reaching out and connecting the volunteers with members of the community.

Upon meeting Marina, an occupational therapist used a collaborative relationship-focused approach (refer to Chapter 12) to identify the primary concerns of Marina and her family. Marina had not received any rehabilitation services since she had been discharged from hospital. She had pressure sores, sensory and motor deficits, complex psychosocial issues that stemmed from her condition and the termination of her relationship with her fiancé and had no regular meaningful occupations.

The occupational therapist assessed environmental factors that could facilitate or hinder Marina's recovery. These factors included but were not limited to, the resources available in the community that could help address Marina's health needs (including prevention of complications and addressing evolving health issues), the home set-up and how this could aid or impede her recovery, the availability and capacity of the family to provide appropriate care and opportunities at home and the community for Marina to re-engage in and/or establish novel valued and meaningful occupations.

The occupational therapist discussed with Marina and her family ways occupational therapy could assist in

addressing those concerns and co-designed a plan (refer to Chapter 19). The family was taught how to position and re-position Marina in bed or the chair to alleviate the pressure sores. The occupational therapist instructed the family members on how to do range of motion exercises, provide wound care and manage spasticity. Further, the family members were taught how to care for themselves, beginning with proper body mechanics when moving or transporting Marina and taking time off from providing care and engaging in rest and recreation.

Possible meaningful occupations, particularly forms of socialisation, were explored. An occupational therapist working in a nearby town was contacted to provide ongoing services for Marina and her family following the departure of the visiting occupational therapy team.

Marina required consults with various professionals for her pressure sores and psychosocial issues. The visiting occupational therapist was able to assess and identify needed resources for Marina. They organised to return in a month with supplies, physiotherapists and a medical doctor for Marina to consult with regarding her medical needs. Recognising that the health needs of Marina were long term, planning and implementing continuous care was conducted with the help of the local speech-language pathologist and other members of the community who were committed to help with Marina's recovery. In particular, a local business organisation was approached to assist Marina and her family with health and other needs. In the following months, the visiting occupational therapist was apprised of developments by the local group through social media.

BOX 47.2
BALAY DULAANAN (PLAYHOUSE) FOR CHILDREN

Cateel is a small town in the province of Davao Oriental on the southern Philippine island of Mindanao. In 2010 it had a population of about 38,000, the largest age group being those between 5 and 9 years old. The primary sources of livelihood were farming (particularly coconut) and trade, with the average monthly family income being below the national average. The poverty level stood at 26%, significantly higher than the 15% targeted by the government and United Nations. The town was also the usual site of encounters between government forces and insurgents (Local Government of Cateel (n.d.).) to align with reference in reference list.

In December 2012, typhoon Bopha struck Cateel. Around 98% of structures and most of the coconut farms were destroyed. Families who were evacuated from at-risk communities were housed in public school buildings.

Children were among those most affected by this disaster. They witnessed family members and friends being caught under the wreckage when their school, then serving as an evacuation site, suddenly collapsed because of the strong winds. Several days after the typhoon, these children loitered around the centre of the town, watching rescue operations, enduring the cold weather and seemingly waiting for something to happen as they observed the change to their town. Consequently, the children missed school for several months as classrooms were either destroyed or used as temporary shelters, not to mention the loss of their school materials. The military was in the town as Martial Law was declared as insurgents threatened to take over the municipality.

Ten days after typhoon Bopha hit Cateel, volunteer occupational therapists visited the area to assist in the

Continued on following page

BOX 47.2
BALAY DULAANAN (PLAYHOUSE) FOR CHILDREN—(*Continued*)

response and rehabilitation efforts. An occupational therapist in the province was contacted by the volunteers to coordinate the work of the volunteers. The engagement of occupational therapists was in three phases:

- Rapid needs assessment;
- Planning and implementation and
- Follow up.

These were implemented through regular weekly visits for the first 2 months, monthly in the next four months and periodically thereafter.

RAPID NEEDS ASSESSMENT

The rapid needs assessment included observing and participating in the people's daily occupations including engaging in games with the children; participating in inter-agency meetings and taking part in casual conversations with adult members of the community. Most of the organisations providing assistance had a time-limited engagement with the community and did not have any long-term plans to sustain their work with the community. Based on the rapid needs assessment, the group of volunteer occupational therapists decided with the community to focus on addressing the needs of the children. In particular, it was agreed that the focus would be on providing the children with safe spaces for play and learning (refer to Chapters 14 and 30).

PLANNING AND IMPLEMENTATION

The occupational therapists established several connections with key organisations in the community to ensure that plans and efforts would have a long-term impact. Coordination was facilitated with the command post at the municipal level, with the school administrator and with the local parish priest, as part of efforts that culminated in setting up Balay Dulaanan (Playhouse).

Balay Dulaanan was conceptualised to be a resource centre that was community-managed. It had a toy and book library aimed at facilitating the coping skills of the children through the occupations of play and learning. School-related activities were included in the programmes since classrooms were destroyed and school materials were damaged or gone. With the help of volunteer teachers, weekly programmes that fostered a learning environment were established in Balay Dulaanan. These programmes transitioned into an after-school programme when, a year or so later, regular classes resumed.

As it was Christmas season, planned activities revolved around themes related to the season. Community members and leaders, family members and the youth were engaged in building Balay Dulaanan. The occupational therapists also collaborated with other professionals in providing training for members of the community in the management of psychosocial issues (refer to Chapters 4,21 and 30).

FOLLOW UP AND CONTINUING COLLABORATION

The occupational therapists, over a period of several months, continued their regular follow-up visits to the community. A year after the disaster, Balay Dulaanan was turned over to the youth parish leaders who became the after-school facilitators and tutors. The centre continues to be managed by the youth group of the local church and currently provides different play and learning activities to almost 500 children in the community. A sense of community was fostered where children were able to share and take care of common possessions such as toys and books reinforcing shared responsibility, cooperation and discipline in the midst of a seemingly chaotic situation in a community that continues the rebuilding process.

The occupational therapists initiated simple activities that facilitated the children's adjustment through the reestablishment of routines and engagement in valued occupations. The occupational therapists played a role in identifying community resources and mechanisms for the sustainability of relevant programmes in postdisaster situations.

BOX 47.3
CRAFTING AND EVOLVING A NATIONAL STRATEGIC PLAN FOR OCCUPATIONAL THERAPY

The Philippines, by virtue of its location and geography – that of being an archipelago and situated in the Pacific Ring of Fire – is exposed to several hazards. It experiences dozens of typhoons annually, is dotted by volcanoes and has several active fault lines. Occupational therapy is a little-known profession in the Philippines, and therefore its role in disaster preparedness and response is even less recognised. Prior to the crafting of the national strategic plan, occupational therapists were rarely, if at all, engaged in DPR initiatives. Disaster preparedness and responses were not part of the entry-level education of occupational therapists. The national association's capacity to effectively conduct or coordinate DPR projects in any part of the country was wanting. There was no mechanism for occupational therapists to engage with each other or external stakeholders in relation to DPR. As such, it was crucial that

Continued on following page

BOX 47.3
CRAFTING AND EVOLVING A NATIONAL STRATEGIC
PLAN FOR OCCUPATIONAL THERAPY —(*Continued*)

a strategic plan was crafted to guide the actions of occupational therapists individually and collectively in this area of practice. The plan was also a way of demonstrating the unique and valuable role of the profession in this area to internal and external stakeholders. The national DPR workshop was held in 2013.

Three primary factors were taken into consideration in the convening of the national workshop:

1. Logistics (including funding and resource persons);
2. Representatives from all relevant sectors and
3. The content and format of the workshop.

Funding was sourced from the national professional association and other government and nongovernment organisations. Resource people included individuals with experience in disaster preparedness and response and those who had experienced the adverse effects of disasters. These people were from both within and outside the occupational therapy profession. To authentically contextualise the outcome of the workshop and ensure the strategic plan was grounded in realities of individuals and communities who have survived disasters and those who have worked with them, a part of the workshop was conducted in an evacuation center that housed some families displaced by a recent typhoon.

The workshop resulted in the formulation of the national strategic plan with four primary objectives:

1. Disseminating information regarding the existence of the strategic plan;
2. Raising the profile of the occupational therapy profession in this area;
3. Identifying entry-level competencies needed by occupational therapists to practice in this area; and
4. Enabling occupational therapists to acquire these competencies.

Although some Filipino occupational therapists had engaged in this practice area, the workshop focused on capacity-building activities to ensure that response to disasters were coordinated and conducted by the national professional association effectively and efficiently (Duque et al., 2013).

It became apparent that a paradigm shift was needed if the profession was to sustain its DPR policies and programmes. Several challenges suggested the need to evolve the strategic plan. Foremost was the fact that there were not enough practitioners to respond to every disaster situation and work on the different projects meant to operationalise the plan. Second, the initiatives were mostly in response to disasters, very few, if any, related to disaster preparedness (Ching & Lazaro, 2019). Finally, practitioners who were expected to engage in DPR activities, themselves became disaster survivors.

The identification of these challenges led to plans on revising and recalibrating the strategic plan. This initiative involved institutionalising the education of occupational therapists in DPR by incorporating it into the required competencies for entry-level education and establishing strategic partnerships with individuals and organisations involved in DPR that shared the profession's values of inclusion, human rights, sustainability and multi-hazard preparedness. Disaster preparedness and response were integrated into the entry-level education of occupational therapists to build a critical mass of practitioners who can engage in this practice area. It is envisioned that all qualified occupational therapists can facilitate disaster preparedness and can lead or participate in disaster responses when necessary. A project related to this was the workshop series, *Handa Kami* (We are ready). Workshops were held in different occupational therapy centres in the country. Participants were taught how to identify hazards and vulnerabilities in their workplaces and communities and determine their level of risks from these hazards and vulnerabilities. Afterwards, they were asked to formulate a preparedness plan for themselves and their respective institutions.

Recognising that resources are limited, individuals and organisations whose values and mission were aligned with those of the profession were identified. Strategic partnerships were forged with these individuals and organisations. This helped ensure that the projects initiated by occupational therapists were sustained even after the therapists had left the community.

In the three practice stories, several hazards were often present, and there was a disproportionate impact of the disasters on the marginalised members of the community. For example, in Marina's story (Box 47.1), the hazards of typhoons, landslides and a house built with substandard materials interacted with her and her family's vulnerability – living in poverty, having an elderly person in the household, poor access to emergency and social services – to raise their level of disaster risk.

In Cateel (Box 47.2), perennial typhoons compounded by poverty, lack of adequate infrastructure to support communities during disasters and lack of preparation, all contributed to the disaster that resulted in the disruption of the occupational lives of the members of the community, particularly the children.

On a national level (Box 47.3), there were two primary risks occupational therapists faced in this practice area – the inability to meaningfully contribute to DPR programmes and policies and occupational therapists being adversely affected by disasters themselves. Becoming disaster survivors somehow negated the capacity of occupational therapists to contribute to DPR efforts. The vulnerability of the profession lies in the lack of preparedness and capacity of occupational therapists themselves and the absence of a strategic framework to capacitate and guide therapists. The national strategic plan was the first step in identifying both the risks and the opportunities the profession faced in this practice area as well as capacitating its members.

The practice stories illustrate how occupational therapists seek an intimate understanding of contexts (and how this understanding evolves) and use this understanding to devise a nuanced, sustainable plan of action. This plan of action not only facilitates the recovery of communities from the effects of disasters, but more importantly, it builds resilience also. For example, in the story of Cateel (Box 47.2), given that the segment of the population most impacted by the disaster was children, the occupational therapists focused their work on this group, taking into consideration their occupational needs (playing and learning) as well as the temporal context (i.e. the Christmas season) in planning projects and activities. The occupational therapists in this story ensured that the gains from the project were sustained over time through a strategic and meaningful collaboration with the community and other organisations.

In each practice story, the occupational therapists worked with the individual and community to co-design goals and plans (refer to Chapter 19). These goals and plans were operationalised and sustained with the individuals and communities. A collaborative review of these plans and goals was eventually carried out to determine if changes were warranted. Finally, transition from occupational therapy was integrated into the plan. This helped build resilience by ensuring that the evolving occupational needs of individuals will be met in the future.

MOVING TOWARDS A DISASTER-PREPARED FUTURE

Due to the impact of climate change and other factors, hazards will be a constant presence in the lives of individuals and collectives. Occupational therapists have a valuable contribution to make to a disaster-prepared future through understanding the hazards, vulnerability and exposure of the profession and of the communities in which they work. Through this understanding and by integrating disaster preparedness into their daily work, occupational therapists can contribute to the mitigation of disaster risks. To this end, it is recommended that:

- Disaster preparedness and response be an integral part of occupational therapists' education and practice. It should cut across all areas of the profession – education, research, practice, advocacy and leadership. Occupational therapists should model disaster preparedness and become advocates within their contexts (e.g. their home, work, community). They should have DPR plans (e.g. emergency kits/bags) at home and at their places of work (refer to Chapter 46 for further information about preparing for disasters).
- DPR strategic plans be formulated at all levels – individual, organisation/community, national – to inform individual and collective actions. These plans need to be periodically reviewed to ensure they remain relevant and sustainable.
- A platform be established for occupational therapists to collaborate at different levels regarding DPR. For example, national occupational therapy associations (and their local chapters) can establish a DPR committee or task force. These committees can then work with committees from other chapters, national associations and external organisations.
- Occupational therapists incorporate principles of sustainability in all practice areas and settings to help mitigate disaster risk (World Federation of Occupational Therapists, 2018).

Occupational therapists are in a strong and unique position to contribute to DPR efforts at different levels and building resilience among those affected by disasters. They need to be capable of both facilitating disaster preparedness in communities as well as responding during and after disasters. Doing so enables them to contribute to sustainable development and social and occupational justice for everyone.

REFERENCES

British Broadcasting Corporation. (2023). *Tonga tsunami sparks "unprecedented disaster", government says*. Retrieved July 30, 2023, from https://www.bbc.co.uk/news/world-asia-60039617. [Accessed July 30, 2023].

Ching, P. E., & Lazaro, R. T. (2019). Preparation, roles, and responsibilities of Filipino occupational therapists in disaster preparedness, response, and recovery. *Disability and Rehabilitation, 43*(9), 1333–1340. https://doi.org/10.1080/09638288.2019.1663945.

Davies, R. (2023). Floods and mudslides after hilary unleashes record rain in California. Retrieved July 30, 2023, from https://floodlist.com/america/usa/floods-hilary-california-august-2023.

Duque, R. L., Ching, P. E., & Bayas, C. (2012). Occupational therapy within layers of disasters, poverty and conflict: A case study. *World Federation of Occupational Therapists Bulletin, 66,* 24–26.

Duque, R. L., Grecia, A., & Ching, P. E. (2013). Development of a national occupational therapy disaster preparedness and response plan: The Philippine experience. *World Federation of Occupational Therapists Bulletin, 68*(1), 26–30. https://doi.org/10.1179/otb.2013.68.1.008.

International Federation of Red Cross and Red Crescent Societies (n.d.). *What is a disaster?* Retrieved July 30, 2023, from https://www.ifrc.org/our-work/disasters-climate-and-crises/what-disaster.

International Federation of Red Cross and Red Crescent Societies (2023a). *Annual Report 2022.* Geneva: Author.

International Federation of Red Cross and Red Crescent Societies (2023b). *World disasters report 2022: Trust, equity and local action.* Geneva: Author.

Local Government of Cateel (n.d.). *Socioeconomic agenda.* Retrieved August 28, 2023, from https://cateel.gov.ph/socio-economic-enterprise/.

Sima, L., Thomas, Y., & Lowrie, D. (2017). Occupational disruption and natural disaster: Finding a 'new normal' in a changed context. *Journal of Occupational Science, 24*(2), 128–139. https://doi.org/10.1080/14427591.2017.1306790.

United Nations Office for Disaster Risk Reduction (n.d.). *DRR and UNDRR's history.* Retrieved July 30, 2023, from https://www.undrr.org/our-work/history#:~:text=1990%2D1999%3A%20The%20International%20Decade%20for%20Natural%20Disaster%20Reduction.

United Nations Office for Disaster Risk Reduction (2007). *Hyogo framework for action: 2005–2015 building the resilience of nations and communities to disasters.* Geneva: Author.

United Nations Office for Disaster Risk Reduction (2015). *Sendai framework for disaster risk reduction 2015-2030.* Geneva: Author.

World Federation of Occupational Therapists (2018). *Sustainability matters: Guiding principles for sustainability in occupational therapy practice, education, and scholarship.* Switzerland: Author.

World Federation of Occupational Therapists (2022). *Disaster preparedness and risk reduction manual.* Switzerland: Author.

48

WELLNESS 2 AGE PROGRAM

KRISTY MAREE ROBSON ■ MELISSA THERESE NOTT

■ ■ ■ ■ ■ ■ ■ ■ ■ ■ ■ ■ ■ ■ ■ ■ ■

CHAPTER OUTLINE

INTRODUCTION

It is well known that globally there is an ageing population, and this will have far-reaching implications for society (Khan, 2019). Some of these implications include direct challenges to health systems due to changing health profiles, increasing demand for health service use, as well as rising health and aged care costs. Additionally, some older people can experience reduced independence and social isolation due to a range of factors, which can impact quality of life and may lead to premature reliance on health and aged care services (Bouaziz et al., 2016). Allied health professionals play an important role in enabling older people to manage the impacts of chronic disease and impairment (Rudnicka et al., 2020). Specifically, occupational therapists can work collaboratively with older people to facilitate engagement in meaningful occupations and support a positive approach to ageing (Mitchell & Walker, 2020).

Wellness in ageing is a multidimensional concept which incorporates the physical, cognitive and social well-being of older people (Rudnicka et al., 2020). The ability to successfully manage and adapt to age-related changes is a key component for supporting occupational participation (Egan & Restall, 2022) (refer to Chapter 11) and sustaining meaningful relationships (Seah et al., 2019). The capability to maintain community and social participation can also minimise the risk of costly hospitalisations (Grimmer et al., 2015), functional decline and reduction in the need for premature transition to residential aged care (Carver et al., 2018). Therefore innovative and person-centred approaches, such as the *Wellness 2 Age Program* can be useful in supporting older people to maintain their ability to undertake activities that are meaningful to them within their home and community, without extensive reliance on health and aged care resources.

It is important to recognise that each older person has unique circumstances and life experiences, and therefore different needs to support their ability to age well. While group-based programs can support older people with maintaining function and facilitating social engagement (De Coninck et al., 2017;

Sherrington et al., 2020), one-size-fits-all approaches do not always consider the individual needs of older people who want to participate in group programs. The *Wellness 2 Age* community-based program has been specifically co-constructed to encourage collaborative relationships through appreciating the nuanced individual needs of older people and is closely aligned to the principles of collaborative relationship-focused occupational therapy (Restall et al., 2022) (refer to Chapter 12).

WELLNESS 2 AGE PROGRAM: INTRODUCING THREE PARTICIPANTS

Before demonstrating how the *Wellness 2 Age Program* effectively supports older community members to maintain or improve occupational participation through an individually tailored, strengths-based approach, three stories from older people who participated in the program are presented (Boxes 48.1–48.3).

BOX 48.1
HELEN

GETTING TO KNOW HELEN

Helen is 73 years old and considers herself to be a 'social butterfly' as she enjoys spending time with her friends, going out for lunch, having coffee and attending her weekly walking group. However, in the last couple of years, she had noticed that it was becoming more difficult to remember things. They were only little things to begin with, but this was still having a major impact on her.

One of Helen's greatest concerns was when she was put on the spot. Helen started to have difficulty remembering her friends' names, and this made her feel very embarrassed. She was so embarrassed that she progressively withdrew from many of her activities for fear of her forgetting her friends' names. Her friends would often ring her and encourage her to come out with them, but she made excuses as to why she could not come. Eventually, her friends stopped calling. Helen became very depressed because she was lonely and socially isolated. She also noticed that because she had stopped going to her walking group, the strength in her legs was declining. All these aspects started to have a significant impact on Helen's overall health and well-being.

HOW THE PROGRAM HELPED HELEN

At the beginning of the program, we spent time working with Helen to determine what specific goals she wanted to focus on throughout the program. Helen identified that she primarily wanted to focus on strategies to assist her memory but also wanted to regain the strength in her legs. Across the 10 weeks, Helen completed a range of activities aligned to these two main goals and learnt targeted strategies that she could continue to use after the program was completed. An example activity that Helen participated in was 'Activities of daily living obstacle course'. Helen achieved Motor Level 3 – Carry tray with teapot and cups while negotiating obstacles and Cognitive Level 3 – Recall specific obstacle course route and manage a phone call distraction part way through the sequence.

We caught up with Helen a couple of months after she finished the program to see how she was going. In her words, she '*was a completely different person*'. She had re-engaged with her friendship group and was back doing her weekly walking program with confidence. Helen continued to use the strategies she had learnt, particularly around memory to support her ongoing engagement within her community. She said, '*I don't know how I can ever thank you for this amazing program, you have truly given me my life back*'.

BOX 48.2
GETTING TO KNOW JOHN

John is 70 years old and plays golf once a week. Being a retired accountant, he is kept busy being on the committee for a number of community-based organisations; he really enjoys this social interaction since giving up work two years ago. John is also a keen gardener and has a large array of fruit trees and a vegetable patch in his backyard.

John found that he was having a few problems with his balance. He has had a few minor falls which he put down to being distracted at the time. Fortunately, to date, he has only sustained minor scrapes and bruising when he has fallen. However, the falls have impacted his confidence, and he was concerned about doing jobs around the house and in his garden as he recently had a close friend badly fracture his hip because of a fall.

HOW THE PROGRAM HELPED JOHN

John's key goal for attending the program was to focus on his balance. He also asked if there were strategies that would improve his concentration as he and his wife were keen to travel overseas, and he did not want to have a fall while travelling in a foreign country. Across the 10 weeks, John completed a range of activities that focused on improving his balance and concentration to reduce his risk of falling. He learnt targeted strategies which he could implement every day to further support his safe mobility around his environment in the community and in novel situations. An example of one activity included in John's program was 'Step it up'. John achieved Motor Level 3 – ascending then descending a longer set of stairs with handrail and then without handrail while performing Cognitive Level 3 – spelling target words forwards and in reverse.

At the end of the program John felt more confident in navigating around his backyard, and he had recommenced his regular gardening activities using the range of strategies he had learnt. He was very excited to tell us that he had booked an overseas trip with his wife.

BOX 48.3
LONI

GETTING TO KNOW LONI

Loni lives alone and does not have any close family nearby. She does not have a strong friendship group, which she puts down to being introverted. Loni has a cat, Pickles, to keep her company, but she often feels lonely and wished she had more friends.

Loni has tried to engage in a couple of groups run through the local community centre, but she often finds that people already know each other, and they tend to stick together, making it difficult for her to meet and talk to people. She finds it difficult to initiate conversation, which is further challenged by her being hard of hearing. Loni has also tried a couple of exercise groups because she wants to keep her fitness up, but she finds large group settings difficult because there is often a lot of background noise which makes it difficult for her to hear instructions.

HOW THE PROGRAM HELPED LONI

Loni's main goal in wanting to join the program was to meet new people and expand her friendship group. She also wanted to learn about strategies to age well. Before starting the program, Loni talked about her challenges in previous group programs such as being an introvert and often just standing at the back of the group because she did not really know anyone. She also talked about the issues related to hearing instructions because of her hearing loss.

The *Wellness 2 Age Program* was specifically designed to enable strong social engagement by pairing participants together within the larger group. Loni found that this approach built her confidence in social engagement due to the structured interactions with others. An activity that Loni enjoyed was the 'Newspaper memory task', requiring participant pairs to walk to the university café while using memory strategies to recall information from

a newspaper article to retell the story to their partner. Having smaller groups or pairs work together on activities within the larger group also assisted Loni to easily hear the activity instructions as the facilitators could go to each individual group or pair to explain what to do.

Within a couple of weeks of starting the program, we noticed that Loni was being invited out to coffee with a group of other females at the end of each of the weekly sessions. At the end of the program, Loni continued to regularly catch up socially with her new friends and they created a walking group together.

OVERVIEW OF THE *WELLNESS 2 AGE PROGRAM*

The program is designed to target older community members who are motivated to remain living at home, by focusing on individualised strategies to build and maintain confidence in performing everyday tasks and activities, thereby supporting independence and engagement within their communities. The *Wellness 2 Age Program* also has a strong focus on translation of strategies into everyday life by explicitly linking learned strategies to home-based activities to create sustainable change within the older person.

Older community-dwelling people were able to self-refer to attend the program which was undertaken at a university-based clinic in a regional area of Australia. The program was advertised as suitable for people over the age of 60 years who were starting to experience some changes in either physical ability or cognitive ability or both. Participants were screened to ensure that they were community dwelling (with or without supports), ambulant (with or without a walking aid) and had sufficient English language skills and cognitive ability to understand verbal instructions in a group setting.

Participants attended 10-weekly group sessions for approximately 60 minutes per session. Each session was facilitated by one or two allied health professionals and up to eight allied health students, including occupational therapy students. Participants identified their individual goals using the Canadian Occupational Performance Measure (COPM) (Law et al., 1990) (refer to Chapter 16) and were then allocated to pairs or small groups with people with similar goals and abilities, with each pair/group working with a student.

Each weekly session involved a short introduction incorporating specific strategies for 10 minutes, completion of two different activities that challenged both motor and cognitive abilities (20 minutes duration for each activity), followed by an end-of-session feedback and review of 10 minutes. Activities undertaken simulated skills integral to daily functional tasks such as balance, mobility and strength, planning, problem solving, attention and memory (Nott et al., 2019).

An example activity with grading that was used in the Program is included in Table 48.1.

TABLE 48.1	
Wellness 2 Age Program **example activity with motor and cognitive grading**	
ACTIVITY	**GARDENING CHALLENGE**
Level	**Motor Challenge**	**Cognitive Challenge**
---	---	---
1	Stand at raised garden bed; move to different sides of garden bed; reach to centre of garden bed.	Recall names of required seeds/seedlings to collect from garden shed (list of 3).
2	Bend to low pots/objects on ground such as tools/watering can.	Plant seeds/seedlings at allocated spacing according to packet direction; use measuring tape for spacing.
3	Walk between garden beds with hose; carry weighted objects such as filled watering can.	Recall sequence for planting (two sequence lists). Plant in allocated sequence.
4	Kneel to ground and stand from kneeling with small pot plant.	Determine companion planting based on information provided in planting guide.

When initially planning the *Wellness 2 Age Program*, careful consideration was given to ensuring that it was designed in a way that enabled a strong, collaborative relationship-focused approach and encouraged occupational participation (Restall & Egan, 2021) (refer to Chapter 12). The *Wellness 2 Age Program* closely aligns with the Canadian Occupational Therapy Inter-Relationship Practice Process (COTIPP) (Restall et al., 2022) (refer to Chapter 12).

Seek to Understand the Context

As part of the development of the *Wellness 2 Age Program*, the team sought to understand what current community-based program were available and how these existing programs met the needs of older people living within the community. Many of the existing programs focused on specific aspects of ageing to support older people. For example, older people can attend exercise programs to improve fitness and balance, falls prevention programs to reduce the risk of falling or memory programs that support cognitive function. However, there are several challenges associated with this approach. Successful ageing is multidimensional and incorporates the ability to maintain physical and cognitive health and social engagement (Rudnicka et al., 2020), therefore targeting only one element to support ageing does not meet all needs. Secondly, many of these community-based programs adopt a deficit model, whereby older people are required to either have an identified diagnosis or injury to be eligible to participate in the program. Thirdly, programs tend to be a snapshot in time, and evidence suggests that unless there are clear translation strategies built into the program to support behavioural change by incorporating learnt strategies, the benefits of the program can diminish rapidly (Close et al., 2005).

Reflect, Critically Reflect and Reason

As part of the design phase, the team reflected on the context and existing evidence and determined that it would be appropriate to develop a new approach to a community-based program that simultaneously targeted multiple aspects of ageing to maximise the potential benefits to participants. Drawing upon existing programs, it was concluded that incorporating a group-based approach was a useful way to ensure specific opportunities could be incorporated to facilitate social interaction and build social connection with others.

There was also a desire to ensure that the program was promoted in a way that older people could clearly identify the potential benefits to participating, as well as incorporating targeted translation strategies to better support older people to continue using the learnt strategies over the long term.

Use Justice, Equity and Right-Based Lenses

It was important to ensure that the *Wellness 2 Age Program* considered equity and justice by removing potential barriers for older people to attend and engage in opportunities to support successful ageing. Common barriers to participation in community-based programs for older people include access and availability of programs, social influences, individual physical barriers and the ability to meet the individual needs of older people (Burton et al., 2017; Franco et al., 2015; Hobson et al., 2019). It was also important that in the design of the program, opportunities for meaningful social engagement were embedded so that all participants had the opportunity to feel included and valued regardless of their abilities.

The health and well-being of rural/regional older people can be significantly impacted by the lack of available services (van Gaans et al., 2018), particularly for individual consultations with allied health professionals. As this program was developed specifically for rural/regional communities, the ability to run a group-based program that incorporated individualised goals and tailored activities with multiple older people at the same time was a key component to promote access to allied health services. This meant that the ability to support older people to successfully age was not just limited to locations where high numbers of health professionals were located.

Connect

The *Wellness 2 Age Program* was intentionally designed and promoted to older community members as a holistic and multi-faceted approach to healthy ageing, involving person-centred strategies to enable wellness and promotion of engagement in meaningful occupations. Language can be a powerful motivator but equally can also influence engagement with health services and programs (Durepos et al., 2022).

Therefore from the very start, the team wanted to build a connection with older community members that was built on a foundation of a strengths-based approach. When initially engaging with potential participants for the program, team members were purposeful in the use of language and approach to build a relationship that not only was person-centred but also encouraged meaningful collaboration between facilitators and participants.

Seek Understanding and Define Purpose

The program was specifically designed to incorporate a 10-minute session at the beginning of each week that was oriented to the program objectives, outlined the purpose of the session and to introduce the relevant strategy the group would be focusing on, regardless of the individual activities they would be undertaking. The deliberate program structure meant that the facilitators were able to effectively connect with group members in a meaningful way to set the scene for each session. This approach also provided individual older people the opportunity to ask questions or seek further clarification on the proposed strategy for that session.

Explore Occupational Participation

Within the program, the team incorporated a range of different standardised outcome measures focused on occupational performance, activities of daily living, quality of life, cognition and mobility. These outcome measures, including the COPM, which supported the development of specific goals for individual participants, aligned to the participants' self-identified strengths and challenges or areas they wanted to focus on improving.

Each program activity was designed to ensure the task was not only fun for participants but also had the right balance by not being too challenging to complete but challenging enough to support improvement and enhance social connection through active engagement. The team was careful to ensure development of a broad range of enjoyable activities so that there was not just variety but also alignment to the overarching goals and strategies. This approach was successful as evidenced by low attrition from the program, and of the few who did leave, most were due to illness.

Trial the Plan, Explore Change and Refine the Plan

At the end of each weekly session, there was scheduled time to focus on feedback from the participants regarding what they liked and did not like in the allocated activities for that session. Sometimes, participants indicated that they found the activity either too easy or too difficult; this provided an opportunity to consider what modifications were needed in subsequent weeks of the program. The weekly feedback session also enabled discussion about what activities participants would like to try in the following week's session. As pairs of participants were undertaking different activities within the one session, typically participants would indicate that a specific activity they had seen another participant do, that looked fun or of benefit, would be of interest to them to try the following week. Additionally, at the very end of each weekly session, there was a focus on recapping the weekly strategy and suggestions on how participants could continue to use the strategy at home during the week ahead to further support the consolidation of new learning.

Co-Design Priorities, Goals, Outcomes and Plans

As the *Wellness 2 Age Program* was specifically designed to focus on individual goals within a group setting, the principles of co-design with the individual older person were an inherent and critical aspect of the program. To further ensure the acceptability and applicability of the program after the pilot trial, the team evaluated the program with older participants to enable the incorporation of any further improvements from the perspective of participants before subsequent offerings of the program were delivered. Out of the eleven pilot participants, seven agreed to be interviewed to explore their experiences of the program. The outcomes from this evaluation identified that participants really valued that the program incorporated multiple aspects of ageing because it enabled participants to have multiple different goals. They also found that the ability to work in pairs/groups within a larger group greatly facilitated their engagement and ability to socially connect. The initial pilot participants also highlighted that the ability to learn new knowledge throughout the program was useful as it enabled them to understand the connection between the activity and how this would help them at home. They emphasised the importance of activities and learnt strategies in the program being easily transferrable to their individual lives so that they could continue using these strategies in the long term. Participants also identified that this aspect could be strengthened by having a range of written materials and resources that they could take away with them at the completion of the program for ongoing reference.

Plan for Transition

The ability to translate strategies learnt within the program to everyday life was a key focus in the development and implementation of the *Wellness 2 Age Program*. For every activity undertaken there was information provided both verbally and written on how this specific activity would assist with occupational participation at home and within the community. In later iterations of the program, and based on feedback, participants were provided with a weekly handbook that outlined weekly at-home activities they could practice to embed the individual strategies and seek clarification on before the end of the program. The team evaluated the perceived long-term impact of the program by interviewing past participants, 12 months after they completed the program. The outcomes of this evaluation identified that the participants perceived that they were able to continue using the learnt strategies over the long term and that the program had a long-term positive impact on cognition, physical mobility and social engagement (Timmermans et al., 2023).

WELLNESS 2 AGE PROGRAM: IMPACT ON THREE PARTICIPANTS

The impact of the *Wellness 2 Age Program* on Helen, Loni and John can be found in Boxes 48.1–48.3.

CONCLUSION

The *Wellness 2 Age Program* is an innovative, community-based program that focuses on simultaneously improving the physical, cognitive and social well-being of older people, through engaging in activities that are meaningful to the individual person. Group-based programs can support older people to maintain functional abilities and facilitate social engagement; however, adopting a one-size-fits-all approach does not consider the individual needs of older participants. Co-design of health programs with program participants ensures that the content, format, implementation and evaluation are appropriate and meaningful to participants. Integrating strengths-based, person-centred program design principles supported autonomy and agency for program participants.

REFERENCES

Bouaziz, W., Lang, P. O., Schmitt, E., Kaltenbach, G., Geny, B., & Vogel, T. (2016). Health benefits of multicomponent training programmes in seniors: A systematic review. *International Journal of Clinical Practice, 70*(7), 520–536. https://doi.org/10.1111/ijcp.12822.

Burton, E., Farrier, K., Lewin, G., Pettigrew, S., Hill, A. M., Airey, P., Bainbridge, L., & Hill, K. D. (2017). Motivators and barriers for older people participating in resistance training: A systematic review. *Journal of Aging and Physical Activity, 25*(2), 311–324. https://doi.org/10.1123/japa.2015-0289.

Carver, L. F., Beamish, R., Phillips, S. P., & Villeneuve, M. (2018). A scoping review: Social participation as a cornerstone of successful aging in place among rural older adults. *Geriatrics, 3*(4), 75. https://doi.org/10.3390/geriatrics3040075.

Close, J. C., Lord, S. L., Menz, H. B., & Sherrington, C. (2005). What is the role of falls? *Best Practice & Research Clinical Rheumatology, 19*(6), 913–935.

De Coninck, L., Bekkering, G. E., Bouckaert, L., Declercq, A., Graff, M. J., & Aertgeerts, B. (2017). Home-and community-based occupational therapy improves functioning in frail older people: A systematic review. *Journal of the American Geriatrics Society, 65*(8), 1863–1869. https://doi.org/10.1111/jgs.14889.

Durepos, P., Sakamoto, M., Alsbury, K., Hewston, P., Borges, J., & Takaoka, A. (2022). Older adults' perceptions of frailty language: A scoping review. *Canadian Journal on Aging, 41*(2), 193–202. https://doi.org/10.1017/S0714980821000180.

Egan, M., & Restall, G. (2022). The Canadian model of occupational participation. In M. Egan & G. Restall, *Promoting occupational participation: Collaborative relationship-focused occupational therapy* (pp. 73–95). Canadian Association of Occupational Therapists.

Franco, M. R., Tong, A., Howard, K., Sherrington, C., Ferreira, P. H., Pinto, R. Z., & Ferreira, M. L. (2015). Older people's perspectives on participation in physical activity: A systematic review and thematic synthesis of qualitative literature. *British Journal of Sports Medicine, 49*(19), 1268–1276. https://doi:10.1136/bjsports-2014-094015.

Grimmer, K., Kay, D., Foot, J., & Pastakia, K. (2015). Consumer views about aging-in-place. *Clinical Interventions in Aging, 10*, 1803–1811. https://doi.org/10.2147/CIA.S90672.

Hobson, N., Dupuis, S. L., Giangregorio, L. M., & Middleton, L. E. (2019). Perceived facilitators and barriers to exercise among older adults with mild cognitive impairment and early dementia. *Journal of Aging and Physical Activity, 28*(2), 208–218. https://doi.org/10.1123/japa.13.1.23.

Khan, H. T. (2019). Population ageing in a globalized world: Risks and dilemmas? *Journal of Evaluation in Clinical Practice, 25*(5), 754–760. https://doi.org/10.1111/jep.13071.

Law, M., Baptiste, S., McColl, M., Opzoomer, A., Polatajko, H., & Pollock, N. (1990). The Canadian occupational performance measure: An outcome measure for occupational therapy. *Canadian Journal of Occupational Therapy, 57*(2), 82–87.

Mitchell, E., & Walker, R. (2020). Global ageing: Successes, challenges and opportunities. *British Journal of Hospital Medicine, 81*(2), 1–9. https://doi.org/10.12968/hmed.2019.0377.

Nott, M. T., Robson, K. M., Murphy, K., Pope, R. P., Cuming, T., & Curtin, M. (2019). Ageing well: Pilot evaluation of a dual-task training program in a rural community. *Australian Journal of Rural Health, 27*(4), 311–316.

Restall, G. J., & Egan, M. Y. (2021). Collaborative relationship-focused occupational therapy: Evolving lexicon and practice. *Canadian Journal of Occupational Therapy, 88*(3), 220–230.

Restall, G., Egan, M., Valavaara, K., Phenix, A., & Sack, C. (2022). Canadian occupational therapy inter-relationship practice process. In M. Egan, & G. Restall (Eds.), *Promoting occupational participation: Collaborative relationship-focused occupational therapy* (p. 122). Canadian Association of Occupational Therapists.

Rudnicka, E., Napierała, P., Podfigurna, A., Męczekalski, B., Smolarczyk, R., & Grymowicz, M. (2020). The world health organization (WHO) approach to healthy ageing. *Maturitas, 139*, 6–11. https://doi.org/10.1016/j.maturitas.2020.05.018.

Seah, B., Kowitlawakul, Y., Jiang, Y., Ang, E., Chokkanathan, S., & Wang, W. (2019). A review on healthy ageing interventions addressing physical, mental and social health of independent community-dwelling older adults. *Geriatric Nursing, 40*(1), 37–50. https://doi-org/10.1016/j.gerinurse.2018.06.002.

Sherrington, C., Fairhall, N., Wallbank, G., Tiedemann, A., Michaleff, Z. A., Howard, K., Clemson, L., Hopewell, S., & Lamb, S. (2020). Exercise for preventing falls in older people living in the community: An abridged Cochrane systematic review. *British Journal of Sports Medicine, 54*(15), 885–891. http://doi.org/10.1136/bjsports-2019-101512.

Timmermans, E., Robson, K., & Curtin, M. (2023). The perceived long-term impact of an ageing well program. *Activities, Adaptation & Aging, 47*(2), 113–132. https://doi.org/10.1080/01924788.2022.2028051.

van Gaans, D., & Dent, E. (2018). Issues of accessibility to health services by older Australians: A review. *Public Health Reviews, 39*(1), 1–16. https://doi.org/10.1186/s40985-018-0097-4.

49

PABLLO AND THEIR DISSIDENCE OF GENDER AND SEXUALITY

JAIME DANIEL LEITE JUNIOR ▪ ROSANA TERESA ONOCKO-CAMPOS

INTRODUCTION

People who experience dissidence of genders and sexualities are those who escape the logic of intelligibility of genders, that is, who destabilise the linearity between sex, gender, sexual practice and desire (Butler, 2013). This concept brings together people identified as lesbian, gay, bisexual, *travesties*, transsexuals, queer, intersex, asexual, pansexual and non-binary, among others (LGBTQIAPN+) categories. This concept goes beyond identity categories, considering those who do not claim any identities for themselves, but also escape cisheteronormative logic (Leite Junior & Lopes, 2022).

Specifically in the Western countries, after colonisation by European countries, people who experience dissidence of genders and sexualities were marked by stigmatisation, and were considered to be expressing genders and sexualities that should be controlled and suppressed. Duarte (2015) provided a historical overview of sexualities in society and described the medical-moral appropriation of sexual behaviours, in which the medical, church and other institutions were violent with people who experienced dissidence of genders and sexualities as this broke with the cisheteronormative ideal.

Durate described how the vilification of people who experience dissident genders and sexualities resulted in many of these people being sent to asylums and prisons. The legacy of this treatment continues to impact the assistance that is offered nowadays as evident by the stigma and distancing of people who experience dissidence of genders and sexualities from public and private places and spaces that should be guaranteeing them citizenship and inclusion. In this sense, professionals, such as occupational therapists, are called on to advocate for change (refer to Chapter 21). Duarte (2011) argues for the need to break with the reproduction of stereotypes when engaging with people who experience dissidence of genders and sexualities, acknowledging the flourishing of the subjectivities and singularities of these people.

There have been achievements in relation to the demands of access to health for people who experience dissident genders and sexualities. At a global level, an important historical milestone was the recognition that homosexuality was not a disease. This recognition led to the removal of 'homosexualism' in 1973 from the Diagnostic and Statistical Manual of Mental Disorders (DSM), published by the American Psychiatric Association (APA). In 1990 'homosexualism' was also removed from the International Classification of Diseases (ICD), a document published by the World Health Organization (WHO) (Back et al., 2019). Presently, there is still debate on the classification of trans identities. Transsexuality is classified in the ICD; it has been moved out of the mental disorders section and included in the section on conditions related to sexual health.

In Brazil, an important milestone was the National Policy for Integral Health of the LGBT Population (LGBT Policy). This policy was 'a watershed for public health policies in Brazil, and a historic milestone in recognising the demands of this vulnerable population' (Brasil, 2013, p. 6). In the introduction to this policy, it is stated that:

> *The LGBT policy marks the recognition of the effects of discrimination and exclusion on the health-disease process of the LGBT population. Its guidelines and objectives are, therefore, focused on changes in the social determination of health, with a view to reducing inequalities related to the health of these social groups.*
>
> *(Brasil, 2013, p. 8)*

There are many challenges with implementing and operationalising the Policy across various health facilities, whether at the municipal, state or federal levels to guarantee a public health system for everyone, that respects the specificities of gender, race/ethnicity, generation, orientation and affective and sexual practices (Brasil, 2013). The commitment of different government bodies, health councils, civil society and social movements is necessary, to ensure systematic monitoring of the everyday routine of services and the implementation of strategies to avoid discrimination against the LGBT population in public health spaces.

Looking specifically at the occupational therapy profession and its possibilities, a scoping review was conducted to explore the production of knowledge about dissident genders and sexualities (Leite Junior & Lopes, 2022). Also, a mix method study was carried out to apprehend the occupational therapy practices in Brazil (Leite Junior, 2024). The findings identified

the necessity of occupational therapy literature providing details of practice to support the work with this population and how best to meet their needs. Considering that, the following practice story provides a description of the strategies implemented to promote the social participation of a young person experiencing dissidence of gender and sexuality.

PABLLO

Pabllo attended a mental health service that specialised in the care of children and adolescents located in a large city in the interior of the state of São Paulo, Brazil. They were 17 years old when we met. Our initial meeting took place in the *ambience*. The ambience differs from a waiting room because is set up to allow observations by health professionals of a person's behaviour and their interactions and relationship with other people in the institution or family members. The first analysis and hypothesis begin with the observations done while people are in the ambience. The ambience is also characterised by the informality, the possibility of the unusual, of encounters between different people. During the period that people are in the ambience waiting for an appointment, they do not see themselves being analysed. This allows them to feel more comfortable, and to be who they are. Often, the observations made in the ambience are discussed with the members of the health professional team and contribute to the strategies of care initially proposed (Santos & Onocko-Campos, 2015).

Building Rapport: Establishing a Collaborative Relationship-Focused Practice

It was at a time when Jaime, the occupational therapist, was responsible for monitoring the ambience, that Pabllo arrived. Pabllo sat in the corner of the room with their head down and only interacted with their cell phone. Pabllo drew Jaime's attention because their presence appeared to be of an 'out of order' body, a dissident person with no similarity to any of the other people in that space. Pabllo's hair was big, and colourful, in a way that made it look like it was not well cared for. Their face at times seemed sad, at times reminiscent of indifference. Pabllo did not interact with anyone else in the ambience. They only interacted with their cell phone and sat with a very hunched posture. Jaime approached Pabllo and said 'hello', but they did not respond.

Jaime persevered in trying to interact with Pabllo and eventually, they responded; however, their eyes never left their cell phone. Jaime continued to encourage an initial conversation, asking about internet topics, like online games, music, among other things that he thought might interest Pabllo. Pabllo exchanged a few words and on occasion briefly gazed at Jaime. After a short time, Pabllo left the room as another worker invited them to participate in an activity. In the following weeks, Jaime used the same strategy to try to stimulate a conversation with Pabllo. Jaime talked about music videos, asked about games, and other things related to the internet universe, anticipating that these would be meaningful interests for Pabllo.

Gradually, Pabllo and Jaime became more connected. Their relationship grew stronger. One time, Pabllo arrived spontaneously talking and telling of their impressions about a new music video released by a 'POP Diva'. They also shared a story they started writing about a character in the online game they were playing.

Pabllo began to feel more comfortable talking with Jaime – who was a gay man and very enthusiastic about queer culture – and they began to talk more about LGBTQIAPN+ culture products, such as Drag Queen's reality shows, the use of slang (the use of slang terms was an important mediator in this relationship as it helped to strengthen the bond between Jaime and Pabllo), ballroom culture, among other things. These subjects began to be the starting point for meetings with Jaime, and they talked about affinities and disagreements, favourite singers, which Drag Queen from the reality show should win, etc.; topics of interest to, and guided by, Pabllo. What seemed like informal conversations was the ambience device operating. Jaime was learning more about Pabllo, based on the way they saw themselves as a person and their history of social participation. Between one comment or another about a pop singer, it was possible to understand a little more about family relationships, the situation of poverty in which they lived and situations of violence they experienced. For example, Pabllo told Jaime what they could and could not watch at home because their parents thought that it was not content that should be watched by a 'man'. Pabllo also said that they needed to go to the

mental health services or go to some other public institution to be able to use the internet, as they were not financially able to pay for the internet at home. As it transpired even if they had the money, they would not be able to have internet where they lived, as it was an 'occupied' place; it was not officially a house intended for housing. They lived in an abandoned room in a public space.

Co-Creating of Goals in Occupational Therapy with Pabllo

Jaime began to realise that as Pabllo spoke of and shared their experiences there was a realisation that the service was a safe space for them to share their story. When they understood that their difference would be respected and could exist in that institution, they seemed more comfortable there. Pabllo began to relax and smile, saying *shades*[1] to the staff and other people in that work setting. As Pabllo's trust in Jaime grew the staff suggested that Jaime integrate officially into Pabllo's health professional team. The health professionals collaboratively talk about possible occupational therapy strategies that may assist them with the social participation challenges they faced (refer to Chapter 19). These occupational therapy strategies focused on everyday life, life projects, experiences, and encourage social participation – targeted by social justice principles (Leite Junior et. al., 2024).

When considering occupational therapy strategies, three resources and social technologies proposed in social occupational therapy (Lopes et al., 2021) were used to frame the approach (refer to Chapter 4):

1. *Individual Territorial Follow-ups.* A resource and social technology that aims to understand the person's everyday and context of life. Through active listening, Jaime sought to delve deeper into Pabllo's history, its paths, its existing social support network and their current conditions.
2. *Articulation of Resources in the Social Field.* This resource and social technology comprised several actions carried out to find resources available in the territory, whether financial, material or emotional ones.

---

[1]Shade is a queer community slang that refers to the act of making fun of another person or some situation in a sarcastic way.

3. *Dynamization of the Support Network*. This resource and social technology are essential to propose a complex and more effective care strategy. Through it, by identifying Pabllo's needs, the services and agencies best placed to assist with meeting each of the needs can be identified and explored.

Social Resources, Technologies and Meaningful Relationships Applied to Social Occupational Therapy Practice

Through the *Individual Territorial Follow-ups*, Pabllo said that they arrived at that mental health service after attempting suicide (there were three attempts in total) and the main trigger for these attempts had been the homophobia they experienced at home. Pabllo's family pressured them often, prohibiting them from expressing themself as they wished. Pabllo often experienced physical and psychological violence and abuse at home. They also spoke about the process of self-knowledge and discovery related to their experiences in relation to their gender and sexuality. Pabllo were experiencing their discovery moment. They did not know how to identify themselves, what is their gender and sexual orientation; but they did indicate that they understood themselves as a pansexual boy at that moment. Pabllo knew very little about the city they lived in, their social network was fragile and limited; they were unable to name friends to go on leisure activities with them. Most of Pabllo's interactions beyond their family and therapeutic spaces took place over the internet.

Based on this information, Jaime and Pabllo talked about amplifying Pabllo's experience, and how it could be beneficial for Pabllo to explore the city and create new connections. Pabllo agreed with these initial propositions and a plan was developed to carry out *Follow-ups* that would take place around the city, to discover new places. These *Follow-ups* led Pabllo and Jaime to activate another technology, the *Articulation of Resources in the Social Field*. In addition to the sensitive listening that took place while exploring the city, new possible places that Pabllo could connect with, learn about and experience were discovered. It was important that Pabllo learnt more about their city, and how to more actively participate in, and engage with, opportunities that arose. This could lead to Pabllo

learning more about themselves and meeting, learning about, and identifying with other young people who experience dissidence of genders and sexualities.

An important social marker that permeated all interventions was economic status. Being from a family in a socially precarious condition, Pabllo did not have income to spend to explore the city. They had a specific number of free bus tickets per week, which were used to go to the mental health service. This increased the layers of complexity, as everything proposed needed to be well with Pabllo's limited expenses; it was not possible to consider interventions that involved other expenses, such as a snack, for example.

Through the *Articulation of Resources in the Social Field*, Jaime learnt about a Vogue group. This group was supported by the city council and focused on providing educational and cultural activities for young people in the city. Anyone who participated received a bus ticket (round trip) and a snack. This support allowed Pabllo to participate in the group. Pabllo was reluctant at first to join the group as they were afraid of feeling exposed and uncomfortable doing many of the activities. However, they agreed to attend one session. Pabllo enjoyed this session and found the other young people who attended the group welcoming.

The *Follow-up* also led to the application of the third social technology, the *Dynamization of the Support Network*. While Pabllo attended the Vogue group, they and Jaime spoke with the relevant social work and education staff. Together with they all talked about Pabllo's situation with the aim of seeking new avenues of support that went beyond the mental healthcare service. It was collaboratively agreed that Pabllo should continue with the Vogue group as it provided them with positive social participation opportunities with a group of peers. Individuals who attended the Vogue group all experienced differences and recognised the possibility of existence while being different. The group was attended by individuals who were poor, dissidents of genders and sexualities, black and with disabilities. All of them were looking for strategies to confront the oppressions that impacted their social participation.

As a result of participating in the Vogue group, Pabllo was invited to attend to a course proposed by the city council about youth policy. The adolescents attending this course would study a range of relevant issues including different notions of youth, policies related to youth, contemporary themes and civil and social rights and duties. The objective of this course was to build a more politically conscious society by training young people to apprehend the course content and then share this understanding with other young people (peer education). To assist the people to participate in this course attendees were offered bus tickets and food; this made it possible for Pabllo to participate.

Through listening to Pabllo, which led to their participation in the Vogue group and attendance at the city council course, they changed from being a person who did not interact with those around them to someone who was becoming comfortable with who they were and their place in the world. This recognition meant that Pabllo went from being someone who lived in silence to a peer educator, responsible for guiding other young people about public policies, rights and duties.

Exploring Discoveries and New Possibilities to Participate

The *Follow-ups* continued to take place, enabling Pabllo to more comfortably participate in a range of activities offered in the city. Pabllo engaged in various groups and training and built another story about the city; experiencing it as a place of care, leisure and learning. Furthermore, through their contact with different people in the city, Pabllo becomes a 'prevention young person'. This was due to another course they attended, which focused on peer guidance, on STI/AIDS prevention. Pabllo also successfully applied for a job that involved assisting people to use computers and the internet. Access to income was important for Pabllo, as it allowed them to have more options to explore the city and develop connections and relationships with other people.

Transition from Occupational Therapy and the Health Service

Pabllo's change and development were partly due to the attentive work that was carried out, taking everyday life in the community as the focus of action and not the closed space of a mental health service. The strategies were inspired by the implementation of the LGBT policy in Brazil. In the policy, there is a focus on the elimination of discrimination and prejudice against LGBT people within health services, and the

prevention, promotion and health recovery to reduce the incident of mental health issues (Brasil, 2013).

Pabllo's willingness to expand their social participation was key to their growth. Escorel and Moreira (2008) discuss the concept of micro-participation, pointing out its instrumental and pedagogical character. It is through these small movements that participatory habits are created that go beyond the family nucleus. From a technical perspective, the micro-participation movements built with Pabllo allowed new projects to be built, expanding their social participation and life repertoire and circulation possibilities. Here, bringing into practice resources linked to the digital universe and LGBTQIAPN+ culture.

Escorel and Moreira (2008) state that there are many reasons to participate, which may be linked to a desire for personal change or even collective motivations. Achieving these objectives depended on various factors including gender, age, education, family relationships and race/ethnicity. Pabllo was a young person, trying to discover themself. As Pabllo was finding themself and becoming more comfortable with their gender and sexuality, they wanted to confront the violence that occurred related to these social markers of difference.

Pabllo's progress was partly in response to their resilience, trust, support network, understanding and self-understanding, criticism and self-criticism (Escorel & Moreira, 2008). Pabllo was able to trust in the institutions and staff working with them. They were also able to experience safety for who they were, and use that space as a place of welcome and support for their transformations and experimentations.

Pabllo still felt fear and uncertainty, but it was no longer an impairment. For example, when Pabllo participated in LGBTQIAPN+ Pride they arranged to attend with friends. Unfortunately, these friends cancelled at the last minute. Pabllo indicated that they thought about returning home but felt they wanted and needed to participate in LGBTQIAPN+ Pride. So, they went, albeit with fear, and they marched and based on that, new encounters became possible.

When planning for the transition from occupational therapy and the mental health service, Pabllo wanted to apply what they learnt in their training as a 'young preventionist' to the mental health service. Pabllo talked about STIs, contraceptive methods and sexuality in general with everyone. It was a very bold desire, given the initially very reserved and shy relationship they had with the other young people in the place. This request demonstrated how far Pabllo had come, how much the encounters with the city, with other people and groups – combined with the other professional interventions that made up their care project – had transformed them.

Pabllo told Jaime several times how their interaction at the mental health service was previously restricted because it was a space for the production of violence. The other young people abused them with looks, laughter, jokes and sayings, all related to their dissidence of genders and sexualities. Pabllo decided that the way they wanted to end their occupational therapy process was to face adversities and be a protagonist to assist with change at the mental health service. So, Pabllo and Jaime made a plan. They both decided to have a 'beauty day', something like a salon/spa and amidst the hair styling and painted nails, to talk about sexualities. A number of staff at the mental health service helped with the organisation of the 'beauty day' and twenty young people participated. It was not easy for Pabllo, even with the support of staff, to guarantee a safe space, as a number of young people who attended behaved disrespectfully. Sometimes Pabllo needed to go out to 'get some air', to reestablish themself, but they persevered and managed to finish what they set out to do.

After the activity, Pabllo asked Jaime to meet for another *Follow-up* in their usual manner, exploring the city. Amidst the shaking of the bus, Pabllo expressed their discomfort regarding the violence they suffered at the service from other young people. They spoke in general but then brought up what happened on the day of the beauty salon/spa activity. Pabllo said of other people who experienced this violence, specifically referring to a young transgender girl. They questioned Jaime, saying that the mental health service needed to build more effective strategies to deal with this violence.

Towards the end of this *Follow-up* Pabllo decided to schedule a meeting with the manager of the mental health service. Pabllo wanted to question her about how the service cared for and promoted health for people who experience dissident genders and sexualities; and what actions would be taken with the people who were aggressors. Through this action, Pabllo was questioning and demanding care from management towards people who experience dissidence of genders and sexualities, attempting to destabilise the vertical logic

of power of institutional functioning and place themself as an active part of social control (Brasil, 2013), an objective guided by the LGBT policy. In a shared way, Pabllo sought co-management paths (Campos, 2013) so that space could expand their actions, enabling abject bodies to find comfort and respect.

For the last occupational therapy session, Pabllo wanted to have their *Follow-up* at a large international coffee shop franchise, located in an upper-class neighborhood. Pabllo was very different, compared to the person Jaime met many months ago. Confident body posture and smiling, they had tried different hair and nail colours and were exploring new styles of clothes. Pabllo told Jaime how much they liked the drink they were drinking and that they could only try it after they were employed. Pabllo spoke about their current everyday life and the fact that the situation at home was still confrontational. However, Pabllo indicated that they felt more able to deal with the situation. They had new resources to talk to their mother, and due to their work did not feel so subordinate. They also started going to nightclubs; another desire they had that was only able to be accomplished after they were employed. They talked with humour about the conflicts they had with friends over taking the bus to the nightclub, and the confusion and stress experienced when deciding the time to leave. They talked about their experiences of falling in love and falling out of love, of liking somebody and this not being reciprocated, of buying a gift for someone for whom they had romantic feelings.

Jaime understood that last occupational therapy appointment was also an opportunity for Pabllo to self-evaluate the care received. They were talking about their growth, new abilities, and new experiences lived. They also recognized their city and community as a possible place to live, build their life, and let their mark on the world.

CONCLUSION

Apprehending Pabllo's reality demanded that health professionals recognise their everyday lives and the violence they experienced due to their gender and sexuality dissidence. From an intersectional lens, it was not possible to think about Pabllo's needs without considering the economic vulnerability in which they were experienced. Collaboratively Pabllo and Jaime found other ways of participating in meaningful activities. This was important as it enabled Pabllo to understand and rediscover themself in the city, leading to the creation and possibilities of experiences and relationships in different spheres of life. It also allowed Pabllo to articulate the assumptions of the LGBT policy and advocate for the health service to become a safe space for other young people who experienced dissidence of genders and sexualities. From an occupational therapy perspective, Jaime's work moved towards the construction of technical actions ethically and politically committed to the redefinition of everyday life, seeking, in a democratic way, social participation.

REFERENCES

Back, J. C., Silva, L. M., Prado, L., & Cyrino, L. A. R. (2019). Despatologização da homossexualidade e transexualidade: revisão integrativa. *Revista Família, Ciclos de Vida e Saúde No Contexto Social (REFACS)*, 7(3), 378–389. https://doi.org/10.18554/refacs.v7i3.3063.

Brasil. (2013). *Política nacional de saúde integral de lésbicas, gays, bissexuais, travestis e transexuais* (p. 32).

Butler, J. (2013). *Problemas de gênero: feminismo e subversão da identidade* (5th ed.). Civilização Brasileira.

Campos, G. W. S. (2013). *Um método para análise e co-gestão de coletivos: a constituição do sujeito, a produção de valor de uso e a democracia em instituições: o método da roda* (4th ed.). HUCITEC.

Duarte, M. J. O. (2011). Diversidade sexual e Política Nacional de Saúde Mental: contribuições pertinentes dos sujeitos insistentes. *Revista Em Pauta, 9*(28), 83–102. https://doi.org/10.12957/rep.2011.2935.

Duarte, M. J. O. (2015). Cuidado de si e diversidade sexual: Capturas, rupturas e resistências na produção de políticas e direitos LGBT no campo da saúde. In A. Rodrigues, C. Dallapicula, & F. R. da Silva (Eds.), *Transposições: Lugares e fronteiras em sexualidade e educação* (pp. 323–349). EDUFES.

Escorel, S., & Moreira, M. R. (2008). Participação social. In L. Giovanella, S. Escorel, L. de V. C. Lobato, J. C. Noronha, & A. I. Carvalho (Eds.), *Políticas e sistema de saúde no Brasil* (pp. 979–1010). Editora FIOCRUZ.

Leite Junior, J. D., Laliberte Rudman, D. & Lopes, R. E. (2024). Alliances between social occupational therapy and critical occupational science: Propositions to mobilize social justice, *Journal of Occupational Science*, 1–17. https://doi.org/10.1080/14427591.2024.2374308.

Leite Junior, J. D., & Lopes, R. E (2022). Dissident genders and sexualities in the occupational therapy peer-reviewed literature: A scoping review. *The American Journal of Occupational Therapy: Official Publication of the American Occupational Therapy Association, 76*(5). https://doi.org/10.5014/AJOT.2022.049322/23908.

Leite Junior, J. D. (2024). "We are talking about letting people who are dying live": professional practices of occupational therapists with people who experience dissidence of genders and sexualities in the brazilian context. Doctoral dissertation, Federal University of São Carlos. https://repositorio.ufscar.br/handle/ufscar/19689.

Lopes, R. E., Malfitano, A. P. S., Silva, C. R., & Borba, P. L. O. (2021). Resources and technologies in social occupational therapy: Action with poor urban youth. In R. E. Lopes, & A. P. S. Malfitano (Eds.), *Social Occupational therapy: theoretical and practical designs* (pp. 169–176). Elsevier.

Santos, R. G. H. S., & Onocko-Campos, R. T. (2015). Ambiência em um CAPS infanto-juvenil: a experiência de um coletivo brincante. *Cadernos Brasileiros de Saúde Mental, 7*(15), 41–52. https://periodicos.ufsc.br/index.php/cbsm/article/view/68516.

50

BUILDING CONNECTIONS AND ACCESSING DIVERSE NETWORKS DURING THE COVID-19 PANDEMIC: NATIONAL AND PROVINCIAL ADVOCACY AND LOBBYING IN SOUTH AFRICA

KASHIFA ABRAHAMS ■ FADIA GAMIELDIEN ■ ROSHAN GALVAAN

INTRODUCTION

Occupational therapy has a vision that promotes health, well-being and social justice for all people through occupation. As occupational therapists, we saw our role during the COVID-19 pandemic as one of advocating for the rights of all citizens to participate fully in their environments of choice. We also drew attention to the rights of marginalised and vulnerable groups as we recognised that there were contextual barriers hindering people's participation.

Kashifa is a qualified occupational therapist and works as a content adviser in the National Parliament of the Republic of South Africa. She serves as an adviser for the Portfolio Committee on Women, Youth and Persons with Disabilities in the National Assembly. Kashifa responded to the pandemic by foregrounding the needs of females, youth, children and persons with

disabilities, who constitute a significant proportion of the population. It was imperative to ensure that the most vulnerable sector of society stayed on the agenda of the key decision-makers in the country within Parliament and Government.

Fadia is an occupational therapist and clinical educator at an academic institution. She actively participates in public mental health service delivery projects, emphasising intersectoral collaboration, health innovation and social engagement. Her passion lies in co-creating knowledge alongside mental health service users, including students in higher education institutions, to enhance her understanding of personal recovery and its role in reshaping services and curricula. As a lifelong learner and disability rights activist, she focuses on creating access to opportunities in living, working, socialising and learning spaces for marginalised communities. She responded to the pandemic as a member of her local civic society in the area where she lives.

Roshan co-leads Inclusive Practices Africa (IPA) at the University of Cape Town. IPA is a research unit with a network of researchers and academic staff aiming to reduce inequalities associated with disability (Box 50.1). Persons with lived experience of disability are part of this group, and all formal communication to Parliament was channelled via IPA. Roshan led this process for IPA, aiming to promote opportunities for disability inclusion.

COVID-19 PANDEMIC IN SOUTH AFRICA

The COVID-19 pandemic impacted societies and healthcare systems internationally, presenting unprecedented challenges. Most countries used stay-at-home and other policies to curtail the spread of the virus, with people allowed varying constraints on their freedom of movement. South Africa experienced one of the most stringent approaches to implementing emergency policies and prolonged lockdown periods, starting on the 22nd March 2020 (Haider et al., 2020). In what was to become regular Sunday night televised announcements, colloquially referred to as national family meetings, the president of South Africa, President Ramaphosa, declared the country to be in a state of disaster and announced that the National Coronavirus Command Council would enforce a 21-day nationwide complete lockdown effective from the end of that week. This was called Alert Level Five as per the Disaster Management Act (No. 57 of 2002). Alert Level 5 restricted movement and commuting within a neighbourhood, city and country coupled with social distancing measures; shopping was limited to a select few essential items; only those deemed essential workers were permitted to commute to work and work at their place of employment; all sport and leisure pursuits in public spaces were prohibited; beaches and public parks were closed – to name a few of the stringent lockdown rules imposed. Two weeks later, the President announced that the complete lockdown would be extended for another month (South African Government, 2020b). This was the first of many extensions, and the country oscillated between Alert Level 4 to 1 between May 2020 and April 2022 (South African

BOX 50.1
INCLUSIVE PRACTICES AFRICA (IPA) MEMBERS

Marlene le Roux is the CEO of Artscape Theatre in Cape Town and a University of Cape Town Disability Studies Alumni. She is a tireless advocate for the rights of persons with disabilities and youth and is a member of the Presidential Task Team on Disability.

Thulani Tshabalala is the CEO of the South African Development Trust and a University of Cape Town Disability Studies Alumni. He is a member of the National Economic Development and Labour Council (NEDLC) as a Disability representative.

Professor Roshan Galvaan, co-leads IPA and is also the Doctoral Programme convenor in the Division of Occupational Therapy, Department of Health and Rehabilitation Sciences, University of Cape Town. She has co-developed community-based approaches to practice, which promote the inclusion of marginalised and excluded groups. Her research, teaching and practice interests include the mental well-being of marginalised groups and populations; occupation-based community development, psychosocial disabilities in higher education and social inclusion.

Professor Harsha Kathard co-leads IPA and, as a previous Head of the Department of Health and Rehabilitation Sciences at the University of Cape Town, supported the development of an inclusive curriculum in the Disability Studies programme from Higher Certificate level to PhD level. She is an NRF-rated scientist who conducts research on disability inclusion in higher education, economy and health systems. She has a special interest in communication disabilities.

Professor Theresa Lorenzo co-leads IPA and is the Doctoral Programme Convenor in the Division of Disability Studies, in the Department of Health and Rehabilitation Sciences, Faculty of Health Sciences, University of Cape Town. She is an NRF-rated scientist. Her research expertise and teaching areas include community-based inclusive development, particularly for youth and females, training community rehabilitation workers, disability inclusion in higher education and monitoring disability-inclusive policy implementation.

Professor Sharon Kleintjes is the Vera Grover Chair and Professor of Intellectual Disability and Head of the Division of Intellectual Disability in the Department of Psychiatry and Mental Health, University of Cape Town. She is an associate member of IPA. Her research interests include public mental health policy and service development, intellectual disability, and recovery from psychosocial disability.

Government, 2020a). The National State of Disaster in South Africa was officially lifted on 5 April 2022.

This decision by the South African Government to enforce a strict lockdown was seen as a decisive measure to save as many lives as possible. The implications of the stringent lockdown impacted the entire population, with the most vulnerable being disproportionately affected. Poverty, gender-based violence, impairments and chronic conditions were compounding factors that exacerbated the adverse effects of the lockdown (Mentor-Lalu, 2022). People who were deemed to not be essential workers were confined to their homes, and people living on the streets were provided with temporary shelter within cities. Without a special permit, nobody was allowed to be outside or drive. Shopping was limited to essential items during an allocated time that was limited, and this could only be done by one adult in a household. Schools were closed and moved to online learning for mostly private schools as public schools did not have the infrastructure and resources to do the same. Day-care centres were closed. Families were confined to their homes. Soup kitchens and school feeding schemes were initially closed, and this massively impacted millions of persons and children living in poverty reliant on these feeding schemes. The South African economy took a huge hit, with many businesses, for example, restaurants, having to close and retrench employees, which deepened poverty in the country.

The ramifications of the state of disaster and lockdown highlighted the need for advocacy and lobbying (refer to Chapter 21), mainly because the occupational participation needs of persons with disabilities were poorly considered. This directly impacted all people doing or not doing, being and becoming. Many services shut down, and many occupational therapy services became inaccessible. It highlighted the rights infringements that occupational therapists needed to consider and begin to grapple with in practice (refer to Chapters 2, 3, 4 and 10). Amnesty International's Annual Report for 2020/21 provided a candid reflection on the protection of human rights during the pandemic (Amnesty International, 2021). The pandemic forced some of us to network and collaborate to find innovative ways to provide services and advocate for those in need by highlighting rights infringements.

Consequently, a handful of academics, disability rights activists, clinicians, civic society organisations, politicians and government officials collaborated as they grappled with addressing the needs of our society's most vulnerable and marginalised people. We had to draw on our collective abilities to establish and nurture connections between different stakeholders during this period. While the lockdown rules limited our contributions to service provision, we had the chance to contribute to policy and law reform actively. The practice stories in this chapter share our journey as we tapped into existing networks and built meaningful connections with different service providers during the pandemic. Further, it describes our lobbying and advocacy efforts at the time to respond to the challenges experienced at community, provincial and national levels.

The pandemic provided us as occupational therapists with opportunities to re-evaluate the implementation of existing policies promoting the rights of persons with disabilities. Occupational therapists have a valuable role in contributing to all aspects of people's lives concerning human occupation (refer to Chapter 6). People's experiences are directly affected by the policies and laws developed for a population group or community. Being open to intersectoral collaborations and multi-sectoral approaches is vital in translating policy into practice. Social justice requires that occupational therapists understand the policy and legislative environment to advocate for effective change and have the skill to build connections and action-diverse networks (refer to Chapters 3, 4 and 21).

The following practice stories show our practical contributions to policy and law reform (refer to Chapters 3, 4 and 21). It involved influencing the country's regulations at the height of the COVID-19 pandemic and lockdown and working directly with Parliament to conduct astute oversight. During the Keynote Address at the 15th Congress of the World Federation of Occupational Therapists, 4–7 May 2010, Santiago, Chile, Galheigo (2010) said: 'Occupational therapists and scientists need to be attentive to human rights issues'. She reflected on the 'need to answer the call for interconnectedness in the present-day complex societies and engage in networking'. The examples discussed in this chapter are practical manifestations of this (Galheigo, 2010). Further information related to this approach can be found in Chapters 4, 14, 21 and 30.

KASHIFA AND IPA'S STORY

With the announcement of the lockdown, I, like many others, recognised the immediate challenges faced by vulnerable populations and the need to address this beyond the medical model. I was part of a small group of stakeholders, including healthcare professionals, disability rights activists, and government officials who met virtually to discuss the exclusion and the need to foreground disability, gender-based violence and youth on the President's agenda. As IPA, we were concerned about how the rights and needs of persons with disabilities were being provisioned for during this time and this prompted us to work with colleagues who shared our concerns. Representing IPA, Roshan led a series of consultations with stakeholders to identify the concerns that needed to be articulated. The group's goal was to ensure that the national government of South Africa did not just consider the needs of people who were ill but also considered the impact of the pandemic with its imposed movement and occupational participation restrictions on the broader population, including those who were marginalised. I also saw it as an opportunity to facilitate the link between occupational therapists and activists with Parliamentarians whose key functions are law reform and oversight. Creating a platform for engagement, networking and collaboration was strategic with the end goal of social justice.

In one of his televised meetings with the South African Nation, President Ramaphosa (South African Government, 2020c) said: 'We are determined to ensure that women, youth and people with disability received particular attention and support'. President Ramaphosa was referring to social impact efforts needed to advance the position of females, youth and persons with disabilities during the pandemic and bolster South Africa's economy in the future. Including persons with disabilities in the President's addresses to the nation was not random; instead, it resulted from intentional, strategic, coordinated advocacy and lobbying efforts spearheaded by the IPA group and myself, who pushed for its inclusion in government discussions and policies. The IPA group included persons with disabilities and took the lead in drafting statements and letters explaining how persons with disabilities were affected by the lockdown measures. By identifying the gaps in policy implementation and explaining how persons with disabilities could be included, clear direction was offered. We understood that working with the State and its various arms was critical to lobbying for change.

We sought opportunities to present our main concerns and offer recommendations on mainstreaming disability and improving access to essential services.

National Lobbying: Understanding the Role of Parliament

In South Africa, 'Parliament's role and outcome is to represent the people and ensure government by the people under the Constitution, as well as represent the provinces in the national sphere of government. The role of Parliament includes promoting the values of human dignity, equality, non-racialism, non-sexism, the supremacy of the Constitution, universal adult suffrage and a multi-party system of democratic government' (Parliament of the Republic of South Africa, n.d.). The South African Parliament is responsible for holding the National Executive to account by assessing the extent to which services, laws and policies are implemented to benefit the people. Identifying a committee in Parliament that oversees the government department responsible for females, youth and persons with disabilities was thus an important strategy for accountability.

Working within a Parliamentary context, it was imperative to link the concerns of the impact of the COVID-19 pandemic and lockdown regulations from people's lived experiences with the Portfolio Committee in order to conduct more effective oversight of government departments. The above letter served as a segway into pursuing this with the Portfolio Committee. As such, I met with the IPA core team (and other key stakeholders to document the concerns and recommendations and arranged a meeting with the chairperson of the Portfolio Committee on Women, Youth and Persons with Disabilities overseeing the Department of Women, Youth and Persons with Disabilities. Our discussions focused on ensuring that the needs of females, youth and persons with disabilities were considered during the pandemic. While there was an acknowledgement of existing legislative and policy frameworks, such as the heavily relied upon White Paper on the Rights of Persons with Disabilities, specific legislation (e.g. Disability Act) related to the impact of COVID-19 on persons with disabilities in South Africa was absent.

Occupational therapists, together with disability activists, could offer insights into the wider impact on

BOX 50.2
EXCERPTS FROM THE LETTER SENT TO THE PRESIDENT OF SOUTH AFRICA

Dear Mr President,
Inclusive Approach for COVID-19 for Persons with Disabilities

'As a part of the Government's strategy to contain COVID-19, we urge you to consider an inclusive strategy for marginalised sectors within the population who are likely to be severely affected, with serious consequences. In particular, we draw attention to Persons with Disabilities who constitute at least 7.5% 1 of our population and particularly those living in impoverished communities. The lessons learnt from the Life Esidemeni tragedy highlighted the human costs that result as a consequence of insufficient attention to and inadequate planning for the health, social and basic needs of Persons with Disabilities. We commend the Government's current initiatives that take into consideration the impact of the lockdown on persons with disabilities. Notwithstanding, there are key issues that require urgent attention and ...'

the occupational participation of people restricted by the lockdown and the pandemic. I facilitated a meeting with the chairperson of the Portfolio Committee on Women, Youth and Persons with Disabilities, where I tabled a letter drafted by IPA (refer to Chapter 21). This letter (Box 50.2) was addressed to the President as well as other role-players such as the Minister, Deputy Minister and the Acting Director General in the Presidency for Women, Youth and Persons with Disabilities, the Minister and the Acting Director General in the Department of Social Development, and the Acting Director General in the Department of Health. This letter raised concerns about persons with disabilities in South Africa in light of the pandemic and the stringent lockdown. Reference was also made to the Life Esidimeni tragedy (Makgoba, 2016), which was still fresh on everyone's minds at the meeting, and parallels were drawn. The tragedy occurred between October 2015 and June 2016 when 1711 mental health service users (MHSUs) with profound intellectual disabilities and severe mental health conditions were transferred from hospital facilities to non-government organisations as part of the deinstitutionalisation process in one of South Africa's provinces (South African Government, 2020c). During this move from institution to community-based care, 144 MHSUs died. Life Esidemeni is cited as an international example of how poor planning, mismanagement and insufficiently resourced implementation plans can result in tragedies (Makgoba, 2016; Mentor-Lalu, 2022). The Life Esidimeni tragedy opened up a discussion on the urgent need to implement a disability-inclusive COVID-19 disaster strategy. The recommendations offered had universal applicability as they articulated key concerns pertaining to persons with disabilities and their families but were also relevant to the broader population.

Some of the key concerns raised in the letter included:

- Females, youth and persons with disabilities were excluded from early discussions with the Government's Corona Virus Council. The regulations did not take into account the gender implications, child rights implications and implications of persons with disabilities.
- People with disabilities had their rights violated. Disability mainstreaming was absent in the promulgation of the policies and laws implemented as part of the government's lockdown regulations.
- Within communities, only those categorised as essential workers were allowed to travel and work. Initially, all public transport ceased, and special permits were issued for those people who needed to drive.
- Schools were closed, and most people had their movements restricted to their homes and immediate neighbourhoods. For caregivers of people with disabilities, it was particularly hard to provide care with no respite options. This disrupted routine placed additional stress on families.
- The limit of exercise to one hour per day posed a problem, especially for females and children in communities where high levels of crime raised safety concerns.

The concerns raised were shared with the deputy minister, who engaged with the President, and the President, in turn, tabled the concerns with the Corona Virus Council. The outcome of this was the President's active inclusion of females, youth and persons with disabilities in his subsequent speeches to the nation during the lockdown period.

Moreover, I advised that the academics advocate and lobby with other Parliamentary Committees (e.g.

Health) and ministers in government at both national and provincial levels. Local examples of difficulties faced by individuals were used to demonstrate how the laws and policies governing the regulations infringed on the rights of persons with disabilities. Within Parliament, the information shared, and examples provided, were used to write a report on the adverse effects of the regulations that the government developed and the need for them to be amended. As illustrated by this practice story, policy shapes practice differently, and occupational therapists must actively engage with potential policy pathways to align policy with the profession's values.

The meeting with the Chairperson Portfolio Committee on Women, Youth and Persons with Disabilities served two purposes. Firstly, to raise awareness through articulating the practical concerns and highlighting how and why constitutional and human rights were being infringed. Importantly, we were also able to offer strategies to address the concerns. To this end, the Chairperson of the Portfolio Committee not only lobbied her colleagues within Parliament about the information she was provided with by the IPA but engaged directly with the Deputy Minister for the Department of Women, Youth and Persons with Disabilities who was tasked with championing disability in the Department. In turn, the Deputy Minister engaged with the President and the Corona Virus Council and then lobbied at that level for change. In addition, the Portfolio Committee submitted a report to amend the lockdown regulations all of which was speared by what had emerged from the discussions held with IPA.

FADIA AND A COMMUNITY-BASED RESPONSE TO THE PANDEMIC

In this practice story, Fadia shares her experiences as an occupational therapist within her community during the pandemic. Fadia was involved in a community-based response to the pandemic, which focused on education, safety, health and food security issues for people in her residential area. She also highlights the difficulties faced by people on chronic medication due to restricted access to healthcare facilities during lockdown.

Lobbying at a Local Level

In March 2020, I responded to an open invitation on social media to join Cape Town Together, a collective of community action networks (CANs) co-constituted by health professionals, teachers, activists and artists (Odendaal, 2021). The CANs aimed to offer community assistance through WhatsApp groups. As an executive member of my area's resident and ratepayers' association, I registered our interest, and the Kensington and Factreton (KenFac) CAN was born. The group later joined forces with an existing non-profit organisation (NPO) and broadened the collaboration to include schools, churches, mosques and other civic organisations. The group aimed to keep the community safe during the pandemic.

I saw my role on the team as facilitating occupational stewardship and collaborative engagement (Rushford, 2015) because I was interested in cultivating resilience in my community while promoting health and well-being during the pandemic. According to Rushford (2015, p. 244), occupational stewardship is a 'twofold process of working within the context and creating occupational spaces for engagement' during times of disaster and development. I understood the interrelationships between people, occupations and the environment, and this helped me guide interventions within the social and relational sphere as the need evolved.

As a collective, KenFac CAN adopted the slogan 'Teamwork makes the dream work', and we offered the following critical activities during the lockdown period:

- **Education**: From the onset, I recognised the need to disseminate fact-checked and verified infographics, government circulars and pamphlets which I sourced from the Department of Health. I then created a WhatsApp group to share educational material and weekly updates with the community. I used hashtags in the messages to connect the content to the topic. A sample of a weekly WhatsApp and Facebook message can be found in Box 50.3.
- **Database and humanitarian relief support**: KenFac CAN submitted the names of 3597 vulnerable households to the Department of Social Development so that they could access humanitarian relief. Due to the absence of government support, we secured sponsorships and donations from sporting groups, religious institutions and

BOX 50.3
SAMPLE OF WEEKLY UPDATE
SENT TO COMMUNITY ON WHATSAPP
AND FACEBOOK

LOCKDOWN DAY 15
  Friday 10 April 2020
  UPDATE KenFac CAN
  Information and Relief Helpline XX XXX (a dedicated cellphone number was assigned)
  Greetings All
  A warm welcome to the newbies in the group. KenFac CAN is a subgroup of the Cape Town Together Community Action Network (CTT CAN). This group was created as a response to COVID-19.
  Please direct all your queries, complaints or compliments to the KenFac CAN Relief Helpline number XXXXXX
  SMS one of these options:
  1. Support (Food, Psychosocial, Special Needs, Elderly, Crime)
  2. Volunteer (Street Committees/Neighbourhood watches)
  3. Donations (Cash, Kind) Sanitisers and Spray Bottles are needed
  4. Skills/Expertise (Admin, IT, Media, Education, Call Centre, CMT, Counselling)
  We have partnered with Maitland and they now have their own CAN group. If you have family, friends or acquaintances in Maitland, please let them know about this.
  Maitland CAN Information and Relief Helpline number XXXXXX
  #anothertwoweeks #socialdistance #practicethepause #dotherightthing #inthistogether #kenfacmatters #nofakenews #2020vision #lovetheyneighbour #spreadlovenotcovid #staysafe #stayhome #belekker #helpyourneighbour #eachoneteachone #2mapart #checkinsafely #everyoneonboard #volunteer #wecandothis #basicneeds #foodwatersafetyeducation #factcheck#kenfaccan,#staysafe, #stopthespread #handupnothandout #notacharity #diversitybreedsexcellence #differentbuttogether
  #differentpeoplecommongoals

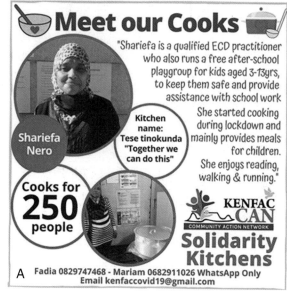

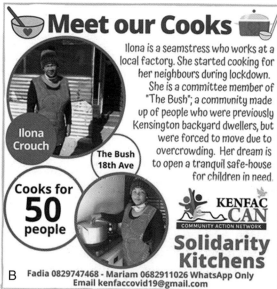

Fig. 50.1 ■ Two samples of the solidarity kitchen flyer. (Courtesy KenFac CAN.)

individuals. We distributed food parcels, bread and meals to almost 21,000 people.

■ **Solidarity kitchens and gardens:** To address the ongoing food insecurity needs of the community, KenFac CAN activated 19 Solidarity kitchens (Fig. 50.1). These kitchens were run by community members who showed initiative and were already cooking for vulnerable children and residents in their vicinity. We supplied the kitchens with enough vegetables and dry ingredients to prepare at least four weekly meals. As part of a sustainability drive to encourage kitchens to grow vegetables and herbs, I secured donations of seeds, fruit trees and gardening equipment (Fig. 50.2). City officials also visited the gardens as there was growing interest in supporting home

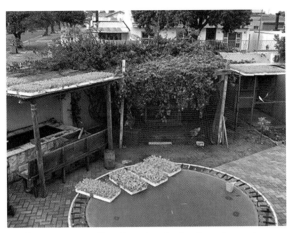

Fig. 50.2 ■ Seedling donation for food garden project.

BOX 50.4

MEDIA COVERAGE ON ACCESS TO THE WATER CRISIS

NEWSPAPER ARTICLE COVERING WATER CRISIS

'Imagine having to lick your school-going child's hands clean just so that he can look presentable at school. Hard to imagine, right? Now try doing this when facing a deadly pandemic.

This is how a Kensington mother from an informal settlement on 18th Avenue in Kensington had to sanitise her child's hands because they didn't have access to running water.

Neville Crouch, a resident and a committee member of the 18th Avenue informal settlement, says no taps and a lack of services from the City of Cape Town is an everyday headache.

Crouch says some residents, who have been living on the open piece of land for many years, were backyard dwellers and have been on the housing database for several years. He says they are finding it especially difficult now with the outbreak of Covid-19'.

From Bantom, K. (2020). Locals suffer water woes. *News24*, June 23, 2020. https://www.news24.com/news24/community-newspaper/peoples-post/locals-suffer-water-woes-20200622.

gardens, but unfortunately, the government did not allocate any resources to the gardeners.

■ **Lobbying for access to water and sanitation:** The KenFac area is socio-economically mixed and has several informal settlements and backyard dwellers who do not have access to water and sanitation. One of the key messages to stop the spread of the coronavirus was handwashing. We held regular meetings with the Department of Water and Sanitation to lobby for water to be delivered to the area, and we secured community media coverage (Box 50.4) on the plight of the residents, which helped to ensure that water was delivered to the area on alternate days. An NPO donated jerry cans to each household in the settlement so that people could safely collect their water (Fig. 50.3). Through ongoing efforts foregrounding access to water as a basic human right, we later managed to have communal taps erected in the informal settlements.

■ **Outreach:** I facilitated a partnership with an animal rescue organisation that provided education, food and pet care to pet owners in informal settlements.

■ **Community engagement:** At the start of the lockdown, a community map was created, and an appeal was made for volunteers to serve on street committees for localised communication since neighbourhood watches were not allowed to operate during the lockdown. In this way, we encouraged people to stay connected through

the: 'Know Your Neighbour, help your neighbour' campaign.

A reflection of the range of activities offered by KenFac CAN is presented in Box 50.5.

Liaison with the Department of Health and Provincial and National Levels

As an occupational therapist, I was acutely aware of the catastrophic impact defaulting on medication could have on those with chronic health conditions. I also knew that contextual barriers could result in people not accessing the help they need when they need it. However, this did not seem to be a consideration within the Department of Health. People with dual diagnoses such as tuberculosis (TB) and HIV/AIDS were deemed complicated cases that could not be seen at the community clinics. Instead, they were required to travel to specialist clinics outside of their residential area, which was expensive and inaccessible due to the financial and transport restrictions. I engaged with the Department of Health and local police to see if we could address these particular needs, along with parolee reintegration issues (refer to Chapter 21). I identified that many

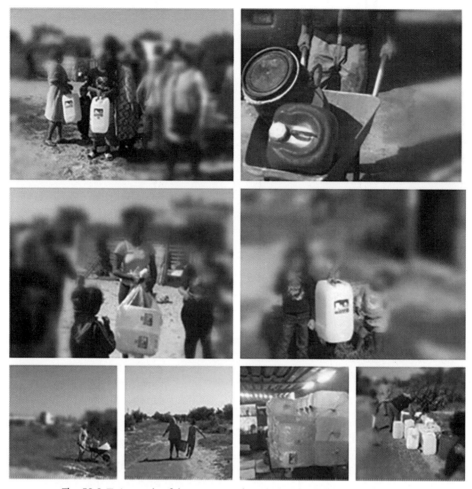

Fig. 50.3 ■ A sample of the water can donation and people collecting water.

individuals on chronic medication were defaulting on their medication due to the imposed lockdown restrictions. As transport was limited and social distancing imposed, it directly impacted access to health care. The dispensing of chronic medication was not decentralised for easy access to people, so many forfeited receiving their medication because they could not commute out of the specified neighbourhood. The regulations did not consider people travelling from one neighbourhood to another where the health care facility was located to access their medication. Parolees under house arrest were also unable to leave their homes to collect their medication. Food insecurity was real, as many people had reduced or no income. When people had no food, non-compliance with medication

increased, compromising treatment regimens and recovery goals.

This prompted me to write letters to national and provincial health authorities, including the Provincial Minister of Health (Western Cape Province), to highlight the negative consequences of the strict lockdown regulations on medication access, especially for people with chronic health conditions such as tuberculosis (TB), HIV/AIDS and chronic diseases of lifestyle. Treatment-resistant tuberculosis was a concern in the Western Cape prior to the pandemic, and restricted access for those with HIV/AIDS exacerbated the issue.

During this process, I considered myself to be a resource agent for others. Through my deliberate efforts to establish connections and build relationships

BOX 50.5
KENFAC CAN: A REFLECTION OF OUR ACTIVITIES

MARCH TO DECEMBER 2020

KENFAC CAN

A REFLECTION OF OUR ACTIVITIES

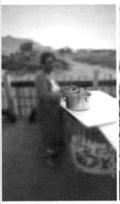
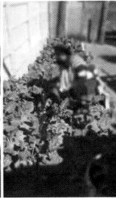
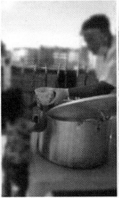
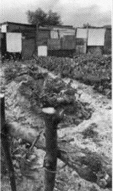

HOW KENFAC CAN BEGAN

On 22 March 2020, President Ramaphosa announced that South Africa would start a 21-day lockdown period from the 26 March 2020, to curb the spread of COVID-19 and thereby flatten the curve. At the same time, the Cape Town Together Community Action Network (CTT CAN), a diverse group of people from all over the city, invited interested parties to join their network.

Local CANs self-organised, took locally relevant action to access resources and coordinate area-specific Neighbourhood activities under the banner CTT CAN.

Some executive members of the KenFac Residents and Rate-payers Association (KFRRA) registered their interest in starting a KenFac CAN to provide support to the Kensington and Factreton community during the COVID-19 crisis.

On the 28 March 2020, Play Sport4Life (PS4L) formed a partnership with KenFac CAN and after that, the collaboration broadened to include schools, other civil organisations, willing individuals, mosques and churches in the area. At the onset, we invited our local ward 56 Councillor to join, and she willingly came on board. The partnership extended to the communities of Maitland and Garden Village.

Given their shared postal codes but vastly different access to resources, the Pinelands CAN "paired" with KenFac CAN and the residents of Pinelands have been generous in supporting the KenFac CAN through donations in cash and kind.

As a collective, KenFac CAN continues seeing to its original vision of keeping the Kensington and Factreton community safe during the COVID-19 pandemic.

We have been overwhelmed by the generosity of spirit bestowed on our society from businesses and community members.

BOX 50.5
KENFAC CAN: A REFLECTION OF OUR ACTIVITIES—(*Continued*)

ACTIVITIES

The admin office and KenFac CAN nerve centre operated from a garage generously gifted to us by a family who could not run their small business under lockdown. They availed their space and resources to us so that we could have a central hub to work from while still being able to employ social distancing and other "keep safe" strategies. Logistics were managed from this "nerve centre".

EDUCATION

As part of educating our community, we shared fact-checked and verified infographics, government circulars and pamphlets via the KenFac CAN WhatsApp chat and social media.

DATA BASE

At the start of lockdown, DSD indicated that they had Humanitarian Relief for COVID-19 vulnerable households.

KenFac CAN undertook to collect information to help people apply for this DSD relief. In May, KenFac CAN submitted the names of 3597 homes "in need" to DSD, Metropole North Office. These households included homeowners, tenants, backyard dwellers and residents of informal settlements.

The houses captured were:
a. Factreton: 1 763
b. Kensington: 701
c. Informal settlements: 862
d. Backyard dwellers: 271

FOOD PARCELS

During data collection and in the absence of DSD or government-funded food security, KenFac CAN launched its Operation Food parcels. Hidayatul Primary School generously offered the use of its premises as a packing warehouse for the food parcel assembly. Through sponsorship drives, fundraising efforts and the generous donations from businesses and communities, KenFac CAN :
· distributed 2 000 food parcels
· distributed 10 562 loaves of bread
· served 40 197 meals
· reached almost 21 000 people.

The first food parcels delivery took place on Saturday, 11 April 2020. KenFac CAN assisted other areas, and 100 parcels were sent to Garden Village and another 100 to Maitland.

All households underwent an assessment of need before a food parcel was allocated to them. This need was based on criteria such as SASSA recipient or not; the number of children in the household; the number of unemployed adults; and people with disabilities. Homes with residents aged 80 years and older were also included as vulnerable groups.

After the KenFac CAN food parcel distribution was concluded, CoCT awarded PS4L funding to

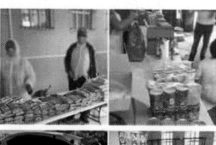
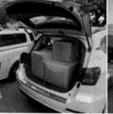
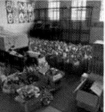

distribute 300 food parcels in the area. A beneficiary list was compiled from the KenFac CAN database and in consultation with the Ward 56 councillor. The database was filtered to highlight those persons who are unemployed and do not receive any grants or other income. The parcels had everything to sustain a family for a month, and 677 Children and 886 adults benefitted.

BOX 50.5
KENFAC CAN: A REFLECTION OF OUR ACTIVITIES—(*Continued*)

FOOD PARCEL DISTRIBUTION

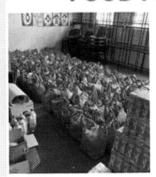

Food parcels were either packed by a food hamper team or donated to KenFac CAN by organisations who needed help distributed it.

Food parcels were allocated to families in need at the nerve centre and then delivered to households by a network of volunteers. These volunteers included members of the food parcel packing team, volunteers from the churches and mosques as well as young Peace Ambassadors from the "Peace Ambassador Network" (PAN).

Volunteers performed their tasks diligently and enthusiastically and were able to field difficult questions around parcel allocation from the community.

LOBBYING FOR ACCESS TO WATER AND SANITATION

KenFac CAN drew attention to the plight of the residents of informal settlements and backyard dwellers to ensure that they had access to water and sanitation. As a result, all informal settlements and backyard dwellers had water delivered to them on alternate days, although this service is not reliable.

The 18th Avenue Informal Settlement, known locally as "die bos", does not have any permanent water and sanitation sources. A truck comes daily to deliver water to the families living there (about 200 people).

Ongoing meetings with the Department of Water and Sanitation have resulted in limited progress on the access to water issue as the 18th Avenue land appears to be disputed land, so there is an unwillingness to recognise it as an informal settlement.

In the space of one week, two Cape Cobras were found in the 18th Avenue Informal Settlement.

A snake handler was called in to remove the snakes, but because there is no refuse collection rats are breeding in the area, and the rats are attracting the snakes.

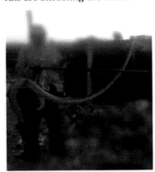

In September, an NPO, Lerato's Hope responded to the plight of the people and donated 100 25l jerry cans to the residents.

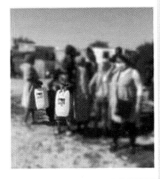

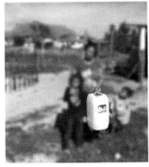

Continued on following page

BOX 50.5
KENFAC CAN: A REFLECTION OF OUR ACTIVITIES—*(Continued)*

SOLIDARITY KITCHENS

During the first part of the lockdown, many people donated hot meals in the area. These meals were distributed to various sites, and the KenFac Response Team was involved in ensuring that everyone adhered to the COVID-19 protocols related to reducing the spread of the virus.

KenFac CAN mapped the "ready to eat" distribution sites while also assessing the safety and dignity issues related to queuing for food. Donations of "ready to serve" pots of food dwindled with the extended lockdown. We thus explored a more sustainable solution to addressing the food security needs of the Kensington and Factreton community. During this period, we activated 19 Solidarity Kitchens across the area. Four became inactive as people returned to work or as their circumstances changed; and currently, we have 15 which have operated consistently since inception. These kitchens are run by community members who showed initiative and were already cooking for vulnerable children and residents in their vicinity. KenFac CAN supplies essential vegetables and dry ingredients every week, and the cooks plan meals for at least four times a week.

One family regularly donates bulk dry ingredients to the kitchens.

The Solidarity Kitchen project requires ongoing fundraising, assistance and support to stay sustainable.

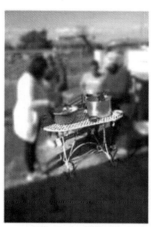 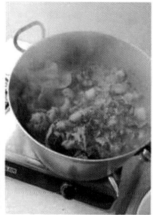 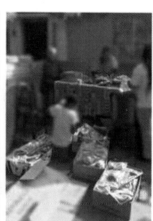

TOWARDS SUSTAINABILITY

On the 16 December, 2020 KenFac CAN and PS4L hosted a *thank you* function in honour of the Solidarity Kitchen cooks for their unselfish service to the KenFac community during the COVID-19 pandemic. Fourteen cooks attended the event, and they were each gifted with a wonderbag and a delicious lunch enjoyed by all. Many cooks met each other for the first time and forged new friendships. KenFac CAN is not a long-term project, but the extended lockdown highlighted community needs in the area that will continue whether or not we are in a pandemic. The enthusiastic networking,

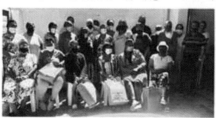

collaborations and bartering between individuals and organisations have seen many new ideas sprouting.

One of these is the expansion of PS4L to include a Community Upliftment Programme (CUP). To ensure the sustainability of the solidarity kitchens, PS4L will adopt eight kitchens as part of the CUP initiative along with other Projects Under Construction.

KENFAC CAN

BOX 50.5
KENFAC CAN: A REFLECTION OF OUR ACTIVITIES—(*Continued*)

SOLIDARITY GARDENS

Given the ongoing food security issues in the country, the Food Growers Network was established to help communities think about growing their food for their pot. In June 2020, we launched 10 Solidarity Kitchens who have keen gardeners and who were interested in starting Solidary Gardens.

The aim is for the community to start growing vegetables and herbs for their meals and for sharing with others.

Pinelands CAN created a group to support the solidarity gardens, and they have been ploughing seeds, plants, expertise and resources into the gardens. The Cape Youth Desk Madrassa also gifted the gardens with fruit trees, and we see the greenery of pomegranate, peach and apricot trees.

City officials visited all the food gardens, and four gardeners were selected to attend the launch of the City's Food

Gardens Project held on the 17 December 2020. The project focuses on supporting home gardens to address food insecurity in vulnerable areas and will launch in January 2021.

CoCT did not include any of the four solidarity gardens from the three informal settlements in the project. Still, we remain convinced of the necessity for food gardens in our community, and we will continue supporting the gardens.

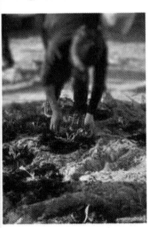
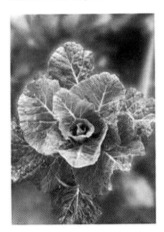
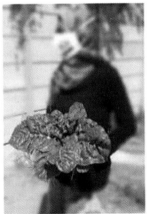

CARING FOR PEOPLE & THEIR PETS

Diesel's Rescue has been doing outreach and education in the informal settlements across the area. There is a significant need for pet care services as many of the animals need to be adequately cared for, sterilised and dewormed. Pet owners have responded well to educational information, but a regular, accessible pet care service is required in the area.

ASSISTING WITH RESEARCH

VPUU did a backyard dweller survey and volunteers in the network were enlisted to assist.

Four cooks were also involved in an energy conservation project where they were asked to survey 50 households and record the type of fuel source for cooking as part of a national research project.

TRAUMA-INFORMED COUNSEL-LING

Subcouncil 15 invited community members to the 2nd round of the Trauma-informed counselling course offered by the organisation R-cubed. The 1st group have completed the training, and group 2 will finish in 2021, God willing.

KENFAC CAN

PAGE 5

Continued on following page

BOX 50.5
KENFAC CAN: A REFLECTION OF OUR ACTIVITIES—(*Continued*)

LIAISON WITH THE DEPT OF HEALTH AND MINISTER OF HEALTH

We have also drawn the Dept. of Health's attention to people with special needs such as the elderly, those living with TB and HIV, people with disabilities and those on chronic medications.

STREET COMMITTEES

At the start of lockdown, a community map was created, and an appeal was made for volunteers to serve on street committees. Since neighbourhood watches were not allowed to operate during the lockdown, this group was seen as a possible means of communicating with the KenFac CAN team and their neighbours if a 'rapid response' was needed in the street.

While this did not take off as envisaged, people have been creative in how they have used it, and Whatsapp neighbourhood watches operating on street block level have been adopted across the area.

LIAISON WITH THE SAFETY AND SECURITY DEPARTMENT

A select group was constituted to respond to the influx of parolees into the area. The parolee group discussed issues related to the wellbeing of the parolees, their families and the KenFac community to which they were returning following their incarceration.

In August 2020, some residents of the 18th Avenue Informal Settlement lost their homes when the land invasion team destroyed it. The Kensington, Factreton and Pinelands residents were once again generous with their donations to assist the displaced families.

DONATIONS

KenFac CAN have received donations in cash and kind from many sources including community sporting organisations, religious institutions, non-profit organisations, schools, clubs, societies, CAN partners and many individuals. KenFac CAN paired with Pinelands CAN, and we have benefitted from weekly donations and support. All these parties have been directly thanked via letters and emails.

APPRECIATION FOR COMMUNITY SUPPORT

We want to maintain dignity and build self-reliance; hence we have not focused on taking photographs of recipients. Where pictures were taken, consent was sought from participants. Photos were taken when they were an occasional requirement of donors or as part of documenting a visual history of the KenFac CAN project. We would like to re-assure the community that all donations have been accounted for and distributed to its intended beneficiaries.

We have been alerted to many social-economic issues such as gender-based violence, the difficulties faced by street workers, burn-related injuries, abandoned babies, inaccessibility of resources to assist with DG grant applications, amongst others. What we have come to learn is that the resources and services to address the mental, physical, financial, spiritual and emotional needs of the KenFac community is insufficient. While many issues were highlighted, the majority remains unresolved.

Despite the hardship faced by people, this pandemic also showed us who the helpers are, and for this, we are incredibly grateful.

with a vast network of service providers, I was able to champion the rights of vulnerable people in my community.

KEY RECOMMENDATIONS THAT WERE IDENTIFIED ACROSS THE TWO PRACTICE STORIES

Reflecting on our efforts to build connections and access diverse networks during the COVID-19 pandemic as illustrated in the practice stories, we offer the following insights:

- An inclusive response to the pandemic was needed as the lockdown restrictions impacted people's mental health, access to health care, livelihood and social interaction.
- Collaboration and coordination with and between government officials and relevant stakeholders was needed to advocate for the rights of vulnerable populations.
- Championing disability rights ensures that government policies and discussions include disability rights as a focal point.
- The intersectionality of issues needs to be acknowledged. Advocacy efforts encompass multiple challenges, such as gender-based violence, children's rights and poverty.
- Understanding Parliamentary processes is needed to raise concerns and advocate for change.
- Understanding Policy and Legislative decisions and how they impact vulnerable populations is essential.
- Occupational therapists have a valuable role to play in policy and law reform thereby actively contributing towards social justice.

CONCLUSION

Occupational therapists in these practice stories played a pivotal role in advocating for social justice, policy change and protection of human rights during the pandemic. We aimed to show that, as occupational therapists, we harnessed our expertise to drive improvements in the lives of vulnerable populations during the COVID-19 pandemic. As occupational therapists, we possess a unique understanding of how human occupation occurs in contexts from which we can effectively advocate for and promote the well-being of individuals and collectives. The practice stories illustrate how intersectoral collaboration efforts were applied to address various challenges faced by youth, females and persons with disabilities. This illustrates how powerful the potential of advocacy is, especially in crisis situations. Working in ways that bring connections across multiple levels of engagement, from local communities to national government, assists in creating systems that are more inclusive. We know that the pandemic has long-term impacts on society, and the challenge now is to learn from the valuable lessons it offered so that we can continue to build a just society for all.

REFERENCES

Amnesty International. (2021). *Amnesty International Report 2020/21: The state of the world's human rights*. https://amnesty.org.

Galheigo, S. M. (2010). *What needs to be done? Occupational therapy responsibilities and challenges regarding human rights*. World Federation of Occupational Therapists XV Congress 4-7 May 2010. Santiago, Chile.

Haider, N., Osman, A. Y., Gadzekpo, A., Akipede, G. O., Asogun, D., Ansumana, R., Lessells, R. J., Khan, P., Hamid, M. M. A., Yeboah-Manu, D., Mboera, L., Shayo, E. H., Mmbaga, B. T., Urassa, M., Musoke, D., Kapata, N., Ferrand, R. A., Kapata, P.-C., Stigler, F., … McCoy, D. (2020). Lockdown measures in response to COVID-19 in nine sub-Saharan African countries. *BMJ Global Health, 5*(10), e003319. https://doi.org/10.1136/bmjgh-2020-003319.

Makgoba, M. (2016). *The report into the 'circumstances surrounding the deaths of mentally ill patients: Gauteng Province' no guns: 94+ silent deaths and still counting*. https://www.sahrc.org.za/home/21/files/Esidimeni%20full%20report.pdf.

Mentor-Lalu, V. (2022). *Through a gendered lens: South Africa's COVID pandemic*. https://za.boell.org/en/2022/05/02/through-gendered-lens-assessing-covids-impact-women-sa.

Odendaal, N. (2021). Recombining place: COVID-19 and community action networks in South Africa. *International Journal of E-Planning Research, 10*(2), 124–131. https://doi.org/10.4018/ijepr.20210401.oa11.

Rushford, N. (2015). Occupational stewardship and collaborative engagement: A practice model. In N. Rushford, & K. Thomas (Eds.), *Disaster and development: An occupational perspective*. Elsevier Health Sciences.

South African Government. (2020a). About alert system. https://www.gov.za/covid-19/about/about-alert-system#:~:text=(c)%20′Alert%20Level%203,a%20low%20health%20system%20readiness.

South African Government. (2020b). President Cyril Ramaphosa: Extension of coronavirus COVID-19 lockdown to the end of April. https://www.gov.za/speeches/president-cyril-rama-phosa-extension-coronavirus-covid-19-lockdown-end-april-9-apr-2020-0000.

South African Government. (2020c). President Cyril Ramaphosa's speech on R500bn rescue package and COVID-19 lockdown ending in phases, 21 April 2020. TimesLIVE. https://www.timeslive.co.za/news/south-africa/2020-04-21-in-full-president-cyril-ramaphosas-speech-on-r500bn-rescue-package-and-covid-19-lockdown-ending-in-phases/.

Parliament of the Republic of South Africa. (n.d.). What Parliament does. https://www.parliament.gov.za/what-parliament-does.

INDEX

Page numbers followed by '*f*' indicate figures, '*t*' indicate tables and '*b*' indicate boxes.